"This encyclopedia of health informa[tion] [is the] most comprehensive on the market. [The combina]tion, technical accuracy and thoroug[hness of SELF] CARE sets it apart from similar guides. It is superbly indexed and illustrated."

Essence

"Detailed discussions of a broad range of gynecological issues and problems. An extremely comprehensive and informative book."

Publishers Weekly

"Exhaustive, thorough . . . A solid, detailed reference."

Kirkus Reviews

"An indispensable handbook of medical information . . . honest, useful, comprehensive, and remarkably up-to-date."

Barbara Seaman, author of
The Doctor's Case Against the Pill

"An invaluable, thorough reference to diseases of the female anatomy."

New York Daily News

Other Avon Books by
Jane Patterson and Lynda Madaras

WOMAN/DOCTOR

WOMANCARE

A GYNECOLOGICAL GUIDE
TO YOUR BODY

NEWLY REVISED, COMPLETELY UPDATED

BY LYNDA MADARAS AND
JANE PATTERSON, M.D., F.A.C.O.G.
WITH PETER SCHICK, M.D., F.A.C.S.

 AVON
PUBLISHERS OF BARD, CAMELOT, DISCUS AND FLARE BOOKS

WOMANCARE: A GYNECOLOGICAL GUIDE TO YOUR BODY is an original publication of Avon Books. This work has never before appeared in book form.

This book was current to the best of the authors' knowledge at publication, but before acting on information herein the consumer should, of course, verify information with the appropriate physician or agency.

AVON BOOKS
A division of
The Hearst Corporation
1790 Broadway
New York, New York 10019

Copyright © 1981, 1984 by Lynda Madaras
Illustrations Copyright © 1981 by Avon Books
Text illustrations by Christine Bondante
Cover design Copyright © 1981 by Roger Whitehouse
Published by arrangement with the author
Library of Congress Catalog Card Number: 80-69608
ISBN: 0-380-87643-4

First Avon Printing, April 1981

AVON TRADEMARK REG. U. S. PAT. OFF. AND IN
OTHER COUNTRIES, MARCA REGISTRADA, HECHO EN
U.S.A.

Printed in the U. S. A.

DON 10 9 8 7 6 5 4 3

DEDICATION

For my mother, Margaret Reiley Vogel, my sister, Carol Vogel Martin, my daughter, Area Madaras, and Pam Rousseau, who is not a member of the family but might as well be.

WOMANCARE

Table of Contents

Table of Contents

Gender: The He, She, It Problem

In the first draft of this book, we used the masculine pronouns *he* and *him* whenever we wanted to refer to the doctor. In the next draft we decided to strike a blow for feminism by using the female pronouns *she* and *her* to refer to the doctor, but since 97 percent of the doctors in the United States are males, this seemed a bit of wishful thinking. Next we tried *he* or *she* and *him* or *her* and then, putting the female first, *she* or *he* and *her* or *him,* but this got a bit too cumbersome. Then we invented some new, neuter pronouns, but how many readers would know what a *shim, herhim, sherm* or any of the other combinations of *her* and *him* meant? In the end we struck a compromise: We simply eliminated most of the *hers* and *hims* and used *s/he* instead of writing *she* or *he*. Not a perfect solution perhaps, but at least it's better than assuming that all doctors are men or pretending that most are women.

Acknowledgments

This book would not have been possible without the generous support of many people, too numerous to mention here. We would, however, like to acknowledge the contributions of certain individuals. Before doing so, we should make it clear that inclusion in these acknowledgments does not necessarily mean that those individuals mentioned agree with the opinions expressed in the book.

Dr. Peter Schick of Brotman Memorial Hospital in Culver City, California, provided invaluable assistance in preparing the information on cancer. We are particularly grateful for his contributions to the section on breast cancer. Diane Burr, a nurse practitioner from South Pasadena, California, made substantial contributions to the section on pregnancy and fertility. Carla Hines of the American Social Health Association assisted in our efforts to gather information on sexually transmitted diseases. Sam Knox, also of the American Social Health Association, was kind enough to review the section on sexually transmitted diseases and offer his comments. Nancy Adess of DES Action shared her expertise, reviewed the sections on DES, vaginal adenosis and clear cell adenocarcinoma and offered many comments. Nancy Kaswell from the Emma Goldman Clinic reviewed a draft of the material on cervical caps and offered valuable criticisms. Dr. Richard Small, a radiologist from Daniel Freedman Hospital in Inglewood, California, was kind enough to answer questions and provide background information on radiation therapy of cancer.

A number of people were helpful in our efforts to gather information on the cervical cap including Dr. James Koch, a physician from Brookline, Massachusetts; Renee Potik, a nurse practitioner from Los Angeles; Jan Scolastico and Lynn Dockworth from the Emma Goldman Clinic; Sarah Brendt, Sandra Malaski and Peg McElroy from the New Hampshire Feminist Women's Health Center; and Dr. Robert Goeppe of the University of Chicago, who, along with Dr. Uwe Freeze, has developed a new type of cervical cap.

Dr. James Heine of Lubbock, Texas, and Dr. Milos Chapvil of the University of Arizona were helpful in our efforts to learn about the cervical sponge. In addition, a number of other members of the medical profession assisted our research efforts, including Dr. James Bouquet, Dr. Anthony Koerner, Dr. Val Davajan, Dr. Gerald Bernstein, Dr. Raymond Kaufman, Dr. John Frey and Dr. Walter Henderson.

Although they were not directly involved in the production of this book, there are some individuals and groups whose work in the field of women's health care provided inspiration, information and direction, including Carol Downer, who introduced us to the concept of speculum self-exam; Rose Kushner, health-care activist and author of *Why Me?*, an outstanding book about breast cancer; Barbara Seaman, health-care activist, coauthor of *Women and the Crisis in Sex Hormones* and author of *Free and Female* and *The Doctor's Case Against the Pill;* the women of the National Women's Health Network, an organization dedicated to improving health care for women; Belita Cowan, feminist activist and Executive Director of the National Women's Health Network; and the women of the Boston Women's Health Collective, authors of *Our Bodies, Ourselves.*

A number of friends provided encouragement and support, assisted our research efforts and read and reviewed sections of the book, including Pam Rousseau, Richard Johnson, Bill Happecook, Patti Pinto, Suzanne Thiele, Peter Tarbox, Pam Rodgers, Annie Sobieski, Jean Madsen, Ann Mulkey, Romaine Alhstrom, Susan Day, Lisa DePalma, Cynthia Pearson, Chris Smith, Sandy Kimball, Clark Bridges, Phil Capobianco, Deborah Capobianco, George Anderson, Carol Depew, David Wright and Leigh Adams.

Without the work of Anita Horvath, Alma Collins, Carole Eden and Gloria Shallcroft, who typed the manuscript, this book, quite literally, could not have been written. The copy-editor on the first edition, Christine Samuels, and the copy-editor on the second edition, Barbara E. Hodgson, also made valuable contributions to the manuscript. We would also like to thank our agent, Harold Moscowitz, and our editors at Avon, Beth Rashbaum and Susan Moldow, for their support and unending patience. Last, but not least, we would like to thank the many women who shared their medical histories and problems with us.

Preface to the Second Edition

In updating the book for this new edition, we found that there were some sections which needed little or no revision; yet other sections needed major rewrites. In certain instances, we added entirely new sections. It would be impossible to mention all the changes in this new edition, but the following are the most significant.

In Chapter Five the section on the long-term effects of the Pill and the possible link between the Pill and cancer has been rewritten. The recent studies suggesting that the Pill may actually protect the user against cancer are reviewed, along with a study indicating that young women using high-potency progesterone pills for extended periods of time may be at increased risk for the development of breast cancer.

The material on the Pill in the reference section on birth control methods has also been revised. Included is information on the newly discovered risks and side effects, and newly recognized noncontraceptive benefits of the Pill such as a lowered incidence of pelvic inflammatory disease (PID).

Important information for the users of the Copper-7 IUD is now included in the section on the IUD. Due to a design flaw in the device's inserter mechanism, some authorities are urging the Food and Drug Administration to withdraw the device. This section also includes new information about a rare form of PID, actinomycosis, which has been found among long-term IUD users, as well as suggestions on how users can protect themselves from actinomycosis.

Because the controversy surrounding spermicides and birth defects received so much coverage in the popular press, we have now covered this controversy in the section on vaginal spermicides.

In the first edition, we mentioned studies of the contraceptive sponge as a future method of birth control. The sponge has now been tested and is available, and we have added a new section on it.

The section on the cervical cap includes new information on cuts and tears of the cervix associated with the Vimule Cap, which some authorities suggest women not wear until more is known.

Because of media coverage of the possible link between vasectomy and subsequent heart and vascular disease, as well as that between vasectomy and impotence, we have included a discussion of these issues. Also, new information on ectopic pregnancies following sterilization and on a recently developed method of sterilization, the Silicon Plug, is now included in the section on female sterilization. A new subsection discussing the effect of repeat abortions on subsequent pregnancies has also been added. Finally, although Ovral, a combined birth control pill, has not been officially approved as a post-coital contraceptive, it is recommended by a number of doctors and clinics as a Morning-After-Pill. New material on Ovral has been added to this section.

Chapter Six appears almost as it did in the first edition, except that the *Symptoms Index* which formerly appeared in the appendix, now appears at the end of the chapter.

Significant revisions have been made in the reference section on diseases. Because a number of readers asked about Gardnerella, another name for the vaginal infection hemophilus, we've included the term in this edition. The major change in this section concerns the treatment of common vaginal infections. Some medications have been proven ineffective; dosage schedules of others have been changed; and in the case of yeast infections, a new home remedy has proven as effective as prescription drugs. The controversial use of a condom as a treatment for cervical dysplasia is now covered in the section on the cervix. Because pelvic inflammatory disease has become increasingly more common, we have expanded the material on PID in the section on the uterus and fallopian tubes. New controversies in the proper treatment of PID are given particular emphasis.

Some doctors are suggesting that women with suspected physiologic cysts of the ovary be put on birth control pills. Our objections to this regime are explained in the revised section on the ovaries. The other major change here concerns the treatment of ovarian cancer, which emphasizes the shift from radiation to chemotherapy as an adjunct to surgery. In the section on the breast, new developments in the treatment of breast cancer are detailed, especially in regard to less disfiguring surgery and the use of certain hormones in addition to chemotherapy. In response to readers' requests for more information on sexually transmissible infections, we have completely revised the section on herpes. Chlamydial infections have now reached almost epidemic proportions, so we have added an entirely new section on chlamydia. Again, readers' requests for more information have prompted revisions of the sections on premenstrual syndrome and menopause. In addition, the material on infertility has been updated to reflect changes in the field.

In the reference section on operations, tests, procedures, and drugs, the portions dealing with the Pap Smear, antibiotics, DES, and estrogen replacement therapy (ERT) have been revised. New material on the seemingly safer hormone replacement therapy (HRT) is included, as is a revised assessment of the risks and benefits of replacement therapy and a new subsection on home pregnancy tests.

We would like to thank the many readers who shared their medical histories with us. Their help was invaluable in preparing this revised edition. We would also like to thank Kathryn Vought, the editor on the second edition, Sharon Shavers, her assistant, Jerold Kappes who assisted in preparing the revised appendices, and Barbara Hodgson, the copy editor on this edition. Special thanks to Claudia Ziroli who prepared illustrations #20 and #24 for this edition.

WOMANCARE

1

How This Book
Came to Be Written

Way back, and it seems like eons ago, when we first conceived the idea behind this book, we wrote what is known in the publishing business as a book proposal. A proposal tells your editor what you're planning to write and is designed to convince the editor that your book fulfills a crying and desperate need and will therefore sell millions of copies.

The primary intent of this book, as we thought of it then, was to teach women how to use a speculum (the medical instrument used by doctors) to examine their own bodies. On the surface the idea of women practicing gynecological self-exam, although it may sound a bit bizarre, is hardly earthshaking. In reality, looking at your own vagina and cervix is about as exciting as looking down your throat. Indeed, in the not-too-distant future, gynecological self-exam will probably be a rather ho-hum topic, a routine matter of personal hygiene, about as controversial as brushing after meals or flossing your teeth. But for the time being, gynecological self-exam remains a rather revolutionary practice, for it brings us up against some basic cultural taboos and makes us confront the negative attitudes about our bodies that have been socialized into us since infancy.

Most women think of their genital organs as unclean, smelly and ugly, which is hardly surprising, since we have been taught to think just that from earliest childhood. The negative images that most women have about these parts of their bodies were formed early on, way back when they were toilet trained, if not before.

Consider the differences between the experience of little boys and that of little girls. Little boys who manage to make it to the bathroom in time, wrestle their pants down and, after taking careful aim, hit the pot are immediately rewarded with lavish praise. In contrast, little girls are told to wipe themselves clean. Equally lavish praise may follow, but for little girls the reflex parental response is "wipe yourself." The implication is clear—that area down there is dirty. Brother, on the other hand doesn't have to wipe himself after he urinates. He just gives his penis a nonchalant shake, with his bare hands, no less, and puts it back in his pants. Little girls must use a wad of protective tissue lest their fingers touch that caustic mess. For women, it is clear right from the beginning that we've got something really unclean between our legs—such a mess, in fact, that we shouldn't even touch it with our bare hands.

As we grow older the message remains unchanged. Boys may gather in groups and stage contests to see who can pee the farthest or write their names in the snow and dot the "i." Size and development of genital organs are gleefully compared. To be sure, many a late bloomer becomes the butt of cruel taunts in the locker room, but at least the matter is openly discussed. For adolescent girls there are no such locker room comparisons of who has the most protruding clitoris, the greatest number of pubic hairs, or whatever (and, as we all know, if it's too terrible to talk about, it's *really* terrible). Girls have long since learned that there is something unclean and hence unmentionable about their genital organs.

The situation continues unchanged into adulthood. Nancy Friday points this out in her book *My Mother, My Self,* when she says: "We all have something to hide. Why else would society build us stalls and cubicles with locks to undress and urinate in, when men are left to get on with it in large, communal, open locker rooms?"[1] The fashion and the cosmetic industries make fortunes exploiting women's insecurity about and dissatisfaction with their bodies. But, Friday argues, it is not really our breasts, thighs or waistlines we are concerned about when we complain that we are ugly (and even the most beautiful woman finds something to complain about). These nagging worries are just displacements; our fears are actually about something more central—our genitals. Complaining about our breasts, calves, thighs and so forth only serves to distract our attention from "that other area that mother would never mention, that had no name, that made her face *distort* with disgust if we got it dirty."[2]

Changing our negative attitudes about our bodies, developing what one psychiatrist has called "genital self-respect," is central to coming to view ourselves as fully acceptable and equal human beings. Or, as Nancy Friday puts it, "Convince woman that her vagina is beautiful and you have the makings of an equal person. I believe this with all my heart."[3]

Practicing self-exam is one way of changing all this, of reversing these negative attitudes. As strange as it may sound to the uninitiated, many women discover that this part of their bodies holds a certain beauty, a beauty, for instance, as delicate as an orchid's, which, unlike other forms of beauty in our culture, can be appreciated for itself, for it does not have to measure up to some Madison Avenue standard of attractiveness.

Practicing gynecological self-exam has other far-reaching consequences. For one thing it challenges the traditional relationship between women and their doctors. Once a woman learns to use a speculum she begins to view doctors differently. She has, literally and figuratively, a whole new perspective on the ritualized practice of the gynecological exam. And the gynecological exam is a highly ritualized phenomenon. It has been compared with the rites performed by medicine men, shamans and priests of supposedly more primitive societies; The supplicant/woman/patient is brought in to be examined by the priest/shaman/holy man/gynecologist. She is depersonalized by the removal of her clothes and/or other marks of personal or tribal identity. The priestly attendant/assistant medicine man/nurse then places her in a vulnerable position, on her knees, flat on the floor or, in our cultural ritual, in the examining table stirrups. The head honcho, in his characteristic garb, then makes an appearance on the scene; the supplicant/patient is draped in the ritual robes—in our culture, the white examining sheet—and the magic rite is performed. But for women who practice self-exam this whole ritual is demystified. Gynecological self-exam is a sure cure for what is often called the M.D.eity syndrome. Belita Cowan first coined the term "M.D.eity" in the early 1970s. Her classic essay, "Death of the M.D.eity," was published in the 1975 edition of *The New Woman's Survival Sourcebook*.

The M.D.eity syndrome is a condition that affects vast numbers of doctors in the United States and generally is transmitted to their all-too-susceptible patients. Perhaps the most characteristic symptom of the M.D.eity syndrome is the use of esoteric and incomprehensible language. A woman appearing before the M.D.eity with an irritating red rash on her inner thighs might, for instance, be told that she has erythema intertrigo, for which the doctor might prescribe an ointment with a multisyllabic Latin name. This too has its purposes. Such a woman might gratefully pay $50 or $75 to learn she had such an impressive-sounding condition that could be cured so easily. But were she to visit a shirt-sleeve doctor who told her that her problem was chafing (a less impressive term for erythema intertrigo) and that she should rub a soothing ointment on her thighs, the woman might, understandably, balk at paying $50, much less $75, for "professional services rendered."

As long as you're not on the short end of the stick the M.D.eity syndrome, with its overblown language and affected postures of authority, has a certain humor. But the syndrome also has its more serious side.

In 1976, 794,000 hysterectomies (an operation in which a woman's uterus is removed) were performed in the United States.[4] Approximately 1,600 women died that year as a result of the operation.[5] But the really upsetting statistic is that, by conservative estimates, some 30 percent to 40 percent, or as many as 300,000, of these operations were unnecessary.[6] Why did 300,000 women risk their lives to have an unnecessary operation? Because the M.D.eity syndrome affects patients as well as doctors. Women too are convinced by the priestly rituals, the medical jargon, the white uniforms, and they fall prey to the delusion that the doctor is an elevated, superior, almost godlike being. The doctor has access to secret knowledge, for s/he can see what we cannot. We have to depend on the doctor for knowledge about this essential part of our bodies. This special knowledge imparts power and gives the doctor control over us, so that when s/he tells us to have our uteri (plural of uterus) removed, far too many of us do not question that judgment. One does not, after all, question the judgment of those in charge. No one wants to find out that the judgments of those one relies on are faulty; the implications of such a finding are far too threatening to our sense of well-being and security.

Self-exam is the first step in changing all this. The knowledge is no longer secret. Practicing self-exam will not magically enable a woman to make sense of all that medical jargon, nor does it take the place of a doctor's examination, but it does begin to demystify the M.D.eity and allow women to deal with their gynecologists in a new way. It is probably a safe bet to say that a woman who practices self-exam will not find herself among the estimated 300,000 women who will have unnecessary hysterectomies this year. She knows too much and is too much in control to allow herself to be manipulated in this way.

This alone was enough to convince us that self-exam was an important topic, vital to every woman. But we had to convince a publishing company of this. Book companies, like most companies, generally are run by men. We were concerned that male readers of our book proposal wouldn't have a gut reaction to it, that it would be difficult for them to understand the impact our book might have on women. So we asked the male readers of our proposal to imagine for a moment that their genital organs were located on their bodies in such a way that they could not see them without making a conscious effort with the aid of a mirror to do so.

"Even then," we continued, "you could only partially see them. In order to see all of them, you would need a special instrument available only to doctors, almost all of whom, not incidentally, are members of the opposite sex. Also imagine that you have grown up in a culture that teaches you that it is nasty and not 'manly' to mention, much less look at or touch, these genital organs. Moreover, these organs have a thin membrane at the orifice that 'nice boys' are cautioned to keep intact for their future wives and to guard from lascivious females who 'only have one thing on their minds.'

"At the age of about 13, you are taken to a female doctor, who drapes you in a white sheet and pokes about in this mysterious area much to your embarrassment and, possibly, pain. Later on, your lovers or wives may familiarize themselves with this part of your body. You may even bear children through it, but you will still never have seen it. From time to time, you are troubled with infections and other ailments in this area, but unless you are especially bold, you are too embarrassed to ask your female doctor any questions. Even if you are so bold, you are too ignorant to ask intelligent questions about this unseen and mysterious part of your body. If, despite all this, you do manange to ask questions, she only pats you on the head and tells you 'not to worry your sweet little head about it, dearie, just do as I say.' ''

To add to their imaginary problems, we asked our male readers to further pretend that they lived in a society in which one of the burning questions of the day is whether or not people equipped with genital organs such as theirs are competent to deal with positions of leadership and power because of the raging hormonal imbalances produced by those never-seen genital organs: ''In this society, you and all other men are conditioned from birth to think of yourself as passive, dependent and weaker than women. As you grow older, though, times change. A Men's Liberation Movement started by some courageous men who feel that biology should not control your destiny gains momentum. At first it seems a bit of a joke, but as the years pass, it begins to exert a pervasive influence on your society. Men, even the most conservative, begin to conceive of themselves and their roles in society differently. Health care, because men by their genital makeup are so dependent on it, becomes a major issue in the liberation movement. Groups of men band together to demand that more men be admitted to medical school and that men be given the legal right to control their reproductive organs. Other groups come together to study and research the working of your still-mysterious body. Numerous books denouncing the women-dominated medical profession are written. Others that teach you how your own body works are published and read by millions of men. Even the effectiveness with which your lovers and wives manipulate these still unseen genitals is scrutinized in print. Then one day, you, with the aid of a mirror, an inexpensive plastic speculum and the latest of these 'male-lib' health-care books, take a look at these genital organs that have caused such a hullabaloo all your life. Imagine how you would feel.''

As it turned out, the editors who read our proposal were, by and large, women, who had no problem whatsoever imagining all of this and recognizing the impact the book might have. So the contracts were signed and work began immediately.

But that was only the beginning and, like all beginnings, was only a glimpse of what lay ahead. Buried in the back of our book proposal was a brief book outline. Not only would this book teach women how to practice self-exam, but because women who practiced self-exam would be in a position (no pun intended) to detect abnormalities and diseases in the earliest stages, when they are more curable, we would also include information on common gynecological problems, the symptoms a woman might notice and the ways in which these conditions might be treated. Because women who practiced self-exam would also have a greater understanding of their bodies and, consequently, new feelings of control and mastery, we thought it would be worthwhile to include information on the barrier methods of birth control—the diaphragm, spermicidal foams and rubbers—which, unlike the Pill and the IUD, are not beset by a host of risks and complications. Women who were familiar with their bodies would, we felt, have more confidence in using these safer, woman-controlled methods of birth control, which are highly reliable when used properly.

All this sounded quite sensible and not too terribly difficult, but as we began to talk with women and to review the available materials about gynecological problems and birth control, it became apparent that the emphasis of our book would have to shift and that the scope would have to enlarge. It became obvious that although gynecological self-exam was important, it was just the first step for women who wanted to gain control over their own bodies.

There were whole shelves of gynecologist-talks-to-the-laywoman books, but the majority of these books provided only the most superficial, Mickey Mouse sort of explanations of gynecological problems. None was of much use in helping a woman navigate her way through the medical marketplace, for even the best of them had a basic fault: They failed to inform women about their options and alternatives. As we talked to more and more women we came to realize that what was really needed was a sort of consumer's guide to gynecology, a book that would let women know what choices existed so that they could make informed decisions about health care and birth control.

Consider, for example, what happened to Susan, who is just one of the many women we came across in the course of writing this book. Susan is 36, divorced and the mother of two children, 12 and 9. It hasn't always been easy for Susan, raising two kids and trying to establish herself in a paying career after years as a homemaker. But when we met Susan things were looking pretty good. Although her job as assistant director at a day-care center wasn't by any stretch of the imagination lucrative, she was making ends meet. And finally, after hectic years of shuffling schedules and juggling the responsibilities of breadwinner, solo parent and homemaker, she was about to complete her thesis and receive her master's degree in early-childhood education.

To add to all this satisfaction was her relationship with a man. The relationship, which was of some years standing, had, after some fits and starts, progressed from friend to lover to live-in roommate. Now, after some serious thought, she and her lover were considering marriage and, more to the point, a baby—which suited Susan, who found mothering a rewarding experience, just fine.

At this time Susan, who neither smokes nor drinks and is conscientious about health matters, went to the doctor for her annual physical, which included a Pap smear, a test that involves collecting cells shed from the cervix

6

and that is used to screen for cervical cancer. Susan's Pap smear showed some irregularities, so she had to return to the doctor for further tests called biopsies, in which a number of tissue specimens are taken from various parts of the cervix. Susan's biopsy specimens were sent to a laboratory, where they were examined by a pathologist, a doctor who specializes in this field of medicine. The biopsy, which gives the pathologist an actual piece of tissue rather than just a few isolated cells to study, confirmed the diagnosis suggested by the Pap smear.

Susan had cervical cancer. Luckily, the doctor told her, she had caught the disease in its earliest stages, for her biopsy indicated that she had carcinoma in situ, a condition in which cells with all the abnormalities of cancer cells are present, but in which there is no sign that the cancer has invaded the surrounding tissue. The doctor told her that her condition was virtually 100 percent curable, but that she would have to have her cervix, uterus and ovaries removed, an operation known as a hysterectomy.

Susan was, understandably, quite shaken. Although it was a relief to know that her condition was curable, the prospect of losing her uterus and her ability to bear children, especially now, when she wanted so much to have another child, was extremely upsetting. Losing her ovaries was especially scary. She knew that having her ovaries removed meant menopause, and even though menopause itself didn't upset her (after all, her mother had never had any problems), she'd heard that having a premature menopause could pose serious health risks.

When she called her mom to tell her the bad news, Susan's mother insisted that she get a second opinion from another doctor. Susan promptly made an appointment with a second doctor and arranged to have her biopsy reports and medical records transferred. After reviewing her records and examining her the second doctor confirmed the diagnosis and again recommended a hysterectomy, although this time the doctor recommended that her ovaries be spared. Reluctantly, Susan allowed herself to be scheduled for surgery.

It just so happened that one of Susan's co-workers, who knew about her situation, also knew about the book we were writing. We had been spreading the word around, hoping to find women who had personally experienced the various conditions we were writing about and who would be willing to read and review what we had written. We had found that women who had gone through the experience of having an illness often had questions or comments that never occur to you until you are faced with the problem. Susan's friend suggested that she contact us.

Anxious to learn all she could about what was happening to her, Susan called the writer half of the gynecologist/writer team that put this book together. By reading the part of the book that deals with carcinoma in situ of the cervix, Susan not only gained a clearer understanding of what was wrong with her but also discovered something that was to prove important to her.

7

What both of her doctors had failed to tell Susan was that there were alternative forms of therapy for her condition. One of these therapies was a relatively new technique known as cryosurgery, which involves destroying the affected cervical tissue by freezing and which doesn't require the removal of any organs. Nor does it affect a woman's ability to conceive or bear children. The other alternative was a procedure known as conization, in which a core of tissue is removed from the center of the cervix, a surgical process somewhat akin to removing a core from the center of an apple. Conization would significantly reduce Susan's chances of being able to have children, but a fair number of women are still able to conceive after the procedure.

There was, however, a catch: Not all women with carcinoma in situ are suitable candidates for these less destructive forms of therapy. We cautioned Susan not to get her hopes up, but we could see she was excited. She was definitely ready for a third opinion. This time Susan saw a gynecologist who was also an experienced cryosurgeon. As it turned out, Susan was an ideal candidate for cryosurgery, although it was necessary to repeat all the diagnostic tests before this was determined. The doctor who originally performed Susan's biopsy had put all the biopsied tissue specimens into the same container when he sent them to the laboratory for analysis, so there was no way of knowing exactly where on the cervix any given tissue sample had originated. Knowing precisely where the tissue samples have come from is a critical factor in determining whether or not a woman is a suitable candidate for cryosurgery. So Susan had to suffer the mental anguish of waiting extra days for the repeat lab tests (not to mention the additional expense involved in repeating the tests).

The lab tests looked good and Susan decided to go ahead with the cryosurgery. Instead of spending a couple of thousand dollars or more and losing her reproductive organs, her ability to have children and a significant amount of time from work, Susan spent less than a hundred dollars, didn't lose any time from work and eventually was able to go ahead with her plans to add to her family.

Why didn't the other doctors tell Susan about cryosurgery? We can't tell you for certain, although the writer half of this book team did try, with Susan's written permission, to find out. Not surprisingly, both doctors refused to discuss the matter. There are a number of possibilities.

Perhaps it was the old M.E.eity syndrome. Doctors do get to thinking of themselves as rather godlike, and gods, having a wider view of things, are, of course, wiser than we mere mortals. Susan was 36 and already had two children. Some population-conscious doctors believe that no one should have more than two children. (Some doctors think that minority women on welfare, in particular, should not have more than two children, but Susan was white and didn't collect welfare, so this was probably not a factor in her case.)

8

Susan was a divorcee and not married, and even in this day and age there are doctors who don't approve of pregnancy in unmarried women and who think they have the right to inflict their unannounced moral judgments on their patients.

Or, their failure to inform Susan of her options and alternatives may have been motivated by some combination of ignorance and greed. The doctors may have known about cryosurgery but may not have had the training, experience and equipment necessary to perform the procedure. Instruction in cryosurgery has only recently been added to the medical-school curriculum for gynecologists. Unless a gynecologist were a fairly recent graduate of medical school, s/he would have had to go back to school, that is, take a special training seminar in the technique. This training takes time and money, and there is also the added financial outlay for the equipment. If the doctor were not skilled in cryosurgery, this might mean referring the woman to another doctor and thereby losing a fee. Doctors' fees for hysterectomies range from about $1,000 to $3,000.

Thanks to the Pap smear, cervical cancer is being discovered in its earliest stages. A doctor with a busy practice might see five to ten patients a year with carcinoma in situ. A doctor who saw ten such patients a year and who charged an average fee of $1,500 for a hysterectomy could be faced with referring away $15,000 worth of business annually. If the doctor's fee were $3,000, referring ten patients might mean a loss of $30,000, a rather hefty chunk of money to forego.

Maybe it was simple ignorance. The first two doctors Susan saw may not have been up to date on the latest techniques. Even though most states have some sort of continuing education requirement designed to keep doctors abreast of the latest developments, these requirements generally are pretty laughable. Attending a few luncheons presided over by a speaker from the medical society can pretty much fulfill these requirements. Or, better yet, a doctor can take one of the numerous cruises to exotic locations that are designed specifically for doctors and offer continuing-education credits sandwiched in between shuffleboard and other shipboard attractions. At any rate, state requirements by no means guarantee that a doctor is up to date, and Susan's doctors might just have been a bit behind the times.

Even if a doctor is a skilled cryosurgeon, s/he still has a financial interest in performing hysterectomies rather than cryosurgery. The cost of cryosurgery runs from about $60 to $150. At $60 per patient, ten patients per year with carcinoma in situ treated by cryosurgery would net the doctor $600, whereas ten hysterectomies at $1,000 per operation would pull in $10,000, a more than tenfold increase in annual income.

This is not to suggest that all doctors are greedy monsters who are eyeing your uterus with dreams of yachts or Aspen condominiums in their heads;

however, the estimated 300,000 unnecessary hysterectomies* performed in the United States each year do give one pause. Still, it is probably a rare doctor who actually sits around and says, "Ah, ha! I think I'll give this woman a hysterectomy and make some extra bucks." The process is somewhat more subtle than that. Doctors, like the rest of us, tend to develop rationalizations for what they do. For instance, a doctor who recommends hysterectomies for carcinoma in situ may argue that cryosurgery is not an adequate form of therapy, that it is too new for its effectiveness to have been conclusively proven.† But how much of this is sincere and how much is rationalizing and self-justifying?

If a doctor were to explain to a woman with carcinoma in situ that there are alternatives but that, personally, s/he did not recommend these forms of treatment, we would not doubt his or her sincerity. But often this is not the case. Neither of the first two doctors that Susan contacted even mentioned that these other forms of therapy existed. In situations like Susan's the financial motivations of a doctor who fails to inform a woman fully of the options available to her are suspect.

Women must realize that this is a "for-profit" medical-care system, which is different from a socialized medical-care system, where doctors are paid a flat salary by the government. In our system there is a financial incentive for doctors to recommend more drastic and hence more profitable treatments. This is not to suggest that medical care under a socialized medical system would be any better or worse; both have their problems, and this is a complex issue beyond the scope of this book. Let it suffice to say that for right now, and for the forseeable future, medical care in the United States will operate on a "for-profit" basis and this undeniably influences the type of health care women receive.

Susan's case is not unusual. In fact, doctors who inform their patients fully of the options available to them and then allow the patient to make her own decisions are the exception rather than the rule. Many gynecologists believe that informing women about their options and letting them make a decision is a waste of time. Their patients, they tell us, don't want to assume responsibility for such decisions. They want the doctor to do it for them. As one doctor put it, "I used to spend time carefully explaining things to my patients. They didn't want to hear it. They wanted me to tell them what to do. So I don't bother with all that anymore. I just tell them what to do. That's what they want, that's what they expect from you."

---

*Unnecessary hysterectomies are those operations in which a healthy uterus is removed. A hysterectomy done for carcinoma in situ would not be considered an unnecessary hysterectomy in the medical sense of the term, even if alternative forms of treatment were available.

†The risk involved in cryosurgery treatment for carcinoma in situ is discussed in greater detail elsewhere in this book. See the index for page numbers.

We don't doubt that there are women who don't want to be informed, who want to leave it all in their doctors' hands. Given the cultural barriers that keep women from knowledge about their bodies, the M.D.eity syndrome and the general sexism in our society, it is not surprising that some women think that they are too incompetent and too ignorant to make decisions about their own bodies. We are so alienated from our bodies that some of us think we cannot even venture opinions—much less make judgments—about what is in our best interests; however, our work with women has convinced us that, given the choice, most women opt for an active role in making decisions about their own bodies. The growing women's health movement is evidence of the fact that women not only want, but are actively demanding, a role in health-care decision making. We suspect that, in reality, doctors who believe that women want decisions made for them enjoy the paternalistic relationship they establish with their patients. There is, after all, a certain ego satisfaction to be derived from playing the M.D.eity. It's also less trouble. No need to waste time bothering with explanations. It's much easier to pat a patient on the head and tell her not to worry about it.

Moreover, many doctors think of women as hysterical, not-terribly-bright creatures who aren't capable of understanding the alternatives, let alone making responsible decisions. It is a popular myth in our society that sexist attitudes are held by truck drivers, construction workers and rednecks. The well-educated doctor is, supposedly, beyond all that. But one has only to take a look at medical textbooks to discover that sexism is rampant in the medical profession. The failure of many doctors to inform women of their options and to include them in decision making stems from their sexist views of women.

Another explanation for why women are not informed of alternative forms of therapy is that many doctors don't see this as their responsibility. They see their job in quite another light. Their function, as they perceive it, is to provide their expert opinion and recommendations for therapy. Medicine, they argue, is a complex, highly technical field. Women don't have the background and knowledge to evaluate intelligently the alternatives available to them. According to this school of thought, that's the doctor's job.

At first glance this point of view seems fairly sound, but these doctors forget one important thing. Experts disagree, and they disagree much more often than most of us outside the field of medicine realize. Susan's case is just one example. There are myriad others. Consider, for example, breast cancer. The same women could consult three different doctors and get three different opinions. Doctor A might recommend a segmental mastectomy, a simple removal of the lump and a segment of the surrounding breast tissue. Doctor B might recommend a modified radical mastectomy, which involves removal of the woman's breast and the lymph nodes in her armpit. Doctor C might recommend a segmental mastectomy with subsequent radiation treatments. None of these doctors could be called a quack. Indeed, each of these procedures is endorsed by topflight doctors at the nation's most renowned medical schools, and the debate about which treatment is best is argued passionately in medical circles—and probably will be for some time to come.

The doctors who argue that women cannot make their own decisions about which form of therapy they should have ignore the fact that there is not uniform agreement among experts. When the experts disagree the decision comes down, as it always must, to one person, the patient herself. In order to make these decisions women need to understand the issues and the options. Then and only then are they in a position to do what they must: Weigh the facts and, depending on their own personal values, make a decision.

Are the issues so complex that women cannot understand them? We think not. In our opinion many doctors have an inflated view of the complexity of what they do. This is not to say that the issues in medical debates are not at times rather convoluted, but the complexities can be simplified so that they can be understood by laywomen without undue distortion.

As we worked with more and more women it became obvious to us that women were not getting the information they needed from their doctors. What was necessary, it seemed to us, was a book that provided this sort of information. Second opinions are fine, and we heartily support them, but as we saw in Susan's case, second opinions are too often just rubber stamps of approvals. Second opinions do not always assure that women will hear the whole story or be informed of all the available options. Thus we began to shift the emphasis and redefine the scope of this book.

We still felt that women needed basic information about their bodies. The first section of this book is designed to provide that information. The following chapter explains the external anatomy of the genital organs and teaches women how to practice gynecological self-exam. Chapter Three discusses the anatomy and function of the breast and teaches women how to breast self-exam. Chapter Four explains the changes that take place in a woman's body over the course of a menstrual cycle and over the course of her lifetime.

The second part of this book discusses birth control, for this is another medical area in which women frequently are misinformed. There is a great deal of bias in the medical profession in regard to birth control. Doctors often push the more dangerous, physician-controlled methods, such as the Pill and the IUD, and downgrade the safer, user-controlled barrier methods, such as the diaphragm, foam and condoms (rubbers). As we explain in Chapter Five, statistics have been used—or rather misused—to create the impression that the Pill and the IUD are vastly more effective than the barrier methods, but this is simply not true. There have been studies of the condom in which the actual-

12

use effectiveness rate was better than the commonly quoted theoretical rate*
for the Pill and the IUD.

This part of the book also includes a reference section that provides detailed
information about the various methods of birth control, so that women can be
well informed when making decisions about this matter.

The third section of this book deals with doctors and disease. Chapter Six
discusses the doctor–patient relationship, how to find a good doctor and how
to get a second opinion. An index of symptoms of the diseases described in
this section and instructions for using the index appear at the end of this chapter.

This section also includes a reference section, which contains information
about virtually all the ills that female flesh is heir to, with descriptions of
causes, symptoms, diagnostic steps and the various treatment options. The
conditions described in this reference section are categorized according to the
organs they affect. Thus, diseases of the breast are found under the heading
The Breast, problems relating to the ovary are discussed under the heading
The Ovary and so forth. There are separate headings for sexually transmissible infections, for problems relating to pregnancy and fertility and for problems related to the menstrual cycle. There is also a separate subdivision that
deals with general information about cancer, but specific information about
cancer of a particular organ is discussed along with the other diseases of that
organ.

Each of the various subdivisions in the reference section on diseases is pref-
aced with a short introduction, which contains valuable general information
about diseases of the particular organ or the set of problems discussed in that
subheading. For instance, the introduction to the section on vaginal diseases
includes information on the prevention and diagnosis of vaginal infections
that applies to *all* the vaginal infections in that section. Rather than repeat that
information in the discussion of each and every vaginal infection, we have included it in the general introduction to vaginal diseases. So be sure to review
the material in the introductions before reading about the specific problem
that interests you.

This reference section is not designed to take the place of your doctor or of
second opinions. Rather, it is designed to provide you with basic information,
so that you will be aware of your options and will have sufficient knowledge
to be able to ask the right questions.

The last section of the book deals with gynecological operations, tests, procedures and drugs. Chapter Seven talks about unnecessary surgery and tests
and explains how to avoid them. Detailed information about the various oper-

---

*The theoretical rate is the effectiveness rate one could expect if that method were used
perfectly, with none of the forgotten pills, broken condoms or other problems that occur in
actual use.

ations, tests and procedures mentioned in other parts of the book is included in the accompanying reference section, along with information about some of the more controversial drugs used in gynecological medicine.

A standard format is used for the descriptions of birth control methods, diseases and operations, tests and procedures, and may include any of the following:

Name: The most widely used name of the birth control method, disease, drug, operation, test or procedure is given at the beginning.

AKA: "AKA" stands for "also known as." There is generally more than one name or term used to refer to any given disease, birth control method, drug, operation, and so on. For example, yeast infections of the vagina may also be referred to as fungus infections, moniliasis and candidiasis, to mention just a few alternate names. We have included all such alternatives in the index so that women will be able to locate the desired information regardless of the name they look under.

Types: This entry, which is found most often in the discussions of gynecological disease, includes a breakdown of the various categories or types of diseases.

Associated Terms: This also appears most often in the discussions of gynecological disease and is a sort of catchall used for terms that are not actually synonyms for a disease or types of the disease but are associated closely with that particular gynecological problem. These too are listed in the index.

The index can also be an important tool in helping you become more fully informed. As mentioned above, you can use it to locate information on a birth control method or a disease, regardless of which of their various names you may know. It may also serve as a sort of dictionary or glossary of terms. Although we have tried to avoid medical jargon, you may at times come across terms that are not familiar to you. If you will then turn to the index, it will direct you to an explanation of the term. In addition, you may also use the index as a sort of guidepost to help you find your way to important, related information. If, for instance, you are reading about a condition that is treated with a hysterectomy, you might want to consult the index and find a page number reference for the discussion of the pros and cons of various types of hysterectomies. By turning to those pages, you would discover that a hysterectomy can involve just the removal of the uterus or removal of the uterus and the ovaries as well. If you require a hysterectomy, will you want your ovaries removed too or will you ask your doctor to spare them? Since some doctors routinely remove the ovaries when doing hysterectomies on women over a certain age, this sort of additional information can be important. We've made the index extensive to enable you to find all relevant information quickly and easily. We encourage you to use it.

Although the index is the main tool we have used to help our readers locate related information, we were concerned that in certain instances it alone might not suffice. There were times, we realized, when no matter how much common sense a reader had, it might not occur to her that she should look in the index for related information or that there was in fact additional material of interest to her elsewhere in the book. We were further concerned that in other instances a reader might not be clear on which term in the index would lead her to the related information she needed. Because of these concerns we devised a cross-reference system. At various points in the text you will see a page number preceded by the word *see* and enclosed in ( ). Related information that may be of interest can be found on the pages given. By using the index *and* the cross-references, you should be able to locate all the information you need to become an informed consumer.

Perhaps we should also mention that metric measurements—centimeters, millimeters, and so forth—generally are used in medical literature and that we have often used them in this book. A list of metric abbreviations and a table that will help you convert measurements to more familiar standards is included in the appendix.

We have tried to organize this book so that the information is easily accessible. We hope that it will help to break down the barriers that make medical information accessible only to members of the medical profession, for we believe that every woman should have access to all available knowledge before making any health-care decision.

You may find that your doctor disagrees with some of the things we have written. Such disagreement is unavoidable, for medicine is not an exact science. You, as a consumer of medical services, have a right to a full explanation of medical controversies before giving your consent for any type of treatment. Only in this way can a woman's consent be truly informed; only then can you weigh the alternatives and make the decision you think is right for you.

Although the medical information in this book represents the most up-to-date findings at the time of writing, some information will need revising before the ink has had a chance to dry, for things change quickly in the field of medicine. We have tried to indicate areas where ongoing research may provide answers or new insights. We hope that there will be revised editions of this book in the future. Nothing would be more helpful in preparing future editions than comments, questions and criticisms from readers. If you have thoughts to share, please contact us by writing to Lynda Madaras, c/o Avon Books, 1790 Broadway, New York, New York 10019.

Gynecological Self-Exam

"A book about what?" squawks our friend and neighbor, whom we'll call Doctor Tom (although he is a doctor, his name is not actually Tom).

"Gynecological self-exam, you know, teaching women how to use a speculum," we repeat, making a mental note to call somebody else next time we want to borrow a medical dictionary. From Tom's reaction, you'd have thought somebody had just called him to say she was writing a book on how to perform brain surgery at home in your spare time and wanted to know if she could borrow his scalpel.

In a few moments Tom, now a man with a mission, is at the front door, medical dictionary in hand. "But it's dangerous," he sputters.

"Dangerous, how?" This stops him cold. "Come on, it's not dangerous; it's not any more dangerous than cleaning your ear with a Q-tip."

"You could puncture your eardrum with a Q-tip," counters Tom, who works in an emergency room and has a flair for medical oddities.

"What could you puncture with a speculum?"

After some hemming and hawing Tom is forced to concede that self-exam isn't dangerous, but now he argues that it's much too difficult. Actually, a speculum is about as difficult to use as a shoehorn or a can opener. An adroit 5-year-old could probably handle the mechanics of it. The thousands of women in the United States who practice self-exam are living proof that it's not too difficult. After a while Tom, who by now has had to concede that self-exam is neither dangerous nor too difficult, comes up with another objection.

"Yes, but what about cancer?"

Cancer? Tom was obviously clutching at straws. He couldn't possibly think that someone could develop cancer as a result of practicing self-exam. As it turned out, Tom's concern was that women who practiced self-exam might come to think that it was no longer necessary to have an annual Pap smear, a test that can detect the presence of cervical cancer before there are any visible signs or obvious symptoms.

We don't believe that women who practice self-exam will come to neglect basic health care; quite the contrary. It seems to us that fear and ignorance, not knowledge, are what keep women from having annual Pap smears, breast exams and general physicals. But just to keep Tom happy, we'll say it: Gynecological self-exam is not meant to be a substitute for going to the doctor. The doctor can perform tests like the Pap smear and other types of examinations that you cannot. Rather, gynecological self-exam is an addition to your regular medical checkups. By practicing self-exam, women can learn to detect abnormalities and seek treatment when diseases are most curable, in their earliest stages, before they become full-blown illnesses. For example, a woman who practices self-exam, is familiar with her own vaginal discharge and knows what is normal for her can detect a vaginal infection (the most common gynecological problem, the chief symptom of which is an increase in vaginal discharge) right away, before the discharge is so copious that it leaks out onto her underclothes. Vaginal infections, although they generally are not serious, can be difficult to get rid of. Not infrequently, they require more than one course of treatment, which means more doctor's visits, lab tests and medications, which can be costly. Women who practice gynecological self-exam can nip these infections in the bud and avoid the necessity for extra courses of treatment, saving themselves time and money.

Not only can gynecological self-exam save you money, but as discussed in the first chapter, it can also change your whole attitude about your body and yourself and about doctors, medical care and your role in making health-care decisions.

Consider one friend's description:

One evening several years ago, a woman I know invited me to attend what I thought was going to be a meeting of a consciousness-raising group. It was, but not in the way I had expected. Instead of the usual rap session, I found a group of women teaching each other to give themselves gynecological self-examinations. My initial reaction was one of acute embarrassment. It was, after all, a fairly bizarre scene. One by one, the women climbed up on the table, inserted plastic speculums and, with the aid of a flashlight and a mirror, took a look at their own cervixes. My curiosity proved stronger than my lingering Victorianism and, when it came my turn, I hopped up on the table too.

As it turns out, looking at your cervix is no big deal. But the first time I did it, my emotional reaction was overwhelming. Here was a part of my own body intimately connected with my sexual identity, my psychological being, my very self, and I had never seen it. Moreover, the men in my life and my all-male string of gynecologists had more experience with this part of my body than I did. My body, and *they* knew more about it than *I* did.

The effect of looking at my cervix was mind-blowing. I had an incredible feeling of personal power and competence. I left that evening, speculum tucked under my arm, walking tall, literally strutting down the street. I knew what was happening. I could take care of business. I was in charge, on top, heavy duty . . . yes, ma'am!

This chapter describes the anatomy of your genital organs and explains how to go about giving yourself a gynecological exam. We hope that taking this guided tour of your own body leaves you feeling equally in charge, on top and heavy duty, yes, ma'am!

Equipment

You will need three pieces of equipment: a mirror, a light source and a speculum. A mirror with a stand is good because you won't have to hold the mirror and thus both of your hands will be free. A makeup mirror with two sides, one of which enlarges your reflection, is also more convenient, but a regular hand mirror will work fine. A gooseneck lamp with a 100-watt light bulb provides a good strong light and is also convenient, since it is adjusted easily to the proper angle and also frees your hands; however, a flashlight will do if you don't happen to have a gooseneck lamp.

The speculum is a little harder to come by. Most doctors use a metal speculum, but this is a fairly expensive piece of equipment. Because these speculums are metal, they can be sterilized after each use and can be used over and over again on the doctor's patients. There are also inexpensive plastic speculums that cost about 50 cents apiece wholesale. These speculums often are used by hospitals and clinics. Because they are plastic and cannot be sterilized by heat, they are intended for one-time use only. It would be unthinkable for a doctor to use these disposable speculums on different patients. You certainly wouldn't want to be examined with a plastic speculum that had been used on another patient, especially someone who had a vaginal disease. However, because your speculum will be used by you and only you, it needn't be heat-sterilized after each use. Your plastic speculum can be used without fear of infection as long as simple sanitary precautions are observed. After each use wash your speculum thoroughly with an antiseptic soap (a number of good ones are available without prescription from the pharmacy) or with isopropyl alcohol, wrap it in plastic and store it in a clean, dry place.

If you are feeling less than certain about sanitary conditions, please remember that millions of women insert diaphragms into their vaginas regularly as a method of birth control, and there is nothing unsanitary about this. As long as simple sanitary rules are observed there is no danger of infection. If at some point you should develop a vaginal infection, you might feel more comfortable switching to a new speculum, but as long as you wash the speculum thoroughly there is no need to discard your old speculum.

Although inexpensive plastic speculums are available, getting hold of one is not always easy. According to a federal law that regulates any instrument inserted into a bodily orifice, a speculum cannot be sold without a doctor's prescription. It is, to say the least, a curious law. You are much more likely to do yourself bodily harm with a Q-tip (perforated eardrums and so forth) than you are with a speculum. Clearly, this law is a legacy of bygone days and old attitudes about women and sexuality.

Sometimes speculums can be bought directly from medical supplies distributors, who are listed in the yellow pages of your telephone book. The largest manufacturer of plastic disposable speculums is Barnett Instruments, a division of C.R. Bard, and their speculum is registered under the trade name Sani-Spec. The Sani-Spec is sold in packages of ten and comes in three sizes—small, medium and large. The sizes vary both in the width and length of the speculum blades. The small and medium Sani-Specs are about the same length, but the small is only half the width of the medium. If you are a virgin, you would probably use a small size. If, however, you are a virgin and are also not used to inserting tampons in your vaginal opening, it may be difficult to insert even the small speculum comfortably. Using tampons for a few months before trying self-exam will widen the vaginal opening and make a speculum exam easier.

Most women can use a medium speculum, especially if they have borne children. If you feel any discomfort on inserting the speculum, you are probably using too large a size. Your doctor can help you if you are uncertain as to size. Special classes in self-help are also given by women's clinics across the country, where you can obtain a speculum and learn how to give yourself an exam. Some of these clinics are listed in the appendix. Some women prefer to learn about self-exam in the group setting provided by these clinics, where there are women with experience in self-exam to help them. Other women prefer doing this with friends, by themselves or with their doctors.

Of course, if your doctor is willing to help, this is the most logical place to obtain your speculum. Not only can s/he write you a prescription or provide you with a plastic speculum, but your doctor can also help you find and identify your cervix, which can be a bit tricky the first time. Unfortunately, not all doctors are receptive to the idea of their patients examining themselves. One woman who got interested in self-exam tells of asking her family doctor, a kindly old gent, who had brought her into the world and who had delivered one of her own children, for a speculum. "He was," she reports, "vaguely horrified. You'd have thought I'd asked him for a scalpel so that I could perform a hysterectomy on myself. Luckily, I had a good relationship with him and was able to talk to him and explain my reasons. He finally came around to my point of view and got me a plastic speculum from the hospital. In fact, he

19

now uses a speculum and mirror with his patients whom he is teaching to use a diaphragm and claims it is ten times easier to teach them now.''

In the course of writing this book we've talked to many doctors, most of whom have been enthusiastic about the idea of self-exam. Some doctors, however, had an initial resistance to the idea. It's a new idea, and like all new ideas it takes some getting used to for some people. One way to find a gynecologist who will be sympathetic to self-exam is to call a women's clinic, a women's center at a local college or university or a free clinic. Such places normally have referral lists of gynecologists who are apt to be more sympathetic to the concept of self-examination. (For more information on finding a doctor, see Chapter Six.)

In any case, once you've managed to get hold of your speculum, spend a few minutes practicing opening and closing it so you are familiar with how it works and are able to operate it smoothly (Illustration 1). Insert the speculum into your body with the duckbill closed, as shown. Once it is inside, clasp the handles together, which opens the duckbill and allows you a view of the walls of your vagina and cervix. To open it wider and lock it in the open position, press down with your thumbs. As you push down you will hear three clicking noises. This clicking is the ratchet mechanism that opens the duckbill wider with each progressive click. The disposable plastic speculum is not a precision instrument. Because it is designed for one-time use, you may find that it tends to stick a bit with repeated use. Don't give up; it's the instrument, not you, that's at fault. With a bit of perseverance and practice you can learn to make it work fairly smoothly.

Exploring Your External Anatomy

Before you insert the speculum and take a look at your internal anatomy, take some time to familiarize yourself with your external genitals, also known as your vulva or, as Granny used to call them, your "private parts."

Illustration 2 will help you recognize and identify the various parts of your external genitals. Some women have told us that these kinds of gynecological drawings are often confusing or misleading. One reason for this is that such drawings typically show only those parts of the female anatomy that doctors are concerned with—the parts that are subject to infection or other ailments. If a feature of the anatomy isn't a typical site of infection or abnormality, then it usually is not named and, for a doctor's purposes, doesn't exist. This can be confusing, especially in regard to the vestibule (see below), where there are several folds and layers of skin that are not shown in gynecological illustrations. Many women, looking at the typical medical illustration, become worried that they have a growth or some spare parts because they are unable to distinguish the medically named features from the unnamed but nonethe-

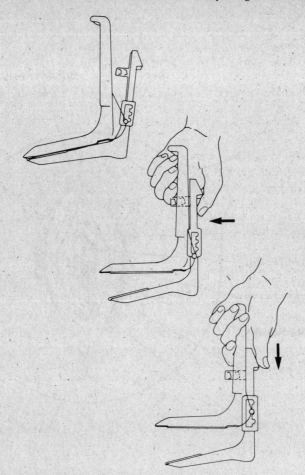

Illustration 1 *Working the Speculum*

less present anatomical features. We have provided more detailed drawings of this area in an attempt to avoid this confusion.

Another reason that it is sometimes difficult to identify parts of your genitals from drawings is that each individual is different. Also, the appearance of your genitals changes in the course of your lifetime. A young girl's genitals do not look the same as a mature woman's. So don't expect to look exactly like the illustration in this book.

However, just as your face has recognizable features (nose, mouth, eyes), so your vulva has identifiable parts that you can learn to recognize. Of course, we are quite used to looking at faces, so it is easy for us to generalize from a stylized drawing of a human face and recognize the salient features on a particular individual. Most of us, however, are not quite so used to looking at

21

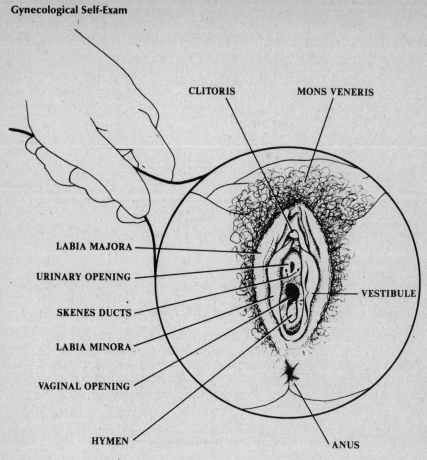

CLITORIS   MONS VENERIS

LABIA MAJORA

URINARY OPENING

SKENES DUCTS

LABIA MINORA

VAGINAL OPENING

VESTIBULE

HYMEN

ANUS

Illustration 2 *External Genitals*

female genitals; therefore, it is not as easy to generalize. Don't worry, though; it is highly unlikely that you are missing any parts, and with a little practice you can learn to recognize the features of your genitals as plainly as you see the nose on your face.

Now, find a quiet place to begin a guided tour of your own body. You might sit on the floor or on a bed, perhaps using pillows to prop up your back so you're comfortable. Bend your knees and spread your legs apart. Position your mirror so that you have a good, clear view of your external genitals.

Mons Veneris

As you look down your body from the position described above you will notice a slight mound that rises between your legs. If you were standing, looking at a wall mirror, it would be a triangular area that in a mature female is cov-

22

ered with short, curly pubic hair. This is called the mons veneris, or "mound of Venus." *Mons* means "little hill" and refers to the pad of fatty tissue that covers your pubic bone.

When you reach puberty the increased output of two hormones, estrogen from the ovaries and androgens from the adrenals, stimulates the growth of pubic hair. Pubic hair tends to be coarse, crisp and curly. The thickness and curliness depend on your racial and genetic background. On some women pubic hair grows up toward the navel and on the inside of the thighs whereas on others it is rather sparse. After menopause, when hormone levels gradually decrease, pubic hair may thin out, become straighter and even turn gray. During sexual excitement the pubic hairs act as a scent trap for the erotically stimulating secretions of scent glands located in the pubic area.

Labia Majora

As you move downward from the mons you will notice that the area covered with pubic hair divides and continues down toward the anus, the rectal opening. The hairy areas on either side of this division are the labia majora or outer lips. These two folds of fatty tissue protect the urinary and reproductive tract openings that lie between them. These outer lips change in size during the course of your life and also vary in size from individual to individual. If you have never had children, these outer lips may actually touch each other. After childbirth many women find that these lips are slightly separated, so that the area between is exposed. If you separate these outer lips with your fingers, you will notice that the insides of them are hairless and are dotted with small, slightly raised bumps, which are oil glands that help keep the area moist. The color of the skin in this area may vary from light pink to brown black.

Labia Minora

If you separate the outer lips, you will see two long ridges or folds of skin. These are the labia minora, or inner lips. They are hairless, sensitive to touch and vary greatly in color and texture from light pink to brown black and from very smooth to very wrinkled. They usually protrude less than the outer lips, although in some women they may actually protrude beyond the outer lips. During sexual excitement they swell and darken in color.

If you follow the inner lips up toward the mons, you will notice that they come together or fuse. The upper fold of this fused portion forms a sort of hood that covers the bud-shaped clitoris and is called the prepuce, clitoral hood or clitoral foreskin. In some women this hood will completely cover the clitoris; in others the clitoris will protrude slightly. The fold of skin that passes beneath the clitoris or may seem to extend from the lower sides of the clitoris is called the frenulum.

23

The labia minora, or inner lips, serve to protect the reproductive and urinary tract openings that lie between them, to lubricate the area with their oil-producing glands and to stimulate the highly sensitive clitoris. Any contact or movement of the inner lips moves the clitoral hood, which in turn stimulates the clitoris as it moves across it.

Clitoris

Now you come to the sexiest part of your anatomy, the clitoris. If you pull back the clitoral hood, you will see a small bud-shaped piece of tissue, the glans clitoris, or the tip of the clitoris, which usually is about the size of an eraser on the end of a pencil. The clitoris is made of erectile tissue, which fills with blood and swells during sexual arousal. As you touch yourself in this area, you may well have pleasurable feelings of sexual excitement.

The rest of the clitoris is hidden from view underneath the surface of the skin. If you press gently just above the clitoral hood in an upward direction toward your mons, you will feel a firm, rubbery, movable cord under the skin. This is the shaft of the clitoris. For some women this is a sexually sensitive area. The rest of the clitoris, including the crura, two wing-shaped extensions of the shaft that spread in wishbonelike fashion and are attached to the pubic bone, and two bundles of erectile tissue called the bulbs of the vestibule, lie too far under the skin and muscle of this area for you to feel. These, along with the rest of the clitoris and a system of connecting veins throughout the pelvis, become firm and filled with blood during sexual arousal and account for the warm, tingling feelings we often experience. Some women experience a similar type of pelvic congestion just before their period, and for some women this creates a heightened sexual desire at that time.

The clitoris is involved directly or indirectly in all female orgasms. Before the pioneering work of Masters and Johnson, two doctors who have done groundbreaking research into female sexual response, it was thought that there were two types of orgasms—vaginal and clitoral. A vaginal orgasm was supposed to be a more mature type of response, whereas a clitoral orgasm was judged to be an "infantile" response to sexual stimulation. Women who experienced orgasms only in response to clitoral stimulation were said to be "frigid," "sexually immature," "less feminine" and "neurotic."

As a result of the clinical work of Masters and Johnson, the so-called vaginal orgasm has been shown to be a myth. All female orgasms are related to the clitoris. Even when an orgasm results from penile penetration, the clitoris is involved, for movement of the inner lips serves to stimulate the clitoris. Also, the vaginal opening lies near the shaft of the clitoris, and the shaft may thus be stimulated orgasmically. For most women, however, penile penetration alone doesn't stimulate the clitoris enough to produce orgasm.

Vestibule

If you separate the inner lips with your fingers, you will be able to see a smooth, boat-shaped area that is called the vestibule. The opening of the urinary tract—the urethral meatus, through which you eliminate liquid wastes, or urine, from your body—is located here. The opening to your reproductive tract, through which you insert a tampon, through which a baby is born and into which the penis is inserted in sexual intercourse, is also located in the vestibule. Two small glands known as Bartholin's glands are located just inside. The ducts of these glands will probably be too small for you to see. They generally are not noticeable except when the duct of the glands becomes blocked and swells as the result of infection. It was once thought that these glands were responsible for lubrication of the vagina during sexual arousal. It is now known that they secrete only a few drops of fluid at this time and that their function is to keep the opening of the vagina moist.

Urethral Meatus

The urethral meatus may be difficult for you to find unless you have the obvious, protruding kind. To find the urethral meatus, start from the clitoris and move down. If you stay in a straight line, the first dimpled area you find will be the urethral meatus. It usually resembles an inverted *v*. You have to stay dead center while you are moving down from your clitoris or you might mistake the ducts of the Skene's glands, two little niches on each side of the urethral meatus, for the urethral opening.

To make certain you have found the urethral meatus, stand in the bathtub or shower, spread your inner and outer lips and position a mirror so you have a clear view of the vestibule; then urinate. This will teach you beyond any shadow of a doubt where your urethral meatus is located. Furthermore, you will learn how the inner lips help to direct your urine flow and that urine does not hurt mirrors. Wash up and get back in position for the rest of your self-exam.

Hymen

As you continue in a downward direction from the urethral meatus you will come to the opening of the vagina. At the entrance you will find the hymen, or maidenhead, as it is sometimes called. It is here that you may have some difficulty making a correspondence between your anatomy and the drawings. This is true for two reasons. First, as indicated by Illustration 3, the appearance of the hymen varies considerably from individual to individual. Moreover, most of us have been taught to think of the hymen as some sort of

25

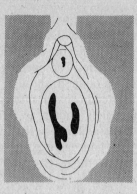 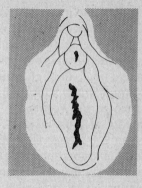

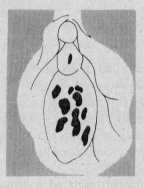 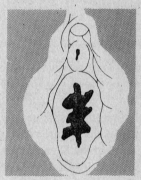

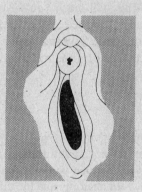 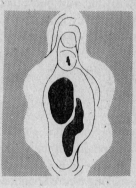

Illustration 3   *Hymen Variations*

disposable plastic seal that is broken the first time we have intercourse (or by some accident) and somehow disappears or dissolves afterward. This is a misconception.

In some women the hymen is a semicircular strip of mucous membrane that fringes the lower edge of the vaginal opening. In some women it encircles the entire rim of the vaginal opening. In still others it may be a semicircular membrane covering the lower half or three-fourths of the vaginal opening. It may have one large opening or several small ones. The variations are endless. In some rare cases it may block the vaginal opening entirely, and it may then become necessary for a doctor to open it to allow for the passage of menstrual flow.

At any rate, the hymen does not break the first time we have intercourse. Rather, it stretches and may tear as it does so, causing some bleeding. And it does not disappear. Irregular fringes or folds of mucous membrane remain and can be seen surrounding the vaginal opening. Some women mistake these irregular bits of membrane for growths of some sort, but they are merely hymenal tissue and are known in medical circles as hymenal caruncles.

Many myths or old wives' tales surround these small bits of tissue. One widespread myth is that a broken or stretched hymen indicates that a woman is no longer a virgin, that is, that she has had sexual intercourse. It is just that—a myth. The hymen may be broken or stretched by exercise, masturbation, a tampon or any number of accidents that can occur in a woman's life. Some women are born with little or no hymen tissue. On the other hand, women with particularly elastic hymens can have intercourse many times and still not tear this tissue.

Vaginal Opening

Just behind the tissue of the hymen lies the opening to the vagina, which is called the vaginal introitus. This opening usually is depicted in illustrations as a gaping black hole, which can be misleading. More than likely you will see folds of flesh rather than a black hole in this area. The folds of flesh are the inner walls of the vagina.

Exploring Your Internal Anatomy

This is the point at which you will begin to explore your internal anatomy. Before you actually insert the speculum, insert a finger or two through your vaginal opening and explore your vaginal cavity.

Vagina

Your vagina, or vaginal cavity, as it is often called in medical textbooks, is a muscular tube about 4 to 5 inches long. The accordionlike walls of your vagina can expand to admit an erect penis and can expand even further during childbirth. In its normal state this muscular tube is collapsed, like an airless balloon, so that the walls of the vagina touch each other.

The walls of the vagina will feel squishy and soft and will mold around your finger. Depending on your age, the stage of your menstrual cycle and how sexually aroused you are, the walls of your vagina may be almost dry to very wet. Your vagina produces continuous secretions that help keep it clean and maintain the acidity of its walls to prevent infections from starting.

If you insert your fingers just inside the opening and push upward on what is called the anterior vaginal wall, you will feel a soft bulge of tissue, which may be particularly sensitive. This is your urethra, the tube that runs from your bladder to the urethral meatus and through which urine flows.

If you slide your fingers more deeply into the vaginal cavity and press on its walls, you will notice that only about the first third of your vagina has any sensation. The upper portion is not very sensitive to your touch, because it has fewer nerve endings.

If you press upward on the walls of your vagina, you may feel the urge to urinate. This is because your bladder lies quite near the vagina (see Illustration 4), and any pressure on the vaginal wall is likely to be felt on the bladder. Likewise, the rectum is located on the underside of the vagina. If you press down on the vaginal walls, you may feel a bump. This is nothing serious, just feces, or waste material, in your rectum.

The vagina is, for all practical purposes, a closed tube. Therefore, a tampon or anything else inserted into your vagina cannot go ''up inside.'' The back wall of the vagina is called the fornix. If you push your fingers along the back wall until you reach the top of your vagina, you will feel the cervix, or the neck of the womb.

Cervix

The cervix is shaped like a rounded cabinet knob and is 1 to 2 inches in diameter. It feels fairly firm, like the tip of your nose, or if you have had children, it may feel as firm as your chin. The firmness/softness of the cervix varies according to what phase of the menstrual cycle you are in. If you have difficulty locating the cervix, bear down as if you were making a bowel movement or bring your knees closer to your chest. Push the cervix around a bit with your fingers, and you will see that it is not a rigid, immovable organ but one with quite a bit of give. In fact, your cervix changes position frequently dur-

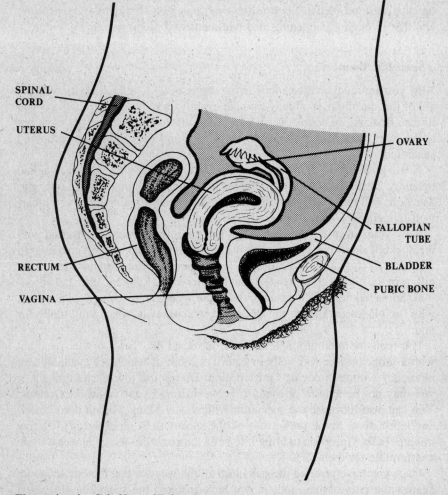

SPINAL
CORD

UTERUS

OVARY

FALLOPIAN
TUBE

RECTUM

BLADDER

PUBIC BONE

VAGINA

Illustration 4 *Side View of Pelvic Structures*

ing different stages of your menstrual cycle and also moves farther back during sexual excitement. So your cervix may not be in the same position each time you examine yourself; however, it is undoubtedly there (unless, of course, it has been removed surgically).

You may be able to feel a small depression or hole or an indented ridge in the center of your cervix. This is the opening to the cervical canal, which leads into the uterus, and is known in medical jargon as the cervical os. In women who have not had children it may be round or oval and about the size of the head of a kitchen match. If you have had children, it may be slightly

29

larger. As we said before, tampons and other objects cannot pass through this opening into the uterus. Sperm, however, can pass through the cervical os, and it is through this opening also that menstrual blood passes.

Speculum Exam

Now you are ready to take a look at the inside of your vaginal cavity with the aid of the speculum. You may find the examination more comfortable if you urinate first and, of course, wash your hands afterward. Assume the same position, with your back propped up by pillows and your knees drawn up and separated.

Next, position the mirror so that you have a clear view of your vaginal opening. Direct the light toward the mirror, not toward your vaginal opening. The light will reflect off the mirror into your vagina so you will have a clear, well-lighted view of the inside of your vagina.

Now you can insert the speculum. The speculum should be inserted with the duckbill sideways, that is, with the blades of the duckbill perpendicular to the floor, as shown in Illustration 5. Then, once the blades are inserted to the hilt, turn the blades up so that they are parallel to the floor and open the speculum. Some women find it easier to insert the speculum in the upright position, with the blades parallel to the floor. Do whichever is most comfortable for you.

If it feels more comfortable for you, lubricate the blades of the speculum with a lubricant like K-Y jelly or Lubrifax, both of which are available at a pharmacy without a doctor's prescription. Do not use too much lubricant or you may not be able to distinguish between it and your vaginal secretions. You can also lubricate the speculum with water. Many women do not need any lubrication. Some prefer to soak the speculum in tepid water for a few minutes before insertion to bring it to body temperature, which makes it more comfortable for them.

Once you have inserted the speculum all the way, so that the blades are up against the pubic bone, and, if you have inserted the speculum sideways, have turned the blades upright, open the speculum by clasping the handles together. Then, with your thumb pushing down on the speculum, lock the speculum in the open position. The speculum locks open in three progressively wider positions. You will hear three clicking noises to correspond to these three positions. Your view will be much better if you open the speculum to its widest position.

Inserting the speculum is apt to be a rather awkward process the first time, indeed the first several times you do it. (Remember the first time you used a tampon!)

Simple mechanics has a lot to do with this awkwardness. Unfortunately, no one has yet devised a speculum to be used by a woman to inspect her own

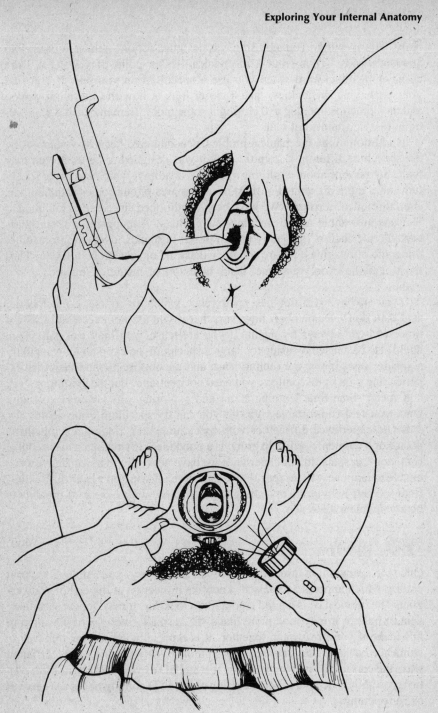

Illustration 5 *Speculum Self-Exam*

body. The speculum you are using was designed for one person to insert into another's body. Thus from a mechanical-design point of view, you'll be doing things backward when you use a speculum on yourself. If you find yourself having difficulties, take a closer look at how the speculum works, and then practice opening and closing it some more. Remember, it's the speculum that's at fault, not you.

In addition to the mechanical problems encountered because you are using the speculum differently from the way it was designed to be used, you may feel a bit nervous about exploring your own anatomy, which can make speculum exam more difficult. For most of us this area of our bodies is unfamiliar, even forbidden, territory. We have been conditioned since early childhood to feel uncomfortable about touching our genitals. Although it is socially acceptable for doctors (generally males) or our husbands/lovers to insert something into our vaginas, we are not given that kind of societal permission. Thus most of us have only a vague, black-hole sort of image of this area of our bodies.

If you are having difficulties, try to relax, which, of course, is much easier said than done. Remember, however, that if you are not successful the first time, you can always try again. If you are tense, you may feel pain. Pain could also be caused by using too large a speculum, and you might want to try a smaller one. If you are feeling tense and uncomfortable and therefore experiencing pain or discomfort, you need not continue. Put the speculum away and spend some time learning about and exploring your external anatomy. Once you feel comfortable with this you can try speculum exam again.

If you experience difficulties with speculum exam, finding a sympathetic doctor or a women's self-help group is a good idea. If you aren't successful at first, don't despair. In our experience we have never found a woman who was unable to learn how to do speculum exam. Even if you don't have difficulties, finding a self-help group or sharing the experience with a group of friends can be a valuable experience.

Finding Your Cervix

Once the speculum is inserted and opened all the way, you can look for your cervix, which appears as a raised, knoblike projection at the end of your vagina. The cervical os is a good landmark to look for. It may appear as a round dent or hole or it may look more like a slit, a smaller version of the slit your lips make if you press them together. It is especially apt to look this way in women who have had children. Illustration 6 shows some of the different ways the cervical os may look. If you use an IUD as your method of birth control, you should be able to see the string of the IUD coming out of the cervical os, or opening.

Some women may have difficulty finding and recognizing the cervix. Med-

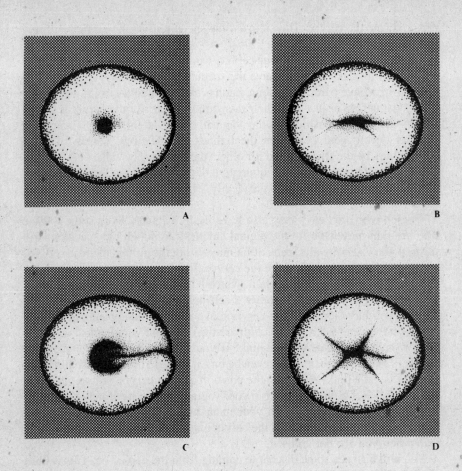

A   B

C   D

Illustration 6   *The Cervix: In a woman who has never borne children (A); in a woman who has borne children (B); in women whose cervixes were torn during childbirth (C and D).*

ical textbooks invariably illustrate the cervix seen through a speculum as if it were on a straight bull's-eye visual path. However, many times this is not the case. The cervix, as we have seen, is a movable organ that is not always in the same place. At various points in your menstrual cycle it may be higher or lower in the vaginal cavity. Moreover, in some women the cervix characteristically may lie a bit to the left or right. If you do not see your cervix immediately, try moving the speculum to the left or right or position it at a higher or lower angle. Changing the position of your body by bringing your knees closer to your chest or bearing down as if you were making a bowel movement may help to bring the cervix into view. Massaging your lower abdomen may also help. If none of this helps, remove the speculum and use your fin-

33

gers to locate the cervix. Then reinsert the speculum, angling it in that direction.

If you still haven't found your cervix, using a larger speculum may help. Also check to make sure you have the speculum open to its widest position. Women who have particularly long vaginas may want to try examining themselves just before or just after their menstrual period, for the cervix is generally at the lowest position in the vaginal cavity at this time. Examining yourself during your period on the lightest day of flow, which for some women may be the first day and for others the last day, can also help because it will be easy to see the blood coming out of the cervical os. On heavier days there may be too much blood to see clearly, but on lighter days it is easy to see the cervical os.

Women who are heavy may also have fleshy vaginas. Even some women who are thin may have fleshy vaginal cavities. Although the speculum will separate the vaginal walls, pads of fat may still bulge around the blades of the speculum, making it hard to see the cervix. Inserting the speculum sideways and using the large-sized speculum, which has wider blades, may help. Here again, finding a doctor or a women's self-help group can be helpful.

Once you have located your cervix make note of the appearance of your cervix and vaginal walls. What color are the tissues of your vaginal walls? In most women the tissue will be pink. If you are pregnant, the cervix might have a faint blue tinge or might even be bright blue. In older women the tissue is apt to be pale pink. Also note the position of your cervix. Is it to the left or to the right? Is it higher or lower in your vagina? The os itself may be more or less open at different stages in your menstrual cycle. You may notice that when you are sexually excited, the cervix may be higher in the cervical canal than when you are not aroused.

You will also see some discharge coming from the cervial os. This is quite natural. The os is the opening to the cervical canal. This canal, which is called the endocervical canal, is about 1 inch long and leads into the uterus. It is lined with tiny, mucus-secreting glands whose secretions change character over the course of your menstrual cycle.

The Uterus, Ovaries and Fallopian Tubes

The uterus (Illustration 7), which is about the size and shape of an inverted pear, is a hollow organ lined with a special type of tissue, called endometrial tissue, that thickens and is shed each month during your menstrual period.

Extending from the upper portion of the uterus on either side are two 4-to-5-inch-long tubes with tiny fingerlike projections on the end. These are the fallopian tubes. Near the ends of each of these tubes on either side of the uterus lie two small organs about the size and shape of a Brazil nut. These are the ovaries. They produce substances called hormones that stimulate the

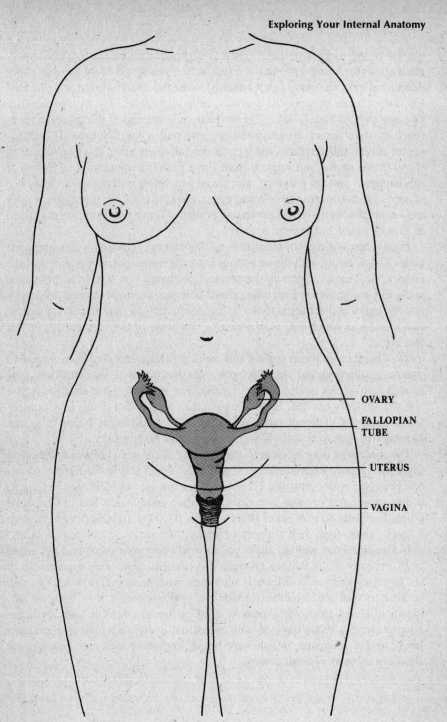

OVARY

FALLOPIAN
TUBE

UTERUS

VAGINA

Illustration 7 *The Uterus, Fallopian Tubes and Ovaries*

uterine lining to grow thicker. They also produce a ripe egg approximately once a month during a woman's reproductive years. Contrary to what many people believe, the ovary is not attached to the fallopian tube but is suspended by its own bands of supporting tissues, called ligaments. The ovary releases a ripe egg every 28 to 32 days. The projections at the end of the fallopian tubes reach out like fingers to grasp the egg and pull it into the tube. If a man's sperm meets and fertilizes the egg in the fallopian tube, the egg may then travel to the uterus and implant itself there in the rich endometrial lining. If this happens, you are pregnant, and the uterine lining will not shed, because it is needed to nourish the developing egg, called the embryo. If pregnancy does not occur, the lining breaks down and is shed. (These processes are discussed in greater detail in Chapter Four.)

Even when you are not menstruating, the uterus is constantly sloughing off cells. These, along with the secretions from the mucus-secreting glands of the endocervical canal, make up the cervical discharge you see. In addition, the walls of your vagina are secreting fluids constantly. These vaginal secretions and the cervical discharges make up the discharge you may see during speculum exam and which you may notice on the blade of the speculum after you remove it.

The character of these vaginal and cervical discharges vary from woman to woman and in each individual woman over the course of her menstrual cycle as well as over the course of her lifetime. The discharge also changes as you become sexually excited. Examining yourself at different points in your menstrual cycle, at different times of the day and at different stages of sexual arousal will help you learn how your particular body works.

The discharge may be clear to milky white in color and thin and watery to thick and creamy in consistency. It will taste, smell and feel different at various points in your menstrual cycle. As you examine yourself note the details of the appearance of your secretions. Are the vaginal walls wet or dry? How much discharge do you have? What color is it? What consistency? How does it smell, taste, feel? Is it slippery or sticky?

In Chapter Four we will show you how to chart your menstrual cycle and keep a record of the various changes that occur in your body each month or so. By doing this you will learn to recognize what is normal for you. You will be able to spot abnormalities or disease, perhaps before they become full-blown illnesses requiring expensive medical treatment. You can also learn how to identify those days of your menstrual cycle on which you are most likely to get pregnant, which may be an important factor in helping you choose a method of birth control.

Other Things You May Notice

Some women may notice small, fluid-filled cysts on the cervix. These are called nabothian cysts and are nothing to worry about. Some women may see a reddish circle around the os or red patches on the cervix. In all probability these are simple cervical erosions or eversions and are discussed in greater detail elsewhere in this book. They are usually nothing to be concerned about. Indeed, about 20 percent of all women are born with cervical eversions. Occasionally, red spots on the cervix will result from something more serious. Don't hesitate to discuss these or any other things you notice with your doctor.

Chapter Six provides information on gynecological conditions, and the Symptoms Index at the end of that chapter contains a list of various signs and symptoms that a woman who is practicing self-exam may notice. If, after you have consulted these sections and read Chapter Four, which details the type of changes you can expect to see over the course of the menstrual cycle, you are still concerned about something you have noticed during speculum exam, feel free to discuss it with your doctor.

You should also feel your vaginal walls and cervix for any lumps, bumps or rough, sandy areas. If, after you have learned what is normal for your body, you are concerned about a possible abnormality, again, don't hesitate to consult your doctor. In all probability s/he will tell you that everything is OK, but this is part of learning about your own body.

Sometimes we are hesitant about discussing a "nonsymptom" or something that is only a vague feeling or apprehension with our doctors. We may fear that the doctor will think we are silly, overly worried or perhaps a bit crazy. But there is nothing wrong with saying to your doctor, "I've learned how to use a speculum and I've noticed (this, that or another thing) and I'm wondering why, or what, or if . . ." If your doctor isn't willing to discuss this with you and answer your questions fully or dismisses you with a pat on the head, assuming a don't-worry-your-pretty-little-head-about-it-dearie attitude, find yourself another doctor.

Removing the Speculum

After you've completed your speculum exam remove the speculum from your vagina. Some women prefer to close the duckbill before removing the speculum by pulling up on the outer rim of the speculum handle. Other women find that it is easier to remove the speculum with the duckbill in the open position. After removal, clean the speculum with antiseptic soap or alcohol, let it dry and store it in a plastic bag in a safe place. Before calling it a day you should also examine your breasts. Breast anatomy and breast self-examination are discussed in the next chapter.

Breast Self-Exam, or How to Save Your Own Life

Breast self-exam (BSE) can save your life and maybe your breast as well. Women who discover breast cancer through BSE have higher survival rates than those whose tumors are detected by the doctor or found only by chance. This is a reflection of the fact that BSE-detected tumors are more likely to be found when the disease is in its early, more curable stages. Studies indicate that deaths from breast cancer might be reduced by as much as 18 percent if women practice BSE regularly.[1] Self-exam is, quite literally, a way to save your own life; yet despite the undisputed value of early detection, relatively few of us practice BSE routinely.

Why don't we? The answer to that question, like the answer to so many questions in the field of women's health care, is complex. First, there's the old it-can't-happen-to-me syndrome. We all prefer to think of breast cancer or, for that matter, any serious problem as something that happens only to other people. But the fact is that 1 of every 14 women in the United States will develop breast cancer at some time in their lives, and three-fourths of these women will die as a result of the disease.[2] The fantasy that breast cancer is something that happens only to other people is just that—a fantasy—at least for the 7 percent of us who actually develop the disease.

To put the whole thing in a less abstract, more personal and concrete way, make a list of women that includes you and the 13 women with whom you have the closest personal contact. Your list might include female relatives, Mom, sisters, daughters, close friends, neighbors, business associates, who-ever. . . . OK, now think about the fact that, statistically, one of the women on your list is going to get breast cancer and odds are three to one that she'll die of it. You may have to mourn the loss of a dearly beloved friend or relative or at least regret the passing of a close acquaintance. Actually, you may not have to worry about the funeral arrangements at all; those you leave behind may have to take care of all that. Also consider that your friend/relative/acquaintance/self could significantly reduce the chances of having to attend the funeral if she simply got into the habit of spending a few minutes a month checking her breasts.

If it sounds like we're trying to push your panic buttons, that's because we are. But we can't step out of the pages of this book and do a personal presentation of our breast-self-exam-can-save-your-life routine. And besides, scare tactics, more than just being a cheap shot, are notoriously ineffective. Perhaps we should try a different approach. How about considering the fact that breast self-exam, in contrast to gynecological self-exam, is a socially acceptable habit. Indeed, it is actively encouraged. Planned Parenthood, the American Cancer Society and other such organizations distribute vast quantities of pamphlets urging women to practice monthly breast exam and explaining how to do so. Part of the reason for this active support of BSE lies in the fact that it has proved to be effective in the early detection of breast cancer.

But more than that, breasts themselves and the idea of touching them are infinitely more acceptable than vulvas, vaginas and cervixes and the idea of touching them, especially when it's the woman herself who's doing the touching. Unlike our vaginas, vulvas and cervixes—or to borrow Granny's phrase, our private parts—breasts are, to put it mildly, quite public. Close-ups of bulging breasts are plastered across billboards, movie marquees and magazine layouts. We are a breast-obsessed culture. From the time we are prepubescent we are inundated with the message that our breasts are an incredibly important part of our anatomies. Most of us got the message early on, standing in junior high gym class, elbows bent and arms winging out at shoulder level, pumping furiously as we chanted:

> *We must! We must!*
> *We must increase our bust!*
> *We may! We may!*
> *We may get big some day!*
> *It's better! It's better!*
> *It's better for the sweater!*

Despite—or perhaps because of—the fact that our breasts are such a public part of our anatomies, many women fail to practice BSE. Often we're afraid of what we'll find. If we find a lump, it could be cancerous and if it's cancerous, that could mean losing a breast. In our culture the breast is so tied up with our notions of sexuality, femininity and our very worth as female people that the thought of losing one immobilizes many of us. Of course, the thought of losing any part of our bodies is a scary notion, especially if we lose it to the big C, cancer. But if 1 out of every 14 of the women in the United States contracted cancer of the thumb and if three-fourths of those who did died of the disease, you can bet that a lot more women would practice monthly thumb self-exam than currently practice BSE.

It is important, then, for women to realize that 80 percent of the breast lumps that are biopsied are not cancerous. Moreover, having breast cancer does not necessarily mean that a woman will lose her breast. Today there are less disfiguring forms of therapy that leave the breast largely intact. Although these methods have not yet proved to be as effective as the older methods, which involve removal of the entire breast, there has been enough convincing preliminary data to suggest this possibility, and large-scale studies to determine the effectiveness of these less disfiguring treatments are now underway. Then, too, great strides have been made in breast reconstruction, so that it is now possible in many cases to create a new breast using plastic surgery techniques. Having breast cancer no longer means that a woman's anatomy will be disfigured forever.

In order to be a candidate for these less radical therapies, a woman's cancer must be discovered in the early stages. Common sense tells you that a woman who practices monthly BSE is 11 times more familiar with her breasts than a doctor who examines them only once a year. More than 90 percent of breast lumps are first discovered by the woman herself, either in the course of routine BSE or by chance, which is why self-exam is so important. The woman who examines her breasts each month has a better chance of discovering the tumor in its early stages. This means that not only is she more likely to save her life but she may also be able to save her breasts.

Some of us are reluctant to examine our breasts because we are not happy with the way they look. If our breasts do not conform to the bulging, airbrushed, blemishless breasts that adorn the pages of *Playboy,* we may think that they are inadequate. Careful examination of our breasts may serve only to remind us of our feelings of inadequacy; hence, we may simply choose to ignore them. But it's important to overcome these feelings. Try to let go of the cultural images of what your breasts should or should not look like and enjoy the uniqueness of your own anatomy. Doing this can be a valuable exercise for your mental and emotional—as well as your medical—health.

Breast self-exam is, then, incredibly important. None of us can afford to let fantasies of invulnerability, fears of losing a breast or feelings of inadequacy deter us from developing this life-saving habit.

Breast Anatomy and Function

Knowing a bit about the anatomy and function of the breast will help you in learning to do breast self-exam. In the center of each breast is the nipple, which is surrounded by a pigmented circular area that is known as the areola (see Illustration 8). The color of the nipple and areola varies from individual to individual, ranging from light pink to deep brown or almost black. The color generally deepens after a woman has had a child. The base of the nipple is ringed with tiny oil-producing glands that help keep the nipple supple. Some women have hairs around the areola.

The nipple is made up of erectile tissue. In some women the nipple is constantly erect; in others the nipple becomes erect only when stimulated by cold, physical contact or sexual activity. The nipple is almost always erect during a woman's orgasm. Most women's nipples protrude beyond the areola, but some women have inverted nipples. This, in and of itself, is not a problem, but if a formerly protruding nipple becomes inverted, this may indicate some underlying disease and should be brought to a doctor's attention.

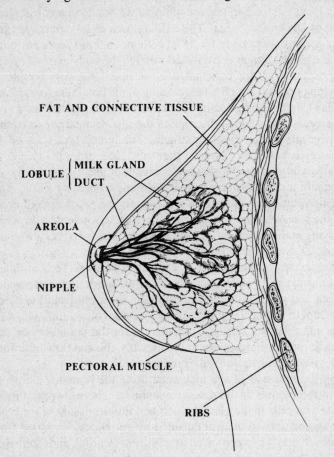

FAT AND CONNECTIVE TISSUE

LOBULE { MILK GLAND
        { DUCT

AREOLA

NIPPLE

PECTORAL MUSCLE

RIBS

Illustration 8   *The Anatomy of the Breast*

The interior of the breast is divided into several sections, called lobes. These lobes are further subdivided into lobules, each of which contains milk-secreting glands cushioned by fat and fibrous connective tissue. An intricate pipeline system of numerous tiny ducts arranged like the branches of a tree carry the milk produced by the glands to the ampulla, a collecting chamber immediately below the nipple. The entire breast is richly supplied with blood vessels.

The connective fibrous tissue attaches the breast to the muscles of the chest wall, which are known as the pectoral muscles. The breast itself contains no muscle tissue. The breast exercises you learned in junior high gym class were designed to develop the pectoral muscles so they would become thick and bulging, creating the impression that the breast was larger. But no amount of exercise will make the breast itself larger.

The pectorals extend up into the armpit area, which in medical circles is referred to as the axillary area. The axillary area also contains lymph nodes. Lymph is a transparent body fluid that is found in tissue spaces throughout the body. Like blood, lymph is circulated through the body in tiny vessels. These lymph passageways are punctuated by accumulations of lymphatic tissue called lymph nodes. Lymph nodes relating to the breast are found in the axilla (the armpit), in the hollow above the collarbone, along the blood vessels beneath the breast bone and at the neck of the ribs. Lymph is part of the body's immunological, disease-fighting system. The lymph nodes act as sieves filtering bacteria, cast-off cells and other substances from the lymph fluid.

The breast also contains sensory nerves that are exceptionally sensitive. They account for the sexual sensitivity of some women's breasts. An infant's sucking also stimulates the nerves and triggers the production of breast milk. In fact, the sensory nerves in the breast are so sensitive that the sound of an infant crying in the next room is sometimes enough to trigger a woman's "let-down" reflex and cause a flow of milk.

The production of breast milk is a complex process. Tens of thousands of tiny cells inside the milk glands absorb basic substances—like water, salts, sugar, fats and small nitrogen-containing molecules—from the bloodstream and use them to synthesize milk. Although actual breast milk is not produced until the infant begins sucking, preparation for the possibility of pregnancy occurs each month. In response to the monthly ebb and flow of hormones the breast begins to gear up for milk production.

During the first half of the menstrual cycle the hormone estrogen is produced by the ovaries in increasing quantities. The estrogen stimulates the growth of new cells in the glands, ducts and fibrous tissues of the breast. This increase in cell activity is accompanied by an increase in blood flow to the breast, which may be experienced as a fullness, warmth and, sometimes, tenderness. At about the middle of the monthly cycle, a ripe egg is released from the ovary, and as a result the second ovarian hormone, progesterone, is released into the bloodstream. The progesterone starts the secreting process in the gland cells. Even this small amount of stimulation can be felt by some women. Part of the swelling and feeling of fullness is caused by an increase in the blood supply, and part of it is caused by a greater amount of fluid seeping into the tissues from the ducts.

If pregnancy does not occur, the hormone levels shift again. The changes that the hormones stimulated in the breast are reversed. New cell growth is slowed and the blood supply to the area is diminished. Secretions and cells are reabsorbed by the body to make room for the new cells and secretions that will be produced during the next menstrual cycle. The swelling of the breast tissues diminishes and the breast softens. If pregnancy does occur, the build-up of the duct, gland and fibrous tissue continues. After delivery another hormone, prolactin, which is produced by the pituitary gland at the base of the brain, is released, and this triggers the actual production of breast milk. As a baby sucks, more prolactin and hence more milk is released. As the baby is weaned, prolactin levels fall and the production of breast milk tapers off.

Breast Self-Exam

Most doctors recommend that women start to practice BSE after they have had their first menstrual period and continue the habit throughout their lives. Because breast cancer is rare in women under age 25, some doctors recommend that women not start BSE until age 25. These doctors believe that if a girl starts BSE at age 13 and practices for so many years without ever finding abnormalities, she will develop a false sense of security and will drop the habit in later years, when it is most important. Personally, we think that BSE should be started at the time of the first menstrual cycle. Although it is true that breast cancer is rare in women under age 25, it does happen. Moreover, there are benign breast conditions that occur in younger women which, although generally not serious in and of themselves, may increase the chances of developing breast cancer later in life. Knowing that she may be at increased risk of developing breast cancer could influence a woman's decisions about methods of birth control. For example, a woman at increased risk might opt to select a method of birth control other than the Pill.* In addition, a young girl having her first period often is living with, or is in close contact with, her mother; if their menstrual cycles are close together, they can practice BSE together, which can be a valuable and special experience for a mother and daughter to share. But regardless of the age at which BSE is begun, it should be continued on a monthly basis for the rest of the woman's life.

*The debate over the relationship between the birth control pill and breast cancer is discussed in more detail in Chapter 5.

Many women become discouraged about their ability to practice self-exam. As we have seen, the breast is an extremely glandular organ. The glands may feel like lumps. At first it is difficult to know what is normal lumpiness and what is abnormal. This is especially difficult for women whose breast tissues are particularly responsive to hormone stimulation, because they are apt to have a periodic increase in the lumpiness and swelling of the breast. Many women have a condition known as fibrocystic disease, which is an exaggeration of the normal, hormone-induced changes in the breast. In its milder forms fibrocystic disease may produce only periodic lumpiness, swelling and breast tenderness. In some cases one or more distinct lumps, sometimes fairly large ones, may be felt as soft, tender, movable lumps in the breast tissue. These lumps may wax and wane with the cyclical ebb and flow of hormones. At other times these lumps may last throughout the menstrual cycle. These persistent lumps require a doctor's attention. Generally, they are simple fibrocystic cysts, collections of secretions and old cells that were not reabsorbed successfully by the body. The doctor may apply a local anesthetic to the breast, attempt to aspirate the contents of the cyst with a needle and examine the aspirated fluid microscopically to rule out the possibility of cancer. The aspiration usually will cause the cyst to collapse; however, these cysts sometimes recur. Women with fibrocystic disease or periodic lumpiness in their breasts should make a chart like the one shown in Illustration 9 to help familiarize themselves with the lumpy areas of their breasts. Any large, definite lumps in the breasts of a woman with a history of fibrocystic disease should be examined by a doctor.

Women with periodic lumpiness in their breasts—in fact all women in their menstruating years—should do BSE at the beginning of their menstrual cycles, that is, right after the menstrual flow stops, for that is when the levels of hormones are lowest and the lumpiness is least noticeable. Younger women who have only recently begun to menstruate often have irregular menstrual cycles. They may go for months at a time without having a period. If this is the case, it's a good idea to pick a certain day, perhaps the first of the month, and do BSE on that day. Women who are no longer menstruating should also set aside a certain day. The first of the month, payday or any significant day will do.

All women, especially those with periodic lumpiness or fibrocystic disease, should enlist their doctors' help in learning to do BSE. This may require more than one doctor's visit. After the doctor examines your breasts repeat the exam yourself. If you find an area that you're not sure about, have the doctor feel it. Explain that you're not sure whether what you feel is normal or abnormal, and ask the doctor to feel the questionable area. It's not always easy to feel comfortable about doing this. We are apt to think that we are taking up the doctor's valuable time with silly, vague, half-formed questions, but BSE is an important, even lifesaving, process, a preventive measure well

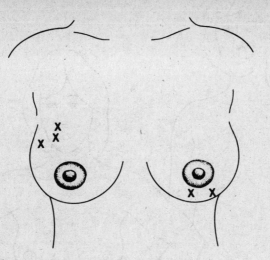

Illustration 9 *Women with fibrocystic disease may want to make a chart like this, with Xs marking the areas where there is periodic lumpiness.*

worth the time and effort of any conscientious doctor. Besides, the doctor is being paid—and being paid handsomely—for his or her time. If your doctor is impatient with your questioning or is otherwise not supportive of your attempts to learn BSE, consider finding yourself another doctor. In fact, if your doctor is a really good one, you won't have to ask for help with BSE. Either the doctor or one of the doctor's staff, perhaps a nurse, should ask you if you practice self-exam and should encourage you to do so, offering help and advice. Studies have shown that one of the most effective means of getting women to practice BSE is to have their doctors actively encourage them to do so.

Part One: Inspection

BSE should be done at a time when you are relaxed and not rushed or distracted. The examination consists of two parts: inspection and palpation, or feeling. To begin the inspection portion, stand in front of a well-lighted mirror and let your arms hang at your sides, as shown in Illustration 10. Note the size and shape of your breasts. No one's breasts are identical to each other, but being familiar with the appearance of each of your breasts will help you spot any changes in subsequent months. Pay attention to the contour of the breast, looking for depressions or bulges. Moles or any dimpled, dark or reddened areas, swellings, sores or areas of the skin with a rough or orange-peel-like texture should be noted. Some women have prominent blue veins in their breasts, which is normal, but changes in the appearance of the veins are im-

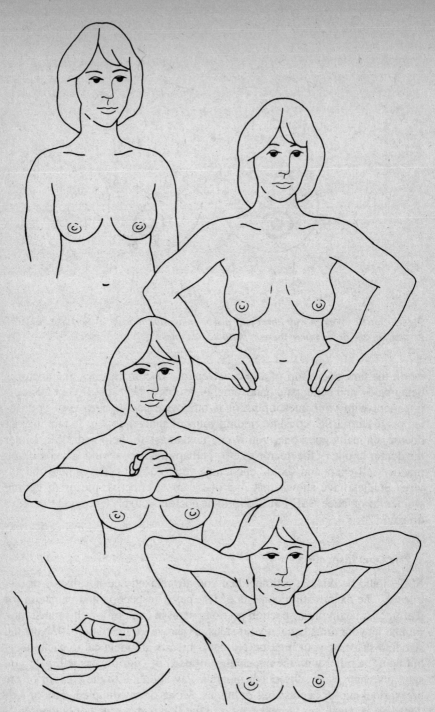

Illustration 10 *Part One—Inspection: Stand in front of a mirror and inspect your breasts in each of the four positions shown here. Finally squeeze each nipple, looking for signs of discharge.*

46

portant. The nipples and areola should also be observed for color changes, scaling, dimpling and retraction. Also note the direction in which the nipples point.

Next, place your hands on your hips, and press inward and down so that the pectorals, the muscles of the upper chest, are contracted. Check to see if the chest muscles contract about the same amount or if any bulging or dimpling appears in this position. While your hands are still on your hips, turn to each side and check again for any dimpling or bulges.

Now put your hands in front of your chest at about heart level, press your palms together and check for muscle contraction, bulges, dimpling and unevenness. Rotate to each side, checking for the same signs. If your breasts are large or hang down, you may have to cup each one to check the undersides of the breast.

Then, raise your arms, flex your elbows and place your hands behind your head. Once again check for dimpling and bulges, rotating to each side and making the same type of check.

This all sounds like a rather elaborate set of gymnastics, but once you have the routine down it's quite simple. To complete the first part of your exam gently squeeze each nipple, looking for signs of discharge. It is not uncommon to have some discharge after childbirth, abortion or miscarriage. A few women have a small amount of discharge at certain phases in their menstrual cycle. Many of us may notice dry, crusted secretions in the cracks of the nipple. This is normal. Some women on birth control pills have a bit of nipple discharge. Discharge is not always a sign of disease, *but any nipple discharge should be brought to a doctor's attention.* In fact, all the signs and symptoms mentioned here deserve a doctor's attention, because any change in the appearance or functioning of the breast is significant.

Part Two: Palpation

This part of the exam is done while you are lying down, as shown in Illustration 11. In this position the breast tissue spreads out against the rib cage and the deeper tissue is easier to feel. Women with large breasts may find that placing a folded towel under the shoulder of the side being examined helps distribute the breast tissue and makes palpation easier and more comfortable. Lotion or oil applied to the fingertips cuts down on skin friction and heightens the sense of touch. Some women do this part of the exam floating on their backs in the bathtub. The soap and water act as lubricants.

To begin, bend one arm and place your hand behind your head. This stretches the chest muscles so that you have a firmer surface to press down on. Use the fatty pads of your fingers rather than the fingertips and, starting on the outside of the breast, using a circular motion, feel the entire breast carefully with the opposite hand. Press down to the chest wall. Women with large breasts may have to hold the breast in place with their other hand, especially

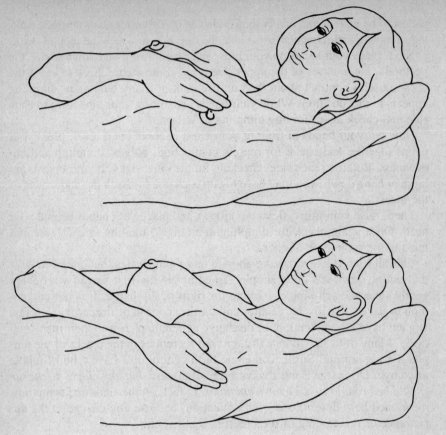

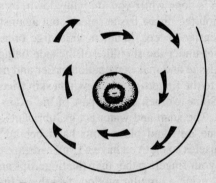

Illustration 11 *Part Two—Palpation: Lie down with one hand behind your head. With your other hand, start on the outside of the breast and, using a circular motion, palpate the entire breast. Repeat on the opposite breast.*

when examining the lower part of the breast, which typically has more fat tissue. Also feel the upper part of the chest wall and the armpit area. Repeat the process on the other side. Women who have had a breast removed should palpate the chest, paying particular attention to the scar area. What you are looking for is any lump or thickening in the breast or enlarged lymph nodes, which may feel like hard, round bumps. This sounds simple, but it's not always easy to learn to recognize lumps. First, the whole process is somewhat akin to feeling for a marble in a plastic bag full of Jell-O. This is why you may have to use two hands, especially on the fatty part of the breast, or else that elusive marble will constantly slide away from the pressure of your fingertips. Second, most women's breasts are not smooth but are rather bumpy. This is especially true of small breasts, which tend to be more glandular than large ones. The upper outer portion of the breast is usually the most lumpy area. In addition to the glands, the ribs, breastbone and underlying muscles can also be mistaken for lumps. Don't hesitate to report any lump, thickening or grainy areas to a doctor. You may think that you feel something, but the sensation is sometimes rather vague. Nonetheless, don't ignore it—see a doctor. It's probably nothing, but investigating your sensations is part of learning self-exam. If it's of any comfort, one of the women who wrote this book (the writer, not the doctor) discovered a suspicious lump and trotted off to the doctor, only to find out that she had discovered her rib. Ah, well, better silly than sorry.

Nothing is to be gained and everything is to be lost by waiting to see if the lump will go away. Any symptom, sign, change in the appearance or feel of the breasts or persistent ache or pain deserves attention.

If, after your first few exams, you feel uncertain about your ability to distinguish what's normal from what's abnormal, don't give up. You'll feel more confident after you've done 50 exams than after you've done only 5. Reading the information on breast diseases in the reference section of this book may be helpful. Find a good doctor and get him or her to assist you. Forge ahead—you *will* get good at BSE, and it just may save your life.

The Monthly Miracle: Menstruation

Each month, deep inside our bodies, the ovary begins, ever so slowly, to turn. A tiny bubble on its surface contains the one egg that has, for some mysterious reason, been chosen out of a field of some 250,000 to ripen that month. The funnel-like opening at the end of the fallopian tube, lined with thousands of undulating cilia, moves toward the ovary, which turns to meet it.

Suddenly, the bubble bursts. Triggered by a spurt of luteinizing hormone, an eloquent chemical messenger from the brain, the ovary contracts sharply and the ripe egg bursts forth. The fringed projections at the end of the fallopian tube reach out like fingers to grasp the ripe ovum and draw it into the narrow tunnel of the tube. In a dreamlike, slow-motion ballet the tiny cilia caress the ripened egg and gently move it along on its 4-inch, 4-day journey to the womb.

Through a precise two-way communication system, so complex that it makes the technology of beaming planetwide transmissions off orbiting satellites look like child's play, the uterus is notified of the impending arrival of the egg and is prepared. The blood vessels in the area swell, flooding the uterus with a rich supply of blood to nourish the soft, spongy tissue of the uterine lining, which will cushion the egg when it arrives. The uterine glands pour forth a banquet of nutriments that will nourish the developing egg. The entire lining of the uterus has thickened to twice its normal depth—a luxurious, rich topsoil in which the egg, if fertilized during its journey through the tube, will implant.

For the first 3 days after its arrival the tiny egg floats freely within the plush uterus. If fertilized, it will embed itself in the uterine lining by the 7th day. Meanwhile, on the surface of the ovary the remnant of the burst bubble, the corpus luteum, which has turned bright yellow in the wake of its explosive spasm, awaits a message from the uterus. While it waits it transmits a continuous stream of chemical messages that direct and sustain the elaborate preparations of the uterus.

If, in the upper reaches of the dark, narrow fallopian tube, no sperm cell meets and joins the egg, the egg will not implant in the uterine wall. The corpus luteum does not receive the message it awaits and ceases transmitting its chemical messages. Without the continued instruction of the corpus luteum the swollen network of blood vessels shrinks, restricting the flow of blood. This deprives the newly grown tissues in the surrounding area of their support and nourishment. Over a period of days the whole structure is dismantled as small pieces of the lining fall away. Within hours of this dismantling the now weakened blood vessels open, a few at a time. Each tiny vessel empties its droplets. More and more droplets are released and the flow of menstrual blood empties the uterus.

It takes approximately 7 days to complete this journey—from the moment the egg bursts out of the ovary and begins to move through the darkness of the tube toward the possibility of the creation of life and the implantation of the fertilized egg in the lush garden of the uterus. It is a journey we all know. It is engraved on our genetic memories and etched inside each tiny molecule of DNA in every cell in our bodies. It is a tale that our species tells over and over again in the ancient archetypal legends of heroic gods and goddesses who traveled from darkness into light and renewed life and in the primal myths of creation that form the basis of all our religions. It is the story of our personal and racial creation. It is indeed a holy story.

We are clearly creatures of incredible lushness, the very source of life. Yet we do not honor our lushness. There are no puberty rites for women. Hardly anywhere in anthropology or in the histories of the kaleidoscope of cultures this planet has spawned are there societies where mothers take their daughters out on moon-full nights to celebrate the ripening of the seeds we carry in our blood-lined wombs.

Instead, both individually and as a culture, we are rather embarrassed about menstruation. Even today, in an era when the most bizarre of sadomasochistic sexual practices are the subject of newspaper headlines, cocktail chitchat and television specials, the natural bodily process of menstruation remains an unmentionable subject. Indeed, when the topic finally did come up on a segment of the well-known TV show *All in the Family,* the network received more letters protesting public mention of "such a thing" than had been received as a result of the airing of any other segment of the controversial show. And this from a show that had broached such topics as premarital sex, racial prejudice, impotence and homosexuality!

There is nothing new. Throughout recorded history, in culture after culture, menstruation has been taboo. The menstruating woman has been regarded as something unholy and unclean. The taboo has taken myriad forms: One must not eat food cooked by a menstruating woman, touch objects she has touched, pronounce her name, look her in the eye, touch her, share sex with her.

Today we no longer believe that a menstruating woman's glance will wither a field of crops. We know her touch won't poison the water in the well and that having sex with her won't make a man's penis fall off. We are no longer banished to menstrual huts as were our ancestral mothers in more primitive societies. But our release from monthly exile does not necessarily represent a more enlightened attitude toward menstruation.

As Nancy Friday suggests in her book *My Mother, My Self,* it is more likely that our release is owing to the fact that as a result of centuries of conditioning we have internalized the menstrual taboo so completely that it is no longer necessary to bother with menstrual huts. Our modern tribe needn't go to such lengths to remove all disturbing reminders of menstruation from its collective consciousness. We do it ourselves with our meticulous, toilet-paper mummification of our bloodied rags as we carefully wrap up and dispose of our used sanitary napkins or tampons. We might drop a used Kleenex in the ashtray without a second thought, but a used Tampax? None of us would think of hiding our toothbrushes under the sink or in the back corners of our bathroom cupboards, yet it is rare to find a box of sanitary napkins prominently displayed next to the deodorants, toothpaste, hair sprays and such that line the bathroom shelves of most homes.

No, the menstrual taboo is not dead. Judging from the resounding silence that surrounds the topic, it is obviously alive and well. And because of this taboo, we are remarkably ignorant about even the most basic facts of menstruation. Most of us couldn't give a coherent explanation of the menstrual cycle to a fifth grader. Our embarrassment and the cultural taboo conspire to keep us ignorant and to make us think of menstruation in largely negative terms. Indeed, we are so embarrassed about menstruation that we can't even call it by its rightful name, relying instead on such negative terms as "the curse" and "falling off the roof." One male reviewer of a book about menstruation put the situation in a particularly telling perspective:

> If men menstruated, they would probably find a way to brag about it. Most likely, they would record it as a spontaneous ejaculation, an excess of vital spirits. Their cup runneth over. Their sexuality superogates. They would see themselves as "spending" blood in a plenitude of conspicuous waste. Blood, after all, is generally considered a good. "Blood" sports used to be a true test of manhood. And at the conclusion of a boy's first hunt, he used to be "blooded." All that is turned around when it is the woman who bleeds. Bleeding is interpreted as a sign of infirmity, inferiority, uncleanliness and irrationality.[1]

It is certainly true that we don't often hear women boasting about their periods. If our tissues swell up with retained water as our periods approach, we don't call it "ripening." Instead, we use a negative term like "bloating." Although it is true that some women experience pain and discomfort at certain periods in their menstrual cycles, it is also true that many women experience extra energy, heightened sexual desire and a general feeling of well-being.

If women are to become informed consumers of medical practice, we must overcome these negative attitudes and cultural taboos about menstruation. No woman can hope to understand what is wrong with her and to evaluate the medical alternatives unless she understands how her body works. The information in the following pages is designed to provide a basic understanding of the workings of the female reproductive system.

Fetal Development

The logical place to begin is, of course, at the beginning—conception. The female egg, the ovum, and the male egg, the sperm, meet and join together, a process known as fertilization. Then the fertilized egg, which at first is called an embryo and later, a fetus, implants in the uterine wall and continues to grow and develop throughout pregnancy, nourished by the rich blood supply to the uterus.

All ova carry what are called X chromosomes. Sperms may have either an X or a Y chromosome. If a sperm carrying an X chromosome joins with the ovum, the baby will be a girl. If the sperm carries a Y chromosome, the baby will be a boy.

The mass of fetal tissue grows larger and divides itself into sections from which specific organs will develop. As early as the 4th week after fertilization there is evidence of a gonad, a specific sex organ, but it is not easy to tell at this point whether the fetus is male or female. By about the 6th or 7th week of fetal life, differentiation of the sex organs becomes apparent. By the fetal age of 3 months, differentiation of the external genital organs is complete.

By 5 months the ovary is recognizable in the female fetus, and by the 5th or 6th month the internal changes that produce the uterus, fallopian tubes and vagina are completely effected. In males the gonad, called the testis, produces a hormone that further influences the development of the fetal tissue. This hormone stimulates the development of the male reproductive organs. The clitoris, under the influence of this hormone, grows larger and becomes a penis. In a sense, a male is a female that has been transformed by hormone stimulation into a male. Contrary to the biblical concept that women derived from Adam's rib, the female seems to be the basic type, and the male, a variation on that basic theme.

At birth the female ovaries contain about 2 million primitive eggs. By age 7

53

about 300,000 remain. Unlike the testis, which continually manufactures new sperm, the ovary contains at birth all the eggs it will ever have and does not manufacture new ones. However, these eggs lie dormant in a sort of state of hibernation throughout childhood, until the time of puberty.

Puberty

Puberty is the phase of the life cycle during which a young woman's reproductive organs mature in size and function. Menarche is the name given to the time when a girl has her first menstrual period, which usually occurs between ages 10 and 16, the average age being about 13. Some experts feel that weight is a more accurate predictor of menarche than age. Most girls menstruate when they reach a body weight of from 92 to 101 pounds.

Menarche is just one of a series of changes that occur during puberty, changes that began to take place a few years earlier. The first changes are invisible. No one knows why or how they occur. Somehow the hypothalamus, the master switch in the brain that controls the body's production of hormones, gets switched on. It then sends substances called gonadotropin releasing factors (GRF) to the pituitary gland, which is located at the base of the brain. In response to this hypothalamic stimulation, the pituitary begins to produce hormones called gonadotropins. The word *gonadotropin* means "acting on the gonads, or sex organs." There are two principal gonadotropins. One of them, called follicle-stimulating hormone, or FSH, travels through the bloodstream to the ovary, where, as its name implies, it stimulates the follicles of the ovary, the sacs inside which the ova, or eggs, have been resting. Specialized cells in these follicular sacs begin to secrete the ovarian hormone estrogen, which helps the eggs to mature. As more and more follicles are stimulated, more estrogen is released into the bloodstream.

By age 8 most girls are producing small amounts of estrogen in their bodies. Over the next few years increasing levels of estrogen and other hormones will cause certain noticeable changes in the girl's body. The first of these is a growth spurt just before puberty. The average girl grows about 2 inches a year after age 2. However, just before puberty this rate doubles. The proportions of the body also change. The head gets larger and the length of the trunk relative to the legs increases. The pelvic bone structure also changes during these years, and fat pads develop over the hips, giving the body a fuller, maturer shape.

The breast also goes through dramatic changes. First, the nipple begins to stand out more. Then, a small mound develops beneath the nipple and the areola, the ring of tissue around the nipple. The areola darkens and continues to enlarge. The breast itself also continues to increase in size until finally, in the mature breast, the areola recedes into the general contour, leaving only the nipple protruding.

The entire vulva also enlarges and changes shape. The outer lips enlarge and tend to cover over the inner lips. The hymen, formerly a thin rim of tissue around the vaginal opening, gets thicker, and the entire vaginal opening looks larger. A fat pad develops under the mons veneris, or "little hill," of the vulva. The skin on the inside of the lips darkens. The clitoris enlarges. Soft, long strands of hair, at first rather sparse and straight but later denser and curlier as well as darker, begin to grow on the lips and mons. Approximately 2 years after the first appearance of the pubic hair, hair also begins to grow in the underarm area.

The internal female organs also undergo changes. The vaginal cavity deepens. The outer layer of tissue on the vaginal walls, formerly only a few cell layers deep, thickens. Vaginal secretions may be noticed for the first time. The entire uterus, both the cervix, or neck, and the fundus, or body, grows larger. The major change is in the fundus. In the years before puberty, the cervix is rather elongated in comparison with the fundus, but during puberty the fundus enlarges until it accounts for three-fourths of the total size of the uterus. The lining of the uterus, called the endometrium, also begins to thicken.

The ovary enlarges in size, and the blood vessels in the area develop. As these vascular channels develop, the hormones from the pituitary begin to have more and more of an impact on the ovary. As more FSH from the pituitary reaches the ovary, increasing numbers of follicles produce more and more estrogen. At first this stimulation is sporadic. The follicles start to grow but then regress. Finally, the amounts of estrogen become more constant. The rising levels of estrogen in the bloodstream affect both the hypothalamus, the control center in the brain, and the pituitary. In the hypothalamus the rising levels of estrogen trigger the release of another hypothalamic GRF called the luteinizing hormone releasing factor (LHRF).* The LHRF travels to the pituitary, where it, along with the direct stimulation of estrogen on the pituitary, causes the pituitary to release a surge of another of its gonadotropins, this one known as luteinizing hormone, or LH.

The LH travels by way of the bloodstream to the ovary, where it causes one of the follicles to burst open and release its egg. The remnants of the burst follicle, which are referred to as the corpus luteum, then begin to secrete the hormone progesterone. The progesterone causes the lining of the uterus, which has already grown thicker as a result of the rising levels of estrogen, to grow even thicker and richer. If pregnancy does not occur, the corpus luteum

*Most current research indicates that there is one gonadotropin releasing factor that releases both LH and FSH. Many scientists think there are actually two, one for each pituitary hormone, although only one has been isolated.

dies and ceases producing progesterone. Without the continued support of the progesterone the uterine lining breaks down and is shed, and the girl has her first menstrual period.

If all this sounds a bit complex, that's because it is. And we've only covered the highlights. The interactions of hormones in the body are not fully understood. Even many practicing doctors don't have a good grasp of what is presently known. The system is a logical one, however, and once you get past the terminology and become familiar with the names of the various hormones and the organs they affect, the whole thing becomes a lot clearer.

Before we consider the workings of the menstrual cycle in the mature female, a word or two about menstrual periods in the early years after menarche and about menopause, the cessation of menstrual periods.

Menstrual periods tend to be rather irregular in the first few years. The interval between periods varies. For instance, the second menstrual period may not occur for 6 months or it might occur in 3 weeks. The amount and duration of bleeding vary too. It usually takes about 40 cycles, or 3 to 4 years, before the pattern is set. Some researchers believe that in the early years of menstruation the girl does not actually release an egg from the ovary, that is, that she doesn't ovulate. Others think that she releases an egg but that no corpus luteum forms from the remnants of the follicular sac. In either case the bleeding that occurs does not result from diminishing levels of progesterone; rather, the lining of the uterus grows so thick from the constant estrogen stimulation that parts of it break off and are shed. In some cases, however, the girl may actually be ovulating and have a functioning corpus luteum, which means that she can get pregnant.

Menopause

"Menopause" is the term used to refer to the time in a woman's life when the monthly cycle gears down and she stops having menstrual periods. It is just one of the events of what is called the "climacteric," a broader term that encompasses menopause and all the other changes taking place at this time in a woman's life.

An incredible amount of nonsense, full of medical inaccuracies, has been written by both doctors and laypeople on the subject of menopause, so perhaps an explanation of the physiological events of this time of life is in order. During menopause the ovaries cease producing eggs (that is, they become anovulatory), so the levels of progesterone and estrogen drop. The pituitary, no longer held in check by the ovarian hormones, produces increasing amounts of FSH and LH in an effort to stimulate the ovary and trigger ovulation.

Typically, the ovary gears down slowly. Women may ovulate one month and have anovulatory cycles the next. Periods may be skipped for a month or two and then start up again. These irregular bleeding patterns are normal and are nothing to be concerned about. If, however, a woman's periods stop for longer than a year and then start again or become heavier than normal, this may be an indication that something is wrong and she should consult a doctor.*

The periods eventually stop altogether. In the past the average age for menopause in U.S. women was 48, but nowadays it is not unusual to find women in their mid-50s who are still menstruating. Some doctors speculate that this may be owing to improved nutrition. There is also some indication that women whose mothers have late menopauses also tend to have late menopauses. Whether this is a hereditary phenomenon or a reflection of the fact that mothers and daughters may tend to have similar patterns of nutrition or other environmental factors is not known.

In addition to the cessation of their menstrual periods, climacteric women may experience other changes, including hot flashes (short episodes of profuse sweating characterized by a feeling of intense heat); a thinning of the vaginal and urinary tissues, which makes them more susceptible to infections and other problems; and osteoporosis, a condition that involves a loss of bone density and may make a person more susceptible to bone fractures. These changes seem to be related to the changing hormone levels.

Although many women experience hot flashes, for most women the problems mentioned above do not present serious difficulties. In the past, women who did experience severe menopausal symptoms were labeled "neurotic" by the medical profession. Medical textbooks often described the typical menopausal patient with severe hot flashes as being a thin, high-strung, emotional and nervous personality type. It's not too surprising that women with severe hot flashes should appear to be psychologically distraught, for hot flashes often occur at night, causing insomnia. Any woman whose sleep is interrupted five or ten times a night might well appear to be high-strung, nervous and emotional. However, her psychological tensions are more likely the result, rather than the cause, of her hot flashes.

It is interesting to reflect on why the thumbnail sketches of the typical woman with menopausal symptoms invariably describe her as being thin. It may turn out that body weight has more to do with the severity of menopausal symptoms than any psychological factor.

Although we are not aware of any research either confirming or denying this theory, it may not be as farfetched as it sounds. Until recently, the fact that some women seem to pass through menopause with virtually unaltered levels of estrogen and continue to produce fairly high levels of it well into old

*For a more detailed description of normal and abnormal menopausal bleeding patterns, see the section on menopause.

age was a puzzle to medical researchers. Now, however, we know that certain substances can be converted into estrogen in the fatty tissues of the body, which may explain, at least in part, why some of these women—presumably the heavier ones—were able to maintain such high postmenopausal estrogen levels. Conversely, perhaps women who are thin and therefore have less of this fatty tissue in which to convert estrogen are more apt to suffer estrogen-related menopausal symptoms, such as hot flashes, than are other, heavier women. Thus rather than being psychiatric in nature, their problems may be related to the amount of fatty tissue in their bodies.

It may also be that, regardless of their body size, women who suffer severe menopausal problems don't produce as much of these other substances that are converted into estrogen in the fatty tissue. But at this point it is impossible to confirm or deny these possibilities, for there has been little in the way of scientific studies of hot flashes. As Barbara Seaman points out in her excellent book *Women and the Crisis in Sex Hormones,* only five studies of hot flashes were recorded in the medical literature in the 70-year period from 1903 to 1973![2]

Despite the fact that so little research has been done on the postmenopausal woman, a wide variety of symptoms has been attributed to the declining levels of estrogen. Indeed, menopause was—and by some doctors still is—considered a deficiency disease. To ''cure'' this deficiency disease, many doctors prescribe estrogen replacement therapy (ERT), which is supposed to keep women from growing old, prevent wrinkling, boost the spirits, ward off depression and keep women slim and sexy, to mention just a few of the benefits claimed for it. ERT does none of these things. As it turns out, what it does do is increase a woman's chances of developing uterine cancer.[3] The pharmaceutical industry has played on women's fears about aging in our youth-worshiping culture and has promoted the widespread use of a dangerous drug. Menopausal women who are considering the use of estrogens should read the sections on menopause and ERT and consider alternative therapies before making a decision about using these drugs.

The Menstrual Cycle in the Mature Woman

Once a woman matures the cycle becomes more regular but never totally regular. All women have some irregularity in their cycles. One month the cycle may be 28 days long, another month it may be 26 or 32 days long. Cycles as short as 20 or 21 days and as long as 35 or 36 days are considered within the normal range. Some women have cycles even longer or shorter than these, and as long as the amount of bleeding is not excessive and the cycles are fairly regular, this usually is not cause for alarm, although any persistent irregularities should be discussed with your doctor.

The classic, medical-textbook menstrual cycle is 28 days long. This does not mean that most women have 28-day cycles; indeed, probably fewer than 10 percent of women in their peak reproductive years have regular 28-day cycles. This 28-day figure was arrived at by measuring the length of the menstrual cycle in a group of women and then dividing the total number of days by the number of women in the group. Thus the majority of women may actually have 31-day or 27-day cycles; the group average can be thrown off by a relatively small number of women with exceptionally long or short cycles. So don't fret if you don't have the classic 28-day cycle; you're not alone.

Many things can cause a woman's cycle to become irregular. The hypothalamus, the brain center that acts as the master switch for the hormone system, is also part of the nervous system and is probably responsible for coordinating the two. Your nervous system collects information from the outside world through your five senses and from the rest of your body as well. The hypothalamus is sensitive to the stimuli collected by the nervous system. Physical and emotional stress can cause menstrual irregularities, probably through the mediation of the hypothalamus. This is undoubtedly a mechanism designed by Mother Nature to prevent us from becoming pregnant when there is already too much stress on our systems.

The intricate relationship between external stimuli picked up by our senses and the menstrual cycle is still largely a mystery. Interestingly, there is now some evidence that our sense of smell may play a role in the timing of our menstrual cycles. It has long been a common piece of womenlore that women who are close friends or who live together tend to menstruate at the same time. This was confirmed in a study done at Harvard University in which the menstrual patterns of women living in a college dormitory were carefully studied.[4] After ruling out other factors, such as common light/dark cycles (light also has an effect on menstrual cycles, at least in some animals) and stress patterns, the researchers speculated that the sense of smell might be a factor in the observed coincidence of menstrual cycles among close friends.

This is not as implausible as it sounds. Scientists have long known that odor particles control the mating and reproductive behaviors of insects. (A squirt of a fertile female moth's odor particles is enough to set all the male moths within a 5-mile radius on the wing.)

The notion that smell stimuli play a role in regulating human menstrual cycles received further support from another study, done in California, in which a female volunteer was asked to wear a tampon on each day of her menstrual cycle.[5] Odor particles were then isolated from each of her tampons by an elaborate process known as gas chromatography. Next, the women involved in the study were divided into two groups, a control group and a test group. Each day all the women were asked to rub cotton pads under their noses. The women in the control group were given odorless pads, but those in the test group were given pads impregnated with the smell particles that had been obtained from the female volunteer. On Day 1 of the study the women in the test group were smelling the odors isolated from the first tampon the volunteer had worn. On the 2nd day they smelled the odors isolated from the volunteer's second tampon, and so on. At the end of 5 months a significant portion of the women in the test group, unlike those in the control group, were menstruating in synch with the female volunteer.

The timing of the menstrual cycle, then, is influenced by a number of factors, many of which we are hardly aware of or understand only dimly. We do know, however, that when variations in the menstrual cycle occur, they are most apt to occur in the first part of the cycle. The menstrual cycle can be divided into four phases. The first phase is the bleeding phase, the time of the actual menstrual flow. The second phase is called the proliferative phase and is dominated by the hormone estrogen. This is followed by the ovulation phase, when the ripe egg is released from the ovary. It is in the first two stages, before ovulation, that variations in cycle length occur. Once ovulation has taken place the fourth stage of the cycle, called the secretory phase, begins and usually lasts for 14 days, after which the menstrual flow starts and the cycle begins again.

The hormones that govern the menstrual cycle are in a constant state of fluctuation. Low levels of all these hormones are produced throughout the menstrual cycle, but these levels are rising and falling constantly, triggering or suppressing levels of the other hormones as they do so. As you can see from Illustration 12, the relationships between these hormones are complex. The ways in which these hormones interact are not fully understood, but let's take a broad look at how these hormones behave during the various phases of the cycle. For convenience, we'll use the classic 28-day cycle, although your cycle will probably vary somewhat.

Phase I: The Bleeding Phase (Days 1–5)

The first day of menstrual flow marks Day 1 of your period and the beginning of the bleeding phase. The bleeding may last from 2 to 8 days—usually between 4 and 6—or an average of 5 days. The total volume of the flow is usually about 4 to 6 tablespoons, or 2 to 3 ounces of blood. Women who have light flows may use as few as one or two menstrual tampons or sanitary pads a day, whereas women with heavy flows might require eight to ten pads a day. (In addition to pads and tampons many women are now using natural sponges, which can be purchased at cosmetic counters. These sponges can be rinsed, wrung out and reused.*) The volume of a woman's flow, incidentally, has nothing to do with her fertility.

*Natural sponges may, however, be associated with certain problems. See the section on toxic shock syndrome for details.

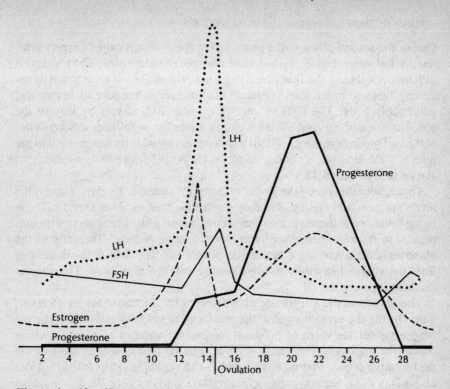

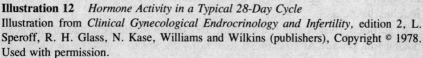

Illustration 12   *Hormone Activity in a Typical 28-Day Cycle*
Illustration from *Clinical Gynecological Endrocrinology and Infertility,* edition 2, L. Speroff, R. H. Glass, N. Kase, Williams and Wilkins (publishers), Copyright © 1978. Used with permission.

The menstrual flow is made up of vaginal and cervical secretions, endometrial tissue and blood. Some women pass clumps of menstrual tissue that look like blood clots, and unless these are excessive this is normal. You may be more apt to notice these clots after you have been lying down for a while, for the blood has been pooling in the upper vagina and has had a chance to form these clotlike clumps of tissue. Menstrual blood has no odor until it comes in contact with air and vaginal bacteria.

During this phase of the cycle the endometrial lining of the uterus sheds most of its thickness until, on the last day of the flow, only the thin innermost level remains. The ovary is producing only small amounts of its hormones, and both progesterone and estrogen are at their lowest levels during this phase.

Phase II: The Proliferative Phase (Days 6–13)

During the second phase of the menstrual cycle, which is called the proliferative, or follicular, phase, the hormone estrogen predominates. The low levels of hormones during the first phase cause the hypothalamus to produce its releasing factors, which then stimulate the pituitary to produce its hormones, particularly FSH. The FSH, along with a little LH, travels by way of the bloodstream to the ovary, where it causes a number of follicles to start to develop and produce estrogen. (If all this is confusing you, try humming it to the tune of "the hip bone's connected to the leg bone" while studying the chart shown in Illustration 13.)

Throughout this phase the levels of estrogen increase. By days 7 and 8 the levels are noticeably rising, and they reach their peak by about Day 13. These rising levels of estrogen act on the uterus, causing the lining to proliferate, that is, to thicken—hence the term "proliferative phase." The cells of the gland and duct tissue of the breast also proliferate. The cells of the tissue that lines the vagina likewise multiply, and the cell layers thicken. The vaginal discharge increases.

The glands in the cervix are also affected by the rising levels of estrogen. During the previous phase the glands were not very active, but the estrogen stimulates them to produce increasing amounts of mucus, which makes the vagina feel increasingly wet. For the first couple of days of the proliferative phase, that is, days 6 and 7, the vagina is apt to feel dry; from about Day 8 the vagina starts to feel wetter, until, on Day 13, this wetness reaches its peak.

In addition to increasing in amount, the secretions also change in character during this phase. At first these secretions are apt to be sticky or pasty and creamy in texture. They may be white. But starting about Day 11 the secretions tend to become thinner, more watery and slippery. By Day 13 the cervical secretions resemble the white of an uncooked egg: clear, gelatinous and slippery. They are also stretchy. If you place a small amount between your thumb and first finger and slowly pull your fingers apart, the mucus will stretch, for some women up to 4 inches. This mucus characteristic, called spinnbarkeit, is usually present just before ovulation (Illustration 14). The secretions are also apt to taste a bit different as ovulation approaches and they become less acid and more alkaline (sugary).

Mother Nature, that consummate designer, never does anything without a purpose, and these changes in cervical secretions have an important function. The thick, pasty, more acid cervical mucus seen in the early days of this phase is hostile to sperm and blocks the entrance to the cervical canal, preventing sperm from moving up into the uterus. But as the character of the mucus is altered by the rising levels of estrogen, it becomes more favorable to the sperm. The formerly acid secretions become more alkaline, which nourishes

The hypothalamus, in response to low levels of estrogen and progesterone, sends its releasing factors to the pituitary gland (A).

The pituitary gland is stimulated by releasing factors to secrete follicle-stimulating hormone (FSH) (B).

Levels of estrogen and progesterone fall steadily after the corpus luteum regresses (E).

The estrogen has stimulated the uterine lining to grown during the proliferative phase. The progesterone then stimulates the uterine lining to secrete nutriments during the secretory phase. When the corpus luteum dies, the lining loses support and sloughs away as the menstrual period (D).

The FSH stimulates the egg follicles in the ovary and they, in turn, produce estrogen which is released into the blood stream in increasing amounts. When the estrogen levels are high enough, the pituitary is stimulated to produce luteinizing hormone (LH), which causes the ripe egg to burst out of the follicle. The remnants of the follicle become the corpus luteum which produces progesterone (C).

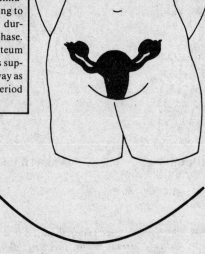

Illustration 13   *The Menstrual Cycle*

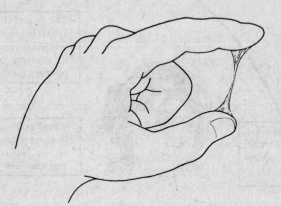

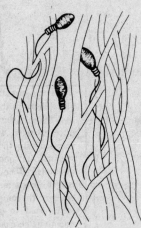

FERTILE MUCUS   INFERTILE MUCUS

Illustration 14 *As ovulation approaches, your cervical mucus becomes slippery and can be stretched into a clear, delicate strand before breaking. Before ovulation the molecules of your mucus have a cross-hatched pattern. During the most fertile part of your cycle, the molecules realign themselves, forming passageways to aid the sperm on their journey to the uterus.*

the sperm. On a microscopic level the molecules of cervical mucus realign themselves. The cross-hatched molecular structure that served as a barrier to sperm is altered, and tubelike passages are formed that help the sperm swim through the cervical canal and into the uterus (see Illustration 14). The cyclical changes in cervical secretions prevent the sperm from getting into the uterus except when the egg is fully ripened. The danger of the egg's being fertilized by weakened ''old'' sperm that have been in the uterus too long or of an older egg's being fertilized by sperm that get into the uterus after ovulation—events that could result in birth defects—is thereby minimized.

The cervix also changes position within the vaginal cavity and becomes softer, and the opening to the cervical canal dilates, all of which make it easier for the sperm to penetrate. Not coincidentally, many women experience an increase in sexual drive during this phase of the menstrual cycle that peaks right before ovulation.

Meanwhile, back in the ovary, certain changes are also taking place. As the egg follicles are stimulated by the FSH from the pituitary, they move toward the surface of the ovary. For some reason only one of these follicles normally continues to develop. The other follicles fail to mature fully and regress. The chosen follicle pushes against the outer capsule of the ovary, stretching the capsule and forming a bubblelike protrusion on the surface of the ovary.

Phase III: Ovulation (Day 14)

During Phase I the rising levels of estrogen reach a certain point and then cause the suppression of the pituitary hormones FSH and LH. When rising levels of one hormone cause a suppression of the production of another hormone, the term ''feedback mechanism'' is used. The feedback mechanism is extremely complex. In the case of estrogen, for instance, we know that it can suppress the production of LH, but we also know that once the estrogen reaches its peak level, it can trigger the release of a spurt of LH. This occurs just before ovulation, and this burst of LH causes the bulging egg follicle on the surface of the ovary to rupture and release its egg (see Illustration 15).

In the mythical 28-day cycle, ovulation is supposed to occur at the midpoint, on Day 14 of the cycle. But even in women with regular cycles there is often a variation of 1 or 2 days either way. Thus a woman with a regular 28-day cycle might ovulate anywhere from Day 12 to Day 16.

The standard textbook 28-day cycle has served to confuse a lot of women about when ovulation occurs. We are often told that ovulation occurs at the midpoint of the cycle, which is fairly accurate for the woman who has a 28-day cycle; however, if a woman has a 36-day cycle, this midpoint would be Day 18. But that probably is not when she ovulates, for the midpoint is not really a guide to calculating the date of ovulation. A more reliable way of figuring your ovulation date would be to count backward 14 days from the first

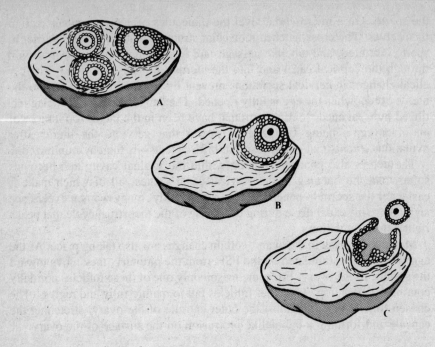

Illustration 15 *The follicles within the ovary are stimulated and begin to develop (A). They migrate toward the surface of the ovary (B). The chosen follicle bursts open and releases its egg at ovulation (C).*

day of your cycle. In other words, the woman with a 36-day cycle probably ovulated on Day 22 (36 − 14 = 22). Because there is often a 2-day variation in ovulation dates, even in women with regularly occurring cycles, a woman with a constant 36-day cycle may have ovulated anywhere from Day 20 to Day 24. Similarly, a woman with a 22-day cycle would have a midpoint of Day 11, but she probably ovulated on Day 8 (22 − 14 = 8) of her cycle or, allowing for the standard 2-day variation, anywhere from Day 6 to Day 10.

Some women are able to pinpoint the time of ovulation because they experience a sharp, cramplike pain at the time of ovulation. This is called mittelschmerz, or middle pain. Some women also experience midcycle bleeding at the time of ovulation, either with or without mittelschmerz. The bleeding is the result of a rapid drop in estrogen levels. The follicle may literally be so shaken up by the act of ovulation that it stops producing hormones for a while. Without the continued support of the hormones, the thickened endometrial lining starts to break down and shed. Such bleeding is usually only a slight spotting that lasts for a few hours, but it may be heavier and persist for a few days. This type of midcycle bleeding is rare, however, and may be the symptom of a more serious problem, so you should report it to your doctor.

In order for pregnancy to occur, a fresh, live sperm must meet and fertilize a live ovum. Actually, a woman can get pregnant only for a period of, at the most, 36 hours a month, for the egg lives for only 12 to 36 hours. But you can get pregnant by having sex up to 72 hours before ovulation and for 36 hours after ovulation. This is because sperm can live for up to 3 days (there is now some evidence that they can survive for as long as 5 days, but it is highly unlikely that a sperm would be vital enough after 3 days to fertilize an egg). If you were to have intercourse 3 days before ovulation, that sperm could still be in your reproductive tract and could fertilize the egg. Likewise, if you had intercourse within 36 hours after ovulation, the sperm could meet and fertilize the egg.

For many of us this business about when ovulation occurs isn't terribly important, but if you're pregnant, have more than one lover and are trying to figure all that out, it could be very important. Similarly, if you're trying to get pregnant or are using a birth control method that requires you to figure out when you ovulated, calculating your ovulation date is of prime importance, for the time preceding and following ovulation is the only time when you can become pregnant.

Just before ovulation the levels of estrogen have reached such a high level that they are no longer suppressing the production of LH by the pituitary. Instead, there is a surge of LH, which triggers the release of the egg from the follicle and initiates the next phase of the cycle.

Phase IV: The Secretory Phase (Days 15–28)

The final phase of the menstrual cycle is the secretory, or luteal, phase. During this phase the remnant of the burst follicle, which is called the corpus luteum, begins to produce the hormone progesterone. The corpus luteum is also producing estrogen, but progesterone production predominates. The preovulation surge of luteinizing hormone from the pituitary is responsible for transforming the burst follicle into the progesterone-producing corpus luteum. Although the egg follicle always contains cells capable of producing progesterone as well as estrogen, it is not until the levels of LH rise to a sufficient degree that these progesterone-producing cells receive the stimulation they need to begin to make significant amounts of this hormone. By Day 16, however, these cells are producing a quantity of progesterone, and they continue to do so throughout the first half of the secretory phase.

One of the major effects of the progesterone is to stimulate the cells in the estrogen-primed endometrial lining of the uterus to secrete nutriments that will nourish the egg if pregnancy should occur—hence the term "secretory phase." The progesterone also initiates the first steps in the secretory process in the milk-producing tissues of the breast, although actual milk production doesn't normally occur until after delivery. This may cause the breast to swell and become tender as progesterone levels reach their peak on about Day 22. From that point on, progesterone levels drop and if the breast tissues have trouble reabsorbing these secretions, you may notice increased tenderness and lumpiness in your breasts in the days preceding your menstrual flow.

As the progesterone levels continue to rise the endometrial lining thickens, reaching its maximum thickness on about Day 21 or 22. After about Day 21 the corpus luteum begins to decline, because the increasing amounts of hormones it produces have forced a decline in luteinizing hormone from the pituitary. Without the pituitary LH the hormone-producing cells in the burst follicle, the corpus luteum, are no longer stimulated. If, however, pregnancy occurs and a fertilized egg implants in the rich endometrial lining, the corpus luteum does not regress. The fertilized egg begins to produce a hormone similar to LH called human chorionic gonadotropin, or HCG. Throughout the first few months of pregnancy the corpus luteum, stimulated by HCG, continues to produce estrogen and progesterone until the fetus and its hormone-producing organ, the placenta, are mature enough to produce these hormones on their own.

In nonpregnant cycles no HCG is produced and the corpus luteum regresses. Without the support of the progesterone the rich secretory endometrium breaks down. The blood vessels shrink, depriving the endometrial tissue of its nourishment, and pieces of tissue begin to fall away. By the end of Day 28 these pieces of tissue are being shed through the cervix, and the menstrual flow (Phase I) of a new cycle has begun (see Illustration 16).

In addition to its effects on the breast and endometrial tissue, progesterone has a number of other effects. Throughout the proliferative and ovulatory phase of the cycle the uterus undergoes mild rhythmic contractions, but within a day or two of ovulation the rising levels of progesterone inhibit these muscle contractions. On about Day 27 or 28 this inhibiting effect is lost and the contractions, which aid the expulsion of menstrual blood, begin again. For some women this resumption of contractions causes cramps just before menstruation, one of the main symptoms of the premenstrual syndrome experienced by many women.

The hormone progesterone is thermogenic, which means that it causes your temperature to rise. Once you have ovulated, your body temperature rises about six-tenths of a degree and generally remains elevated for a number of days. The cervical mucus is also affected by progesterone. In this phase it tends to be scant, thick and pasty. On a microscopic level the molecules realign themselves once again. The molecular tubes or tunnels that aided the sperm on their journey into the uterus are again replaced by the cross-hatched type of structure that blocks the sperm and prevents them from moving into the uterus.

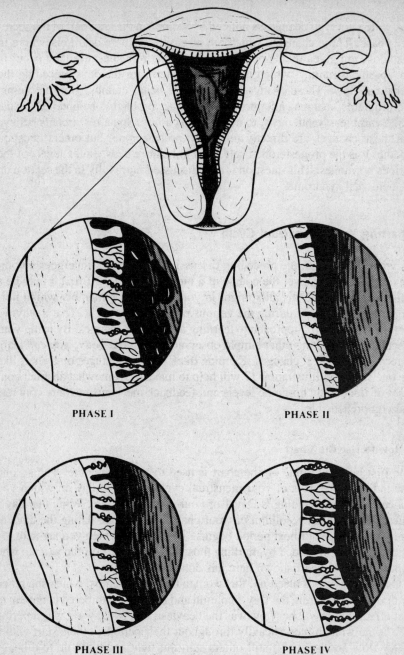

PHASE I

PHASE II

PHASE III

PHASE IV

Illustration 16 *Phase I: The lining of the uterus is shed. Phase II: The lining grows thicker. Phase III: The lining is about 2 mm thick at the time of ovulation. Phase IV: The lining begins to secrete nutriments.*

A wide variety of changes is noticed by women in the later half of the secretory phase. These changes, which are discussed in more detail elsewhere in this book, are given the name premenstrual syndrome because they occur in the "premenstruum," which is the medical term for the days preceding the menstrual flow. These changes may include acne, cramps, skin problems, eye problems, asthma, allergies, urinary tract problems, heightened sexual desire and breast tenderness, to mention just a few. Some researchers believe that these changes are directly related to progesterone, but others question whether it is the progesterone itself or an imbalance between the levels of the various hormones. This question is also discussed more fully in the section on premenstrual syndrome.

Charting Your Menstrual Cycle

As you can tell from the preceding discussion, your body undergoes a complex set of changes over the course of a menstrual cycle. At first it may be a little difficult to get this all straight in your mind and remember which hormones are doing what during the various phase of your cycle. That's why we prefer a "hands-on" approach to learning about these changes. By using your speculum and making other simple observations of your body, you can learn to recognize cyclical changes. Keeping track of these changes on a chart like the one shown in Illustration 17 will help to make the somewhat abstract concepts of fluctuating hormone levels and feedback mechanisms more concrete and comprehensible.

How to Use the Chart

The first horizontal line on the chart is used to record the date. The second line indicates the days of your menstrual cycle. The first day on which you notice menstrual bleeding is Day 1 of your menstrual cycle. Write that day's date above the Day 1 column on your chart and continue dating the days of your cycle until your next period begins. The days on which you are actually bleeding can be recorded by marking those days with an X as the woman who kept the sample chart shown here has done.

On the first day of bleeding, this woman had mild cramps, which she noted by drawing a line from the Day 1 column and making a numbered comment to that effect. On Day 2 her flow was the heaviest, and by Day 4 it was tapering off. Some women bleed heavily throughout their periods; others start with a heavy flow and taper off; still others start out light and build up to a heavy flow. There are numerous individual patterns of menstrual bleeding. You may find that yours is fairly constant or that it changes from month to month.

70

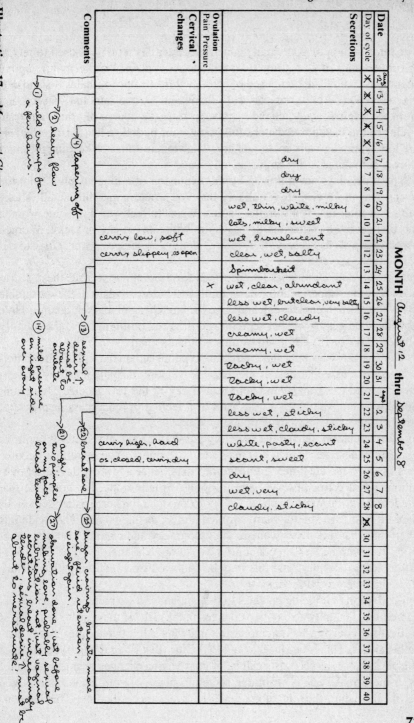

MENSTRUAL CYCLE CHART

MONTH August 12 thru September 8

Illustration 17 Menstrual Chart

Vaginal Secretions

The third section of your chart, which is headed Secretions, is used to record information about your vaginal secretions. As explained earlier, your vaginal secretions, which are composed of cells shed from your vaginal walls and cervix, secretions from your cervical glands and a small amount of secretion from the vaginal walls, change character over the course of your menstrual cycle. In the days immediately following your period, when estrogen levels are low, your vagina is apt to feel dry. The woman who was keeping the chart shown here noted 3 dry days, days 6, 7 and 8.

These dry days are followed by the expulsion of a mucous plug from the opening of the cervix. It is unlikely that you would notice this small, sticky plug, but after its expulsion the vagina begins to feel wet. For some women the first secretions after the dry days are white and sticky or tacky. Women use such words as *creamy, wet, milky, cloudy, abundant, scant, pasty* to describe these secretions.

As ovulation approaches and estrogen levels continue to rise, these secretions become slipperier and clearer until, just before ovulation, they resemble the white of an uncooked egg and have the stretchy spinnbarkeit quality. Note how the changes in vaginal secretions during the proliferative and ovulatory phases (days 6–14) are noted on this woman's chart.

The woman who kept the chart also experienced a sharp pain, the mittelschmerz discussed earlier, at the time of ovulation that she noted by placing an X on the chart under the appropriate day in the row labeled Ovulation. Some women experience a mild pain or a feeling of tenderness or pressure; others do not have any ovulation symptoms.

After ovulation, during the secretory phase, the vaginal secretions continue to undergo changes, which you may be able to notice. The secretions become less slippery and creamier. Some women experience a few dry days after ovulation, when estrogen levels are dropping. Progesterone, the hormone that predominates during this phase, is apt to produce thicker, pastier secretions that are hostile to sperm. Many women notice, as the woman who made this chart did, that they have whitish, sticky or tacky and creamy or pasty secretions that become less abundant after ovulation. The first few days after ovulation are usually dry, and this may be followed by a random pattern of dry days interspersed with sticky days.

In addition to noticing changes in the amount and character of your vaginal secretions, you may also notice changes in the taste of these secretions. Most of the time your vagina is apt to taste somewhat salty, but at times it may taste rather sweet. This is because the acid/alkaline (that is, acid/sugar) balance, or the pH balance, as scientists call it, of your vagina changes over the course of your menstrual cycle. During the secretory phase of your cycle, as estrogen levels are rising, the vagina gradually becomes more alkaline. This happens for two reasons. First, the estrogen not only stimulates greater quantities of cervical secretions, but the secretions it stimulates have greater amounts of sugar in them. Second, the estrogen also causes changes in the composition of the cells that make up the vaginal wall, causing the sugar content of these cells to increase. As we noted earlier in the discussion of the secretory phase, the rising levels of estrogen also cause the cells that make up tissues of the vaginal walls to multiply and thicken. As they do so, greater numbers of cells are shed from the vaginal walls. As these vaginal cells are shed and break down, they release their sugar and this also makes the secretions more alkaline. For some women this gives a sweet taste to their secretions that is especially noticeable just before ovulation. Conversely, some women notice a more acid or salty taste at this time. This quality depends on the woman's personal body chemistry.

Each of us has bacteria that normally live in our vaginas. These bacteria, which are called lactobacilli, or Döderlein's bacilli, are essential to maintaining vaginal health. As the vaginal secretions become more alkaline, these bacteria, which thrive on sugar, multiply. They eat the sugar and secrete a mild acid. This restores the acid balance to the vagina and keeps disease-causing organisms, which prefer sugary environments, from thriving. Women whose lactobacilli are very active and get to work right away will notice an acid taste in their vaginas when the sugar content of the secretions increases. Others will note a sugary taste for a while. The mechanism of the acid/alkaline balance of the vagina is not well understood, but we do know that some women experience a distinctly acid, salty taste or a particularly sweet taste at certain points in their cycles. Note how our chart women recorded these taste changes on days 10, 12 and 25.

For those of you who are having qualms about the sanitary aspects of tasting your vaginal secretions, remember that your vagina is probably a less infectious environment than your mouth. Of course, if you had an infection in your mouth or a cold sore on your lips, you would want to take precautions. The same is true of your vagina. If you have an abnormal discharge (abnormal in terms of unusual color, texture, odor or amount), you may have an infection and so should not taste your secretions. For instance, it is theoretically possible for a couple engaging in oral-genital sex to transmit a yeast infection from the woman's vagina to the mouth of her partner. In order for this to happen, the woman would have to have a roaring yeast infection and we have never seen this. Still it is possible to orally pass some of the sexually transmissible infections, such as herpes, gonorrhea or syphilis, from one person to another, so if you have an infection of any type or think you may have been exposed to one of these diseases, let common sense prevail and don't do any tasting.

There is a great deal of variation in the pattern of vaginal secretions that different women notice. Your individual pattern may change from month to month. Women who use birth control pills will probably not notice cyclical changes in their vaginal secretions, for the synthetic hormones in the Pill alter the body's normal fluctuations in hormone levels. Similarly, women who have anovulatory cycles, that is, cycles in which they don't actually ovulate, also will not have the usual sort of hormone fluctuations and may not notice changes in their secretions. Anovulatory cycles often occur in women who have just begun to menstruate and in women approaching menopause. They also occur in women with certain gynecological conditions and, on occasion, in all women. Some women, even though they have normal ovulatory cycles, do not notice these changes in secretions.

Women who use spermicidal foams, creams or jellies for birth control may have difficulty in distinguishing between their secretions and the spermicide. Sexual activity can also make it difficult to observe the quality and quantity of your secretions. When you become sexually excited your vagina produces lubrication that has a stretchy quality similar to the spinnbarkeit type of secretion seen just before ovulation. Moreover, ejaculate, or "come," deposited in the vagina when a man has an orgasm can also obscure the true nature of your secretions. One way to avoid these confusions is to examine yourself when you are not feeling sexually aroused. If you have had sex the previous night, especially if you use spermicidal creams, foams or jellies, wait until late the next afternoon or evening to allow time for the ejaculate or spermicides to leak out of the vagina before making your observations.

Having a vaginal or cervical infection can also alter the character and amount of your cervical secretions. Infections can cause a change in the color, the texture, the amount and the odor of your secretions. By becoming familiar with your normal secretions you will be able to recognize abnormalities and seek treatment for infections early, when they are easiest to treat.

It is not necessary to perform speculum exam each day in order to keep a chart like this. Some women can tell the wet/dry condition of their vagina merely by observing; others feel the vaginal lips; still others insert a finger into the vaginal cavity to get a sample of secretions.

Recording Cervical Changes

The fluctuating hormone levels throughout your cycle also have an effect on the position of your cervix. Around the time of ovulation, when you are most fertile, the cervix is high in the vaginal cavity; when you are not fertile, it tends to occupy a position lower in the vaginal canal. You may notice that speculum exam is easier during these infertile days, when the cervix is lower and therefore easier to find.

If you practice speculum self-exam at these times, you may also notice other changes in your cervix. For instance, during the fertile times, when the cervix is higher in the canal, it is apt to feel softer (like your fingertip) and the cervical os, the opening to your cervical canal, is apt to be more widely dilated. The whole surface of the cervix may be shiny and feel slippery. When the cervix is lower in the canal, it tends to feel firmer (like the tip of your nose or chin), the os will be closed and the shiny appearance and slippery feeling of the cervix won't be as noticeable. Your os is likely to be dilated again just before your period begins, and the cervix may be lower in the canal at that time. You can record these changes in the section of the chart marked Cervical Changes.

Comments

The last section of the chart, the one labeled Comments, can be used to record other changes that you may notice over the course of your menstrual cycle. Individual patterns vary considerably, and many women are not able to find consistent patterns. But if you record the physical and emotional changes that you experience over the course of your cycle, you may begin to note certain characteristic patterns.

Perhaps a few words about emotional changes and phases of the menstrual cycle are in order. Many women experience emotional changes that seem to be related to the phases of the menstrual cycle. The feminist movement has shied away from this topic, perhaps because feminists fear that this will feed into the cultural stereotype of women as creatures subject to raging hormonal imbalances who are unfit to hold positions of leadership in society because they suffer from periodic bouts of emotional instability. The truth of the matter is that beyond the folklore about "women on the rag," we know little about emotions, moods and phases of the menstrual cycle.

The small body of supposedly scientific research that has been done consists of studies analyzing groups of women who have attempted suicide and committed murder or other crimes to see if there was a correlation with a specific phase of their menstrual cycle. The assumption behind these studies is that women become unhinged emotionally at certain points in their cycle. Some of these studies "prove" that these things happen more often during the bleeding phase; others "prove" that they happen more often in the days preceding menstruation; still others find no correlation.[6] So much for raging hormonal imbalances. . . .

The fact remains that many women do notice changes of mood that seem to be related to their cycles. Given the negative attitude about menstruation in our culture, it is not surprising that we generally hear about these negative emotional changes. This is not to suggest that women who experience depression, irritability or other negative emotions are merely responding to the general cultural attitude about menstruation. There may be a very real physiologic basis for their feelings. But what we do want to point out is that many women also experience positive emotional changes during this time—

75

increase in sexual desire, extra energy, a generally elevated mood, for example—and yet we hear little about these things. So if you are noting emotional responses on your menstrual chart, be aware of this bias and record the positive changes as well as any negative ones.

In addition to emotional changes you may note a number of other variations in yourself, including increased sexual drive, different levels of energy, a craving for sweets, changed sleep patterns, weight gain and acne or clearing of the skin, to mention just a few. Any of the changes listed in the discussion of the secretory phase may be noted. Recording such observations in the comment section of your chart will help you to learn more about your particular body cycles and rhythms.

The Value of Keeping a Chart

In addition to helping you learn to understand the workings of the menstrual cycle, these charts can be useful in other ways. An expanded version of the chart that includes a daily body temperature record can be used as a method of birth control or to determine the optimum time for intercourse if you are trying to become pregnant. This is discussed in detail in the section on birth control methods under the heading Natural Family Planning.

An accurate history of your menstrual cycles can be especially important if you develop certain gynecological problems and may aid your doctor in diagnosis. Knowledge of the length of your cycles and whether or not they are regular may be an important factor in your choice of a method of birth control. Familiarity with your vaginal discharges and the appearance of your cervix can help you spot abnormalities and diseases in their earliest stages, when they are most curable.

Perhaps even more important is the fact that the chart can help you learn more about your body's rhythms and cycles. Once you have this sort of knowledge you are in a much better position to wend your way through the medical marketplace, to make informed decisions about birth control and health care. Armed with knowledge about your body you are not likely to fall prey to an unnecessary hysterectomy or other form of medical mistreatment.

Birth Control:
The Statistical Lie

Mark Twain probably wasn't thinking about birth control when he made the above observation, but it certainly applies. Statistics have been used, or rather misused, to create false impressions about birth control, in particular about the relative effectiveness of the various methods. Somewhere, somehow, somebody has managed to pull the wool over everybody's eyes.

In order to understand the statistical lies told about birth control effectiveness, a few definitions are in order. Basically, there are two types of effectiveness rates, theoretical effectiveness rates and actual-use effectiveness rates. The theoretical effectiveness rate is just that—a theory. It tells us how many women would probably get pregnant if that method of birth control were used correctly and consistently, without mistakes: if, for instance, the Pill were taken at the same time every day and no pills were ever missed or if the diaphragm were inserted correctly each and every time a woman had intercourse. The actual-use effectiveness rate, on the other hand, includes all the mistakes. It is based on studies of groups of women who actually used that particular method over a period of time. The actual-use effectiveness rate is less impressive than the theoretical rate, for it reflects all the method failures—condoms that break, diaphragms that slip out of place, IUDs that are expelled unknowingly—and all the user failures—the women who forget to take their pills or who don't use the foam or diaphragm each time they have sex.

Both actual-use and theoretical rates are given in terms of a group of 100 women using that method for a year. If a method is said to be 98 percent effective, this means that 98 out of 100 women using that method for a year would not get pregnant, but 2 would. If a method is said to have a failure rate of 2 per 100 woman-years of use, this means that we could expect that 2 women out of a group of 100 using this method for a year would get pregnant.

Most U.S. women are laboring under the misconception that, in terms of effectiveness, the Pill and the IUD are vastly superior to the older barrier methods, such as the diaphragm, the condom, spermicides or foam. But, as we shall see, t'aint necessarily so.

This whole issue of effectiveness deserves careful consideration, for as everybody knows, or should know by now, deciding which method of birth control to use is a game of trade-offs. There is no perfect method, so we have to deal with what's available. Basically, there are three cards in the deck: safety, convenience and effectiveness. Each of us must shuffle the cards, arrange our hands according to our priorities and pick a method from the pile. It often seems like a no-win game, for no matter which method we choose, we win some but we also lose some.

The Safety vs. Convenience Trade-Off

Methods like the Pill and the IUD, which have the worst safety records, are more convenient. All we have to do is swallow a little tablet once a day or, in the case of the IUD, have the doctor insert a small plastic device into the uterus. What could be easier? On the other hand, the older barrier methods of birth control—diaphragms, spermicides or condoms—are undeniably safer; one doesn't hear about women who die of heart attacks (Pill complication) or massive pelvic infections (IUD complication) because they used one of the barrier methods. But the barrier methods are messy and, as anyone who's ever chased a springing diaphragm around the bathroom or tried to unroll a condom the wrong way at the critical moment knows, they are definitely less convenient to use. With them there's clearly a trade-off between convenience and safety.

In the past, many women felt comfortable about choosing convenience over safety. The Pill and the IUD were the most widely used forms of birth control. But over the years this has begun to change. The ever-growing list of known and suspected side effects and complications from the IUD and the Pill (a list that now contains some 50-odd items) have made many women reconsider the safety vs. convenience trade-off. The fact that the list of complications and side effects keeps growing and that neither the Pill nor the IUD has been around long enough for anyone to judge its long-term effects has contributed to our uneasiness about the safety of these methods.

The Long-Term Effects

The biggest concern about the long-term effects has centered on the Pill and the possibility that the Pill might, in the long run, cause cancer in at least some of the women who have used it. The Pill and its possible link to cancer has been one of the most widely researched and hotly debated topics in modern medicine. In fact, there has been so much controversy and conflicting information that it is hard to make heads or tails of the issue. When the Pill first came out, in the early 1960s, we were told that it was perfectly safe and harmless. Then in the seventies we began to hear all sorts of scary stories about scientific studies linking the Pill to cancer, and as a result a lot of us stopped using it. As we moved into the eighties the scene shifted again, and we were told that not only did the Pill *not* cause cancer but it might also protect us from getting cancer. Encouraged by this news, some of us renewed our Pill prescriptions. But almost before the ink on the prescriptions was dry, we were presented by another set of studies indicating that the Pill does, after all, cause cancer.

In order to make sense out of all this contradiction and controversy it helps to know a bit about the history of the whole issue. The Pill first came on the market in 1960, and as we have said, it was touted as being safe and harmless. But before the decade was out, studies documenting the increased risk of heart attacks, blood clots, strokes, gallbladder disease, liver tumors and other problems in Pill users began to appear in medical journals.[1] These problems generally were attributed to the hormone estrogen in the Pill, but the other Pill hormone, progesterone, was also suspect.[2]

Once the studies documenting these immediate, short-term hazards of the Pill began to appear, questions about the possible effects of long-term use, in particular about cancer, were raised in the medical community and in the popular press. A number of early studies failed to show an increased risk of cancer in Pill users, but critics of these studies pointed out that cancer is a slow, growing disease. Those who were concerned about the possible link between the Pill and cancer argued that it would take, at the very best, 20 years before a large enough number of women had been using the Pill for a sufficiently long period to allow detection of any cancerous effects the Pill might have.

Pill critics also pointed to studies of laboratory animals in which both estrogen use and progesterone use were linked to the development of cancerous tumors.[3] Things began to look particularly bad for the Pill as we moved into the seventies. In 1971 it was discovered that the daughters of women who had taken a synthetic estrogen known as diethylstilbestrol (DES) during their pregnancies in order to prevent miscarriages were at greater risk of developing a rare form of vaginal cancer.[4] The risk was small, but it clearly was related to the mother's use of estrogen.* Some data also suggested that DES mothers might be at greater risk of developing breast and other cancers.[5] DES is a different estrogen than that used in the Pill, but this link between estrogen and cancer in humans made many doctors and women leery of the Pill.

In 1975 a study was published showing that women who took estrogen for menopausal symptoms, such as hot flashes, were at greater risk of developing uterine cancer.[6] Other studies confirmed that menopausal women who took estrogen had a 4.5 to 13.9 times greater chance of developing uterine cancer than women who do not use estrogen.[7] No one knew what implications, if any, this would have for younger women who were taking lower doses of estrogen in the Pill, but these studies added to the uneasiness about the Pill.

Then, in 1976, one type of birth control pill, the sequential pill, had to be withdrawn from the market because of the development of uterine cancer in some of the women who were using it.[8] Needless to say, this added to the concern about the pills that were still on the market.

Researchers continued to study the Pill throughout the seventies. Many researchers who were concerned about the Pill and breast cancer studied the relationship between the two. There was no proof that estrogen can act as a "seed" for breast cancer. But there was ample reason to believe that estrogen may act as a "fertilizer," accelerating the growth of certain preexisting breast cancers. Some breast cancers have "estrogen receptors" that make them responsive to stimulation by estrogen produced in the body. What is the effect of synthetic estrogen in the Pill on estrogen-sensitive cancers in the breast? If a woman with an undetected estrogen-sensitive cancer of the breast takes the Pill, will her cancer grow more rapidly or be more likely to spread to other parts of her body faster? Because 1 out of 14 women in the United States will develop breast cancer, and because 40 percent to 60 percent of them will have estrogen receptors, these are important questions. Unfortunately, they cannot be answered at this time. But both Pill "fans" and Pill critics agree that women who have had breast cancer or indeed any cancer of the female organs should not take the Pill. And many doctors believe that women with family histories of breast cancer (mother, sister, aunt, grandmother) should not take the Pill.

Studies done in the late seventies indicated that Pill users are less likely to develop benign (noncancerous) breast disease than are other women.[9] Because having a benign breast disease increases one's statistical chances of developing breast cancer, it was hoped that this lower incidence of benign breast disease might mean a lower incidence of breast cancer in Pill users. However, other studies done at about the same time were not as encouraging. One study indicated that women who already had benign breast disease when they

*Other abnormalities have since been discovered in both daughters and sons of women who took DES. For more information, *see* pp. 808–18.

started on the Pill, or those who did develop benign breast disease despite the Pill, may be more likely to develop breast cancer.[10] The findings of one disturbing study suggested that women who took estrogen for menopausal symptoms may, after a lapse of some 15 years, be at greater risk of developing breast cancer.[11] This association held true regardless of how long the women took the estrogen, but the study only involved a small number of women, so it was impossible to say whether the results of this study were valid or merely a statistical fluke. As the seventies drew to a close there were no studies indicating that women on the Pill were more apt to develop breast cancer, but there were a number of unanswered questions and considerable reason for concern about a possible link between estrogen and breast cancer.

During the seventies, researchers also looked at the possible relationship between cervical cancer and the Pill. Most of these studies failed to show any link between the two; however, the follow-up time in these studies was often limited.[12] Then a longer-term study indicated that women who have a cervical condition known as dysplasia, which is sometimes a precursor to cervical cancer, were more likely to have their dysplasia progress to cancer if they used the Pill.[13] Thus by the end of the decade there was also considerable reason for concern about this form of cancer and the Pill.

Also in the seventies conflicting evidence about the possible relationship between the Pill and skin cancer came to light. Most studies failed to show a connection, but a few hinted at one.[14]

None of the studies done in the seventies *proved* a connection between the Pill and any type of cancer. But the studies of laboratory animals, the DES scandal, the link between menopausal estrogen and cancer, the withdrawal of the sequential pill and the possibility of a link with cervical and skin cancer all contributed to a considerable lack of confidence in the Pill. More women (and doctors) became uneasy about the Pill. Pill sales declined markedly.

Then, in the early eighties, the public image of the Pill got a face-lifting. The concerns raised in the seventies were all but forgotten in the flood of articles in women's magazines and the popular press claiming that the Pill did not increase a woman's chance of developing breast cancer, and that Pill use may actually make a woman less likely to develop ovarian or uterine cancer. Most of these articles were based on two studies: one from Kaiser-Permanente Hospital, in Walnut Creek, California, and one from the Centers for Disease Control (CDC), in Atlanta, Georgia.[15] Although much of what was said in these articles was accurate, some of it was misleading.

Take, for example, the findings concerning ovarian cancer. Both studies indicated that Pill users were less likely to develop ovarian cancer. The CDC study showed that, compared with women who had never used the Pill, Pill users were at less than two-thirds the risk of developing ovarian cancer. Pill critics were not surprised that the Pill was associated with a decreased risk of ovarian cancer. Most cancer of the ovary arises from the ovarian epithelium, the outer skin of the ovary. Because the hormones in the Pill inhibit ovulation, there is less activity and cell change in the ovarian epithelium of Pill users and hence less cancer.

What was misleading about the articles in the popular media was that they were often published under Pill-protects-against-cancer sorts of titles, giving the impression that the Pill had been shown to be protective against *all* forms of cancer, which, as we shall see, is not true. Such articles also failed to point out several other facts. For one thing, ovarian cancer is relatively uncommon. About 18,000 new cases are diagnosed each year compared with 100,000 new cases of breast cancer.[16] When selecting a method of birth control, women must always weigh the risks against the benefits, and certainly the noncontraceptive benefits, such as a protection against ovarian cancer, should be considered in any risk/benefit assessment. But Pill critics have argued that the benefit of protection against ovarian cancer should not be weighed too heavily, because it is a relatively uncommon type of cancer.

Another point that these optimistic articles in the popular press generally failed to mention was that the researchers who did these studies showed only that the protective effect of the Pill continued for about 10 years after the woman had stopped using the Pill. But 10 years after discontinuing use of the Pill will users still have a decreased risk of developing ovarian cancer? This question is significant, because most of the women who develop ovarian cancer are well past menopause. Most of them, even if they had been using the Pill, would have stopped doing so more than 10 years before their cancers developed. The protective effect of the Pill in relation to ovarian cancer may, then, only be meaningful for the small percentage of women who develop ovarian cancer at unusually early ages. Thus Pill critics again caution women about being overly impressed by the studies showing a decreased risk of developing ovarian cancer. The articles that appeared in the popular magazines generally reported only the results of the studies, without explaining the reservations the Pill critics had, which gave women misleading impressions.

Both studies also indicated a decreased risk of uterine cancer developing in Pill users. This protective effect of the Pill was also not surprising to some of the Pill critics, for many researchers believe that it is not estrogen per se that causes uterine cancer, but what scientists call ''unopposed estrogen.'' Unopposed estrogen is estrogen stimulation that is not opposed or counterbalanced by progesterone, which normally is produced in greater quantities in the second half of the menstrual cycle, after ovulation. The women who were taking estrogen for menopausal symptoms were, of course, no longer ovulating and producing progesterone. Therefore, the estrogen they were taking was unopposed estrogen, which is what led to a higher incidence of uterine cancer in menopausal women. Also, the hormones in the Pill cause Pill users to have less growth and cell change in the lining of the uterus each month (which is why Pill users generally have scantier menstrual periods). Because there is less activity, there is also less chance for cancer, and for many researchers this explains the lower incidence of uterine cancer in Pill users. Thus, at least to some critics, the finding that the combined birth control pills, which contain both estrogen and progesterone, protect against uterine cancer was not a great surprise.

Not everyone agrees with this line of reasoning. Some researchers think that any estrogen, unopposed or otherwise, may be a factor in uterine cancer (for details, see the section on Uterine Cancer). These researchers and others question the notion that it is the Pill itself that accounts for the lowered rates of uterine cancer in Pill users in studies like those done at Walnut Creek and by the CDC. Their reasoning goes like this. A large number of women in the United States have a disease called polycystic ovary disease, or Stein-Leventhal syndrome. Women who have this condition do not ovulate. Unless they are treated for the condition they are subject to unopposed estrogen. It has long been known that women with polycystic ovaries are at high risk of developing uterine cancer unless the condition is treated. One of the most common ways to treat the condition is to put the woman on birth control pills. The question then arises, Was the lower incidence of uterine cancer in these studies a reflection of the Pill or of the fact that a lot of Pill users in the studies had polycystic ovaries? In other words, if all the women who had polycystic ovaries were eliminated from the studies, would the rates of uterine cancer still be lower in Pill users? We do not know the answer to this question. Again, most of the articles in the popular press simply reported the optimistic news about the lower incidence of uterine cancer, without discussing the reservations that Pill critics had about the meaning of the studies.

The studies also showed that women on the Pill were not any more likely to develop breast cancer than were women who did not use the Pill. These encouraging results also received a great deal of publicity along the lines of the-Pill-does-not-cause-breast-cancer, which, of course, was good news for many women who had been concerned about this issue. But here again, the reports in the popular media were somewhat misleading. True, the studies did not indicate an increased risk of breast cancer among Pill users. But, like ovarian cancer, breast cancer generally occurs in older women. The Pill became available only in the early sixties. Women who were in their early 20s or 30s when the Pill first came out and who started using it then are just now reaching their 40s and 50s. Because breast cancer generally occurs in women who are older than 50, studies that do not include a significant number of Pill users over age 50 or 55 cannot really tell us a whole lot about breast cancer and the Pill.

Although the studies that were done in the early eighties have given us some encouraging news about the Pill and cancer, they have not, as the popular press sometimes leads us to believe, proved that the Pill does not cause cancer or that it provides meaningful protection against some forms of cancer.

Women should know that, in addition to the encouraging news, the Walnut Creek study also provided some discouraging news about the Pill and cancer. Although these findings did not receive the same publicity as the more optimistic findings, the fact is that the study found a higher incidence of cervical cancer in women who had used the Pill, especially in those under age 40, as well as a higher incidence of skin cancer. The researchers explained the higher rates of skin cancer by suggesting that the Pill users in the study might have been more apt to sunbathe than the nonusers might have been. Because exposure to the sun is known to increase the risk of skin cancer, the researchers theorized that it was sunlight exposure and not the Pill that had led to the higher incidence of skin cancer. However, we question the validity of this reasoning. Nothing in the data suggested that women who use the Pill are either more likely or less likely to sunbathe than are women who do not use the Pill. Moreover, it has long been known that the Pill may affect the pigment cells in the skin. In fact, some users develop chloasma, a condition in which areas of the skin darken. To think that the Pill might have some cancerous effects on the melanin (pigment-producing) cells in the skin is not all that farfetched. The finding in the Walnut Creek study of a higher incidence of melanoma, cancer of the melanin-producing skin cells, may, as researchers theorize, be owing to a propensity for sunbathing in Pill users, but it seems equally possible, if not more likely, that it may be owing to the Pill itself.

The finding of a higher incidence of cervical cancer in Pill users in the Walnut Creek study also received little attention in the popular press. The researchers who conducted the study also found that the Pill users had a greater degree of sexual activity than the nonusers. Because a greater degree of sexual activity (multiple sexual partners, starting sexual activity at a young age) increases a woman's chances of developing cervical cancer (for details, see the section on Cervical Cancer), the researchers theorized that it may have been this factor, rather than something about the Pill, that accounted for the higher rates. They may be right, but the studies indicating that women with a precancerous condition of the cervix were more likely to have that condition develop into cancer if they used the Pill[17] may indicate that it might be something about the Pill that increases a user's chance of developing cervical cancer.

It is interesting to speculate why these negative findings in the Walnut Creek study received so little publicity. Barbara Seaman, health-care activist and author of such books as *The Doctor's Case Against the Pill* and *Women and the Crisis in Sex Hormones*, has discussed this very issue.[18] She pointed out that the drug company which funded the study also hired a public relations/advertising firm to publicize the study, a fact she became aware of when an employee of the firm sent her some intercompany memos outlining the strategy for downplaying these aspects of the study.

At any rate, the studies done in the early eighties, although encouraging in some respects, did not exonerate the Pill. Nevertheless, because of the wide-spread—albeit misleading—publicity that these studies received, public confidence in the Pill improved markedly over what it had been in the seventies. But in 1983 articles about two recent studies that seriously undermined this newfound confidence in the Pill appeared in *Lancet,* the prestigious English medical journal. One of the studies dealt with the Pill and cervical cancer.[19] This study was longer term (10 years follow-up) than many of the previous studies were. It showed a higher incidence of cervical cancer and precancerous cervical diseases, such as dysplasia and carcinoma in situ, in Pill users as compared with IUD users, and that the likelihood of developing one of these conditions increases the longer the woman uses the Pill. The researchers did not collect information about risk factors, such as degree of sexual activity, from *all* the women in the study, but they did collect such data from some of the women. The differences in degree of sexual activity between the IUD users and the Pill users were not significant, but the researchers pointed out that without exact information from all the women, no one can say conclusively that the Pill was responsible for the higher incidence of precancerous and cancerous cervical disease in Pill users. But the researchers did make a strong recommendation that Pill users, especially those who are on the Pill for longer than 4 years, have frequent Pap smears, a test that can detect cervical cancer in its earliest, most curable stages.

The second study dealt with breast cancer and the Pill.[20] Findings showed that long-term use of pills with a high progesterone content before age 25 increased a woman's chance of developing breast cancer. The researchers also concluded that long-term use of low-progesterone-content pills before age 25 appeared "to increase breast cancer risk little or not at all."[21] They further stated that use of high-progesterone-content pills after age 25 "may also carry some added breast cancer risk" but concluded that more study is needed to determine the extent of the risk.[22]

The pills that the authors of this study considered suspect were those with a "progesterone potency" of 5 or higher. "Progesterone potency" is the important term here, for it is not the actual amount of progesterone in the pill that counts. Different progesterones have different potencies. Table 1 lists the progesterone potency of some birth control pills. If you are taking a pill with a potency of 5 or higher, you might ask your doctor to prescribe another brand of pills (or another method of birth control). If the pill you are taking does not appear in this table, ask your doctor what the progesterone potency of your pill is. If it is higher than 5, you may want to switch brands. If you are young and have been using these pills for a number of years, do not panic. Not all the women in the study using these pills develop breast cancer. Moreover, this is only *one* study. This finding has not been confirmed by other studies. Also, the statistical methods used in the study have been severely criticized. This study *does not* prove that taking high potency progesterone pills increases your risk for

Table 1
Progesterone Potency of Birth Control Pills[23]

Brand Name	Progesterone Potency
*Ovulen	15.0
*Demulen	15.0
*Ovral	15.0
*Enovid 10	10.7
*Norinyl 10	10.7
*Ortho-Novum 10	10.0
*Lo/Ovral	9.0
*Enovid 5	5.4
*Norlestrin 2.5	5.0
Zorane 1.5/30	3.0
Enovid-E	2.7
Ortho-Novum 2	2.0
Norlestrin 1	2.0
Loestrin 1/20	2.0
Zorane 1/20	2.0
Norinyl 1 + 80	1.0
Ortho-Novum 1/80	1.0
Noriday-1	1.0
Ortho-Novum 1/50	1.0
Brevicon	.5
Modicon	.5
Micronov	.35

*Potency of 5 or higher.

breast cancer. More studies are needed. However, if you are a young woman and have been using high potency pills for a number of years, you may want to consider switching brands. Also be sure to have breast exams regularly and to practice self-exam monthly.

The studies done to date on the subject of the Pill and cancer do offer some encouraging news about ovarian and endometrial cancer in Pill users. And, with the exception of this latest study on high potency progesterone pills, and the study of post menopausal women mentioned earlier, the studies of women using the Pill have uniformly failed to show any increased likelihood of their getting cancer.[24] The data on skin and cervical cancer is not so good. But as it stands now, the possibility that the Pill may increase the chances of getting some forms of cancer in some of the women who have used it cannot be denied. More studies and more time are needed before we can make firm conclusions about the relationship between the Pill and cancer.

Safety

So far we have been talking about *possible* problems. There are, in addition, definite, clearly documented complications and side effects associated with use of the Pill and the IUD. Fatal and nonfatal heart attacks, strokes, liver tumors, gallbladder disease, high blood pressure and diabetes are just a few of the health problems in which the Pill has been said to be a factor.[24] The IUD has also caused the death of a number of women. One IUD in particular, the Dalkon Shield, the tail (the strings that protrude through the cervix into the vaginal cavity) of which was twined like a candlewick, apparently served as a ladder that allowed disease-causing organisms to ascend into the uterus. It was later banned after being implicated in the deaths of some young women.[25] Other types of IUDs have also been associated with death, sterility and serious illnesses.[26]

When reports of Pill- and IUD-related deaths and complications first began to appear in the medical literature and the popular press, advocates of these birth control methods were quick to point out that, despite the risks, these methods were still safer than pregnancy. The chances of dying as a result of using an IUD or the Pill were considerably lower than the chances of dying of a complication related to pregnancy.

Many women have objected to looking at things from this point of view, however. If the Pill and the IUD were the only methods of birth control available, comparisons of pregnancy versus Pill or IUD risks might be relevant. But the IUD and the Pill are not the only methods available; there are other, safer methods that should be considered in estimates of comparative risks.

Moreover, we now know that the Pill and the IUD are not safer than pregnancy for certain groups of women. Table 2 shows the leading causes of death in American women aged 15 to 44 years. Table 3 shows the deaths associated with birth control and pregnancy complications in these age-groups. In the 40-to-44-year-old age-group, women who use the Pill *and* who smoke are more likely to die from Pill complications than from pregnancy complications.

These tables tell us that for younger women the risks of birth-control–related deaths are relatively small. (Of course, this is all relative; the risks don't seem so small if you're the one who dies.) For all age-groups the safest method of birth control is a barrier method, with a backup abortion should the method fail. Women under age 30 are more likely to die as a result of a traffic accident (the second most common cause of death in women of all ages) than as a result of birth control complications. After age 30 the likelihood of dying as the result of a Pill complication for users who smoke ap-

Table 2
Leading Causes of Death: U.S. Women Aged 15 to 44

Cause	Deaths per 100,000 Women per Year
All causes	91.20
Cancer	18.80
Motor vehicle accidents	14.50
Heart disease	7.25
Suicide	6.95
All other accidents	6.50
Homicide	5.70
Stroke	3.95
All other causes	Less than 3 per 100,000 each

SOURCE: Mortality Statistics Branch, Division of Vital Statistics, National Center for Health Statistics, US Department of Health, Education and Welfare.

proaches the risk of dying in a traffic accident, and by age 40, Pill users who smoke are more likely to die as a result of a Pill complication than in a traffic accident. Because of the risks reflected in these charts, many doctors no longer prescribe the Pill for women over 30 who smoke; others won't prescribe it for women over 40, regardless of whether or not they smoke; and no one should prescribe the Pill for smokers over age 40.

These safety features include only the risks of death from complications that have been clearly documented. They do not reflect possible complications. Five or ten years ago safety figures for the IUD and the Pill especially looked a lot better than they do today. Back then we didn't realize the risks involved for women, or how dramatically they increased for Pill users over 40. What will these safety figures look like in another 5 or 10 years? Only time will tell.

These figures reflect only death rates. Although the IUD is safer than the Pill in terms of risk of death, each year as many as 1 in every 300 IUD users will have IUD-related complications serious enough to require hospitalization.[27] These complications generally involve perforation of the uterus by an IUD or an IUD-related infection, both of which often can be treated successfully without further difficulty. At other times these complications may cause infertility, constant pelvic pain and recurring episodes of pelvic inflammatory disease.

Table 2
Birth Control and Risk of Death

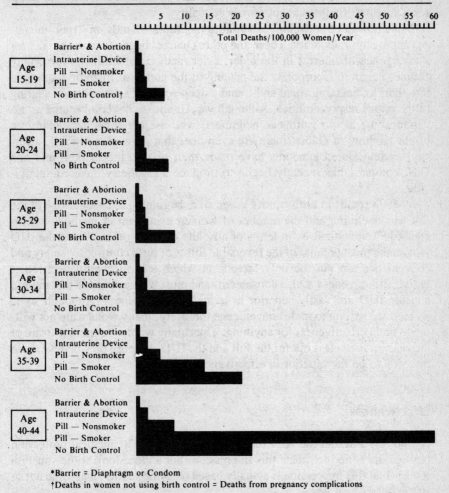

*Barrier = Diaphragm or Condom
†Deaths in women not using birth control = Deaths from pregnancy complications

SOURCE: FDA-approved package insert

Reexamining the Safety vs. Convenience Trade-Off

In light of the new information about relative risks and possible long-term effects, informed women began to reconsider the safety vs. convenience trade-off. Many women thought that it was high time to overhaul old images and attitudes about lovemaking anyhow. The fuzzy, romantic fantasies of swooning passion and orgasmic ecstasy on which most of us were weaned and that, of course, couldn't be interrupted by anything so prosaic as inserting a diaphragm, were due for replacement, especially in light of Masters and Johnson's research findings about female sexuality.

Women began to develop, or admit to having, a "hands-on" (pun-intended) approach to sexuality. These and other changes began to pave the way for a resurgence of interest in the older, safer methods of birth control. Many couples began to incorporate the placing of the condom, foam or diaphragm into their lovemaking ritual and found a deep sense of satisfaction in sharing birth control responsibilities. Although we Americans haven't become as adventuresome as our European neighbors, who use condoms that come in a bright rainbow of colors (there are even ones that glow in the dark!), a few shy, pastel-colored condoms have made their way to the market, and one U.S. company has recently begun to produce a raspberry-flavored spermicide.

By 1978 trends in birth control usage were beginning to change. Use of the Pill was declining and the number of women using barrier methods has increased.[28] Nevertheless, in terms of absolute numbers, the Pill and the IUD remain the most popular of the reversible forms of birth control, for safety and convenience are not the only factors on which a birth control decision is based. Effectiveness is also considered, and most women believe that the Pill and the IUD are vastly superior in terms of effectiveness. Although some women are willing to trade convenience for safety, many women are not willing to trade effectiveness for anything. Thus many women, although aware of the risks, nonetheless opt for the Pill and the IUD, because they believe these methods to be far superior in effectiveness.

Effectiveness

But are the Pill and the IUD really more effective? The medical profession has certainly tried to create this impression, but a close look at the situation reveals that this impression is actually based on some subtle—and some not so subtle—statistical lies.

One way in which women are hoodwinked into thinking that the Pill and the IUD are more effective than the barrier methods involves the misuse of both the theoretical effectiveness rate and the actual-use effectiveness rate. Studies have shown that medical professionals, when informing women about birth control, tend to quote theoretical effectiveness rates for the Pill and the IUD and actual-use effectiveness rates for the barrier methods.[29] Not only that, but they also often quote figures that are better than the theoretical rates for the Pill and IUD and that are worse than the actual-use effectiveness rates for the barrier methods. Hardly a fair comparison!

Theoretical rates are an example of the bias against barrier methods, for the way in which they are determined begins, on examination, to seem like a bit of a mystery. It is easy to see how one could come up with a theoretical rate for a device like the IUD or for the Pill. One could insert the IUD and check the woman regularly to make sure that it had not been expelled or hadn't perforated the uterus and then get a pretty good idea of its theoretical effectiveness rate. With the Pill, one could run a study in which it was administered to women each day at the same time and again come up with a good idea of its theoretical effectiveness rate. But how does one establish a theoretical rate for the condom, the diaphragm or foam? One could, we suppose, assign to every woman in the study a researcher who would check the placement of the diaphragm before each act of intercourse. Although this has certain comic possibilities, it is hardly a practical experiment. So the solution seems to involve pulling a figure out of a hat and calling it the theoretical rate. The theoretical failure rate commonly quoted for foam is three pregnancies per 100 woman-years of use.[30] Yet there are foam studies with actual-use failure rates of 1.55 per 100 woman-years of use,[31] so it does not make sense to say that the theoretical failure rate is 3. Many birth control experts feel that theoretical rates are meaningless and should be disregarded. We agree.

When comparing the effectiveness of various birth control methods the important figures to look at are the actual-use effectiveness rates. But here again we run into statistical shenanigans. The Food and Drug Administration (FDA) publishes a pamphlet entitled *Contraception: Comparing the Options* that is the official word on birth control.[32] It too is biased heavily against the barrier methods, telling us that we can expect anywhere from 3 to 36 pregnancies in a group of 100 condom users in a year. The idea of 36 pregnancies is hardly reassuring. Given a figure like this, no one who seriously wanted to prevent conception would use a condom.

Yet the facts behind these statistics tell a very different story. As it turns out, the figure of 36 pregnancies is taken from a study done in West Virginia in 1942[33]—and how applicable is a study done almost 40 years ago to today's situation? For one thing, the quality of condoms has improved dramatically since the time of the West Virginia study. Traditionally, the objection to condoms was that they decreased sexual pleasure for men. Using a condom was likened to taking a shower with a raincoat on. In the past this reputation was probably well deserved, but with the advent of latex rubber, condoms became much thinner and far more pleasant to use. As a result, they are used much more now than previously.

Moreover, condom manufacturers today must meet strict quality control standards. Each batch must be tested for pinholes and other defects. Some manufacturers even test each condom individually, although this is a fairly recent innovation. Condoms manufactured in the forties did not have to meet such rigorous quality-control standards. The fact that condoms in the forties were not tested for manufacturing defects and were unpleasingly thick undoubtedly accounts for the high pregnancy rates.

91

The time during which the study was done may also have been a factor in the high pregnancy rates. Published in 1942, the actual study probably took place a year or two before. The United States was about to enter a war, men were being drafted left and right and a lot of young men undoubtedly were in a hurry to become family men before they were grabbed up. Of course it's impossible to say whether any of the men in the West Virginia study had draft evasion on their minds, but given this possibility and the fact that the condoms used were not quality controlled and were rather primitive forerunners of the modern condom, the study hardly seems applicable to today's situation. More to the point would be studies done using the new, quality-tested, latex rubber condoms or, better yet, the natural-skin condoms, which allow for better heat transfer and superior sensitivity. One of the most recent studies of condom effectiveness, cited in the prestigious work *Contraceptive Technology* (Emory University), was a study done in 1975 with an actual-use failure rate of only 0.83, which is better than the *theoretical* effectiveness rate of the Minipill and within a few tenths of a percentage point of the *theoretical* rate for the regular Pill.[34] But these effectiveness rates are not reflected in the FDA's official 3-to-36-pregnancy failure rate for the condom.

The FDA figures are supposedly an objective and fair representation of the data available in the medical literature. Yet the FDA's effectiveness rates for the rhythm method are derived, in part, from studies done years ago on a group of Tongan women.[35] Again, how applicable are the results of a study done in a South Sea island community whose cultural attitudes about pregnancy and sense of urgency about birth control may be very different from ours? If the FDA's figures are a fair presentation of the available data, why is a rate of only one pregnancy per 100 woman-years of use cited for the Pill when in fact there are reports in the medical literature in which actual-use failure rates for the Pill are as high as 25 percent?[36] If studies of South Sea Islanders and of men using condoms that bear about as much similarity to today's condoms as a Model T bears to a Mustang are going to be included, in all fairness the FDA pamphlet should tell us to expect anywhere from 1 to 25 pregnancies among women using the Pill for a year. But it doesn't.

Why does the medical profession downgrade the barrier methods? Why does the FDA present such biased effectiveness statistics? There are a number of plausible explanations.

First, back in the fifties and early sixties, when the Pill and the IUD first made their debut, Americans were having a love affair with technology. Science had ushered in the era of gadgets galore. With just the flick of the switch and a push of the button, we could automatically wash the dishes, dispose of the garbage, brush our teeth, Osterize the morning juice, remotely tune our TVs and open the garage door. If that wasn't sufficient testimony to the incredible efficiency of modern technology, one had only to consider the seemingly endless array of consumable, disposable, throw-away convenience products that were rolling off production lines across the nation. To top it all off, we counted backwards from 10, pushed a button, launched a rocket and landed a man on the moon. If science and technology could perform such miracles, certainly they could produce wonderfully effective methods of birth control.

Less than a decade later, knee-deep in nonbiodegradable garbage and choking on industrial pollution, many of us were wondering whether the new era of technology was such a dandy thing after all. But that was later on; at the time when the IUD and the Pill first appeared on the scene, Americans still possessed an incredibly naive faith. Science and technology were in effect the new gods, and one does not question the efficacy of the gods—or look a gift horse in the mouth.

In the era of gadgetry and man-on-the-moon technology it simply was not believable that age-old methods like the diaphragm and the condom could be as effective as the wondrous new man-made chemicals that could stop a woman' s body from ovulating or the clever plastic doodad that could prevent a fertile egg from implanting in the womb. We were so busy admiring our technological accomplishments that we never stopped to take an objective look at the realities of the situation.

Besides, the birthrate was declining, a phenomenon attributed to the widespread use of the Pill and the IUD. But here again the facts were ignored by technology-bedazzled family planners. In actual fact, the lowest birthrate the United States ever experienced was in 1930, long before either the Pill or the IUD was available.[37] This fact *could* be interpreted as a sign of the efficiency of the barrier methods—the only birth control options available at that time.

On the other hand, the low birthrate might not have been a reflection of their efficiency at all. Perhaps the Depression depressed people's sex drives as well as the economy. Maybe people simply didn't have sex very often; this certainly could account for the low birthrate. In the same vein, perhaps the lower birthrate that occurred during the time of widespread use of the Pill and the IUD was also just a coincidence. Were the Pill and the IUD really responsible for the lower birthrate, or were factors like the legalization of abortion, the opening up of jobs for women, improvements in infant and child survival (because most children now live to maturity, women no longer have ''replacement'' children for those they once expected would die) more directly responsible? Without a clear answer to this question we can hardly consider lower birthrates a testimony to the effectiveness of the Pill and the IUD.

Yet the myth that the Pill and the IUD are vastly superior methods of birth control persists and is supported actively by doctors. Doctors consider themselves scientists and are perhaps especially apt to place faith in the wonders wrought by science. Then too the Pill and the IUD appeared on the scene at a time when abortion was still illegal. All too often doctors were forced to deal with the aftermath of illegal abortions. Then along came two methods that

93

were so easy and carefree to use that consistent and proper usage seemed assured. Understandably, doctors who had watched women die as a result of back-alley abortions didn't cast too critical an eye on the statistical data concerning the effectiveness of these new birth control methods.

Abortions are now legal, but despite this fact doctors still tend to downgrade barrier methods. A less benevolent explanation for their continued putdown of these methods has been suggested by Barbara Seaman: It is easier to push a prescription for the Pill across the desk than to take the time to fit a diaphragm carefully and teach a woman how to use it. It's also more profitable. The diaphragm takes more of the doctor's time and does not involve the annual or semiannual checkup that women on the Pill must have. In addition, during the heyday of the Pill and the IUD in the 1960s, many medical schools dropped diaphragm fitting from their curricula, so that many doctors today do not know how to fit one correctly.

The other major barrier methods are not physician controlled. Condoms and foam can be purchased at pharmacies without a doctor's prescription. Perhaps both ego (the doctor's assumption that anything that only s/he can provide is better than anything a woman can do for herself) and financial considerations have contributed to doctors' tendencies to downgrade barrier methods.

Sexism is also a factor. Many doctors think women are too dumb to learn how to use the barrier methods, so they downgrade the effectiveness of these methods, hoping to convince women to use the Pill and the IUD instead.

An overwhelming cultural ignorance about their bodies is imposed on women. We are taught from early childhood to believe that someone other than ourselves has the knowledge, the expertise and the right to control our reproductive organs. But the barrier methods are childishly simple to use, and anyone with a modicum of knowledge about how her body works can be taught to use these methods if the person doing the teaching speaks the same language.

We are not being facetious when we add the qualification that the teacher must speak the woman's language. A number of studies of barrier methods involved women who did not speak the same language as the people who were conducting the study. Follow-ups of some studies of foam effectiveness in which the failure rates were unacceptably high have shown that some women used the foam after making love or applied it to the outer genitals instead of to the inner vaginal cavity.[38] Not surprisingly, the studies showing the best rates for the barrier methods are those in which the women in the study were taught how to use the method by someone of the same racial or ethnic background who spoke the same language.

Pharmaceutical companies have also played a role in creating the impression that the IUD and the Pill are vastly superior methods of birth control. Birth control is, after all, a big business. About 325 million monthly cycles of oral contraceptives were sold in 1977.[39] Retail prices for a single monthly cycle may run from $5 to $10. Not all the money goes back to the manufacturer, but a hefty chunk of it does. The IUD is also a profitable item, retailing to doctors for $15 to $25. It is not as profitable as the Pill, but when you consider that the device contains only a few cents worth of materials, the profit margin isn't bad.

A diaphragm, on the other hand, sells for $5 to $10 and, with proper care, may last for years. Although foam and condoms are consumable items, supplies of which must be replenished constantly, they are used only when they are needed, unlike the Pill, which must be taken every day regardless of whether or not a woman is having intercourse.

About half of the dozen or so major worldwide manufacturers of the Pill are U.S. companies. A couple of large U.S. pharmaceutical companies make IUDs. These companies have spent considerable sums of money to advertise their products in medical journals, promoting the notion that these methods of birth control are superior to other methods. Doctors, primed by their faith in technology, by their financial and ego interests and by biased statistics from the FDA, have been all too willing to accept these advertising claims and pass erroneous information about relative effectiveness rates on to their women patients.

The fact that the FDA's official statistics on birth control are biased against the barrier methods and favor the methods promoted heavily by the pharmaceutical industry will not come as a shock to women who are active in the health-care movement. The FDA is the government agency responsible for regulating the drug industry, and their performance of their regulatory duties has come under sharp criticism. Although the agency does a stunning job of stamping out snake-oil salesmen and other small-time quacks, their track record as far as regulation of the major drug companies is somewhat less admirable. To cite just one example, it took at least 7 months for the FDA to act on the unquestionable proof it had about the relationship between the synthetic estrogen DES and cancer.[40] Having the FDA regulate the drug industry has been compared to having the fox guard the chicken coop. As Barbara Seaman points out in her fine book *Women and the Crisis in Sex Hormones,* it is not unusual for officials in the FDA to wind up as executives in the drug industry after leaving their government posts.[41]

Regardless of the reasons, one thing is clear: Women in the United States have been receiving biased information about birth control effectiveness from both their doctors and the FDA, the very sources women should be able to rely on for objective facts.

What is the truth of the matter? How do the various methods of birth control compare in terms of effectiveness? No one knows. Unfortunately, there has never been a well-designed, sound, scientific study comparing the different methods, nor is it likely that one will be done, for such a study would be impractical, if not downright impossible. First, such a study would require a number of different groups of women, each of which would use one of the methods for a period of time. The women in the different groups would have to be matched carefully. They would all have to have had at least one child, thus indicating that they were indeed fertile, and they would have to be matched according to age, because 25-year-old women are much more fertile than 35-year-old women. All the women's sexual partners would each have to have fathered at least one child, indicating that they too were fertile. The women would have to have intercourse about the same number of times per week. They would also have to be matched in regard to their intentions, for studies have shown that couples who are using birth control with the intention of merely postponing pregnancy are much less successful at birth control, regardless of the method used, than are couples who have completed their families and don't intend to have any children in the future. The study would also have to involve large numbers of women in order to be statistically significant. The differences in actual-use effectiveness rates, if indeed there are any, are going to be small ones, and the laws of statistics tell us that when we are looking for large differences between groups, only relatively small numbers of people have to be studied. But when we are looking for more refined data and smaller differences, large numbers of participants are necessary in order for the statistics to be valid.

In addition, the study would have to be randomized, which means that the participants could not choose which method of birth control they were to use but would be assigned a method at random. Randomization would be necessary in order to prevent bias; otherwise, the fact that more motivated users might tend to pick a certain method could bias the results of the study. Finding large groups of well-matched subjects who would be willing to use a birth control method assigned to them at random would be—to say the least—rather difficult.

Lacking such a study, the best that can be done is to hunt through the medical literature and catalog the highest and lowest use effectiveness rates that have been reported. Table 4 lists the highest and lowest rates we have been able to find. We think that some of the low figures are probably not too meaningful. For instance, the lowest condom rate of 64 percent comes from the

Table 4
High and Low Effectiveness Rates Reported in the Medical Literature

Method	Highest (%)	Lowest (%)
Pill	99 +	75
IUD	99 +	91.7
Condom	99 +	64
Foam	99 +	60
Diaphragm	98.6	80.3

1942 study discussed earlier. The high rates may be a bit more meaningful, for they represent results that can be expected from highly motivated users who are conscientious about using the method. Depending on your own motivations, you can expect to fall somewhere between these two extremes.

As you can see from looking at Table 4, there is less-than-1-percent difference in actual-use effectiveness rates when these methods are used in the best of circumstances, that is, when used by women who have been well educated about the method and who are highly motivated. These facts will probably come as a surprise to most women, for as we have seen, women are rarely informed about the high effectiveness rates of the barrier methods. Instead, we are fed a collection of statistical lies, with two serious consequences.

First, the widely held but erroneous belief that methods like the Pill are vastly superior has slowed research into the development of barrier methods that could be even more effective and more convenient to use. Research funds have been funneled into the development of hormonal, Pill-type methods and improvements on the IUD that, it is hoped, will result in their having fewer side effects, thus lowering their high discontinuation rates (large numbers of both IUD users and Pill users stop using these methods within the first year because of their side effects). Only a minuscule amount has been allocated to the development of barrier methods. Yet it is not beyond the scope of technology to develop a longer-lasting spermicide that could be inserted several hours before intercourse so that the spontaneity of the sex act would not be interrupted (one of the major drawbacks to the use of spermicides and diaphragms).

The Effectiveness vs. Safety Trade-Off

Unfortunately, the bias against the barrier methods has delayed their development. Misinformation about barrier-method effectiveness has also had the unfortunate effect, as we pointed out earlier, of causing many women who are led astray by the statistical lies about birth-control effectiveness to opt for the more dangerous Pill and IUD. Current trends in birth control usage are changing, however, and the Pill and the IUD are declining in popularity.

Many couples who are concerned about safety yet want maximum effectiveness have chosen sterilization—either tubal ligation for females or vasectomy for males. In fact, sterilization is now the most widely used method of birth control for married couples in their 30s.[42] Although vasectomy appears to be a simple operation with few serious side effects, there has been some concern about the fact that a number of vasectomized men develop antibodies to their own sperm.[43] Antibodies are substances produced by the body

97

to attack germs and other foreign bodies. The long-term effects of this irregularity in the body's immune response is not known.

Female sterilization, despite the nickname of "Band-Aid surgery" given to certain sterilization procedures, is major surgery that has serious potential complications, including death. The risks are small, but they do exist. Moreover, some recent studies indicate that women who have been sterilized have subsequent menstrual pain and excessive menstrual bleeding, as well as higher rates of hysterectomies and premature menopause than do nonsterilized women.[44]

Thus although sterilization is undeniably the most effective method of birth control, it carries some risks and may have long-term effects whose ultimate impact on a person's health is unknown. In light of this, many men and women are rethinking sterilization decisions. We cannot help but believe that objective information about the effectiveness of barrier methods might be an influential factor for those considering sterilization.

As you may have gathered by now, we are fans of the barrier methods and encourage their use. On the other hand, we are not what we call "no freaks"—medical professionals who refuse to prescribe the Pill or the IUD. Our basic belief is that every woman should be informed of the facts and then allowed to make her own decisions. If a woman is aware of the facts and chooses the Pill or the IUD, we support her right to make that decision and would not deny her access to the option she chooses. But we believe it is vital that she be well informed before making that decision. In the following reference section, we provide detailed information about each of the major methods: the Pill, the Mini-pill, the IUD, the diaphragm, spermicides, the condom, the contraceptive sponge, the cervical cap, sterilization, abortion and postcoital contraception. We also include a section on natural family planning, a method of birth control that depends on a woman's learning to recognize when she is fertile and abstaining from intercourse during that time. This method may be particularly suitable for women who practice speculum self-exam. We do not include information on withdrawal, or coitus interruptus, in which the man withdraws before ejaculation, or on breastfeeding as methods of birth control because both of these methods are notoriously ineffective.

Reference Section:
Birth Control Methods

BIRTH CONTROL PILLS

AKA: the Pill, oral contraceptives, OCs

Types: combined pill or estrogen/progestin pill
Mini-pill or progestin-only pill

Birth control pills are tablets containing synthetic (man-made) hormones similar to the ones made by a woman's ovaries. Two types of birth control pills are presently marketed in the United States: the combination pill, which contains both synthetic progesterone (progestin) and synthetic estrogen, and the Minipill, or progestin-only pill, which does not contain estrogen.

The Pill works by preventing the ovary from maturing an egg and releasing it at ovulation. By taking a daily dose of hormones, a woman's normal cyclical fluctuations in hormonal levels are stopped and the complex feedback mechanism that controls ovulation is interrupted. As you may recall from Chapter Four, the low levels of the ovarian hormones in the early part of the cycle stimulate the hypothalamus to produce its releasing factors, which in turn causes the pituitary to release two essential hormones, FSH, the follicle-stimulating hormone, and LH, the luteinizing hormone. The FSH acts on the egg-containing follicular sacs in the ovary, causing the eggs to mature. As they do so, the cells lining the inside of the sacs produce estrogen. Once the levels of estrogen are high enough they trigger a spurt of LH, which causes the ripe egg to burst out of the ovary at ovulation.

The combined pill prevents this from happening by providing a daily dose

99

of estrogen that is high enough to prevent the triggering of the hypothalamus and, indirectly, of the pituitary, which therefore doesn't produce FSH. Without FSH there are no mature eggs, so fertilization cannot occur.

The Mini-pill doesn't contain estrogen and doesn't suppress the pituitary hormones completely, but the constant daily dose of progestin blocks or at least blunts the surge of LH. The majority of Mini-pill users, then, don't ovulate. A significant proportion do, but pregnancy is nonetheless prevented, for the Mini-pill also works in the following ways.

The progestin in both the Mini-pill and the combination pill alters the character of the mucus secreted by the glands in the cervix. Normally, the cervical mucus becomes more alkaline (sugary) at the time of ovulation, which nourishes the sperm. On a microscopic level the molecules of the mucus realign themselves, forming tunnels to aid the sperm on their journey into the uterus. After ovulation, when the hormone progesterone is produced by the remnant of the burst follicular sac (the corpus luteum), the cervical mucus becomes hostile to sperm—more acidic and thicker, with a cross-hatched molecular structure that blocks the sperm (see Illustration 14). The progestin—synthetic progesterone—in birth control pills has the same effect on the cervical mucus.

The uterine lining is also altered by the hormone stimulation of the Pill. Normally, the estrogen in the first part of the cycle stimulates the development of the uterine lining. The process is then completed by the progesterone in the second half of the cycle. With the combined pill and its continual stimulation of both estrogen and progesterone, there is not the normal alternation between the two hormones that is necessary in order for a uterine lining that is capable of nourishing a fertilized egg to develop. Similarly, the continual progestin stimulation of the Mini-pill alters the endometrial lining, making it impossible for a fertilized egg to implant in the uterus.

The hormones in both the combined pill and the Mini-pill may also change the normal contractions of the fallopian tube, which help the fertilized egg move through the tube into the uterus. In order to develop properly the egg must spend a certain amount of time in the tube, nourished by special tubal secretions. The Pill speeds up the tubal contractions, so that the egg reaches the uterus before it has matured properly. Therefore, it cannot implant successfully in the uterine wall.

Effectiveness

We are often told that the pills are 99 percent or "practically 100 percent" effective. This is a theoretical effectiveness rate for combined pills containing at least 50 micrograms (mcg) of estrogen. Pills containing 35 mcg or less have a slightly lower theoretical rate of about 98 percent to 99 percent. Mini-pills have a theoretical rate of about 97 percent.

100

Actual-use effectiveness rates may be considerably lower, for these rates reflect all the user failures, that is, forgotten pills. Actual-use effectiveness rates for the Mini-pill range from 87 percent to 97 percent.[1] Actual-use effectiveness rates of 90 percent to 96 percent are generally quoted for the combined pill,[2] although rates as low as 75 percent have been reported.[3]

How to Use the Pill

Combination pills come in 21- and 28-day packs and are numbered sequentially. Starting with pill number 1, you take one pill a day until the pack is completed. With the 21-day pack you have 7 days in which you do not take any pills and during which you will have your menstrual period. On the 8th day you open a new 21-day pack and take the first pill from that pack. With the 28-day pack there are no "days off." The last seven pills in the 28-day pack are "blanks" containing sugar and iron but no hormones. During the days when you are taking the "blanks" you should have your menstrual period. After you complete a 28-day pack, open a new pack the next day and take the first pill from the new pack.

When you initially begin using combined pills, start your first pack in one of these three ways: (1) Take the first pill from your pack on the first Sunday after your period begins; (2) take the first pill from your pack on the 5th day after your period begins; or (3) take the first pill from your pack on the 1st day you begin menstrual bleeding during your menstrual cycle. We usually recommend #1, the first-pill-on-the-first-Sunday approach, because nowadays most pills come in packs that not only number the pills 1 through 21 or 28, but also label the pills with the days of the week on which they are to be taken. In such packs the first pill is labeled "Sunday," the second, "Monday," and so on. Because of this it is less confusing to start on a Sunday.

If you are using Mini-pills, you take a pill every day for as long as you want to prevent conception. There are no off days; you must take the Mini-pill during the time of your menstrual flow as well. To start on Mini-pills, take the first one on Day 1 of your menstrual period.

☐ Do not start on pills if there is any chance that you might be pregnant. If your menstrual period seemed too light, too early or too late, tell your doctor.

☐ Try to take the pill at about the same time each day. This is especially important if you are taking Mini-pills or if you experience "spotting" (see below).

☐ Before you take your pill each day, check to see that you've taken your pill for the previous day. If you miss one combination pill, take two the next day. Take the missed pill as soon as you remember it and take your regular pill for that day at the usual time. If you don't remember it until

101

you go to take your regular pill for that day, take the missed pill and your regular pill for that day at the same time. If you are on Mini-pills, use another method of birth control in addition to the Mini-pill until your next period starts. (This is not necessary if you are using the combination pill.)*

☐ If you miss two pills, take two each day for 2 days until you are caught up. Take the first missed pill as soon as you remember it and your regular pill for that day at the usual time. Take the second forgotten pill along with your regular pill at the normal time on the following day. Use a back-up method of birth control until your next period starts.

☐ If you miss three or more pills, stop using your pills until you have your period. If you are using combination pills, start a new pack as you normally would after your period starts. If you are using Mini-pills, begin a new pack on the first day of your period. Use a back-up method as soon as you discontinue the pills and continue to use the back-up method for 2 weeks after you have started your new pack.

☐ If you lose, damage or run out of pills, call your doctor. You can usually arrange for a refill with a telephone call so you won't have to interrupt your pill schedule. Many family-planning clinics, such as Planned Parenthood, will provide emergency refills if you are traveling or are unable to reach your doctor.

☐ If you have nausea, try taking your pill with dinner or in the evening. If you vomit within 1 hour of taking a pill, take another from a separate pack. If you have a bout of severe diarrhea, this may interfere with your body's absorption of the pill, making it less effective. Consult your doctor, as you may need to use another method of birth control as a back-up measure during that cycle.

☐ If you are on combination pills and want to alter your menstrual cycle to avoid having your period at a certain time (during vacation, for example), you can change your cycle length by taking as many as seven additional pills (one pill per day) or by discarding one or two from your regular pack. Your period should start about 48 hours after you take your last pill. Regardless of whether you've brought your period on 2 days early or have delayed it for 7 days, you must allow for your usual 7 no-hormone days before starting your new pack.

☐ If you are using combination pills and do not have a period during your 7 no-hormone days and are *absolutely sure* you have taken all your pills correctly there is little likelihood that you could be pregnant, so most doctors recommend that you go ahead and start your new pack as scheduled. We think that this advice is acceptable for women who do

---

*Some doctors recommend using a second method of birth control even if you've only missed one combination pill.

not have religious or moral objections to abortion. But if you would not have an abortion under any circumstances—because there *is* a slight chance of being pregnant—you should use another method of birth control and have a pregnancy test before starting a new pack, since there is evidence that use of hormones during pregnancy can cause birth defects. If you have missed a period and are *not* sure that you have taken your pills correctly, there is a greater chance that you are pregnant. Stop taking the pills and see your doctor for testing. Similarly, if you miss two periods, regardless of whether or not you have taken your pills correctly, also stop the pills and see your doctor.

☐ If you are taking Mini-pills and do not have a period within 45 days of your last period, stop taking the pills and see your doctor for pregnancy testing.

☐ If you have spotting or bleeding while you are taking combination pills, continue on your pill schedule. This bleeding will usually stop after a few days and is not uncommon during the first couple of months of Pill usage. But if the bleeding is heavier than the bleeding you have on the heaviest days of your period, if you soak more than three sanitary napkins in an hour or if the spotting continues for more than one cycle, call your doctor so that s/he can examine you to rule out the possibility that the spotting is being caused by something other than the Pill. If you are using Mini-pills and have persistent spotting, you will also need to discuss this with your doctor. If you have a fever or abdominal pain along with the spotting, call your doctor at once, as you may have an infection or other serious problem.

☐ If you develop any of the following danger signs, see your doctor right away:

* Chest pain	* Dizziness or faintness
* Shortness of breath	* Muscle weakness or numbness
* Unusual coughing	* Speech disturbance
* Pain in the legs	* Vision changes or loss of vision
* Severe headache	* Severe depression
* Breast lump	* Yellowing of the skin

☐ Because there is some evidence that certain drugs, including antibiotics such as ampicillin; sulfa drugs; antihistamines (both prescription and over-the-counter varieties); tranquilizers like Librium; some antidepressants; sedatives like phenobarbital and some drugs taken for epilepsy, tuberculosis and arthritis, can decrease the effectiveness of birth control pills, you should discuss this with your doctor. You may have to switch to another method or use a back-up method while you are taking these drugs.

☐ Pills can also interact with insulin, anticoagulants, certain tranquilizers

103

such as Valium, Demerol (a pain medication) and tuberculin skin tests. Pills can alter the results of laboratory tests, so be sure to tell the doctor that you are a Pill user, even if you are being tested for a totally unrelated problem.

Advantages

An important advantage to the Pill is that, with the exception of sterilization, it offers a most effective method of birth control if used properly. Another advantage is that it does not interfere with the spontaneity of lovemaking.

Pills offer other benefits in addition to contraception. For many women the greatest advantage of the Pill is that it offers them freedom from heavy bleeding and painful menstrual cramps. With the Pill, periods are regular, light and predictable. The Pill also allows women to manipulate their periods to allow for vacations or other such events in their schedules.

Many women find that the Pill improves acne. The incidence of benign breast disease[4] and rheumatoid arthritis[5] is lower among Pill users. Because the Pill suppresses ovulation, the incidence of certain ovarian cysts,[6] ectopic pregnancies[7] and mittelschmerz (ovulation pain) is lower among Pill users.* Because menstrual blood loss is reduced, deficiency anemia is less common in Pill users.[8]

One important advantage of the Pill that has recently come to light is that Pill users are less likely to develop pelvic inflammatory disease (PID) than are nonusers.[9] This finding is important, because PID can be a serious, even life-threatening disease. PID is often a complication of gonorrhea and other sexually transmissible infections. It has become increasingly common in recent years and is one of the leading causes of infertility (see pp. 393–401). The fact that the Pill offers protection against PID is a real plus for women who have multiple sex partners and are therefore at increased risk of developing gonorrhea and other sexually transmissible infections that can lead to PID.

The media has recently been full of articles suggesting that the Pill might protect a woman from developing certain types of cancer, such as ovarian cancer and uterine cancer. However, there has been some controversy as to whether this is true (see pp. 79–86).

Problems and Disadvantages

As more time has passed and greater numbers of women have used the Pill, our knowledge about side effects and complications has grown considerably.

*Chances of developing an ectopic pregnancy may be increased by the Mini-pill.

There are now more than 50 side effects and complications that may be associated with Pill usage. In some cases the association between Pill usage and a side effect or complication has been clearly established. In other cases the evidence for a cause-effect relationship is strong but not conclusive. In still others the relationship is only speculative. There may also be other as yet undiscovered side effects and complications. Research is still being done. Something that is thought to be a possible complication today may be either confirmed or refuted in the future. For example, blood-clotting disorders, which are responsible for most Pill-related deaths, were at one time only a suspected complication. There was no proof that Pill usage increased a woman's risk of developing such disorders. But today that relationship has been well documented. Women who choose to use oral contraceptives should keep up to date on the latest findings.

Some Pill-related problems are thought to be associated specifically with the estrogen in the Pill, and some with the progestin, but often it is not possible to say which hormone is responsible. The Mini-pill generally is considered safer than the combination pill, but most of the side effects and complications listed below may be caused by either type.

Changes in the Menstrual Cycle

The menstrual period usually becomes shorter, and the blood flow is usually lighter. Normally, the uterine lining is built up by the rising levels of ovarian hormones at different points in the cycle. Because women on the Pill do not experience these same peaks of hormone production, they don't build up as much of a lining; hence there is less menstrual flow. Pill users may experience spotting or bleeding between periods, which is called breakthrough bleeding. This happens because there is not enough hormone present to maintain the endometrial lining, so some of it sloughs off. This may also happen if you miss a pill. Such bleeding does not mean that the contraceptive effect is not working, however. It is most common in the first few months of Pill use, as the uterus is adjusting to altered hormone levels. If it persists, you should see a doctor.

Some women on the Pill cease to have menstrual periods and/or do not resume menstruation after discontinuing its use, a condition known as amenorrhea. Between 1 percent and 3 percent of Pill users fail to resume normal menstruation within 6 months after discontinuing Pill use.[10] This is most likely to happen to women who had menstrual irregularities before going on the Pill.

Many women experience relief from menstrual cramps on the Pill because ovulation no longer occurs. Many also experience relief of premenstrual syndrome symptoms; for other women, however, menstrual cramps and other menstrual symptoms may be intensified by the Pill.

Breast Tenderness and Swelling

Breast tenderness and swelling are not uncommon side effects. Sometimes this problem passes after 1 or 2 months, but it may persist.

Skin Changes

A Pill high in estrogen often improves acne; the Mini-pill or a Pill high in progestins may increase skin oiliness. Some women have an allergic reaction to the Pill and break out in skin rashes; others become more sensitive to sunlight (become sunburned more easily, for example). The Pill may affect the pigment (color) cells of the skin and a few women develop a condition called chloasma, in which areas of the skin darken. The Pill may possibly play a role in skin cancer (see Chapter Five for details).

Vaginal Discharge

The estrogen in the Pill may cause an increase in vaginal discharge. The Pill also alters the acid/alkaline balance of the vagina, making the vaginal environment more conducive to yeast organisms. Women on the Pill seem to be particularly susceptible to yeast infections. They may be more susceptible to gonorrhea as well, but their gonorrhea is less likely to develop into pelvic inflammatory disease.

Weight Gain, Bloating, Fluid Retention, Headaches, Nausea and Vomiting

These symptoms are common side effects in Pill users. For some women they are not serious problems; for others they are and cause these women to discontinue using the Pill.

Cervical Problems

Cervical erosions and eversions are more common in Pill users. In one large-scale study Pill users had a rate of cervical erosion and ulcerations of 9.4 per 1,000, whereas diaphragm users had a rate of 4.82 and IUD users, 3.03 per 1,000.[11] The Pill has also been implicated in cervical cancer (see Chapter Five).

Bronchitis and Viral Infections

Women who use the Pill have higher rates of bronchitis and of virus infections like flu, chicken pox and colds.[12] The reason for these increased rates is not known. Some theorize that because the Pill decreases the level of infection-fighting gamma globulin protein in the blood, users are more susceptible to illness. On the other hand, some argue that perhaps Pill users are more likely to have intercourse with greater frequency and are therefore exposed to more disease-causing organisms.

Urinary Tract Infections

Some reports indicate that women on the Pill are more susceptible to urinary tract infections, that is, bladder and kidney infections. Some women report relief of chronic urinary tract infections after discontinuing the Pill.

Fibroid Tumors

Fibroid tumors, benign tumors of the uterus affecting perhaps as many as one in every five women, are estrogen-sensitive, and their growth may be stimulated by the estrogen in the Pill. Although these tumors are benign, they can cause problems if they grow large and may necessitate a hysterectomy.

Sex Drive

Reports of the Pill's effect on sex drive are contradictory. Some women report an increase, some a decrease; others don't notice any change. Some researchers point to studies showing that many women experience an increase in sex drive at the time of ovulation and theorize that the Pill's suppression of ovulation might account for a lessened sex drive.

Bowel Disease

Women who use the Pill may be at increased risk of developing inflammatory bowel disease.[13] Since the Pill came into popular use, there has been a significant increase in a bowel disease known as Crohn's disease in women of childbearing age. There has not been a similar increase of the disease among men. Since the adverse effects of the Pill have become more widely known, there has been a decrease in Pill use in several countries. The incidence of bowel disease in young women has also decreased in these countries. The risk of developing inflammatory bowel disease, the most common types of which are Crohn's disease and ulcerative colitis, were shown to be 1.5 to 2 times greater in Pill users. At this point, the connection, if indeed there is one, is considered speculative.

Caffeine

There is some data to suggest that Pill users eliminate caffeine from their bodies only about half as efficiently as nonusers, which may mean that they accumulate caffeine in their bodies.[14] Whether or not caffeine is harmful is still a subject of debate. Some think caffeine is implicated in insomnia, anxiety, breast disorders, bladder cancer and heart disease; others dispute this. Still, it may be a wise idea for Pill users to cut back on their intake of caffeine.

Dental Problems

Some Pill users experience swelling and inflammation of the gums. If a user already has gingivitis, a gum disease whose chief symptom is bleeding from the gums, the condition may worsen.[15]

Circulatory Disorders

Women who use birth control pills are at greater risk of developing circulatory disorders, such as abnormal blood clotting, heart attack and stroke. Whether it is the estrogen or the progestin in the Pill that is responsible is not clear. Most Pill-related deaths result from circulatory disorders.

Several types of clotting disorders have been associated with Pill usage, including:

Thrombophlebitis: This is a condition in which plugs, clots or pieces of blood are attached to the wall of a vein or artery. These clots may become detached and travel to other parts of the body, in which case they are called emboli, and can cause crippling or even fatal complications, depending on where they lodge. Symptoms include a knot or swelling and heat or redness in the calf or thigh.

Pulmonary embolism: If a clot travels to the lung, it may cause a heart attack. Symptoms include chest pain, cough and shortness of breath.

Myocardial infarction: This blood-clot–related heart attack can produce such symptoms as chest pain, pain in the left arm and shoulder, difficulty in breathing and weakness.

Cerebral infarction: Also called a stroke, this blood clot in the brain can cause headaches, numbness, weakness, visual problems and intellectual impairment.

Retinal vein thrombosis: This is a blood clot in the eye, which can cause such symptoms as loss of vision and headaches.

Pelvic vein thrombosis: This is a blood clot in the pelvic veins that may produce lower-abdominal pain and cramps.

Any of these conditions may have serious or fatal consequences. The Pill definitely increases the risk of developing these conditions. For instance, for Pill users aged 15 to 34 the risk of death from a circulatory disorder is about 1 in 12,000 per year, whereas for nonusers it is only about 1 in 50,000. The risk of hospitalization for a clotting disorder is also increased. Nonusers aged 20 to 44 have about a 1 in 20,000 risk, whereas Pill users have a 1 in 2,000 risk, a tenfold increase.

The use of oral contraceptives may double the risk of heart attack. That's bad enough, but if a woman is both a Pill user and a smoker, her chances of having a heart attack are even greater. Such women are five times more likely to have a heart attack than users who do not smoke and ten times more likely to have a heart attack than women who neither smoke nor use the Pill. Age is also a factor in this risk equation. If you are a Pill user between ages 30 and 39, you have a 1 in 10,000 chance each year of having a fatal heart attack if you smoke and a 1 in 50,000 chance if you are a user but don't smoke, as compared with a 1 in 100,000 chance for women who do not smoke or use the Pill. For older women the odds are more frightening. In the 40-to-44-year-old age-group a woman who neither uses the Pill nor smokes has a 1 in 14,000 chance of having a fatal heart attack, but if a woman both uses the Pill and smokes, her chances are 1 in 1,700. For this reason women who are smokers or are over 35 (some say 40) should not use this method of birth control. Risk also seems to increase for women who have used the Pill for 5 years or more, so some doctors limit the years of Pill usage. The risks continue as long as you use the Pill and may continue for some time afterward as well.

In addition to blood-clotting disorders, women who take the Pill are twice as likely as nonusers to have a stroke from a ruptured blood vessel in the brain.

A good deal of the data we have on increased risk of these sorts of problems in Pill users was gathered before the new, low-dose pills were available. Researchers are hopeful that these risks will decrease as more women switch to low-dose pills. Indeed, according to the results in one recent, widely publicized study done at the Kaiser-Permanente Health Facility in Walnut Creek, California, there was no overall increase in the risk of heart attacks (myocardial infarctions) among young, healthy, nonsmoking Pill users as compared with nonusers.[16] However, the validity of this study has been widely questioned by women's health-care activists, for example, Barbara Seaman, who points out that relatively few women in the study were currently using the Pill.

Women on the Pill, especially smokers, should be aware of the danger signs of circulatory disorders (see above) and should consult their doctors immediately if they develop any of these signs.

Because there is a four- to sixfold increase in the development of postsurgical blood clots in Pill users, the Pill should be discontinued at least 4 weeks before surgery when possible.

Gallbladder Disease

A number of studies have documented the fact that Pill users are at increased risk of developing gallbladder disease. In one study an increased risk was evident after 2 years of use and doubled after 4 or 5 years of use. In another study increased risk was apparent between 6 and 12 months of use. However, another study has recently challenged these studies and has indicated that the risk may be much smaller than previously thought.[17]

Liver Problems

Women who use birth control pills are at increased risk of developing benign liver tumors. It is not clear whether this is solely an estrogen effect or whether both estrogen and progestin are to blame. Although these tumors are noncancerous, they have been known to rupture and cause death. Cancerous liver tumors have also been reported in women taking the Pill, but whether these rare cancerous tumors actually occur more commonly in Pill users is unknown.

Women who have a history of jaundice, a liver disorder that leads to an accumulation of yellow pigment in the eyes and skin and thus gives the skin a yellow tinge, may get jaundice again if they take the Pill. Because the liver is responsible for breaking down estrogen and eliminating it from the body, women with impaired liver function should not use the Pill.

High Blood Pressure

Large studies involving thousands of women have indicated that 5 percent to 7 percent of all women on the Pill will develop abnormally high blood pressure, a condition known as hypertension, which puts a woman at higher risk of heart attacks and a type of stroke caused by ruptured blood vessels in the brain. Although only 5 percent to 7 percent develop hypertension, many women on the Pill experience some elevation of blood pressure. The long-term effects of having elevated blood pressure that is still within the normal range are not known. The blood pressure usually reverts to normal within 6 months after discontinuation of the Pill, but there is some evidence that some of the changes associated with Pill-related high blood pressure may persist, at least in some women.

Certain women are more prone to Pill-related hypertension: those with a family history of hypertension, women over 40 and overweight women. Black women in general are more prone to hypertension; whether they are more prone to develop hypertension when on the Pill than white women are is not known. There are contradictory reports as to whether women with a history of toxemia, a type of hypertension that occurs during pregnancy, are more prone to develop a rise in blood pressure if they use the Pill.

All women on the Pill should have their blood pressure checked once every 6 to 12 months.

Birth Defects

The Pill is not 100 percent effective and women do not always use it consistently and correctly. As a result, pregnancies do occur in Pill users, and such women may unwittingly continue taking the Pill for a month or longer before they realize they are pregnant. Some of these women will decide to have an abortion, but some may wish to continue the pregnancy. Those who wish to continue should have complete information about the relationship between the hormones in the Pill and birth defects. Unfortunately, this is a controversial topic and clear-cut information is not available.

The concern about Pill use in early pregnancy and the possibility of birth defects was first raised when it was discovered that some of the offspring of women who, when they were pregnant, took another type of hormone, the estrogen DES, developed cancer and other abnormalities later in life as a result of their mothers' use of DES.* Even children whose mothers took small amounts of DES for a short time developed problems. DES, however, is a different estrogen than the one used in the Pill, and there is no evidence to date indicating that DES-type problems occur in the offspring of women who took the Pill during pregnancy. But it was many years before the DES problems became apparent, so there is still concern among some doctors.

Results of studies of birth defects in the offspring of women who took the Pill during pregnancy have been contradictory. Some have shown an increase in defects; others have not.[18] The reason for these contradictory results is probably owing to the fact that any increased risk that may exist is probably a small one that would not become obvious unless large numbers of women are studied. Because relatively few women who are on the Pill become pregnant and an even smaller number decide to continue pregnancy, studies involving large numbers of women have not been possible. There have been studies indicating a twofold increased risk in women who took the Pill during pregnancy,[19] which sounds pretty scary. But the chance of having a deformed infant is so low anyhow that even doubling the risk is still a very minor problem. For some women even a small increase in risk would be intolerable; for others the small increase in risk may be worth taking, especially if they have strong feelings about abortion or if they are especially desirous of having a child.

Not only may the risks of birth defects increase if the Pill is taken during

*For details, see the section on DES.

111

pregnancy, but there is also evidence that taking birth control pills *before* pregnancy can also cause problems in the embryo. One study showed an increase in a rare type of chromosomal aberration in the aborted embryos of women who conceived within 3 months of discontinuing the Pill.

Recent studies have refuted the claim that hormones taken *before* conception can cause birth defects or higher rates of miscarriages.[20,21,22] Despite these new, more favorable reports most doctors still suggest that women who stop the Pill in order to become pregnant use another form of contraception for 3 months before they attempt to conceive.

Because pills have been implicated in birth defects, these hormones should never be taken during pregnancy. Women who miss one or more pills during a cycle and then don't have a period after the last pill, should get a pregnancy test before starting a new box of pills. If a woman takes a pill accidentally after becoming pregnant, she should consider the possibility of abortion.

Ectopic Pregnancy

The likelihood of ectopic pregnancy, in which the fertilized egg implants in the fallopian tube or some other inappropriate location, is higher if you become pregnant while using the Mini-pill. Ectopic pregnancies can have serious complications, including death. Because routine pregnancy tests may fail to detect an ectopic pregnancy, any Mini-pill user who suspects pregnancy should insist on the most sensitive type of pregnancy test (p. 788).

Infertility

As noted earlier, some women do not resume normal ovulation and menstruation after discontinuing the Pill. One study suggested that temporary infertility may be a problem for some Pill users who have never had previous pregnancies.[23] After 30 months the former Pill users had 5 percent fewer pregnancies than former users of other methods of contraception; however, after 40 months there was no difference between the groups. A delay of 40 months, or about 3⅓ years, might not be a significant problem for a woman in her 20s, but because the chances of conception decrease and the chances of birth defects increase as a woman grows older, this might be a problem for a woman in her 30s.

Breast Milk

The use of birth control pills may reduce the quantity and quality of breast milk. Small amounts of Pill hormones have been found in the breast milk of nursing mothers using oral contraceptives. The effect of these hormones on the infant is unknown, so it is suggested that nursing mothers not take the Pill.

Depression

Some Pill users experience depression. Studies designed to investigate the relationship between the Pill and depression have produced contradictory results. Some studies, including one of the largest and most thorough studies ever done, reported a 30 percent increase in depression in oral contraceptive users. Other studies have reported a decrease in depression, and still others have failed to find any difference in the incidence of depression between users and nonusers.

The depression experienced by some Pill users may be related to the fact that some Pill users are deficient in vitamin B_6. Depression may subside when such women take supplementary vitamin B_6.

Thyroid Gland

The Pill can cause changes in the results of some of the tests used to measure thyroid function. Although these test results are altered, the thyroid gland itself is apparently not affected, for other, more sensitive thyroid tests do not indicate changes in its function.

Pituitary Tumors

There has been some evidence that estrogen in the Pill can, if not cause, at least stimulate the growth of preexisting benign tumors in the pituitary gland.[24] As many as 5 percent to 10 percent of the population probably have microscopic pituitary tumors that never become large enough to cause problems. Some studies indicate that if a woman with a microscopic pituitary tumor takes the Pill, tumor growth may be stimulated and the tumor may eventually require treatment. A recent study, however, has cast doubt on the idea that Pill use is associated with an increase in pituitary tumors.[25]

Eye Problems

The Pill, on rare occasions, has caused inflammation of the optic nerve, loss of vision, double vision, pain and swelling. Because the Pill causes fluid retention, the shape of the eyeball may be altered, with the result that some women who use the Pill may have to have their contact lens prescriptions changed; other women find that they çan't use contacts at all.

Lipid Content

The Pill alters many metabolic and chemical processes in the blood. Lipid content, for instance, is increased. Lipids are potentially harmful chemical substances that are found in the blood. Fatty acids, cholesterol, phospholipids and triglycerides are all lipids that may be affected by the Pill. It has been theorized that these substances contribute to arteriosclerosis, or hardening of the arteries, which makes the arteries more prone to blockage by a blood clot and may account, in part, for the blood-clotting problems experienced by Pill users.

Vitamin and Mineral Metabolism

The Pill may affect the way in which the body uses vitamins and minerals. Studies of Pill users have indicated deficiencies in folic acid, trace minerals, riboflavin, thiamine and vitamins B_6 B_{12}, C and E.[26,27,28] As noted earlier, in some Pill users depression has been relieved by the use of a vitamin B supplement. Some doctors prescribe vitamin supplements for Pill users.

On the other hand, the Pill increases the levels of certain other nutriments. Vitamin K levels, for instance, are higher in some Pill users. Because vitamin K influences blood-clotting factors, some researchers have linked these higher levels of K to the blood-clotting disorders that are the source of most Pill-related deaths.

Sugar Metabolism and Diabetes

The Pill alters the way in which the body metabolizes sugar. Women who are on the Pill and have previously had normal test results may develop abnormal glucose tolerance, or sugar tolerance, tests like those of women who have diabetes, a disease in which the body cannot metabolize sugar properly. These women do not have the symptoms of diabetes, but no one knows what the long-term effects of this stress on the body will be. Test results usually return to normal after the Pill is discontinued; in a few cases, abnormal test results have persisted.

Because of the Pill's effect on blood sugar levels, most doctors will not prescribe the Pill for women who have borderline test results before going on the Pill.

Cancer

The Pill may protect against some forms of cancer, such as ovarian and uterine cancer, but may increase the risk of developing breast, cervical and skin cancer. For important information on these topics, see The Long-Term Effects in Chapter Five.

Contraindications

A contraindication is a medical condition that makes the use of a certain type of drug or form of treatment inadvisable. Because of the controversy that has surrounded the Pill, there is a good deal of disagreement as to who should and shouldn't use birth control pills. The following list of contraindications is divided into three parts: absolute contraindications, with which all doctors would agree; strong contraindications, with which most doctors would agree; and relative contraindications, with which many, but not all doctors, would agree. Because the combination pill contains estrogen, it is sometimes contraindicated where the Mini-pill would not be.

Absolute Contraindications (women with these conditions should definitely not take the Pill)

- [ ] Blood-clotting disorders, such as thrombophlebitis and pulmonary embolism
- [ ] Heart attack, stroke or angina (heart pain)
- [ ] Impaired liver function, hepatic adenoma (liver tumor)
- [ ] Coronary artery disease
- [ ] Known or suspected cancer of the breast, uterus, cervix, ovaries, vagina or elsewhere in the female reproductive tract.
- [ ] Pregnancy or suspected pregnancy

Strong Contraindications (women with these conditions who take the Pill may be vulnerable to serious health problems)

- [ ] Pregnancy within the past 10 to 14 days, including childbirth, abortion or miscarriage
- [ ] History of severe headaches
- [ ] High blood pressure now or during pregnancy in the past
- [ ] Diabetes or a strong family history of diabetes
- [ ] Gallbladder disease or gallbladder surgery now or in the past
- [ ] Jaundice during pregnancy in the past, a condition known as cholestasis or Gilbert's disease
- [ ] Mononucleosis now or in the recent past
- [ ] Sickle-cell disease
- [ ] Undiagnosed abnormal uterine bleeding
- [ ] Major surgery planned in the next month
- [ ] Leg casts or major injury to the lower leg

☐ Fibrocystic breast disease or fibroadenoma of the breast, abnormal breast X-rays in the past, or close family history of breast cancer.
☐ Age 35 to 40 or older
☐ Heavy smoker (15+cigarettes a day)
☐ Cervical dysplasia

Relative Contraindications (women with these conditions may want to avoid the Pill)

☐ History of serious heart or kidney disease
☐ History of heavy smoking
☐ Failure to have established regular menstrual cycles or history of irregular menstrual patterns
☐ Breast-feeding
☐ Five or more years of Pill use
☐ Previous exposure to DES-type drugs
☐ Fibroids (tumors of the uterus)
☐ Severe asthma
☐ Severe varicose veins
☐ Epilepsy
☐ Serious depression or suicidal feelings
☐ History of hepatitis
☐ History of hair loss or chloasma (darkening of the facial skin during previous pregnancy or Pill use)
☐ Sickle-cell trait
☐ High cholesterol levels
☐ Recurrent urinary tract infections
☐ Weight gain of more than 10 pounds while on the Pill
☐ Termination of a term pregnancy within the past 10 to 14 days

INTRAUTERINE DEVICE

AKA: IUD, loop

Types: Lippes Loop
Copper-7
Copper-T
Progestasert or Progesterone-T

The intrauterine device, or IUD (Illustration 18), is a small plastic device that is inserted into the uterus by a doctor or trained medical person. It prevents pregnancy as long as it remains in place. Most types of IUD may be left in the uterus for a considerable period and should be removed only by a doctor or trained medical person.

How the IUD Works

Despite the fact that the IUD has been around for some time, no one is quite sure how it works. One theory is that the IUD irritates the uterus so much that it triggers the body's defense mechanisms, which literally "eat up" either the sperm or the fertilized egg. Another theory is that the fertilized egg may not be able to attach itself to the irritated uterine lining. Still another theory holds that the IUD works by mechanically dislodging the implanted egg, a sort of miniabortion. There is also the theory that the IUD somehow speeds up the movement of the egg through the fallopian tube. Because the time the egg spends moving through the tube is critical to its proper development, too short a time in the tube will result in an egg too immature to implant successfully in the uterine wall.

Types

Several types of IUD are currently available, including the Lippes Loop; the Copper-7, or Gravigard; the Copper-T, or Tatum T; and the Progestasert, or Progesterone-T. Until recently, the Saf-T-Coil was also available. Although there were no special problems with the safety or effectiveness of the Saf-T-Coil, the manufacturer has stopped producing it because so few were sold.

The original IUDs were made of nonmedicated plastic. Later types included copper or a synthetic form of the hormone progesterone (progestin) embedded in the plastic. Because copper has sperm-killing effects, it was added to the Copper-7 and the Copper-T to enhance their contraceptive capabilities. Also, it was thought that the copper would relax uterine contractions and therefore relieve cramping. Progestin was added because it changed the character of the cervical secretions (see p. 67), making it difficult for the sperm to pass through the cervix and into the uterus, and because it was thought that progestin would reduce the bleeding problems associated with IUDs.

Three other types of IUD—the Majzlin Spring, the Birnberg Bow and the Dalkon Shield—were formerly available in the United States but have now been withdrawn from the market because they were associated with some of the serious problems discussed below.

117

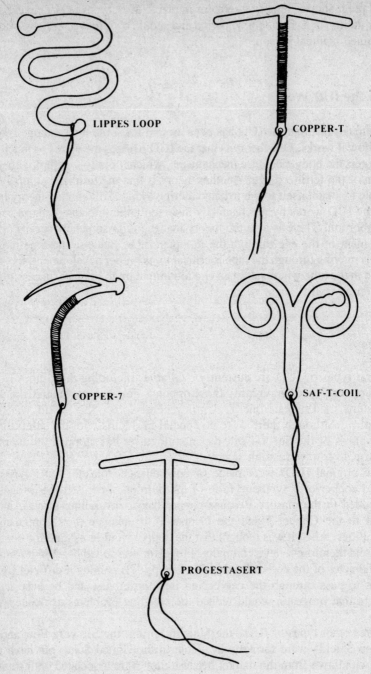

Illustration 18   *Types of IUD*

The Dalkon Shield

The Dalkon Shield has received the most publicity. The device was withdrawn after a somewhat lengthy battle between the manufacturer, the Food and Drug Administration (FDA) and women's health-care activists.[29] It was thought that the strings of this particular IUD, which were intertwined like a candlewick, served as a ladder to permit disease-causing organisms to travel up the strings into the uterus, causing serious pelvic infection that necessitated hysterectomy in some women and resulted in infertility and even death in others. The results of recent studies have indicated that women who use the Dalkon Shield are more susceptible to pelvic infections than they would be if they used other IUDs. These problems may occur even if the woman has worn the Shield successfully for many years.[30]

When the bad news about the Dalkon Shield first became public, Planned Parenthood encouraged all women under its care who wore the Shield to have the device removed. Many gynecologists throughout the United States have not followed this policy, so many American women still have Dalkon Shields in place. Any woman who has a Dalkon Shield should contact her doctor or a Planned Parenthood clinic. It is our policy to explain the situation to women who have Dalkon Shields or other banned devices and to encourage removal. Most women who are apprised of the facts decide to have their shields removed.

The Dalkon Shield is not the only IUD that has raised doubts in the medical community. The use of the progesterone devices, which seem to be associated with higher rates of ectopic pregnancies—that is, pregnancies that implant in the fallopian tube or other abnormal location—has been questioned.[31] The Lippes Loop also came under scrutiny at the time of the Dalkon Shield investigations; however, the FDA did not consider the data sufficient to ban the loop as well.[32] The Copper-7 has also been criticized because of the design of the mechanism used to insert it (*see* p. 128). Some authorities believe that the Copper-7 should be recalled and that the device should not be used until the mechanism is redesigned.[33]

The National Women's Health Network has established a registry for IUD-related problems. Women who have suffered such problems can contact the Network by writing to NWHN, 2025 I Street NW, Suite 105, Washington, DC 20006.

Effectiveness

The effectiveness rates quoted by the FDA tell us that somewhere between one and six pregnancies will occur in a group of 100 women using the IUD for a year.[34]* For some types of IUD this figure may be as low as two to three pregnancies per 100 woman-years of use.[35] Although the rates of effectiveness seem to vary, depending on which particular device is used, it is hard to evaluate relative effectiveness, because the women in these various studies are not well matched in terms of age, background, proven fertility and other important factors.

This is the one method of birth control in which the theoretical rate most closely matches the actual-use rate, for there is no pill to take each day, no diaphragm and foam or condom to put into place. The failures occur because the woman has an ectopic pregnancy, the IUD has been expelled without the woman's knowing it or the device has perforated the uterus or has simply not done its job. The failures are method failures, not user failures.

Insertion

The IUD must be inserted by a doctor or other medical person trained specifically to do so. It is important to have an experienced person insert the IUD, for incorrect insertion can cause the IUD to perforate, that is, to make a hole in the uterus. Unfortunately, it is difficult for a woman to be sure that the person who is inserting the IUD is experienced. Even if she goes to a family-planning clinic or a Planned Parenthood clinic, where IUD insertion is done frequently, it might be her lot to get an intern who has relatively little experience. One rule of thumb is to not accept an IUD from someone who tries to talk you out of that method of birth control, for their negative attitude, although perhaps justifiable, will probably mean that they don't insert IUDs routinely.

A thorough medical history and physical exam must be done before insertion to rule out the possibility of undiagnosed pregnancy or disease or abnormality of the uterus, all of which could cause serious complications if an IUD were inserted.

The doctor then determines the position, shape and depth of the uterus with an instrument called a uterine sound. This step should not be ignored, for it is important in preventing perforations of the uterus (see below).

Once all of this has been done and the cervix has been washed with an antiseptic solution, the IUD is retracted back into an inserter tube, which is a hollow tube with about the same diameter as a straw. The tube is gently pushed through the cervical os, the opening into the uterus. The IUD is then released from the inserter tube (Illustration 19). If the cervical opening is narrow, it may be necessary to dilate it with a special instrument before insertion.

Insertion may be painful. The degree of pain varies from woman to

*For an explanation of birth-control effectiveness terminology, see Chapter Five.

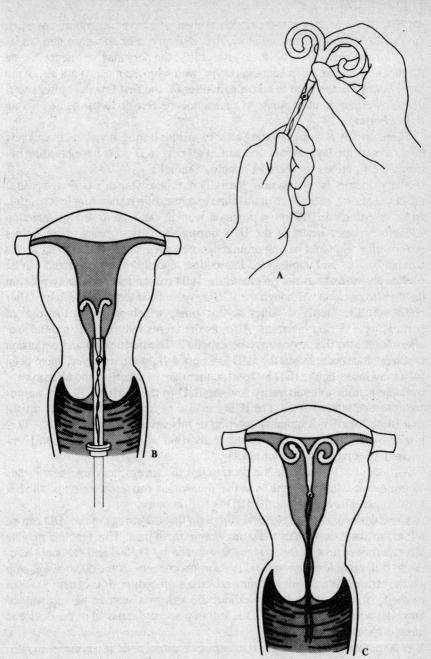

Illustration 19   *Insertion of the IUD: The IUD is placed inside the inserter tube (A). The tube is inserted through the cervix into the uterus (B). The IUD is released into the uterus and the inserter tube withdrawn (C).*

121

woman. There usually is less pain for women who have had children or when the device is inserted immediately after delivery. For some women, especially for women who have never given birth, the pain may be intense. Some doctors inject a painkiller into the cervix, which blocks most, if not all, of the pain. Some women need to take a painkiller for the first few days after insertion. A woman should arrange to have someone else drive her home after an IUD insertion.

There usually is some bleeding after insertion, lasting anywhere from a few hours to several days. About one-half of all new IUD users have bleeding between their periods for the first couple of months.

Many doctors favor inserting the IUD during a woman's period, because the cervical os is more open at this time and insertion is therefore less painful. Also, inserting an IUD into a pregnant woman can lead to serious infection and miscarriage. Inserting the IUD during the period means there is less chance of a woman's having an undiagnosed pregnancy. But as long as the woman has not had unprotected intercourse since her last period and can be reasonably sure she is not pregnant, the IUD can be inserted at any point in the menstrual cycle. Although the IUD can also be inserted immediately after childbirth, the uterus is softer at this time, which increases the risk of perforating it during insertion. Also, as the uterus returns to its normal size after childbirth, the device may be expelled. The perforation and expulsion problems that occur when the IUD is inserted right after delivery have been solved by inserting the IUD by hand, rather than by inserter, and by using absorbable sutures to temporarily sew the IUD to the uterine wall (the sutures are absorbed after awhile). The IUD can also be inserted immediately after a first-trimester (first 3 months) abortion or miscarriage. But when the IUD is inserted right after a second-trimester abortion, the rate of expulsion is increased by a factor of five or ten.[36]

After the IUD is inserted the doctor clips the strings, leaving a few inches of string protruding from the os so that the woman can feel the strings with her fingers and thus check that the IUD is still in place.

Some women's sexual partners complain that the strings of the IUD can be felt or, in some cases, that the strings cause them pain. This problem may be alleviated over time as the strings are softened by vaginal and cervical secretions. If the problem persists and is a serious concern, some doctors will snip off the strings. We do not recommend such a procedure. It is better to switch methods of birth control, for without the strings a woman has no way of knowing whether or not the IUD is still in place and removal of the device is more difficult.

It is important to check the IUD strings regularly—at least once a month, right after the menstrual cycle (when expulsion is more likely), and preferably more often, especially during the first few months, when expulsion rates are highest. The strings should also be checked anytime the woman experiences unusual cramps, as this may be a sign of expulsion or perforation. Checking is important, for if the strings cannot be felt, this may mean that the IUD has been expelled, that it has become embedded in the uterine wall or that it has perforated the uterus, which can lead to an unwanted pregnancy or other serious problems (see below). Women should practice feeling for the string before leaving the clinic or doctor's office.

A change of string length is also important. If the strings suddenly seem longer, this indicates that the IUD is too low in the uterine cavity* —possibly embedded in the cervix or in the process of expelling itself— and if so, is less effective in preventing pregnancy. Shortened strings may mean that the IUD is embedded in the uterus or is in the process of perforating the uterus.

The cost of IUD insertion may run anywhere from a low of around $10 at a family-planning clinic to a high of $100 at a Park Avenue gynecologist's office.

How Long Should an IUD Be Left in Place?

Another area of controversy surrounding the IUD concerns the question of how long the device should be left in place. It is generally agreed that the Progestasert should be replaced every year, because the progestin becomes depleted. The manufacturers recommend that the copper devices be replaced every 3 years because of copper depletion. But recent studies have indicated that the copper remains effective for 4 years, so this recommendation may change in the future.[37] Because the act of insertion itself carries the risk of perforation and pelvic infection, it is generally recommended that other types of IUD not be removed unless there are problems or the woman wishes to become pregnant or use another method of birth control.

Women should make sure they know which type of IUD they have and how often it should be replaced.

Advantages and Benefits

The chief advantage of the IUD is its convenience; there is no pill to remember to take. It is put in once and can remain in place for a considerable amount of time. It does not require any interruption of lovemaking, as do the condoms, diaphragm and foam. In addition to its convenience, the IUD is also highly effective.

*Except at times with the Copper-7; see p. 128 for details.

Problems and Disadvantages

A number of problems are involved in using the IUD. It may be acceptable for women who aren't exposed to sexually transmissible infections and who have all the children they want, but for other women, other methods may be preferable.

Contraindications

Not all women can tolerate an IUD, and certain women should not use one. There is some difference of opinion among doctors as to what these contraindications are, so not all doctors will agree with the following list:

- ☐ Gonorrhea or any other acute infection of the organs of the pelvic cavity
- ☐ Known or suspected pregnancy
- ☐ Abnormal uterine bleeding
- ☐ Known or suspected cancer of the pelvic organs
- ☐ Severe obstruction of the cervical canal
- ☐ Certain congenital deformities of the uterus
- ☐ Certain heart diseases involving the valves
- ☐ Fibroid tumors of the uterus
- ☐ Use of anticoagulants
- ☐ Sickle cell disease
- ☐ Anemia
- ☐ Small uterus (less than 6.5 cm)
- ☐ History of pelvic infection
- ☐ Multiple sex partners
- ☐ History of ectopic pregnancy
- ☐ Endometriosis
- ☐ Endometrial polyps
- ☐ Impaired response to infection (diabetes,* steroid therapy)
- ☐ Heavy menstrual flow†
- ☐ Severe cramps†
- ☐ Known or suspected allergy to copper ‡
- ☐ Desire to have children in the future

*Women with diabetes may also have higher failure rates with the IUD.
†The Progestasert may be therapeutic.
‡Some doctors have the woman tape a penny to her forearm the night before insertion of an IUD. If there is skin discoloration, the woman may have copper allergy and should not use a copper IUD.

Safety

One of the biggest concerns with the IUD is safety. The FDA's official estimate is that the mortality (death rate) from the IUD is between 1 and 10 deaths per 1 million woman-years of use.[38] Although the odds of even 10 per 1 million do not seem too risky, the odds on complications serious enough to require hospitalization are less reassuring, ranging from 1 in 300 to 1 in 100 per year.[39] Moreover, this figure includes only complications serious enough to necessitate hospitalization. If complications not requiring hospitalization were added, the figures would be much higher.

Women who develop any of the following symptoms should consult their doctors right away:

- ☐ Period late, no period
- ☐ Abdominal pain
- ☐ Fever, chills
- ☐ Foul-smelling or unusually profuse vaginal discharge
- ☐ Spotting, unusually heavy periods, clots

Bleeding and Menstrual Cramps

The most common problem for IUD users is increased menstrual bleeding, often accompanied by cramplike discomfort or lower-back pain. This increased bleeding may take the form of a greater volume of flow, longer menstrual periods and/or spotting between periods. Between 5 percent and 15 percent of all IUD users have their IUDs removed within 12 months because of these types of problems.[40]

The amount of blood lost may increase as much as two- or threefold for some women. The blood loss is related to the type of IUD being used. The copper devices increase the bleeding, but not as much as the Loop, Saf-T-Coil and other nonmedicated IUDs. Progestin-releasing IUDs do not increase the overall volume of flow and in some cases may even decrease it, at least temporarily, but they may prolong the length of the menstrual period.[41]

Some evidence suggests that women with heavier-than-normal periods before IUD insertion experience a smaller increase in bleeding after IUD insertion than do other women.[42] In some cases there may even be a decrease in bleeding. So, whereas some doctors think women with heavy periods should not use IUDs, others, with this evidence in mind, believe that IUDs are an acceptable form of contraception for such women.

The length of the menstrual period is also prolonged, anywhere from one-half day to 4 days, depending on which study you read and which IUD is used. Some researchers now believe that the progestin devices are more likely to prolong periods.

Bleeding between periods may occur with any type of IUD but, again, seems to be somewhat more frequent with the progestin devices. Such bleeding usually is of the spotting type.

IUDs have also been associated with increased menstrual pain, which usually takes the form of increased cramplike pain in the lower abdomen and back. Such pain is thought to be associated with the contractions caused by the uterus as it attempts to expel the foreign body. In some cases the Progestasert relieves cramps.

Because of prolonged and heavier periods, anemia may be a problem for IUD users. Some doctors recommend iron supplements for IUD users for at least 3 months each year.[43] We feel that a woman who becomes anemic as a result of blood loss from her IUD should have the IUD removed and use another method of birth control.

Vaginal Discharge and Infection

IUD users tend to have a characteristic discharge that is watery, mucuslike and odorless. It causes no itching or burning and is believed to be caused by the IUD strings stimulating the mucus glands in the cervix.

Women who wear IUDs may be more susceptible to the common vaginal infections, which, although not serious, can be extremely bothersome.

Pelvic Inflammatory Disease

Pelvic inflammatory disease (PID) is the most serious IUD complication, accounting for the majority of IUD-related deaths and hospitalizations. PID is an infection of the uterus and tubes that can have severe, even fatal, consequences and that can result in infertility. It is caused by gonorrhea, *E. coli*, actinomyceses, and other germs in the vagina that get up into the normally sterile uterus and tubes. Women who have IUDs are three to five times more likely to get PID than are nonusers.[44] The risk is thought to be greatest in the first few months after insertion, probably because germs from the vagina were introduced into the uterus during insertion. Anyone who has gonorrhea or another infection, or even thinks she may have been exposed to such germs, should not have an IUD inserted until she has had tests to rule out the presence of infection.

Although it is more common in the first months of IUD use, PID can occur at any time. No one knows why PID is more prevalent in IUD users. Some authorities believe the IUD sets up a chronic inflammation that makes the uterus less able to defend itself against infection. Others think that the strings of the IUD act as a ladder, enabling germs to ascend from the vagina into the uterus. In fact, some researchers are considering the use of the "tailless" IUD (common in countries like China) to help cut down on PID. But, as explained on pp. 122–123, the "tailless" IUD creates other problems.

A woman who has multiple sexual partners is more likely to develop PID than a woman who has only one partner, because there are more opportunities for disease-causing organisms to enter her body. Because using the IUD also increases PID risk, many doctors think that the IUD should not be used by women who have multiple sexual partners. Since the IUD increases the chance of developing PID significantly and since even one attack of PID may cause infertility, most doctors are reluctant to insert an IUD in a woman who may want to have children in the future. A woman who has an IUD should familiarize herself with the symptoms of PID (see p. 397) and should consult her doctor immediately if she develops any of these symptoms. If she does develop PID, she should have her IUD removed *immediately* (see p. 398).

There has been a great deal of concern recently about the relationship between the IUD and an organism called actinomyces, which can cause a rare but especially serious form of PID known as actinomycosis.[45] Actinomyces sometimes show up on the Pap smears or vaginal cultures taken from women wearing IUDs, even though the women have no symptoms. Although actinomyces can appear in any IUD user, they are more commonly found in women who have worn the device for longer than 3 years.

If a woman has symptoms of actinomycosis PID (low-grade and diffuse abdominal pain, night chills and sweats, weight loss, odorous vaginal discharge, bleeding between periods, dramatic increase in menstrual bleeding) and actinomyces in her Pap smear, everyone agrees that the IUD should be removed and the woman should be treated with antibiotics. But there is considerable disagreement about what to do with a woman who has actinomyces in her Pap smear but has no symptoms of disease. Some doctors who are concerned that the actinomyces eventually will cause PID, remove the IUD and treat the woman with antibiotics. Others think that simply removing the IUD will get rid of the actinomyces. The Pap smear is repeated in a few weeks. In most women the actinomyces disappear from the Pap smear in 1 or 2 months without antibiotics. Still other doctors leave the IUD in place, and watch the woman in case she develops symptoms.

Because actinomyces are easily mistaken for other organisms, some doctors have the Pap smears of asymptomatic women repeated before deciding what, if any, action to take.[46]

Because the likelihood of harboring these organisms increases with the length of IUD use, some researchers have gone so far as to recommend that all IUDs be replaced every 3 years. The prevailing view at this time, however, opposes routine removal and reinsertion, for the act of reinserting poses risks of perforation, expulsion and PID that outweigh the possible benefits of cutting down on the relatively rare cases of actinomycosis/PID.[47]

Women who have IUDs, especially those who have been wearing them for longer than 3 years, should ask their doctors to note on their annual Pap smear that they are IUD users and to specify that the laboratory look for actinomyces. Some doctors suggest that long-term users have cultures taken from inside the cervical canal as well.

Expulsion and Perforation

Another problem with the IUD is that some women's bodies don't tolerate the IUD very well and the device is expelled, either partially or completely. Between 5 percent and 20 percent of IUD users will have expelled the device after 1 year.[48] Symptoms of expulsion may include unusual vaginal discharge, cramping or pain, spotting between periods or after intercourse, pain on intercourse (for the woman or her partner), lengthening of the strings (possibly a partial expulsion), absence of the strings (possibly a complete expulsion), feeling the hard IUD at the opening to the cervix or in the vagina or passage of the IUD itself from the vagina. Sometimes the woman is aware that the IUD has been expelled, but in about 20 percent of the cases she is not.[49] Because the expulsion rate is highest in the first few months after insertion, many doctors recommend use of foam and condoms, the diaphragm or another back-up method during that time.

Women who use the Copper-7 IUD should be aware of special problems that are associated with the strings in this device. Unlike the strings in other types of IUD, the Copper-7 strings do not go down through the inserter tube but instead are looped over the top of the tube. This means that a length of string can get caught on the upper arm of the IUD during insertion (see Illustration 20). If this loop works itself off the upper arm, the woman may notice that her strings are getting longer. Her doctor, figuring that the string got caught up during insertion and is just working loose, may cut the string a bit shorter. This is inconvenient for the woman, necessitating a second office visit. But more serious than this is the possibility that the increase in string length is actually owing to a partial expulsion. If this is the case, the woman may then become pregnant, and pregnancy in IUD users may cause special problems (see both The IUD and Ectopic Pregnancy and IUDs and Pregnancy below). Additional problems are associated with the Copper-7. The loop of string may remain caught over the upper arm of the device. When the device is removed the process of pulling on the string exerts force on the upper arm, distorting it. In such cases, removal may be extremely painful and may even necessitate hospitalization. Also, some authorities theorize that the Copper-7 string's being on the outside of the inserter tube is a potential means of introducing bacteria into the cervical canal at the

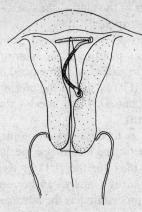

Illustration 20 *Copper-7 with loop of string caught over the upper arm of the device.*

time of insertion, as the string is dragged up through the cervical canal. For this reason we do not recommend that the Copper-7 be used until this design flaw is corrected.

The IUD may also perforate the uterus, either partially or completely, and can move out into the pelvic cavity, where it may cause problems. Some authorities think that perforation occurs only at insertion, even though this may not be evident for quite some time, and that it results from faulty technique on the part of the inserter. Others believe that perforation can occur at any time and even with the most conscientious of inserters. It is hard to say how often perforations occur, because many times there aren't any obvious symptoms. Some studies estimate a rate of 2 perforations per 1,000 insertions, whereas others report a rate as high as 8.7 per 1,000.[50] To help avoid perforations, always insist that the uterus be sounded (measured) before insertion.

If the IUD is expelled or perforates the uterine wall, the woman is, of course, susceptible to pregnancy. The first step in dealing with a missing IUD is to do a pregnancy test. The problems of the IUD in pregnancy are discussed below. If the pregnancy test is negative and the woman knows for certain that the device has been expelled, she may choose to have the IUD replaced or select another method of birth control. The problem arises when the strings are no longer visible and it is not clear whether the IUD has been expelled, whether the strings have merely been drawn up into the uterus or whether the device has perforated the uterus.

There are a number of ways in which a doctor can check to see if the IUD is still in the uterus. After injecting anesthetic into the cervix the doctor can insert a special instrument into the uterus to feel for the IUD. Most of the time, if the IUD is still in the uterus, it can be located and the string pulled back

129

down, but if the IUD is not in the uterus, the doctor doesn't know whether it has perforated or has been expelled.

Another alternative is to do an ultrasound examination, which, like an X-ray, is a method of taking pictures of the interior of the body, although it does not involve exposure to radiation. Ultrasound is painless and can tell the doctor whether or not the IUD is still in the uterus or pelvic cavity, but the procedure is expensive (about $75) and doesn't retrieve the strings, should the IUD still be in the uterus.

Still another alternative is to do a hysteroscopic examination, which involves using a local anesthetic and inserting a specialized viewing instrument into the uterine cavity to look for the IUD or signs of perforation. If the IUD is in the uterus, the string usually can be retrieved at the time of the hysteroscopic exam. This procedure has the advantage of direct visualization and string retrieval but is new and not yet widely available.

Yet another alternative is to locate the IUD by X-ray, with a probe or a second IUD inserted into the cervix. The X-ray will confirm the presence of the IUD and its relationship to the probe or second IUD will help the doctor decide whether or not the IUD is still within the uterus. (Remember, the uterus is soft tissue and will not show up on an X-ray.*) This alternative might be suggested if the doctor suspects perforation, has been unable to find the IUD by probing or thinks the IUD may have moved out of the pelvic cavity.

If these methods fail to locate the IUD, the woman can safely assume the device was expelled without her knowing it. If the device is still within the uterus, the woman has the choice of having the device removed or leaving it within the uterus. There is some controversy about what to do if the device has perforated the uterus. Devices with copper or progestin embedded in them *must* be removed, because these substances can irritate the pelvic cavity. Similarly, it is universally agreed that certain closed devices (no longer marketed) that have perforated the uterine wall must be removed, because they can obstruct the bowel. We believe that any perforated device should be removed, because the IUD could cause an infection to flare up any time the woman's general resistance to infection is lowered. Moreover, there has been evidence that all devices, closed or open, can cause obstruction and perforation of other organs. Although most doctors favor removal, there are, nonetheless, still some doctors who think it's all right to leave an IUD that has perforated the uterus in the pelvic cavity unless it starts to cause problems. A woman whose doctor doesn't counsel removal would be wise to seek a second opinion (*see* p. 238).

Most of the time an IUD that has perforated the uterus can be recovered by laparoscopy, a procedure in which a small incision is made in the abdomen and a tubelike viewing instrument, a laparoscope, is inserted to locate the

*Some of the early models of the Dalkon Shield do not show up on X-rays.

IUD. A tool for removing the IUD can be passed through the tube. If the IUD is not located in a place accessible by laparoscopy, a more major form of surgery must be done.

The IUD and Ectopic Pregnancy

Another controversy centers around the IUD and the ectopic pregnancy, that is, a pregnancy in which the fertilized egg implants outside the uterus, usually within the fallopian tube. An ectopic pregnancy is a potentially life-threatening situation that, when diagnosed, calls for immediate surgery.

When pregnancy occurs in an IUD user she has roughly a seven to ten times greater chance of having an ectopic pregnancy; that is, approximately 1 in 30 pregnancies of IUD users will be ectopic as compared with 1 in 125 pregnancies of nonusers.[51]

All women who wear an IUD should consult their doctors if they miss a menstrual period and should be alert to the possibility of an ectopic pregnancy (*see* p. 685), the symptoms of which include abdominal pain and bleeding. Unfortunately, these symptoms may be caused by either the IUD itself or a number of other gynecological problems. In fact, IUD users with ectopic pregnancies are often misdiagnosed on the first visit to their doctors. This delay in diagnosis is important, because the larger the fetus grows, the greater the chance that the fallopian tube will rupture, causing a medical emergency that could result in sterility or even death.

The higher ratio of ectopic to uterine pregnancies in IUD users could be explained in a number of ways, and this is where the controversy arises. Some authorities have argued that this higher ratio simply reflects the fact that the IUD, although it does a fairly good job of preventing uterine pregnancies, doesn't do very well when it comes to preventing ectopic pregnancies. Others think that the IUD actually causes ectopic pregnancies, by so inflaming the uterine lining that the fertilized egg is forced to find another place to implant.[52]

Strong and convincing arguments are made on both sides, and at this point there is not enough good, clear-cut data to settle the debate. Should it be decided that the IUD causes ectopic pregnancies, it would be unwise for any woman to use the IUD as a method of birth control. Some doctors believe that until the final verdict is in, women with histories of ectopic pregnancies should not use an IUD. Other doctors are particularly reluctant to use the Progestasert IUD, which some studies have implicated as being associated with particularly high rates of ectopic pregnancies.[53]

Still other doctors believe that because of the increased risk of ectopic pregnancy and of PID, both of which can result in sterility, women who have never had children and who, according to some studies, are therefore more at risk for these sorts of problems than users who have had children, should not

131

use the IUD if they hope some day to conceive. (*See* IUD and Subsequent Fertility below.) Still other doctors think that the chances of ectopic pregnancy, especially of ectopic pregnancies that result in death or permanent effects on fertility, are so low that the IUD, which is so convenient to use, is worth the risk. This risk/convenience trade-off is one each woman must weigh for herself.

IUDs and Pregnancy

If the IUD does fail while remaining in place and the woman becomes pregnant, there are other reasons for concern besides the possibility of an ectopic pregnancy. About 50 percent of women who continue their pregnancies with IUDs in place will have a miscarriage, which can be an emergency situation.[54] This is about three times the normal rate. If the IUD is removed, this cuts the risk of miscarriage to 25 percent.

The question of septic abortion (that is, infected miscarriages) and the IUD must also be considered. In the early seventies attention was focused on a small number of deaths caused by septic abortion in IUD users. A survey conducted by an FDA committee uncovered 289 cases of septic midtrimester abortion in IUD users, including 21 deaths.[55] A later analysis of data collected between 1972 and 1974 showed that of the 50 women in the United States who died of spontaneous abortions, 23 were IUD users.[56] The news of these septic abortion deaths led to the withdrawal of the Dalkon Shield, a device that, at the time, was thought to be particularly associated with such deaths. However, some researchers have questioned whether the attention focused on the Dalkon Shield might not have obscured the fact that septic abortion, with the risk of death, apparently can occur with any IUD.[57] Indeed, of the 50 percent of pregnant IUD users who miscarry, as many as 95 percent may show signs of septic abortion.[58]

There is also some evidence that the continued presence of an IUD increases the risk of premature delivery[59] and stillbirth.[60] There has been some concern expressed about the copper and progestin IUDs being close to the developing fetus. There has been some evidence that *progestin* may also cause birth defects; however, no deformities have been reported in the small number of infants born after exposure to a Progestasert IUD.[61] There has been a report of two copper-IUD users, both of whom gave birth to infants with limb deficiencies, but it is not clear that these birth defects were related to the IUD.[62] Another study showed no limb deformities and only one minor vocal cord abnormality.[63] The final verdict is not yet in, for the number of infants thus far born under such conditions is too small to make any definite judgments.

Until fairly recently most doctors recommended leaving the IUD in place if the woman wished to continue the pregnancy; however, with the information now available about increased rates of miscarriage and septic abortions and the possibility of premature labor, birth defects and stillbirths, doctors now advise that the IUD be removed if the strings are still visible or that an abortion be considered if the strings are not visible.

If the strings are still visible, there generally isn't a problem, for the IUD can usually be removed without disturbing the pregnancy. Although removal can cause a miscarriage, the increased risk of miscarriage from this procedure is more than offset by the increased risk of miscarriage and other problems if pregnancy is continued with the IUD in place. Sometimes the strings will be visible but the IUD won't come out, or the strings will break off, making removal impossible. In such cases doctors recommend that the woman consider abortion.

If a pregnant woman whose IUD strings are missing or whose IUD strings break off during removal does have an abortion, the contents of the uterus will be examined. If the IUD is found, no further treatment is necessary. If the IUD is not found, the question of whether it was expelled or has perforated the uterus remains, and the doctor may do one of the procedures described previously.

Although abortion should be considered if the strings are not visible (especially if the woman has a Dalkon Shield), a woman who would like to avoid abortion on the chance that the IUD was expelled without her knowing it might choose to have an ultrasound exam to see if the device is still in the body. If no IUD is visible, she can assume the device was expelled and continue her pregnancy without worrying. Since ultrasound does not involve radiation, there is no problem about radiation exposure to the fetus, although there have been some questions about the possible effects of ultrasound on a fetus. In this instance, when a decision about abortion is being made, the benefits probably outweigh the theoretical risks of ultrasound.

Women who are opposed to abortion and choose to continue the pregnancy with the IUD in place should be followed carefully and alerted to the signs of impending miscarriage (*see* p. 675). Such women should also know that the combination of an infection and pregnancy is potentially fatal for an IUD user when the IUD is still in place. They should also know that such infections may begin with nothing more than mild, flulike symptoms, such as fever, headaches, nausea, vomiting and muscle aches.

IUD and Subsequent Fertility

Still another area of controversy is the question of the effect of an IUD on a woman's ability to become pregnant after the IUD has been removed. We have already discussed the relationship of pelvic inflammatory disease and ectopic pregnancies to the IUD. Both of these conditions can cause infertility.

For this reason some doctors have been reluctant to prescribe IUDs for women who have never had children.

Even beyond the question of pelvic inflammatory disease and ectopic pregnancy, there has been some debate about IUDs and fertility. There are basically three points of view in this controversy. The first holds that there is no effect on subsequent fertility. This has been the generally accepted viewpoint, based on a number of studies, including large-scale studies done in 1970 and 1971.[64]

The second viewpoint holds that although women who use IUDs may be slower to achieve pregnancy after removal, the overwhelming majority eventually do recover their fertility. This point of view is supported by a study done in England in 1978 with smaller groups of women.[65] The study showed that 48.7 percent of 258 women who had had their IUDs removed in order to get pregnant had not given birth after 12 months as compared with 29.4 percent of 1,085 women who had abandoned diaphragms or other traditional methods. After 3½ years, however, only one former IUD user (0.4 percent) as compared with 13 women from the other group (0.8 percent) had not given birth.

The third viewpoint holds that the longer a woman wears her IUD, the less chance she has of getting pregnant after removal of the IUD as compared with a group of nonusers of the same age. This viewpoint is supported by a large study of former IUD users done in Taiwan in 1977, which followed women for a period of 6 to 9 years and showed a significant decrease in fertility among former IUD users even in the absence of obvious pelvic inflammatory disease when compared with nonusers of the same age.[66] This was particularly true of women over age 30 at the time of removal who had been using the IUD for longer than 3 years.

This question obviously needs more study before it can be resolved. In the meantime, women who are using the IUD to delay pregnancy rather than to prevent it altogether, especially long-term users over age 30, should consider the possibility of reduced fertility after IUD use when weighing the various birth control possibilities.

Removal of an IUD

The IUD should be removed right after menopause. Delaying removal could cause problems, because the uterus gets smaller after menopause and the IUD could become embedded.

If a woman decides to have her IUD removed before menopause, she should not have it removed in the middle of her cycle, as conception may have occurred just before removal. With the IUD gone the fertilized egg could then implant in the uterus. (If the IUD is being removed for emergency reasons, such as pelvic inflammatory disease, this rule need not apply.) If a woman *is* planning to have the IUD removed at midcycle, she should use a second method of birth control, such as foam and condoms, for at least 5 days before removal.

IUD and Cancer

None of the studies done on IUD users has demonstrated any link between IUDs and cancer. However, some critics of the IUD argue that cancer is a slowly developing disease and that sufficient time has not yet elapsed for cancerous effects to be obvious.

DIAPHRAGM

Types: coil spring
       flat spring
       arcing
       bowbent

A diaphragm is a shallow cup of thin latex rubber with a rim of flexible metal that is also covered by rubber. It looks like a rounded lid or dome and is about 3 inches in diameter. After sperm-killing cream or jelly is placed inside the dome, the diaphragm is inserted into the vagina, before intercourse.

The diaphragm works in two ways. First, when inserted correctly, it fits into the top of the vagina, up around the cervix, covering the cervix so that it forms a mechanical barrier to block the sperm. Second, it holds the spermicidal cream or jelly up against the cervix, so that any sperm that do manage to swim up around the rim and into the diaphragm are killed before they can reach the cervical opening.

Types

Diaphragms are available in various diameters, or sizes, and in a number of varieties. Ideally, a woman should have a chance to try the different types, because some women will find one type more comfortable or easier to use than another. Women with certain physical irregularities or medical problems, such as a tipped uterus, cystocele, rectocele or poor vaginal muscle tone, may require diaphragms that are specially fitted to their anatomies.

The latest innovation is the disposable diaphragm, intended for one-time use. It is available in the same sizes as regular diaphragms and comes packaged with an application of spermicidal jelly.

Spermicides

The diaphragm should be used with a spermicidal cream or jelly. Some spermicidal creams and jellies are made to be used specifically with a diaphragm; others are made to be used alone. The spermicides manufactured to be used alone may be stronger than those made to be used with a diaphragm, so some authorities think it makes sense to also use these stronger spermicides with a diaphragm.

If the choice is between jellies and creams, it may be a matter of individual taste. But Masters and Johnson have shown that creams, when used alone, disperse better than jellies.[67] Whether this makes any difference when the creams or jellies are used with a diaphragm is still a question. Some women, on the basis of what is known, prefer to use the creams.

You needn't use a spermicide that is manufactured by the same company that manufactures your diaphragm. Try various products until you discover which is most pleasing to you.

Some women find that they can use the diaphragm successfully without a spermicide, but this is not recommended at present, because too little is known. We do know that the upper two-thirds of the vagina balloons during intercourse. This ballooning can cause the diaphragm to slip, especially when the woman is in the superior position (on top) or when the couple experiences simultaneous orgasm. By using a cream or jelly with the diaphragm, there is still some protection should one of these situations occur. If a diaphragm with spermicide is too objectionable, a woman would probably do better to try another method of birth control.

Effectiveness

When fitted and used correctly the diaphragm can have an effectiveness rate on par with that of the Pill and the IUD.

The official FDA figures on diaphragm effectiveness rates tell us to expect anywhere from 2 to 20 pregnancies per 100 women using the diaphragm for a year.[68] Unfortunately, these odds are rather wide-ranging, with a spread of from about 1 in 5 chances to 1 in 50. A woman concerned about the possible side effects of the Pill and the IUD, a woman willing to trade off an increased risk of pregnancy or abortion for greater long-term safety or a woman whose sexual contacts are infrequent might be willing to accept a 1-out-of-50 set of odds, but 1 out of 5 would probably be unacceptable to anyone who seriously wanted to prevent conception. It is necessary to take a closer look at the effectiveness rates and the studies from which they are derived in order to figure out whether you, as a particular individual, are more likely to have the 1 in 50 chance of getting pregnant—or the 1 in 5 chance.

When considering these studies it must be remembered that even when there were 20 women who got pregnant, there were 80 who did not. What makes the difference? Why does the method work for some and not for others?

First, there are problems with the method itself. That is, even if you used your diaphragm each and every time you had intercourse, you still might get pregnant. This is owing to a number of factors:

☐ Your diaphragm may not have been fitted correctly, you may have lost or gained more than 10 pounds or you may have had a child, miscarriage or abortion that has affected your fit.

☐ Your diaphragm may have a manufacturing defect (unlikely). Or you may have made a hole in it when removing it or cared for it incorrectly, resulting in leaks or in deterioration of the rubber.

☐ Your diaphragm may have become dislodged during intercourse, because the vagina expands during orgasm. As noted earlier, this expansion is more of a problem when the woman is on top during intercourse or when the couple experiences orgasm at the same time. Dislodgment also may occur when there are multiple mountings, that is, when the penis slips out and is reinserted, either accidentally or deliberately, during lovemaking.

But when one looks at the studies closely, it becomes apparent that, despite these possible drawbacks, the diaphragm can be highly effective.

As it turns out, the critical factors seem to be the age of the woman, how long she has used the diaphragm, proper instruction in its use, correct fit and whether or not she has completed her family or is using the diaphragm merely to delay pregnancy (that is, her motivation). In a large study done in England in 1974, more than 4,000 diaphragm users were tested for a combined number of months of use that totaled more than 70,000 months. This large-scale, long-term study came up with the 2.4 failure rate per 100 woman-years of use.[69] This study was limited, however, to women over age 25 who had been instructed carefully in diaphragm use and fitted carefully and who had used the method for at least 5 months before being included in the study. When the data from this study was further analyzed it showed failure rates as low as 1.1 per 100 women for women aged 35 to 39; 4.1, for women aged 25 to 29; and 1.4, for women who had been using the diaphragm for 5 years. In 1976 the largest study ever done in the United States showed rates as low as 1.9 per 100 women under age 18* to a high of 3 per 100 women aged 30 to 34.[70]

---

*This low rate for women under age 18 may be a reflection of the fact that although women in this age-group menstruate, some are not actually producing eggs and therefore cannot get pregnant.

Fitting a Diaphragm

A diaphragm requires a doctor's prescription. The initial kit, which comes with a diaphragm case and a small tube of spermicide, costs about $5 to $10. The doctor's visit can run anywhere from $10 to $75, depending on whether you get the diaphragm at a clinic or from a private doctor.

A diaphragm should be fitted by someone who is well trained and experienced. This person need not be a doctor. A paramedic, nurse, nurse practitioner or other medical personnel can fit a diaphragm and often have more time to help you learn how to use it correctly.

Most diaphragms vary in size by only about 1 inch, but these small variations are critical. Correct fit is important, because too small a diaphragm may slip out of place when the upper part of the vagina swells during sexual excitation. Too large a diaphragm may buckle or lie vertically in the vaginal canal, leaving the cervix uncovered and causing discomfort.

The fitter estimates the proper diaphragm size by inserting two fingers into the vagina and determining the distance between the pubic bone and the cervix. Then a sample diaphragm is inserted. The fitter should also insert the next larger and next smaller sizes to make sure there is a correct fit.

Once the fitter has selected the correct size, the woman should practice inserting the diaphragm herself. The fitter should then check to see if the diaphragm has been inserted correctly and should recheck the fit, as the woman may be less tense after having practiced, which could affect the sizing. Some clinicians use fitting rings—diaphragms with the dome cut out—for fitting or for practicing insertion. But the woman should insist that an actual diaphragm be used to ensure proper fit and to make sure she knows how to insert the actual diaphragm correctly.

If you are a virgin, it might be wise to use another method of birth control, like foam or condoms, for a while before having a diaphragm fitted, because sexual intercourse tends to enlarge the vaginal cavity.

If you were particularly tense or uptight during your fitting, as many women are, it is especially important to have the fit rechecked after you've practiced and before you've left the office, or to arrange a second visit after you have practiced at home with your diaphragm, for nervousness may have made you tighten your vaginal muscles, thus altering the normal contours of your vagina.

If you have decided that the diaphragm is the method, or one of the methods, you would like to use for birth control, scout around for a doctor who is a diaphragm enthusiast and who has had a good deal of experience in fitting them. Since the Pill and the IUD came into vogue, instruction in the techniques of fitting a diaphragm was dropped from many medical school curriculums. Because correct fitting is so important to successful diaphragm use and because many doctors tend to downgrade the effectiveness of the diaphragm, it is important to find a diaphragm "fan," who is much more likely to be experienced with them, when making your choice. Never have a diaphragm fitted by a doctor who has tried to talk you out of using this method of birth control.

How to Use the Diaphragm (Illustration 21)

☐ Put about a tablespoon of spermicidal cream into the cup of your diaphragm. Apply a thin film on the inside of the rim. Some women coat the outside of the diaphragm as well, for extra safety.

☐ Pinch the opposite sides of the rim together so that the diaphragm folds in the middle.

☐ The diaphragm can be inserted while you are in a number of positions: sitting on the edge of a chair, lying flat on your back with knees bent, squatting or propping one leg up on a toilet or chair. If you are standing, the diaphragm is inserted almost horizontally; if you are lying down, it is inserted almost vertically.

☐ The diaphragm is pushed up along the back wall of the vagina as far as possible. This ensures that it is covering the cervix. It should then move into place, fitting snugly against the pubic bone in the front. Make sure the cervix is covered by feeling for it beneath the rubber dome of the diaphragm. (Your cervix feels like a knoblike projection and is firm, like the tip of your nose.)

☐ The manufacturers and many doctors advise that the diaphragm should not be inserted more than 2 hours before intercourse. Some doctors allow early insertion. Recommendations vary between 2 and 12 hours. In one major study, participants were allowed to insert the diaphragm as many as 6 hours before intercourse, and a 3-pregnancies-per-100-women effectiveness rate was still achieved.[71] Until we know more about how long the spermicide stays active, 2 hours is probably the safest. We feel comfortable with the 6-hour rule. But if you occasionally find yourself needing to insert the diaphragm earlier than this, remember that inserting it earlier is better than forgetting contraception altogether.

☐ Check your diaphragm for holes and tears before inserting.

☐ If your partner is going to ejaculate a second time, most doctors recommend using a second application of spermicide. Do not remove the diaphragm; simply insert a second applicator of cream or jelly (foam may be used) into the vagina before the second ejaculation. Others believe that a second application of spermicide is unnecessary unless several hours have elapsed between the first and second ejaculations.

☐ Leave the diaphragm in for at least 8 hours after intercourse. After

139

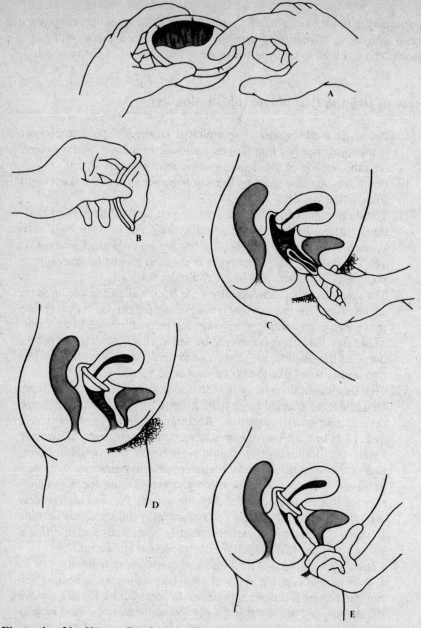

Illustration 21 *Using a Diaphragm: Place spermicide in the dome of the diaphragm, and rub it on the dome and the rim (A). Fold the diaphragm so the rims are touching (B). Insert the diaphragm into the vagina (C). Guide it along the back wall of the vagina until it covers the cervix (D). Use your finger to check that the cervix is under the dome of the diaphragm (E).*

removal, wash it with mild soap, dry and store. Failure to clean the diaphragm thoroughly could lead to recurrent yeast infections. Do not use talc or perfumed powders on your diaphragm, as this could harm the rubber and irritate the vagina.

☐ Do not use petroleum jelly (Vaseline) as a lubricant with the diaphragm, as this could harm the rubber. K-Y jelly or spermicide may be used as a lubricant.

Advantages and Benefits

When fitted and used correctly the diaphragm has a high rate of reliability. Not one hospitalization or death has ever been related to the diaphragm. This method is particularly well suited for women who have sex only infrequently, especially as compared with the IUD and the Pill, which must be worn or taken even if a woman is not having sex very often.

There are no long-term effects on fertility, and a woman may use a diaphragm during breast-feeding without worrying about its effect on her milk.

There seems to be a lower incidence of both cervical and vaginal infections and of sexually transmissible infections in women who use the diaphragm.[72] This lower incidence may be owing to the antibacterial effect of the spermicide or to the mechanical protection provided by the diaphragm. Studies have shown that cervical cancer, which may be associated with herpes type II (*see* p. 376), is less common in women who use the diaphragm.[73]

Women who experience an upsurge in their sexual desire at the time of menstruation like the diaphragm because it catches the menstrual blood and makes sex at that time less messy. Others like the diaphragm because they involve their mates in the insertion of the diaphragm and find that sharing the responsibility for birth control is very satisfying.

Disadvantages and Problems

Some women cannot wear a diaphragm because of their particular anatomies or because of poor muscle tone in the vagina. The following conditions may also make it impossible for a woman to use a diaphragm:

☐ Prolapse of the uterus
☐ Fistulas
☐ Severe cystocele or rectocele
☐ Severe retroversion or anteflexion of the uterus
☐ Septate vagina

Some women experience cramps and pressure on the bladder or rectum when the diaphragm is left in place for 8 or more hours after intercourse, as recommended. A smaller size or a different type of diaphragm may correct the problem, but if it persists, the woman should use a different method of birth control.

There is some evidence that women who use diaphragms are more apt to develop urinary tract infections.[74] It is theorized that the pressure of the diaphragm on the bladder or on the urethra causes this increased susceptibility to infection. A smaller-sized diaphragm may eliminate the problem, but women who have repeated infections should use a different method of birth control.

In addition, in certain rather rare cases a woman or her partner may be allergic to the latex rubber or to the spermicides. Changing brands of spermicide may help. Some men complain that they dislike the sensation of hitting up against the diaphragm during intercourse, but this is not usually a problem if the diaphragm is fitted correctly.

Some women find the diaphragm too messy, too inconvenient or too distasteful to use. Women who don't like to touch their genitals may find that using a plastic inserter makes this method of birth control more acceptable. Other women claim that this method interferes with the spontaneity of their sex lives. Some couples incorporate the placement of the diaphragm into the lovemaking ritual so that spontaneity is not compromised.

If a couple tends to reach orgasm simultaneously and prefers the woman-superior position or if the man tends to slip out during intercourse or prefers to withdraw and reenter (multiple mounting), the diaphragm is more likely to become dislodged and is probably less effective as a means of contraception.

Couples who enjoy oral-genital sex sometimes find the taste of spermicides unpleasant. They may engage in oral-genital lovemaking and then insert the diaphragm, but if the partners become intensely excited by this form of foreplay, the diaphragm may be forgotten.

Other than an occasional allergic reaction, there have been no adverse effects attributed to the spermicides used with the diaphragms. The results of some studies have even indicated that spermicides may be antibacterial and may promote vaginal health.[75] In the past there has been some question about certain spermicides that included a compound containing mercury, but these compounds are no longer used. Even though the spermicide may be anti-infective, a diaphragm left in too long may cause irritation and a smelly discharge, but these conditions usually clear up by themselves. To prevent these conditions, remove the diaphragm at least every 24 to 36 hours, and wash and dry it thoroughly before reinserting it.

There has been some concern about spermicides and the possibility of birth defects. This is discussed in the next section, Vaginal Spermicides.

There has also been some concern that leaving a diaphragm in for longer than 24 hours could make a woman more susceptible to toxic shock syndrome

(TSS), but studies have not shown that women who use the diaphragm are more apt to develop TSS (*see* p. 651).

VAGINAL SPERMICIDES

AKA: spermicides or topical contraceptives

Types: contraceptive foam
contraceptive tablets
contraceptive cream
contraceptive jelly

Vaginal spermicides are chemical mixtures containing a base material and a sperm-killing agent. They are inserted into the vagina just before intercourse. They work in two ways: by coating the cervix and forming a mechanical barrier, so that the sperm cannot pass into the uterus, and by killing the sperm within the vagina. There are basically three kinds of spermicide available: foams, creams and jellies. The creams and jellies are used with a diaphragm or a cervical cap. Although some manufacturers advertise their creams and jellies to be used alone, we do not recommend this procedure. While they are excellent when used with a diaphragm or cup, the creams and jellies simply don't disperse and cover the cervix as well as the foam does.[76]

Types

Foam is available in two forms: in an aerosol spray can and in tablets (suppositories) that are inserted into the vagina before intercourse. The vaginal secretions activate the tablets and the foam is released (a process somewhat akin to dropping an Alka-Seltzer into a glass of water). We do not recommend use of the tablets, as studies have shown that the tablets do not always dissolve completely.[77]

A special note should be added here about the Encare Oval, a new and highly advertised foam tablet that is well packaged and easy to use. The effectiveness rates cited by the Encare Oval manufacturers, which are extremely high—on a par with the Pill—are based on studies derived from what one diplomatic source discreetly called a ''very unconventional study design.''[78] Our personal experience, having performed a number of abortions on women who were relying on the Encare Oval, make us skeptical about their effectiveness and we don't recommend them.

Effectiveness

Foam, like all the barrier methods of birth control, has a bad reputation as far as effectiveness goes. One study conducted in Puerto Rico with a group of low-income women indicated that 29 out of 100 women using this method for a year would get pregnant.[79] Yet, other studies have reported rates as low as 1.5 pregnancies per 100 woman-years of use.[80] The wide variance in rates may have to do with the fact that the studies with high failure rates were done with non-English-speaking women, teenagers and others who had not been instructed properly in the use of foam.[81] Some of these women reported jumping up and applying the spermicide immediately after intercourse. Others applied the foam to the outside—not the inside—of their bodies. Moreover, many of these less successful studies were done with women who did not specifically choose to use the foam. With those who actively decide that foam is the method they want to use, the results are, not surprisingly, much superior. One such study, which included more than 3,000 women who were "medically indigent" (that is, low-income) and who were chronically unsuccessful at birth control, showed a pregnancy rate of only 4 per 100 women.[82] Moreover, these women were told that the foam could be inserted as long as 3 hours before intercourse, which is a couple of hours more than most manufacturers recommend (see below). The results might have been even better had the product been used according to the manufacturer's directions, although perhaps the freedom to insert the foam before intercourse contributed to better rates. A critical difference between this and other studies is that the staff administering the study came from the same background as the women in the study, spoke their language and presumably understood their life-styles and problems.

Also, many of the studies that yielded high pregnancy rates involved women who wanted to delay, rather than prevent, pregnancy. Other studies have shown that there is a great deal of difference in the effectiveness of any birth control method, depending on whether the users' intentions are to merely delay pregnancy until a later date or to prevent pregnancy, either because their families are complete or because they absolutely do not want children.[83] One study conducted among couples who firmly did not want children showed a failure rate of 1 percent for the Pill, 7 percent for foam, and 6 percent and 7 percent for the diaphragm and condom, respectively.[84] The latest study, published in 1979, involved 326 "affluent, well-educated and highly motivated" women, all of whom were instructed carefully by private physicians and followed-up at regular intervals.[85] The results of this study showed 0.3 pregnancies per 100 woman-years of use. If the foam is used with a condom, the effectiveness rate should be even higher.

The upshot of all of this seems to be that foam is an extremely effective method of birth control. Its effectiveness can be on a par with that of the Pill if it is used correctly.

How to Use Foam

First things first—read the directions that come with the foam. Unfortunately, these directions often leave much to be desired, so we've devised a set of our own:

☐ Most instructions will include a line like "Shake the can." Really shake it—at least 20 times. This will make the foam about the consistency of shaving cream, so that it is more effective. Shaking vigorously will also assure an even distribution of the spermicide, which tends to settle on the bottom of the container.

☐ Most foams come with a plastic plunger and tube device that works like a tampon. In most cases the applicator tube is filled by pressing down or by tilting it over the nozzle on the container of foam. The foam is released into the tube by pulling the plunger back as far as possible, so that it is ready to insert. Foam can get a bit messy at this point, because it takes a light touch and good timing to remove the applicator before it fills and the excess foam spurts out every which way.

☐ The applicator is then inserted into the vagina right away, preferably while you are lying down. It should be inserted as far as it can go (about 3 or 4 inches), withdrawn about a half-inch or an inch and the plunger pressed down to release the foam. The reason for the partial withdrawal is to assure that the foam is being deposited on or near the cervix (which protrudes from the top of the vaginal cavity) and not on the back wall of the vagina (*see* Illustration 22).

☐ Push slowly while pressing the plunger in, so that the bubbles have a better chance of spreading evenly over the cervix and vaginal walls.

☐ The applicator should be withdrawn without pulling the plunger out to avoid sucking some of the foam back into the applicator.

☐ Women who have had children or have had abortions sometimes use 2—rather than 1—applicatorsful of foam, because in such women the opening of the cervix is larger. Some women use extra foam around the time of ovulation.

☐ Brands like Delfen and Koromex have applicators that hold only 5 cc of foam, so some clinics recommend that women who use these brands use 2 applicatorsful of foam.

☐ The foam should be inserted as close to the time of actual intercourse as possible. Some authorities say the bubbles go flat within 15 minutes to

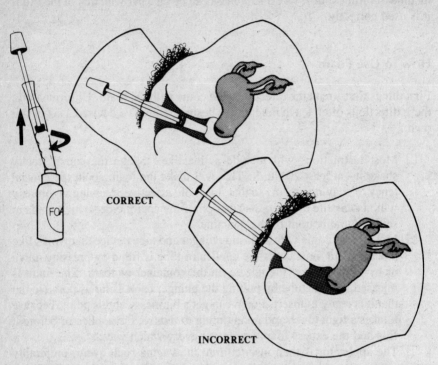

CORRECT

INCORRECT

Illustration 22 *Inserting foam: Insert the foam applicator deep into the vagina so that the foam will cover your cervix.*

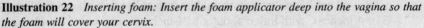

a half hour. Some researchers have allowed insertion as long as 3 hours ahead with good results, but the consensus is that insertion no more than 1 hour before intercourse is optimal.

☐ An additional applicator of foam should be inserted before each act of intercourse. Each dose has the capacity to kill the amount of sperm deposited each time a man ejaculates, or comes, but it may not be strong enough to be effective a second time. Then, too, if an hour has passed, the bubbles may have fizzled out, making a second application necessary.

☐ If the woman gets up or goes to the bathroom after application but before intercourse, she should insert another application because some foam may have been lost. After intercourse, getting up poses no problem because the spermicide has done its work.

☐ The applicator should be washed with water and a mild soap. It should not be boiled because it is made of soft plastic, and sterilization is not necessary anyway. Some women keep a glass of water handy and drop the applicator into it. In any case the applicator need not be washed immediately.

☐ Do not douche for 8 hours afterward. This may dilute the foam and force any sperm that are still alive up into the womb.

☐ Although the foam won't stain and dries or dissolves within a few hours, some women use a sanitary napkin to catch the foam that sometimes leaks out after intercourse. A tampon should not be used for this purpose.

Buying Contraceptive Foam

Contraceptive foam is available in drugstores and some grocery stores. There is no law regulating how old you must be to buy foam. Most of the time the foam can be found sitting on the store shelves. If not, ask for it by one of the brand names listed below. Be sure that the product you are buying is contraceptive foam and not one of the feminine hygiene products (douches, deodorants and such) that are often on the shelves right next to the contraceptive foams. Foam is also available by mail in an unmarked envelope from Population Services, Inc., 105 North Columbia Street, Chapel Hill, North Carolina 27514 (919-929-7195).

Contraceptive foam deteriorates over time and has a shelf life of 3 years. Most brands are now dated for freshness, but for some manufacturers this is a recent innovation, so you may find older, undated boxes. Shop for a dated brand that has an expiration date and check to make sure you have a fresh batch.

The cost of foam ranges from about 20 cents to 40 cents per application, which can get rather expensive if you have an active sex life. However, using foam does not require initial or follow-up doctor's visits. Also, foam is used only when it is needed, unlike the Pill, for example, which is taken every day. Moreover, the user does not run the risks of costly complications (except perhaps the cost of pregnancy or abortion should the method fail).

A number of types of foam are available:

☐ Emko Contraceptive Foam: Available in 30- and 60-application containers. The foam can be purchased in a starter kit, which includes an applicator and carrying purse, or in the slightly less expensive refill kits, which come without an applicator. A dosage cup that lets you know how much foam is left in the container comes with all except the 30-application refill kit; however, the cup from the other kit will fit. This is an important feature, because it prevents you from getting an incomplete dose or from suddenly discovering that you've run out.

☐ Emko Pre-Fil Contraceptive Foam: Available in a 25-to-30-application kit, which comes with an applicator and a carrying purse, or a 50-to-60-application refill kit. The Pre-Fil foam is in liquid form until the plunger is depressed. This means that the applicator can be filled ahead of time so that lovemaking need not be interrupted by the somewhat messy and more time-consuming process of filling the applicator.

☐ Because Contraceptor: This is also an Emko product. It contains six applications in one easy-to-use, tampon-sized applicator.

☐ Koromex II Contraceptive Foam: Manufactured by Holland-Rantos, it is available in 30- and 60-application containers, again with applicator and purse or refill kits.

☐ Delfen Contraceptive Foam: Manufactured by Ortho Pharmaceutical, it comes in a starter kit, which includes an applicator, a purse and a container that holds about 20 applications, or in refills in either the 20- or 50-application size.

☐ Dalkon Contraceptive Foam: Made by the A. H. Robins Company, it comes in a starter kit, which contains an applicator, carrying purse and 35 applications of foam. Refills, holding 90 applications, are also available. Like the Emko products, Dalkon has a built-in device that lets you know how much foam is left.

☐ Couple's Choice: This kit contains both foam and condoms and is marketed by Youngs Drug Products, Inc. Included in the kit are 12 ribbed Trojan condoms and a container of Koromex foam. The cost is less than if these items were purchased separately.

Advantages and Benefits

One of the biggest advantages that foam has in comparison with methods like the Pill and the IUD is that no one has ever died as a result of using foam. Occasionally, there may be an allergic reaction, but this can usually be cured by switching to another brand.

Foam does not require a doctor's exam, prescription, supervision or follow-up. It is readily available in drugstores and grocery stores. Unlike the Pill or the IUD, which are used on a day-to-day basis, foam is used only when intercourse is going to take place. Also, its use does not involve a device like the cervical cap or the diaphragm.

Foam is effective against venereal disease and common vaginal infections.[86,87] It doesn't offer 100 percent protection, but it does reduce your chances of getting such infections. There is also some evidence to suggest that spermicides provide some protection against the development of precancerous and cancerous conditions in the cervix.[88]

Contraceptive foam is often used during the first several months of IUD use. It is good to keep some around in case you stop, run out of or forget to take your pills. It is also a good backup in case your IUD is expelled or a condom breaks (insert several applicators of foam immediately). Foam is also used by some women at midcycle to increase the effectiveness of an IUD or condom. Because many doctors recommend that a woman should not try to become pregnant for the first few months after stopping the Pill (*see* p. 111), foam may be useful at these times.

Foam is also relied on by diaphragm users who have intercourse a second time, but some professionals think that the contraceptive jellies or creams are better, fearing that the foam will weaken the rubber of the diaphragm.

Disadvantages and Problems

The biggest drawback to foam as a contraceptive is the fact that it must be applied just before intercourse and thus interrupts lovemaking. Some couples overcome this problem by using a prepared type of foam, so that they aren't bothered by having to fill the applicator. Other couples incorporate the insertion of the foam into their lovemaking. Because the foams have an unpleasant taste, couples who enjoy oral-genital contact must apply the foam after oral sex and may not care to resume this form of lovemaking once the foam has been inserted.

Some women find that the foam provides too much lubrication and, consequently, reduces their sexual pleasure. On the other hand, women who produce only a minimal amount of lubrication may prefer foam for this very reason.

There has been some theoretical concern that spermicides might cause birth defects. A spermicide could possibly cripple, but not kill, a sperm, and that damaged sperm could cause a defective pregnancy. Or, perhaps spermicide could get into the uterus of a woman who used it in early pregnancy, before she realized she was pregnant, and cause a birth defect. Until recently, these concerns were only theoretical; no real evidence supported a link between spermicides and birth defects. Some authorities still believe there is no evidence, but others point to a new study linking spermicides and birth defects.[89]

This study, which received a great deal of publicity in the popular press, looked at the infants of 4,655 women, of whom 763 had filled a prescription for spermicide within 600 days of delivery. Among the 763 spermicide users, there were 17 babies with birth defects, a rate of 2.2 percent. Among the 3,902 nonusers, there were 39 babies with birth defects, a rate of 1.1 percent. In other words, the rate for presumed users of spermicides was twice as high as the rate for nonusers.

But researchers have pointed out that some other things need to be considered.[90] For example, the national rate of birth defects is 2.1 percent. There was no single, well-defined type of defect among the children of the users. It

149

was not determined that the users were actually using spermicides at the time they got pregnant. It was not determined whether the prescriptions that were filled were actually used. Also, since this study came out another major study, which did not have some of the flaws this study had, indicated that there was no increased risk of birth defects.[91] Based on what is now known, most authorities are not too concerned about the possible link.

CONDOMS

AKA: rubbers, prophylactics, safes, French letters, sheaths, skins, trojans

A condom is a sheath made from thin rubber or lamb's gut that fits over the erect penis in a glovelike fashion. Placed on the erect penis just before intercourse, the condom acts as a barrier that prevents the sperm from entering the vagina. Some condoms have a plain end; others have a special receptacle at the tip to contain the sperm after the man ejaculates, or comes. The rubber at the open end of the condom is thicker, forming an elastic ring that keeps the condom from slipping off the penis. The condoms available in the United States are available in only one size, but since they are considerably elastic, one size is supposed to fit all.

Types

There are three types of condoms: those made from a basic grade of latex rubber; those made from a thinner grade of latex; and those made from the intestines of sheep, which are called skin condoms. Skin condoms are more expensive, but many men prefer them because they transmit body heat much as human skin does and therefore permit more sensitivity. Many men object to using a condom, likening it to "taking a shower with a raincoat on"; however, when questioned, many such men will admit that they have never used one or have not used one for many, many years. A number of men, once they've tried them, find that the new condoms, either skins or those made from a thinner grade of latex, provide a natural feeling.

Latex condoms are available either dry or lubricated and with either a dry or wet lubricant. Most users prefer the lubricated varieties, because they replace the natural secretions from the penis that are blocked by the condom, thereby facilitating entry and cutting down on the penile or vaginal irritation that is sometimes experienced with the nonlubricated variety. Some users complain about the medicinal odor of some of the wet lubricants and prefer the dry lubricants, which are odorless and slippery rather than wet. A new type of condom that is lubricated with a spermicide and may provide extra contraceptive protection (the Ramses Extra) has come on the market recently.

Most condoms are colorless—opaque or transparent—but recently U.S. companies, following the lead of foreign manufacturers, have been marketing colored condoms. In some countries even glow-in-the-dark condoms are available, but the more adventuresome in the United States who would like to try them out will have to wait until a U.S. company manufactures them, because the thinner foreign condoms do not meet U.S. standards.

Condoms are also available with ribbed and textured surfaces and with "ticklers" on the end. Such extras are advertised as being sensually pleasing to women (if that's what "drive her wild" is supposed to mean); however, we've yet to meet a woman who has noticed the difference.

The lamb's gut, or skin, condoms are lubricated with a special oily substance that makes them cling to the penis for a snug fit. Still, they don't fit as snugly as the latex type, which makes some first-time users worry that these condoms will fall off. But despite their seeming looseness they don't. Although many men find that the skin condom enhances penile sensation, others find that the oily, lubricating substance makes them messier to put on.

Effectiveness

Condoms, like other barrier methods of birth control, have long been downgraded as being ineffective, but a look at the facts provides a different picture.

The highest rates of condom contraceptive failure are quoted as being 36 pregnancies per 100 woman-years of use.[92] This study, however, was done in 1942. We have already discussed the problems with this study in Chapter Five. A study done in 1969 recorded actual-use rates of 3.1 pregnancies per 100 woman-years;[93] rates as low as 0.83 have been recorded in one study.[94] The big factor is, of course, motivation. If the condom is used correctly, each and every time a couple has intercourse, it is a highly effective method of birth control.

Using contraceptive foam with the condom increases effectiveness. Using the new condoms that are lubricated with spermicide may also increase effectiveness, but the new condoms may not be as effective as the condom/foam combination.

Using Condoms

Condoms, it's true, are simple devices, but they can be a bit tricky the first time because the directions that come with the condoms (if there are any) tend to be brief and leave a lot to be desired. We've created our own expanded version:

- [ ] The condom purchased years ago by a young boy in junior high school (with high hopes) and carried around in his wallet to impress his friends won't be too useful, because body heat tends to deteriorate the rubber, and even the best-sealed condoms, carefully stored away from heat, should be discarded after 2 (some say 5) years. Condoms should be stored in a cool, dry place, away from heat and sunlight.

- [ ] Dry condoms, which may irritate the vaginas of women who don't have a lot of lubrication, should never be lubricated with Vaseline or petroleum jelly, because this tends to deteriorate the rubber. Lubrication will help prevent tearing, and spermicidal foam, cream or jelly will lubricate with the additional advantage of adding extra contraception. Saliva works well but is said to increase the chances of contracting vaginal yeast infections.

- [ ] Although this may seem obvious, especially to anyone who has tried it another way, the condom can be placed on the penis only after the man is sexually aroused and his penis is at least semi-erect. If lubrication is desired, it should be applied after the condom is in place.

- [ ] Most condoms come prerolled. They are usually rolled around the firm rubber-ring end. Unless the condom is placed over the tip of the penis and unrolled the reverse way, it will not move smoothly down the shaft of the penis and will become bound up after unrolling an inch or so. Unroll the condom about ½ inch and then place it on the penis (see Illustration 23).

- [ ] Some condoms come with a tip at the end to collect the semen. If yours doesn't, leave about a half inch of free space between the tip of the penis and the closed end of the condom, making sure that the air is squeezed out of the tip or half inch of space. This is done so that the come will collect in this area and not be forced down the shaft of the penis, around the rolled end of the condom, possibly finding its way into the vagina. Some manufacturers claim that the tip or half inch of extra space prevents the condom from "bursting" when the man comes, but this somewhat exaggerated suggestion is probably wishful thinking.

- [ ] The condom should be unrolled all the way, to the base of the penis, if possible. That way, even if semen does leak down the shaft, it is unlikely that it could travel all the way back up the condom to the top of the vagina and cause a pregnancy.

- [ ] Uncircumcised males should pull the foreskin back from the end of the penis before putting on the condom.

- [ ] The condom should be used each time a couple has intercourse and

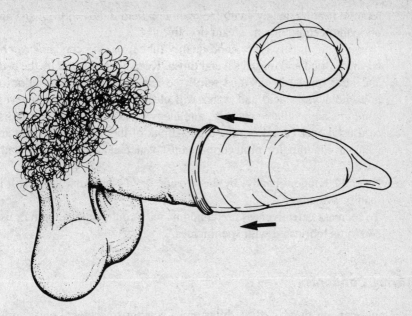

Illustration 23   *The Condom: Unroll the condom on the erect penis, leaving space at the end for semen to collect.*

should be placed on the penis before any contact with the vagina. Some couples begin actual intercourse without the condom, the game plan being to withdraw before orgasm. Needless to say, the game doesn't always go according to plan, and the condom may be forgotten until it's too late. Besides, many authorities believe that even the small numbers of sperm that leak from the penis before orgasm can cause pregnancy.

☐ The penis should be withdrawn as soon as possible after intercourse, because with most men the penis becomes smaller and softer soon after climax, which might allow semen to leak out of the open end or allow the condom to slip off the penis into the vagina. Hold the condom firmly at the base of the penis when withdrawing so that semen won't be spilled in or near the vagina. This is particularly important for women who have little vaginal lubrication. Pulling out too abruptly may cause the condom to slip off or allow the semen to escape.

☐ The vagina should not come in contact with the penis after it has been withdrawn, since there still might be live sperm on the penis. If you have multiple intercourse, a fresh condom should be used each time.

☐ If the condom breaks (which may happen if the woman's vagina is not lubricated sufficiently) or slips off in the vagina (which may happen with condoms that are lubricated on both the inside and the outside),

153

remove it immediately (with the open end held tightly closed) and apply contraceptive foam, cream or jelly.

☐ If you're the thrifty type, good-quality rubber or skin condoms can be washed, dried and reused several times. Keep a jar of water by the bed, and later on wash, dry and reroll the condom. A dilute solution of household boric acid and water will clean skin condoms. However, condoms are available cheaply, and many couples find it easier to discard used ones (not down the toilet—think of the fishies!).* If you are using a condom for protection against venereal ·disease, use it only once.

☐ Keep the condom handy, by the bedside or in your purse, so that it is readily available.

☐ To increase effectiveness use condoms with contraceptive foam or use condoms lubricated with spermicides.

Buying Condoms

Condoms can be purchased at drugstores, vending machines, and family planning and Planned Parenthood clinics or through mail order. The prices run from about 20 cents to 80 cents per condom, depending on which kind you buy (natural skins are the most expensive), whether you buy them in packages of 3, 12 or economy-sized (6 dozen, the cheapest way to buy them) and whether you buy them in a discount or regular drugstore.

Since the Supreme Court decision of 1977, there are no laws prohibiting minors from buying condoms or drugstore owners from displaying them prominently.[95] Sales, not surprisingly, have risen accordingly.[96] Women are making up a larger share of the market, 20 percent according to some estimates, which probably reflects dissatisfaction with the riskier forms of birth control and a growing awareness of the protection against venereal disease that the condom provides.

There is some controversy as to the quality of condoms that are purchased through vending machines. All condoms must pass strict quality control standards, but over time and under conditions of heat or direct sunlight, the quality of the materials deteriorates. Some authorities think that vending machines may contain condoms that are over the generally accepted usefulness age of 2 years. Other authorities point out that nobody would be in the vending machine business if it took that long to turn a profit. The key factor may be whether or not the condoms are stored in hermetically sealed foil

*Believe it or not, dead fish, apparently strangled by condoms, have been found floating on the surface of the water!

packages. But if you have to dust off the machine in order to insert your coin, you probably ought to do your condom shopping elsewhere.

Condoms may also be purchased by mail, in an unmarked envelope, from Population Planning, 105 N. Columbia Street, Department GW-1, Chapel Hill, North Carolina 27514.

Varieties and Brands

Most drugstores have open displays of condoms, usually near the cash register, but ask if you can't locate them. Salespeople may ask what size you want. If so, they are inquiring about whether you want a 3-pack, a 12-pack or a 72-pack, since the condoms themselves come in only one size. The list below, which includes some of the popular brands, will help you make your selection and know what to ask for.

Wet Lubrication: Trojan Brand Guardian and Trojan-enz Lubricated

Dry Lubrication: Trojan Plus, Conceptrol Dry-Lubricated, Trojan Ribbed

Nonlubricated: Trojans, Trojan-enz (with reservoir tip), NuForm Nonlubricated, Ramses Nonlubricated (plain end), Sheik Nonlubricated

Lubricated with Spermicide: Ramses Extra

Fitted Condoms (Body Hugging) with Reservoir Tip: Trojans Plus (dry lubrication, golden colored), Conceptrol Shields (nonlubricated or dry lubricated, transparent)

Ribbed and/or Flared: Excita (flared end, ribbed surface), Nuform Lubricated (flared end, allows for freedom of movement within condom), Trojan Ribbed (golden and transparent)

Natural Skin: Fourex Skins Capsule Pack (lubricated inside and out, comes in blue capsule), Trojan Brand Natural Lamb (lubricated, rolled)

Colored Condoms: Trojan Plus (golden, dry lubrication), Fiesta (pink, yellow, green and black, lubricated)

Condoms Packaged with Foam: Couple's Choice (cheaper than buying foam and condoms separately)

Advantages and Benefits

The condom has many advantages. It is relatively inexpensive and highly reliable when used consistently. It is readily available and doesn't require a medical examination, supervision, prescription or follow-up. This is particularly important to teenagers who are uncertain about approaching their family doctors about birth control, fearing that their confidence will not be kept. The condom is light, compact and disposable, another feature of value to teenagers who are worried about their parents knowing about their sexual activity.

There are no side effects other than an occasional, minor allergic reaction to the latex or lubricant. The condom is easy to use and totally reversible; that is, if pregnancy is desired, one need only to discontinue use without fear of reduced fertility or birth defects.

The condom may be a particularly good idea for those men who cannot maintain an erection during intercourse. The rim of the condom may have a slight tourniquet effect, helping them to prolong the erection. Because of decreased sensitivity, the condom may also be helpful in cases of premature ejaculation.

Some women have allergic reactions to their partners' sperm that can cause medical problems for them. Such cases are rare, and a condom can help the situation. In fact, couples suffering from infertility for this reason are sometimes treated by using a condom for a few months to decrease the woman's allergic response.

Perhaps the most important advantage to the condom is its role in the prevention of sexually transmissible infections. Unless there is leakage of the semen during withdrawal, the condom is highly effective in preventing gonorrhea. There is also some protection against syphilis, venereal warts, trichomoniasis and herpes, but less so because these organisms may enter through the unprotected outer lips of the vulva or from the man's scrotum. Studies of the incidence of these diseases among men who use condoms versus those who don't support this decrease in risk,[97] and other studies, like those correlating the rise in condom sales in Sweden with the drop in disease rates, help to confirm it.[98] The protective factor in the case of herpes is especially important, because there is evidence linking herpes to cervical cancer (*see* p. 376). And there are now studies indicating a lower incidence of cervical cancer in women whose partners use condoms.[99] One recent study indicated that condom use may actually help to improve the condition of women who have abnormal Pap smears or precancerous conditions of the cervix.[100]

Condom use during pregnancy may help protect against amnionic fluid infections that sometimes occur late in pregnancy.[101]

For some women the fact that using condoms means that the man is sharing the responsibility for birth control is important. The act of placing the condom can become part of lovemaking. It is a way for a sexual partner to demonstrate his care and concern for a woman by protecting her from the risks associated with other forms of birth control, such as the Pill and the IUD. In long-term relationships this demonstrated element of caring can be particularly important. In shorter-term relationships, in which you may not know if you'll be having intercourse or not, condoms may be convenient. If you don't know your sex partner well enough to trust that he'll have a condom with him, it makes sense to carry one with you. It may be hard for some of us to pull out a condom and suggest that our partner use it, but given the fact that we are in the midst of an epidemic of gonorrhea and herpes, such a practice makes a good deal of sense.

Disadvantages

One disadvantage to the condom is that it has such a bad (although undeserved) reputation for effectiveness. Many women who are planning to use this method may fail to do so at the last minute, figuring, "Oh, well, it doesn't work very well anyhow, so I might as well not bother." This is not true: The condom is highly effective, but its biggest disadvantage is that it must be placed on the erect penis just before intercourse. For some of us, remembering to use it and interrupting our lovemaking to place it on the penis is a problem. Keeping them handy, in our wallets, pocketbooks or by the bed, and making the placement of the condom part of our lovemaking can help.

From a man's point of view, the condom's most serious drawback is decreased penile sensitivity. Trying the new, thinner latex condoms or the more natural, heat-transferring skin condoms may alleviate this problem.

In rare cases there may be an allergic reaction to the latex rubber. This reaction is usually milder in women so affected than in men and can often be dealt with by switching brands or using dry condoms. In the case of couples with an active sex life the cost of natural-skin condoms may also be a problem.

CONTRACEPTIVE SPONGE

AKA: The Sponge, cervical sponge, vaginal sponge, collatex sponge, spermicidal sponge, Today Vaginal Contraceptive Sponge

The contraceptive sponge, which is a newly approved birth control device, is not to be confused with the menstrual sponges some women use to absorb their menstrual flow. Menstrual sponges have no contraceptive effect and are not designed to prevent pregnancy. The contraceptive sponge, marketed under the name Today Contraceptive Sponge, is a round, white sponge that is impregnated with spermicide. (*See* Illustration 24). It has a cuplike depression in its center and is about 1½ to 2 inches in diameter. The sponge is moistened and inserted into the top of the vagina before intercourse. It works to prevent pregnancy in three ways: (1) like the diaphragm, it mechanically blocks the sperm's passage into the cervix and uterus; (2) the spermicide in the sponge kills sperm; (3) the absorbent material of the sponge soaks up the sperm.

The sponge, which has been called "the female equivalent of the condom," is a one-size-fits-all, disposable method of birth control that can be purchased over the counter for about the same price as a high-quality condom. It can be inserted as long as 24 hours before intercourse, so it does not

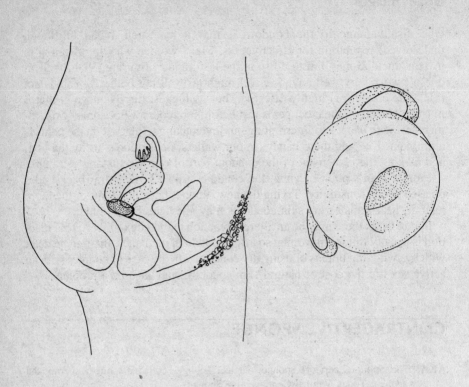

Illustration 24   *Contraceptive Sponge*

have the problem of interrupting the spontaneity of lovemaking that other barrier methods have. However, as explained below, it does have drawbacks that other barrier methods do not have.

Effectiveness

The sponge is said to be "about as effective as the diaphragm."[102] But this statement is a bit misleading. Studies in which the participants were highly motivated and carefully instructed in diaphragm use have yielded 98.6 percent effectiveness rates.[103] The sponge, on the other hand, has only yielded 86 percent to 92 percent effectiveness in the manufacturers' studies and rates ranging from 8.7 to 14.1 pregnancies per 100 woman-years in international and domestic tests.[104] Perhaps the women in these tests were not as highly motivated or carefully instructed in use of the method as were the women in the best of the diaphragm tests. It may be that further tests with such participants will yield effectiveness rates for the sponge that are as high as the diaphragm rates. On the other hand, perhaps the pregnancies that occur with the sponge are owing to method failure rather than user failure, and the effectiveness rates will remain the same regardless of how conscientious, how motivated or how carefully instructed the sponge users are. At the present time, however, it is misleading to say that the sponge is as effective as the diaphragm. Still, it is a convenient method with many advantages, so a 92 percent effectiveness rate—the best reported effectiveness rate—may be acceptable for some women.

How to Use the Sponge

The sponges have a loop for removal on the underside and come in individually wrapped packages. To use, take the sponge out of the package and moisten with water. Be sure to moisten it well, as this is necessary to activate the spermicide. Then, fold the sponge in half so the removal loop is on the outside and the cuplike depression is on the inside, in the same way you would fold a diaphragm for insertion (*see* Illustration 21). Next, push the sponge up into the top of the vagina. The cuplike depression covers the cervix, and the vaginal walls hold it in place. The sponge is expandable and pliable and does not have to be "locked" into place, as does the diaphragm. It molds to the contours of the woman's vaginal anatomy. According to the manufacturer, the sponge even accommodates itself to the expansion of the upper third of the vagina during sexual arousal (*see* p. 136), making its chances of being dislodged during intercourse less likely than with the diaphragm. The manufacturer further claims that even if the sponge is dislodged, the spermicide and the sponge's absorbency will still protect against pregnancy.

Once inserted, the sponge provides continuous contraceptive protection for 24 hours. It can therefore be inserted many hours before intercourse. If a woman's partner is going to ejaculate again, there is no need to insert more spermicide, as there is with the diaphragm or foam. The spermicide in the sponge is effective for 24 hours, regardless of how many times the man ejaculates.

The sponge must be left in place for at least 6 hours after the last act of intercourse. To remove the sponge, simply pull on the removal loop, and the sponge will come right out, just as a tampon comes out when you pull on the string. After removal the sponge should be thrown away; it should not be reused. Sponges should not be flushed down the toilet, as they may clog the plumbing.

The sponge's manufacturer originally planned to market the sponge as the "2-Day" sponge, which could be left in place for 48 hours. Laboratory tests indicated that the slowly released spermicide would remain effective for 48 hours. But in the actual-use effectiveness tests, women generally removed the sponge after 24 hours, perhaps because they did not need contraceptive protection any longer, perhaps because of odor problems from leaving it in longer or perhaps because they were in the habit of removing tampons at least that frequently. At any rate, because so many women in the effectiveness tests removed it after 24 hours, the FDA would not approve it for 48-hour use.[105] Therefore, the manufacturer changed the name of the sponge and recommended that it be removed after 24 hours.* If future tests prove the sponge is effective for 48 hours, this recommendation may change.

Advantages and Benefits

The chief advantage of the sponge is convenience. Because it can be inserted as long as 24 hours before intercourse, it does not interrupt the spontaneity of lovemaking, as do the diaphragm, condom, foam or other barrier methods. It only costs about a dollar, can be purchased without a doctor's prescription and lasts for 24 hours, regardless of how often you have intercourse during that time (again, unlike the other barrier methods).

Because it contains spermicide the sponge probably has the same advantages as vaginal spermicides (*see* pp. 148–149), such as protection against sexually transmissible infections and cervical cancer. Unlike the Pill or the IUD, it has not been shown to cause serious complications or side effects. Also, unlike the Pill or the IUD, which are based on a day-to-day usage, the sponge is used only when you plan to have intercourse.

Disadvantages and Problems

The sponge has only recently come on the market, so drugstores and grocery stores in your area may not yet have it in stock. If you have a problem getting sponges, contact Planned Parenthood or other family-planning clinics or write to the manufacturer (Vorhauer Laboratories, Inc., 130 McCormick Avenue, Bldg. 104, Costa Mesa, California 92626) to find out where you can buy sponges.

The best effectiveness rates reported so far are not as good as the best rates for other barrier methods. Because most sponge-related pregnancies occur in the first 3 months of use, some authorities suggest using a back-up method in the first months of sponge use.

*During the effectiveness tests the sponge was sometimes called the "Secure Vaginal Contraceptive Sponge."

Some couples find that the taste of the spermicide in the sponge is unpleasant, which is a problem for couples who like oral-genital sex. Some couples find that the spermicide provides too much lubrication, which cuts down on sexual pleasure. (Conversely, some find the extra lubrication a plus.) Some women have allergic reactions to spermicides, and any itching or burning associated with the spermicide in the sponge should be reported to the doctor. Just as it is uncommon for a woman to be allergic to the material used in the diaphragm or condom, so it is uncommon for a woman to be allergic to the sponge material.

Women with certain problems, such as prolapse of the uterus or vagina, cannot use sponges.

The biggest drawback to sponge usage are the concerns voiced by two consumer groups* who have petitioned the FDA to withdraw approval of the sponge pending further tests.[106] The concerns of these groups center around two possibilities. The first is that the sponge may lead to toxic shock syndrome (TSS), which is based on the fact that tampons—devices also left in the vagina for considerable periods—can cause TSS. The manufacturer counters this possible TSS/sponge connection by pointing to the laboratory studies showing that the sponge kills the organism that is presently thought to cause TSS.[107] However, recently there were 5 cases of TSS in women using the contraceptive sponge. Although these five cases alone don't prove a connection between the two, there is at least some reason to think that the sponge may be associated with TSS.

The second, more serious possibility the consumers groups have voiced centers around the polyurethane in the sponge.[108] Polyurethane has been shown to cause cancerous lesions in mice. The FDA is now reconsidering approval in light of these objections. New information should be forthcoming, but it is unlikely that the FDA will withdraw approval. To confirm or deny possible cancer effect from the sponge could take many years of use by large numbers of women.

Women who are particularly concerned about the theoretical possibility of the polyurethane causing long-term cancerous effects might want to avoid the sponge until more is known. Indeed, women who want to use the safest method of birth control might want to consider natural family planning (see below).

*The two consumer groups are the Associated Pharmacologists and Toxicologists (Washington, D.C.) and the Empire State Consumer Association (Rochester, N.Y.).

CERVICAL CAP

AKA: birth control pessary

The cervical cap is a device that looks like a thimble for a giant-sized finger. It fits right over the cervix and is held in place by suction. The cap works by mechanically blocking the sperm and by acting as a holder for spermicides (the same type used with the diaphragm), which are put into the cervical cap before insertion. The cervix swells slightly from the pressure of the cap and forms an airtight seal. It is believed that this allows the spermicide to stay active for a considerable period. Therefore, the cap can be inserted well in advance of intercourse and may be left in place for a number of days.

The cap is made of firm rubber and is widest at its open end, which has a thick, semirigid rim. The two types of cap presently available are the "Prentif" Cavity Rim Cap and the Vimule Cap, which come in a number of sizes.

At the present time the cervical caps used for birth control are manufactured only in England, so they are not widely used in the United States.* They were manufactured in the United States during the late fifties and early sixties; however, the popularity of the Pill and the IUD eclipsed the cervical cap. Since there was not sufficient demand, the manufacturer stopped making the device. With the growing evidence of the side effects and consequences of the Pill and the IUD, there has been a renewed interest in the cervical cap, which, unlike the other barrier methods of birth control, doesn't require insertion immediately before intercourse.

Little is known about the cervical cap, and there are a number of unanswered questions about its effectiveness, use and safety. It is not known, for instance, how long the spermicide inside the cap remains effective. There is also some question as to how much, if any, spermicide should be put inside the cap and how long the cap can be worn without changing it. The cap appears to be much safer than the Pill and the IUD, however, and much less intrusive to use than the diaphragm, condom or foam. For these reasons it has been championed by concerned doctors and women who are active in the health-care movement.

---

*A device that is also called a cervical cap and that is used to treat infertility problems is manufactured in the United States, but it is not designed to be used for birth control.

Effectiveness

According to the Planned Parenthood Federation of America, the cervical cap is about as effective as a diaphragm.[109] Some authorities believe that the cervical cap may be more effective than the diaphragm. Because it fits right on the cervix, they think that the cap is less susceptible to being dislodged during intercourse, as sometimes happens with the diaphragm when the upper portion of the vagina expands during sexual excitement. Others believe that the cap may be more easily dislodged.

Valid effectiveness rates are not available, because no large-scale, long-term studies have been done. The last major study was done in 1953 on a group of 143 women using old-style plastic caps.[110] The overall use effectiveness rate in this study was 7.6 pregnancies per 100 woman-years of use, which included the women who used the cap incorrectly, inconsistently or not at all. For those women who claimed to have used the cap regularly and correctly, the rate was 3.2 pregnancies per 100 women using the cap for 1 year. Some of these failures might have resulted from the cap's having been dislodged during intercourse, which is less likely to happen with today's rubber caps, since their suction grip is tighter than that of the plastic caps used in this study. Moreover, the researchers could not follow up on all the women that they fitted with caps. Those who became pregnant might have been more likely to stay in contact with the doctor than those who did not, and this may have biased the effectiveness rates.

An informal, unpublished study of 165 women fitted with caps found that 6 of the women became pregnant, all during the first 2 months of use.[111] In other words, about 96 percent of the women fitted did not become pregnant. Studies are now being done to evaluate the cap's effectiveness, so more data may soon be available.

Fitting a Cervical Cap

Correct fit is essential, and although the person doing the fitting does not have to be a doctor, special training is required. Unfortunately, very few people in the United States have been trained to fit cervical caps. Fees vary, but many doctors charge more to fit caps than to fit diaphragms, because correct fitting and instruction in use require more of the doctor's time. The person fitting the cap will first look at the cervix with a speculum to determine its size. After selecting the proper cap, the fitter places it on the cervix and checks the suction to make sure that the cap fits correctly. Caps a size larger and a size smaller than the one selected should be tried as well in order to ensure the best fit.

After the cap has been fitted the woman should practice inserting and removing it until both she and the person doing the fitting are confident that she has mastered the process. The woman should not be aware of the cap once it is in place.

Some women, approximately 20 percent, cannot wear caps. Women with deep cervical lacerations or extremely long or extremely short cervixes can't be fitted with cervical caps. Some doctors believe that women with cervical erosions or eversions, especially those that are congenital rather than ac-quired, should not wear cervical caps. Others think that the cap may actually aid in healing erosions. Women who have erosions and who use the cap should practice gynecological self-exam so that they can monitor the effect of the cap on their cervixes and discontinue use if their condition worsens. Such women may not want to leave the cap in as long (that is, they may want to use it the same way you'd use a diaphragm) until the erosions heal.

Some women's cervixes change size over the course of the menstrual cy-cle. This cervical swelling is usually rather slight, and most authorities be-lieve that it shouldn't cause any problems. Others think that perhaps some women should have two caps, one to be worn at the time of ovulation and the other to be worn during the rest of the month.

Women with active cervical or vaginal infections should not be fitted for a cap until the infection is cleared up, since the infection might cause the cervix to swell, resulting in an incorrect fit.

Childbirth, miscarriage or abortion can alter the cervix; the cap should be refitted after any of these occurrences. Even though it might become slightly discolored, if the cap is cared for properly it will be good for a number of years.

How to Use the Cervical Cap

Before the cap is inserted (Illustration 25) it should be from one-third to two-thirds filled with spermicide. The same spermicides that are used with a dia-phragm can be used with the cap, although some doctors argue that creams are preferable to jellies because they last longer in the cap. Some authorities recommend that the cap be one-third full, because they feel that too much spermicide will affect the suction. Others favor the cap being two-thirds full, believing that the moisture from the spermicide tightens the seal and makes for better suction. Some authorities recommend that the spermicide be smeared around the inside rim as well, but others have found that this causes the cap to become dislodged.

The cap can be inserted in a number of positions. Some women like to stand up, with one foot raised and resting on a chair, bathtub or bed. Other women like to squat or to recline halfway.

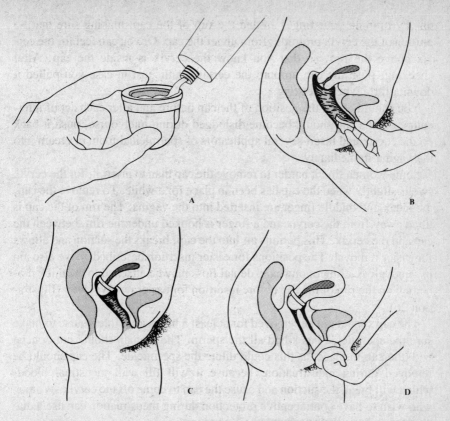

Illustration 25 *Inserting the Cervical Cap: The spermicide is placed in the cap (A), inserted into the vagina (B), guided along the back wall of the vagina and fitted over the cervix (C). Use your finger to feel for the cervix under the cap (D).*

The cap is compressed between the thumb and forefinger of one hand, while the other hand spreads the lips of the vagina apart. The cap, with the open end first, is then inserted into the vagina and slid along the back wall until it reaches the top of the vaginal cavity. Use one or two fingers, whichever is easiest for you. Care must be taken not to spill the spermicide out of the cap. The cap is then released and pushed onto the cervix.

If you have difficulty reaching your cervix, squat and bear down as if you were having a bowel movement or push down on the abdomen above the pubic hair. These maneuvers will bring the cervix to a lower position.

The cervix will not fill the cap completely. The extra space in the dome of the cap will hold the spermicide and cervical secretions. This extra space may collapse or it may not, but either way, suction is not affected.

After inserting the cap, check to see that the cervix is covered. You can do

165

this by running your finger around the rim of the cap, making sure that no portion of the cervix protrudes from under the cap. Or you can feel for the cervix above the rim, so that you know the cervix is inside the cap. After checking, push the cap up onto the cervix again, just in case you pulled it down a little when checking.

You should check the position of the cap before and after each act of intercourse. If the cap should become dislodged during intercourse, push it back on the cervix and insert several applicators of spermicidal foam or cream into the vagina immediately.

Some women find it harder to remove the cap than to insert it, for the cervix swells slightly when the cap has been in place for a while. To remove the cap, the index and middle finger are inserted into the vagina. The rim of the cap is tilted away from the cervix and a finger is hooked under the rim, between the cap and the cervix. This permits air into the cap, breaks the suction and allows for easier removal. The positions for easier insertion described above also aid in removal. A string of unwaxed dental floss may be attached to the thick rubber tab on the rim of the cap before insertion for easier removal later (Illustration 26).

The cap should not be removed for at least 8 hours after intercourse to make sure the spermicide has killed all the sperm. The woman should not douche with the cap in place, as this could dilute the spermicide. The cap should be removed during menstruation, because it will fill with menstrual blood, which will break the suction and cause the cap to come off the cervix. Women who wish to have contraceptive protection during menstruation can use a diaphragm or have their partners use a condom.

The cap should be inserted at least a half hour before intercourse to allow time for cervical swelling and the formation of the suction seal. Exactly how long before intercourse the cap can be inserted is a matter of debate. It is thought that the airtight seal created by the cap helps the spermicide to remain

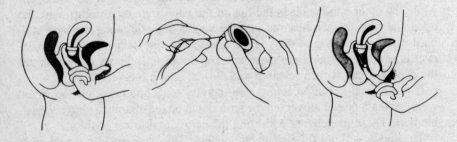

Illustration 26   *Removing the Cervical Cap: Hook your finger over the edge of the rim to break the suction. Some women attach a piece of dental floss to the rubber ridge to aid in removal.*

effective for a longer time than it does with the diaphragm. Some doctors allow as long as 7 days, provided that the first time the woman uses the cap she removes it after 3 days and checks to see that it is still at least one-third full of spermicide. If it is, she then refills the cap to two-thirds full and checks it again after 5 days. If the cap remains at least one-third full, she repeats the process after 7 days. (Always use a condom as back-up protection during this ''checking period.'') If the cap is still one-third full, her maximum time for leaving the cap in place would be 7 days; if it is not, her maximum time would be shorter. The time the cap is left in place should not exceed 7 days, for the effectiveness of the spermicide after that is questionable. Many cap fitters believe that the cap should not be left in place for longer than 3 days; others say 5 days. Still others don't think it is necessary to use spermicide at all.

Some women use the cap in the same way a diaphragm is used, except that they insert it several hours or even a day or so before intercourse. Other women like to take the cap out every day or every other day. They think that replacing the spermicide gives them more protection and that washing the cap is more hygienic. Some women develop odor problems if the cap is left in for longer than 24 hours; others can go 3, 5 or even 7 days without developing odors. If odors do develop, the cap can be washed with soap and water or vinegar or soaked in a solution of dilute lemon juice or alcohol. Some women add a drop of chlorophyll to the inside of the cap before insertion to prevent odor problems.

Removing the cap also allows the cervical secretions to flow freely, which may prevent vaginal infections. Although some doctors believe that the cap can be refilled and reinserted immediately, some women like to leave it out for at least several hours to give the cervical secretions a chance to flow.

Once the cap has been removed it should be washed in soap and water, patted dry with a towel and, if it isn't going to be replaced immediately, stored in a clean, safe place. The cap should never be boiled. It can be soaked for 15 minutes in alcohol or vinegar to prevent odors. Dusting with cornstarch makes the cap last longer. Talc should not be used, for it could be irritating and is not water soluble, so it can't be washed off easily. Vaseline, cold cream or other greasy products should not be used with the cap, because they will deteriorate the rubber. A water-soluble, nongreasy lubricant like K-Y jelly or spermicide, which can be purchased without a doctor's prescription, can be used if lubrication for intercourse is desired.

Disadvantages and Problems

One problem with the cap is availability. The cap is not approved as a birth control device. The FDA classifies it as an investigational device, and the dispensing of caps is limited to the relatively small number of facilities and individuals who have applied to the FDA and been granted an IDE (investigational device exemption). Women who cannot find a women's health center, college health service, public clinic or private doctor in their area who has an IDE can write to the FDA (HFK-470 Bureau of Medical Devices, FDA, 8757 Georgia Avenue, Silver Spring, Maryland 20910) and request a list of IDEs granted for the cervical cap.

Another problem is that about 20 percent of the women whose particular anatomies do not conform to the caps presently available cannot be fitted for caps.

In some rare cases there may be an allergic reaction to the material that the cap is made from or to the spermicide. Changing brands can usually solve allergy problems.

Some women's sexual partners complain that they can feel the cap if they thrust deeply, and in some cases this causes some discomfort for the man. This probably results from the penis's hitting the little tab of thick rubber on the rim of the cap and can sometimes be avoided by making sure the tab is facing backward, so that the penis doesn't hit it.

Although some clinics report high effectiveness rates and a high level of satisfaction among users, other clinics report high discontinuation rates.[112] Some women have difficulty inserting or removing the cap. This, of course, limits the usefulness of the cervical cap for such women.

The effectiveness rates for the cap have not been clearly established. Since the pregnancies that do occur with the cap seem more likely to occur in the first 2 months, some cervical cap fitters recommend that women use extra spermicide in the vagina or that the man wear a condom at least around the woman's ovulation time (*see* p. 65) for the first 2 months.

In one study some users of the Vimule cap developed cervical and vaginal abrasions, probably from the sharp edges on the rim of the cap.[113] Women in the study who used Cavity Rim caps did not have this problem. No one knows what sorts of long-term problems, if any, such abrasions and lacerations might cause. But women should be aware that these problems exist for some Vimule cap users, and that some authorities believe that these caps should not be used until more is known.

In another study the majority of women who left the cap in for longer than 3 days developed a vaginal discharge and odor, so some researchers think the cap should not be left in for longer than 3 days.[114]

Although no one is too concerned about using the cap pretty much as you would use a diaphragm, some researchers are concerned about leaving the cap in for 3, 5 or 7 days at a stretch and then replacing it again right away. The degree to which the normal, constant downward flow of the cervical mucus may be altered is unknown. Some doctors worry that keeping the mucus up next to the cervix instead of flowing down the vaginal walls might foster bacterial growth on the cervix, causing infections. One study did show inflammatory changes in the Pap smears of half the cap users in the study, but the women in the study had worn the cap continuously for $2\frac{1}{2}$ weeks.[115] There is no evidence that shorter-term use of 3 to 7 days causes such problems.

Because of the concern that obstructing the mucus flow could lead to problems, and because of the problems with fitting about 20 percent of women, Dr. Robert Goeppe and Dr. Uwe Fresse have developed a custom-fitted cap with a one-way valve that obstructs sperm but permits the flow of cervical and menstrual secretions.[116] A wax impression of the woman's cervix is made, and a special machine laminates a silicone cap in a matter of minutes. The developers hope that women will be able to wear the cap for months without having to remove it. The Contracap, as it is called, is now being tested for safety and effectiveness. The initial results look good, so in the not-too-distant future a cervical cap that alleviates many of the disadvantages and problems associated with the present cap may be available.[117]

Advantages

The cap can be inserted well in advance of intercourse and left in the vagina for a number of days, so there is no need to interrupt the spontaneity of lovemaking in order to insert the cap. This convenience also means that the cap is less likely to be forgotten, as might be the case with the condom, diaphragm or spermicidal foam.

Since the vagina is not full of spermicide (as it is with the diaphragm), oral-genital lovemaking is more pleasant than with the diaphragm.

The cap is inexpensive, probably quite effective when used properly and safe. Although there have been a few minor side effects, the cap has not caused a single death. It can be used by many women whose anatomies preclude the use of the diaphragm.

NATURAL FAMILY PLANNING

AKA: NFP, periodic abstinence, fertility awareness method, FAM, natural or organic birth control, cooperative birth control

Associated Terms: rhythm, or calendar rhythm, method; cervical mucus, or Billing's, method; basal body temperature, BBT, or thermal method

Natural family planning (NFP) can be used either to prevent pregnancy or to maximize the chances of conceiving for those women who want to get pregnant. Women can get pregnant only during a certain period of time in each cycle, and that period generally occurs about 2 weeks before the onset of the next menstrual flow. Women who use this method of birth control learn to determine when they are fertile and either abstain from intercourse during this time or use another method of contraception.

NFP is based on certain biological facts:

- ☐ Ovulation occurs quite consistently about 14 days before the next menstrual period begins, regardless of the length of your menstrual cycle.
- ☐ There is occasionally a 2-day variance either way, so ovulation may occur 12 to 16 days before the first day of the menstrual flow.
- ☐ Sperm are capable of surviving for 3 days or, according to some experts, for 5 days.
- ☐ The female ova live for only 12 to 24 hours or, according to some experts, for 36 hours.
- ☐ Once ovulation has occurred, the hormone progesterone is produced in increasing amounts, which causes a rise in body temperature.
- ☐ The character of the cervical mucus undergoes changes both before and after ovulation.

Because a woman can get pregnant for only a certain amount of time before and after ovulation, NFP depends on two factors: (1) predicting when ovulation will occur, so that a woman can avoid intercourse before ovulation for the 3 (some say 5) days of the sperm's lifespan; and (2) being able to recognize when ovulation has occurred, so that a woman knows when it is safe to resume intercourse. The days before ovulation, when a woman is infertile and it is therefore safe for her to have intercourse, are called the early safe days, and the days after ovulation, when she is again infertile, are called the late safe days.

NFP encompasses three methods for predicting when ovulation will occur and recognizing when it has happened: the rhythm method, the basal body temperature chart and the cervical mucus method. (**IMPORTANT NOTE:** The following information is only a *basic* description of NFP. You will need more instruction from a trained counselor to use this method effectively. What you learn from a trained counselor may differ in specific details from what is described below. Rely on what you learn from your counselor, and do not use this method until you have been carefully instructed by a trained counselor.)

The Rhythm Method

The rhythm method can be used alone, without the other components of NFP, but unless safe days are calculated by the strictest method (see below), it is not a dependable method of birth control (*see* Effectiveness below). It can be used to calculate both early and late safe days, but unless a woman is using only this method, the late safe days are not as important, for NFP provides other ways of determining these days.

Calculating Early Safe Days

In order to use the rhythm method you must know the length of your menstrual cycles for the previous 6 to 12 months. To calculate your early safe days, subtract 14 days from the length of your shortest cycle, since ovulation usually occurs 14 days before the first day of the following cycle. Now, subtract 2 more days just in case, as sometimes happens, you have ovulated 16 days before the first day of your next cycle. Next, subtract 3 more days to allow for the life span of the sperm, since sperm deposited before ovulation could still be alive in your reproductive tract 3 days later. There is some evidence that sperm have a life span of 5 days, so if you want to be extra careful subtract 5 days. Altogether you will be subtracting 19 days (or 21 days if you're figuring on a 5-day sperm life span) from the length of your shortest cycle. The resultant figure will be the last of the early days of your cycle on which you can safely have intercourse.

This can be expressed in the following formula:

$$(S = \text{the length of your shortest cycle})$$
$$S - 19 = \text{last of the early safe days}$$
$$\text{or}$$
$$S - 21 = \text{last of the early safe days}$$

Table 5 lists the safe days for various cycle lengths. Example: Jeanenne's shortest menstrual cycle in the past 12 cycles was 25 days long. Subtracting 14 days puts her at Day 11, the day on which she probably ovulated. Subtracting 2 more days puts her on Day 9, the earliest she is likely to have ovulated. Subtracting 3 more days to allow for the life span of the sperm would put her at Day 6. If she allowed for a 5-day sperm life span, that would put her at Day 4.

Table 5
Early and Late Safe Days as Calculated by the Rhythm Method

If your shortest cycle has been:	The last of your early safe days would be:	The first of your late safe days would be:
21	Day 2	Day 11
22	Day 3	Day 12
23	Day 4	Day 13
24	Day 5	Day 14
25	Day 6	Day 15
26	Day 7	Day 16
27	Day 8	Day 17
28	Day 9	Day 18
29	Day 10	Day 19
30	Day 11	Day 20
31	Day 12	Day 21
32	Day 13	Day 22
33	Day 14	Day 23
34	Day 15	Day 24
35	Day 16	Day 25
36	Day 17	Day 26

$$S-19 = \text{last of the early safe days}$$
$$25-19 = \text{Day 6}$$

or

$$S-21 = \text{last of the early safe days}$$
$$25-21 = \text{Day 4}$$

Using the rhythm method, Jeanenne could safely have intercourse from Day 1 (the first day of her menstrual flow) to Day 4 or Day 6 without using any protection.

Calculating Late Safe Days

To calculate the late safe days of the cycle, subtract 14 days from the length of your longest cycle. Then, add 2 days to that figure in case you actually ovulated 12 days before the first day of the following cycle. Next, add 1 more day to allow for the 24-hour life span of the ova. Some authorities believe that the ova can survive for 36 hours and suggest adding 2 days. If, to be safe, you have added 2 days to allow for the life span of the sperm, you would then be subtracting a total of 10 days from your longest cycle. If, however, you are using the rhythm method in conjunction with other NFP techniques, this is not necessary, since there are other more accurate ways of determining postovulatory safe days.

These calculations can be stated in the following formula:

$$(L = \text{the length of the longest cycle})$$
$$L-10 = \text{the first late safe day}$$

Table 5 lists the safe days for various cycle lengths. Example: Jeanenne's longest cycle was 31 days. Subtracting 14 days would put her at Day 17, the day she probably ovulated. Adding 2 days just in case, as sometimes happens, she ovulated 12 days, instead of 14 days, before would put her at Day 19. Adding 1 more day to allow for the life span of the ova would put her at Day 20, the last day of her cycle during which she would be fertile:

$$L-10 = \text{the first of the late safe days}$$
$$31-10 = \text{Day 21}$$

So Jeanenne could resume unprotected intercourse on Day 21.

The Strictest Method

There is another method of calculating early safe days that is quite simple: no days before ovulation are considered safe. In Jeanenne's case this would mean that she could have unprotected intercourse only from Day 21 of her cycle on. If she had a 25-day cycle, she could have unprotected intercourse for the last 5 days of that cycle. If she had a 31-day cycle, she could have unprotected intercourse for the last 11 days of her cycle. If a woman is using other methods of birth control on her unsafe days, this might be acceptable and has the advantage of greatly increasing the effectiveness of the method (see below), but for women who are abstaining on their unsafe or fertile days, this method of calculating, which would severely restrict sexual activity, might be too limiting.

Basal Body Temperature

The basal body temperature, the temperature of the body at complete rest, drops about 24 hours before ovulation in 50 percent to 60 percent of women and then rises and generally stays elevated throughout the rest of the cycle. Thus your basal body temperature may indicate when ovulation is about to occur. Because it provides only a one-day warning, it cannot be used to calculate early safe days, since sperm can survive in the reproductive tract for 3 or, possibly, 5 days. It may, however, indicate that ovulation has occurred and is therefore of use in calculating late safe days.

In order to determine your late safe days by this method, you will need a chart like the one shown in Illustration 27, which is available at pharmacies (or you can make your own with graph paper), and a thermometer. Either an oral or a rectal thermometer may be used, and the temperature may be taken orally, rectally or vaginally. Do not switch back and forth, as there may be a variation of a degree or two that could make the chart difficult to interpret.

A standard fever thermometer, which runs from 94° to 108°F and has a mark every two-tenths of a degree, can be used, but most women prefer to use a basal body temperature thermometer (BBT), which runs from 95° to 100° and is marked off in tenths of a degree, making it easier to read. BBTs can be purchased at a pharmacy without a prescription.

Taking and Recording Your Basal Body Temperature

The temperature reading must be taken first thing in the morning, before you get out of bed, smoke a cigarette, talk or do anything else. Your basal body temperature is the temperature of your body at complete rest. Even slight activity may cause a rise in temperature. Shake your thermometer down the night before (some authorities say the energy required to do this is negligible but suggest that you do it then to guard against breaking the thermometer in the early, groggy hours of the morning).

After leaving the thermometer in your mouth (or rectum or vagina) for about 5 minutes, take it out, read your temperature and record it on the chart.

It is not necessary to record your temperature on the first few days of your cycle, while you are still bleeding. Mark those days with an X, as shown in Illustration 27. Start to record your temperature as soon as the menstrual flow stops.

Once you have read your temperature, record it on the chart by making a dot where the vertical date column joins the horizontal temperature column. Connect the dots with straight lines, as shown. If you occasionally miss a day, make a note on the chart. Likewise, if you are forced out of bed before taking your temperature (a ringing phone, a crying child or whatever) or are unable to or have forgotten to take your temperature, note this on the chart.

Interpreting the Chart

The chart shown in Illustration 27 is an easy one to interpret. Yours is apt to be more complex, but for now, consider this chart. The Xs indicate the days of the menstrual flow. The first temperature of 97.6°F was recorded on Day

174

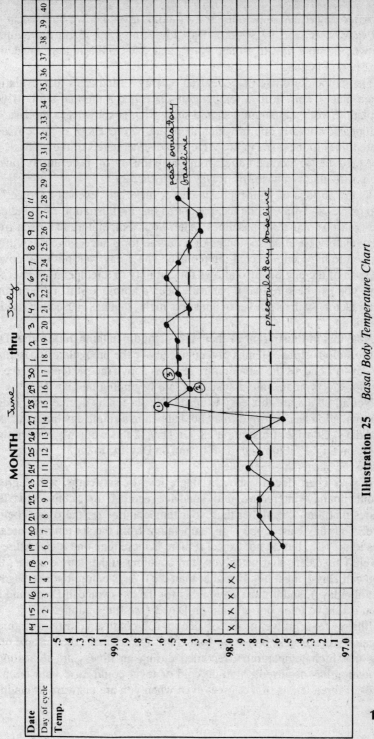

Illustration 25 *Basal Body Temperature Chart*

6. After Day 6 the temperature sort of jumps up and down but basically stays between 97.6° and 97.9° until Day 15. From Day 15 on the temperature shows a definite rise, to around 98.6°, and stays in this higher range until the next period begins.

The temperature rise that occurred on Day 15 indicates that ovulation has taken place. This shift in temperatures is called a thermal shift. If you are ovulating, your temperature should show what is known as a biphasic curve. A biphasic curve is one in which there are two levels or distinct areas. The dotted lines in the chart indicate the two distinct levels of the biphasic curve. The preovulatory temperature, from Day 6 to Day 14, is definitely lower than the postovulatory phase, from Day 16 to Day 29.

To get an idea of your biphasic curve, make an "eyeball average" of the two phases and draw a line like the dotted line in Illustration 27 to indicate the pre- and postovulatory baselines. After your temperature has risen from the preovulatory baseline six-tenths of a degree for 3 successive days, it is safe for you to have unprotected intercourse. The 3-day wait not only covers the lifespan of the egg but also allows for certainty of a temperature rise. After 3 days you can be sure that it has truly been a hormone shift rather than some other factor, such as a fever or a restless night, that has caused the rise in temperature.

Note that in Illustration 27 there is a slight dip in temperature after Day 15, but this dip is still six-tenths of a degree above the preovulatory baseline, and on days 17 and 18 the temperature remains above the six-tenth degree range. So, for this woman, intercourse was safe beginning on Day 18.

Not all charts are this easy to read. The six-tenths-degree rise, indicating that ovulation has occurred, may not happen in a single day but may take several days. Consider Illustration 28. On Day 12 this woman's temperature was 97.7; on Day 13 it jumped to 98.0, and on Day 14, to 98.3°. It took 2 days to make the six-tenths-degree leap.

If your chart doesn't show a single leap of six-tenths of a degree, you should not have intercourse until you have recorded three consecutive temperatures that are .4°F higher than your temperatures for the 6 days before the rise. You may cancel one high temperature from the six temperatures previous to the rise, but do not cancel if there is more than one temperature at that level. This means that when you start counting higher temperatures, the day you call Day 1 must be .4° higher than the 6 days before the rise began (or 5 out of 6 days), and it must stay higher for the days you call Day 2 and Day 3. You can have intercourse again on Day 3 (*see* Illustration 29).

Illness, fever, travel or use of alcohol can confuse your temperature readings. If you are sick, note it on your chart. Do not make the mistake of thinking that high temperatures recorded during an illness are indications that ovulation has occurred. A slight cold or fever could raise your temperature two- or three-tenths of a degree, even when you are unaware of having a fe-

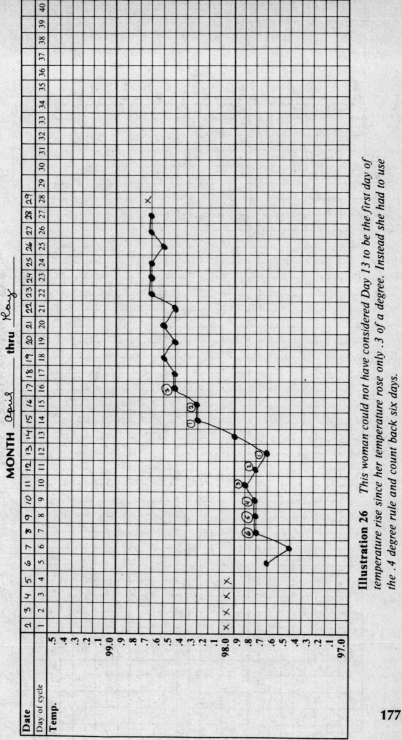

Illustration 26 *This woman could not have considered Day 13 to be the first day of temperature rise since her temperature rose only .3 of a degree. Instead she had to use the .4 degree rule and count back six days.*

177

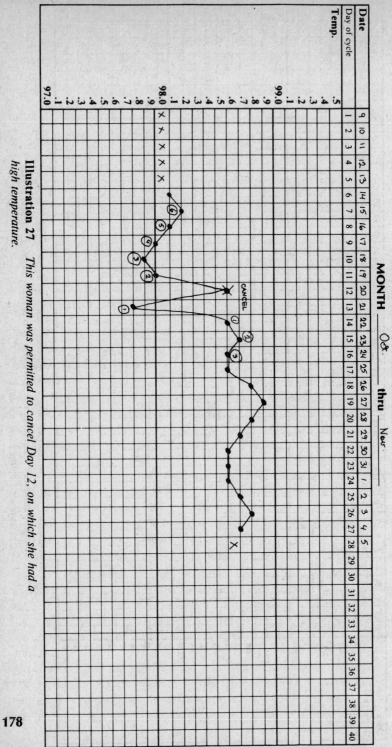

BASAL TEMPERATURE CHART

MONTH ___ Oct. ___ thru ___ Nov. ___

Illustration 27   *This woman was permitted to cancel Day 12, on which she had a high temperature.*

178

ver. You should not have intercourse for 3 days after you are *sure* your illness has passed. Remember also that illness during one cycle can cause early or late ovulation during the following cycle, so be especially careful during the subsequent cycle. You might, for instance, want to use the strictest calendar rhythm method and not calculate any early safe days the following month.

The Cervical Mucus Method

The cervical mucus method can be used to predict when ovulation will occur and to confirm BBT evidence that ovulation has taken place. As explained in Chapter Four, mucus secreted by the cervical glands changes over the course of the cycle. In the early days of the cycle, when estrogen levels are low, the secretions are scant and the vagina is dry. As ovulation approaches and estrogen levels rise, the cervical secretions become more abundant and the vagina feels increasingly wet. The character of the secretions also changes from a dry, pasty, tacky texture, gradually becoming creamier, until just before ovulation, when it changes to a slippery, thinner, more watery type of mucus. The pasty, thick secretions are rather acid and hostile to sperm. On a molecular level, the structure of this type of mucus is crosshatched and prevents sperm from passing through the cervix into the uterus. The more abundant, thinner secretions that occur later, just before ovulation, are more alkaline and favorable to sperm. The molecules that make up the mucus have rearranged themselves to form tubes, or tunnels, to facilitate the sperm's passage through the cervix (see the illustrations on p. 64). This type of mucus is the most fertile and can be stretched between your thumb and forefinger into a clear, shimmering, delicate strand or thread before breaking. The term "spinnbarkeit," or spinn, is used to refer to this type of mucus.

Illustration 30 shows the four types of mucus conditions you may notice over the course of your menstrual cycle. For purposes of this method of birth control, there are two types of mucus: fertile and infertile. The only time the mucus can be considered infertile is in condition I (Dry), when the vaginal opening is dry. No one is certain whether Condition II (Early Mucus) is fertile or not, so it must be considered as fertile mucus for purposes of birth control.

The Mucus Cycle

The mucus cycle in most women works something like this: Day 1 through Day 5 there is bleeding from the menstrual period. Right after the period, secretions are almost absent and the vagina feels dry. These 2, 3 or more dry days are followed by the expulsion of a mucous plug from the opening of the cervix. The small, sticky plug may not be noticed, but after its expulsion the vaginal lips feel wet. For some women the first mucus after the dry days is

179

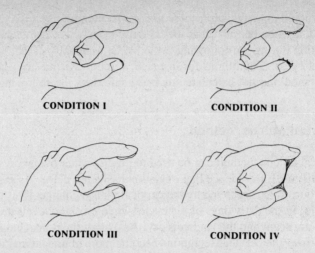

CONDITION I   CONDITION II

CONDITION III   CONDITION IV

Illustration 30 *Condition I: dry, infertile mucus; Condition II: pasty, tacky mucus, possibly fertile; Condition III: slippery, wet, fertile mucus; Condition IV: spinnbarkeit, very fertile. Intercourse is safe only during Condition I.*

white and sticky or tacky. Although this creamy mucus is probably not fertile, it can quickly change to slippery, fertile mucus. (Besides, "probably not fertile" is not too reassuring when you're talking about birth control, so it should be considered fertile.) By the day of ovulation or the day preceding it the mucus takes on the classic spinn character. Its appearance has been compared to the white of an uncooked egg—somewhat gelatinous, slippery and translucent.

After ovulation the secretions become creamier and less slippery. Some women have dry days after ovulation; others have a more variable pattern that changes from dry to wet to creamy. Illustration 31 indicates a typical mucus cycle.

Observing Your Mucus Cycle

Each woman is different, and your pattern may not correspond to the typical pattern described above. Women with very short cycles may not have any dry days after menstruation. Those with long cycles may have 5 or 6 dry days. Some women never see spinn mucus. Before relying on this method you should observe your patterns for at least 6 months.

You will need to keep a daily record of your secretions. Some women can observe their mucus symptoms by merely noting a feeling of wetness or dryness. Others touch the inner lips of the vagina or note the discharge on their underclothes. Still others insert a finger into the vagina and take a sample of

MENSTRUAL CHART

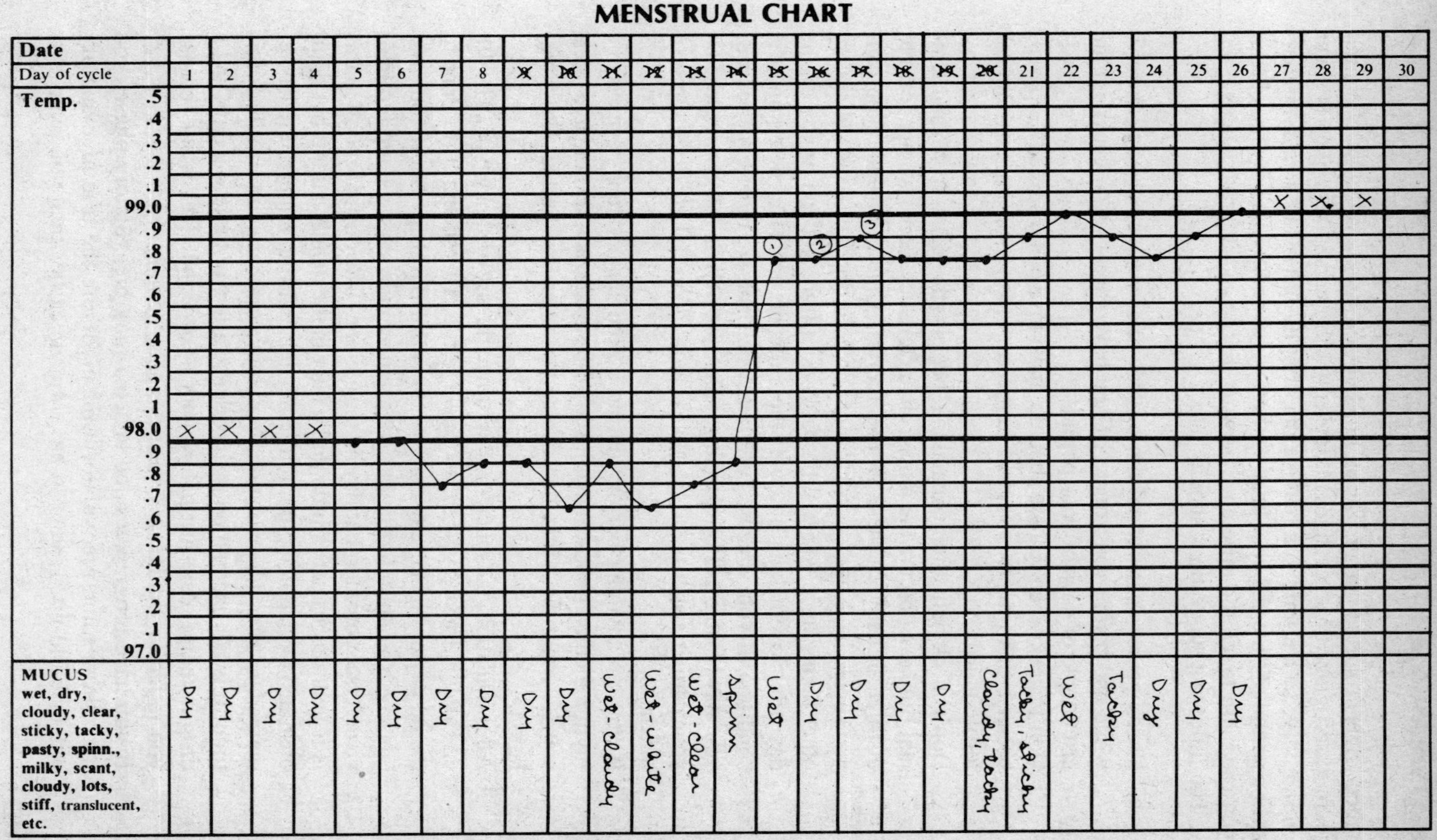
Date
Day of cycle
1 2 3 4 5 6 7 8 9 10 11 12 13 14 15 16 17 18 19 20 21 22 23 24 25 26 27 28 29 30
Temp.
.5 .4 .3 .2 .1 99.0 .9 .8 .7 .6 .5 .4 .3 .2 .1 98.0 .9 .8 .7 .6 .5 .4 .3 .2 .1 97.0
MUCUS
wet, dry, cloudy, clear, sticky, tacky, pasty, spinn., milky, scant, cloudy, lots, stiff, translucent, etc.
Dry
Dry
Dry
Dry
Dry
Dry
Dry
Dry
Dry
Dry
Wet-cloudy
Wet-white
Wet-clear
spinn
Wet
Dry
Dry
Dry
Dry
Cloudy, tacky
Tacky, sticky
Wet
Tacky
Dry
Dry
Dry

Illustration 29 *Chart combining BBT, Rhythm and Cervical Mucus Methods*

mucus right from the cervix. If you practice self-exam, you will be able to learn to recognize these changes more easily. Of course, the vagina is never entirely dry, so the term is a relative one, but by observing your symptoms over a period of time and coordinating them with the BBT and rhythm charts, you can learn to tell the difference between fertile and infertile mucus.

The following suggestions should help:

☐ Check your mucus several times a day after you've been awake for a while and before you urinate. If you have short cycles, check on the last couple of days of your period.

☐ Don't check when you are about to make love or are sexually aroused, because this produces vaginal lubrication that could be mistaken for fertile mucus.

☐ Don't check right after lovemaking, because the man's sperm and seminal fluid can obscure the mucus characteristics. Some women learn to distinguish between these two secretions. Unless, or until, you can, you should have intercourse at night on your dry days—and only every other night, since you will probably be a little wet and drippy on the day after lovemaking and will therefore be unable to determine the condition of your mucus. Later on, when you are more experienced, you may be able to stop skipping a day, but only if you always lose all your partner's sperm and ejaculate before noon and are dry the rest of the day.

☐ If you are anything but dry during a preovulatory time, even if the rhythm method indicates that it should be a safe day, do not have intercourse; your mucus may be warning you of an unexpected, early ovulation.

☐ After ovulation, the mucus will return to the dry or sticky type. The 4th day after it dries up you are no longer fertile. This should correspond to the 3d day of higher temperatures on your BBT chart. But if your mucus says you are infertile and your temperature says you are fertile or vice versa, consider that day an unsafe one. The one exception to this is if your mucus gets a little milky later in the month, after it has demonstrated ovulation (spinn, fertile mucus) and your temperature has remained up after this ovulation. You may consider yourself safe at this time. It is not uncommon to experience a few of these wet days and a drop in temperature just before your next period. This is not because you're fertile, but because your period is coming.

☐ If you have long cycles and hence a long preovulatory phase, you may show some preovulatory mucus before the true preovulatory mucus build-up. If you do have mucus earlier than you expect it, don't have unprotected intercourse on that day and for 3 days after you become dry again. Then you can go back to having intercourse every other night, as long as the rhythm method indicates that it is a safe day.

☐ After your temperature and mucus have both demonstrated that ovulation has occurred two days previously, you can resume having intercourse every day, if you choose, until the end of your cycle. Any mucus you might have from then on is not fertile.

Recording and Interpreting Your Mucus Symptoms

You can record your mucus symptoms on a chart like the one shown in Illustration 31. Use descriptive words like creamy, wet, white, clear, sticky, slippery, spinn, milky, scant, cloudy, profuse or translucent.

The cervical mucus method can be used alone. This is particularly valuable for nursing mothers and women approaching menopause whose BBT charts are apt to be rather meaningless, since they may not be ovulating regularly.

Effectiveness

Unfortunately, there are no good studies of how the rhythm, BBT and cervical mucus methods work when used in combination. The calendar rhythm method used alone has produced rates ranging from 14 to 47 pregnancies per 100 woman-years of use. The BBT method has produced rates ranging from less than 1 to 20 pregnancies per 100 woman-years of use. The mucus method has produced pregnancy rates ranging from 1 to 25 pregnancies per 100 woman-years of use. Using the BBT and having intercourse only on the late safe days after ovulation has occurred has produced rates ranging from 1 to 7 pregnancies per 100 woman-years of use.[118] The combination of all three methods would undoubtedly improve these figures.

How to Use Natural Family Planning

NFP can be used in two ways: by abstaining from sex on the unsafe days or by using one of the barrier methods, such as foam, diaphragms, condoms or cervical caps on the unsafe days. Women who choose to use NFP in combination with a barrier method on unsafe days should be aware that the effectiveness of the barrier methods may be significantly reduced when they are not used consistently during each act of intercourse. Nonetheless, some women who dislike these barrier methods are willing to compromise on effectiveness as long as some days of unprotected intercourse are available to them during each cycle. We would encourage women who decide to use NFP in this manner to calculate their early safe days by the strictest calendar method and not have unprotected intercourse until after ovulation has occurred.

In order to use NFP you should mark off your early safe days as calculated by the calendar rhythm method on a chart, as shown in Illustration 31. This woman's shortest cycle in the previous 9 months was 27 days long. She allowed for a sperm life span of 3 days in making her calculations, so her last early safe day would be Day 8. Her longest cycle was 31 days, so the first of her late safe days would be Day 21. The intervening days were marked off with Xs on the line marked Days of the Cycle.

Next, record your mucus and temperature observations each day. This woman had dry days until Day 10. But she could not have intercourse after Day 8, since that was the last of her safe days according to her calendar rhythm calculations. If she had noticed fertile mucus before Day 8, she would likewise have had to discontinue having unprotected intercourse. If any of the methods indicate that an early day is an unsafe day, you should discontinue unprotected intercourse.

This woman had a temperature jump on Day 15, and her temperature remained high for 3 days, so she was able to resume intercourse on Day 17. In calculating late safe days you may ignore the calendar rhythm days and resume unprotected intercourse after you have recorded three high temperatures. If, however, your cervical mucus shows signs of spinn or maximum wetness on that day, you may not resume intercourse. If, on the temperature rise day that you call Day 1, you still have spinn mucus or a lot of wetness, wait until the spinn has gone or the wetness has dried up before counting Day 1. If your mucus indicates fertility but your temperature chart indicates a safe day, do not have unprotected intercourse. Similarly, if your temperature indicates not safe but your mucus says safe, do not have unprotected intercourse.

Using this method may seem rather difficult, but people who use it claim that it becomes automatic once it is incorporated into the daily routine. We recommend that couples who are interested in this method not rely solely on the instructions given in this or any other book. It is best to have personal instruction from a doctor, medical professional or couples who have practiced the method successfully. We suggest that people who are interested in information about NFP and training in the use of this method contact Natural Family Planning Federation of America, Inc., Suite A, 1221 Massachusetts Avenue NW, Washington, DC 20005 or Planned Parenthood. Some chapters of Planned Parenthood offer classes in NFP; contact your local chapter for information.

Advantages

NFP is completely safe. It poses no threat to the user's health and has no effect on long-term fertility. NFP is inexpensive and is acceptable to the Catholic Church and religious groups that are opposed to other methods of contraception.

NFP enables women to tune in on their cyclical patterns and to learn more about how their bodies work. It may open couples up to alternative forms of sexual pleasuring on the days when intercourse is not safe. It does not require the use of any apparatus, such as an IUD, or harmful medications, such as the Pill, and is a completely natural, organic method of birth control.

Disadvantages and Problems

Some people find the extra time and attention required to keep these charts too bothersome. Other people have schedules that are too irregular or too hectic to allow them to incorporate this method of birth control into their life-styles.

Another problem is that you must accumulate at least 2 months of records and charts before you begin to use this method of birth control. The Pill, which alters normal BBT curves and cervical mucus patterns, cannot be used during the time you are establishing your charts and records. Using spermicides either with or without a diaphragm may present difficulties in establishing the cervical mucus patterns. IUDs can also distort cervical mucus patterns. This leaves only the condom, the strict calendar method or abstinence as birth control choices during the months you are learning to establish your cycles.

Douching, infection, semen and lubrications can make it difficult to recognize cervical mucus patterns. Some women do not have recognizable cervical mucus or BBT patterns.

There has been some concern that women using this method might have a higher rate of birth defects.[119] Intercourse is avoided before and after ovulation, but should ovulation occur unusually early or late, the egg or sperm involved might not be a fresh one. Studies on laboratory animals have shown that the rate of birth defects is higher in such pregnancies.[120] In addition, the incidence of birth defects is higher among Catholics than among Protestants.[121] Neither of these facts proves that couples using the rhythm method are more likely to give birth to abnormal infants should the method fail. Moreover, chances of such a pregnancy occurring are reduced when the BBT and cervical mucus methods are combined with the rhythm method. Still, the possibility of increased risk of birth defects should be considered by couples using NFP.

VASECTOMY

AKA: male sterilization

Vasectomy, or male sterilization, is a surgical procedure in which the vasa deferentia, the internal tubes that carry sperm from the testes to the penis, are severed. It is considered a permanent, irreversible form of birth control, although in some cases it has been possible to perform corrective surgery to restore a man's fertility. The severed tubes can be rejoined in 40 percent to 90 percent of cases (this figure varies according to which type of vasectomy was performed and the skill of the surgeon doing the repair), but not all these men will actually be fertile again. One study involving small numbers of men who were particularly likely candidates found that 69 percent of the men were successfully able to impregnate their partners after corrective surgery. Other studies have reported considerably lower rates. In the largest study the success rate after corrective surgery was only about 19 percent.[122]

There are also sperm banks where sperm can be frozen and stored. More than 500 normal infants have been born as a result of using frozen semen, the greatest success being with sperm stored less than 6 months, although pregnancy has been achieved using sperm stored for as long as 10 years.[123] Most investigators, however, question the viability of sperm stored longer than 3 years. Moreover, sperm banks are hard to find and several have gone bankrupt or closed for lack of financial success. Any man considering a vasectomy should not count on the possibility of reversing the operation or of using frozen sperm specimens.

It may be difficult for a young man, especially a single one who has never fathered any children, to find a doctor willing to perform a vasectomy on him. The Association of Voluntary Sterilization (708 Third Avenue, New York, New York 10017) has a referral service.

Finding an experienced doctor to perform the vasectomy is important. Many of the complications—although these are rare—can be prevented by having the operation performed by an experienced doctor.

Effectiveness

Although vasectomy is not completely foolproof (studies in the late sixties reported failure rates as high as 4 per 100), today, with improved techniques, the failure rates are less than 1 per 100.[124] When failure does occur it is most often because the cut ends of the tube have rejoined. Occasionally, when the procedure is done by an inexperienced doctor, the wrong structure is cut or the ends of the tubes are not tied or clipped tightly, permitting sperm to leak through. In some instances a man will have more than two vasa deferentia (singular form, vas deferens), and thus one may be missed. Because some sperm remain in the tubes and it takes a number of ejaculations before all the sperm are cleared out, unprotected coitus before two consecutive negative sperm counts could also cause pregnancy.

Procedure

Vasectomy is a minor surgical procedure that takes about 15 minutes and can be done in a doctor's office under local anesthetic. Fees range from about $150 to $300.

The scrotal area is shaved, a local anesthetic is injected and either one or two small incisions are made, as shown in Illustration 32. Next, each of the vasa deferentia is located, pulled out through the incision and cut. The loose ends are then tied, burned or clipped. Most doctors remove a small portion of the vas to assure that the loose ends will be kept apart and won't grow back together. The incision in the scrotum is closed with absorbable sutures that dissolve in 7 to 10 days.

After a successful vasectomy the sperm produced in the testes are blocked from passing beyond the point of the operation. These sperm simply dissolve. Because sperm accounts for only 10 percent of a man's ejaculate, or come, the volume of ejaculation is not noticeably affected.

There may be some slight problems after the vasectomy. Skin discoloration—a bruise—is common and is caused by blood seepage. This usually occurs in the scrotal area but may involve the penis or, less frequently, the groin and inner thighs. There may be some associated swelling. Ice packs should be applied to the area for at least 4 hours after the operation. Neither of these complications requires any special treatment, and both subside within a few days or, at the most, a few weeks.

Although seldom severe, there may be pain or discomfort either when the local anesthetic is injected, when the vas is pulled into view or when the procedure is over. Pain sometimes occurs during the first intercourse after vasectomy, and in some cases it may persist for a few months during both erection and ejaculation. Ice packs will help reduce the initial discomfort, swelling and bruising. Aspirin can be taken for pain. Hot sitz baths taken four times a day will help promote healing and relieve discomfort. One week after the procedure there should be a postoperative checkup so the doctor can be sure that everything is healing properly.

Most men experience a moderate amount of pain and discomfort on the day of surgery and on the day after. A man should not plan to drive himself home after a vasectomy. Returning to work is not advised for 3 days after the vasectomy if the man has a sedentary job, or for 7 days if he performs manual labor. Strenuous activity should be avoided for at least a week. It's a good idea to wear an athletic supporter day and night for the first 48 hours and thereafter as long as it is more comfortable to wear it than not to wear it. Sexual intercourse may be resumed after 2 or 3 days, as long as it feels comfortable to do so.

After the procedure there are still some sperm left in the vasa deferentia and seminal vesicles (the sperm "storage tanks") that must be emptied before a man can rely on his vasectomy for contraception. It can take anywhere from 6 to 20 ejaculations to empty all the active sperm. Most doctors will ask a man to bring a sample of sperm after 8 to 10 ejaculations and then a second one after another series of ejaculations. Not until two negative ejaculation samples can a man consider himself sterile, and other forms of birth control must be used until this is accomplished.

In addition to the minor problems of pain, bruising and swelling mentioned earlier, there are other possible complications from the vasectomy. A hematoma, a mass of clotted blood, may form in the scrotal area. This occurs in less than 4 percent of all vasectomies.[125] and can be prevented by careful surgery and by avoiding heavy straining for several days after the vasectomy. Most small hematomas reabsorb spontaneously. Ice packs can usually be used to treat those that do not. In less than 1 percent of the cases it becomes necessary to reopen the scrotum, drain off the blood and tie off the bleeding vessel.

Infections, ranging from superficial skin infections to deeper ones, occur in less than 1 percent of the cases[126] and can usually be prevented by proper surgical sterilization by the doctor and cleanliness on the part of the man; however, a man should not shower or bathe for the first 2 days after vasectomy. Antibiotics and bed rest can be used to treat these rare cases of infection. Other rare complications include adhesions (scar tissue), hydrocele (a collection of fluid around the testes owing to surgical injury), orchitis (inflammation of the testes), epididymitis (inflammation and tenderness near the testes) and sperm granuloma (generally small and harmless accumulations of "leaked" sperm, which, in rare instances, may become infected). Some of these complications have no symptoms, whereas others require antibiotics and bed rest or, in some cases, minor surgery. If a man experiences a fever over 100°F, bleeding from the incision site and/or excessive pain and swelling, he should contact his doctor.

It is interesting but hardly surprising that although these relatively minor complications associated with vasectomy are given a great deal of attention in both medical and lay literature on the subject, complications of similar importance (for example, bruising and subsequent infection of incision scars) are never even mentioned in most discussion of female sterilization procedures.

Advantages and Benefits

Vasectomy is the simplest, cheapest, safest, most effective method* of birth control. There have been no significant long-term side effects, although many millions of operations have been done. The complications rate is low, only 2 percent to 4 percent, and most of these are short term and minor.[127] The operation takes only about 15 minutes and, in most cases, can be performed in the doctor's office.

Disadvantages and Problems

In addition to the minor problems of swelling, bruises and pain and the rare complications (generally short term and minor) mentioned earlier, there are several other disadvantages and problems associated with vasectomies.

First of all, not all men can have vasectomies. Men with previous hernia surgery; a thick, tough scrotum; a fixed, undescended testis; a hydrocele (collection of fluid around the testis) or a varicocele (varicose vein) are not good candidates for vasectomy. Any local infections or problems should, of course, be cleared up before the vasectomy is attempted.

Moreover, about one-half to one-third of all vasectomied men develop antibodies to sperm, that is, their own bodies produce an immunity that inhibits sperm activity.[128] Although similar antibodies have been found in normal fertile men, they are more common in infertile men and in men who have had vasectomies. There is some controversy as to the importance of these sperm antibodies. The immunological response of the human body is not well understood. Although there is no such evidence to date, some authorities theorize that sperm antibodies may attack something other than sperm and note that other irregularities in the immune system have been associated with such con-

*Actually, hysterectomy, or removal of a woman's uterus, is slightly more effective, but we do not recommend such a major operation for the sole purpose of birth control.

ditions as arthritis. Time will tell whether vasectomized men develop a higher incidence of immunological disorders in old age.

Although the majority of men who have had vasectomies report an improvement in their sex lives (probably owing to freedom from fear of pregnancy and the hassle of other methods of birth control), a small number of men experience a decline in their sex drive or inability to achieve and/or maintain an erection.[129] Most authorities believe that this relatively uncommon problem is psychological and can be prevented by careful preoperative counseling to make sure that the man is not harboring such fears about the vasectomy. Another problem with vasectomies is that, in rare cases, the partner of the sterilized man may experience a decrease in sex drive. For such women the act of intercourse may be so tied up with conception that once pregnancy is no longer a possibility, sex becomes less pleasurable. Again, preoperative counseling involving the partner might help to prevent this problem.

Studies of vasectomized men have only rarely indicated that impotence (inability to achieve and maintain an erection) is a problem for vasectomized men. One recent study, however, has raised the possibility that there may be a long-term link with impotence and vasectomy.[130] This study was conducted with 42 men being evaluated for impotency problems. Although the study was not concerned with vasectomy per se, about 33 percent (14) of the men had had vasectomies, many of which had been performed 20 or more years earlier. A control group of men without impotency problems had only a 9.8 percent rate of vasectomy. The question, then, arises, Why was the percentage of men with vasectomies in the impotency group more than three times as high as that in the general population? Is there something about a vasectomy that could lead to impotency? Although short-term studies have not detected impotency problems, would longer-term studies reveal a link with impotency and vasectomy? Most researchers do not think so, pointing to the fact that this study involved only small numbers of men; that the impotent, vasectomized men may have other factors that caused their impotence; and that vasectomized men may be more apt to take better care of their health and thus be more likely to seek help for an impotency problem. They also point to a study of more than 4,385 vasectomized men who had had their vasectomies performed more than 10 years earlier.[131] The incidence of sexual problems in the men in this study was no higher than in the control group of nonvasectomized men. More studies are needed, however, before we can say with certainty that there is no link between impotence and vasectomy in at least a certain portion of men.

Another area of concern involves atherosclerosis and vasectomy. Two studies done on monkeys indicated that vasectomized monkeys had more extensive and severe atherosclerosis than did nonvasectomized monkeys.[132] Because atherosclerosis is linked with heart disease, these studies raised a great deal of concern. Several studies done on vasectomized men have failed to reveal the same type of problem found in the monkeys, but the studies done thus far on humans may not have been long term enough or involved large enough numbers of men to allow us to conclude that there is no link between vasectomy and atherosclerosis in humans. Still, the general consensus among researchers seems to be that there is little threat of vasectomy leading to heart disease. No one is recommending that vasectomies *not* be performed; however, some researchers are suggesting that men who are at high risk of developing heart disease (those who smoke; who have high blood pressure, family or personal histories of heart disease, high cholesterol levels, diabetes; who are overweight) might want to wait until there is more information about vasectomy and atherosclerosis before undergoing vasectomies.

FEMALE STERILIZATION

AKA: tying the tubes, tubal ligation, tubal sterilization

Types: minilaparotomy, or Pomeroy technique
laparoscopic sterilization, Band-Aid sterilization or
belly-button surgery
colpotomy

Female sterilization is a method of birth control that involves removing or blocking some portion of the female reproductive tract. In the past, hysterectomy, an operation that removes the uterus, tubes and sometimes the ovaries as well, was a standard procedure for the sterilization of a woman. Although hysterectomies are, unfortunately, still done by some doctors for the sole purpose of sterilization, we do not recommend them. Federal funds can no longer be used for such hysterectomies. Hysterectomies have considerably higher complication rates, anywhere from 10 to 100 times higher, than the less radical procedures now available. Even though the risks facing a young, healthy woman are not all that great, hysterectomy is more expensive, requires a longer recovery time and may be more difficult to adjust to emotionally than the other types of sterilization. Any woman whose doctor suggests a hysterectomy for sterilization should read the section on hysterectomy carefully and should seek a second medical opinion (*see* p. 238) before consenting to the operation.

Less drastic procedures, which involve blocking or cutting the fallopian tubes, have recently been developed and have become increasingly popular.

191

Indeed, for married couples over age 30, sterilization has become the most commonly used method of birth control in the United States.

Sterilization Abuse

Women who are considering sterilization, especially minority and low-income women, should be aware of the controversy surrounding sterilization abuse. Since 1970 female sterilization has increased almost threefold, and poor and minority women are heavily overrepresented. Twenty percent of the married black women in the United States have been sterilized versus 7 percent of the married white women. Fourteen percent of native American women have been sterilized. In Puerto Rico one-third of all women of childbearing age have been sterilized. The United States has widely financed and promoted sterilizations in Third World countries as well.[133]

Consent forms have been pushed at women in the throes of labor and at women under the influence of anesthetics and drugs. In some cases written consent was not even obtained or women were mistakenly led to believe that the operation was not permanent and that their tubes could be untied sometime in the future. Other women were told that they would die if the procedure was not done. Still other women have been forced into sterilization by being threatened with having their welfare benefits cut off.[134]

A number of doctors believe that overpopulation has become such a problem that, for them, it is acceptable practice to trick or coerce women into being sterilized. Indeed, a survey that polled gynecologists in four major cities indicated that 94 percent of the doctors responding favored compulsory sterilization for welfare mothers with three or more illegitimate children.[135] Women who are interested in learning more about sterilization abuse and how to prevent it can contact the Committee to End Sterilization Abuse, CESA, Box A244, Cooper Station, New York, New York 10003.

Making the Decision

Every woman considering sterilization should know that it is a permanent method of birth control. It means that she could not have children in the future. Although there have been some cases in which the tubes were repaired after sterilization, these reparative operations involve risks and are usually unsuccessful. At present no dependably reversible form of sterilization exists, even though some people mistakenly believe that certain types of rings or clip sterilizations are easily reversible. A woman should never have a sterilization procedure done with the idea that it can be fixed later on. Both she and her partner, if she has one, must be certain that permanent sterilization is what they want.

A woman should also know that at any point she has the right to change her mind about having the procedure done—even after she has signed the consent form—and that no one can deprive her of any benefits, such as welfare or medical payments, because she has refused the operation.

Through the efforts of female health-care activists and doctors concerned about sterilization abuse, certain rules for sterilization operations funded by the federal government have now been established. First, you must be at least 21 years of age. You must wait at least 30 days after you have signed the consent form to have the operation, except in some special instances, such as premature delivery or emergency abdominal surgery that takes place at least 72 hours after the consent is obtained. (This is done to prevent unnecessary second surgeries.) Also, a woman's consent to sterilization cannot be obtained while she is in the hospital for childbirth or abortion or under the influence of alcohol or any other substance that might affect her state of awareness. A woman may, if she chooses, bring someone with her when she signs the consent form. The consent form is effective for 180 days from the date on which it is signed. If a woman has questions or if something is not clear to her, she has the right to have all her questions answered and to have a translator available if she speaks a foreign language.

Although sterilization has sometimes been forced on minority and poor women, many white, middle-class women have had difficulty finding a doctor who will perform the operation on them. It is no longer necessary for a woman to have the legal consent of her husband in order to be sterilized. Still, some doctors are reluctant to perform sterilizations on such women, especially if they have no children and sometimes even if they already have two or three children. Any woman having difficulty finding a doctor to perform a sterilization operation can contact a local Planned Parenthood or Zero Population Growth office or can write or call the Association for Voluntary Sterilization, 14 West 40th Street, New York, New York 10018 (212-524-2344).

Couples considering sterilization should know that despite the publicity surrounding so-called Band-Aid sterilization, female sterilization is a major surgical procedure with significantly higher risks, more potentially serious complications and higher costs than the male sterilization procedure, vasectomy. A couple considering sterilization should seek counseling on both methods before they make their final decision.

193

Effectiveness

Other than abstinence, that is, not having intercourse at all, sterilization is the most effective method of birth control. Surprising as it may seem, however, it is not 100 percent effective. If failure does occur, it is usually because the woman was already pregnant at the time of the sterilization, the tubes have grown back together or a ligament rather than a tube was cut or tied off. But these are rather uncommon occurrences, and the failure rates for all the various methods of sterilization are said to be about 0.04 percent.[136] Certain techniques have a slightly higher rate than others, but pregnancy rates for all forms of sterilization are lower than those obtained with any other method of birth control.

Methods of Sterilization

Tubal sterilization procedures, which interrupt the fallopian tube, are now the preferred methods for female sterilization. Traditionally, this has involved ligation (tying of the tube), which may be accompanied by excision (cutting away) of a piece of the tube. More recently, electric coagulation (burning), elastic bands and rings and/or clips have been used to close the tubes.

Tubal sterilization can be done by either a vaginal or abdominal route or approach, depending on how the doctor decides to get at the tubes to close them off. In the vaginal approaches, such as colpotomy and culdoscopy, an incision is made in the vagina. But the vaginal approaches have higher complication rates, so the abdominal approaches are more commonly used. If your doctor proposes a vaginal approach, be sure to ask why and to seek a second opinion if the answer isn't satisfactory. The two most widely used abdominal approaches are the minilaparotomy, involving an incision in the abdomen, and the laparoscopic tubal ligation, which makes use of another special viewing instrument, the laparoscope.

Before Surgery

Before the operation the doctor will take a detailed medical history, which should include complete information about previous problems with anesthesia, bleeding disorders, allergies and any medications currently being taken. Any history of sexually transmissible infections, pelvic infections or previous surgery should also be noted, for any of these conditions may result in pelvic scar tissue or adhesions that could complicate certain methods of performing tubal sterilization. Most doctors recommend that IUDs be removed before surgery to decrease the chances of infection. The Pill, which increases the risk of blood clots, should be discontinued for at least a month before surgery, and another form of contraception should be used. A complete physical to identify any medical conditions that might alter the decision about surgery or anesthesia, is also done before surgery. A gynecological exam is given to identify pelvic disease, such as fibroids, that might complicate surgery or indicate the need for alternative surgery. Laboratory tests, including a Pap smear, which should be normal, a blood count and urinalysis, are done. Although not all doctors do it, it is a good precaution to have preoperative bleeding and clotting-time tests done and to have a specimen of blood held in the blood bank in case transfusion is needed during surgery. We also recommend chest X-rays, even if a woman is having a local anesthetic, in case some complications during the operation should require a general anesthetic. The chest X-ray will rule out possibly dangerous conditions that could contraindicate general anesthesia.

Before the operation the area where the incision is to be made is scrubbed with an antiseptic solution. If the approach is abdominal, the area is shaved, and if the incision is to be made near the pubic hair, most or all of the pubic hair will be shaved to prevent infection. All food, solids and liquids are prohibited for 8 hours before surgery so that the stomach will be empty in case an emergency occurs and a general anesthetic is required. Some doctors will also order a preoperative enema. In some cases the doctor will empty the bladder by way of a tube known as a catheter before surgery. This makes some forms of sterilization operations easier for the doctor. However, the introduction of the tubal catheter also increases the chance of postoperative urinary tract infection, so some doctors will merely have the woman empty the bladder herself immediately before the operation.

Either a local or a general anesthetic can be used for most tubal ligations. If a general anesthetic is used, a tube is inserted down the throat after the woman is put to sleep, which will help the anesthesiologist control her breathing. Local anesthetics may be injected into the incision site. Although there may be a slight prick from the first injection, subsequent injections can't be felt; however, there may be some discomfort when the fallopian tubes are pulled into view by the doctor. Spinal anesthetic, which temporarily immobilizes the legs, or, preferably, epidural anesthetic, which allows for movement of the legs, may also be used in some tubal sterilization procedures. The anesthetic is injected into the lower back so that there is no pain at the operative site but the woman will still be awake. The epidural doesn't have the disadvantage of the excruciating headache that sometimes follows the spinal, but the epidural

195

is more difficult to administer and not all anesthesiologists are equally skilled at it.

If a general anesthetic is used, about a half hour before surgery a shot is given that contains a tranquilizer and a drug that dries up secretions in the mouth and throat that might cause breathing problems. Even if only a local anesthetic is planned, the drug to dry up secretions may still be given in case serious bleeding complications necessitating prolonged surgery occur and a general anesthetic is then needed. Because of the possibility of complications that might require a general anesthetic, some doctors feel that the anesthesiologist should be at hand during the operation. This is particularly important in a laparoscopic tubal ligation, even if it is done under a local anesthetic.

Either a local or general anesthetic can be used for most sterilizations; however, even though a general anesthetic involves more risks, most doctors prefer it, since if emergency surgery is required, there is no time lost giving a woman a general anesthetic and inserting the tube into the windpipe. Moreover, some doctors think that a woman is apt to move when the tubes are grasped if she has only had a local anesthetic, which could lead to complications in the operation.

Laparoscopic Tubal Ligation

As mentioned earlier, there are a number of different techniques for tubal sterilization. In recent years the laparoscopic tubal ligation (*see* Illustration 33), also called Band-Aid sterilization, has become increasingly popular. The laparoscope is a lighted viewing instrument that can be inserted into the abdomen and used to locate the fallopian tubes. After the anesthetic is given, a tiny incision is made at the bottom of the navel. Next, a long, thin needle is inserted into the abdomen. The needle is then attached to a tube, which in turn is connected to a machine containing either carbon dioxide or nitrous oxide gas. The gas is run through the tubing into the abdominal cavity until the abdomen is so swollen and firm that it sounds like a drum when tapped. The gas moves the intestines out of the way and makes it easier for the doctor to see the pelvic organs and to close off the tubes without injuring any other tissue. If only a local anesthetic is used, the woman may experience a feeling of bloating and mild to moderate discomfort as the abdomen fills with gas.

An instrument known as a trocar, which is enclosed in a special sleeve, is then inserted through the incision. The trocar is removed, leaving the special tubelike sleeve in place. When the trocar is removed an audible *whoosh* of gas may be heard. After the trocar has been removed the laparoscope is inserted through the sleeve, and the light source and gas tub-

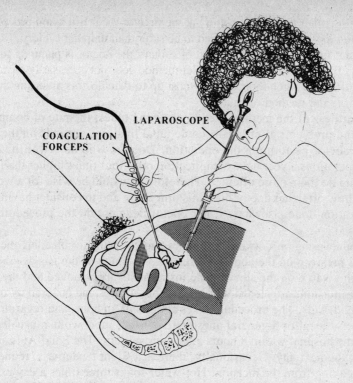

Illustration 33 *Laparoscopic Tubal Ligation*

ing are attached to it. Most doctors then make a second incision lower in the abdomen and insert a smaller trocar in a sleeve. The electric coagulation tool (if coagulation is the method used to close the tubes, see below) is inserted through this sleeve. If a local anesthetic is being used, more anesthetic is first injected, but even with adequate local anesthetic the woman is likely to feel more discomfort from this incision than from the first incision. Other doctors use only one incision, and the coagulation equipment is introduced through this incision as well.

The fallopian tube is then grasped with the forceps of the coagulation tool. Once the doctor is sure that the intestines or other tissues are not near the tube and in danger of being accidentally burned, s/he pushes a button or pedal that activates the electric current from the electric cautery machine. The short burst of electricity causes the fallopian tube to burn and turn white. The doctor may then pull slightly on the forceps to break the tube in half. Some doctors prefer to burn the fallopian tube in several locations rather than pulling on it to separate the pieces. A new type of cautery, bipolar cautery, is used by some doctors and has cut down on the dangers

197

of burning other tissue (see below) at the time of the sterilization procedure. Because bipolar cautery has proved to be safer than unipolar cautery, women may want to inquire which method of cautery the doctor is planning to use. The fact that a doctor uses the unipolar method does not necessarily mean that s/he will not do a good job, but the most up-to-date doctors are using the superior, bipolar method of cautery.

Regardless of the method used to close the tubes, the rate of complications and problems after laparoscopic tubal ligations depends on the skill of the doctor performing the operation. Doctors who do fewer than 100 such operations a year have complication rates four times higher than doctors who do them more often.[137] Therefore, it would be wise for a woman to ask how often her doctor does this procedure and to consider having her sterilization done elsewhere if her doctor does not do the procedure frequently.

After severing or blocking both tubes and checking for bleeding the doctor, by pressing on the abdomen, releases as much of the gas as s/he can through a valve on the sleeve. The instruments are removed and the incision or incisions are closed with absorbable sutures and covered by one or two Band-Aids. The procedure takes about half an hour, and regardless of whether a local or a general anesthetic is used, most women usually can leave the hospital within 8 hours after their surgery. The Band-Aids are removed the next day. Occasionally, there is a slight tenderness, redness or fluid leaking from the incision. Hot-water soaks three times a day usually will clear this up.

Minilaparotomy

Another abdominal procedure, the minilaparotomy (Illustration 34), or minilap, involves inserting an instrument through the cervix and into the uterine cavity in order to push the uterus up against the lower wall of the abdomen. An abdominal incision is made directly over the top of the elevated uterus, and the tubes are then brought into view. Next, the doctor cuts, ties, burns or clips the tubes. A special instrument that looks like a small vaginal speculum may be inserted through the incision to help the doctor see the tubes. This operation also takes about 30 minutes, and the hospital stay usually is less than 24 hours.

Colpotomy and Culdoscopy

Vaginal tubal ligation (Illustration 35) can be performed by colpotomy. "Colpotomy" is a term used to refer to any operation in which an inci-

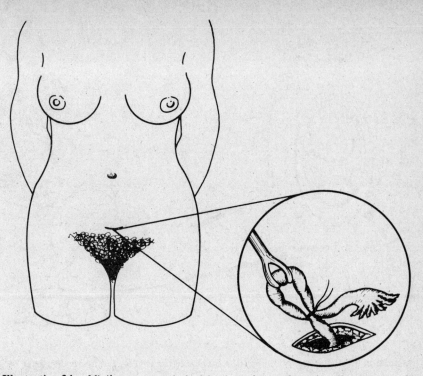

Illustration 34   *Minilaparotomy: An incision is made just above the pubic-hair line. The tube is pulled through the incision. A loop of the tube is sutured shut with the Pomeroy technique and then the top part of the loop is cut away.*

sion is made in the vagina just below the cervix. Once this is done the tubes may be brought out through the incision and then tied. The incision is then stitched up. The procedure takes about half an hour. This operation has the advantage of not leaving any visible abdominal scar. After the operation the woman usually can go home on the same day, but this is not always possible.

Women who have enlarged uteri, which includes all women who have just given birth, cannot have this operation, for the tubes would be too far away to be reached through the vaginal incision. If the woman has had previous abdominal surgery or has a history of pelvic inflammatory disease, there may be too much scar tissue for the colpotomy to be done safely. It is also easier to do this operation on women who have had children previously.

The problem with this method is that the complication rate is about twice as high as with abdominal tubal ligations. The complications (see below) can include bleeding, acute chronic pelvic infection, chronic pelvic pain

199

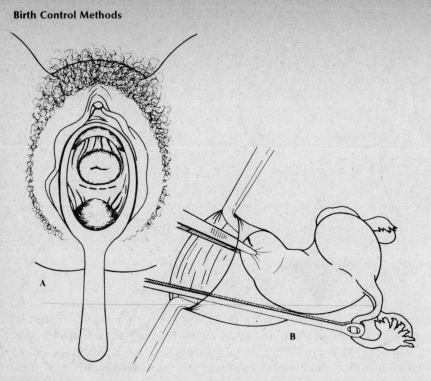

Illustration 35 *Colpotomy: An incision is made in the vagina, just below the cervix (A). The cervix is lifted up and held steady while a grasping instrument is used to locate the tubes (B).*

and chronic pain on intercourse, even when the operation is done by a well-trained, experienced gynecologist. In the hands of a novice the complication rates may be extremely high. When complications do develop they are potentially more serious than those following abdominal tubal ligation, and the postoperative pregnancy rates are slightly higher.

Culdoscopy, the other vaginal approach, requires a great deal of skill and experience on the part of the doctor. Since laparoscopy has been developed, this method of sterilization is rarely used anymore.

Methods for Closing Off the Tubes

With laparoscopic procedures the tubes usually are coagulated (burned). Because this method sometimes involves serious complications, some doctors have recently been using rings, clips or bands instead. Although this avoids the risks associated with coagulation, these devices may not be as effective in preventing future pregnancies. Coagulation is never used for vaginal approaches. Usually, the Pomeroy technique is used for colpotomy or laparotomy. The Pomeroy technique involves elevating a knuckle of the tube (*see* Illustration 34) and tying a suture just below the knuckle. By the time the suture is absorbed, several weeks later, the two stumps have healed, leaving a gap in the tube.

After Surgery

Most women experience some pelvic pain and discomfort after surgery. There may be abdominal and shoulder pain resulting from gas and air pressing on abdominal organs or on the diaphragm, but this shouldn't last longer than 24 to 48 hours. There may be soreness around the incision site. With the vaginal procedures, sexual intercourse is prohibited for 3 to 4 weeks to give the incision time to heal. For the abdominal procedures, intercourse can be resumed whenever the woman feels comfortable, usually within a week. Even if a local anesthetic has been used and a less extensive procedure has been done, the woman should not plan to drive herself home afterward, and she will need to rest for at least 24 hours. She should not expect to resume regular activities for a minimum of 2 to 3 days or, in some cases, for a week or so and should avoid straining or lifting heavy objects for at least 1 week. The doctor will have specific instructions about bathing, showering, intercourse and the use of tampons.

The stitches do not require removal, for they will dissolve themselves. There should be a follow-up appointment, however, within a month, so that the doctor can check the incision and healing process. If a woman develops any of the following symptoms, she should contact her doctor immediately, for they may be signs that one of the more serious complications described below has occurred: fever greater than 100°F, fainting spells, abdominal pain that is persistent or increasing after 12 hours and bleeding from the incision site.

Advantages and Benefits

Sterilization is the most effective method of birth control. For many women, freedom from the fear of pregnancy and the bother of contraception means increased sexual enjoyment. Although sterilization may cost anywhere from $700 to $2,000—or even more—assuming there are no major complications, this is a one-time expense. There may be some questions about the long-term effects of sterilization on the menstrual cycle, but these effects are not thought to be as serious as those that may be encountered with some other methods, such as the Pill.

Disadvantages and Problems

The most obvious disadvantage with sterilization is that it must be considered a permanent, irreversible method of birth control. It is important to get good counseling and to consider the question thoroughly before having the sterilization operation. In one study, 30 percent of the sterilized women later regretted their decision.[138] One question that might be helpful for a mother contemplating sterilization is to consider whether she would want more children if something happened to her existing children. Other women might ask themselves if they were to marry or remarry, would they then want to start a family?

Aside from the common postoperative problems of pain and discomfort described above, there are sometimes more serious consequences from sterilization. Despite the nickname of Band-Aid sterilization, which implies a minor surgical procedure, sterilization is a major operation. Although the risks of death are low, they do exist. The use of general anesthetic always carries risks. In addition, arteries may be punctured, and blood clots and heart attacks can occur. The overall death rate for women undergoing sterilizations is between 1 and 10 deaths per 100,000.[139]

Aside from death, other serious complications, such as the burning of surrounding tissue, puncture of the bowel or other organs, cardiac arrest, hemorrhage, infection and chronic pelvic pain can also be complications of sterilization. Some women continue to have pelvic pain for months or years after surgery. The pain is usually localized in the area of the tubes and is described as a tugging, drawing sensation. It is often associated with intercourse or sudden changes in position that stretch the pelvic muscles.

Sterilization has a psychological effect as well. Feelings of depression are not uncommon. Most women recover within weeks; however, some stay depressed and mournful.

Sterilization is not 100 percent effective. As many as 8 women in 1,000 who are sterilized will subsequently get pregnant.[140] Such pregnancies are often ectopic, especially those that occur more than a year after the sterilization.[141] Ectopic pregnancy can be a life-threatening situation and may be especially dangerous in sterilized women, because doctors frequently fail to diagnose the ectopic because the woman has been sterilized.[142] Women should be aware that pregnancy can occur even after sterilization and should familiarize themselves with the symptoms of ectopic pregnancy (*see* pp. 685–88) so they will not be misdiagnosed should they develop an ectopic.

Of the 8 per 1,000 sterilizations that are followed by pregnancy, 2 or 3 are owing to the fact that the woman was already pregnant at the time of sterilization.[143] Women should not undergo sterilization if they think there is any chance they might be pregnant. Women who have had their IUDs removed or who have gone off the Pill in preparation for their sterilization procedures should be sure to use another method of birth control while they are awaiting their procedures. It is a good idea to have a pregnancy test of the most sensitive type (*see* pp. 788–92) before sterilization, but even the most sensitive of tests cannot detect a pregnancy less than a week old. Some doctors routinely do D&Cs (removal of the uterine lining) on women being sterilized in hopes of removing undiagnosed pregnancies. We do not think this is a good idea because (1) only 2 or 3 women per 1,000 have undiagnosed pregnancies at the time of sterilization, which means that the other 997 or 998 women would be undergoing a needless D&C; (2) in a very early pregnancy the fertilized egg may still be in the tube, so removing the lining would not help; and (3) D&Cs done in very early pregnancies do not always remove the fertilized egg.[144] If a woman's doctor recommends a D&C as part of her sterilization, she would do well to question the wisdom of this procedure.

Another problem with sterilization is the possibility of menstrual problems following the procedure. A study done in 1974 compared the menstrual bleeding patterns of two groups of women, one of which had been sterilized by laparoscopic tubal ligation and the other by laparotomy, with a third group of women whose husbands had been sterilized.[145] Thirty-nine percent of the women sterilized by laparoscopy had increased menstrual blood loss, and another 21 percent had increased menstrual pain. A year after the operation, 7.4 percent of the women who had had laparoscopic sterilizations had to have hysterectomies, compared with only 5.4 percent of those who had had the older minilaparotomy, tube-tying method and 1.4 percent of the control group, whose husbands had been sterilized.

There are several problems with this study. First, it was a retrospective study. Retrospective means ''looking back.'' Information about menstrual pain and amount of menstrual flow came from what women remembered about their periods before the procedure. It asked subjective questions, like ''more or less pain?'' and ''more or less blood flow?'' According to another group of critics, the study fails to take into account the fact that these women may have used different forms of birth control before the sterilization. Perhaps it was the long-term effects of the previous birth control method that were responsible for the subsequent differences. Obviously, a better study than this one is needed; still, the fact that there was a striking difference between the laparoscopic group, the laparotomy group, and the nonsterilized group, both in terms of bleeding, pain problems and in the higher hysterectomy rates, raises some serious questions about sterilization and its long-term effects. It may be that the blood supply to the ovary is damaged during the operation, especially with the laparoscopic sterilization and cautery. But this is mere speculation. We are not even sure that a negative effect exists, much less what causes it. We do know that some

203

women who have been sterilized have had premature menopause, which is probably caused by damage to the blood supply of the ovaries at the time of operation, but how frequent this effect is and whether it is actually connected to a sterilization procedure remain to be determined.

Another problem with sterilization is that not all women are candidates for the procedure. A woman with a history of pelvic inflammatory disease, endometriosis or any condition that leaves a good deal of scar tissue in the abdominal cavity may not be suitable for sterilization. Likewise, large fibroids and certain ovarian cysts make some methods of tubal sterilization impossible for some women.

The Silicone Plug

A new method of sterilization that is now being tested and that will probably be available in the not-too-distant future is the silicone plug. This method involves the injection of silicone rubber into the fallopian tubes. The silicone forms a plug in the tube and blocks sperm from moving into the tubes and fertilizing the female egg (ovum). Unlike other methods of blocking or cutting off the tubes, the plug does not involve an incision or surgery. The procedure can be done in a doctor's office or a clinic. A local anesthetic, a paracervical block, is given, and a hysteroscope, a lighted, periscope-type viewing instrument, is inserted through the cervical canal into the uterus. The doctor then locates the openings to the fallopian tubes at the top of the uterus. Silicone rubber is injected through a special instrument into each of the tubes. After 5 to 7 minutes the silicone hardens and forms a plug that conforms to the shape of the tube. X-rays are then taken to make sure that the plug is placed correctly. Unlike other methods of sterilization, the recovery time is very short. The woman can go about her business as soon as the procedure is over. Because the method is still experimental and may have to be redone if it does not "take" the first time, women are advised to use another method of birth control for the first 3 months after this procedure and must return to the doctor for repeat X-rays after 3 months and at 6-month intervals for the next 2 years. As the method is tested more extensively, it may be that such frequent follow-up visits will not be necessary.

This method is cheaper than other tubal sterilization methods, does not require surgery and such extensive anesthesia, does not require a recovery time and may be more reversible than other sterilization methods. The plug does not adhere to the tissue so, theoretically, the plug can be easily removed by hysteroscopy. The woman could have it removed should she change her mind about sterilization and want to get pregnant. But the method is only experimental, so its reversibility has not yet been proved.

Early experiments have not proved the plug to be as effective as other methods of tubal sterilization, and women have gotten pregnant despite having plugs injected. Moreover, there is some concern about the possibility of the plug leading to increased rates of ectopic pregnancy and pelvic inflammatory disease as well as questions about the long-term effect of the silicone rubber on the tubes. The method offers many advantages, but it is still experimental. At this point neither its safety nor its effectiveness has been proved. Although the FDA might conceivably OK this method if current tests prove it to be effective, many years of use and study are necessary before we can be assured of its safety.

ABORTION

AKA: induced abortion, therapeutic abortion, TAB

Types: vacuum abortion, early abortion or suction curettage
menstrual extraction, very early abortion, menstrual regulation or menstrual induction
dilation and evacuation, or D&E
amniocentesis abortion or infusion or instillation abortion
prostaglandin suppository abortion
hysterectomy
hysterotomy

Abortion is the deliberate removal of fetal tissue from the uterus. Elsewhere in this book we discuss spontaneous abortions, or miscarriages. Here we are concerned with therapeutic abortions, that is, the deliberate removal of fetal tissue in order to terminate a pregnancy.

There is a rather widespread misunderstanding about abortion. Many people, women and doctors alike, are apt to think that a woman who has an abortion has been careless or irresponsible about birth control. Women who have more than one abortion are often viewed as having some deep-seated psychological problem. These attitudes betray an ignorance of the facts. No method of birth control is 100 percent effective, which means that any woman, no matter how conscientious, is liable to face the problem of an unplanned pregnancy at some time in her life.

Consider, for example, what would happen in a group of 100 women who were using a method of birth control with a theoretical effectiveness rate of 98 percent. As we explained in Chapter Five, birth control rates are given in terms of 100 women using that method for a year. A 98 percent theoretical effectiveness rate means that in the course of a year 98 of those 100 women would not get pregnant, but 2 would, simply because their method failed to do its job even though they used it consistently and correctly. Women have an average of 35 years of fertility during their lifetimes. Over a period of 35 years this could mean as many as 70 unplanned pregnancies in a group of 100 women! Women faced with an abortion decision should be aware of these facts and should not allow themselves to be made to feel that they have been careless and irresponsible. Although some women who have repeated abortions may not practice proper birth control methods or may have psychological problems, repeat abortions are also statistically inevitable.

Legal Status

In 1973 the Supreme Court handed down a landmark decision that legalized abortion.[146] The Court ruled that during the first trimester (the first 12 weeks of pregnancy),* decisions regarding abortion are a private matter between a woman and her doctor and that neither the state nor the federal government can place restrictions on how, when or where an abortion procedure is done. During the second trimester (the second 12 weeks of pregnancy) a state may impose regulations designed to protect a woman's health. For instance, an individual state can require that second-trimester abortions be done only in licensed hospitals. According to the same Supreme Court decision, an individual state can also place restrictions on or even outlaw abortions after the second trimester, when fetal viability begins (the time after which a fetus might possibly survive outside the womb), except when the mother's life or health is in danger. (Viability occurs at 24 weeks or, according to some, at 26 weeks. In other words, some fetuses who are born as early as 24 to 26 weeks of pregnancy might be able to live if they were given special care.) The Supreme Court decision did not automatically overrule all state laws regarding abortion—at least not those covering late abortions—so in some states late abortions may be difficult to obtain.

There has been considerable opposition to this Supreme Court decision, and the groups who are opposed to the legalization of abortion, called Right-to-Life groups, have worked hard to have these laws weakened or reversed, because they believe that abortion is morally wrong.[147] Their efforts have met with considerable success. In 1977 the Supreme Court decided that states had the right to prohibit payment for abortion for poor women receiving state medical assistance. More recently, regulations written for federally funded medical programs have prohibited abortion payments except in cases of rape, incest or risk to the mother's life. Many military dependents no longer have insurance coverage for abortion.

The Right-to-Lifers believe that abortion, regardless of the viability of the fetus, is morally wrong, the equivalent of murder. They want to protect the

---

*The duration of a pregnancy is measured by counting from the first day of the last menstrual cycle, even though conception probably didn't take place for a couple of weeks after that.

206

rights of the unborn. The groups who support the legalization of abortion, Pro-Choice groups, believe that a woman must have the legal right to control her own reproductive organs and to decide what happens inside her own body. They point to the fact that before legalization, millions of women were having illegal abortions, often under dangerous conditions, and that many of these women lost their lives needlessly. Pro-Choicers believe that abortion is a moral decision but one that must be made by the individual woman. They argue that no group of people has the right to inflict its personal moral judgments on others by legally restricting abortion.

We too believe that abortion should remain legalized. Unless the Supreme Court reverses its decisions or a constitutional amendment outlawing abortion is passed, the procedure will remain a legal one. There is, however, a strong movement to pass such a constitutional amendment. Women who want abortion to remain legalized should be aware of this and of the fact that their silence on this issue could allow a vocal minority to change the legal status of abortion. Women interested in working to assure their legal right to abortion can contact Abortion Action Coalition, Box 2727, Boston, Massachusetts 02208.

Legally, a woman need not have the consent of her spouse, her parents or anyone else in order to have an abortion.[148] There are, however, some clinics and hospitals that require the husband's or parent's signature before they will provide treatment. This is more likely to happen with late abortions. In such cases a woman may either provide the required signatures, seek treatment elsewhere or take legal action.

Making the Decision

A woman who is pregnant has three basic options:

1. She can have an abortion.
2. She can have the baby and keep it.
3. She can have the baby and give it up for adoption.*

Many times this decision is difficult for a woman to make. In most cases there is not much time in which to decide. By the time most women discover that they are pregnant, they are already 4 to 6 weeks pregnant. Although there are now special tests that can detect pregnancy within 22 to 24 days of the last

*A cooperative community group known as The Farm (Summertown, Tennessee 38483) has offered to help any woman who is thinking about abortion to deliver her baby by natural childbirth for free. If the woman decides to keep the baby, she may; otherwise they will raise the child for her. If the woman ever decides that she wants the baby back, she can have it. The Farm midwives offer this alternative to the limit of their ability to provide good care.

menstrual period, the standard test is not accurate until about 6 weeks. Since the less risky, simpler abortion procedures must be done before 12 weeks, only a month is usually allowed for decision making.

A woman is likely to have ambivalent feelings when making this difficult decision about whether or not to have an abortion. The first step for her is to find out for certain if she is pregnant. This can be done through her regular doctor, a public health clinic or Planned Parenthood. Planned Parenthood has chapters throughout the country that provide testing, counseling and abortion referrals.

A good, reputable counselor will not try to influence a woman's decision but will help her by providing information about her options, by arranging for adoption or medical assistance while she is pregnant and afterward (if she should choose to keep the child) and by giving information about abortion procedures and other important facts.

Somewhere between 5 percent and 6 percent of the women who at first decide on abortion change their minds before they actually have the abortion. For this reason it is suggested that the counseling and the actual abortion do not take place on the same day.

There may be medical factors that will influence the decision. Now that abortion has been legalized and it is possible to detect certain defects early in pregnancy by analyzing a sample of fluid from the amniotic sac that surrounds the fetus (a procedure known as amniocentesis), more women are having abortions to terminate defective pregnancies.

Any woman who is age 35 or older, has already borne a child with a birth defect, has a personal or family history of birth defects or whose sex partners have such a history should have genetic counseling to determine whether or not she is a candidate for amniocentesis. Your doctor can obtain a free directory of federally supported genetics centers from the National Foundation for the March of Dimes, Box 2000, White Plains, New York 10602.

Many pregnant teenagers wonder whether or not they should involve their parents in the decision-making process. They are reluctant to upset their parents or are afraid that their parents will be angry with them. Despite these fears many teenagers find that their parents are supportive and helpful in terms of finances and in finding good medical care. Parental consent, however, is not legally required for pregnancy care or for abortion, and many teenagers handle these problems on their own.

Test and Examinations Before Abortion

All women should have a pregnancy test before undergoing an abortion. Although this seems obvious, there have been cases where women were referred to abortion clinics solely on the basis of the fact that they had missed one or more menstrual periods.

It is a good idea to have the pregnancy test performed at a qualified laboratory and not at the clinic or facility where the abortion will be done. There have been cases where women's health-care activists who were investigating abortion clinics deliberately submitted male urine samples to a number of clinics. Some of these clinics actually told these women that they were pregnant and offered to schedule abortion surgery for them. You can see why it can be important for women to have independent pregnancy testing.

Many doctors and clinics do a routine test for gonorrhea on all women undergoing abortions. If you think that you might have been exposed to gonorrhea, insist on having this test before the abortion. If you do have gonorrhea and go ahead with an abortion, there is a good chance that the gonorrhea may spread beyond the cervix and into the uterus and tubes. This can cause pelvic inflammatory disease, which can have serious and even fatal consequences.

You also should have your blood pressure taken and blood tests made to check for anemia and to find out whether you have Rh-negative blood or Rh-positive blood. Most women have Rh-positive blood, which doesn't cause any problems. But if a woman with Rh-negative blood becomes pregnant with an Rh-positive fetus, the Rh-positive cells from the fetus could enter her bloodstream during abortion, delivery or miscarriage. Because the mother's blood is Rh-negative, this may cause an antibody reaction. Antibodies are protein substances that are part of the body's immune system. They attack "foreign invaders" in the body, which, in this case, would be the Rh-positive blood cells from the fetus. If an Rh-negative woman develops these antibodies, they will attack the blood cells of the fetus during each succeeding pregnancy, possibly causing severe jaundice and fetal death.

A vaccine that will prevent the antibody reaction can now be given to the mother within 36 to 72 hours after delivery, miscarriage or abortion. After a full-term delivery the decision as to whether or not to give this vaccine is based on a sampling of the baby's blood. If the baby's blood is negative, there is no need for the drug. But if the baby's blood is positive, the drug is given. It should be given to all women whose blood is Rh-negative after abortion or miscarriage. At one time the vaccine wasn't given to Rh-negative women who had early therapeutic abortions, but studies reported in the medical literature indicated that even in early abortions there is a small chance of the mother's developing antibodies. Now the vaccine is given in these cases as well. Women who are having therapeutic abortions should ask about their blood type, whether the vaccine will be necessary and, if so, whether the cost of the vaccine ($35 to $55) is included in the price of the abortion.

Urine tests and chest X-rays may also be done, especially if you are having a general, rather than a local, anesthetic. Some doctors and clinics give preoperative enemas or shave the pubic hair, neither of which is necessary.

The doctor should do a pelvic exam and take a medical history to find out if you have a history of heart disease, blood-clotting disorders, epilepsy, adverse drug reactions or other medical problems that could influence how the abortion is done. The pelvic exam and the date of your last period will help the doctor decide how advanced the pregnancy is, which will also influence the choice of procedure. Some doctors or clinics do a routine Pap smear on all women undergoing abortion. You should be prepared to make two visits to the doctor or the clinic, one for tests and one for the abortion.

You should not eat or drink anything for 8 hours before the abortion, regardless of whether you are having a local or a general anesthetic. Some doctors allow a woman to eat a light breakfast if a local is planned, but we don't think this is a good idea. If complications necessitating a general anesthetic do occur, food or liquids in the stomach could be regurgitated, causing respiratory problems. If a woman is having a general anesthetic, she may be given a preoperative shot of a drug called atropine to dry up secretions in her mouth and throat, so that she doesn't choke on them. If a local anesthetic is planned, she may be given a shot of tranquilizer before the abortion.

Early Vacuum Abortion (4–12 Weeks)

In a vacuum abortion, or suction curettage (Illustration 36), a tube attached to a suction device is inserted through the cervix into the uterus. Suction is then applied and the contents of the uterus are gently vacuumed. This abortion procedure is the one that is used most widely.

It may be done using either a local or a general anesthetic. Most clinics prefer a local anesthetic because it is safer, but there have been deaths associated with locals as well.

The general anesthetic has the advantage of completely blocking any pain. Women may experience some pain with a local, but most consider the pain to be tolerable. Not all abortion facilities offer a choice between the two types of anesthetic, so if you are adamant about having a general, this may be a factor to consider in deciding where to have the procedure done (see below).

The doctor first performs a bimanual pelvic exam. A speculum is inserted, and the cervix is cleaned with swabs that have been dipped in an antiseptic solution. The doctor then steadies the cervix with a special clamplike device called a tenaculum.

If a local anesthetic is used, it is injected into the cervix and the ligaments that support the uterus. The anesthetic usually takes effect in a few seconds. Some women experience a numbness in the mouth or fingertips after the injection, but these reactions usually subside in 2 to 3 minutes. Some women feel a pinprick sensation when the local anesthetic is injected, or a mild cramping; others don't feel anything.

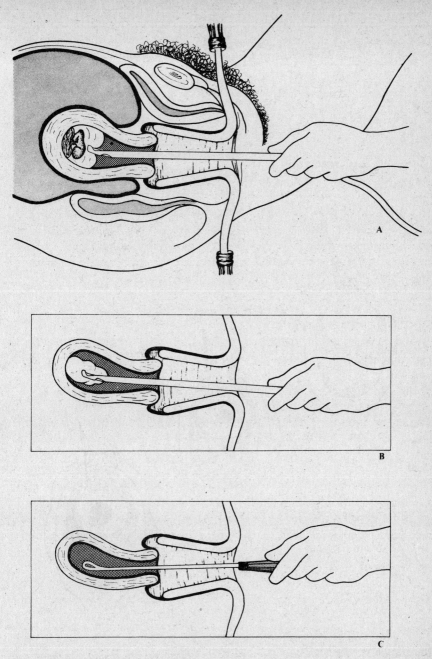

Illustration 36 *Dilation: A tenaculum steadies the cervix, and rods of increasing diameter are used to dilate it.*

211

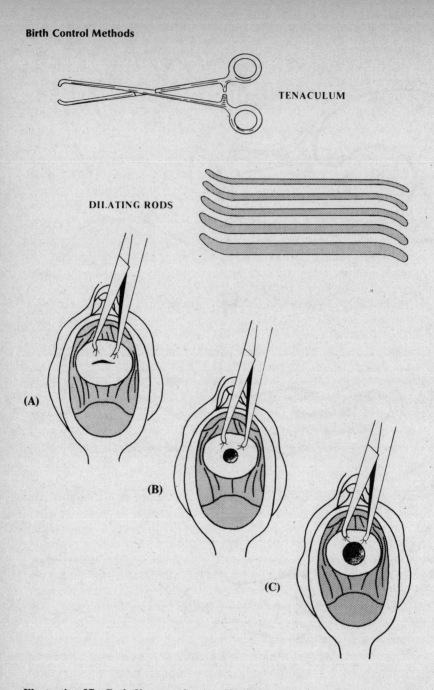

TENACULUM

DILATING RODS

(A)

(B)

(C)

Illustration 37 *Early Vacuum Abortion: Vaginal retractors are used to keep the vagina open, and the suction tube is inserted through the dilated cervix into the uterus (A). The contents of the uterus are vacuumed out (B). A curette may be used to ensure that all of the contents of the uterus have been removed (C).*

The anesthetic takes effect in 5 to 10 minutes, and the doctor then gently pulls the cervix to straighten it. Next, the opening to the cervix is dilated by the insertion of metal rods of increasing width until the os, the opening to the cervical canal, is open wide enough to accommodate an appropriate-sized vacuum tube (Illustration 37).

For abortions that are done in the first 8 weeks, a tube called a cannula, 6 mm in diameter, is generally used. After 8 weeks a tube with a diameter equal to or 2 mm less than the number of weeks of pregnancy is used. Most doctors think that these larger tubes, called curettes, should never exceed 12 mm. Some doctors have used larger ones to abort pregnancies of more than 12 weeks' duration. However, most abortion experts believe that the risks of uterine perforation, bleeding complications, cervical injuries or subsequent cervical incompetence—a condition in which the cervix opens up too early in the pregnancy, causing a miscarriage—are increased by use of a curette larger than 12 mm. This belief is based on studies in which uteri removed surgically for other reasons were dilated with various size curettes and then examined microscopically for signs of damage.[149] The researchers found that there was no evidence of tissue damage with dilators less than 8 mm in size. In almost 50 percent of the uteri tested there was some evidence of tissue damage with dilation of 9 mm to 11 mm. Although there is some question about the applicability of data obtained on surgically removed uteri to processes that occur in live uterine tissue, the point is obvious: The smaller the diameter, the better. Women should ask their doctors what size dilators and tubes will be used. If the answer is a 9-mm dilator for a pregnancy of 7 weeks' duration, for example, or a dilator larger than 12 mm at any time, find another doctor or clinic.

Some doctors prefer to use laminaria, rods made of sterilized seaweed, rather than metal dilators to open the cervix. The rods are inserted into the cervix either the night before or several hours before the abortion. The rods swell up with fluid, gently dilating the cervix. This gradual dilation over a period of hours seems to be associated with lower risk for uterine perforation, bleeding complications, cervical injury or cervical incompetence. Some doctors fear that the use of laminaria may cause a higher rate of infection, however, because the cervix is open for a longer time, allowing more disease-causing organisms to enter the uterus. This is more likely to be a problem with rods left in place for longer than 24 hours before the abortion. Also, on rare occasions the rods will cause a spontaneous abortion.[150]

The rods, which look like brown tampons, may come out before or at the time of the abortion. Be sure to save them to show to the doctor if they come out beforehand, since on occasion they are inserted too far into the cervix and move up into the uterus. X-rays may then be necessary to locate them so that they can be removed.

Most women experience a mild cramping sensation when the laminaria rods are inserted. Such cramping may persist for hours, and some women

213

have reported severe cramping. Studies comparing metal dilators and laminaria rods are now underway. Women should discuss these two methods of cervical dilation with their doctors, obtaining up-to-date information before making a decision.

After the cervix has been dilated and the vacuum tube inserted, the tube is attached to a suction machine. The suction machine, the sound of which you will probably hear, is turned on and the tube is moved around in the uterine cavity until its contents have been suctioned out. After the vacuuming begins, women who have had locals may feel a slight tugging sensation. Toward the end of the procedure the uterus contracts sharply. The procedure takes 3 to 5 minutes. Some doctors then insert a curette instrument into the uterus to check it for retained tissue or abnormalities.

Most women experience strong cramping sensations that may last for 2 to 20 minutes. Pain medication may be given. Women who have had locals can usually get up and walk to the recovery room. Some women experience nausea and cramping for a half hour or so, but most can leave in 1 or 2 hours. If a general anesthetic has been used, the recovery time may be longer. You should plan to have someone help you home.

Many doctors give six tablets of ergotrate to be taken every 4 hours for 24 hours. This drug helps to keep the uterus contracted and diminishes the amount of bleeding. There may be some cramping after you take each tablet. Since the drug tends to elevate the blood pressure, it cannot be used by women with high blood pressure.

Most women experience some bleeding and cramps for the first 2 weeks. The blood may be dark and occasionally contain a clot. The bleeding may stop, and begin again a few days later. Using four to five pads a day for 10 days after the abortion and light spotting for up to 4 weeks is not unusual; however, soaking two pads with bright red blood in an hour or less, passing several clots over a short period or experiencing bleeding for 2 days in a row that is heavier than the heaviest day of bleeding during your normal period may be an indication that something is wrong, and should be reported to the doctor. In addition, severe cramps that begin a day after the abortion, or hives and rashes, or a green or foul-smelling vaginal discharge, or burning or frequency of urination should be reported to the doctor. Take your temperature each day for a week, and call your doctor if it reaches 100°F or more. If you are taking Tylenol or aspirin for pain, take your temperature before you take the pain tablet. If you do not have a period within 50 days, or if pregnancy symptoms, such as nausea and breast tenderness, persist, see your doctor. Always schedule a follow-up exam 2 to 3 weeks after the abortion, even if you are feeling fine.

You should rest the day of the abortion, but most women can return to work the next day. Avoid douching or intercourse for a week, and use napkins, not tampons, for the 1st week or so.

Fertility returns rapidly. Your next normal period should begin in 4 to 6 weeks. Sixty percent of women ovulate within the first 25 days, so contraception must be used right away.

Deciding Where to Have a Vacuum Abortion

Suction abortions can be performed in a doctor's office, an abortion clinic or a hospital. Several studies have shown that complication rates are lower when early abortions are performed in an abortion clinic rather than a hospital.[151] This may be because local rather than general anesthetics are generally used in doctors' offices and in clinics.

Abortions done in a doctor's office or a clinic are usually less expensive. Having the abortion done in the office of a doctor whom they know and feel comfortable with is an important factor for some women, but it may be slightly more expensive than an abortion clinic. Moreover, doctors working in clinics perform large numbers of abortions and become quite proficient at them.

If the pregnancy is beyond 11 weeks, many doctors prefer a hospital setting, because occasionally there are bleeding complications necessitating transfusion when the uterus is this large. Women with fibroid tumors and congenital abnormalities of the uterus may have to have their abortions done in a hospital. Likewise, high-risk women—those with heart disease, blood-clotting disorders, chronic debilitating diseases and anemia—are often treated in a hospital.

Choosing the right doctor or clinic is important. We talk about choosing a doctor in more detail in Chapter Six. Having a board-certified gynecologist is important. Although the family doctor or a general surgeon might be competent to perform an abortion, a board-certified gynecologist is apt to do a better job should complications occur.

If you are planning to have your abortion done at an abortion clinic, you will want to make sure that the clinic is a good one. After abortion became legal a number of clinics were set up for the sole purpose of performing abortions. Although the majority of them provide excellent care, there are definitely some substandard ones. One way to locate a good clinic is to contact your local Planned Parenthood chapter. Some Planned Parenthood chapters provide first-trimester abortions, and these clinics must meet rigid standards. In addition, those chapters that don't provide abortions can refer you to a doctor or a clinic in the area. The doctors and clinics on their referral list have usually been inspected by a representative from Planned Parenthood, and they also get follow-up evaluations from women who have been referred to these doctors or clinics. If treatment is below par, the doctor or clinic doesn't stay on the referral list for long. Other family planning clinics may also have such referral lists. Be sure to ask whether the facilities on their list have been personally inspected and whether follow-up evaluation has been done. Women's health clinics are another excellent source for referrals. These groups often have referral lists that are carefully and scrupulously evaluated.

No matter where you have your abortion done, be sure that there is a 24-hour emergency telephone number so that you can reach a doctor in case complications develop. It is crucial that the clinic or doctor you choose be able to provide immediate access to a hospital should a medical emergency arise. There should be a hospital within a 10-minute drive and more important, the doctor performing your abortion should have staff privileges at that hospital. Be sure to inquire about this when choosing a facility or doctor.

Cost may also be a consideration. Prices range from $125 to about $300, but this could change if inflationary trends continue. There may be an extra charge for a general anesthetic, Rh vaccine or IUD insertion.

Complications

The complication rates vary according to the duration of the pregnancy. The earlier the abortion is done, the safer it is. Problems that may arise include infection, excessive bleeding, injury to the cervix, perforation of the uterus or other organs, adverse drug reactions and incomplete abortion, in which some of the fetal tissue is left in the uterus.

Mortality figures vary in different studies, but one of the largest and most complete studies reported a death rate of less than 1 per 100,000 for abortions performed within the first 8 weeks, 1.9 per 100,000 in the first 9 to 10 weeks and 4.1 in the first 11 to 12 weeks.[152] After that point, procedures that carry higher mortality (see below) are required.

There is some evidence to indicate that women who have more than one abortion may have problems with future pregnancies. (*see* p. 224).

Other Early Abortion Procedures
(see also Postcoital Contraception below)

Some doctors perform a D&C instead of an early vacuum suction abortion, but this may involve more blood loss and more pain and has a higher rate of complications. If your doctor does not have access to suction equipment, find one who does.

Menstrual Extraction

Menstrual extraction is a procedure similar to vacuum abortion, only a syringe rather than a vacuum machine is generally used and it is usually not necessary to dilate the cervix. In the past, when pregnancy tests were not accurate until 6 weeks, this method was used on women whose periods were slightly overdue who thought they might be pregnant. Now that there are special pregnancy tests that can be accurate within 1 day of a missed period, it is no longer necessary for a woman to undergo this procedure without really knowing whether or not she is pregnant. Many doctors no longer perform menstrual extraction, since there is a greater likelihood that the procedure will not succeed in removing all the fetal tissue.

Menstrual extraction does have advantages. It may not require dilation or an anesthetic, although some women do find the procedure quite painful. It is usually less expensive than an early vacuum abortion, and women can usually leave the doctor's office within a half hour. It is important to have a follow-up visit within 3 weeks to make sure that the pregnancy was indeed terminated and that no complications have developed.

Some women involved in the health-care movement are strong advocates of menstrual extraction. Women in certain self-help groups have developed their own equipment and learned to perform this operation on one another. Since an anesthetic is not required and the cervix is not dilated, this procedure can be done quite simply. A flexible plastic tube is inserted through the os. Gentle suction is applied with a syringe and the menstrual lining is removed, along with the products of conception—if the woman was pregnant (*see* Illustration 38). Some women extract their menses on a regular basis, regardless of whether they suspect pregnancy, claiming that to do so relieves menstrual cramps. Advocates of menstrual extraction also believe that it is important for women to develop such simple, do-it-yourself methods in case there is an abortion backlash and abortion again becomes illegal. We do not recommend that women have this procedure done on a regular basis. No one knows what the effect of continually removing the lining of the uterus in this manner will be. Nor do we recommend that women perform this procedure on one another. There is always a risk of uterine perforation, cervical injury and infection with this procedure, even when it is performed by experienced personnel in approved medical facilities. Moreover, we feel that political action is a more effective way of safeguarding the legal right to abortion.

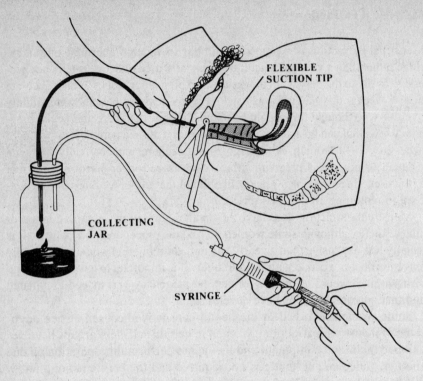

Illustration 38 *Menstrual Extraction: The flexible suction tube is inserted into the uterus. A vacuum is created by drawing on the syringe, and the contents of the uterus are sucked into the collection jar.*

Dilation and Evacuation Abortion (13–20 Weeks)

Dilation and evacuation (D&E) is a combination of the suction curettage done in early abortions and a surgical procedure in which a sharp curette is used to remove any remaining fetal tissue. The curette is necessary because of the larger volume of fetal tissue. A general anesthetic is usually required, and the cervix must be more widely dilated (12 to 14 mm or more) than with an early vacuum abortion. The procedure also takes longer (20 to 30 minutes). Otherwise, from the woman's point of view, the procedure and recovery are similar to the early vacuum abortion.

Some doctors perform this procedure beyond 20 weeks, even up to 24 weeks, but many doctors feel the amniocentesis abortion described below is preferable after 20 weeks; however, studies are now underway to evaluate the D&E, and recommendations may change in the future.

D&E is a relatively new procedure. Because suction curettage alone will not usually suffice after 12 weeks, owing to the greater volume of fetal tissue, and because amniocentesis abortion cannot be performed before 16 weeks (see below), it used to be that women over 12 weeks would have to wait until 16 weeks to have their abortion, which sometimes was emotionally devastating. Although the D&E involves higher complication rates than an earlier abortion, studies have shown that for a pregnancy of 13 to 20 weeks, it is the safest procedure.[153]

Amniocentesis Abortion (16–24 Weeks)

Amniocentesis (Illustration 39) is a procedure whereby a hollow needle is inserted into the fluid-filled amniotic sac that surrounds the developing fetus. As mentioned earlier, fluid may be withdrawn from the sac and analyzed in order to detect certain birth defects. In an amniocentesis abortion a drug that causes fetal death is injected into the sac. Fetal death is followed by a series of uterine contractions, which causes the expulsion of the fetal tissues.

Amniocentesis cannot be done before 16 weeks because before that time the amniotic sac does not contain enough fluid for the procedure to be done safely.

This procedure must be done in the hospital. It involves more risk than earlier abortions, and emergency facilities must be on hand in case complications occur. A local anesthetic is used, for the woman must be wide awake and fully alert so that she can report any unusual sensations to the doctor.

Before the procedure the woman is asked to urinate so that her bladder is not distended. This cuts down on the chances of accidentally puncturing the bladder when the needle is inserted. The doctor then examines the abdomen and locates the top of the uterus. A small area of skin may be shaved, and the area is then washed with an antiseptic solution. A local anesthetic is injected into the area, which may cause a brief stinging feeling. A long, hollow needle is then inserted through the anesthetized skin and the uterine muscle. Most women experience pressure and some discomfort when this is done, but the discomfort subsides once the needle is in place.

Some doctors insert a narrow, flexible plastic tube called a catheter through the needle and then withdraw the needle, leaving the tube in place. This practice has advantages and disadvantages. The advantage is that the tube can be taped to the abdomen and left in place, so that if abortion does not occur within 48 hours, reinjection of the fluid is easier and less painful. On the other hand, leaving the tube in place increases the chance of infection. Since the majority of women will not require a second injection, many doctors don't use the tube.

Regardless of whether the needle or tube is used, some of the amniotic fluid

219

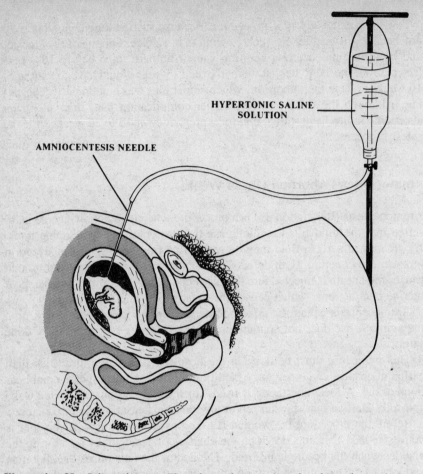

HYPERTONIC SALINE
SOLUTION

AMNIOCENTESIS NEEDLE

Illustration 39 *Saline Abortion: The saline solution is introduced into the amniotic sac
through the amniocentesis needle.*

is withdrawn and the drug is introduced into the sac. Many women note a
slight sense of fullness or pressure at this time, which is normal; however,
any feeling of pain or warmth should be reported to the doctor immediately.

If a needle is used, it is then withdrawn and the puncture is covered with a
Band-Aid. If the tube is used, it is closed off and taped to the abdomen. Experiments in which the fluid is introduced through the cervix rather than the
abdomen have been tried, but this method has proved to be less satisfactory
and is done only in special cases.

Some doctors insert one or two laminaria rods (described above) into the
cervical canal after the amniocentesis procedure. Some doctors insert the laminaria 14 to 19 hours before the procedure. The point of inserting the lamina-

ria is to dilate the cervix and thus to avoid tearing the cervix when the fetal tissue is expelled from the uterus. It has also been shown to shorten the time between the injection of the solution and the expulsion of the fetus. Although the insertion of laminaria rods 14 to 19 hours before the procedure assures that the cervix will be well dilated by the time the fetal tissue is expelled, the longer they are in place, the greater the chance of disease-causing organisms moving past the cervix and into the sterile uterus. If the laminaria rods are inserted right after the amniocentesis procedure, there may not be enough time before the expulsion of the fetal tissue to allow for sufficient dilation of the cervix but there is less chance of infection. Other doctors believe that the cervical dilation that occurs naturally once the fetus dies is sufficient, so they do not use rods.[154]

After the amniocentesis procedure the woman is usually returned to her hospital room. Uterine contractions, similar to labor pains, usually begin within 6 to 8 hours; however, the contractions may begin earlier than this or later.

Some doctors give an injection of oxytocin, a drug that causes uterine contractions. Again, this has advantages and disadvantages. It shortens the time between the amniocentesis procedure and the expulsion of the fetus, which reduces the chances of infection and of the placenta being retained (see below). However, it increases bleeding complications, especially in women with certain blood disorders. The drug sometimes causes fluid retention, which if untreated can cause serious complications, including coma and convulsions. (If the drug is used, all fluid intake and output must be monitored carefully.) Some doctors use it routinely, whereas others prefer to reserve use of it for cases where the contractions are not strong enough and don't seem to be progressing rapidly enough.

The length of time between the amniocentesis procedure and the expulsion of the fetus varies considerably. In most cases expulsion takes place within 24 to 36 hours, and 93 percent of the women undergoing this procedure will abort within 72 hours.[155]

Most women experience an increasing sense of fullness and pressure as the time for expulsion of the fetus approaches. The degree of pain a woman feels may be slight, moderate or intense. Pain medication can be given. Since the fetus is relatively small, the expulsion itself is usually not painful and doesn't normally require the incision at the vaginal opening (an episiotomy) that is frequently used in the delivery of a full-term pregnancy.

A member of the nursing staff may be with you when the expulsion occurs, or it may happen before the nurse arrives. You should be prepared for the fact that the fetus is recognizable at this stage of development. The nurse will usually handle the situation, so that you will not see the tissue. You may prefer not to look, should expulsion occur before she arrives. On the other hand, some women feel a strong need to see the actual fetus, finding that this makes it easier for them to deal with the emotional aspects of the situation. If you are among the latter, you should make your wishes known beforehand, as most nurses have been trained to conceal the fetus from you.

In three out of four cases the expulsion of the fetus is followed shortly by the expulsion of the placenta, but sometimes it is necessary for the doctor to remove the placenta. This may be accomplished by pressing on the abdomen or by the use of a blunt grasping instrument. If these techniques don't work, a D&C may be required.

After expulsion the woman usually remains in the hospital for at least 3 or 4 hours. The length of the hospital stay varies, depending on the time between the amniocentesis and the expulsion. Some clinics will send a woman home after the amniocentesis procedure, telling her to return once contractions have begun, but this is a questionable practice, and a woman should seek treatment elsewhere if her doctor or clinic suggests this.

Risks and Complications

The risks and complications involved in amniocentesis abortions depend somewhat on the drug used to cause fetal death. Any of the following substances may be used: urea, a concentrated solution of nitrogen waste products excreted by the kidney; prostaglandins, a class of hormones; and saline, a concentrated salt solution. Saline is the most widely used, but some doctors now prefer prostaglandins. The use of urea is a fairly recent innovation, so there have not been as many abortions done using this substance. Each solution has its own particular advantages and disadvantages, and there have not yet been a sufficient number of prostaglandin and urea abortions done for conclusive comparisons to be made.

Infection, excessive bleeding and injury to the cervix can occur with any type of amniocentesis procedure. The complications may be serious enough to be fatal. The mortality for saline abortions is about 15.2 per 100,000 cases.[156] Most of these deaths result from infection; however, complications may also occur if the saline is not injected properly. If the saline is injected into the muscle wall of the uterus, this may cause death of the tissue and necessitate a hysterectomy. If the saline is accidentally injected into the abdomen, there is usually instant, severe pain, but this stops when the saline is discontinued. If the saline is injected into a blood vessel, it can cause instant death, although rarely is the reaction that severe. Indications of saline in a blood vessel include headache, restlessness, numbness and a feeling of warmth.

Prostaglandins are associated with a shorter interval between amniocentesis and expulsion of the fetus but with a higher incidence of the fetus being born alive and not expiring until shortly afterward. The mortality for the woman appears to be lower—about 10.5 per 100,000—than with saline, but there is a higher proportion of cervical injuries.[157] As many as 50 percent to 75 percent of women experience vomiting, nausea or diarrhea.

The complications associated with improper injection are less severe, even if the prostaglandins are injected into a blood vessel. Many doctors now feel that prostaglandins are safer than saline.

Urea is thought to be safer and to have less serious complication rates than either saline or prostaglandins. There is less vomiting, nausea and diarrhea than with prostaglandins and there are fewer clotting problems than with saline.[158] So far there have been no reports of live births. Bleeding may occur, but so far, these problems have not required transfusions. Infection is infrequent and can usually be treated with antibiotics. The rate of cervical injuries may be lower than with prostaglandins. Unfortunately, urea usually involves a longer time interval before the fetus is expelled and is less potent than saline or prostaglandins. Oxytocin or the use of a second dose of prostaglandins may be required.[159]

Prostaglandin Vaginal Suppositories

Vaginal suppositories of prostaglandins, inserted every 3 to 4 hours, have recently been used to induce abortion. This method is new and has not been widely used. It can cause extreme nausea, intense contractions, diarrhea and fever. It is also associated with relatively high rates of incomplete abortions necessitating immediate D&C's. Since prostaglandins are hormones and all their effects are not yet understood, it is too early to evaluate this method accurately.

Hysterectomy and Hysterotomy

Hysterectomy, an operation whereby the uterus is removed, is rarely used anymore for abortion purposes. It may, however, be used for women who have serious medical problems that prevent them from having an amniocentesis abortion. But since it is a major operation and since we now have alternative procedures, it should be used for abortion only on this and other rare occasions.

Hysterotomy is an operation whereby an incision is made in the uterus through which the fetal contents are removed. It is a sort of mini-cesarean section. Again, the operation is rarely used today and is reserved for special cases.

Look to the Future

Many questions about abortion procedures still need to be answered. The safety of the D&E versus the amniocentesis abortion, the use of contraction-stimulating drugs, the proper method of cervical dilation, the possibility of using prostaglandin suppositories in early abortions, the choice of medications in second-trimester abortions—all these issues are being studied, so watch for future developments in this area.

Abortion and Subsequent Pregnancies

In the past it was thought that having repeat abortions would not affect a woman's subsequent pregnancies. Although reports from other countries indicated that women who had had repeat abortions were more likely to have miscarriages, premature births, infants with lower-than-normal birth weights and other problems,[160] it was believed that inferior medical care and abortion procedures in those countries probably accounted for these problems. However, the findings of some recent studies in the United States indicate that women who have had previous abortions might be more likely to have problems with subsequent pregnancies. One study shows a two- to threefold increased risk of miscarriage in women who have had two or more abortions.[161] Other studies indicate a higher rate of premature births, infants with low birth weights and ectopic pregnancies in women who have had repeat abortions.[162] But it is unclear whether the repeat abortion itself or other factors, such as cigarette smoking, infection complications after the abortion or the type of procedure used to do the abortion—rather than the number of abortions—actually accounted for these problems.[163]

At the present time, then, we cannot say for certain what effect abortion has on subsequent pregnancies. More studies are needed. But because research has indicated that earlier suction abortions are less likely to result in these problems,[164] women should try to have their abortions as early as possible, before 12 weeks, when the suction method can be used. There is also some indication that using laminaria rods instead of mechanical dilators reduces the risk of future pregnancy problems,[165] so women who may want to have children in the future, especially those undergoing repeat abortions, should ask their doctors about the use of lamanaria rods, particularly if their cervices must be dilated beyond 11 mm. Such women should also avoid smoking during subsequent pregnancies. Because there is also some indication that getting pregnant soon after an abortion increases the likelihood of these problems,[166] women who have had prior abortions and want to carry their next pregnancy to term should wait awhile before getting pregnant again. Precisely how long has not been determined, so women should discuss this with their doctors.

Until we know more about how abortion affects subsequent pregnancies, some doctors are recommending that women who have had one or more abortions and who may wish to have children in the future "place greater emphasis on the effectiveness, rather than on the safety, of her contraceptive method,"[167] that is, that they use the Pill, rather than one of the barrier methods. Others suggest that such women might want to combine two barrier methods, such as the diaphragm and condoms or condoms and foam, so she will have less likelihood of getting pregnant until she is ready to have a child.[168]

POSTCOITAL CONTRACEPTION

Types: morning-after pill (MAP)
morning-after IUD
menstrual extraction, menstrual regulation or menstrual induction

Coitus means "intercourse," and postcoital contraception is a method of birth control that is used after a woman has had unprotected intercourse, because she has been raped, has forgotten to use birth control, has used it incorrectly or has used a method that has failed (broken condom, expelled IUD, etc.).

There are basically three methods of postcoital contraception now available: the morning-after pill, the morning-after IUD and menstrual extraction. The first two methods must be used within a few days of the unprotected intercourse. The third may be used around the time of the missed period.

There is some controversy about the use of postcoital contraception. The chance of becoming pregnant from a single act of intercourse may be as little as 2 percent and is probably no higher than 30 percent,[169] even if you have intercourse at the most fertile time of the month (*see* p. 65). The postcoital methods all involve certain risks, and in some cases their effectiveness has been questioned or has not been confirmed, so some doctors recommend that women wait until a pregnancy test can confirm the pregnancy before doing anything. The newest pregnancy tests can be accurate in about 22 days after the last menstrual period, so women can find out whether they are pregnant quickly and can then have an abortion if they so desire. However, many women don't want to wait. They may prefer to take the risks without awaiting confirmation of pregnancy. Also, some women who have moral or religious objections to abortion prefer

225

postcoital contraception, which may be viewed as preventing implantation of the egg rather than as actual abortion.

Before making a decision about how to deal with unprotected intercourse, read the following material as well as the above information on abortion and discuss the alternatives with a doctor. In making your decision you will want to weigh the relative risks and benefits of each course of action against the probability of your actually being pregnant. Remember that your chances of getting pregnant are between 2 percent and 30 percent, with the chances being greater if the unprotected intercourse occurred near ovulation. If you are over 30 to 35 years of age, your chances of being pregnant are less than those of a woman who is in her 20s, the peak age for fertility. Similarly, if you are in your early teens, your chances are lower than if you were in your 30s.

We personally do not encourage the use of postcoital contraception and recommend that women wait and have pregnancy tests to make sure they are actually pregnant before taking any action. Women should remember that postcoital contraception is an emergency measure and is meant only for one-time protection. They should start using a regular method of birth control immediately.

The Morning-After Pill (MAP)

A synthetic estrogen, DES, has been approved by the FDA for use as a morning-after pill in emergency cases. Five pills of 5 mg each must be taken twice a day for 5 days, beginning within 72 hours (preferably within 24 hours) of the unprotected intercourse, in order for the drug to be effective. Even then there is some question about its effectiveness. Although most studies have indicated that DES is effective as a postcoital contraceptive, one study of rape victims who had been given DES has raised serious questions.[170] In this study the rate of pregnancies was about the same as that in similar groups that had not been given DES.

It is theorized that DES works (if indeed it does work) by altering the endometrial lining of the uterus in such a way that a fertilized egg cannot implant or survive. Some experts theorize that DES interferes with pregnancy by slowing down or speeding up the passage of the fertilized egg through the fallopian tube.

One problem with the massive doses of DES required for postcoital contraception is the fact that these doses (50 times what the body normally produces) cause nausea as well as vomiting in 16 percent to 25 percent of the women who take the drug. Many doctors therefore prescribe an antinausea medication to be taken 1 hour before taking DES. If vomiting occurs within 4 hours, another dose of DES must be taken, since there is a chance that not all the DES in the first pills was absorbed.[171]

With DES, more than 7 out of 10 women experience one of the following problems: nausea and vomiting, headaches, menstrual irregularities and breast tenderness. Some women may also experience vaginal spotting, dizziness, diarrhea, increased vaginal discharge, cramps or bloating. Only about one-third of the women who take DES as a postcoital contraceptive are symptom-free. About 20 percent of the women who take DES have unusually heavy, unusually light or delayed menstrual periods. A late or light menstrual period does not mean that the DES has failed, but women whose periods are more than 2 weeks late should have pregnancy tests to rule out this possibility.[172]

If pregnancy does occur, despite MAP treatment, the chances are greater that the pregnancy will be an ectopic pregnancy, a condition in which the egg implants in the tube or some other abnormal location and that can have serious consequences, including infertility and death. It is not clear whether this increased rate of ectopic pregnancies is because the MAP is more effective in preventing uterine pregnancies than ectopic pregnancies or because the MAP actually contributes to ectopic pregnancies by slowing down fallopian tube contractions.[173]

DES has been implicated in reproductive tract abnormalities and cancer in the offspring of the women who used this drug during pregnancy. (*see* p. 808). Because DES has caused the development of cancer in some of the daughters of the women who took it during pregnancy as well as other serious problems in both DES sons and daughters, many doctors recommend that the drug should not be taken by women who would not consider abortion if the drug were not effective and pregnancy ensued. Nor should the drug be taken by women who are themselves DES daughters.

Because of the problems associated with DES, researchers have investigated the use of other estrogens and of progestins as morning-after pills. The most promising results have been with the use of Ovral, a combined birth control pill. Studies indicate that it is as effective as DES and has a lower rate of side effects.[174] As a morning-after pill, Ovral is taken in two doses: two tablets within 24 to 72 hours of the unprotected intercourse and then two more tablets 12 hours later. Nausea may still be a problem, but taking the pills with food is helpful in some cases. If vomiting occurs within an hour of taking the medicine, the woman should take a second dose along with an antinausea medication.

If the woman's menstrual period does not start within 3 weeks of taking DES or Ovral as a morning-after pill, she should see her doctor for pregnancy testing. If a woman *is* pregnant, despite having taken Ovral as a morning-after pill, and wishes to continue the pregnancy rather than have an abortion, her situation is probably not as serious as it would be had she taken DES. Although there has been some concern that birth control pills taken during pregnancy might have adverse effects on the fetus (*see* p. 111), Ovral has not been associated with cancer and other abnormalities found in the offspring of women who took DES during pregnancy.

Both DES and Ovral can cause any of the side effects associated with birth control pills (*see* pp. 104–14); the same contraindications to the use of the Pill (*see* p. 115) apply to the use of DES and Ovral as morning-after pills. Both drugs contain estrogen, which has been associated with strokes, blood clots and heart attacks. If a woman develops any of the following symptoms while taking DES or Ovral, she should not take any more pills and should call her doctor IMMEDIATELY:

*severe headaches	*severe leg pains
*dizziness	*blurred vision
*numbness in arms or legs	*chest pain
*shortness of breath	*abdominal pain
*loss of vision	*sensation of flashing lights

Despite the fact that the FDA has approved DES as a morning-after pill, the major manufacturer of DES, in its package insert, warns that DES *should not* be used as a postcoital contraceptive. The company apparently thinks (as we do) that its use as a postcoital contraceptive is too dangerous and with this disclaimer is seeking to avoid future lawsuits. Nonetheless, private physicians and many college and university health centers have continued to prescribe DES as a postcoital contraceptive. Ovral has not been approved by the FDA as a morning-after pill. But many doctors believe that it is preferable to DES because of the lower incidence of side effects and the decreased likelihood of harmful effects on the fetus if the pregnancy continues. Although there is no evidence that Ovral taken as a morning-after pill is not harmful, thousands of women use Ovral as a regular contraceptive. When such women forget a pill or two they are advised (as all pill users are; *see* pp. 101–02) to double up on pills, taking the missed pill along with the regular pill, and if they have missed two pills, to take two at their regularly scheduled time the next day. So far, there has not been any indication that taking Ovral in these doses causes risks any greater than the general risks associated with taking any regular-dose pill.

The Postcoital IUD[175]

The IUD has also been used as a method of postcoital contraception. So far, only the copper IUD has been tested for this purpose, and only on a relatively small number of women. These tests have indicated that the copper IUDs are highly effective when used in this manner, but larger numbers of women must be studied before firm conclusions can be drawn.[176]

The postcoital insertion of the copper IUD apparently prevents the implantation of the fertilized egg in the uterine wall. Because implantation takes place about 6 days after ovulation, researchers have inserted the copper IUDs as long as 6 days after unprotected intercourse, but most experts believe that the sooner the IUD is inserted, the better.

The copper IUDs were chosen for testing because the effect of the metal begins almost immediately after insertion of the device. Other, noncopper IUDs may take several days or weeks to reach maximum effectiveness and may therefore be less effective when used postcoitally.

The postcoital IUD has some advantages in comparison with the morning-after pill. Although IUD insertion may have side effects, such as pain and bleeding, and may cause perforation and other complications (*see* pp. 125–31), there usually isn't any nausea or vomiting. Moreover, once the IUD has been inserted it provides protection against future pregnancies as well. The postcoital IUD is probably a better choice for women who would leave it in place and would continue to rely on the IUD as a method of birth control.

If pregnancy should occur after IUD insertion, removal of the device or abortion is advisable, because pregnancy with an IUD in place involves risk to both the fetus and the mother (*see* p. 132–33).

Postcoital contraception with an IUD does have definite drawbacks. The usual contraindications to the IUD should be observed (*see* p. 124). The risks and problems normally associated with IUD use also apply to postcoital IUD use. Many doctors will not insert an IUD except during the menstrual flow (they believe that complications like expulsion and perforation are thereby minimized), so they do not use the IUD postcoitally. In addition, the postcoital IUD is not a wise choice for rape victims or women who have multiple sex partners. The chances that such women have been exposed to gonorrhea or other infections are simply too great. Inserting an IUD with one of these diseases could cause pelvic inflammatory disease (PID), a condition that can have serious and even fatal consequences. (Because the risk of PID is greater in IUD users, some authorities recommend the removal of an IUD inserted as a postcoital contraceptive within 2 months if the woman is at especially high risk for developing PID.)

Menstrual Extraction

Menstrual extraction (*see* p. 217) is an office procedure in which the uterine lining is removed by suction. It is performed at about the time the menstrual period is normally expected. Before the advent of today's pregnancy tests, which are accurate within a day or so of the missed period, this procedure was done on women who had had unprotected intercourse and feared that they might be pregnant. Now that such tests are available, this procedure is not widely used. The advantages and drawbacks of menstrual extraction are discussed in greater detail in the section on abortion.

Dealing with Doctors, or How to Survive in the Medical Marketplace

In November 1979 the Commonwealth of Massachusetts signed a bill into law.[1] In some ways it was a pretty silly law, hard to implement, probably impossible to enforce and subject to such a variety of interpretations that it will undoubtedly enrich the lives of dozens of lawyers for years to come if anyone ever tries to file a suit based on it. Still, it was a gesture, and gestures like this one do have a certain significance.

The law says, among other things, that a doctor must inform a woman with breast cancer of "all alternative treatments that are medically viable." Although we're not lawyers, it seems to us that the hook, the catch-22 in this law, lies in the words "medically viable." A doctor who performed a modified radical mastectomy† on a woman with breast cancer without telling her of the availability of other, less disfiguring treatments, like a simple removal of the lump‡ could be sued under this law. However, the doctor could make a defense by arguing that, in his or her opinion, anything less than a modified radical mastectomy was not a viable medical alternative. At present it's a moot point medically—and probably legally as well.

By making this criticism of the Massachusetts law, we aren't trying to rain on anybody's parade, and we certainly aren't intending to belittle the efforts of the dedicated souls who must have worked like maniacs to push the bill

†Modified radical: same as a radical mastectomy, except that chest muscles are not removed.
‡Lumpectomy: removal of the cancerous lump; breast left largely intact.

231

into law. They deserve our undying (pun intended) gratitude, for although the law may not offer a completely solid legal recourse to women whose doctors fail to inform them about treatment options, the law is nonetheless a public and legal statement of the responsibility of the physician. It marks the beginning of the end for the M.D.eity.

The M.D.eity and the Doctor/Patient Relationship

[He] got past the nurses by impersonating a doctor. All he did was clip four ballpoint pens on his vest pocket and march in looking preoccupied.

—Lois Gould, *Such Good Friends,* 1970

In the introduction we talked about the M.D.eity syndrome and poked a bit of fun at the pomposity of doctors, and quite rightly so, for as we also pointed out, the M.D.eity syndrome, which allows to doctors the status of at least a minor god, also has its distinctly unfunny side: the some 300,000 unnecessary hysterectomies performed in the United States each year, for instance.[2] And hysterectomies are just one example; gynecological medicine is full of them. What woman doesn't have a gynecological atrocity tale to tell about a woman who was misdiagnosed, mistreated, misinformed, maimed or mangled by her doctor?

In all fairness to doctors (and we do want to be fair to them; after all, one of us *is* a doctor), not all these gynecological horror stories are to be believed, for gynecologists are dealing with sex and reproduction, two extremely sensitive issues. Moreover, most gynecologists are men. In this era of women's liberation any man trying to deal with a woman on the issues of sex and reproduction in the framework of what had traditionally been an authoritarian, paternalistic relationship between women and doctors—well, it's not surprising that he doesn't always come up smelling like a rose.

Yet even if you discount the horror stories, it's undeniably obvious that there are basic problems with the way in which many doctors relate to patients, which is what the Massachusetts law is an attempt to remedy. The M.D.eity syndrome has reached epidemic proportions. Many, if not most doctors, have convinced themselves that they—and not the patient—should have the final say when it comes to making treatment decisions, so they feel that there is really no point in the patient's bothering her pretty little head about other options. These doctors would oppose the spirit of the Massachusetts law. They don't believe it's their job to inform women of "all the alternative treatments that are medically viable," so that she can make her own

232

decision. They, the experts, the M.D.eities, by virtue of their special knowledge and training, are the only ones qualified to make these decisions. As one noted breast cancer specialist explains:

Every woman with breast cancer must make the only decision she is capable of making. . . . She must choose which physician will be responsible for her treatment; she cannot choose which treatment to have. She must rely completely on the good judgment of the physician in whom she has confidence.

—Philip Strax, M.D., in *Early Detection: Breast Cancer Is Curable,* 1974

According to Dr. Strax's philosophy, a woman who goes to a modified radical mastectomy proponent must have a modified radical; if she ends up at the office of a remove-the-lump-and-radiate-the-breast fan, she must be radiated; and if she happens on a lumpectomy advocate, she must have a lumpectomy. *She* can't choose what treatment to have; she has to trust her doctor.

Peculiar advice. Do you suppose Dr. Strax buys a car this way—if he winds up at a Cadillac dealer, he buys a Cadillac, at a Volkswagen dealer, a Volkswagen?

However strange Dr. Strax's advice may seem, he is by no means an isolated crackpot on the fringes of the medical world. We'd be willing to bet that his views are shared by most card-carrying members of the AMA. In the context of all this it seems rather petty to criticize the Massachusetts law because it isn't the most airtight legal construct ever devised. Indeed, one is tempted to advocate the passage of similar laws in all states, laws that would require doctors to inform women of all the viable medical alternatives not just for breast cancer but for all diseases.

But laws alone can't right what's wrong with the doctor/patient relationship. They can't change the hierarchical, authoritarian mode of relating that characterizes most medical training programs, where the medical residents, or "the boys," as they are called by "the king," the chief resident, vie for interesting patients so they can score "brownie points" and maybe, someday, make it to the top of the heap and get to be the chief themselves. (These descriptive phrases are lifted from Dr. William Nolen's best-seller, *The Making of a Surgeon,* a saga of medical training that alternates between sounding like the story of a bunch of adolescent boys working out their personality problems and the melodrama of a Prussian Army training camp.)

Nor can the law legislate away sexism in the medical profession. As long as most of the women in a doctor's life are nurses, who are viewed not as partners on the health-care team but as subordinates, it's going to be tough to get

233

doctors to deal with their women patients on an equal footing, where the patient is seen as having a right to make her own health-care decisions.

Perhaps we're painting too black a picture. There are plenty of good doctors out there, doctors who are committed to a patient's right to know, who are well informed about the latest developments and who don't dismiss women's complaints as "psychogenic." You just have to know how to go about finding them.

Finding a Doctor

Most of us spend more time choosing a new dress than we do choosing a doctor. Although we would never dream of asking a friend to recommend a new dress and then calling the store and ordering it sent out to our house sight unseen, we might very well ask a friend for the name of a doctor and just call to make an appointment, without thinking any more about it.

This is another consequence of the M.D.eity syndrome. Just because a person has an M.D. after his or her name, we assume that s/he is competent. Moreover, the idea of shopping around, of comparative buying, is definitely a consumer's notion, and women patients are not encouraged to think of themselves as consumers. We may hire an architect or a lawyer, but one does not "hire" a doctor. Indeed, we are apt to consider ourselves lucky if we manage to get an appointment, particularly if the doctor is highly recommended.

So begin your search for a doctor at the beginning: by collecting the names of doctors to interview for the job of being your doctor. Remember, just like the butcher, the baker, the candlestick maker or anyone else in the business of selling their services or goods, the doctor is in the business of selling his or her services—in this case, medical care. The doctor is in your employ. You are his or her client, and this holds true whether the doctor is being paid directly by you, by your insurance company or by a state or federal medical-care program.

An excellent source of names of prospective doctors is a hospital scrub nurse. These nurses work in the operating room, right alongside the doctors. They have an inside track, know who's good and who isn't and are generally pretty open about sharing that information. Similarly, an anesthesiologist (a doctor who administers anesthesia) or an anesthetist (a nurse or specially trained person who administers anesthesia) is an excellent source of information. In some areas of the country, women's health groups have files of consumer comments and ratings of doctors in the area. These can be invaluable and can save you a lot of time by steering you away from the less-than-adequate doctors and toward those that have the qualities and qualifications you are looking for.

Board-Certification

Once you have some possibilities, check these doctors' credentials. Evaluating credentials is only part of the process of choosing a doctor, but such credentials are important factors to consider. One important credential is board-certification. Certification boards are private, nonprofit organizations that offer certification to doctors who meet their standards. There are individual boards for each of the various medical specialties, including general surgery, pediatrics, psychiatry, family practice, obstetrics (childbirth) and gynecology. There are also subspecialties. A surgeon might, for example, specialize in plastic surgery or vascular surgery. Gynecology and obstetrics, or OB/GYN, also has subspecialties, including fertility, gynecologic oncology (cancer of the female reproductive organs) and perinatology (difficult or high-risk pregnancies).

Once a gynecologist has completed residency training, s/he may take written examinations administered by the board. After practicing medicine for at least 2 years, s/he submits records of all hospital cases to the board for review. Members of the board, which is made up of top-notch gynecologists, then conduct oral examinations. If the written and oral examinations and the review of the hospital cases are satisfactory, the board certifies the doctor.

Not all doctors are board-certified. You may hear the term "board-eligible." This means that the doctor has completed the necessary training but is not yet certified. A young gynecologist who has not yet completed the requisite 2 years of medical practice would be board-eligible. There has been a movement recently to restrict the use of the term, for some doctors who have long since completed their residencies and the required 2 years of practice continue to call themselves board-eligible even though they have either failed to pass the requirements for certification or don't even intend to try for it. If a doctor claims to be board-eligible, ask how long s/he has been board-eligible and be skeptical if s/he has been eligible for a number of years.

There are many good doctors who are not board-certified, and board-certification does not guarantee competency. But a doctor who is board-certified has subjected himself or herself to the rigorous testing required for certification, and his or her technical skill and experience have been evaluated by experts in the field and judged to be outstanding.

You can check your doctor's qualifications in *The Directory of Medical Specialists,* which gives detailed information, including where the doctor trained, membership in professional societies, appointments to medical schools, hospital affiliations and specialties. All doctors listed in this directory are board-certified. *The American Medical Directory* also gives information about doctors' credentials but lists only those doctors who are members

235

of the American Medical Society, regardless of whether they are board-certified. Many public libraries have these books, as do most medical libraries. If you can't get hold of a copy, you can call your local or state health department or medical society and ask whether or not the doctor you are considering is board-certified.

Most people outside the medical profession are not aware of the process of board-certification, but it is widely recognized as a sign of competency within the profession. You can bet that when doctors or their families are operated on, the operations are performed by board-certified surgeons.

In addition to board-certification, there are other factors to consider, including:

Where the doctor served his or her internship and residency: The most coveted intern and residency programs are those associated with university medical schools, for the top-notch doctors work in these hospitals and a wide variety of patients are referred there for care. A doctor who has trained at a university hospital generally has had the opportunity to work under the most skilled doctors in the field and has had more experience with a wider variety of cases than doctors who train at less prestigious hospitals.

Hospital affiliations: Doctors are granted staff privileges at hospitals. The quality of the hospitals with which the doctor is affiliated is important. The most prestigious types of hospital affiliations are with hospitals associated with medical schools. Hospitals are accredited by the Joint Committee on Hospital Accreditation (JCHA). It is preferable that your doctor be affiliated with an accredited hospital. The size of the hospital is also a factor. Generally, hospitals with 200 or more beds are better equipped than smaller hospitals.

Membership in professional societies: Membership in professional societies like the *American College of Gynecologists and Obstetricians* that offer conferences, workshops and other continuing education programs are an indication of a doctor's interest in keeping up-to-date and well informed on developments in his or her specialty. If a gynecologist is not only a member, but also a fellow of the American College of Gynecologists and Obstetricians, this means that his or her colleagues have accorded the gynecologist special recognition.

Personal style (also known as bedside manner): Your gut reaction to the doctor is of utmost importance. A string of impressive credentials after a doctor's name doesn't mean a thing if you can't communicate. A doctor you feel comfortable with, even if his or her credentials aren't as impressive, is a better choice. On the other hand, don't let a charming bedside manner obscure a lack of experience, training or skill.

Health Care for Gay Women

Lesbians face special difficulties in finding a doctor with whom they can communicate openly. Many doctors have prejudices about lesbians and consider any sexual preference that is not strictly heterosexual a sign of a deep-seated psychological disturbance. Thus many lesbians are in a quandary. If they tell their doctors they are gay, they are apt to be put down, lectured, treated with scorn or horror and referred to a psychiatrist. One woman we saw who was having abnormal vaginal bleeding told her doctor that she was a lesbian. He referred her to a psychiatrist and, in his preoccupation with "curing" her of her "problem," neglected the symptom that had brought her to him in the first place. When she finally came to us it was too late; her undiagnosed vaginal bleeding turned out to be cancer of the endometrial lining.

If, on the other hand, a gay woman doesn't tell her doctor that she is a lesbian, her symptoms are apt to be attributed to conditions related to pregnancy or to diseases like gonorrhea, which lesbians rarely develop. Valuable time is lost and needless expense incurred in ruling out diagnostic possibilities that she, because she is a lesbian, is not subject to.

Women's centers and lesbian groups may be able to refer such women to doctors who will treat them in a nonjudgmental way. A group of doctors sympathetic to the health-care problems of both gay women and gay men has recently established a referral service in San Francisco and in the Los Angeles area. (In the San Francisco area, contact Bay Area Physicians for Human Rights, P.O. Box 14546, San Francisco, California 94114, 415–673–3189; in the Los Angeles area, contact Southern California Physicians for Human Rights, 7985 Santa Monica Boulevard, Suite 109, Los Angeles, California 90046, 213–658–6261.)

The Nurse Practitioner

All women looking for good health care should be aware of the emerging role of a new health-care professional, the nurse practitioner. Many gynecologists are taking advantage of the services of nurse practitioners, who are nurses with special training who can perform many of the routine services usually performed by doctors. In our experience, nurse practitioners provide excellent care. Their time is less expensive, so they usually have more time to spend explaining things and answering questions. Indeed, they are often better at explaining things to the layperson than doctors are, so don't feel slighted if you spend more time with one of them than with the doctor. In fact, if your doctor incorporates nurse practitioners into his or her office staff, this is a sign that you've found yourself a forward-thinking gynecologist, one who is probably not so caught up in the M.D.eity syndrome.

Second Opinions

Even if you manage to find an absolute wonder of a gynecologist, one who walks on water, you should still consider getting a second opinion before consenting to any form of treatment for a serious illness. Doctors, even the top-notch ones, disagree, and you owe it to yourself to get all the facts and many points of view before making a decision.

Of course, getting a second opinion falls into the easier-said-than-done category. It is hard for many women to say, "I'd like a second opinion before deciding, so don't write out that prescription or don't schedule me for surgery yet." Let's face it, most of us have difficulty switching hairdressers or garage mechanics, let alone switching M.D.eities. Even though on an objective, rational level all that a second opinion means is that you want more information before making a decision, the implication is that you are somehow not satisfied with or are distrustful of your doctor.

Undoubtedly, an up-front, honest approach is best. But if you find yourself unable to do this, you've got a couple of other options. You can always shift the responsibility by saying, "My mother, my husband (or somebody else in charge of my life) insists that I get a second opinion." Given most gynecologists' view of women, you'll probably find your doctor is remarkably accepting of the notion that someone other than you is doing your thinking for you and is making your decisions. It feeds right into the view of women patients expressed in the quote from Dr. Strax above. Perhaps you're copping out a bit this way, but if you've got a serious medical problem, the paramount thing at this point is to obtain quality medical care. First things first; you can sort out your inabilities to be assertive later on.

Another option is to simply pocket the prescription or hedge about scheduling the surgery date and beat a hasty retreat from the office. Then schedule a second appointment and simply call your first doctor's office later, speaking to the secretary and getting her to arrange to have the necessary medical records sent to the second doctor. Again, this is not the most up-front way of dealing with the situation, but if that's what you need to do, it's perfectly OK.

When making your appointment with the second doctor just say that you've been diagnosed as having such and such a condition and that you'd like a second opinion or consultation before you make any decisions. You should ask what medical records, test results and so forth the doctor would like to see before consulting with you and arrange to have these available for him or her at the time of your appointment (*see* Your Medical Records below).

When you see the second doctor, explain your medical history, your problem and symptoms and what diagnostic tests have been done (the results of which he or she should now have). The natural impulse in this situation is for you to say something along the lines of ''So my doctor recommended such and such; however, I want a second opinion before going ahead.'' If that's your impulse, stifle it. We recommend that you not mention the first doctor's opinion, even though it may be stated in the medical records transferred to the second doctor. If it's not stated, your second doctor is likely to ask you what your first doctor said or recommended. If so, simply say, ''Before discussing that, I'd like to hear what you have to say.''

The reason for this rather secretive approach is that too often the second opinion will simply be a rubber stamp of approval. ''Professional ethics'' dictate that your second doctor not malign the opinions or professional competency of your original doctor. It is considered extremely tacky in the medical profession for doctors to ''steal'' one another's patients. (In our opinion extreme tackiness enters the situation when a doctor fails to tell a patient that another doctor has, in his or her opinion, misdiagnosed, misinformed or mistreated a patient, but ethics are always situational, and what any given person sees as ethical depends on his or her particular point of view.) By approaching the matter in this fashion you are letting the second doctor off the hook and decreasing the chances that the second opinion will merely be a polite affirmation of the first doctor's recommendations.

Many of the medical books written for a lay audience pay lip service to the idea of obtaining second opinions and suggest that you find a doctor for a second consultation by asking the first doctor for a referral. Perhaps it is putting it too strongly to say that this is like asking the fox for advice about guarding the chicken coop. Still, asking the first doctor to recommend a second-opinion doctor and expecting to thereby obtain an unbiased, objective opinion seems a bit foolish.

We suggest that a woman go about getting a second opinion in the same way that we suggested she find a doctor in the first place—by asking for referrals from a number of sources, checking the doctor's credentials and then interviewing him or her. One excellent source for second opinions is a university hospital outpatient clinic. If you live near one of these institutions, call the gynecology department or the women's clinic and ask for a consultation.

If you have been diagnosed as having a specific problem for which there are alternative treatments (see below), you may want to ask if the doctor you are consulting for a second opinion is equipped or trained to perform or provide alternatives to what your first doctor has recommended. If, for example, you have been diagnosed as having carcinoma in situ of the cervix and your first doctor has recommended a hysterectomy, you might ask if the second doctor has cryosurgery equipment. If you are under age 35–40 and your first

239

doctor has recommended a total hysterectomy (removal of the uterus *and* ovaries) for a benign disease, you might ask the second doctor whether s/he recommends simply removing the uterus or whether s/he routinely removes the ovaries in all women in your age-group. But you must be cagey in wording your questions. The standard response to such questions is, "I'll have to see you to answer that," and it's a fair response. No doctor can be expected to make a diagnosis, recommend treatment or give a second opinion over the phone. If, however, you phrase your question along these lines: "Doctor, I am 36 and have been diagnosed as having (some benign disease) and am considering a hysterectomy. Of course, I want a second opinion before surgery and would like to make an appointment for a consultation. I realize you can't tell me much before you have reviewed my medical records and examined me, but I would like to know, just in general, do you ever consider sparing the ovaries in a woman my age, assuming of course this is possible, or do you feel it's better, as a rule, to take them out?"

Some doctors will still refuse to answer your question. Most will still hedge a bit, but you can often get at least some indication as to whether they would or would not consider sparing the ovaries. By asking such questions of the doctor when making your consultation appointment, you can make sure that you will be getting a second opinion from someone who will at least consider another point of view on your case.

So far we've been talking about situations in which getting a second opinion is a fairly easy matter. Things get a bit trickier if you're already in the hospital. If you know ahead of time that you're going into the hospital to have a hysterectomy or whatever, the time to get a second opinion is, of course, *before* you are admitted. But you may not always know ahead of time. For example, a woman might be hospitalized in order to receive intravenous (IV) antibiotics to treat pelvic inflammatory disease, an infection that can affect the uterus, fallopian tubes, ovaries and other pelvic organs. If the antibiotics don't work, the doctor might suggest a hysterectomy.

In such cases you can get a second opinion in one of two ways. The first option is to check yourself out of the hospital and seek a second opinion. This is not always possible. The other alternative, having the second doctor see you in the hospital, may be more feasible. The second doctor must be on staff at the hospital or have consulting privileges there. Most hospitals have some sort of patient adviser or social worker who can help you arrange for a second opinion, or the head nurse may be able to supply you with a list of such doctors.

Getting a second opinion becomes even more complex when the disease involved is a cancerous one. This is discussed in detail under the heading Cancer in the reference section. If you have been diagnosed as having cancer or there is even a possibility that you may have cancer, be sure to read that section.

240

The cost of a consultation varies but is often surprisingly inexpensive. Many medical and insurance companies and government medical programs will cover the costs of a second opinion, but you may want to check your coverage first, since some companies or government programs still do not do so.

Your Medical Records

In some states the laws have clearly established that a patient has a right to her own medical records. Yet even in these states a woman may have difficulty getting the doctor to release her records to her. They will, however, release your records to another doctor, so you may have to ask the doctor you are consulting to call and request that your records be transferred.

Dealing with Doctors/How to Use This Book

Regardless of whether you are seeking a first or a second opinion or are merely having a routine check-up, there are certain things to keep in mind when you are consulting a doctor. Of primary importance is the fact that *you* are paying the doctor, directly or indirectly, and that by virtue of this simple fact, you have certain rights and a certain amount of consumer power. If you are paying the doctor directly, this fact may be obvious.

If, however, like the majority of Americans, you are employed by a company that provides medical benefits or are receiving state or federal medical aid, you may not feel that you are actually paying the doctor. If it's your company that is providing medical coverage, you may think that you are fortunate to be employed by an organization generous enough to offer its employees such extra benefits. You may believe that your employer provides this as an extra, added attraction, a "freebie." This is not true. When you receive benefits they are in lieu of extra salary. Instead of paying you a wage that would allow you to seek medical care at your own expense, the company that employs you has made a deal with an insurance company. By insuring all its employees with the company, the employer is able to get insurance at a group rate that is much cheaper than it would be for an individual. So your medical coverage is not a gift bestowed on you out of the kindness of the corporate heart; it is part of the wages you earn for the work that you do. If you are paying your doctor indirectly, through a medical insurance plan, it is still you who are paying the doctor and you have the same consumer power as if you were paying directly out of your own pocket.

If you are receiving medical aid from the state or federal government, you are still paying the doctor and you have the same rights as if you were paying out of your pocket. Our national social programs—food stamps, welfare pay-

241

ments, medical assistance and the like—are attempts to compensate for the inequities created by racism, sexism and ageism in our society. Contrary to the popular image of the welfare recipient as a shiftless, lazy person unwilling to work, the typical recipient is a single mother with children under school age who cannot find a job that will pay her enough money to allow her to feed, house and clothe her family as well as pay for child care. The elderly and the disabled are also typical recipients. Such people have a right to medical care; it should not be considered a gift. Your doctor is paid by the government for the services s/he provides you—and paid well. The doctor does not receive money unless you "pay" him or her with your medical voucher. Again, even though you are paying the doctor indirectly, you have the same rights as people who pay for medical care directly.

Your Medical Rights and Duties

Now that we've got that important point out of the way, what exactly are your medical rights? First and foremost, you deserve a clear explanation of what is wrong and why, at least to the best of the doctor's ability to give you that information. There are gaps in our medical knowledge, and many times a doctor will not be able to diagnose what is wrong.

The It's-All-in-Your-Head-Dearie Diagnosis

In cases where medical information is less than perfect, you have the right to an honest "I-don't-know" reply from your doctor, although you may not get it. It has long been a medical custom for doctors to attribute diseases for which they are unable to find a cause or cure to "psychogenic factors," the old it's-all-in-your-head-dearie diagnosis. M.D.eities do not like to admit to not knowing, so they fall back on the old I-can't-figure-out-what's-wrong-with-you-so-you-must-be-crazy switcheroo, projecting their problem onto you. Throughout the reference section on diseases we have tried to alert women to situations in which they may run into these sorts of reactions from doctors.

If your doctor suggests that your symptoms are psychosomatic or refers you to a psychologist or psychiatrist, consider this bit of advice carefully. Has the doctor fully evaluated you medically? In the section on menstrual disorders we talk about a woman who had severe nausea and vomiting during her period each month. Her doctor couldn't figure out what was wrong, decided the woman was neurotic and referred her to a psychiatrist. After months of exploring "her rejection of her female role" with her male therapist, this woman saw a second gynecologist, who didn't dismiss her symptoms. Instead, the doctor took a look at the woman's pelvis with the aid of a special viewing instrument called a laparoscope, which is inserted into the body through an incision in the abdomen. As it turned out, this woman's problem was not in her head but in her pelvis. She had a condition known as endometriosis, and once it was treated, her symptoms disappeared.

Use the symptoms index at the end of this chapter. Read the sections on the possible diseases that could be causing your symptoms, and check to see that your doctor has done all the diagnostic tests to rule out the various possibilities. Although psychotherapy can be valuable for anyone, you should not let symptoms that may be caused by a medical problem that needs attention be diagnosed as psychosomatic, especially if your medical condition has not been fully evaluated.

Other Medical Rights

Along with the right to a clear explanation of your problems, you also have a right to an explanation of all the treatment options available. Here again, you may not get it. If you have been diagnosed as having a specific problem, look up that disease in the reference section of this book. Find out if there are alternative treatments. Ask your doctor about the possibility of using these other forms of therapy in your case. The questions listed in Chapter Seven may be particularly helpful. And always get a second opinion before submitting to any form of treatment for a serious problem.

Your doctor may disagree with the opinions expressed in this book or may recommend a form of treatment different from the ones outlined here. This is to be expected and certainly doesn't mean that your doctor is wrong. New discoveries are being made all the time, and there may have been advancements in the forms of treatment for your condition since this book was written. In addition, the particulars of your case may rule out a specific mode of therapy for you.

This book cannot be used to diagnose or recommend treatment. Rather, it is intended to make you aware of the existing options and to provide enough information to allow you to ask questions and to evaluate your alternatives. If your doctor disagrees with us, that's fine, but remember, you have the right to a full explanation of his or her point of view. If all you get as a reply to your questions is a because-I'm-the-Doctor-and-I-say-so response, find another doctor.

Similarly, you have the right to a full explanation of any tests the doctor may order. Again, the questions listed in Chapter Seven will be helpful. You may find that your doctor is not terribly pleased with your asking all these questions. If you balk at following orders, you may be made to feel that you are being "difficult," that you are a troublesome sort of person or that you are being silly and overly cautious. Well, so what if you are. If, according to some estimates, 30 percent of the X-rays done in the United States each year are unnecessary, women are quite right to refuse to follow their doctors' orders blindly and submit to all these tests.

Your Responsibility

Along with these rights come certain responsibilities. You must assume responsibility for being informed about the basic workings of the female body. If, for instance, you don't know how the menstrual cycle works, it's unrealistic to expect the doctor to explain why you've stopped having menstrual periods and the various tests s/he wants to do or the various methods of treating your condition. This is where this book comes in; use it to inform yourself. Once you have been diagnosed, read the section on your disease carefully, and make notes so that you will remember your questions. Take this book along with you when you see the doctor so you will be able to refer to the appropriate section if the need arises.

If you are confronted with the possibility of a serious disease, you may want to ask a family member or friend to read the section as well and help you frame your questions. Our experience has been that women diagnosed as having something seriously wrong, for example, cancer, are often so shaken and upset that they find it difficult to absorb all the necessary information. A relative or friend may be better able to do this.

When you see the doctor, take notes so that you will be able to refer to them later on. You may also want to bring a friend or relative along with you when you see the doctor. Women's groups often have volunteers who serve as patient advocates and who are usually well informed. They will visit the doctor with you. Having another person along can be particularly valuable. It's more difficult to communicate and receive information when you're upset, and having a friend along assures that you will clearly understand what is being said to you.

A Word About References

As explained in Chapter One, the diseases and conditions described in the following reference section are organized according to the organs that they affect. There are separate subsections for the vulva, the vagina, the cervix, the uterus and fallopian tubes, the ovaries and the breast. In addition, there are separate subsections that deal with problems related to pregnancy and fertility, the menstrual cycle and sexually transmissible infections, as well as a section giving general background information on cancer. At the back of the book you will find a list of references.

We have relied on two main sources in preparing this reference section, *Novak's Textbook of Gynecology*, 9th ed., by Edmund R. Novak, M.D., Georgeanna Seegar Jones, M.D. and Howard W. Jones, Jr., M.D. (Baltimore: Williams & Wilkins, 1975), and *Gynecology,* 2d ed., by Langdon Parsons, M.D., and Sheldon C. Sommers, M.D. (Philadelphia: W.B. Saunders, 1978). These are the two most widely used gynecological texts. Facts and figures given in our text are, unless otherwise noted, derived from these two sources, although to avoid littering the pages with footnotes, we have not cited them explicitly. When other sources were used, appropriate references are given.

SYMPTOMS INDEX

Most medical books, including those written for lay readers and those written for professionals, aren't very helpful if you have a particular symptom and want to know what diseases could be causing that symptom. To find the cause of a symptom you must either have a fairly good idea of which diseases could cause the symptom in the first place or devote hours to a difficult and frustrating search through the text. To remedy this situation we have included the following Symptoms Index.

This index is by no means complete, for gynecological diseases can produce a wide variety of symptoms. To catalog all of them would be impossible. Also, some of the symptoms produced by gynecological diseases are "nonspecific." For example, a number of the conditions described in this book can cause a fever. Fever is a "nonspecific" symptom that can be caused by a wide variety of diseases, some of which have no relation to a woman's reproductive organs. For practical reasons we have limited this index to the following categories of symptoms:

☐ Symptoms Related to the Vulva
  Itching, Burning and/or Rashes on the Vulva
  Sores, Lumps or Growths on the Vulva
  White Patches on, or a White Appearance of, the Vulvar Skin
☐ Symptoms Related to the Vagina
  Growths, Lumps or Protrusions on the Vaginal Walls or at the Vaginal Opening
  Sores or Red Areas on the Vaginal Walls
  Painful or Difficult Intercourse
  Vaginal Discharges
☐ Symptoms Related to the Cervix
  Changes in the Shape of the Cervical Os
  Growths or Clumps of Tissue Protruding Through the Cervical Opening
  Sores, Cysts, Lumps, Red or White Areas on the Cervix, or Other Abnormalities in the Appearance of the Cervix

☐ Symptoms Related to the Breast
  Breast Lumps and Other Abnormalities in the Shape, Feel, and Appearance of the Breast
  Nipple Discharge
  Painful Breasts
☐ Symptoms Related to the Menstrual Cycle
  Abnormally Heavy or Prolonged Menstrual Periods, Bleeding or Spotting Between Periods or Abnormally Long or Short Intervals Between Periods
  Missed Periods or the Absence of Menstruation
  Hot Flashes and Symptoms that Occur at the Time of Menopause
  Menstrual Cramps
  Premenstrual Pain, Weight Gain, Breast Tenderness, Mood Changes and Other Symptoms that Occur in Relation to the Menstrual Cycle
☐ Infertility and Sterility
☐ Abdominal or Pelvic Pain
☐ Vaginal Bleeding

This index is not meant to take the place of the doctor. Don't fool yourself into thinking that you can diagnose or treat yourself, for accurate diagnosis usually is not based on the presence of a single symptom. The exact nature of the symptom, the presence or absence of other symptoms, the medical history and the findings of physical exams and laboratory tests may be necessary. If, for example, you have a nipple discharge, the doctor will want to examine the discharge microscopically. If s/he finds that the discharge is composed of breast milk, s/he will want to proceed differently from the way s/he would if the discharge were composed of pus. If you have a milky nipple discharge, the doctor will want to pay close attention to your medical history, especially to your childbirth experiences. If your milky discharge is accompanied by an absence of menstrual periods, the presence of this symptom will also aid the doctor in diagnosis. Many factors, then, come into play, and a simple index like this one cannot hope to cover the complexities in diagnosis. It can, however, help you to identify a group of possible causes for your symptom and to become well informed about the possibilities and the necessity for certain diagnostic procedures.

Symptoms Related to the Vulva

Itching, Burning and/or Rashes on the Vulva

Itching and burning or rashes on the vulva can be caused by inadequate ventilation of the area because of wearing panty hose or tight clothing or by allergies to vaginal deodorant sprays, soaps, perfumed powders or the material in your underclothes. The majority of vulvar itching, burning and rashes

are related to vaginal discharges from some form of vaginitis (*see* pp. 298–305) or sexually transmissible infections (*see* pp. 556–62). Less frequently, other forms of vulvitis or other problems may cause these symptoms.
Any of the following diseases may give rise to vulvar itching or burning:

Vulvitis (*see* p. 265)
Postmenopausal vulvitis (*see* p. 270)
Vulvar folliculitis (*see* p. 271)
Hidradenitis (*see* pp. 271–72)
Vulvar dystrophy (*see* p. 282)
Preinvasive cancer of the vulva (*see* p. 286)
Invasive cancer of the vulva (*see* p. 289)
Trich (*see* pp. 306–7)
Yeast infections (*see* p. 313)
Hemophilus (*see* p. 317)
Nonspecific vaginitis (*see* p. 319)
Postmenopausal vaginitis (*see* p. 319)
Cervicitis (*see* p. 351)
Pelvic inflammatory disease (*see* pp. 393–401)
Gonorrhea (*see* p. 562)
Herpes (*see* p. 569)
Chlamydial infections (*see* p. 579)
Syphilis (*see* p. 582)
Crabs (*see* p. 587)
Genital warts (*see* p. 590)
Granuloma inguinale (*see* p. 592)
Chancroid (*see* p. 593)
Lymphopathia venereum (*see* p. 594)
Other sexually transmissible infections (*see* pp. 595–97)
Allergies to vaginal spermicides or the materials used in diaphragms, condoms, contraceptive sponges or cervical caps (*see* pp. 135–69)

Sores, Lumps, or Growths on the Vulva

The skin of the vulva, like the skin anywhere else on the body, is subject to a number of sores, lumps and bumps. Any of the diseases that cause itching and burning (see above) can lead to scratching, which in turn can lead to rashes and the formation of vesicles, or pimplelike blisters. In addition, a number of sexually transmissible infections, vulvar diseases and other conditions can cause sores, lumps, or growths on the vulva, such as:

Vulvar folliculitis (*see* p. 271)
Hidradenitis (*see* p. 271)
Bartholinitis (*see* pp. 272–73)
Skenitis (*see* pp. 274–75)

247

Circulatory diseases of the vulva (*see* p. 275)
Vulvar cysts (*see* pp. 279–80)
Benign solid tumors of the vulva (*see* pp. 280–82)
Vulvar dystrophy (*see* pp. 282–83)
Preinvasive cancer of the vulva (*see* p. 286)
Invasive cancer of the vulva (*see* p. 290)
Endometriosis (*see* pp. 403–6)
Herpes (*see* pp. 570–71)
Syphilis (*see* pp. 583–85)
Genital warts (*see* p. 590)
Granuloma inguinale (*see* p. 592)
Chancroid (*see* p. 593)
Lymphopathia venereum (*see* p. 594)
Other sexually transmissible infections (*see* pp. 595–97)

White Patches on, or a White Appearance of, the Vulvar Skin

White patches on, or a whitish hue to, the vulvar skin can be caused by any of the diseases that can cause itching, burning and rashes of the vulvar skin (see above). The itching, burning and rashes may lead to scratching, which can result in a white appearance of the vulvar skin. In addition, the following diseases can cause this symptom:

Postmenopausal vulvitis (*see* p. 270)
Depigmentation (*see* pp. 277–78)
Vulvar dystrophy (*see* p. 283)
Preinvasive cancer of the vulva (*see* pp. 286–89)
Invasive cancer of the vulva (*see* pp. 289–97)
Yeast infections (*see* p. 314)

Symptoms Related to the Vagina

Growths, Lumps or Protrusions on the Vaginal Wall or at the Vaginal Opening

A number of conditions can cause these symptoms, including:

Bartholinitis (*see* p. 273)
Skenitis (*see* pp. 274–75)
Imperforate hymen (*see* pp. 276–77)
Vulvar cysts at the vaginal opening (*see* pp. 279–80)
Benign solid tumors of the vulva located at the vaginal opening (*see* pp. 280–82)
Preinvasive cancer of the vulva (*see* pp. 286–89)
Cancer of the vulva located at the vaginal opening (*see* pp. 289–97)

248

Cystocele and urethrocele (*see* pp. 324–25)
Rectocele and enterocele (*see* pp. 327–28)
Benign tumors of the vagina (*see* pp. 334–35)
Clear cell adenocarcinoma (*see* p. 340)
Cancer of the vagina (*see* p. 343)
Endometriosis (*see* pp. 403–6)
Prolapse of the uterus, vagina and cervix (*see* p. 429)
Genital warts (*see* p. 590)
Other sexually transmissible infections (*see* pp. 595–97)

Sores or Red Areas on the Vaginal Walls

Women who practice vaginal self-exam may notice sores or red areas on the vaginal walls. These usually are related to such infectious diseases as vaginitis (*see* pp. 298–305) or sexually transmissible infections (*see* pp. 556–97). Other conditions can also cause these symptoms. Any of the following conditions may be responsible:

Trich (*see* pp. 306–7)
Yeast infections (*see* p. 314)
Hemophilus (*see* p. 318)
Nonspecific vaginitis (*see* p. 319)
Postmenopausal vaginitis (*see* p. 319)
Lacerations of the vagina (*see* p. 322)
Fistulas (*see* p. 330)
Vaginal adenosis (*see* pp. 336–37)
Clear cell adenocarcinoma (*see* p. 340)
Cancer of the vagina (*see* p. 343)
Gonorrhea (*see* p. 563)
Herpes (*see* pp. 570–71)
Chlamydial infections (*see* p. 580)
Syphilis (*see* pp. 583–85)
Granuloma inguinale (*see* p. 592)
Chancroid (*see* p. 593)
Lymphopathia venereum (*see* p. 594)
Toxic shock syndrome (*see* pp. 651–53)
Allergies to vaginal spermicides or the materials used in diaphragms, condoms, contraceptive sponges or cervical caps (*see* pp. 135–69)

Painful or Difficult Intercourse

The medical term for painful or difficult intercourse is "dyspareunia." Painful intercourse may be associated with attempts to place the penis in the vagina or with deep thrusting during intercourse.

The vulvar, vaginal or cervical tissues may become inflamed, and friction from the penis may further irritate these tissues. Any of the following conditions may cause inflammation of the vulvar, vaginal or cervical tissues and make intercourse painful:

Vulvitis (*see* p. 265)
Postmenopausal vulvitis (*see* p. 270)
Hidradenitis (*see* pp. 271–72)
Bartholinitis (*see* pp. 272–73)
Skenitis (*see* pp. 274–75)
Vulvar dystrophy (*see* p. 283)
Trich (*see* pp. 307–8)
Yeast infections (*see* p. 314)
Hemophilus (*see* p. 318)
Nonspecific vaginitis (*see* p. 319)
Postmenopausal vaginitis (*see* p. 319)
Cervicitis (*see* pp. 352–54)
Gonorrhea (*see* pp. 563–65)
Herpes (*see* pp. 570–71)
Chlamydial infections (*see* p. 580)
Syphilis (*see* pp. 583–85)
Genital warts (*see* p. 590)
Granuloma inguinale (*see* p. 592)
Chancroid (*see* p. 593)
Lymphopathia venereum (*see* p. 594)
Other sexually transmissible infections (*see* pp. 595–97)
Allergies to the materials used in diaphragms, condoms, contraceptive
    sponges and cervical caps or to vaginal spermicides (*see* pp. 135–69)

Painful intercourse may also be caused by anatomical abnormalities, such as:

Imperforate hymen (*see* pp. 276–77)
Vaginal stenosis (*see* p. 321)
Congenital absence of the lower part of the vagina (*see* p. 332)
Transverse vaginal septum (*see* p. 332)
Septate vagina (*see* p. 332)
Tipped uterus (*see* pp. 425–26)

Infections of the urinary tract may also make intercourse painful. If a woman has not been sufficiently aroused and lubricated before intercourse, the penis may irritate the dry tissues. Also, when a woman is aroused the uterus and ovaries move to a slightly higher position in the pelvis. If a woman is not sufficiently aroused, the penis may jar these organs on deep thrusting, causing pain.

Any benign (noncancerous) tumor or cyst or any of the precancerous or cancerous conditions of the pelvic organs can cause difficult or painful intercourse, including:

Vulvar cysts (*see* pp. 279–80)
Benign solid tumors of the vulva (*see* pp. 280–82)
Vulvar dystrophy (*see* pp. 282–86)
Preinvasive cancer of the vulva (*see* pp. 286–89)
Invasive cancer of the vulva (*see* pp. 289–97)
Benign tumors of the vagina (*see* pp. 334–35)
Vaginal adenosis (*see* pp. 335–40)
Clear cell adenocarcinoma (*see* pp. 340–42)
Cancer of the vagina (*see* pp. 342–49)
Cervical dysplasia (*see* pp. 367–72)
Carcinoma in situ (*see* pp. 372–75)
Cervical cancer (*see* pp. 375–91)
Uterine fibroids (*see* pp. 431–39)
Benign tumors of the fallopian tubes (*see* pp. 440–41)
Uterine cancer (*see* pp. 445–59)
Cancer of the fallopian tubes (*see* pp. 459–61)
Physiologic cysts (*see* pp. 468–71)
Benign ovarian tumors (*see* pp. 476–84)
Functioning ovarian tumors (*see* pp. 485–87)
Ovarian cancer (*see* pp. 487–99)
    Other gynecological conditions that may cause difficult or painful intercourse include:

Circulatory diseases of the vulva (*see* p. 275)
Vaginal stenosis (*see* pp. 320–22)
Lacerations of the vagina, vulva and perineum (*see* pp. 322–23)
Cystocele and urethrocele (*see* pp. 323–26)
Rectocele and enterocele (*see* pp. 326–28)
Vaginismus (*see* p. 329)
Fistulas (*see* pp. 329–31)
Cervical polyps (*see* pp. 357–59)
Cervical lacerations (*see* pp. 361–62)
Pelvic inflammatory disease (*see* pp. 393–401)
Endometriosis (*see* pp. 402–414)
Prolapse of the uterus, vagina and cervix (*see* pp. 427–30)
Endometrial polyps (*see* pp. 439–440)
Ectopic pregnancy (*see* pp. 683–92)
    Pain on intercourse may also be caused by an intrauterine device that is in the process of being expelled (*see* pp. 128–31) or by an incorrectly fitted diaphragm (*see* pp. 135–42).

Vaginal Discharge

It is normal to have some vaginal discharge. Normal vaginal discharge tends to be clear to somewhat milky and may leave a slightly yellow stain on the underclothes. The texture, consistency and amount of the vaginal discharge varies according to the stage of the menstrual cycle and the state of sexual excitement. Becoming familiar with your vaginal discharge will help you to recognize abnormal discharges.

The most common cause of vaginal discharge is vaginitis (*see* pp. 298–99). The nature of the discharge may give a clue as to what type of vaginitis you have. For instance, trich (*see* pp. 307–8) tends to produce a discharge with a yellow or green tinge, although it may also be gray or white. The trich discharge is apt to be thin and watery, although in mixed infections it may be thick and creamy. It is often frothy (that is, it has tiny bubbles in it) and tends to smell rather fishy. Yeast infections (*see* p. 314) often cause a cottage-cheese-like discharge—a white discharge that is watery, with thick, curdlike clumps of cheesy material. It often smells like fermenting yeast. Hemophilus (*see* p. 318) discharge tends to be abundant and smell bad. It may look like a thin, gray, flour paste. Any of these discharges may cause itching and burning of the external genitals.

Although the various types of vaginitis tend to have characteristic appearances, appearances can be deceiving. Another organism may be responsible, or the infection may be a mixed one. The symptoms of one form of vaginitis may mask those of another. Any form of vaginitis, cervical infection, pelvic infection or sexually transmissible infection can cause abnormal vaginal discharges, including:

Trich (*see* pp. 307–8)
Yeast infections (*see* p. 314)
Hemophilus (*see* p. 318)
Nonspecific vaginitis (*see* p. 319)
Postmenopausal vaginitis (*see* p. 319)
Cervicitis (*see* p. 352)
Cervical erosions (*see* p. 356)
Pelvic inflammatory disease (*see* p. 397)
Gonorrhea (*see* p. 564)
Herpes (*see* p. 570)
Chlamydial infections (*see* p. 580)
Syphilis (*see* p. 583)
Genital warts (*see* p. 590)
Granuloma inguinale (*see* p. 592)

Chancroid (*see* p. 593)
Lymphopathia venereum (*see* p. 594)
Other sexually transmissible infections (*see* pp. 595–97)

In addition to infections, other conditions can cause an abnormal vaginal discharge, including any of the following:

Vaginal adenosis (*see* pp. 336–37)
Clear cell adenocarcinoma (*see* p. 340)
Cancer of the vagina (*see* p. 343)
Cervical polyps (*see* p. 358)
Cervical dysplasia (*see* pp. 367–72)
Carcinoma in situ (*see* p. 373)
Cervical cancer (*see* p. 378)
Uterine fibroids (*see* p. 434)
Endometrial polyps (*see* p. 439)
Uterine cancer (*see* p. 449)
Cancer of the fallopian tubes (*see* p. 460)

An object left in the vagina too long (tampon, diaphragm, cervical cap, pessary) can cause a foul-smelling discharge. The strings of an IUD may irritate the cervical glands, causing an increase in the amount of vaginal discharge. The hormones in the Pill can stimulate the cervical glands and may also result in an increase in vaginal discharge. Some women have a brown discharge at the end of their menstrual cycle. This discharge is old blood still being shed.

If the vaginal discharge has a pink or brown tinge, this may indicate that there is blood in the discharge (*see* Vaginal Bleeding below).

Vaginal Bleeding

Women normally experience bleeding from the vagina about once a month, when they are having their menstrual periods. A woman's menstrual bleeding may be abnormally heavy, her period may be prolonged. The interval between periods may be unusually long or short, or she may have spotting or bleeding between periods. Irregularities in menstrual bleeding are discussed below, under the heading Symptoms Related to the Menstrual Cycle.

A woman may also experience bleeding from the vagina that is not associated with her menstrual period. Some of the possible causes of this type of abnormal bleeding are listed on p. 637 of the reference section on diseases under the heading Abnormal Uterine Bleeding.

Sometimes women experience painful or difficult intercourse, and this pain is sometimes accompanied by bleeding (see Painful or Difficult Intercourse above).

In addition, the following conditions may cause vaginal bleeding:

Lacerations of the vagina, vulva and perineum (*see* pp. 294–95)
Fistulas (*see* pp. 302–4)
Vaginal adenosis (*see* pp. 335–40)
Clear cell adenocarcinoma (*see* pp. 340–42)
Cancer of the vagina (*see* pp. 342–49)
Cervical lacerations (*see* pp. 361–62)
Lacerations in Vimule Cervical Cap users (*see* p. 168)
An IUD that is in the process of perforating the uterus or being expelled (*see* pp. 128–31)

Symptoms Related to the Cervix

Changes in the Shape of the Cervical Os

The cervical os may change in appearance, but this is not necessarily a sign that something is wrong, for the os changes over the course of the menstrual cycle and over the course of a woman's lifetime. At the time of ovulation and the time of the menstrual flow, the os is apt to be more dilated. Before childbirth the os usually appears as a small, round indentation in the center of the cervix. After childbirth it is apt to look more like a short, vertical slit. Other variations in the shape of the os of an otherwise normal cervix may be caused by growths or clumps protruding through the os (see below) or to any of the following conditions:

Cervical lacerations (*see* pp. 361–62)
Cervical stenosis (*see* pp. 364–65)
An IUD in the process of being expelled (*see* pp. 128–31)

Growths or Clumps of Tissue Protruding Through the Cervical Opening

Women who practice speculum self-exam may see clumps of tissue or growths protruding through the cervix. Conditions that can cause this include:

Cervical polyps (*see* pp. 357–59)
Cervical cancer (*see* pp. 378–79)
Pedunculated submucus or cervical fibroids (*see* pp. 433–35)
Endometrial polyps (*see* p. 439)
Uterine cancer (*see* p. 445)
Miscarriage (*see* p. 673)
Cervical ectopic pregnancy (*see* p. 691)
Trophoblastic disease (*see* p. 692)

Sores, Cysts, Lumps, Red or White Areas or Other Abnormalities in the Appearance of the Cervix

Women who practice self-exam may notice sores, cysts, lumps, red or white areas or other abnormalities in the appearance of the cervix. Most often these are the result of infections of the vagina and cervix, sexually transmissible infections or cervical erosions and eversions. Any of the following conditions may result in these symptoms:

Trich (*see* p. 307)
Yeast infections (*see* p. 314)
Hemophilus (*see* p. 318)
Nonspecific vaginitis (*see* p. 319)
Postmenopausal vaginitis (*see* p. 319)
Fistulas (*see* p. 330)
Cervicitis (*see* pp. 352–54)
Cervical erosions and eversions (*see* p. 355)
Nabothian cysts (*see* pp. 360–61)
Cervical lacerations (*see* pp. 361–62)
Leukoplakia (*see* p. 366)
Cervical dysplasia (*see* pp. 367–68)
Carcinoma in situ (*see* p. 373)
Cervical cancer (*see* p. 379)
Pelvic inflammatory disease (*see* p. 397)
Gonorrhea (*see* p. 564)
Herpes (*see* p. 570)
Chlamydial infections (*see* p. 580)
Syphilis (*see* p. 584)
Granuloma inguinale (*see* p. 592)
Chancroid (*see* p. 593)
Lymphopathia venereum (*see* p. 594)
Allergy to spermicides or to the materials used in condoms, diaphragms, contraceptive sponges or cervical caps (*see* pp. 142, 156, 161, 168)

Symptoms Related to the Breast

Breast Lumps and Other Abnormalities in the Shape, Feel, or Appearance of the Breast

A lump or thickening in the breast is an important symptom. In addition, the following signs or symptoms in the breast deserve attention:

- ☐ A depressed or bulging area in the skin or any change in the shape or symmetry of the breast
- ☐ A thickening on the skin of the breast that may feel warm
- ☐ Dilated veins in the breast. Some women normally have visible blue veins in their breasts; however, the appearance of such veins in a woman who has not had them previously or a change in the appearance of such veins in a woman who has previously had them calls for medical attention.
- ☐ A change in the texture or color of the skin of the breast. The appearance of areas of skin with the texture of an orange peel, a condition known as peau d'orange, is particularly important.
- ☐ Any change in the condition of the nipple or the areola. Changes in the size or shape, skin texture or direction in which the nipple points, retraction of the nipple, cracks in the nipple or scaling of the skin around the nipple are important.
- ☐ Discharge from the nipple (see Nipple Discharge below)
- ☐ A lump in the axilla (armpit)
- ☐ A sore on the breast or nipple that does not heal
- ☐ Hot, swollen or sore breast
- ☐ Unusual ache or pain that persists

These signs and symptoms may be caused by either a benign or malignant condition, such as:

Cystic disease of the breast (*see* p. 505)
Mastitis (*see* p. 507)
Fat necrosis (*see* pp. 508–9)
Fibroadenomas (*see* pp. 509–10)
Cystosarcoma phyllodes (*see* p. 511)
Lipomas and other benign, soft tumors of the breast (*see* p. 512)
Intraductal papillomas (*see* p. 512)
Mammary duct ectasia (*see* p. 513)
Breast cancer (*see* p. 523)
Sore breasts may be caused by any of these conditions. In addition, pregnancy and premenstrual syndrome may cause the breast to feel sore.

Nipple Discharge

Nipple discharge is sometimes, but not always, a sign that something is wrong. On occasion, newborn babies secrete milk from the breast. The same kind of secretions may occur at puberty, and some women produce a milky secretion at certain points in their menstrual cycles. These types of secretion may be caused by temporary hormone fluctuations and may therefore not be anything serious. Some women, especially those that have had more than one child, secrete breast milk during pregnancy. Women who are breast-feeding may have a spontaneous trickle or even a flow of breast milk at times when the infant is not actually sucking on the nipple. Although this may be distressing, it generally is not a sign of disease. Some women produce breast milk even when they are not pregnant or breast-feeding, and this condition, known as galactorrhea, may result from a serious underlying problem.

In addition to milk, a number of other types of discharge may be expressed or may flow spontaneously from the nipple. The color, texture and consistency of these discharges vary. Red, brown or black discharges may indicate that either fresh or old blood is present in the discharge. The discharge may also be white, green, yellow or gray. A number of breast diseases may be responsible for nipple discharges, including:

Cystic disease (*see* p. 503)
Mastitis (*see* p. 507)
Intraductal papillomas (*see* p. 512)
Mammary duct ectasia (*see* p. 513)
Breast cancer (*see* p. 523)

Symptoms Related to the Menstrual Cycle

Abnormally Heavy or Prolonged Menstrual Periods, Spotting or Bleeding Between Periods or Abnormally Short or Long Intervals Between Periods

Irregularities in menstrual bleeding may occur at the time of puberty. The periods may be spaced irregularly or may be unusually heavy or light. These irregularities are normal during this period of life, when the menstrual cycle is just gearing up. Unless the bleeding is especially profuse (soaking more than six to eight pads or tampons a day) there is no need for concern, since it takes a few years for most girls' periods to become regular.

Irregularities in menstrual bleeding also occur at the end of the reproductive cycle, during menopause, when a woman's menstrual cycle is gearing down.

Some women menstruate normally until they come to an abrupt stop; others experience a gradual decrease in the volume of flow and longer times in between periods; still others have irregularly spaced periods interspersed with times when they have normal periods. All these patterns are considered normal. If, however, there is a heavy, gushing flow, if periods last longer than usual, if periods occur more frequently than every 21 days or if bleeding starts again a year or more after the last period, this may be a sign that something is wrong.

Irregular menstrual periods may also occur in women during their menstruating years. The length of the cycle and the duration and amount of the flow may vary from month to month, even in a normal, healthy woman. But persistent or severe abnormalities may be a sign that something is wrong.

Spotting or bleeding between the periods and other types of abnormal bleeding may occur in any age-group and may or may not be serious.

There are a wide variety of conditions that can cause these symptoms. These causes are discussed under the heading Abnormal Uterine Bleeding (*see* pp. 635–640), and a chart of causes is included there (*see* p. 637).

Missed Periods or the Absence of Menstruation

Missed periods or the absence of menstruation is called amenorrhea. If a girl hasn't had her first period by the expected age, she is said to have primary amenorrhea. If a woman who has previously menstruated stops having her periods, she is said to have secondary amenorrhea. Secondary amenorrhea happens when a woman is pregnant, for a time after childbirth, especially if a woman is breast-feeding, and, of course, at menopause. Occasionally, a non-pregnant, premenopausal woman will experience amenorrhea even though there is nothing wrong with her. However, if two or three periods in a row are missed, the woman should consult a doctor, for missed periods may be a symptom of disease.

Amenorrhea may be a symptom of disease, but it is not a disease itself. Because amenorrhea may be the symptom of a number of underlying diseases, some of which are not strictly gynecological in nature, diagnosis is largely a process of elimination. We have included a discussion of amenorrhea (*see* pp. 615–635) in the reference section on diseases. A chart on the possible causes of this symptom is given there (*see* p. 617).

Hot Flashes and Symptoms that Occur at the Time of Menopause

Hot flashes, or flushes, are intense sensations of heat that are not uncommon among women who are experiencing a natural or a premature menopause (*see* pp. 649–50). Some women experience hot flashes temporarily after hysterectomy, even if the ovaries have not been removed. The cause is unknown. Possible causes for hot flashes, osteoporosis, the drying of urinary and vaginal tissues, depression, changes in sex drive and other symptoms that may occur at the time of menopause are discussed under the heading Menopausal Changes (*see* pp. 642–49).

Menstrual Cramps

Menstrual cramps are not uncommon; almost every woman experiences them at some time in her life. Sometimes the cramps are the result of a specific underlying disease. Sometimes no cause can be found. Although menstrual cramps are a symptom and not a disease, we have included a section on menstrual cramps (*see* pp. 609–15) in the reference section on disease. Possible causes for this symptom are detailed there.

Premenstrual Pain, Weight Gain, Breast Tenderness, Mood Changes and Other Symptoms that Occur in Relation to the Menstrual Cycle

Women experience a wide variety of symptoms in relation to their menstrual cycles. Most of these occur in the days preceding the menstrual cycle, so these symptoms are termed "premenstrual syndrome," or PMS, for short. There are many theories to explain PMS. A description of the types of symptoms associated with PMS and possible causes are given under the heading Premenstrual Syndrome (*see* pp. 600–609)

Infertility and Sterility

These conditions are often thought of as diseases in and of themselves, for the inability to get pregnant is what causes a woman to seek medical help. Actually, these conditions are the symptom or aftermath of some underlying disease or abnormality. Although these conditions are, in a sense, symptoms, we have devoted a section in the reference section on diseases to these conditions. Detailed information about the possible causes is given there under the heading Infertility and Sterility (*see* pp. 659–72).

Abdominal or Pelvic Pain

Abdominal or pelvic pain may be a symptom of literally hundreds of conditions that have nothing to do with gynecological problems, including kidney stones and gallstones, urinary tract problems, appendicitis, ulcers and other gastric disturbances, benign or malignant tumors, colitis and other infections in the abdominal cavity, to name a few. The following gynecological conditions described in this book can cause abdominal pain:

Cervical cancer (*see* pp. 378–79)
Pelvic inflammatory disease (*see* p. 397)
Endometriosis (*see* pp. 403–6)
Adenomyosis (*see* pp. 415–16)
Uterine fibroids (*see* pp. 433–36)
Endometrial polyps (*see* pp. 439–40)
Benign tumors of the fallopian tubes (*see* pp. 440–41)
Uterine cancer (*see* p. 449)
Cancer of the fallopian tubes (*see* p. 460)
Physiologic ovarian cysts (*see* p. 469)
Polycystic ovarian disease (*see* pp. 472–73)
Benign ovarian tumors (*see* pp. 476–78)
Functioning ovarian tumors (*see* pp. 485–87)
Ovarian cancer (*see* p. 489)
Premenstrual syndrome (*see* p. 601)
Menstrual cramps (*see* p. 610)
Miscarriage (*see* pp. 675–76)
Ectopic pregnancy (*see* pp. 685–88)
Trophoblastic disease (*see* pp. 694–95)
Ovulation (*see* pp. 65–66)
Intrauterine device (*see* pp. 125–26)

Reference Section: Diseases

The Vulva

The Vagina

The Cervix

The Uterus and the Fallopian Tubes

The Ovaries

The Breast

Sexually Transmissible Infections

Problems Related to the Menstrual Cycle

Problems Related to Pregnancy and Fertility

Cancer

The Vulva

The anatomy of the vulva is illustrated and described in Chapter Two. Reviewing the information in that chapter will help you to understand the vulvar diseases described in the following pages.

Most of the diseases and conditions described in this section are skin diseases, for the skin of the vulva, just like the skin elsewhere on the body, is subject to all sorts of lumps, bumps, pimples and inflammations.

Vulvitis

The vulva is particularly susceptible to inflammations because the area is frequently warm, and moisture there is trapped by clothing. This warm, moist environment is a perfect breeding ground for infection. Moreover, the vulva is subject to a number of irritants, including vaginal and menstrual discharge, sanitary napkins, vaginal deodorants, perfumed soaps, powders, the laundry soap used to wash undergarments and so forth. Additionally, the chemicals used in the manufacture of synthetic undergarments may dissolve because of the heat in the area, also irritating the vulva. "Vulvitis" is the general term used to describe these inflammations, and the various types of vulvitis are described in the first part of this section.

Other Vulvar Problems

In addition to vulvitis, a number of other inflammations of the vulva, including postmenopausal vulvitis; vulvar folliculitis, an infection of the hair follicles; hidradenitis, an infection of the sweat glands; bartholinitis and skenitis, infections of the Bartholin's and Skene's glands, respectively; and vulvar dystrophies, are included in the following pages. Circulatory diseases of the vulva and congenital and acquired abnormalities are also discussed. Both cystic and solid benign vulvar tumors as well as malignant and premalignant tumors are considered as well.

In addition to the problems discussed in this section there are other conditions that can cause the same or similiar symptoms. These include sexually transmissible infections, common vaginal infections, genital tuberculosis, endometriosis, lacerations of the vulva and vagina and congenital abnormalities of the ovary.

Vulvar Biopsies

Any itching, sore, lump, swelling, red or white areas—indeed, any abnormality of the vulvar skin that persists after treatment or that does not go away in 3 or 4 weeks, requires medical attention. Even as serious a disease as invasive vulvar cancer may produce no more than an itching in its early stages. Too often these symptoms are not given sufficient attention by the woman or her doctor. Yet any chronic irritation of the vulva requires attention, for if untreated it could lead to vulvar cancer. Therefore, any persistent itching, inflamed areas, lumps or sores that do not respond to medical treatment deserve a vulvar biopsy.

In the majority of cases the vulvar biopsy is a simple office procedure that can be done under a local anesthetic. Many doctors will, however, hospitalize a woman and may even use a general anesthetic. This is more dangerous for the woman, since any general anesthetic involves a risk, however slight, of serious complications—and in some cases fatal ones. It is also more costly and inconvenient. A few doctors will argue that hospitalization is necessary because of the risk of excessive bleeding, but the most widely respected experts believe that the biopsy should be done in the office. Perhaps the fact that a biopsy done in a hospital and using a general anesthetic is more lucrative for the doctor explains why these procedures are sometimes done there. At any rate, if your doctor proposes to do the procedure in the hospital, and especially if s/he proposes to use a general anesthetic, insist that the reasons be made clear to you. If you are not satisfied with the answers, remember that you have the right to seek a second opinion.

The vulvar biopsy involves cutting samples of tissue that are sent to a lab for microscopic evaluation. A tissue sample of any obvious sores or lumps will be collected. The doctor may also paint the vulva with a stain called toluidine blue. This stain is then washed off with a slightly acidic solution. A sample should be taken of any areas that retain the blue stain. This process helps the doctor locate affected areas that cannot be seen with the naked eye. This is important, for invasive cancer may be lurking at the edges of an area affected by some other, more obvious disease. Without the staining this more serious condition might go undetected until it was too late.

The biopsy may also include a colposcopic exam. The colposcope is a magnifying instrument that can be used to examine the vulva (and also the vagina and cervix). With the colposcope the doctor can see abnormal areas that might be missed by the staining method. Although the use of a colposcope is not as critical in vulvar biopsy as it is in cervical biopsy, it is still an important tool; however, many doctors believe that a good magnifying glass is equally effective for vulvar biopsies.

VULVITIS

AKA: vulvar dermatitis

Types: chronic dermatitis, eczema or chronic eczemoid dermatitis
allergic vulvitis, contact dermatitis, drug eruption or dermatitis medicamentosus
seborrhea or seborrheic dermatitis
intertrigo, erythema intertrigo or chafing
vulvovaginitis or secondary vulvitis
tinea cruris
diabetic vulvitis
neurodermatitis

The term "dermatitis" in its broadest sense refers to any inflammation of the skin. When these sorts of irritations occur on the vulva the term "vulvitis" or "vulvar dermatitis" is used. Vulvitis may be caused by bacteria, fungus, injury, allergic substances or other irritating factors.

Symptoms

Vulvitis is characterized by itching, redness and swelling. The itching is usually followed by scratching; then, if they weren't already there to start with, symptoms like swelling, redness, irritation, oozing, crusting and scaling may appear. In some forms, fluid-filled blisters called vesicles may appear. Scratching may cause the vesicles to break open. Pus formation, crusting and scaling may then follow. There may be secondary infection. The scratching may also thicken the skin and give it a white appearance that could be mistaken for vulvar dystrophy. As bothersome as this all may be, it is generally not serious in terms of general health.

Types

Vulvitis may be acute—sudden in onset and lasting for a relatively short time—or chronic—slow in progressing and lasting for a long time. The terms "eczema" and "chronic eczemoid dermatitis" are sometimes used to refer to chronic dermatitis. Chronic dermatitis commonly affects postmenopausal women in whom a drop in estrogen production causes a thinning and drying out of the vulvar tissues. Minute cracks in the surface of the skin then make the area more susceptible to inflammations, a condition known as atrophic, or senile, vulvitis. There are many different types of vulvitis and a great deal of overlapping in the classifications of these various types by different writers. It would probably take a whole book just to sort through it all; however, the major types are described below.

Allergic Vulvitis

Allergic vulvitis refers to an irritation of the skin of the vulva that results from an allergy to either a natural or synthetic substance. Sometimes the offending substance actually comes in contact with the vulva, in which case the term "contact dermatitis" is used. Vaginal deodorants, sanitary napkins, perfumed soaps, cosmetic powders, laundry detergents and the chemicals in synthetic materials are frequently responsible for allergic reactions. In addition, synthetic undergarments and panty hose create an environment that will contribute to any existing vulvar irritation. Menstrual blood, feces and other normal bodily secretions may on occasion cause contact dermatitis.

Medications, either those applied directly to the vulvar area or ones taken by mouth or injection, may cause allergic vulvitis. Such terms as "drug eruption" and—if you prefer medical jargon—"dermatitis medicamentosus" are used to describe this type of allergic vulvitis. These reactions may involve the skin in various other parts of the body or may affect only the vulva and the surrounding area. Interestingly, allergic vulvitis caused by drugs often occurs without fever, joint pains and that sick-all-over feeling that usually accompany drug reactions.

The allergic vulvitis reaction may not appear immediately after exposure to the allergen. In some cases it may be delayed for some time; but normally, the reaction appears within 2 to 4 days. The reaction does not always occur at the first exposure; sometimes the sensitivity develops only after repeated exposure.

The symptoms range from a mild redness to severe swelling. Itching is almost always present, which leads to scratching, which in turn may lead to the formation of tiny blisters and the sequence of events described above.

Seborrhea

Seborrhea, or seborrheic dermatitis, is related to an overproduction of the sebaceous (oil-producing) glands located in the vulva. The reason for this overproduction is not known. Seborrhea can occur in the hairy areas of the vulva as well as on the inside of the vulvar lips. Other areas of the body where there are concentrations of sebaceous glands, such as the scalp, ears and underarms, are apt to be affected at the same time. It is more likely to occur in overweight people. In the typical case there are greasy, yellow scales covering the glands.

Intertrigo

"Intertrigo" refers to any acute, superficial inflammation of opposing skin surfaces. The condition is also referred to as "erythema intertrigo," which is an even more pompous term for what most of us call chafing. It is caused by moisture, warmth and friction from opposing skin surfaces rubbing together. The labia are subject to this kind of chafing, as are the inner thighs, the anal region, the underarms, the spaces between the fingers and toes and the area under the breasts. Women who are overweight, have diabetes or perspire profusely in hot weather are more likely to be bothered with intertrigo. Like all forms of vulvitis, this condition, although it is not serious, can become quite uncomfortable, causing redness, itching and burning, especially if the skin is rubbed raw. In more extreme cases the skin may thicken and turn white, in which case the condition may be incorrectly diagnosed as vulvar dystrophy. Monilial and bacterial infections are common complications. If these should occur, treatment of these infections is combined with local treatment to relieve symptoms. Preventive measures include regular use of nonirritating dusting powder and, for overweight women, losing weight. Here again, wearing cotton underwear rather than synthetics and wearing loose clothing rather than tight garments will help prevent the condition.

Secondary Vulvitis

The terms "vulvovaginitis" and "secondary vulvitis" are used to refer to those irritations of the vulvar skin that are secondary to vaginal infections, cervicitis or various sexually transmissible infections. The symptoms will depend on the nature of the primary infection. Treatment consists of curing the primary infection that is creating the irritating discharge, and applying various creams and lotions to soothe the irritated vulva and relieve the itching.

Tinea Cruris

In some cases certain fungi may cause vulvar dermatitis. These may be secondary to fungal vaginal infections or may exist solely on the vulva. Tinea cruris is a fungus infection that can affect the upper inner thighs, the vulva, anus and buttocks. It begins as a small red circular patch that has small bumps, pimples or blisters on its outer edges. Sometimes it heals in the center as the edges continue to spread outward. It is contagious and has been known to spread rapidly through schools, prisons and similar institutions. Treatment consists of keeping the area dry and application of antifungal lotions and powders during the day and creams at night. If the condition persists or recurs, oral antifungal medication may be used.

Diabetic Vulvitis

Irritation of the vulva may also occur in women who have diabetes, a disease in which the body is unable to process certain vital nutriments. In this case the term "diabetic vulvitis" is used. Women with undetected diabetes may complain of itching and burning before there are any observable changes in the skin of the vulva. Eventually, the vulvar skin takes on a beefy-red color and looks extremely irritated. Local treatment without diagnosis and treatment of the underlying diabetic condition will not do much to alleviate the irritation.

Neurodermatitis

Just as it is often hard to identify the exact nature and cause of acne on the face, it may be difficult to diagnose irritations of the vulvar skin. Thus we have the term "neurodermatitis," which is a sort of scapegoat diagnosis. A puzzling case may be diagnosed as neurodermatitis, a condition that is said to have "a large psychogenic component"—it's "nerves," it's psychosomatic or the old it's-all-in-your-head-dearie diagnosis.

In some medical textbooks, neurodermatitis of the vulva is said to be common "in women whose life situations create sexual frustrations, such as widows and divorcees."[1] The itching associated with it is said to be worse at night than during the day, when, according to one medical text, "her thoughts are diverted from her genital organs." Such texts often fail to mention the fact that itching from insect bites, drug eruptions and other forms of dermatitis also tend to be worse at night.

Undoubtedly, some women do develop vulvitis as a result of psychological problems, just as some people develop nervous tics or break out in hives as a result of "nerves." Perhaps in the largest sense all disease is basically psychological in origin, for we have yet to figure out why, when two seemingly

268

healthy, robust individuals are exposed to the same bacteria, one gets sick and the other one doesn't. Be that as it may, the diagnosis of neurodermatitis is often not accurate. It would be much better for the doctor to simply tell a woman that s/he is unable to find a cause for her condition, rather than falling back on the standard medical ploy, I-can't-figure-out-what's-wrong-with-you-so-you-must-be-crazy. Not only is it unfair to manipulate a woman in this way, but also the anxiety created by implying that a woman is psychologically disturbed is counterproductive and contributes nothing to the healing process. In the absence of obvious psychological disturbances, women should be wary of accepting a diagnosis of neurodermatitis and should insist on a thorough investigation of their symptoms.

Treatment

Whatever the cause of vulvitis—insect bites, vaginal infections, drug reactions, vaginal sprays and so forth—the treatment basically is the same. The aim of treatment is to eliminate the causative factor, when possible, and to alleviate the symptoms, particularly the itching, since unchecked it will lead to even more intense itching and bothersome complications. There is a tendency to overtreat, coating the area with creams, lotions and ointments that in turn cause irritations. The simplest treatments, applied locally, are the best.

If the vulvitis is caused by a vaginal infection, any treatment applied to the vaginal canal should also be applied to the irritated vulva. If diabetes is the associated disease, the diabetes and the often-accompanying vaginal fungus infection must be treated as well as the vulvitis.

Cleanliness, hot boric acid compresses and hot sitz baths may be helpful. After compresses or sitz baths the area should be gently patted dry with soft linen or cotton and allowed to dry in the air. Then and only then should drying powders (nonirritating ones) be applied. Calamine lotion, available without prescription at pharmacies, will help alleviate the itching. Cortisone creams may be prescribed if the itching is particularly severe.

In cases of chronic vulvitis, that is, vulvitis that recurs or that is resistant to cure, a vulvar biopsy should be done to rule out the possibility that a more serious type of cancerous or precancerous disease is present. This biopsy can be done in the doctor's office using a local anesthetic. If the doctor proposes hospitalization and a general anesthetic, be sure to read the discussion of vulvar biopsy in the introduction to this section.

POSTMENOPAUSAL VULVITIS

AKA: senile atrophy, atrophic vulvitis

To atrophy means "to wither." It is a normal part of aging. Older women who are past menopause or younger women who for one reason or another no longer have functioning ovaries will notice changes in the appearance of the vulva. Without the stimulation of hormones, the skin becomes less elastic, the layer of fat beneath the skin may be lost, the labia majora and labia minora (large and small lips) and even the clitoris may shrink. The skin may become dry and smooth, and pubic hair becomes sparse. Some women's skin thickens to a leathery consistency and becomes brown and splotched in color. The atrophic skin is thin and easily irritated. Minute breaks or cracks in the surface of the skin may occur, and these may be the site of a low-grade bacterial infection.

Symptoms

Itching, which may become intense, is the primary symptom. The itching leads, of course, to scratching, which only irritates the vulva more, creating sores and red, irritated areas. Intense scratching may cause the skin in the area to turn white.

Treatment

The simplest form of therapy is the best. The area should be kept cool, dry and clean. Cold compressions will help relieve the itching. Drying agents or lotions should be avoided, as they may aggravate the itching. A lubricating cream may be applied, and antibiotic creams may be used to combat infection.

If the condition persists or tends to recur, estrogen replacement therapy (ERT), either orally or as a locally applied cream, may be prescribed. ERT should, however, be used with caution, for it has been implicated in various forms of cancer.[2] Women should carefully weigh the risks and benefits of ERT before accepting this form of treatment.

Women should also be hesitant about accepting treatment over the telephone or without a thorough examination. Too many times the doctor just assumes the itching or sores are a manifestation of postmenopausal vulvitis, but these same symptoms may also be caused by vulvar cancer. In cases of persistent symptoms this possibility must be ruled out by a vulvar biopsy. If a vulvar biospy is required, be sure to read the discussion of vulvar biopsy given in the introduction to vulvar diseases.

VULVAR FOLLICULITIS

Types: folliculitis
      furunculosis

Associated Terms: carbuncles, or boils

Vulvar folliculitis is an infection of the hair follicles of the vulva. Certain bacteria, usually staphylococcus, are prone to attack the hair follicles in the vulvar region because it is difficult to keep this area dry. Depending on the depth of penetration, the woman may have either a superficial infection of the follicles—folliculitis—or a deep one—furunculosis. This type of infection is particularly common in women who have diabetes.

Symptoms and Treatment

If the infection is superficial, small pimples pierced by a shaft of hair are seen. These pimples tend to break and crust over. Soap-and-water cleansing and the application of antibiotic ointments are all that is needed to clear up these superficial infections.

If the infection is deep-seated, carbuncles, or boils, may be formed. Treatment involves hot salt packs to promote drainage of the infected follicles or, if necessary, incisions to drain the carbuncles and infected areas. Antibiotics are then given by mouth, rather than locally by ointment. Usually penicillin is given, although some doctors will examine the pus microscopically so that they can select a more specific antibiotic.

HIDRADENITIS

Types: acute hidradenitis
      Fox-Fordyce disease or chronic hidradenitis

Hidradenitis is an infection of the apocrine (sweat) glands, which are located around the nipples and in the underarm and vulvar areas. If the vulva is infected, these other areas are likely to be affected as well.

Symptoms and Treatment

The symptoms may cause considerable discomfort. There may be intolerable itching and pain, and there are generally a number of boils on the skin.

271

If treatment in the acute stage is not successful, the disease may progress to the chronic stage, which is known as Fox-Fordyce disease and is characterized by even more intense itching and pain. The vulva may be dotted with fine, slightly raised, pimplelike growths or large boils.

Oral contraceptives, which modify the secretions of the apocrine glands, may be used to control the disease and cut down on recurrences. In some instances it may be necessary to remove the infected skin. In the most extreme cases a vulvectomy—removal of all or part of the vulva—and plastic surgery involving skin grafting may be necessary.

BARTHOLINITIS

AKA: Bartholin's adenitis

Associated Terms: Bartholin's abscess, Bartholin's cyst

Bartholinitis is an infection of the Bartholin's glands (Illustration 40). These glands lie right inside the vaginal opening on either side and secrete a fluid that keeps the vagina moist. In most women they are not noticeable unless they become infected.

Most cases of bartholinitis are caused by gonococcus, the bacteria that causes gonorrhea, but other organisms can also cause this infection. The dis-

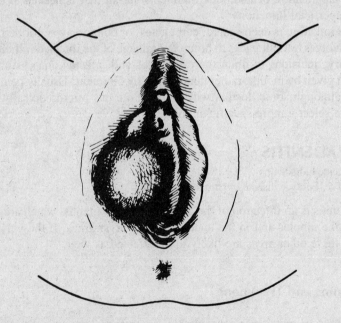

Illustration 40 *Bartholin's Cyst*

ease may be acute or it may progress to a chronic state, punctuated by occasional acute flare-ups.

Symptoms

The skin around the opening of the gland may be red and swollen. The opening to the gland may be partially or totally obstructed. If the gland is open, pus mixed with glandular secretions may ooze out or be milked out by gentle pressure. If the duct is closed up, a collection of pus known as a Bartholin's abscess may form. The abscess is usually hot, swollen and tender. As the infection progresses the overlying skin and the tissues around the bottom of the gland may become involved, and the whole labia may become swollen.

A woman with bartholinitis is usually intensely miserable and has difficulty sitting and walking. Surgical incision and drainage may be performed for relief, although sometimes spontaneous rupture of the abscess will occur.

The symptoms during the acute stage—the swelling and discomfort—are more local than general. The temperature may be only moderately elevated. After the pus is drained away the symptoms subside promptly. Then the disease may enter the chronic stage. The gland itself usually is not too seriously injured by the acute infection, but the duct may be partially or totally obstructed by scarring. Thus the gland's secretions cannot be released, and one or two Bartholin's cysts, full of these retained secretions, may develop. These cysts vary in size and may even get as large as a hen's egg. The cysts, as opposed to the abscesses, generally are not painful. Depending on the size of the cyst, a woman may be unaware of the cyst or it may interfere with intercourse and become a nuisance.

Treatment

The treatment for acute bartholinitis usually consists of bed rest, sufficient painkillers to relieve the discomfort, ice packs or hot sitz baths and some form of antibiotic therapy. If an abscess has formed, antibiotics alone may not be enough and the doctor may have to cut and drain the abscess.

If Bartholin's cysts are large enough to cause bothersome symptoms, they will require treatment but not while there is active, acute infection. Some doctors will treat these cysts by cutting, draining and cauterizing (burning) with electricity or with chemicals; others will treat the problem by removing the contents of the cyst by needle and replacing them with a penicillin solution. Still others will cut open the cyst, drain its contents and keep the cup open until it starts to heal from the inside out, a process known as marsupialization that usually can be performed in the doctor's office. Still others will remove the entire cyst surgically, but not until the acute infection or flare-up has subsided. If large or recurring abscesses have formed, these may be treated in the same way. In some cases it may be necessary to drain a large abscess even though there is acute infection. However, draining usually is not enough, for these abscesses will tend to recur unless removed surgically.

SKENITIS

AKA: infection of the Skene's glands

Types: acute skenitis
        chronic skenitis

The openings to the Skene's glands are two small slits located on either side of the opening of the urinary tract. These glands secrete a small amount of fluid that helps keep the urinary opening moist. The disease can be acute or chronic. If the disease-causing organisms retreat deep into the gland tissue, or if infected areas become walled off by a hardened, fibrous substance manufactured by the surrounding healthy tissue as a defense mechanism, the organisms cannot be reached by antibodies and the disease becomes chronic. It may persist for months, with occasional acute flare-ups.

Cause

Acute skenitis is often caused by gonococci, the organisms that cause gonorrhea; however, other organisms may also be responsible. Sometimes chronic skenitis is the result of gonococci that have resisted treatment. In most cases the gonococci have been killed but have paved the way for other bacteria that are responsible for the chronic skenitis. In the rare cases where gonococcus is responsible for chronic skenitis, the woman may pass gonorrhea on to her sex partners even though she shows no laboratory evidence of gonorrhea.

Symptoms

Pus can often be seen oozing from the openings of the glands or can be milked from the glands by gentle pressure. The openings of the glands may be red, hard, swollen and tender. Abscesses—collections of pus—may form on one or both sides and may be swollen and painful.

Skenitis is often associated with infections of the urethra, the tube that leads from the bladder to the urinary opening. Infection in the urethra spreads easily to these glands because of their proximity and vice versa. Thus there

274

may be a frequent and urgent need to urinate, and urination may be accompanied by pain and burning.

Treatment

If pus can be milked from the glands, it should be examined microscopically to determine what specific organism is causing the infection so that a specific antibiotic can be given. If no pus is present, a broad spectrum of antibiotics is given. However, if the disease has progressed to its chronic stage, often the only way to get rid of the infection is to destroy the glands by electric cautery.

CIRCULATORY DISEASES OF THE VULVA

AKA: varices, varicose veins

Circulatory diseases may occur anywhere in the body, including the vulva. The most common of the circulatory diseases affecting the vulva is varicose veins, or varices, which are swollen, twisted, enlarged veins.

Symptoms

Circulatory diseases of the vulva usually affect the outer lips and usually occur on only one side. Like varicose veins elsewhere in the body, veins here may swell up with blood, especially when the woman is standing, and tend to empty and become smaller when she is lying down. They may become extremely large, and although it is not common, they may even burst, causing bleeding. Usually, the dilated veins appear as a group of small, purple elevations, although they may occur singly as well. Varices may be caused by pressure on the veins from pregnancy or a large tumor; however, no specific cause can be identified in most cases. Other circulatory diseases that may cause swelling of the vulva usually are secondary in nature (which means they are the result of or are associated with some other condition that already exists). Generally, the only time that varicose veins on the vulva become symptomatic is during pregnancy, when they cause burning and pain.

Treatment

There is no specific treatment other than resting in a prone position as necessary. The varices regress after pregnancy. In rare cases surgery may be necessary.

275

CONGENITAL AND ACQUIRED ABNORMALITIES OF THE VULVAR ANATOMY

Types: imperforate hymen
absence of the hymen
double vulva
depigmentation, leukoderma or vitiligo
agglutination of the labia
clitoral hypertrophy
lacerations of the vulva

Associated Terms: hydrometrocolpos, hematocolpos, hematocolpometra, hematosalpinx

Abnormalities of the anatomy of the vulva may be either congenital (that is, birth defects) or acquired as a result of an injury or accident that occurred after birth.

Imperforate Hymen

Congenital abnormalities of the vulva are rare. Of the ones that do occur, the imperforate hymen is the most common. Normally, the hymen, the thin strip of tissue that surrounds the vaginal opening, has one or more openings through which vaginal, cervical and menstrual fluids may pass. If there are no openings, as is the case with imperforate hymen, these fluids cannot escape and build up inside the body.

This condition may be discovered in infancy. Sometimes a mother's hormones are strong enough to activate the newborn's uterus and vagina, causing the infant to pass vaginal secretions and possibly a bit of blood. If this happens in a child whose hymen is imperforate, these secretions can't pass through, and the hymen may be seen bulging at the vaginal opening. In some cases the backup of fluids will cause the infant's vagina and uterus to swell up and may be confused with the presence of a tumor.

Most of the time this condition is not discovered until failure to menstruate brings a young girl to the doctor. The girl may actually have started to menstruate and may have cyclic menstrual symptoms like cramps, pain in the lower abdomen, backache and so forth. On examining her the doctor finds that she has indeed been menstruating but has an imperforate hymen, so none of the blood has escaped. If she hasn't yet menstruated, there may still be a buildup of clear mucus.

There are a number of names for these conditions. A buildup of the watery mucus in the vagina and uterus is called a hydrometrocolpos. If blood has backed up in the vagina, the condition is called a hematocolpos, and if the uterus is also involved, it is called a hematocolpometra. If things really get filled up, the tubes too distend with blood, a condition known as hemato-salpinx. The doctor may be able to see a bulging hymen, which has a blue tinge because of the accumulated blood. These conditions can cause swelling and pain, especially at the time of the menstrual period. It's amazing how large an accumulation can build up with relatively little discomfort. In extreme cases the blood may back up through the fallopian tubes and spill into the pelvic cavity. Since the tissue that lines the pelvic cavity is extremely sensitive to blood, this can cause great irritation and pain. There may be associated pelvic endometriosis, a condition in which the menstrual tissue implants and grows on the ovaries and other abnormal locations, causing a variety of problems.

The treatment for an imperforate hymen involves making an incision in the hymen. If there is backed-up blood, this must be drained away. An antibiotic usually is given, since the old blood is a perfect environment in which infection can develop. In some extreme cases, where the retained menstrual blood has filled the vagina and uterus and has spilled into the pelvic cavity, causing great pain and irritation, the doctor may have to perform abdominal surgery to drain the blood from the cavity and the fallopian tubes. Normally, simple incision and draining will correct the problem.

Absence of the Hymen/Double Vulva

Some girls are born without hymens, although this is so common as to hardly be considered an abnormality. Such a situation causes no diseases or medical problems. It is also possible, although incredibly rare, to be born with a double vulva, which is associated with certain congenital vaginal and uterine abnormalities.

Depigmentation

A pigment is a substance that imparts color. The pigment of our skins gives us our characteristic skin color; absence of pigment makes the skin white. Some people are born without pigment in certain areas of their body or with a condition that causes them to lose pigment at some point in their lives (usually in the late teens and early 20s). This congenital condition is referred to as leukoderma. The lack of pigmentation may also be acquired as the result of a chronic infection or an injury, for instance, scarring resulting from an X-ray burn. Acquired loss of pigmentation is referred to as vitiligo.

Both vitiligo and leukoderma can occur on the vulva and can produce white patches on the skin. The condition in and of itself is not serious, is not common and usually doesn't require treatment. It is mentioned here because it can be the cause of a white appearance of the vulva that could be confused with the white patches that are symptoms of other, more serious vulvar problems.

Agglutination of the Labia

Although it is not a congenital abnormality, the condition known as agglutination of the labia often is discussed under this heading in medical textbooks. In this condition the lips—labia minora and/or labia majora—are fused or stuck together. This is rare and much more likely to occur in children than in adults, although it is seen occasionally in adults with gonorrhea. The labia are fused together as a result of a mild childhood inflammatory process that may have been so mild that it passed unnoticed. Sometimes the fusion is so great that it prevents normal urination. Treatment consists of surgical separation of the labia and the use of petroleum jelly or estrogen creams to prevent the labia from sticking together again.

Clitoral Hypertrophy

The labia may be fused together or other vulvar abnormalities may occur as a result of certain congenital abnormalities involving the chromosomes, as in hermaphroditism, a condition in which the sexual tissues and structures of both male and female are present in the same person. Abnormalities in the appearance of the external genitals might also include a clitoris that resembles the tip of a penis, a condition known as clitoral hypertrophy. This condition may be caused by certain types of hormone therapy in adults. These sorts of abnormalities may also be caused by hormones the mother took during pregnancy. Treatment for these vulvar abnormalities may include surgery and/or hormone therapy.

Abnormalities in the normal anatomy of the vulva may also result from injury. These are discussed under the heading Lacerations of the Vulva, Perineum, and Vulva.

VULVAR CYSTS

Types: endometrial cysts
Bartholin's duct cysts
sebaceous cysts
mucinous cysts
wolffian duct cysts
cyst of the canal of Nuck

A number of varieties of benign (noncancerous) cysts can appear on the vulva. They appear as soft, fluid-filled, bluish swellings or bumps. Two of these, the endometrial cyst and the Bartholin's cyst, are discussed elsewhere.

Sebaceous Cyst

One of the most common of these vulvar cysts is the sebaceous cyst, which is the result of the blockage of the sebaceous, or oil-producing, glands that dot the skin of the vulvar area. These cysts are filled with a cheesy, oily material. They are prone to infection and abscesses (collections of pus surrounded by inflamed tissue). If they are small and cause no symptoms, they don't require treatment. If they are large enough to be bothersome, they may need to be removed by simple surgery, using a local anesthetic.

Mucinous Cyst

Mucinous cysts occasionally appear near the urinary openings or on the inner surfaces of the small lips. They are probably the result of a displacement of cellular elements in the early stages of embryonic development. They develop in various sizes and may be pedunculated, that is, connected to the surrounding tissue by a pedicle, or stem of tissue. Some small cysts that appear at the vaginal opening and are classified as mucinous are probably related to the minor glands that exist in the vestibule, the smooth, boat-shaped area between the small, or inner, lips. Again, these may not require treatment unless they are large enough to be bothersome or become infected.

Wolffian Duct Cysts and Cysts of the Canal of Nuck

Wolffian duct cysts, which are also the result of an early embryonic developmental problem, rarely appear on the vulva, but if they attain any size, they may protrude through the vaginal opening. Likewise, an even more uncommon cyst, the cyst of the canal of Nuck, which also results from abnormalities in the developing embryo, may appear on the vulva. They usually don't require treatment unless they become large enough to cause problems, in which case they are removed.

BENIGN SOLID TUMORS OF THE VULVA

Types: fibroma, lipoma, lipoma fibrosum, fibrolipoma, myoma, leiomyoma, leiofibroma or leiomyofibroma
neorofibroma
granular cell myoblastoma
angioma (hemangioma, senile hemangioma, lymphangioma, angiokeratoma)
hidradenoma
nevus (plural: nevi), or mole

The vulva is subject to a number of lumps and bumps. The general medical word for such lumps and bumps—for any kind of localized swelling—is *tumor*. Such tumors may be cancerous or noncancerous. Noncancerous tumors are called benign tumors, and these may be either solid or cystic.

A number of solid benign tumors can appear on the vulva. Some of them have the potential of becoming cancerous, so they must be watched carefully. Others, although benign, may mimic the appearance of cancer and so must be removed or biopsied and examined microscopically to rule out that possibility. Still others may be associated with one of the sexually transmissible infections, and even if they go away, the disease itself will still need treatment. Some of the more common benign vulvar tumors are described below.

Fibromas

Fibromas, lipomas, fibrolipomas and leiomyofibromas are all tumors that can appear on the vulva as well as other parts of the body. Fibromas arise from fibrous tissue; lipomas, from fatty tissue; fibrolipomas, from a combination of the two; and leiomyofibromas, from smooth muscle and fibrous tissue. They are usually of small or moderate size and can be felt as firm to soft, movable lumps under the skin. They cannot be distinguished from one another except by microscopic examination. They are rarely noticed unless they grow large and become pedunculated, which means that they have grown a stem, or pedicle, by which they are attached to the surrounding tissue. On occasion they may grow extremely large and become so pedunculated that they dangle between the legs. The fibroma, in particular, is a favorite of medical-textbook writers who, with the spirit of proud fishermen taking snapshots of their biggest catches, always include at least a half-page illustration of a Dr. Buckner's classic (1851) vulvar fibroma, which weighed 268 pounds.

In some cases the underlying skin may become ulcerated (form an open sore), and if this happens, the fibroma may be confused with vulvar cancer, perhaps necessitating a biopsy. Unless treated, fibromas usually continue to grow and may become a nuisance. Treatment consists of surgical removal.

Neurofibromas

Neurofibromas are tumors arising from certain tissues that sheath the nerve fibers. They may appear as small, single, flabby, brown red, pedunculated tumors or as a number of brown spots. They usually are a local symptom of a central nervous system disease known as von Recklinghausen's disease. Since they do not produce symptoms or cause inconvenience because of their small size, they do not require removal unless they become so numerous that they are bothersome.

Granular Cell Myoblastoma

The granular cell myoblastoma appears as a nontender swelling of no great size in and around the vulva as well as on other parts of the body. Sometimes the surface of the lump ulcerates, mimicking the appearance of certain forms of cancer, so that it must be cut out and examined microscopically to rule out this possibility. The doctor will cut a wide margin of tissue, since it is not clearly separate from surrounding tissue.

Angiomas

Angiomas are tumors that involve dilation of the blood vessels (hemangioma) or lymph vessels (lymphangioma). They often are congenital and may appear as raised, strawberry-colored birthmarks. Occasionally, these may be irritated in infants by diapers and urine, but they usually don't require treatment and usually regress as the child grows. Hemangiomas may appear as a cluster of deep purple little bumps and may extend upward into the vaginal canal, causing considerable alteration in the normal anatomy, which can sometimes lead to problems. They can, for instance, cause maternal bleeding during delivery. If they are small and asymptomatic, no treatment is necessary, but if they are large and cause problems, they must be removed. Yet another form is the senile hemangiomata—dark red blue, small nodules that frequently are seen in the vulvar area of postmenopausal women, although they may occur in other age-groups as well. Sometimes these blood-filled tumors, because of their exposed position, may bleed, but this can easily be controlled by removing the hemangioma. Still another variety of angioma, the angiokeratoma, may appear on the vulva as single or multiple wartlike, red brown (occasionally blue black) tumors. Sometimes they may leak a bit, producing bloody stains on the underwear. They may increase in size during pregnancy owing to pressure on the veins. They often are misdiagnosed as moles, warts or hemangiomas. They may cause alarm when they swell during pregnancy or bleed, since this type of change in a wartlike growth is also associated with cancer. A biopsy may be necessary if these types of changes occur.

Hidradenoma

Hidradenomas are tumors of the vulvar sweat glands and often appear as pea-sized swellings on the vulvar area. In some cases the overlying skin may be red, grainy and sorelike, perhaps with slight bleeding. In such instances they may mimic the appearance of vulvar cancer. Most of the time there are no bothersome symptoms, but they may itch. Treatment consists of simple surgical removal, because in rare cases they have become cancerous.

Nevus

The nevus is, in layman's terms, a mole. It may be flush with the skin or raised above it. It may be about the color of the surrounding skin, have a slightly tan hue or be quite dark. If it has been present since birth, it may darken around the time of puberty. Nevi usually are benign and don't produce any symptoms but must be watched carefully, for moles anywhere on the body, and particularly those in the vulvar area, have the potential of becoming cancerous. If a nevus in the vulvar area shows any sign of change (increase in size, change in color or a tendency to bleed), it should be biopsied, that is, cut out, along with a wide margin of surrounding tissue and examined microscopically. Fortunately, the wide cutting may also provide a cure should the nevus turn out to be cancerous.

VULVAR DYSTROPHY

Types: leukoplakia, leukoplakia vulvitis or leukoplakia vulvae
hyperplastic dystrophy
lichen sclerosus, lichen sclerosus et atrophicus
kraurosis vulvae
mixed dystrophy

The term "vulvar dystrophy" refers to a group of diseases that causes abnormal changes in the skin of the vulva. In the past, such terms as "leukoplakia," "kraurosis vulvae," "lichen sclerosus" and "lichen sclerosus et atrophicus'' were used to refer to these diseases. These terms caused a great deal of confusion, for they frequently were misused. Part of the confusion was owing to the fact that these diseases can all cause itching and white patches on the vulvar skin, so that microscopic examination usually is necessary to differentiate between them. Moreover, doctors use the terms differently. A few years ago, in an effort to clarify things, the powers-that-be reclassified these diseases under the general term "dystrophy."[3] Dystrophies were broken down into three groups: lichen sclerosus ("lichen" because of the similarity to lichens, the white patches that grow on rocks); hyperplastic (used to describe an increase in the number of cells in a given area) and mixed (including primarily lichen sclerosus but also including hyperplastic areas). Knowing what kind you have is important, for a few types of dystrophy are percursors of cancer.

Incidence

Vulvar dystrophies usually appear in the postmenopausal woman; however, at times they may appear in younger women. Lichen sclerosus has even been found in young children.

Symptoms

The vulvar dystrophies may take on a wide variety of appearances. They may start out as a dry, thick, red, swollen area of skin, but as the disease progresses the red changes to an opaque white. Small, white pimples may dot the surface of the skin. These pimples may group together to form white, raised patches. The layer of fat under the lips of the vulva may be lost, and the lips may flatten out. In the case of lichen sclerosus the skin tends to have a dry, thin, white, parchment surface. In kraurosis vulvae, which most experts believe is not a separate disease but just a more advanced stage of lichen sclerosus, the skin may become thin and shiny, the lips and clitoris may shrink and the vaginal opening may become constricted. Not all women have bothersome symptoms, but the white areas do tend to crack and cause minute fissures. If this happens, there is apt to be itching and subsequent burning sensations. Secondary infection may occur, the whole vulva may become swollen and intercourse may be painful because of the narrowing of the vaginal opening.

Diagnosis

Diagnosis of vulvar dystrophies involves a vulvar biopsy, a simple office procedure that can be done under a local anesthetic. Many doctors will hospital-

283

ize a patient and use a general anesthetic. This is not necessary in the majority of cases and involves needless risk and expense. The vulvar biopsy is discussed in greater detail in the general introduction to this section.

The biopsy is vitally important, for more serious conditions—like carcinoma in situ of the vulva and invasive cancer of the vulva—can both produce similar white patches. Moreover, there seems to be some relationship between cancer of the vulva and vulvar dystrophies, and the biopsy will help to determine if any cancerous or precancerous cells are present.

Vulvar Dystrophy and Cancer

When the first studies of vulvar dystrophy were done it was noted that many women who had vulvar cancer also had the white patches characteristic of vulvar dystrophy. Reports on how often the two conditions coexist varied widely. Figures ranged from 12 percent to 80 percent.[4] This variation probably resulted from the confusion caused by misuse of the old terminology.

At any rate, since the initial studies had indicated that a high percentage of vulvar cancers were associated with white patches, it was decided on this basis that the white patches were a precursor to cancer. To prevent the later development of cancer, then, it became common practice to do a "skinning" vulvectomy, an operation that involves removing the outer layers of vulvar skin. Eventually, the question was raised by some researchers as to whether these white patches were really precursors to cancer or whether cancerous tissue wasn't just more conducive to their growth. Which came first, the cancer or the white patches? Further studies were done to evaluate this question and showed that although the white patches might be present in women with cancer, the majority of these white lesions did not go on to become cancerous.[5]

Under the revamped classifications the category of hyperplastic and mixed dystrophies was broken down into two groupings, based on the results of a biopsy: those that have atypical cells and those that don't. The small number of cancers that do develop in women who have vulvar dystrophies are most likely to develop in women who have these atypical cells in their biopsies. Probably less than 5 percent of all vulvar dystrophies go on to become cancer, although some authorities will place this figure at 10 percent.[6] The experts in the field now think that vulvectomy should be done only in those cases in which atypical cells are present in the biopsy. Unfortunately, it takes a while for this information to filter down from the experts. As one authority in the field, Dr. Raymond Kaufman, explains:

Frequently patients would be seen by their gynecologists with so-called white lesions of the vulva, and these patients would be treated rather radically by having their vulva removed to act as a prophylaxis [preventive measure] against the development of carcinoma. And I'd say to this day, this is still very commonly done and it's not uncommon at all that I'll receive a set of slides to review in a patient with lichen sclerosus, the game plan being to do a vulvectomy on this patient, to go ahead and cure the disease process. Well, first of all, it's not necessary. Second of all, it probably doesn't cure the disease process because these changes will generally recur even after vulvectomy in the vast majority of cases.[7]

Treatment

Vulvectomy, then, is no longer the treatment of choice for vulvar dystrophies, except in cases where biopsy has shown premalignant changes. There are now less radical treatments available. These treatments are also more effective, for, as Dr. Kaufman points out, many of the vulvar dystrophies, especially lichen sclerosus, tend to recur after vulvectomy.

First, contributing factors should be eliminated. If, for instance, a woman has a vaginal infection or uses certain powders, deodorants, perfumes or wears tight jeans or synthetic undergarments that keep moisture from evaporating or that contain irritating chemicals, these factors should be eliminated before treatment of the dystrophy. Eliminating these possible contributing factors will help alleviate the symptoms and changes in the vulva that are seen in dystrophies.

The symptoms should also be treated, not only so that the woman is more comfortable, but also because any irritated lesion on the vulva has the potential of becoming malignant. If there is swelling in the area, the doctor may prescribe cold boral solutions to help reduce the swelling and relieve the itching. If a woman has hyperplastic dystrophy, the doctor may prescribe cortisone in the form of cream or lotion to be applied three to four times a day to relieve itching. Once the itching and, consequently, the scratching is stopped, the white patches will also subside in most cases. If a woman has lichen sclerosus, the doctor may prescribe testosterone propionate, an ointment that frequently is useful. This is applied two to three times a day to relieve the itching and the appearance of the white patches. If a woman has the white patches but no distressing symptoms, treatment usually is not necessary as long as she remains symptom free.

If the treatments described above do not relieve the itching enough to stop the woman from scratching, the doctor will try more extreme forms of treatment. S/he might inject an alcohol solution into the skin of the vulva in several spots within the infected area. This may relieve the symptoms for several months, but it is a last-resort treatment, for it may be followed by sloughing of cells in the vulvar area. Another drastic treatment involves incisions or cuts in the area of the labia or lips to disrupt the sensory nerves. This treatment is employed only in cases where there is extremely severe itching.

Follow-up treatment for any woman with vulvar dystrophy consists of periodic biopsies every 6 months or every year, depending on the severity of the symptoms. This way the doctor can spot any atypical changes and detect any cancer that might occur right away.

PREINVASIVE CANCER OF THE VULVA*

AKA: noninvasive cancer, carcinoma in situ, intraepithelial cancer or Stage O carcinoma of the vulva

Types: Bowen's disease
Paget's disease
erythroplasia of Queyrat

The diseases described here involve abnormal changes in the cells of the tissue that make up the skin of the vulva. The very early stages of these diseases are akin to cervical dysplasia, that is, they are considered the first step in a process of abnormal changes that may or may not lead to cancer. When the cells have all the characteristics of cancer, except that there is no evidence that they have invaded beyond the skin layer to involve the lower tissues, the terms "carcinoma in situ," "intraepithelial cancer" and "Stage O carcinoma of the vulva" are used to describe these conditions.

Types

The term "carcinoma in situ," which means "cancer that is in place," often is used synonomously with the term "Bowen's disease." Most authorities classify another of these preinvasive diseases, which has the exotic name erythroplasia of Queyrat, as a specific type of carcinoma in situ. A third type of preinvasive disease, Paget's disease, is considered by some to be a separate category, whereas others lump all these conditions under the heading carcinoma in situ. Sometimes it is difficult to distinguish among them, even under a microscope. There is a good deal of debate among pathologists as to the classification of these conditions, and different terminology may be used by different pathologists. This is another reason why good communication between the doctor and the pathologist, to ensure that they are both using the terms in the same way, is important.

*The reader is also referred to the general discussion of cancer and to the following section on invasive cancer.

Bowen's Disease

Bowen's disease is not peculiar to the vulva but may precede invasive skin cancers anywhere on the body. The disease tends to precede invasive cancer of the vulva and has a slow growth rate. Women with Bowen's disease have an average age of 49 as compared with 63 for invasive vulvar cancer. Approximately one-third of the women with untreated carcinoma in situ will either develop or already have an invasive cancer.

The disease may show up as red, raised areas with a grainlike surface or as shallow, open sores. If the growth is softened by the moisture often present in the vulvar area, it may appear as a white patch. Itching is a common symptom.

Bowen's disease tends to occur in areas where vulvar dystrophies have developed and is more likely to develop when the vulvar dystrophies have extended into the vagina. Although the symptoms may appear in only one area, microscopic examination of tissue taken from other, nonsymptomatic areas of the vulva will often show evidence of the disease.

Erythroplasia of Queyrat

Erythroplasia of Queyrat is a rare condition, most often seen on the penis, but it may affect the vulva as well. It appears as a red, velvety patch, which may have a finely granular surface resembling the surface of a strawberry. Here again, itching is a common symptom. Under the microscope it may resemble Bowen's disease, but its appearance and the fact that it arises only on mucous membranes may help to distinguish it. It may appear in a single area, but like Bowen's disease, it may also exist in other areas without obvious signs. The growth rate is slow, although it may be somewhat faster than in Bowen's disease.

Paget's Disease

Paget's disease is another rare precancerous growth that can occur on other parts of the body as well. It occurs in the apocrine (sweat) glands of the vulva. It usually appears in women in their 50s and 60s, rarely in younger women. About 25 percent of the cases are associated with underlying invasive cancer.

This disease appears as red, clearly separated areas interspersed with white patches. The red areas may be ulcerated (that is, have formed sores) and "weep." Occasionally, these weeping sores will crust over. There often is intense itching.

Because it is a rare disease, many times the biopsied material is misdiagnosed by the pathologist. It may be confused with Bowen's disease or with truly invasive forms of cancer. If there is no cancer in the underlying sweat gland system, the disease does not spread, or metastasize. But it does tend to recur later, even when the tissue left behind has not shown any microscopic evidence of the disease.

Diagnosis

All these diseases are diagnosed by vulvar biopsy, which is described in the general introduction on vulvar diseases. Vulvar biopsy usually is a simple office procedure involving a local anesthetic. If the doctor proposes hospitalization and a general anesthetic for the biopsy, be sure to read the introduction to this section carefully.

Treatment

There is some disagreement as to which is the best method of treatment once it has been established that one of these preinvasive conditions exists. Some doctors will merely remove the affected area and a wide area of surrounding tissue. Most experts, however, consider this an inadequate form of treatment, for the disease in most cases is multicentric, that is, although it appears to be confined to one area, there may be other microscopic diseased areas throughout the vulva. Thus most doctors will do a "skinning" vulvectomy, an operation in which the outer layers of vulvar tissue are removed. They believe that the entire substructure of the vulvar skin has "gone wrong" and merely cutting off the affected areas is not sufficient, for the disease will only recur later. If the recurrence is not caught in time, it could become invasive cancer and spread to adjacent tissue or regional lymph nodes, which then requires more extensive surgery—and may be fatal. Some doctors are experimenting with cryosurgery (freezing), but long-term results are not yet available.[8]

Other doctors have advocated chemotherapy instead of surgery for treatment of carcinoma in situ. However, the chemotherapy used to treat these conditions, which is given in the form of a cream called FU-5, is extremely painful and is associated with a high rate of recurrence and complications,[9] so most experts think that surgical vulvectomy is preferable. Any woman whose doctor proposes chemotherapy would do well to seek a second opinion (*see* p. 238).

In the case of pregnancy the doctor may delay treatment until after delivery, for a few cases of carcinoma in situ of the vulva have been shown to regress spontaneously after pregnancy.[10]

Women who have had a preinvasive type of vulvar cancer will need to have careful follow-up for the rest of their lives.

INVASIVE CANCER OF THE VULVA*

Types: epidermoid carcinoma
basal cell carcinoma
malignant melanoma
adenocarcinoma or cancer of the Bartholin's gland

Invasive cancer of the vulva is uncommon but occurs often enough to account for about 3 percent to 5 percent of all cancers of the female genital organs.[11] The majority of vulvar cancers involve a type of tissue known as epidermal tissue. More rarely, cancer of the vulva may be of a type known as basal cell cancer. Yet another rare type is melanoma of the vulva, which may arise from moles. Occasionally, cancer will arise in the Bartholin's glands.

Incidence

Cancer of the vulva most often occurs in elderly women. The majority are in their 60s, but a third of the women are in their 70s.[12] The disease can, however, occur in younger women, and about 15 percent of the cases occur in women under age 40.[13]

Causes

The cause of invasive cancer, like the cause of all cancers, is unknown. However, there seem to be certain predisposing factors.[14] Failure of the ovaries to produce estrogen as a result of natural, surgical or radiation-induced menopause is one such factor. Most women who have the disease are postmenopausal, and in younger ones who do develop it there usually is a history of early ovarian failure. There seems to be some association with venereal diseases, such as syphilis, lymphopathia venereum and granuloma inguinale, but this is not clearly established. Here again, the younger women who develop invasive vulvar cancer are more likely to have histories of such diseases. Vulvar dystrophy is also associated with vulvar cancer.

*Anyone reading this section should first read the background information on cancer (*see* p. 699).

Symptoms

Although the symptoms may appear only on one side or area of the vulva, vulvar cancer usually is multicentric, that is, the cancer generally will exist in more than one area. The most common symptom is itching, although this is not universally present. There often is a lump that does not disappear. Less frequently, instead of a lump, the tumor is a raised sore that does not heal. Most of the time the lump or sore first appears on the inner or outer lips. Sometimes these tumors first appear on the clitoris or fourchette (the area below the vaginal opening, where the lower edges of the vulvar lips meet), but in most cases these areas become involved only as the disease spreads. The lumps or sores may be solitary or multiple.

The skin covering the tumor almost always ulcerates (forms an open sore) as the cancer progresses; however, the lump may sometimes remain firm and hard, with an intact skin covering. If this occurs and the lump is located on the side of the vaginal opening, it may be mistaken for a chronically infected Bartholin's gland.

Once the tumor has ulcerated the area may become tender and painful. The pain may result from exposed nerve endings or from the infection that frequently affects the ulceration. Urination is likely to be accompanied by intense burning as the urine passes over the open sore. Vulvar cancer, incidentally, is one of the few types of cancer in which the cancer itself produces symptoms of pain and tenderness. The pain worsens as the disease progresses. The ulcerated lump may also produce some bleeding, but this usually is rather slight. If the ulceration is extensive, there may be a bothersome discharge.

There may also be a good deal of swelling of the vulvar tissue. If the cancer is associated with one of the vulvar dystrophies, white patches and other symptoms associated with dystrophies may also be present.

The growth may spread up into the vagina. In advanced cases the urethra and the area between the anus and vaginal opening may also be ulcerated. When the disease spreads beyond the local area it usually is by way of the lymph nodes, and these too may be swollen.

A certain rare type of vulvar cancer may develop from a mole. The mole may be dark or skin-colored, and the symptoms of this form of cancer, which tends to be more deadly, are itching and, sometimes, bleeding. Any change in the appearance of such moles should be considered a suspicious symptom.

Spread

Cancer of the vulva usually spreads by direct invasion and/or by way of the lymph system. In most cases the cancer spreads to the lymph nodes in the groin and from there to the pelvic lymph nodes. In rare instances cancer is found in the more distant pelvic nodes even though none has been found in the lymph nodes in the groin. Some authorities believe that in these rare cases the woman actually did have cancer in the groin nodes, but the cancer was missed by the pathologist who examined the removed groin nodes.

Diagnosis

The early symptoms may be so slight—just itching and soreness—that the woman hesitates to see a doctor. Most growths are fairly large, 4 cm or more, before a woman consults the doctor. Then too the diagnosis is sometimes delayed by the doctor's failure to biopsy the lump or sore until the disease has progressed to a more extensive stage. The fact that the vulvar area is sensitive and tends to bleed freely may explain in part the doctor's reluctance to biopsy vulvar tissue. Moreover, doctors are taught that cancerous lumps and sores are painless. Even though vulvar cancer is an exception to this rule, many doctors have a sort of mental block that prevents them from doing biopsies on the often painful lump or sores of the vulva. This is especially true when the patient is younger and is therefore less likely to have vulvar cancer. Since vulvar cancer as well as any number of infections may produce lumps and bumps with a wide variety of appearances, it is a risky business for a doctor to decide on the basis of appearance alone that the lump isn't cancerous. Any vulvar ulceration or lump that doesn't disappear within 3 to 4 weeks should be biopsied.

The biopsy should, with rare exceptions, be an office procedure, requiring only a local anesthetic. See the discussion of vulvar biopsies in the general introduction to vulvar diseases if your doctor suggests hospitalization and/or general anesthetic.

Once the presence of cancer has been confirmed by biopsy, routine tests to detect metastasis (*see* p. 714) are done to rule out the possibility that the cancer has spread to other parts of the body.

Careful attention is also given to the lymph nodes. These will be carefully palpated (felt) by the doctor. If the doctor feels unusually enlarged lymph nodes and/or lymph nodes that are not freely movable, s/he will suspect that cancer has already spread to these areas, although infection can cause these symptoms too. Even in cases where the feel and appearance of the lymph nodes are not suspicious, cancer may be present. In addition to careful palpation the doctor may do a lymphangiogram, an X-ray examination of the lymph nodes, in order to make a more accurate estimate of the possibility of cancer there, but this test is not entirely reliable and is rarely used.

The visible cancerous area or areas will be measured carefully, for tumors that are larger than 2 cm in diameter have a much greater likelihood of lymph node involvement.

Staging

Table 6 outlines the staging scheme for vulvar cancer.[15] The size of the cancer is important in Stage I and II, as is the condition of the lymph nodes. The lymph nodes in the groin will be removed and examined by the pathologist at the time of operation, but the doctor's estimate of the possibility of groin node involvement before the operation may be important in decisions about how to treat the pelvic lymph nodes (see below). The doctor's physical exam and the results of tests to detect metastasis will help in classifying Stage III and Stage IV cases.

Table 6
Staging Scheme for Cancer of the Vulva

Stage O:	Carcinoma in situ
Stage I:	Cancer confined to the vulva, 2 cm or less in diameter. No suspicious lymph nodes.
Stage II:	Same as above, only the cancer is larger than 2 cm in diameter. No suspicious lymph nodes.
Stage III:	Cancer of any size that has (1) spread to the urethra, all or part of the vagina, the area between the vaginal opening and the anus and/or the anus itself; (2) and/or suspicious lymph nodes.
Stage IV, A and B:	Cancer of any size that has infiltrated (A) the bladder and/or rectum; and/or (B) cancer that is fixed to the bone and/or has metastasized to distant sites.

Treatment[16]

The treatment of Stage O vulvar cancer is discussed elsewhere. Here we are concerned only with invasive vulvar cancer—stages I, II, III and IV. Since 90 percent to 95 percent of all vulvar cancers are of a type known as squamous cell cancers, the following discussion centers around treatment of this type of vulvar cancer. Other rare forms are mentioned only briefly.

The aim of treatment in these cases is to remove the actual tumor, the surrounding areas where microscopic cancer may be lurking and the lymph passageways and nodes that may be involved.

Vulvectomy

Simply removing the tumor itself would not suffice, for vulvar cancer tends to be multicentric, that is, to have many points of origin. The entire vulva must be removed, an operation known as a vulvectomy. To do anything less than a total vulvectomy would be taking too great a chance of leaving behind microscopic areas of cancer that could metastasize before they were discovered.

There is some debate about how extensive the total vulvectomy should be. Some doctors think that it is acceptable in certain instances to do an operation that allows for what is known in surgical circles as "primary closure," in which enough skin remains to close over the operative wound. If primary closure is not possible, skin grafting (removing skin from other areas of the body and transplanting it to the wound area) must be done. Other doctors believe that doing a vulvectomy that allows for primary closure, although it offers better cosmetic results and superior healing, is too dangerous, since it is associated with higher rates of recurrence. This is one issue that women with vulvar cancer interviewing prospective doctors might wish to discuss and to seek second opinions regarding.

Although radiation therapy theoretically could be effective in treating cancer in the immediate area of the vulva, this generally is not done, for tissues in this area are extremely sensitive to radiation. Doses of radiation high enough to destroy the cancer would cause too much damage to these tissues. In certain cases, where a woman is in such poor health that the general anesthetic required for surgery would pose too great a threat to her life, removal of the tumor alone under local anesthetic and/or radiation therapy may be used. Since this results in lower cure rates, surgery is done whenever possible. In certain cases, where the tumor is too large to be removed surgically, radiation treatment may be given before surgery, in order to reduce the tumor to the point where it can be removed surgically. Most of the time, however, the vulvar area is not radiated.

Another instance in which surgery might not be done is in Stage IV cases, when the disease has spread to the bones or other distant areas. In these cases the surgery will not improve a woman's chances of survival, so there is no point in subjecting her to the risks and discomforts of surgery. An exception would be the woman with Stage IVB disease who has intense itching and heavy discharge. In her case a partial vulvectomy may be helpful in relieving the symptoms and making her more comfortable.

Inguinal Lymphadenectomy

In most cases the surgery will also involve removal of the lymph nodes in the groin, a procedure known as inguinal lymphadenectomy. Even if there is no suggestion that these lymph nodes are involved before surgery, they must be removed, for even in Stage IA cases there is a chance that microscopic areas of cancer may be lurking in these nodes. The only way to find out is to remove them and examine them microscopically.

There is a tendency among some doctors to do the vulvectomy and not to remove the lymph nodes as well if there are no symptoms of swelling, especially when, as is often the case, the woman is elderly. Such doctors may delay the treatment of the lymph nodes until the woman actually develops the swelling in the nodes that indicates that cancer may be present. This is considered a dangerous course of action by most experts, for cancer is sometimes present even though there is no swelling. By waiting for signs of swelling the woman's best chance for a cure is lost. Sometimes, in women who have such poor general health that the more prolonged and taxing operation of lymph node removal would be too much of a strain, even the experts concede that the more radical surgery should not be done. However, most of these experts caution against this modification of surgery on the basis of age alone. Although some surgeons argue that the elderly patient won't live long enough to justify subjecting her to the risks of extended surgery, most experts believe that the facts don't justify this line of thinking. They believe that it is unfair to do less-than-adequate surgery, which will jeopardize her long-term chances of survival, just because she is elderly. Many times a team approach to surgery is used. One doctor does the vulvectomy, and the other removes the lymph nodes. This allows for a faster operation and less anesthesia time; hence there is less risk.

In certain specialized cases, removal of the lymph nodes in the groin may be omitted. Carcinoma in situ and some rare types of cancer, for instance, one known as basal cell carcinoma, don't require removal, for the nodes are rarely, if ever, involved in the disease process. Many doctors believe that certain early invasive cancers in which the depth of invasion is less than 5 mm (some would say 3 mm) and in which the tumor cells are low grade (*see* p. 714) don't require lymph node removal.

It is possible to survive without lymph node surgery, but survival rates generally are improved when the lymph nodes in the groin are removed.

Pelvic Lymphadenectomy

The pelvic nodes may also be removed, by a procedure known as a pelvic lymphadenectomy. Here again, removal makes the operation more extensive, requiring longer anesthesia time, and therefore the risk is greater. The rate of complications is significantly higher as well. There has been a good deal of uncertainty about when it is worthwhile to remove these pelvic lymph nodes.

If the woman is a good enough surgical risk to allow for vulvectomy and removal of the lymph nodes in the groin, the surgeon will send the removed groin nodes to the pathology lab for analysis by frozen section. If the pathologist sends back word that the groin nodes are cancer-free, most surgeons will not remove the pelvic nodes. Although some doctors favor removal of the pelvic nodes even if the groin nodes are negative, the majority of doctors would consider this unnecessary and to involve too many extra risks and complications to be worthwhile.

If the pathologist's report indicates that the groin nodes are positive, the situation is a bit more complex. Just because the groin nodes have cancer in them does not necessarily mean that the pelvic ones do. Although vulvar cancer spreads from the original site to the immediately adjacent groin lymph nodes relatively quickly, it then seems to slow down. It apparently remains in the groin nodes for some time before spreading to the pelvic nodes. It is thought that only about 16 percent of women in whom the pathologist has found cancer in the groin nodes will have cancer in the pelvic nodes. An estimated 20 percent to 25 percent of women with pelvic node metastases can be cured. But this means that only 20 percent to 25 percent of the 16 percent who have positive pelvic nodes, that is, only 3 percent to 4 percent of those women with cancerous groin nodes, would benefit from having their pelvic lymph nodes removed. To remove the pelvic lymph nodes in all women with negative groin nodes doesn't then seem justifiable to many doctors. Still other doctors will remove these nodes routinely.

Some authorities recently have adopted special criteria for deciding whether or not to remove the pelvic nodes. Some studies have shown that those women who, on the basis of the pathologist's report, were shown to have positive lymph nodes in the groin *and* who also have had suspicious-appearing nodes in the groin before surgery are the ones most likely to have positive pelvic nodes.[17] If the nodes did not appear suspicious before surgery and cancer was found only during the pathologist's microscopic examination, there is little chance that the pelvic nodes are involved. Sometimes, however, the pelvic nodes can be cancerous even if the groin nodes do not appear suspicious before surgery.

The groin lymph system narrows down to one specific node called Cloquet's node before branching out to the pelvic network of lymph passageways. This key node may be removed by the surgeon and subjected to frozen-section analysis. If it tests positive, the woman may require removal of the pelvic nodes, regardless of the appearance of the groin nodes before surgery. Many doctors, then, will remove the pelvic nodes only if the woman has positive groin nodes both by frozen-section analysis and by the doctor's clinical opinion preoperatively, and/or if the Cloquet's node is found to have cancer by frozen-section analysis at the time of surgery.

The question of pelvic lymph node removal is a problematic one and opinions, even among experts, differ. Every woman has the right to a full discussion of her doctor's operative plans. She should know what nodes the doctor plans to remove, how these decisions will be made and on what basis. She should know, given her particular state of health, what the possible risks and complications of less extensive or more extensive surgery are. Second opinions (*see* p. 238) are, of course, in order.

Pelvic Exenteration

In certain advanced cases a partial or total pelvic exenteration may be combined with vulvectomy and pelvic/inguinal lymphadenectomy. Total pelvic exenteration involves removal of the vulva, vagina, uterus, tubes, ovaries, supporting and connective tissue, urethra, bladder and/or rectum. Partial exenteration involves the removal of only some of these organs. If the bladder, urethra and/or rectum are removed, new openings are constructed surgically and waste products are collected in plastic bags. This is an extensive operation and can be done only in cases where the woman is in good health. It is not done in Stage IVB cases, where the disease has spread to distant sites in the body, for it would not result in improved survival. However, in women who are good candidates for this type of extensive surgery, 50 percent to 75 percent success rates in controlling the disease have been reported.[18] Even if it does not result in absolute cure, it can prolong life significantly.

Radiation Therapy

As discussed earlier, radiation therapy generally is not used to treat cancer in the vulvar area; however, in recent years there has been a great deal of interest in using radiation instead of or in conjunction with lymphadenectomy to treat the groin and pelvic nodes. Since the vulvar area is not radiated directly, the problem of excessive damage to these radiation-sensitive tissues does not arise. Proponents of this form of therapy believe that there would be fewer risks and complications than with lymphadenectomy. At the present time we simply do not know enough to say conclusively whether radiation would or would not be superior to lymphadenectomy.

Some doctors will use radiation therapy to treat women who refuse or are not candidates for pelvic exenteration. But here again, there is the problem of radiation damage to the sensitive bladder and rectum. Radiation therapy may be used to treat recurrent cancer.

Radiation has also been used in palliation, that is, in treatment designed to relieve symptoms and make the woman more comfortable. This may be done in certain cases of distant metastases, but many doctors question palliative value in treating the vulvar area. They think that the radiation does little to relieve symptoms, that it may actually shorten the woman's life span and that the aftereffects of the radiation cause so much pain and discomfort that it is not worthwhile to use it. Here again, women have the right to a full discussion of the benefits and risks of radiation therapy in their particular case and to second opinions or consultations as needed.

Chemotherapy

Chemotherapy is used only on an experimental basis. Although there have been a few reports of limited success in controlling vulvar cancer, most results have been disappointing.[19]

Recurrent Cancer and Follow-up

All women with vulvar cancer must be followed for life in order to detect recurrences and the cancers that such women frequently develop in their other female organs.

Survival Rates

Surgery is only possible in about three-quarters of the women with vulvar cancer, and survival rates are lower for those who are inoperable. Table 7 gives survival statistics by stage.

Table 7
Five-Year Survival Rates for Squamous Cancer of the Vulva

Stage	Survival %
I	85
II	58
III	24
IV	0

SOURCE: Adapted from J.L. Benedet et al., "Squamous Carcinoma of the Vulva: Results of Treatment 1930–1976, *American Journal of Obstetrics and Gynecology* 134:2 (May 15, 1979):201–7.

The Vagina

The anatomy of the vagina is described and illustrated in Chapter Two. The changes that occur in the vagina over the course of the menstrual cycle and during a woman's lifetime are discussed in Chapter Four. In this section we are concerned with vaginal diseases.

Vaginitis

The first few diseases discussed in this section are forms of vaginitis. The term vaginitis is a broad one, used to refer to any inflammation of the vagina. The chief symptom of vaginitis is excessive vaginal discharge, which may smell bad and cause itching.

A certain amount of vaginal discharge is normal, for the discharge helps to cleanse the vagina and keep it healthy. The discharge is made up of secretions from the glands of the cervix and vaginal walls and cells shed from the uterus, cervix and walls of the vagina. The amount and character of this discharge changes over the course of the menstrual cycle and over the course of a woman's lifetime. It also varies from individual to individual. Most of the time the discharge is clear or milky white, moderate in quantity, thin or watery in consistency and has a mild odor. It may leave a slightly yellowish stain on underclothes. Women who practice self-exam and are familiar with their own discharges can detect abnormal discharges and seek treatment for vaginitis in the earliest stages of the disease, when it is easiest to treat.

Vaginitis is associated with changes in the normal acid/alkaline balance of

298

the vagina. Most of the time the vaginal secretions are rather acidic. Scientists measure acidity on a relative scale called the pH scale that looks like this:

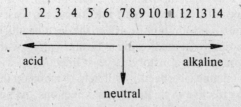

The scale runs from 1 to 14, and 7 represents a neutral condition, that is, neither alkaline (sugary) nor acidic. The average pH of the vagina of a woman in her reproductive years is usually about 4.5 to 5.0. Most disease-causing organisms prefer a more alkaline environment. For instance, trichomonads, the culprits responsible for trich, one of the most common forms of vaginitis, thrive best in a pH of 4.9 to 7.5. Monilia, the organisms responsible for yeast infections, prefer a pH of about 5.4. Gonococci, the bacteria that cause gonorrhea, and streptococci, other disease-causing organisms, do best at a pH of 7.4.

The protective, slightly acidic environment of the vagina is maintained by bacteria known as lactobaccilli, or Döderlein's bacilli, that normally live in the vagina. Without them the vagina would be quite alkaline, for the cervical secretions and the cells that are constantly being shed from the vaginal walls are alkaline. The cells of the vaginal wall contain large amounts of a sugar known as glycogen. This sugar is derived from carbohydrates taken into the body when sugars and starches are eaten. As the cells of the vaginal wall are shed and break down, releasing their alkaline glycogen, the lactobaccilli convert the sugar to a weak acid known as lactic acid.

The pH of the vagina changes over the course of the menstrual cycle. It is most alkaline at the time of ovulation, when levels of estrogen are highest. The cervical secretions are then more abundant, and there are greater numbers of sugar-rich vaginal cells. Symptoms of vaginitis, which are sometimes cyclical—appearing for a while and then subsiding, only to appear again—are apt to manifest themselves or to be particularly intense at the time of ovulation. The pH of the vagina also changes after menopause. Typically, the vagina of a postmenopausal woman has a pH of about 7.0. This change in pH, coupled with the fact that after menopause the vaginal walls become thinner and are easily irritated—a condition known as postmenopausal vaginitis— explains why postmenopausal women are so prone to vaginal infections.

There are a number of other things that can alter the vaginal pH, making the vagina more alkaline and more susceptible to infection. Sometimes antibiotics prescribed to combat infections elsewhere in the body also destroy the lactobacilli. Then, disease-causing organisms that may already have been present but were held in check by the acid environment of the vagina or that are introduced into the body at this time, thrive in the vaginal environment, which has become more alkaline without the lactobacilli. Women taking antibiotics are thus especially prone to yeast infections, for yeasts are frequently present in the vagina and antibiotics affect the lactobacilli but not yeasts. Some doctors prescribe yeast medication to be taken along with the antibiotic, especially if the woman has a history of yeast infections.

Yogurt, which contains lactobacilli, will help to maintain the acidity of the vagina, and is also effective in treating yeast infections and nonspecific vaginitis.[1] A spermicide or medicine applicator can be used to insert the yogurt into the vagina. Eating yogurt will help, but inserting a couple of applicatorsful of yogurt once or twice a day and again at bedtime during the course of antibiotic treatment will be even more helpful in preventing infections. Using a tampon to help keep the yogurt in the vagina or a sanitary napkin to catch the yogurt that may leak out is a good idea.

In order to be effective the yogurt must contain live lactobacilli. Most of the yogurt sold in the grocery store has been pasteurized after the lactobacilli were added. Because the heat from the pasteurization process destroys the lactobacilli, it is important to find yogurt that has not been pasteurized or that was pasteurized before the addition of the lactobacilli. Health-food stores often carry this type of yogurt. It is also possible to purchase yogurt culture and make your own.

Birth control pills also alter vaginal chemistry. Not only do the extra hormones in the bloodstream stimulate the cervical glands to produce more secretion, but the Pill also changes the chemical composition of the vaginal cells. This makes the vagina more alkaline and more susceptible to yeast infections. This is especially true for women who are taking high-dose estrogen pills containing more than 0.05 mg of estrogen per pill. In fact, the Pill makes the vagina so alkaline that some women who take the Pill are troubled by recurrent yeast infections. Such women may have to discontinue use of the Pill in order to clear up their yeast infection. The Pill may also make a woman more susceptible to gonorrhea (although gonorrhea in Pill users is *less* likely to develop into pelvic inflammatory disease).

Pregnant women may also have more alkaline vaginas, for during pregnancy, hormone levels are higher and the vaginal changes that result are similar to those created by birth control pills. It is often difficult for pregnant women to get rid of a vaginal infection.

Women with diabetes, a disease in which the body is not able to metabolize nutrients properly and which causes high levels of sugar in the body, also tend to have more alkaline vaginal environments. Their vaginal cells have high levels of glycogen, and they are, therefore, particularly susceptible to yeast infections.

Excessive douching can also alter the vaginal pH. Although the value of the douches that are sometimes prescribed as part of the treatment of vaginitis is not questioned, many doctors think that douching as a routine hygiene measure is not a good idea, because it can alter the acid/alkaline balance, making the woman more susceptible to infection. In addition, the chemicals used in many of the commercially available douche mixes may irritate the vagina. Most women who douche do so because they are concerned about odor. Sexual activity, emotional changes and the stage of the menstrual cycle can all cause changes in the composition and hence the odor of vaginal secretions, but vaginal odor usually emanates from the outer genital organs. Improper wiping with toilet tissue can trap urine and feces in the vulvar lips and cause odor. Hot weather and inadequate ventilation of the genital organs because of tight clothing or synthetic undergarments (which trap air and moisture) also contribute to the problem. Daily washing of the genitals with soap and water will usually eliminate any odors, and such routine hygiene is preferable to disturbing the pH balance of the vagina with commercial douche preparations.

Some doctors advise women who use tampons to douche at the end of their menstrual periods, because leaving a tampon in for an extended period of time may trap the menstrual blood and vaginal discharges, creating odor. But women who use tampons should change them frequently to avoid this problem, rather than douching. Pregnant women should never douche, since the douche water could be forced up into the uterus and cause an infection, miscarriage or fetal death.

Women who do douche should not do so more than twice a week and should avoid commercial douche preparations. Two tablespoons of white vinegar diluted in a quart of warm water is a less-expensive alternative and one that closely mimics the pH of the vagina. Bag-type douches are usually more effective than syringe-type douches (Illustration 41). Douching equipment should not be shared, because infection can be transmitted by a douche nozzle that has not been properly cleansed. Before douching you should inspect the nozzle for cracks, which could injure the vaginal tissues or harbor infection. The nozzle should be washed thoroughly with soap and hot water but should not be boiled, since the nozzles are usually made of plastic, which could melt at high temperatures.

To douche, lie on your back in the tub or shower with the douche bag about 1 foot above your hips. The higher the bag, the more forceful the flow of water into the vagina, but too much pressure could injure the vaginal tissues or force bacteria or other disease-causing organisms up into the normally sterile environment of the uterus.

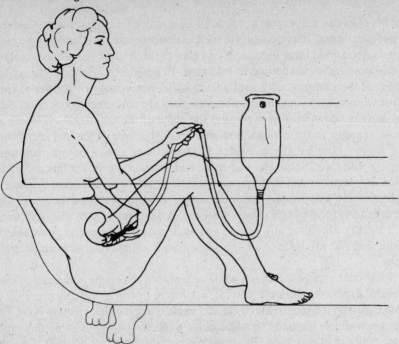

Illustration 41 *Douching*

Prevention

Vaginitis is generally not serious in terms of general health, but it is often hard to get rid of and recurrences are common. Prevention is the best form of treatment. The following suggestions will help to prevent vaginitis:

- ☐ Take care of yourself! Being run down, not getting enough sleep and eating improperly make you more susceptible.
- ☐ Avoid eating sugars and starches and thereby creating an alkaline vaginal environment. Include yogurt in your diet, and if you are especially susceptible to yeast infection or take birth control pills, you may want to apply yogurt to your vagina, especially around ovulation, when your pH rises.
- ☐ Insert applicatorsful of yogurt into the vagina a couple of times a day if you are taking an antibiotic. Or, if you have a history of yeast infections, ask the doctor to prescribe yeast medication to be taken along with the antibiotic.
- ☐ Avoid douching.
- ☐ If you use a diaphragm, don't leave it in place longer than necessary, for this can cause vaginal odor in some women.

302

☐ Use condoms if you have more than one sexual partner or are starting a sexual relationship with a new partner, as these two factors make you more prone to infections.

☐ Always wipe from the front to the back to avoid spreading bacteria from the bowel into the vagina.

☐ Wear cotton underpants; avoid synthetic undergarments, pantyhose and tight pants.

☐ Avoid using feminine hygiene sprays, perfumed soaps and other such products that can irritate the vulva and vaginal opening and also mask odors that are one of the signs of vaginitis.

Diagnosis and Treatment

Practicing self-exam regularly will make you familiar with your own discharge and help you to learn what is normal for you at various points in your menstrual cycle. Vaginitis can be detected in its earliest stages, before the infection has gotten to the point where the discharge is so profuse that it is leaking out of the vaginal opening and causing burning, itching and redness of the external genitals. Some women who are familiar with their own bodies use yogurt at the first sign of vaginitis and this often clears up the infection and avoids the expense and inconvenience of a doctor's visit and medications, but this could be a risky practice. Any woman who does this must be absolutely positive that she has not been exposed to gonorrhea. We know of one woman who practiced self-exam and noticed an unusual discharge that looked like the classic yeast infection discharge. She had a long history of yeast infections, so she used yogurt for a week and her discharge returned to normal. As it turned out, the woman didn't have a yeast infection at all; she had gonorrhea. Gonorrhea is often asymptomatic in its early stages or there may be minimal symptoms, one of which is a slight vaginal discharge. These early symptoms may subside even though the infection has not gone away. This woman's discharge did subside, although it didn't do so because of the yogurt, for yogurt is not effective against gonorrhea. Luckily, this woman went to the doctor a couple of weeks later for her yearly checkup, which included a gonorrhea culture. Her gonorrhea was therefore detected and treated. If it had not been caught, it could have had serious consequences, including pelvic inflammatory disease, sterility, and perhaps even death. This woman had only one sexual partner, and her sexual partner was supposedly having sex only with her. He wasn't, and she got gonorrhea.

Any woman who is having heterosexual sex and notices an unusual discharge should consider the possibility that she has gonorrhea and should ask that a gonorrhea culture be done. Women should also insist that the doctor do a wet smear. A wet smear takes only a few minutes. With a speculum in place the doctor takes a sample of the discharge. The discharge is then smeared across a glass slide and viewed under a microscope.

The organisms responsible for most forms of vaginitis are easily identified by way of the wet smear. Some doctors don't do a wet smear. They may think that they can diagnose the type of vaginitis just by looking at the discharge. Although it is true that each form of discharge has its characteristic appearance and odor, it is easy to be fooled. For one thing, it is not at all unusual to have two infections at the same time. In these cases of mixed infections the symptoms of one form of vaginitis may mask the symptoms of the other. Each type of vaginitis requires its own specific medication. If a woman had trich *and* yeast infection, the medication used to treat the trich wouldn't be effective against the yeast, and her yeast infection would persist. She would return to the doctor, who might assume her trich was still present and prescribe another round of medicine for it. A wet smear will avoid such confusion. But do not douche before going to the doctor, for this can alter the results of a wet smear or other tests.

If you have vaginitis, your sexual partner may need to be treated as well. And you should use condoms until the infection clears up or you may constantly reinfect each other, even if you are both taking the medication.

It is important to take all the medication that is prescribed. Too many times women will discontinue the medication as soon as the symptoms disappear, but the stronger organisms that have not yet succumbed to the medication remain. They will eventually reproduce until their numbers are sufficient to produce symptoms. Then you've got a recurrence of the infection that will be harder to cure, since the new infection will be caused by the offspring of the stronger, more drug-resistant organisms.

Sometimes women with vaginal infections, such as trich, yeast or hemophilus are given prescriptions for sulfa creams or suppositories, but such medications are *not* the best treatment for these infections. In fact, a special committee of the Food and Drug Administration recently concluded that creams and suppositories whose major ingredients are sulfanilamide or sulfisoxazole are not effective against these infections.[2] Such medications are sold under brand names like AVC Cream or Suppositories, Vagimide Cream, Vaginal Sulfa Cream, Vaginal Sulfa Suppositories, Cantri Vaginal Cream, Vagilia Cream or Suppositories, Sulfa Tablets and Koro-Sulf Vaginal Cream. If your doctor prescribes one of these medications, be sure to question this treatment and to ask for a more effective form of therapy.

Another type of medication frequently prescribed for trich, yeast and hemophilus, known as triple sulfa creams, which contain sulfabenzamide, sulfacetamide and sulfathiazole, are ineffective for trich and yeast and their effectiveness against hemophilus and nonspecific vaginitis is also questionable.[3] Triple sulfa creams are sold under brand names like Sultrin, Trysul and Triple Sulfa Cream. Again, if your doctor prescribes one of these drugs, insist on a medication of proven effectiveness, such as one of those described in the sections on various types of vaginitis in the following pages.

Anatomical Abnormalities

Although vaginitis is the most common type of vaginal problem, there are other problems that can affect the vagina. One group of problems involves alterations of the normal anatomy of the vagina. The vaginal canal may become smaller and less elastic, a condition known as vaginal stenosis. The opening of the vaginal canal may be disturbed as a result of injury. This sort of problem is discussed under the heading Lacerations of the Vagina, Vulva and Perineum. Sometimes because of a muscle weakness or defect in the vaginal wall, the bladder or urethra may sag and bulge into the vaginal wall. If this happens, the woman has either a cystocele or urethrocele. Similarly, a portion of the rectum or intestines may bulge into the vagina, conditions known as rectocele or entrocele. A woman may also experience involuntary spasms of the vaginal muscles, a condition known as vaginismus. Another distortion in the normal vaginal anatomy is the fistula, a condition in which there are abnormal connections or passageways between the vagina and the urinary tract or the vagina and the rectum. A woman may also be born with a vagina whose anatomy is abnormal. This problem is discussed under the heading Congenital Abnormalities of the Vagina.

DES-Related Problems

One type of congenital abnormality of the vagina that has received considerable attention in recent years occurs in the daughters of women who took certain synthetic hormones during their pregnancies. This is discussed under the headings Vaginal Adenosis and Clear Cell Adenocarcinoma. Many DES daughters are not aware of the fact that they have been exposed. All women should read the discussion of DES on pp. 808–18.

Benign and Malignant Tumors

Lastly, the vagina may be the site of tumors, either benign or cancerous. Both benign and malignant tumors are discussed below.

TRICH

AKA: trichomonas vaginitis, trichomoniasis, trichomonosis, TV

Trich, or TV, is a form of vaginitis. Important information about the cause, diagnosis and treatment of vaginitis is given in the introduction to this section, so be sure to read that material as well as the information below.

Incidence

The exact incidence of TV is hard to determine because many women carry the organisms without having any symptoms. Various studies have reported that anywhere from 20 percent to 65 percent examined have the organisms in their vaginas even though they have no symptoms. It is estimated that 15 percent of these women will become symptomatic. TV is, then, a widespread disease.

Cause and Transmission

TV is caused by a microscopic organism whose scientific name is *Trichomonas vaginalis*. This organism does not normally inhabit the vagina or any other area of the human body. Since the disease may be asymptomatic, it is possible for a woman to carry the organism for many years without ever knowing she has trichs in her body. Some doctors think that additional organisms, for instance, streptococci, must also be present in order to produce symptoms. Some authorities believe that emotional stress and strain may be responsible for a flare-up, persistence or recurrence of symptoms.

Trichs are usually introduced into the vagina by sexual intercourse. There is circumstantial evidence that the disease can be passed by non-sexual contact, as the organisms have been cultured from Bakelite toilet seats, washcloths and the wooden benches of washrooms at room temperature after 24 hours, but it has thus far been impossible to actually prove that the disease is transmitted in nonsexual ways. Most authorities think that the majority of cases of TV are transmitted through sexual intercourse.

Anyone who gets TV is likely to wonder, "Who did I get it from?" Sometimes this question may be hard to answer. First, there is the possibility, although it is probably a pretty remote one, that the transmission *was* nonsexual. Second, there is the possibility that a woman could have been harboring the trichs for some time, for years even, without knowing it. Emotional stress, a general lowered resistance or changes in the vaginal pH can cause the disease to suddenly become symptomatic. Even if a woman has had many wet smears done for other infections, it is still possible that she may have had TV for quite some time. The wet smear would have shown the presence of the trichs, but there are some doctors who do not inform the woman that trichs are present unless she is symptomatic. The third possibility is that although the trichs were in her body for some time, the other organisms that some experts believe must also be present to produce symptoms may not have been there.

Symptoms

As mentioned above, many women are asymptomatic and it is also possible for the disease to be present for quite some time before the symptoms appear. Sometimes the symptoms are cyclical in nature, appearing for a few days and then disappearing for a month or even for many months. In the great majority of cases, it is thought that the symptoms appear within 4 to 28 days of the infected contact. The symptoms may be mild or very severe. Since other diseases, especially gonorrhea, yeast infections and hemophilus, often occur along with trich, symptoms of these diseases may also be present.

In some cases the only symptom may be a vaginal discharge. The discharge is usually yellow-white or green-yellow but may be white or gray. The discharge is usually thin and watery, but in case of mixed infections it may be thick and creamy. It tends to be frothy, that is, to have little bubbles in it (caused by fermentation of the trichs) and to smell bad.

The vaginal opening may be red and sore owing to irritation from the discharge. There is apt to be itching and burning, especially on urination. Sexual intercourse may be painful. In extreme cases the whole vulvar area and even the inside of the thighs and/or the anus may be irritated.

The symptoms of TV are likely to be more severe just before and just after the menstrual period. This may be because the vagina is more alkaline (as opposed to acidic) at this time, and trichs thrive in an alkaline environment. Pregnant women, whose vaginal environments are also apt to be more alkaline, are particularly susceptible and may have more severe symptoms. The introduction to this section discussed acid/alkaline balance and vaginal infections in more detail.

On speculum exam it may be possible to see a pool of the typical thin, green-yellow, bubbly discharge around the cervix. The walls of the vagina may be quite red. In severe cases the upper walls and cervix may be covered with strawberrylike red patches.

Men rarely suffer symptoms; however, some men may notice a burning after ejaculation or urination. There may be a slight moistness on the tip of the penis and some itching. Trichs do not survive well on the male sex organs, although on uncircumcised men the area under the foreskin may afford an environment conducive to the trichs. Such men may notice a discharge from this area.

Diagnosis

Sometimes the symptoms are so characteristic that the diagnosis is obvious. However, even if the classic symptoms are present, a woman should insist that the diagnosis be confirmed by a microscopic examination of the vaginal discharge—by a wet smear—for other diseases are frequently present along with TV, and the treatment for TV may not be effective against these other diseases. A wet smear precludes the problem of unnecessary or ineffective treatment.

Because the discharge may be heavy and tends to smell bad, many women douche before going to the doctor. This should not be done, for it may flush out a large number of trichs and cause a negative wet smear, even though trichs may still be present and will multiply, causing symptoms again later. Sometimes women who are familiar with their discharges will note a slight increase or an unpleasant odor in the early stages of TV. In very early cases a doctor, seeing none of the signs of TV and not noticing an unusual odor or unusual discharge, might be reluctant to do a smear. One woman reported that her doctor told her, "Some vaginal odor is normal," in response to her complaint. When, at her insistence, he reluctantly did a wet smear he found trichs. Women who notice unusual symptoms should insist on having appropriate tests done.

The smear is not always entirely accurate. Trichs may be present and yet be missed. In doubtful cases or when the symptoms lead the doctor to suspect that other diseases are present, it is possible to grow the trichs in a special culture, but this takes some time and is more costly, so the culture is not routinely used to diagnose TV. (If there is even a remote chance that you might have gonorrhea, it is probably a good idea to have a gonorrhea culture done as well, since the two diseases often coexist.)

Women should be aware that some doctors, finding trichs in routine wet smears, will not even bother to tell asymptomatic women. Such doctors also don't believe in treating the disease if it is asymptomatic. However, even if a woman isn't symptomatic, she is still able to pass the trichs on through intercourse. It is important to communicate with your doctor on this issue and to make it clear that you want access to any information s/he has about your body. Other doctors think that if a woman has a population of trichs in her vagina large enough to show up on a wet smear, she is likely to become symptomatic in the future and should be treated.

TV occasionally shows up as an incidental finding on a routine Pap smear.

As long as a woman has no symptoms, the majority of doctors will not treat trich when it is discovered only as an incidental finding on a Pap. The drug used to combat TV is a potent one, and they believe that if the trichs haven't shown up on a wet smear and aren't producing symptoms, it is better to rely on the body's own defenses to keep the problem in check.

TV can also cause an abnormal Pap smear. The pathologist's report will usually say that "inflammatory cells" are present. This is nothing to worry about, since the Pap will revert to normal once the TV is cleared up. However, on rare occasions TV will cause changes in the Pap smear that mimic dysplasia, a possibly precancerous condition. Any woman with trich who has an abnormal Pap smear should have the smear repeated after 3 months. A Pap smear falsely indicating dysplasia in a woman with TV will revert to normal after the TV is treated. But if true dysplasia is present the dysplasia will persist, despite the treatment for TV.

Treatment

In the United States, TV is usually treated with metronidazole, which is sold under brand names such as Flagyl. Metronidazole can be used by most people and doesn't usually produce severe side effects; however, the drug is contraindicated (that is, should not be taken by) for certain people.[4] Obviously, anyone who has had a previous allergic reaction should not take the drug. People who have certain blood diseases cannot take it because it can cause a temporary decrease in white blood cell count. People taking certain types of anticoagulant drugs should not take metronidazole because the two drugs can interact in dangerous ways. People who have active disease in the central nervous system should not take it because there is some evidence that the drug may affect the central nervous system. The drug is officially contraindicated for women in the first 3 months of pregnancy, for it can cross the placental barrier and enter the fetal circulation system. Although it has not been shown to cause birth defects in either animal or human studies, there is not sufficient data available to rule out the possibility. Moreover, there is some evidence that metronidazole can cause both cancerous and noncancerous tumors (see below). Since it can produce tumors and affect the central nervous system, many doctors believe that it should not be used in pregnant women at all, regardless of the stage of pregnancy. Since the drug is secreted in breast milk, a nursing mother taking the drug must discontinue breast-feeding for a while.

Metronidazole can cause adverse reactions in some people. Nausea, sometimes accompanied by headaches, loss of appetite, occasionally vomiting,

309

diarrhea, abdominal cramping and constipation are the most common complaints. A person taking metronidazole should not drink alcohol, for drinking can aggravate the reaction, and a few authorities recommend abstaining for 3 days after treatment too.

A metallic taste is not uncommon. Other adverse effects associated with the drug include a furry tongue; dryness of the mouth, vulva and vagina; nasal congestion; itching; hives; painful urination; painful intercourse; a sense of pelvic pressure; fever; decreased sex drive; pus in the urine; excessive urine; inability to control urine flow; inflammations of the bladder and the rectum; confusion; irritability; depression; weakness; insomnia; dizziness; lack of co-ordination and even convulsive seizures. Pain in the joints or numbness of the arms, legs and hands are important side effects, because these sorts of effects have persisted even after the drug was discontinued in some people who had taken metronidazole for a long time. If any of these side effects appear, the medicine should be discontinued, the symptoms reported to the doctor and possible alternative treatments discussed.

Women taking metronidazole are more apt to get yeast infections, because the acid/alkaline balance of the vagina is altered. Prevention of such yeast infections is discussed in the general introduction to vaginal diseases (*see* p. 302).

Although Searle, the company that sells Flagyl, has asserted over the years that Flagyl does not cause cancer, in 1972 an article in the *Journal of the National Cancer Institute (JNCI)* reported the results of an experiment in which a greater number of cancerous and noncancerous tumors appeared in a group of mice given the drug as compared with a control group.[5] This led to a reexamination of the data Searle had provided to the Food and Drug Administration. The reexamination was apparently necessary, for as it turned out, the original Searle rat data confirmed the *JNCI* findings.

Since that time other studies have been done that showed an increase in the incidence of various tumors in rats, particularly breast tumors.[6] Two other studies done on hamsters, however, were reported as negative.[7] Moreover, the animal studies have been criticized, because in some of them the animals were given the drug every day for their entire lives. Even in the studies where the animals were given metronidazole intermittently, critics point out that the dosages were rather high. More recent studies of the urine excreted by people taking the drug have shown some evidence that the drug has the power to cause mutations in bacteria.[8] The implications this may hold for human cancer are not yet known.

The dosage was originally one 250-mg tablet three times a day for ten days; however, many people stopped taking the drug as soon as the symptoms cleared up, often after only 2 or 3 days. This led to a high rate of recurrence of the disease owing to insufficient dosage, so shorter dosage schedules with higher-dose tablets were tried. The Food and Drug Administration (FDA) next approved a schedule of one 250-mg tablet three times a day for 7 days. Some doctors give 500 mg two times a day for 5 days, whereas others believe that 250 mg three times a day for 3 days is sufficient. These two alternatives seem to work about as well. In recent experiments the drug was given in a single eight-tablet (2-g) dose or split into a double dose of four tablets each taken in the same day. This dosage schedule has now been approved by the FDA. Some researchers report cure rates as high as 90 percent, whereas others report rates as low as 56 percent. It is unclear why there should be such a variance in rates. It has been suggested that the studies that yielded high cure rates may have had inadequate follow-up and recurrences may have been missed. At any rate, there may be more intense side effects with these high-level doses. Indeed, in our experience, people taking this much metronidazole are apt to get quite sick and to vomit up the medication, thus necessitating another course.

Some cases of TV do not respond to metronidazole. There has been some suggestion in recent articles that the drug is not as effective as it once was. Whereas metronidazole provided a 97 percent cure rate in 1967, the results now being recorded are not as good and may be as low as 74 percent. This may be caused by the development of a stronger strain of trichs or it may be that the bacteria that often accompany TV tend to inactivate the drug. If the latter proves to be true, an antibiotic may be given along with metronidazole in the future. In either case, larger doses may someday be necessary.

A new drug, nitrimidazone, which is sold in Great Britain under the brand names Naxogin and Minerazole and which is about as effective as metronidazole (indeed, possibly more effective in single-dose therapy), has recently been used to treat TV. It is not yet sold in the United States, so information as to its possible side effects is not readily available; however, it would not be surprising if the drug were available in the United States in the not-too-distant future.

In about 25 percent of the people treated, there will be a recurrence of the disease. This may be owing to reinfection or to failure of the drug to destroy all the trichs. If the metronidazole is taken a second time, there should be a waiting period of 4 to 6 weeks before the second course, to allow the white blood cell count, which may be depressed by the drug, to return to normal.

Other drugs can be used to treat trich in pregnant women or others who cannot use the drug, but the cure rates for these are not as high as with metronidazole. Antibiotics in the form of Aureomycin or Terramycin* given orally have met with some success. We also use Betadine. Sulfa creams are *not* an effective medication (*see* p. 304).

Douches of 5 tablespoonsful of ordinary vinegar to 2 quarts of water may be used in the treatment of TV. The douches will make the vagina more acidic so that the trichs have trouble surviving. The douches often help to cut down on the symptoms; however, they are not likely to cure the disease, for it is virtually impossible to flush out all the trichs that may be lurking in the recesses of the vaginal folds and some may survive despite the acidity. Keeping the vulvar area dry, using cotton underpants instead of synthetic garments (which trap moisture) and avoiding the use of powders, ointments and sprays will also cut down on the severity of symptoms.

Some doctors prohibit intercourse during the treatment period; others allow intercourse as long as the man wears a condom. The point of prohibiting or protecting intercourse is to prevent the woman from being reinfected and the man from picking it up.

Still another debate centers around whether or not male partners should be treated.[9] Some doctors will write out extra prescriptions for the women's sexual partners; others will not. Some will prescribe for one, two or even three partners, but they may be reluctant to write out a larger number of prescriptions. There are basically two schools of thought on the issue. Those who won't prescribe for the male partner say that since there are contraindications to the drug, they are reluctant to prescribe without interviewing the man concerning the possibility of his being at risk. They also point out that the man may not actually have the disease and that the drugs should be given only when disease is actually present, to prevent things like acquired resistance and side effects. Moreover, some doctors believe that the organisms do not survive well on the penis and will die out without treatment. Those who do prescribe for the unseen male sexual partner do so because they fear that he, who is likely to be asymptomatic, may not bother to go to a doctor for diagnosis and may reinfect his partner or pass it on to another woman. They question how quickly and thoroughly the organisms die out on the man and point to the high recurrence rate. Untreated men, they think, are too often responsible for reinfection. The Centers for Disease Control recommend treatment of the male partner, even if he is asymptomatic.

---

*Terramycin should not be used by pregnant women (*see* p. 795).

YEAST INFECTIONS

AKA: fungus infections, candidiasis, moniliasis, vaginal thrush, fungus vaginitis

Associated terms: *Monilia vaginitis, Candida vaginitis, Candida albicans, Monilia albicans*

Yeast infections, which are called by a number of different names, are not serious, but they can be bothersome. They are often hard to get rid of and recurrences are common. In addition to the information given here, the general introduction to vaginal diseases (*see* p. 298) contains important information about yeast infections.

Incidence

Yeast infections are common. They tend to occur more frequently during the menstrual years, when, under the influence of the monthly ebb and flow of hormones, the vagina provides a rich environment for their growth.

Cause and Transmission

Yeast infections are thought to be caused by a fungus of the yeast family known as *Candida albicans*. Some authorities believe that other, similar organisms may be responsible for the milder forms of the disease.

The organism may be passed through sexual intercourse. A man may give the disease to a woman; however, he is much more likely to get it from her than to give it to her. Nonsexual methods of transfer—douche nozzles, washcloths, etc.—may explain how the organism is originally introduced into the vagina. It is present in the feces of between 17 percent and 40 percent of all people, so careless wiping may also explain how the organism gets into the vagina. *Candidae* are apparently normal inhabitants of the vagina in many women. They usually don't cause any problems. The mere presence of the organisms doesn't mean that there will be symptoms of infection. *Candidae* only seem to cause problems when the environment of the vagina is disturbed. They do not thrive in the normally acid vaginal environment, preferring a more alkaline environment. If, however, the vagina does become more alkaline, they will multiply. Taking antibiotics, douching, eating a lot of carbohydrates, having diabetes, being pregnant and using oral contraceptives may alter the normal acidic vaginal pH.

313

Chemotherapy or radiation therapy used to treat cancer may make a woman more susceptible, probably because they weaken the body's immunological system. Some women seem to have deficient immunological systems, which makes them more prone to yeast infections.

Symptoms

The symptoms vary somewhat from woman to woman and may be similar to those of trich. There may be discharge, burning, itching, localized soreness and pain. Women with yeast infections often complain of a frequent need to urinate and of painful intercourse.

The most common symptom is a vaginal discharge, which tends to be less abundant than with trich. The characteristic discharge is white, thin and watery, with thick, curdlike chunks of a white, cheesy substance that gives the discharge a cottage-cheese-like appearance. The discharge may have a disagreeable odor, which some women liken to fermenting yeast. The symptoms tend to be worse just before and after the menstrual period, when the vagina is usually more alkaline. On speculum exam, the walls of the vagina may appear red and swollen. There may be chunks of white discharge, which, in some cases, adhere firmly to the vaginal walls.

If the discharge is profuse, it can cause an itchy rash on the external genitals. The vulva can be affected as well and may be dry, red, swollen and tender to the touch. If the infection is widespread, the whole vulva may take on a white appearance. Itching, of course, can cause scratching, which makes the area even more irritated and swollen and can lead to a secondary infection. There may be soreness or pain in the whole genital area. As mentioned earlier, intercourse can become very painful. There may also be pain when urine passes over the red, raw tissues.

Diagnosis

Many times the symptoms alone will be enough to make an accurate diagnosis; however, the doctor should also do a wet smear, for in 35 percent of cases there is an associated infection.[10] Hemophilus and trich often go hand in hand with yeast infections. Moreover, the second infection may be masked by the symptoms of the yeast infection and will go undetected unless a microscopic examination is made. Many doctors ignore this vital step, but it is essential. If a woman is treated only for a yeast infection, she will not get rid of the second infection. If she comes back in a week complaining, the doctor may not bother to do another microscopic examination, and she may get treated for the yeast infection all over again. The second infection, when finally recognized, may require an antibiotic, which in turn could provoke another yeast flare-up. It's best, then, to take the medications simultaneously. Women should always insist on a wet smear before accepting treatment.

The diagnosis can also be made by growing a culture. This is done by spreading a bit of the discharge on a special substance that is favorable to the growth of *Candida*. In 4 or 5 days, patches of the fungus can be seen growing in the culture dish. Some doctors question the value of this, since *Candida albicans* often exists in the vagina and will, therefore, "grow out" on the culture even in women who are not having problems. Other doctors think that the extent of culture growth is indicative of a heavier than normal concentration of *Candidae*. The value of doing a culture is, then, debatable. Fortunately, most infections can be diagnosed accurately with a simple wet smear.

The culture that is done to diagnose gonorrhea will also tell the doctor whether or not a yeast infection is present. One danger in diagnosis is that a woman with a yeast infection will be diagnosed by way of a wet smear, and her doctor, assuming that the yeast infection alone is responsible for her discharge, will fail to investigate the possibility that the woman also needs a gonorrhea culture. This is especially likely to happen to middle-class women or other women who the doctor considers "nice girls," the theory being, of course, that "nice girls" don't get gonorrhea. Unfortunately, the gonococcus is not such a moralistic organism; it thrives as well in "nice girls" as it does in "wanton women." So if you have a discharge and have slept with someone who might possibly have given you gonorrhea (which means just about anybody), you should also have a gonorrhea culture.

Treatment

In the past, gentian violet, a rather messy, purple-staining medication, was used to treat yeast infections. The gentian violet was painted on the vagina and cervix by the doctor. This was supplemented with gentian violet tablets or creams inserted into the vagina daily by the woman over a period of days. Although gentian violet is still used by some doctors, especially for recurrent cases, new antifungal drugs, such as miconazole (Monistat) and clotrimazole (Gyne-Lotrimin), inserted into the vagina daily at bedtime for seven days, or nystatin (Mycostatin, Nystatin, etc.), used for 14 days, are now the medications officially approved by the Food and Drug Administration (FDA).[11] Higher doses of some of these drugs, given over a 3-day period, have also been approved by the FDA. The results of a number of recent studies have indicated that a single, high-dose (500-mg) treatment of clotrimazole is as effective as both a 200-mg dose daily for 3 days and a 100-mg dose daily for 4 to 6 days.[12]* In the future, then, shorter-term, heavier-dose treatments may be approved by the FDA.

The medication should be kept in the refrigerator. While a woman is using a medication, she may want to wear a sanitary napkin to protect her clothing, especially if her doctor recommends (as some do) that the medicine be used once during the day as well as at bedtime. She should continue to use the medication even if she starts menstruating during treatment and should also use all the medication prescribed, even if the symptoms subside. A second round of medication may be necessary to cure the problem. If the drug does not work, or if you have a recurrence after taking the medication, or if your doctor suspects that the gastrointestinal tract and feces are infected, s/he may also prescribe oral medication. Women who have a recurrence after using a vaginal cream or suppository should ask their doctors about using oral medication. Women troubled by frequent recurrences may need to be tested for diabetes.

An interesting development in the treatment of yeast infections is that, according to some scientific studies, certain traditional home remedies have proved to be as effective as doctor-prescribed medications. As mentioned in the introduction to this section (*see* p. 300), yeast has been shown to be effective in treating this form of vaginitis. Boric acid powder capsules have also recently proved to be effective in treating yeast infections.[13] In one of these studies some of the women were given size 0 gelatin capsules containing 600 mg of boric acid powder to insert into their vaginas. (Both the powder and the capsules can be purchased in pharmacies and some health-food stores for about 31 cents per capsule.) The other women in the study were treated with vaginal capsules of nystatin, which is more expensive and messier to use. The women using the boric acid had a 92 percent cure rate after 7 to 10 days as compared with a 64 percent cure rate for the women using nystatin.

Women who wish to use boric acid powder capsules should insert the size 0 gelatin capsules into their vaginas once a day for a week and then twice a week for 3 more weeks. Women troubled by recurrent yeast infections may want to use the capsules once a week when they are ovulating, using antibiotics, or showing early signs of a recurrence. However, women who are trying not only to treat but also to diagnose their own possible yeast infections should read the material on p. 303 carefully. Unless you can be quite sure that you have only a yeast infection and not a mixed infection (*see* p. 303), or possibly gonorrhea as well, you should not try these home remedies until you have had the diagnosis of yeast infection confirmed by a doctor.

Women with yeast infections should not accept prescriptions for sulfa creams or sulfa vaginal suppositories, as these are not as effective as the treatments described above (*see* p. 304).

Many women feel uncomfortable having intercourse during treatment, and

*Pregnant women should use the 4 to 6 day treatment regime.

some doctors tell patients to refrain from intercourse during this time because they believe it further irritates the area. Other doctors, especially in cases where the symptoms are mild, simply suggest that the man use a condom to prevent the penis from becoming irritated or likewise infected. Men, however, are much less likely to have problems with fungus infections since their genitals don't provide the same kind of warm, wet environment conducive to growth of the fungus that the vagina does. Still, in cases where a woman has a stubborn case that is not responding to treatment, the doctor may suspect that the man is harboring the *Candidae* and is constantly reinfecting her, and s/he will want to check him as well.

Treating pregnant women is sometimes difficult because their alkaline vaginal environment is conducive to fungus growth. Successful treatment may have to wait until after delivery. Some doctors think it's especially important to treat pregnant women who are about to deliver, even if they have little or nothing in the way of symptoms, so that the baby doesn't get the fungus infection (thrush) in his or her mouth and throat during delivery. Other doctors point out that thrush is fairly uncommon and easily cured, so they don't treat asymptomatic pregnant women even if they find a lot of *Candidae*. Still others treat such a woman because they think she will probably become symptomatic.

Sometimes it is difficult to treat women who are using birth control pills. Use of the Pill may have to be discontinued while they are being treated.

Some doctors prescribe prophylactic (preventive) medication. For instance, women who have a history of yeast infections might be given yeast medication to take along with an antibiotic. This is discussed more fully in the introduction to this section (*see* p.p. 299–300). For women in whom recurrences are serious problems, some doctors prescribe medication in advance. Then, at the first sign of a symptom, the woman can begin the course of medication prescribed by the doctor. Or, she could use the yeast or boric acid powder treatments described above. Thus she is able to catch the infection in its earliest stages, when it is easiest to cure.

HEMOPHILUS

AKA: Hemophilus vaginitis, nonspecific vaginitis, *H. vaginalis, Corynebacterium vaginalis, Gardnerella vaginalis, Gardnerella*

Hemophilus is a common form of vaginal infection. In the past, hemophilus infections were called nonspecific vaginitis, but it is now known that many of these nonspecific cases are caused by *Hemophilus* bacteria. Indeed, some authorities argue that *all* cases of nonspecific vaginitis, at least during the reproductive years, are actually hemophilus infections. Many doctors have recently begun to refer to hemophilus as *Gardnerella*. Others use the terms *Corynebacterium vaginalis* or *H. vaginalis*.

317

Incidence

The incidence is hard to determine, since some women may not have symptoms; however, it is generally agreed that hemophili are a common cause of vaginitis. Hemophilus infections don't usually occur before puberty or after menopause, for without estrogen stimulation of the vaginal tissues, the vaginal environment is not rich enough to support the growth of these organisms.

Cause and Transmission

The infection is caused by the organism *Hemophilus vaginalis,* which likes moist places and is killed by drying. The hemophilus don't survive well in the normal vaginal environment. In order for them to thrive the normal acid/ alkaline balance of the vagina must be disturbed. This is discussed more fully in the introduction to this section (*see* p. 299). Although it is possible to acquire the infection from douche nozzles, toilet seats, washcloths and other, similar sources, the most common method of acquiring and transmitting the disease is through sexual intercourse.

Symptoms

As many as 75 percent of women are without symptoms in the early stages of the disease. The most common symptom is an increase in vaginal discharge. Typically, the discharge looks like a thin flour paste, has a grayish hue, and tends to smell quite bad. There may be burning and itching of the external genitals, but this is less likely to happen with hemophilus than with TV or yeast infections.

Hemophilus may occur with other forms of vaginitis, so symptoms of these diseases may also be present. For instance, about 25 percent of women with trich will also have hemophilus.[14]

Diagnosis

The diagnosis of hemophilus can be made with a wet smear or a culture. Because the wet smear is cheaper and quicker, it is routinely used; however, the culture may be used in a questionable or stubborn case. As explained in the introduction to this section, (*see* p. 303), specific diagnosis is important, particularly in mixed infections. For instance, if a woman also has a yeast infection and is treated only for the yeast, her hemophilus will not be cured. The persistence of the smelly discharge may be interpreted as a persistence of the yeast infection. Another round of yeast medication may then be given, again to no avail. Specific diagnosis, by way of a wet smear, is therefore essential.

Treatment

Hemophilus responds well to such oral antibiotics as ampicillin and tetracycline.* Because the use of antibiotics causes yeast infections in some women, susceptible women should take the precautions described in the introduction to this section.

Such antibiotics are preferable to vaginal sulfa medications which, although widely prescribed, have *not* been shown effective (*see* p. 304). Metronidazole (*see* pp. 309–12) has also recently been used to treat hemophilus, and the drug is now approved for this use by the Food and Drug Administration.

Sexual intercourse is either prohibited or a condom must be used. This prevents further irritation of the vagina and the possibility of passing the infection back and forth.

NONSPECIFIC VAGINITIS

AKA: *see* Hemophilus above

There is some controversy about the use of the term "nonspecific vaginitis." Some doctors think that all nonspecific vaginitis that occurs during the reproductive years is caused by hemophilus and that the term should be reserved for cases of vaginitis occurring in prepubescent girls and postmenopausal women. Others feel that other organisms besides *Hemophilus* may be responsible for nonspecific vaginitis. At any rate, the symptoms are generally the same as those of any form of vaginitis: increase in vaginal discharge, soreness, itching and burning. The diagnostic procedure is also the same: a wet smear or, in confusing or stubborn cases, a culture to rule out one of the specific forms of vaginitis like trich, yeast infection or hemophilus. Treatment is described under Hemophilus above.

POSTMENOPAUSAL VAGINITIS

AKA: senile atrophy of the vagina, atrophic vaginitis
Associated Terms: adhesive vaginitis

After menopause, when the tissues of the vagina are no longer stimulated by estrogen from the ovaries, the walls of the vagina become smooth, dry, shiny

*See pp. 795–96.

and less elastic. The vaginal secretions are scant, so there is little lubrication. The entire vaginal canal shrinks. In some women the walls of the vagina may stick to each other, a condition known as adhesive vaginitis. Tiny sores may appear on the vaginal walls, causing a slightly blood-tinged discharge. There may be a burning or itching feeling or a general soreness in the vagina, and intercourse may be painful. The dried-out skin is prone to injury and minute cracks, which may become secondarily infected and cause nonspecific vaginitis. Postmenopausal vaginitis is often associated with postmenopausal vulvitis.

Treatment

If there is a secondary infection, this is cleared up with antibiotics. Estrogen, given either by mouth or as a locally applied cream, will usually return the vagina to its premenopausal state and eliminate symptoms; however, estrogen replacement therapy (*see* p. 797) has been implicated in the development of cancer, so it must be used with caution. Sometimes less drastic treatments, such as vinegar douches and a well-balanced diet—especially one rich in vitamin A and vitamin B complexes—may help. Regular sexual activity stimulates blood flow to the area, helps keep these tissues supple, and helps to prevent postmenopausal vaginitis. If adhesions form, they can usually be broken up easily by carefully dilating the vaginal canal. This is done by gently probing the vaginal canal with a finger or two and is best done by the woman herself, although the doctor can also do it.

VAGINAL STENOSIS

AKA: narrowing of the vaginal canal

The term "stenosis" means "a narrowing" or "stricture." In women with vaginal stenosis the vaginal canal becomes smaller and narrower.

Causes

Sometimes vaginal stenosis is a natural part of the aging process. After menopause, estrogen levels are diminished. Without estrogen stimulation the vaginal canal and opening become smaller. The vagina loses its elasticity as the blood supply to these tissues is diminished, and the elastic tissue is replaced by fibrous tissue. The skin becomes thinner and drier. Vaginal stenosis also occurs in younger women whose ovaries have been surgically removed or irradiated, or in women who, for some other reason, have a premature menopause.

Radiation treatment for cancer can also cause vaginal stenosis, partly because the ovaries are often sterilized, which brings on premature menopause, and partly because there is damage and scarring from the radiation itself. Before abortion was legalized it was not uncommon to find cases of vaginal stenosis in women who had put caustic substances, such as lye, into their vaginas in an attempt to abort themselves. Fortunately, thanks to liberalized abortion laws, this type of vaginal stenosis is a medical rarity today. Sometimes stenosis occurs after vaginal surgery; for example, a radical hysterectomy, in which the upper third of the vagina is removed along with the uterus, shortens the vagina and may leave scar tissue that further narrows the vaginal cavity. Lacerations of the vagina, that is, injuries received as a result of rape or accidents, can also cause scar tissue and vaginal stenosis.

Symptoms

Vaginal stenosis can cause pain or difficulty with intercourse. In women who have had high doses of radiation therapy, the vagina may become so stenotic that intercourse is extremely painful or downright impossible. The vagina is apt to be rather dry, a common problem for postmenopausal women, which can also cause painful intercourse. Postmenopausal women with bothersome stenosis may also have postmenopausal vaginitis. If minute cracks occur in the drier vaginal tissue, such women may also be susceptible to other forms of vaginitis, particularly nonspecific vaginitis.

Diagnosis

The diagnosis of vaginal stenosis is made on the basis of the symptoms and a physical examination and in light of a history that includes menopause (natural, surgical or radiation-induced), radiation treatment, vaginal surgery, rape or injury.

Treatment

The type of treatment for vaginal stenosis depends on the cause and the severity of the condition. In mild cases the use of a vaginal lubricant like K-Y Lubricating Jelly, which is available without a prescription from pharmacies (and is also greaseless, water soluble and nonstaining), will relieve the difficulties or discomfort associated with intercourse.

321

Extreme cases of postmenopausal stenosis can be effectively treated by giving estrogen replacement therapy, either orally or by locally applied creams. The estrogen will thicken the vaginal tissues and restore tissue elasticity; however, estrogen has been associated with an increased risk of certain types of cancer (*see* p. 448) and cannot be used by some women. We suggest that a woman try some of the alternative treatments for menopausal therapy (*see* p. 649) before resorting to estrogen.

Unfortunately, there is little that can be done for women who have stenosis resulting from radiation therapy. For those women who have had vaginal surgery or injury, it is often possible to create an adequate vagina using plastic surgery techniques, but after radiation therapy, the tissues are usually too thin and heal too poorly to allow for this.

LACERATIONS OF THE VAGINA, VULVA OR PERINEUM

AKA: tears or stretching of the vagina, vulva or perineum

Associated Terms: relaxation of the vaginal outlet

Lacerations or tears of the vagina, vulva or perineum (the area between the vagina and anus) may be the result of surgery, accidental injuries, rape or insertion of an object into the vaginal canal with or without consent. For instance, a hymen may be torn as the result of rape, and the tear may extend into the vaginal canal or perineum. A woman may also fall on a sharp object that projects into the vaginal canal. More often such lacerations result from difficult childbirth or abortion. Women who have exceptionally large infants, rigid or unyielding tissues, small or unprepared vaginal canals, forceful spontaneous deliveries or complicated labors that necessitate instruments are more likely to have lacerations.

Symptoms and Treatment

Bleeding may be profuse and, in rare instances, fatal, but this is not usually the case. Such occurrences may result in a hematoma or a localized collection of blood, but generally this is reabsorbed by the body and seldom becomes infected or forms abscesses. Treatment usually consists of the application of hot packs and sitz baths.

For the most part, lacerations of the perineum or vaginal wall heal quickly and do not require suturing; however, excessive bleeding must be controlled, and larger tears, especially those acquired in childbirth or abortion, should be repaired.

Sometimes the tear involves the underlying muscle structure; at other times the lacerations may occur under the surface of the skin, in which case stretching is probably a better word to describe the condition.

Lacerations are generally not serious in and of themselves; however, over time they may contribute to muscle weakness and thereby contribute to relaxation of the vaginal outlet. The vaginal opening has been compared to the mouth, one being a horizontal opening and the other, a vertical opening. Both have a fixed upper portion and a movable lower portion. If the muscles that control the movable portion are injured or weaken with age, the opening no longer closes snugly. Relaxation of the vaginal outlet is often associated with other forms of genital relaxation, such as uterine prolapse, cystocele and rectocele.

If the tears are extensive, they may extend all the way from the vagina to the anus, exposing the mucous lining of the rectum. If the muscles are torn or stretched to an extreme, it might become impossible for such a woman to control her bowel movements. In such cases, surgical repair may be required.

CYSTOCELE AND URETHROCELE

AKA: fallen, or prolapsed, bladder, or vesicocele; fallen, or prolapsed, urethra

Associated Terms: stress incontinence

A cystocele (Illustration 42) is a condition in which the bladder drops down from its normal position and bulges into the vagina. A urethrocele is similar, only it is the urethra, the tube that connects the bladder to the urinary opening, that is involved. These conditions are usually associated with a general relaxation of the muscles and tissues that support the pelvic organs. They may result from a congenital defect in the supportive tissue and muscle or from an injury, usually one connected with childbirth. Over time what started as a weakness can become an actual defect. The muscle and tissue can become so stretched and thin that the fibers separate and a hole is created. The process is somewhat akin to wearing a hole through the heel of a sock. The bladder or urethra is no longer held firmly in its proper place, sags down next to the vagina and eventually bulges into the vaginal wall. These conditions occur most frequently in older women or in women who have had many children, which lends support to the theory that these conditions are caused by tears and injuries during childbirth. At times they occur in women who have never had children, so it is thought that an inherited muscle weakness or some other type of injury may also be involved.

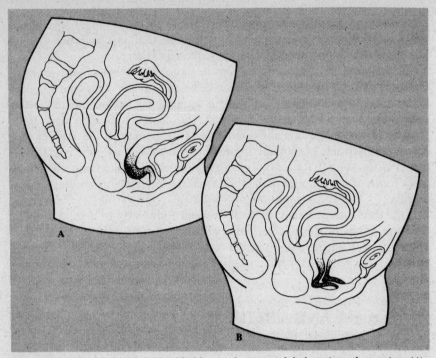

Illustration 42   *Cystocele: The bladder prolapses and bulges into the vagina (A). Urethrocele: The urethra, the tube that conducts urine, prolapses and bulges into the vagina (B).*

Symptoms

A woman with cystocele or urethrocele may not have any symptoms; however, she may complain of a sense of pelvic fullness or a discomfort when bearing down. It may feel as if her pelvic organs are dropping out. She may sense or feel a bulge in the wall of the vagina that is nearest to the bladder and urethra. She may actually see the bulge at the vaginal opening.

The symptoms are often aggravated by long hours of standing. If the cystocele or urethrocele is small, there is rarely more than minor discomfort, but if the descent of the bladder or urethra is extreme, it may be uncomfortable to sit down and difficult to walk. If the cystocele or urethrocele is large, it may even protrude through the vaginal opening. In rare instances the tissue that covers the bladder or urethra may be stretched so thin that its exposure to the vaginal secretions will result in an ulcer, an irritated sore that produces a discharge or bleeding, but bleeding is only rarely a symptom.

If the back part of the bladder drops below the neck of the bladder, there may be mechanical difficulties in completely emptying the bladder. Urinary frequency owing to the diminished capacity of the bladder may occur. The woman may feel she has to urinate even though she has just done so. The urine that stays in the bladder quickly stagnates and provides an excellent environment for bacteria. Thus urinary infections with symptoms like painful and frequent urination may develop.

With the urethrocele, since the position of the bladder in relation to the bladder neck is altered, the muscle at the base of the bladder that controls the flow of urine may be disturbed. It may be difficult to control the urine, and sudden movements like coughs and sneezes may result in leaks of urine, a situation referred to as stress incontinence.

Diagnosis

In the majority of cases these conditions are not difficult to diagnose. The doctor can feel or even see a round, soft elastic bulge if the woman coughs or strains, especially if she is standing up. The bulge can easily be pushed back into its proper place. Occasionally, the cystocele may be so small as to be hidden, especially if the woman is lying down. If so, the doctor may ask her to strain downward as s/he presses against the area or to stand up for the exam. On rare occasions, the cystocele will be evident only when the woman is relaxed under anesthesia. Diagnosis is usually an easy matter, for there are only a few rare vaginal cysts whose presence could be mistaken for a cystocele.

Treatment

If a cystocele or urethrocele is small, or even only moderately large, and a woman has little in the way of symptoms and no repeated bouts with cystitis or urinary infections, there is no rush for treatment. This is especially true if a woman is young and plans to have more children, because the surgical repair job is often destroyed by childbirth and subsequent repair jobs might not be as successful. But if a woman has distressing symptoms and recurring urinary tract infections, or if the cystocele or urethrocele is enlarging, the doctor will repair the defect surgically, even if it is a small one. A larger one, even if it isn't producing symptoms, will require treatment, for chances are that it will eventually cause symptoms. Repairing the defect before it gets larger and the muscles weaker will result in better long-term results.

Sometimes surgery can be avoided. A series of exercises that involve alternately tightening and relaxing the muscles involved may be helpful in less severe cases. In order to know which muscles need exercise a woman should practice stopping the flow of urine midstream. These are the same muscles that help support the pelvic organs. The exercise consists of tightening these muscles and holding for 3 seconds. (Don't push down as if making a bowel movement; rather, tighten and pull the genitals together.) This exercise should be done about 200 times over the course of the day (work up to this point gradually). It takes a couple of months to get results, but doing these exercises can help avoid discomfort and the need for surgery in future years.

Some doctors prescribe estrogen replacement therapy (ERT), which will thicken the lining of the vagina and the urinary tract. ERT will not cure the problem, but it may alleviate symptoms. ERT, however, has been implicated in cancer and must be used with caution.

The surgical repair of a cystocele or urethrocele is called vaginal repair, plastic surgery or cystocele repair. It is done through a vaginal incision. The bladder is pushed back into its normal position and sewn in place. The back wall of the vagina may also be repaired if the woman has a rectocele or if the tissue is so stretched and torn that a rectocele is likely to occur in the future.

The results of vaginal repair are reasonably good; however, the doctor cannot promise that it will relieve stress incontinence, which continues to be a problem for about 20 percent of the women who have the operation. If the stress incontinence is not cured and is creating serious problems, another operation, done through an abdominal incision, in which the surgeon changes the angle of the bladder opening, may be undertaken. This procedure involves more risks and complications and is successful in about 50 percent of the cases.

RECTOCELE AND ENTEROCELE

AKA: prolapse of the rectum, prolapse of the small intestines

A rectocele (Illustration 43) is a condition in which part of the rectum bulges into the back wall of the vagina. An enterocele is a condition that involves a weakness higher up in the vagina in which part of the small intestine may bulge into the back wall of the vagina. Because the rectum is located below the small intestine, the rectocele is usually felt in the lower portion of the vaginal wall.

Causes and Incidence

Both conditions result from a weakness in the tissues that support the organs and hold them in place. As the result of pregnancy and childbirth—especially prolonged and complicated labors and deliveries—aging or, sometimes, a congenital or inherent weakness in the supportive tissues, the organs involved begin to sag. They slip down and press against the rear wall of the va-

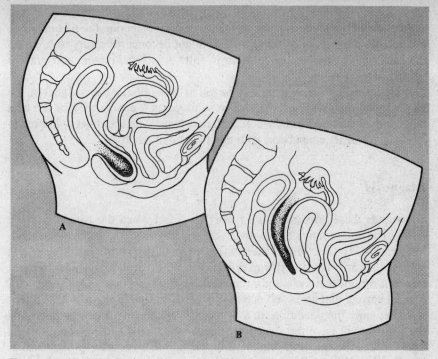

Ilustration 43 *Rectocele: The rectum prolapses and bulges into the back wall of the vagina (A). Enterocele: Part of the small intestine prolapses and bulges into the vagina (B).*

gina. Slowly, over time, a defect or even a hole is opened in the vaginal wall, and a section of the rectum or small intestines may bulge into the vaginal vault. These conditions are usually associated with a general relaxation of the pelvic organs and may occur together. It is rare to find only a rectocele; usually this condition is associated with a cystocele; lacerations of the vagina, vulva or perineum; some degree of uterine prolapse or relaxation of the vaginal opening.

It is unusual to find either of these conditions in women who have never had children. When it does occur in such women it results from a congenital defect in the vaginal wall or in the supporting tissues. It most often affects older, postmenopausal women.

Symptoms

The rectocele causes little discomfort. Women with this condition may, however, complain of some pain or discomfort when bearing down or be aware of a bulge in the vagina. If the rectocele is large, it may protrude through the

327

vaginal opening. There may be difficulty in fully emptying the rectum when moving the bowels. In extreme cases it might become necessary to press on the back wall of the vagina in order to fully empty the rectum and prevent constipation.

With the enterocele, a bulge may be felt in the vagina, but it is higher on the vaginal wall than with a rectocele. In some cases it can be seen or felt as a bulge immediately behind the cervix. It may expand and contract with breathing because of its connection with the abdominal cavity.

Diagnosis

Sometimes these conditions are harder to detect when the patient is lying down. The doctor may need to do the examination with the patient in a standing position. The doctor will insert a finger into the rectum and into the vagina and ask the patient to bear down. Sometimes it is difficult to tell the difference between a high rectocele and an enterocele. It is important that the doctor make a correct diagnosis and determine whether a bulge is a rectocele or enterocele, since the operation for a rectocele will not correct an enterocele and the woman will have the same bulge after treatment. A doctor may shine a light into the rectum. If the bulge inside the vagina is not thereby illuminated, the doctor will suspect an enterocele.

Treatment

Because a small rectocele causes little trouble, it doesn't usually require treatment and is ignored unless surgery is being done to correct some related condition, like prolapse of the uterus, a cystocele or urethrocele or a bothersome enterocele. If an abdominal hysterectomy is being done for some reason, it is a good idea to correct large rectoceles at the same time, even if they aren't causing problems, for many times women who were previously unaware of the rectocele will start to have symptoms once the uterus has been removed. The larger rectoceles, especially those that cause problems with elimination, should be repaired surgically.

The enterocele is somewhat more serious. The loop of intestine may swell and get caught in the bulge that protrudes into the vagina. If the blood supply of the intestinal loop is cut off, the hernia becomes strangulated, which may result in gangrene that could in turn lead to death. Prompt surgical attention and a proper repair job are necessary with all enteroceles.

VAGINISMUS

AKA: spasms of the vaginal muscles

Vaginismus is a condition characterized by involuntary contraction of the vaginal muscles. Most doctors believe the problem is a psychological one, but some cases may result from congenital abnormalities of the vagina, imperforate hymen, vaginal stenosis or a particularly rigid and unyielding hymen. If one of these conditions is present, intercourse or the introduction of a speculum, a finger or, for that matter, anything into the vaginal cavity will cause such pain that the muscles contract sharply. The muscles may spasm so tightly that intercourse is painful or downright impossible.

Diagnosis and Treatment

Diagnosis involves eliminating any of the physiologic conditions that can cause the problem. If the problem seems to be psychological in origin, there may be a history of rape, repression or a lack of education about sexual matters that has led to fear of intercourse. Psychological counseling may be in order, as well as basic sexual education. The woman is taught to explore her own genitals, gradually relaxing her vagina by inserting a finger or two. The woman's sexual partner may need education about sexual foreplay and the need for vaginal lubrication before insertion of the penis.

FISTULAS

AKA: genital fistula

Types: urinary fistula, bladder fistula, vesicovaginal fistula or vesicouterine fistula
urethra fistula or urethrovaginal fistula
ureter fistula or ureterovaginal fistula
rectal fistula, vaginal-fecal fistula or bowel fistula

A genital fistula is an abnormal passageway or connection between the genital organs and the urinary tract or intestinal tract. The vagina or, in some cases, the uterus may be involved. There are a number of types of fistulas, depending on where the abnormal connection is located. A fistula between the bladder and vagina is a vesicovaginal fistula; between the uterus and bladder, a vesicouterine fistula; between the urethra (the tube that conducts urine from the bladder to the outside of the body) and the vagina, a urethrovaginal fistula; between a ureter (one of the tubes that conducts fluid from the kidneys to the bladder) and the vagina, a ureterovaginal fistula. When the intestinal tract and bowels are involved, the connection is called a rectal, bowel or vaginal-fecal fistula.

329

Cause

In the past, most fistulas were the result of prolonged and difficult childbirth or the improper use of forceps. As obstetrical care has improved, the incidence of childbirth-related fistulas has declined. However, increases in major surgery, more complex and risky procedures and the use of radiation for dealing with gynecological problems has led to a considerable increase in the incidence of surgically or radiation-induced genital fistulas. Fistulas may also result from the destruction of tissues by malignant tumors or ulcers (open sores) caused by foreign bodies, especially vaginal pessaries used to treat cystoceles and uterine prolapse. When the vagina and rectum are involved in the fistula, granuloma inguinale may be the cause.

Symptoms

The most common symptom of urinary fistulas, which involve the vagina and the organs of the urinary system, is leakage of urine from the vagina. With small fistulas this may be only a slight dribble and may be more noticeable when the body is in certain positions. In other cases the flow of urine may be constant and profuse. In fact, in extreme cases, all urine leaves the body through the vagina and none through the urethral meatus, the normal opening to the urinary tract. The vagina, vulva and surrounding areas may become irritated and there is often an unpleasant ammonialike odor. Unless careful hygiene measures are taken, the fistula may become encrusted with mineral deposits, adding to the irritation. Fistulas that involve the rectum or bowels and vaginal canal may be so slight that only a small amount of fecal matter or gas gets into the vagina, and this may be a problem only when the stools are especially soft. If, however, such a fistula is large, there is bound to be considerable irritation as well as an offensive odor, not to mention possible infection.

Diagnosis

The diagnosis of a urinary fistula is usually fairly simple, although if it has occurred as the result of an operation, the usual postoperative vaginal discharge may confuse the issue. Determining the nature and location of a fistula is not always easy, however. Sometimes after an operation or childbirth the muscle that controls the flow of urine becomes too weak and urine is leaked. At first glance this can be mistaken for a fistula. In most cases, however, the doctor can see a fistula on speculum exam or feel it during a bimanual pelvic exam. Small, highly placed fistulas may require special diagnostic techniques involving colored water or air placed into the bladder. This will help the doctor decide whether the bladder, or the tube that leads from the bladder to the opening, is involved.

Treatment

Small urinary fistulas, unless they are the result of malignant disease, may, on rare occasions, close up by themselves. Urinary antiseptics and the temporary use of a tube called a catheter to drain the urine from the body will sometimes help this natural healing process, but most of the time surgical repair is necessary. Unfortunately, it is best to wait 4 to 6 months after the fistula has occurred, if it was surgically induced, to give the recently operated-on tissues a chance to get back to normal. Because this delay can be disturbing to a woman with a fistula, some doctors use cortisone to cut down on the waiting period. Antibiotics and local soothing treatments may also be given.

If there is a great deal of damage to the urinary tract, the doctor may have to perform a nephrostomy, an operation whereby a direct opening from the kidney to the outside of the body, bypassing the rest of the urinary system, is created. Although most of the time if this is done it is as a temporary solution to allow tissue to heal before attempting surgical repair, it is also done when surgical repair of the fistula is unsuccessful or impossible.

Like the urinary fistula, a fistula involving the bowels or rectum and vagina can usually be repaired surgically; but in some cases, especially in ones caused by malignant disease or radiation, this is not possible. A colostomy, an operation that results in the contents of the bowels being emptied directly into a bag attached to the outside of the body, may then be necessary. Sometimes the colostomy is done as a temporary measure to allow the irritated tissues to heal before attempting surgery. Certain special X-ray techniques, such as a barium enema, may be used to pinpoint the location of a vaginal-fecal fistula. If the fistula is a "high" one involving the intestines, it must be treated promptly, without the usual waiting period, because the contents of the intestines could be pouring into the vagina.

CONGENITAL ABNORMALITIES OF THE VAGINA

Types: absence, or atresia, of the vagina
    transverse vaginal septum
    double, or separate, vagina, or vaginal partitioning
    vaginal adenosis
    vaginal ridges

The middle and upper vagina are formed from two tubelike organs in the developing embryo called müllerian ducts. The lower portion of the vagina develops from the same embryonic tissue as the bladder. Sometimes there are irregularities in the normal process whereby these embryonic tissues grow and fuse together to become properly functioning organs. Some of these irregularities in development of the vagina are related to more serious situations, where sexual characteristics of both sexes appear in the same individual. These are discussed under the heading Congenital Abnormalities of the Ovary.

Certain vaginal abnormalities may occur in women whose mothers took hormones during pregnancy. These hormones may produce such congenital abnormalities as vaginal adenosis, a condition in which gland cells are present in the vagina and raised ridges of tissue appear on the vaginal wall. These abnormalities are discussed more fully under the headings Vaginal Adenosis and DES.

Symptoms and Diagnosis

Atresia, the most extreme form of congenital vaginal abnormality, is the partial or total absence of the vagina. The external genital organs, the vulvar lips, clitoris and so forth, may be normal in appearance. Sometimes the lower part of the vaginal canal is present but usually only as a shallow depression. In typical cases of atresia the uterus, the middle and upper portions of the vagina and sometimes the fallopian tubes are missing. The ovaries are often normal. There may be some rudimentary development of the uterus, and in some very rare cases the uterus is actually present and functioning, which means its lining swells and is shed each month, which is a source of trouble, because there is no opening through which the menstrual discharge can escape.

Another type of abnormality of the vagina is called a transverse vaginal septum. In this condition there is a septum, or a wall of tissue, that runs crosswise through the vagina, usually at the junction of the middle and upper third of the vagina, although it can occur at other points. The transverse vaginal septum may be confused with partial absence of the vagina, because the doctor can easily mistake the wall of tissue for the roof of a partial vagina. Sometimes this wall of tissue will have openings in it through which the menstrual blood and vaginal and cervical discharges can pass; at other times it will be solid, with no openings through which these secretions can pass.

There is also the double, or septate, vagina, which usually occurs with a double uterus. A double vagina may also occur with normal uterus and tubes. There may also be a double vagina, double cervix and single uterus. The septum that divides the double vagina is longitudinal (going up and down) as opposed to transverse (going across). It may be partial or it may extend all the way to the vaginal opening. In some cases the wall of tissue may be off-center and fused to one of the vaginal walls, so that one side of the divided vagina is closed off.

Congenital absence, transverse septums and double vaginas are sometimes recognized in infancy, but usually it is not until a girl menstruates or attempts intercourse that these problems become apparent. Sometimes these abnormalities become apparent in strange ways. A young woman might come to the doctor wondering why tampons don't control her menstrual flow and she has to wear sanitary napkins. On investigation the doctor may find that she has a double vagina and therefore the tampon, which has, of course, been inserted into only one vagina, hasn't absorbed all the menstrual flow.

If there is a transverse vaginal septum without any openings, the menstrual blood will continue to collect. A young girl may seek medical attention because she has never menstruated. She may be having periodic menstrual symptoms, cramps, headaches and so forth but no blood, and this may lead her to seek medical help. Or, the buildup of menstrual blood may lead to a swelling and pain in the abdomen. Again, this may bring her to a doctor.

A double, or septate, vagina may cause pain on intercourse, because the penis hits the wall of tissue that separates the double vagina. In the case of a transverse septum the same kind of pain on intercourse can occur. Or, if a woman has a transverse septum or partial atresia with some sort of lower vaginal opening, she may come to the doctor complaining of pain and difficulty on intercourse, because the penis cannot penetrate her vagina. Sometimes the double vagina will be constructed in such a way that the woman can have intercourse. Then the abnormality may not be discovered unless she has a child, when it will usually become apparent during labor and delivery.

If the double vagina is off-center and fused so that one portion of it is closed off, vaginal secretions and menstrual blood may collect on the closed-off side, resulting in swelling and pain and possibly an infection owing to the retained menstrual blood. For a description of the problems related to the retention of menstrual blood, see the information on imperforate hymen under the heading Congenital Abnormalities of the Vulva.

Treatment

Treatment of a double vagina or transverse vaginal septum that is causing symptoms or problems in childbirth is rather simple but bloody, consisting of surgical removal of the barrier. If menstrual blood has been retained, the doctor will usually prescribe an antibiotic to prevent infection after the operation. It is important to drain all the old retained blood, because it is a perfect breeding ground for germs. In some rare cases the old blood will have backed up into the uterus and spilled out the tubes into the pelvic cavity, causing such pain and irritation that abdominal surgery is necessary to drain off all the old blood. There may be associated endometriosis, a condition in which the tissue that lines the uterus is found in abnormal locations.

If a child is discovered to have an absent or partially absent vagina, this is usually not treated right away. If the child has normal ovaries and uterus, at puberty a vagina can be created by plastic surgery so that the menstrual blood will be able to escape. If the uterus is absent, the plastic surgery may be delayed until the woman wants to have it done for purposes of intercourse. Because there's no need to worry about a buildup of menstrual discharge and because the surgically created vagina must be kept open by frequent intercourse or manual dilation, it's best to wait until a woman does intend to have intercourse.

BENIGN TUMORS OF THE VAGINA

Types: inclusion cysts
Gartner's duct cysts
endometrial cysts
condyloma acuminatum, genital warts or venereal warts
fibroids

Associated Terms: vaginal polyps

There are a number of benign tumors that can affect the vagina. In medicalese the term "tumor," in its broadest sense, means "swelling." "Benign," of course, means "noncancerous."

Benign tumors of the vagina fall into one of two categories: cystic or solid. The most common cystic tumors are inclusion and Gartner's cysts. Endometriosis, a condition that can create blood-filled cysts, may also affect the vagina. Similarly, condyloma acuminatum, fibroids and vaginal adenosis may form tumors or swellings in the vagina. Some of these tumors may take the form of polyps—teardrop-shaped growths on a stem. The polyps may also be formed as the result of the body's attempts to heal itself (see the section on Cervical Polyps for details). Generally, the benign tumors that affect the vagina can be treated by simple surgical removal. Most of these benign vaginal tumors are discussed in more detail under other headings, so only the most common benign vaginal cysts will be discussed here.

Inclusion Cysts

Inclusion cysts are found at the lower end of the vagina. They are caused by the inclusion of little tags of skin beneath the surface of the skin, usually as the result of imperfect healing of surgical scars or of tears or lacerations acquired during childbirth or through injury. Occasionally, such cysts may be found at the top of the vagina near a hysterectomy scar. They are usually small, only a few centimeters in size, and the contents are usually rather cheeselike. If they are causing problems, they may be removed surgically, but if they are small and are not bothersome, no treatment is necessary.

Gartner's Cysts

Gartner's cysts arise from the remnants of an embryonic organ called Gartner's duct and are the most common form of vaginal tumor. They may either be small or become so large as to bulge from the vaginal outlet. Treatment is the same as for inclusion cysts.

VAGINAL ADENOSIS

Associated Terms: cockscomb, pseudopolypoid, rim, collar or hooded cervix

Vaginal adenosis is a condition in which the glandular tissue that normally lines the inside of the cervical canal is found in the vaginal cavity—on the vaginal walls and vaginal portion of the cervix. In a sense it is an advanced degree of cervical eversion, a condition in which this glandular tissue is found on the vaginal portion of the cervix but not on the vaginal walls. Having vaginal adenosis would be like having the tissue that lines the inside of the mouth growing out onto the lips and face. Although the tissue might be healthy, it would be abnormally placed.

Cause

Most cases of vaginal adenosis are associated with certain hormones taken during pregnancy by the mothers of the girls and women who have this condition. Beginning in 1940 the synthetic hormone DES and DES-type drugs were given to millions of pregnant women in the United States to help prevent miscarriage, premature birth and other pregnancy problems. It has since been shown that these drugs were of no use in preventing miscarriage or premature deliveries.[15] By 1971 the tragic consequences of this widespread, ill-advised use of hormones became apparent, when a small number of the daughters of these women developed a rare form of vaginal cancer, clear cell adenocarcinoma.[16] Further investigation indicated that other, less serious cervical, vaginal and uterine abnormalities were also more common among DES daughters; that DES sons may also have problems[17] and that the mothers themselves may be at increased risk for certain types of cancer.[18] The DES

335

problem is discussed in greater detail under the heading DES; here we are concerned with only one type of DES-related abnormality: vaginal adenosis.

Sometime during the first 20 weeks of pregnancy the female fetal tissue undergoes changes that are critical to the subsequent development of the upper vagina, cervix, fallopian tubes and uterus. If all goes well, the mature woman will have a vagina and outer cervix that are covered by pink tissue known as squamous cell tissue. The inner cervical canal will be composed of red columnar tissue that contains mucus-producing glands. The point where these two tissues meet, known as the transformation zone, or the squamocolumnar junction, will lie in the area of the cervical os, the opening to the cervical canal. In women who have vaginal adenosis this orderly arrangement of tissue types is disturbed. The squamocolumnar junction is not located at the cervical os. Thus the columnar-type tissue, with its gland cells, extends out over the vaginal portion of the cervix (as in a cervical eversion) and, in many cases, well into the vagina, where it does not belong. In this manner, then, glandular tissue appears in the vagina in women with vaginal adenosis. The condition becomes obvious in the years before and during puberty, when the abnormal tissue is stimulated to new growth by the rising levels of estrogen.

It now appears that the dosage of the hormone given to the person's mother need not have been prolonged or excessive for the abnormality to occur. Indeed, abnormalities have appeared with dosages as low as 1.5 mg. In one known instance the drug was given for only a few days.[19]

Incidence

Vaginal adenosis is not a new disease. Reports of it have appeared in the medical literature since the late 1800s. It can occur even when there is no history of the mother's having taken a DES-type drug, but it is rather uncommon.

Studies of the daughters of DES mothers show that anywhere from 30 percent to 90 percent of them will have adenosis.[20] The wide variance in these percentages may be at least partially accounted for by the fact that the mothers took the drug at different times in their pregnancies. One study showed incidence rates for adenosis of 73 percent in daughters who had been exposed during the first 8 weeks of pregnancy and 7 percent in those who had been exposed later than 17 weeks.[21] Adenosis seems to result only when the hormone is administered before the 4th month of pregnancy.

Symptoms

Vaginal adenosis usually does not produce any obvious symptoms. Some women, however, do have an increase in vaginal discharge or irregular bleed-

336

ing and some report having pain on intercourse. The vaginal discharge may be scant or quite profuse. Adenosis tends to occur in young girls in whom bleeding patterns are often quite irregular. Thus in girls of this age-group, the irregular bleeding caused by adenosis may be mistaken for this more usual sort of menstrual irregularity.

The vaginal walls or cervix may have red patches that may feel sandy or rough and may bleed easily when touched. There may be ridges of tissue across the vagina or a wall of tissue that partially or totally divides the vagina, a condition known as a septate vagina. Cysts formed in the improperly located glands may give a nodular or lumpy feeling to the vaginal walls.

The cervix also may appear abnormal. Cervical erosions or eversions may be present. There may be transverse ridges of tissue running across the cervix. The cervix often has an unusual appearance, for which a wide variety of terms, including ''hooded,'' ''cockscomb,'' pseudopolypoid,'' ''rim'' and ''collar,'' have been coined.

Recent studies have shown that DES daughters may have other abnormalities. Cervical abnormalities that result in cervical imcompetence, which in turn causes miscarriages between the 18th and 32d week of pregnancy, have been noted in DES daughters.[22] Uterine abnormalities, in particular a shortened or ''T-shaped'' uterus, have been attributed to DES exposure and may also occur with adenosis.[23] The ultimate effect of the abnormalities on the fertility of these women is not yet known, but very recent studies suggest that DES daughters are more likely to have difficulty getting pregnant and carrying a pregnancy to full-term live delivery.[24]

Vaginal Adenosis and Cancer

The biggest concern about vaginal adenosis is its relationship to cancer. Indeed, the whole controversy about DES began in 1970, when an alert physician, Dr. Arthur Herbst, and his colleagues reported seven cases of a rare form of vaginal cancer—clear cell adenocarcinoma—in women 15 to 22 years of age.[25] Until this time there had been only three reported cases of this rare cancer in women under age 35. After a year of careful investigation the linkup between DES exposure and the cancers was made. This led to the establishment of a worldwide tumor registry to which such cancers could be reported. Some 300 to 400 cases have been recorded thus far. The overwhelming majority of the young women who developed the disease also had vaginal adenosis.[26]

The cancer findings led to attempts to screen females who were known to have been, or thought to have been, exposed to DES. As mentioned earlier, a number of these DES daughters were then found to have vaginal adenosis. Not all DES daughters have vaginal adenosis. Of those who do only a small percentage have thus far developed cancer. Most experts feel that the risk of developing cancer in women definitely known to have been exposed is around 1 in 1,000.[27] But the accuracy of this estimate is questionable; the actual risk may be much higher or much lower.

Those who argue that the estimate is too low think that we are just seeing the tip of the iceberg, and that as time passes we will be seeing more of this type of cancer. Those who say the estimate is too high point to the fact that the peak incidence of clear cell adenocarcinoma in DES daughters occurs around age 19, and after that it seems to taper off.

Other experts fear that DES daughters with adenosis may be at increased risk of developing not just this rare form of vaginal cancer but also of developing the more common cervical cancer.[28] Part of their concern comes from the fact that most cancers of the cervix arise in the region of the squamocolumnar junction. The simple fact that in DES women with adenosis this junction is not confined to the area of the os, but may extend over the surface of the cervix and down into the vagina, means that there is a wider transformation zone and thus a wider surface area of tissue with a potential for the development of cancer. The least serious of these cervical cancers, carcinoma in situ, most commonly occurs in women in their 30s and 40s. Again, some experts believe that not enough time may have elapsed for us to see the whole iceberg.[29]

Alarming recent studies have indicated that DES-exposed women may have a higher incidence rate (as much as a fivefold increase) of a condition known as cervical dysplasia, an abnormality of the cells of the cervix that is thought by most experts to be the first step in a series of changes that eventually leads to cervical cancer.[30] Other researchers have disputed this finding of an increase in cervical dysplasia.[31] They argue that the cell changes seen in these DES daughters are not owing to cervical dysplasia, but to a totally noncancerous process known as squamous metaplasia. Squamous metaplasia is a developmental process in which the more differentiated, more sophisticated, misplaced glandular tissue in the vaginal walls is being replaced by the less differentiated, less sophisticated, glandless squamous cell tissue that belongs in the vaginal cavity. In other words, the cell changes being labeled cervical dysplasia are not abnormal, precancerous changes but actually cell changes occurring as a result of a natural developmental process. In short, the vaginal adenosis is being healed spontaneously. These doctors point to studies that have shown that in women over age 30, 80 percent of the adenosis was replaced with squamous tissue. From these findings they postulate that the majority of women with adenosis will go on to spontaneous resolution of the adenosis in their 30s. They believe that only a small percentage will develop true cervical dysplasia, carcinoma in situ of the cervix or invasive cervical cancer in this process. Let's hope that they are right. At any rate, studies now being done should yield important information on this topic. One way to keep abreast of the research being done in this area is to join DES Action (*see* p. 818) and to read their excellent newsletter.

Diagnosis and Follow-Up

Careful diagnosis and follow-up of DES-exposed women, especially those with adenosis, is vitally important. This crucial diagnosis and follow-up should be done by doctors experienced in DES exposure who have access to the special equipment that may be required. The diagnostic procedures and follow-up programs are discussed in detail under the heading DES.

Because it is not known how often vaginal adenosis will progress to cancer and because many cases may spontaneously resolve themselves without treatment, most experts think that the best treatment is careful follow-up, unless, of course, cancerous or precancerous changes are found, in which case treatment for the cancer is indicated.

When the news of the relationship between DES exposure, adenosis and cancer first broke, some doctors performed a rather radical form of preventive surgery—removal of the vagina, with, if possible, plastic surgery to provide a functional vagina. This type of operation, a vaginectomy, is now considered far too radical a treatment by the majority of experts. Any woman whose doctor proposes this treatment for noncancerous adenosis should definitely seek another medical opinion.

Some doctors will cut, freeze (cryosurgery) or burn (electric cautery) away the area of adenosis, a process that may necessitate hospitalization. Laser treatment to destroy affected areas has also been advocated. In some instances the doctor may do the tissue removal in the office, and if the areas of adenosis are extensive, this may be done in gradual stages so that adhesions and scar tissue will not form. While some well-respected physicians advocate this form of treatment—removal of the adenosis—there has been a great deal of debate about it. The majority of doctors consider it unnecessary, the rare exception being made for the woman who has severe discharge and severe pain on intercourse.

There is some indication that the jellies used with diaphragms, which help make the vagina more acidic, may have a healing effect on the adenosis. In addition, the problem of increased vaginal discharge, which affects some 15 percent of DES daughters, seems to respond favorably to these products; thus some doctors prescribe spermicides or similar products for their patients.

Birth control pills that contain estrogen have been prescribed for DES daughters both for contraceptive purposes and to control menstrual irregularities, but many doctors question the wisdom of giving estrogen in any form to DES daughters or mothers.

The general consensus of medical opinion at this time seems to be that DES daughters don't require specific treatment beyond careful follow-up. What constitutes careful follow-up is debatable, however. This issue is also discussed under the heading DES.

CLEAR CELL ADENOCARCINOMA*

AKA: DES-related cancer

Clear cell adenocarcinoma is a rare disease. Before 1970 the few cases of vaginal clear cell adenocarcinoma that were found occurred primarily in postmenopausal women; however, since that time somewhere between 300 and 400 cases of clear cell adenocarcinoma have been reported, the majority of them occurring in young women and girls in their teens.[32] The upsurge in the disease is related to a synthetic hormone, DES, that was given to pregnant women in the United States from 1940 to 1971.[33] The daughters of these women are at risk of developing this rare form of cancer.

Cause, Symptoms and Diagnosis

The cause of the disease, the symptoms it produces and the methods of diagnosis have been discussed in the section on vaginal adenosis. Related information is discussed in the section on DES.

Treatment

The types of treatment available and the considerations involved in deciding which is the best type of therapy for clear cell adenocarcinoma are basically the same as those for other forms of vaginal cancer; however, the fact that it strikes young women and that it may, with careful follow-up of DES daughters, be found at an earlier stage than most vaginal cancers influences the choice of treatment.

Most other cases of vaginal cancer are treated by radiation therapy. For a number of reasons, however, most experts prefer to use surgery to treat clear cell adenocarcinoma, which generally occurs in younger women. First of all, although we know that exposure to radiation can cause cancer as well as cure it, radiation-caused cancer takes many years to develop. For women in their 60s and 70s the possibility that the radiation therapy may actually cause cancer in another 10 or 20 years is not so much of a consideration. But for the younger woman this possibility is much more threatening, because she has an expected lifespan of another 50 years.

Moreover, although radiation is preferred in older women because their

*See also the general discussion of cancer and the discussion of vaginal cancer.

general poor health and associated diseases may either prevent surgery altogether or at least cause much higher complication rates, younger women, whose general health is usually better, can expect fewer complications. Another factor is that surgery, even extensive surgery, allows for preservation of the ovaries. Here again, since most cases of vaginal cancer occur in older, postmenopausal women, the destruction of the ovaries is not a significant factor. But in younger women, destruction of the ovaries leads to premature menopause, which carries certain risks. The preservation of the vagina is a factor as well. Radiation will leave the vagina intact, but most of the time radiation, especially external radiation, will result in a vagina that is so dry and constricted that sexual intercourse is painful or impossible. In surgery the vagina, as well as the uterus, cervix, lymph nodes and surrounding tissue, may be removed, but it is possible to reconstruct the vagina using skin grafts and specialized surgical techniques that will allow for intercourse and orgasm. Once radiation has been given, however, it is not possible to perform plastic surgery and create a functioning vagina.

Little if any attention has been given to sexual response in women after this type of surgery. The personal reports we have received from a few individual DES daughters indicate a range of sexual responses. The clitoris remains intact and orgasm is reported by many. Others feel so demoralized and shaken by their experience and the surgery that they cannot bring themselves to relate sexually; others find sex is difficult, painful and unsatisfying after the surgery.

Effectiveness of surgery versus radiation is, of course, an important factor. The survival rate for the small number of patients who have been treated thus far is about 75 percent, regardless of whether radiation or surgery was used.[34] But not enough time has elapsed to accurately compare survival rates. Since the survival rates for surgery versus radiation as treatment of adenocarcinoma are thus far the same, surgery, which allows for the creation of a functioning vagina as well as ovarian preservation and doesn't involve long-term radiation risks, is the treatment of choice in most experts' minds.* As more time passes this may change.

The choices are difficult ones, and it may be some time before more information about the best treatment is available. Women who have clear cell adenocarcinoma of the cervix should be treated by experts and should have opinions from doctors who favor radiation as well as from those who favor surgery. One way to contact experts in the field is through the DESAD projects set up by the National Cancer Institute to monitor women exposed to DES-type drugs. They are listed in Table 31 (*see* p. 812). DES Action (*see* p.

*For further information on therapy, see Note 35 in the references that appear at the end of the book.

818), a national organization of people concerned about DES, is also an excellent source of medical information.

CANCER OF THE VAGINA*

AKA: carcinoma of the vagina

Types: squamous cell cancer
adenocarcinoma
sarcoma
melanoma
sarcoma botryoides

Cancer of the vagina may originate in the vagina itself or it may appear as the result of direct extension of cancer of the adjacent organs, such as the cervix, vulva or uterus. It may also appear as the result of metastasis (spread) from a tumor growing at a distant site in the body. Sometimes it is hard to tell whether the cancer is primary—originating in the vagina—or secondary—the result of direct invasion of metastases. In the following discussion we are concerned mainly with primary cancer.

Types

Most vaginal cancers are squamous cell cancers, arising from the squamous cell tissues of the vaginal walls. Occasionally, adenocarcinomas, cancer arising from gland tissue, will occur in the vagina. When these rare adenocarcinomas appear in young women there is usually a history of their mothers' having taken synthetic hormones, like DES, during pregnancy. This unusual form of vaginal cancer is discussed under the heading Clear Cell Adenocarcinoma. Other rare forms of vaginal cancer include sarcoma, melanoma and sarcoma botryoides, which, unlike other forms of vaginal cancer, usually affects children.

Incidence and Risk Factors

Primarily vaginal cancer is a rare form of cancer accounting for only about 1 to 2 percent of all female genital cancers.[36] It is estimated that for every case of vaginal cancer there are 45 cases of cervical cancer and 3 cases of vulvar cancer.

Vaginal cancer is usually a disease of older women. Approximately 70 percent of the cases occur in women over age 50. The peak incidence occurs in

*Anyone reading this section should first read the general discussion of cancer and cancer terminology.

women between ages 60 and 70; however, the disease has been reported in younger women and even in infancy.[37] As noted above, a certain form of vaginal cancer related to DES exposure occurs in young women (ages 7 to 29).

Risk factors such as those associated with cervical or breast cancer have not proved significant in vaginal cancer. Ethnic background, previous pregnancies and childbirth, marital status, sexual history, family history and genetic factors appear to be unimportant.

Cause

The cause of vaginal cancer, like the cause of all forms of cancer, is unknown.

Symptoms

Vaginal cancer may not produce any symptoms, especially in the early stages. Indeed, approximately 5 percent to 10 percent of those women diagnosed as having vaginal cancer, even some with cancer in advanced stages, are entirely asymptomatic.[38] When symptoms do occur they may be so slight that they are hardly noticed. If symptoms do occur, the three most common ones are vaginal bleeding, vaginal discharge and pain.

The bleeding may take the form of slight bleeding or staining, prolonged or profuse menstrual periods, contact-type bleeding, or spotting, such as after intercourse or douching. About 60 percent of the women diagnosed as having vaginal cancer will have a history of one of these types of painless vaginal bleeding.

There may be an increase in vaginal discharge. It may be watery, brown and cause itching. About 20 percent of the women with vaginal cancer will have this symptom, either with or without the vaginal bleeding.[39]

Bladder pain, pain on urination and frequent need to urinate may be symptoms in the early stage but are more common in the later stages of the disease. Vaginal pain, pressure in the rectum, pain on moving the bowels and constipation may also occur. About 5 percent of women with the disease will first come to the doctor with symptoms of pain.[40] As the disease progresses and spreads to the bladder and rectum, pain and irregularities in bowel movements and urination are more common. Fistulas, openings or holes connecting the vagina and the bladder and/or rectum, are frequent complications.

A visible tumor or open sore can sometimes be seen on speculum exam but usually only in the late stages of the disease. A lump or hardened area can sometimes be felt on the vaginal walls. The lymph nodes in the area may become swollen.

Diagnosis

Unfortunately, bothersome symptoms often fail to appear until the disease is fairly well advanced. Even though there may be symptoms of discharge, itching and bleeding, they are often not severe enough to cause the woman to seek medical help. Since the disease most often occurs in women who are no longer menstruating, the symptoms of bleeding between periods or prolonged, profuse menstrual periods are not relevant clues for most women who have this disease. All such women may notice is a slight staining after intercourse or douching. The doctor, too, is often to blame for the lack of prompt diagnosis. Because symptoms like itching or vaginal discharge are not uncommon in women in this age-group an are more often caused by postmenopausal vaginitis, too often doctors prescribe for these symptoms over the telephone or without giving the woman a thorough examination. Women should insist on a complete physical and gynecological exam and not accept a telephone diagnosis or cursory examination.

Sometimes a routine Pap smear will detect vaginal cancer, but it is not as useful a tool in screening for vaginal cancer as it is in cervical cancer, for the usual Pap smear does not take cell samples from the entire vaginal cavity. A special four-quadrant Pap smear, which takes cell samples from the vaginal walls, may be done to detect vaginal cancer, but because this involves a considerably more involved laboratory analysis, this test is not done in routine examinations.

Determining the stage of the disease involves a careful bimanual pelvic exam and palpation (feeling) of the vagina, which may be done under a general anesthetic so that the woman is totally relaxed, allowing the doctor to feel the vaginal walls and pelvic area thoroughly. Generous biopsy specimens are taken from areas that appear suspicious when stained with a special dye. The vagina may be examined with a special magnifying instrument called a colposcope. Biopsy specimens may be taken from the cervix as well. In some cases a cervical biopsy will be done to eliminate the possibility of cervical cancer. Such biopsies are done by conization, a process in which a central core of tissue is removed from the cervix. Endometrial biopsies or even a D&C may be done to eliminate the possibility of uterine cancer.

Cystourethroscopy, a procedure in which a special viewing instrument is used to examine the urinary tract, and proctosigmoidoscopy, a procedure in which a viewing instrument is used to examine the rectum, will usually be done while the woman is under anesthesia so that the doctor can decide about the possibility of bladder or rectal involvement and can stage the disease more accurately. In addition, other standard tests to assess local invasion and distant spread of the disease are done. The lymph nodes in the area are carefully felt, and biopsy specimens of the suspicious ones are collected and examined during surgery to determine whether or not they need to be treated.

Staging

Vaginal cancer can range from precancerous cell abnormalities called dysplasia to frankly invasive cancer that has spread to the lymph nodes, adjacent organs like the rectum and bladder or distant organs.

Because vaginal cancer is a rare disease, a clear-cut classification scheme on which to base treatment and compare the results of various therapies has been difficult to establish; however, the staging system outlined in Table 8 is now widely used.[41]

Table 8
Clinical Staging Scheme for Vaginal Cancer

Stage O:	Carcinoma in situ ("cancer that is in place") or intraepithelial carcinoma; cancer in which cancerous-type cells are present but in which there is no evidence, microscopic or otherwise, to indicate invasion.
Stage I:	The cancer is limited to the vaginal wall.
Stage II:	The cancer has invaded the subvaginal tissues but has not extended to the pelvic wall.
Stage III:	The cancer has extended to the pelvic wall.
Stage IVA:	The bladder and/or rectum is involved.
Stage IVB:	The cancer has spread beyond the pelvis, that is, there are distant metastases, or spread of the cancer to distant organs.

Treatment

The treatment of vaginal cancer is complicated by the fact that the vagina is located between the bladder and the rectum. Because the bladder and the rectum are extremely sensitive to radiation, massive doses of X-ray cannot be given. The fact that there is only a thin wall of tissue separating the organs means that surgical removal of the cancer along with adequate margins (cancer-free areas) of adjacent tissue may not be possible.

Treatment may be given by radiation, surgery or a combination of the two. A comparison of surgery and radiation therapy brings out some important differences. Except for a few instances when there are superficial cancers or small tumors in the upper vagina, or in certain cases of recurrent cancer, the surgery that must be done is quite extensive, requiring pelvic exenteration, an operation in which the uterus, tubes, ovaries, vagina, bladder and/or rectum are removed and urinary and/or bowel wastes are collected in plastic bags attached to the outside of the body. The age and physical condition of most women who have vaginal cancer and the loss of these organs makes this surgery impractical in many cases. Although serious complications may result from radiation therapy, it generally offers less overall risk and a better chance of perserving bladder, rectal and vaginal function.

Radiation Therapy

The majority of women are treated by radiation. Radiation is often effective in this area, for it can be administered through the vagina, which makes possible direct contact with the tumor, without having to pass through normal tissue to get at it.[42]

The radiation may be administered in a number of ways, depending on the size of the tumor, its location and the extent of the spread:

☐ Radioactive implants, either in the form of intracavity implants—radiation sources placed in the vagina and possibly the uterus as well, for specified amounts of time—or interstitial radiation—needles filled with radioactive substances that are inserted directly into the tumor

☐ External beam therapy—X-ray beams directed toward the vagina from outside the body

☐ Transvaginal cone therapy—an X-ray beam directed into the vagina

When the cancer is located in the upper third of the vagina the treatment plan closely resembles that used for cervical cancer. If the invasion of the vaginal tissue is less than 1 cm in depth, a single dose, applied by inserting the source of radiation into the vagina, may be all that is necessary. If the cancer is deeper, external beam therapy is also necessary.

In most Stage I and Stage II cases both external beam therapy and internal radiation are used. External beam therapy is usually given first. This will shrink the vaginal tumor and make it more receptive to subsequent internal radiation. It is hoped that it will also succeed in killing any cancer that has spread beyond the vagina into the surrounding tissues and lymph nodes. External beam therapy that succeeds in shrinking the tumor is usually followed by implants in the vagina and the uterus. In some cases, particularly if the tumor has not been sufficiently reduced by the external beam therapy or has widely spread into the immediately adjacent tissues, interstitial radiation by way of needles may be used instead of intracavity implants.

If the cancer is located near the vaginal opening, external beam therapy will probably not be used, because the vulva would also be radiated, and vulvar tissues are easily destroyed by radiation. Instead, interstitial radiation or transvaginal cone therapy is generally used for early-stage cancers in this location.

In Stage III, external therapy is more important, for the external beam can reach a wider area than the implants or needles, which are designed primarily to kill the central tumor and are not as effective in killing the cancer that has spread beyond the vagina into surrounding tissues and into the lymph nodes. Thus a large external dose is given to the whole pelvic area over a period of weeks. This may be followed by lower external doses given directly over the tumor area or by interstitial radiation by way of needles planted directly into the tumor area.

Stage IV therapy is similar to that used for Stage III; however, in cases where the rectum and/or bladder are bound by adhesions to the vagina or where the disease is too widespread for any hope of cure, lower doses of radiation are given in hopes of providing palliation, or relief of symptoms. Although the dose is not high enough to kill all the cancer cells, it may reduce the pain, lessen the discharge and help stop the bleeding. The dose is low enough to avoid radiation damage to the radiation-sensitive bladder and rectum.

Surgery

Sometimes surgery is used to treat vaginal cancer, either alone, as primary treatment, or in combination with radiation. If vaginal cancer recurs after a full course of radiation, surgery, usually pelvic exenteration, rather than reirradiation offers the best chance of a cure. In certain Stage IV cases where the vagina is bound by adhesions to the bladder and/or rectum, so that it is impossible to give high enough doses of radiation to kill all the cancer without undue damage to these organs, radical surgery—pelvic exenteration—sometimes in conjunction with lower-dose external beam therapy, may remove the central cancer and may be worth the risks involved and the unpleasant aftereffects (the plastic bags for bodily wastes). This is one of those instances in which more than one medical opinion is of critical importance.

Other instances in which surgery might be used include small Stage I cancers (those confined to the vaginal wall), Stage O cancers (carcinoma in situ) and certain Stage II cancers in which the tumor is in the upper third of the vagina. For small Stage I cancers, surgery can be as effective as radiation. If a Stage O or Stage I cancer is found after previous radiation treatment for cervical or uterine cancer, surgery rather than more irradiation is done. Surgery in these cases would include a radical hysterectomy, removal of the pelvic nodes and total or partial vaginectomy (if the cancer is in only the upper third). If there hasn't been previous radiation treatment for cancer, some doctors prefer surgery in such cases, while others prefer radiation. Women should hear opinions from both sides, and here again, a team approach to treating cancer is of utmost importance.

Stage O

In the past few years, treatment of Stage O, carcinoma in situ, that is, cancer that is locally confined, has been reappraised because of evidence that the disease grows slowly and because it usually occurs in younger women in whom the sexual function is considered to be more important.* Radical forms of surgery and extensive radiation both destroy the vagina, so less-radical surgery and less-extensive radiation are now used.

Cryosurgery, removal of the cancerous areas by freezing, or removal by excision (cutting away) have been tried.[43] Cryosurgery results appear to be good. There is none of the scarring or contracting of the vagina, a condition known as vaginal stenosis, that can occur with radiation or with surgery. However, these methods should not be used unless a staining and biopsy of suspicious areas have been done with the aid of a colposcope. A "blind" biopsy, one done without the aid of the colposcope, is not sufficient if cryosurgery or local incision is planned. The danger in this more conservative therapy lies in the fact that vaginal cancer tends to be multicentric—to have more than one point of origin. Other areas of cancer might exist that are not yet advanced enough to be recognized. The doctor must be satisfied that the cancer is clearly in situ (in place) and not invasive before these less-radical methods can be attempted.

So far, treatment by cryosurgery seems to be effective; however, such cases have been followed for only about 3 years. More time is needed before the results can be judged accurately.

Laser beam therapy has also been used in the treatment of Stage O cancer.[44] With laser therapy there is not the same degree of mutilating scar formation that there is with radiation therapy, and injury to the bladder and rectum can be avoided. Thus it is regarded by some as superior to radiation therapy as well as to cryosurgery or local incision for the treatment of this stage of cancer. Although several institutions are experimenting with laser surgery, the technique is not widely available. Too few cases have been followed for too short a period for an accurate assessment of its effectiveness.

Treatment of vaginal cancer must be highly individualized according to the size, type and location of the cancer, the age of the woman and the importance she attaches to preserving a functioning vagina. The basic principles in treatment have been outlined here, but these principles must be adapted to

*This is not to say that preserving sexual function is not important to older women, just that the medical profession recognizes it to be more important in younger women.

meet the specific situation. A doctor may recommend a treatment plan different from the ones outlined here, perhaps because of the particulars of the case or because new information has become available since the time of this writing. However, the material outlined here covers the usual therapy plans. If the doctor disagrees, the woman has the right to have his or her reasoning explained in language she can understand. She also has the right to seek other medical opinions (*see* page 238). Because of the rarity of vaginal cancer, it is especially important that women with this condition find specialists who have had experience with this particular form of cancer.

Chemotherapy

Experiments with chemotherapy have not produced any increase in survival rates. Any relief of symptoms provided by chemotherapy has unfortunately brought considerable risk to the patient. The dosage, in order to be effective, is too close to the lethal dose, and the side effects have so far negated any benefits obtained. New approaches to chemotherapy are constantly being developed, however, so at some time in the future, chemotherapy may become an important part of the treatment program.[45]

Survival Rates

Survival rates, of course, vary with the stage of the disease. Table 9 lists, stage by stage, the range of 5-year survival rates reported for vaginal cancer treatment by radiation.

Table 9
Five-Year Survival Rates for Vaginal Cancers Treated by Radiation*

Stage	Percent
I	69–83
II	41–68
III	27–40
IV	0–14
Overall	46–52

*SOURCE: Data for this table were condensed from survival data from three separate institutions: A.M. Anderson Hospital, Washington University and the University of Maryland. See Robert D. Hilgers, M.D., "Squamous Cell Carcinoma of the Vagina," *Surgical Clinics of North America*, vol. 58 (Feb. 1978), pp. 25–38.

The anatomy of the cervix is described in Chapter Two, and details about how it functions at various points in the menstrual cycle are discussed in Chapter Four. But in order to understand the disease processes that can take place in the cervix, it is necessary to understand the cellular makeup of this organ. The external portion of the cervix, the part that protrudes into the vaginal cavity, is covered by pink tissue known as squamous cell epithelium. The cervical canal, which leads into the uterus, is lined with red, columnar epithelium, which contains mucus-secreting glands. Normally, the squamous cell tissue and the columnar tissue meet at the cervical os, the opening to the cervical canal. The area where these two types of epithelial tissue meet is called the transformation zone, or the squamocolumnar junction.

Sometimes these two tissues do not meet at the cervical os. If the cervical canal becomes infected—a condition known as cervicitis—the columnar tissue may swell and protrude out of the cervical canal onto the vaginal portion of the cervix. This is known as cervical eversion and is discussed under the second heading in this section, along with cervical erosion, a condition in which the pink squamous tissue is eroded away by sores.

At other times, tears or injuries to the cervix can cause cervical eversion, and this is discussed under the heading Cervical Lacerations. About 20 percent of women are born with cervical eversions in which the squamous and columnar tissue meet somewhere other than the opening of the cervical os. This does not usually cause any problems; however, some women with congenital cervical eversion have the condition because their mothers took a synthetic hormone, such as DES, during their pregnancies. This is discussed under the heading Congenital Abnormalities of the Cervix.

In addition to these disturbances in the normal cellular makeup of the cervix, the squamocolumnar junction may also be the site of more serious problems. Cancerous and precancerous conditions of the cervix often arise in the area of the squamocolumnar junction. Luckily, this junction is readily accessible, and a simple screening test known as the Pap smear, whereby cells from the cervix are collected and studied microscopically, can detect cancerous and precancerous conditions in their earliest stages. Every woman should have a Pap smear regularly. (*see* pp. 783–87).

Along with the conditions discussed above, this section also includes information on cervical cysts and cervical polyps, both of which may follow a case of cervicitis. Cervical stenosis, a blockage of the cervical canal that can be caused by cervical infections or other problems, is also discussed in the following pages. A description of a condition known as cervical incompetence, in which the cervix dilates prematurely during pregnancy, is also included.

CERVICITIS
AKA: inflammations of the cervix or cervical canal

Types: acute cervicitis
chronic cervicitis
endocervicitis

"Cervicitis" is the term used to describe a variety of inflammations of the cervix. The condition may be acute or chronic and may be caused in a variety of ways. In most cases it is associated with other, more general infections of the vaginal cavity or the female organs. For instance, pelvic inflammatory disease, especially when it involves the fallopian tubes, is often accompanied by cervicitis. Any of the common vaginal infections can involve the cervix. Acute and chronic gonorrhea, as well as many of the other sexually transmissible infections, can also affect the cervix. In some cases, however, only the cervix is affected, without involving the vagina or other pelvic organs.

Some authorities believe that many times cervicitis results from infections caused by tears or lacerations of the cervix, which can occur during childbirth. Other authorities think that such injuries are only rarely associated with cervicitis. This confusion stems from the fact that after such injuries the cervix may heal in such a way that it looks red, raw and irritated. But this irritated appearance may not be owing to infection at all, but to the simple fact that on soft internal tissues like the cervix, scar tissue tends to have this unusual appearance. Some doctors on seeing such scar tissue will do a culture or wet smear, find bacteria present and decide that a woman has a case of cervicitis. The bacteria found in many such instances, however, are normal inhabi-

351

tants of the vaginal cavity. Their presence does not necessarily mean that disease is present.

If such doctors also see what they consider to be an abnormal amount of cervical discharge, they consider this further evidence of infection. However, as any woman who practices regular self-exam knows, the amount and character of cervical discharge varies, depending on the phase of the menstrual cycle. It also varies from individual to individual. Thus a doctor who sees scar tissue from a cervical laceration that gives the impression of infection; what appears to be an abnormal amount of discharge (even though, in fact, for that woman, in that particular phase of her cycle, it may be quite normal); and test results showing bacteria may decide that this is a case of cervicitis that needs treatment. Other doctors, aware of these confusions, do not consider such women to have cervicitis unless they complain of an unusual discharge.

In most bona fide cases of cervicitis, when the external, vaginal part of the cervix is involved, the cervical canal—the passageway between the vaginal cavity and the uterus—is also infected. Sometimes the cervical canal will be inflamed without any obvious problems on the external, vaginal portion of the canal, and this is known as endocervicitis.

Symptoms of Acute Cervicitis

The disease may be either acute or chronic. The chief symptom of acute cervicitis is a discharge from the cervical os. The discharge may be abundant and pus filled and may vary in color from clear to gray, white or even yellow, depending on the type of infection. If the infection is caused by gonoccocus, the cervical discharge is apt to be profuse, and usually the urinary tract, Skene's glands and/or Bartholin's glands are also infected. If these other organs are involved, there may also be associated symptoms like urinary frequency and urgency, and pain. If the cervicitis is associated with one of the common vaginal infections, the discharge is also apt to be profuse, and there may be burning and itching of the external genitals. On those rare occasions when the cervicitis is associated with lacerations and injury and the only bacteria found are the normal vaginal inhabitants, the discharge is less heavy and irritation to the external genitals is likely to be minimal or absent. Sometimes acute cervicitis will produce general systemic symptoms, such as fever, as a result of the white cells in the body attempting to fight off the infection, but this is not usually the case.

In acute cervicitis the cervix may look quite abnormal. It may be swollen, with red, irritated-looking areas. If the cervicitis is associated with a vaginal infection or sexually transmissible infection, there may be other symptoms associated with these diseases. A syphilis chancre, for instance, may be present. In the case of trichomoniasis the characteristic strawberrylike patches may cover the cervix. If moniliasis is the culprit, the cervix may be white. There may be a reddish ring or halo around the cervical opening or red sores on the surface of the cervix. These are called cervical erosions or eversions and may be associated with chronic cervicitis as well (see below).

Treatment of Acute Cervicitis

Because cervicitis may be caused by a number of different organisms, treatment depends on identifying the specific organism and selecting an appropriate antibiotic or sulfa drug. Cautery (destroying the infected tissue by chemical or electrical means) or cryosurgery (destroying the tissue by freezing) should never be done in the case of acute cervicitis, for this could cause the disease to spread to other organs.

Care must be taken to keep the area clean so that the infection won't spread. Intercourse is prohibited. If the infection is severe and there are general systemic reactions, such as fever or urinary problems, these should be treated as well and the woman should be confined to bed with plenty of fluids to drink.

Symptoms of Chronic Cervicitis

Acute cervicitis can become chronic. This frequently happens when gonococci are the infecting organisms. It may not even be possible to detect any gonococci in a smear of culture, and if such is the case, the woman may be an asymptomatic carrier of the disease. Chronic cervicitis may also be associated with lacerations or injuries caused during abortion, rape, childbirth or surgery. Here again, it may not be possible to detect any specific bacteria other than the normal vaginal bacteria. In such cases, cervicitis should be treated only when the woman herself feels that there is an abnormal discharge.

Chronic cervicitis doesn't look as extreme as acute cervicitis and does not look the same in all cases. In some instances the cervix may appear to be normal on its vaginal surface, but the cervical canal is thickened and produces a white pus. Sometimes the entire cervix becomes swollen and barrel-shaped.

In other cases the top layers of the tissues of the cervix have eroded away owing to the irritation of the discharge. There will be a reddish area or sores, called erosions, around the os, just as in acute cervicitis. At times these reddish areas will be slightly raised, with tiny nipplelike protrusions, and this is known as papillary cervical erosion.

If the chronic cervicitis is associated with lacerations owing to injury during childbirth or, as is much more likely, to an abortion, the cervix is likely to be quite swollen. Under such conditions the infected and swollen mucous membrane lining of the canal often rolls out, much like the lining of a sleeve that is too long for the outer cloth. This condition is known as cervical eversion. The area around the os is red and angry looking and is apt to be thicker and to cover a wider area than an erosion. Like an erosion, this sort of eversion may bleed easily on the slightest contact.

In an attempt to heal and repair itself, the surrounding tissue proliferates and attempts to grow over the eroded or everted areas. In the course of this natural repair the mucus glands in the inflamed tissue may be pinched off, forming nabothian cysts. In other cases the overgrowth of the repair process may lead to the formation of teardrop-shaped growths known as cervical polyps.

In addition to these changes in the cervix, chronic cervicitis also produces a thick, gelatinlike, mucous discharge that may have quite a bit of pus in it and may be white or yellow. Often a mucous plug fills the cervical os and is difficult to dislodge.

There is apt to be a slight, irregular staining-type of contact bleeding, especially when polyps, erosions or eversions are present. There may be pain on intercourse if the penis pushes against the tense, rigid cervix. Backache is a common complaint, because the disease-fighting lymph system for the cervix drains back along the rear supporting ligaments that hold the uterus in place, which may also explain the sense of pelvic heaviness that many women report. Urinary symptoms are not uncommon, since the bladder is so close by. Many cases of "honeymoon bladder" are probably the result of vigorous intercourse that has stirred up a low-grade infection in the cervix and bladder. Any attempt to treat the bladder problem without treating the cervix is unlikely to succeed.

Cervical infections have also been implicated in fertility problems. A thick discharge from an irritated cervix may affect the sperm or block its passage through the cervical canal. Long-standing cervical infection may affect the monthly ferning pattern of the cervical mucus (*see* p. 62), which creates pathways that aid the sperm in its passage to the uterus, thereby making conception impossible. The polyps associated with cervicitis may also cause problems with fertility if they mechanically block the passage of the sperm.

Diagnosis

Diagnosis of cervicitis depends on a history of previous disease or injury, the presence of an irritating discharge and the particular appearance of the cervix. Cultures and wet smears must be done to identify the organism causing the cervicitis. Pap smears and biopsies may be in order to eliminate the possibility of cancer, since the appearance of the cervix and the symptoms of cervicitis may mimic cervical cancer.

Treatment

Although antibiotics may be effective for acute cases, they are often not successful in cases of chronic cervicitis. In such cases, then, the infected tissues must be destroyed either by electric cautery or, preferably, cryosurgery. Cryosurgery is more comfortable and has fewer complications. Unfortunately, not all doctors have the equipment or skill to perform cryosurgery.

CERVICAL EROSION AND CERVICAL EVERSION

AKA: ectropion

Associated Terms: congenital erosion, congenital eversion

Erosion and eversion (Illustration 44) are terms used to describe certain conditions of the cervix. The term "ectropion" is sometimes used instead of "eversion." There is a great deal of confusion about the terms and some medical writers use them differently. As if that weren't enough confusion, there is also a great deal of controversy about what causes these conditions, whether or not they need treatment and, if so, what constitutes proper treatment.

In the case of an eversion the columnar tissue that lines the cervical canal is pushed to the outer, vaginal portion of the cervix. Just as the lining of a sleeve that is too long will hang out beyond the edge of the sleeve, so the angry-looking, red columnar tissue will protrude beyond the os. There is usually a ringlike shape to the eversion, or it at least seems to follow the contours of the os. Some women are born with this trait, in which case the term "congenital

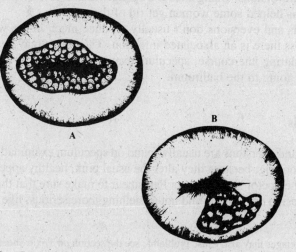

Illustration 44 *Cervical Eversion (A) and Cervical Erosion (B)*

355

eversion'' is used. Some writers use the term "congenital erosion" even though it is an eversion they are actually talking about. An infection of the cervical canal, endocervicitis, can also cause the swollen, irritated columnar tissue to pout out of the os, particularly when there are tears or lacerations of the cervix caused by childbirth, abortion, rape or injury.

An erosion, as the name implies, means that some of the cells on the surface of the os have been worn away and the raw surface of the cervix is exposed, just as happens when there is a graze on the skin of the outside of the body. Such sores look like dark pink or red spots on the cervix. An estimated 95 percent of all women will have an erosion on the cervix sometime in their lives. An erosion may be associated with a white discharge that may have an unpleasant odor. If the erosion is infected, there may be a slightly blood-tinged discharge. Sometimes, especially in the case of cervicitis, the erosion too may seem ring-shaped, forming a soft halo of redness around the os, and it may be mistaken for an eversion. At other times the erosion looks more like a separate little sore or graze on the skin and there is not a definite border between the redness and the normal pink tissue.

Causes

Some doctors believe that the Pill and the IUD string, as well as cervicitis, can cause these two conditions, but other doctors dispute this. It is thought that intercourse may also be a factor in erosions. Some women are born with eversions. It has recently been discovered that women whose mothers took certain hormones (see the section on DES) during pregnancy are apt to have congenital eversions. Using a natural sponge instead of a tampon during their periods has helped some women get rid of their erosions.*

Erosions and eversions don't usually produce much in the way of symptoms unless there is an associated infection. Then there may be contact-type bleeding during intercourse, speculum exam, or douching or even on straining when going to the bathroom.

Diagnosis

Erosions and eversions are usually found on speculum examination. They can be scary looking, because they alter the usual pink, healthy appearance of the cervix. The doctor should take a Pap smear to make sure that the process is a simple erosion or eversion and not something more serious, like cervical cancer.

*Natural sponges may also cause problems; see the section on Toxic Shock Syndrome for details.

Treatment

Some doctors treat erosions and eversions with drugs; however, unless there is an infection such treatment doesn't really affect these conditions. Other doctors will destroy the eroded, everted tissue by means of electric cautery or by freezing the tissue off with cryosurgery. This too is of questionable value. Some doctors justify the expense, inconvenience and discomfort of such treatment by saying that they fear that erosions and eversions are related to cervical cancer. Although it is true that cervical cancer often arises in conjunction with erosions, and less frequently with eversions, it is also true that the majority of women with erosions and eversions never get cancer. It is our opinion, then, that any suspicious-looking sore or reddened area on the cervix should be examined by Pap smear and, possibly, a cervical biopsy. If such areas turn out to be benign, no treatment is necessary.

CERVICAL POLYPS

AKA: growths in the cervical canal

Types: decidual polyps

Polyps (Illustration 45) are small protrusions that grow from a mucous membrane. Cervical polyps are tubular or tear-shaped growths with little stems that grow from the mucous membranes of the cervical canal. In rare instances they may grow from the surface of the vaginal part of the cervix. Although polyps are abnormal growths, they are benign. Only in rare instances is cancer found in a polyp.

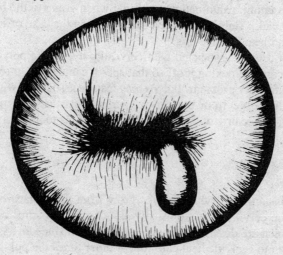

Illustration 45   *Cervical Polyp*

357

Causes

Cervical polyps are often the result of the body's attempt to heal itself after an infection of the cervix. The tissue around the infected area proliferates, growing new cells in an attempt to heal and cover over the raw, inflamed tissue. Sometimes the tissue may become so overgrown that clumps of excess tissue—polyps—are formed. In some cases the tissue irritates the cervical canal, which contracts in an effort to rid itself of the clumps of tissue. Thus the tissue gets dislodged from its primary position, and a stem, called a pedicule, is formed, with a tubular or tear-shaped clump of tissue at its end.

Polyps may also be formed during pregnancy, when hormonal excess provides too much stimulation and provokes a similar overgrowth of tissue. They are found more frequently in women who take birth control pills.

Symptoms

Polyps are usually bright pink or red and somewhat spongy; however, the rare varieties that grow on the vaginal portion of the cervix tend to be firmer and paler. They can occur singly or multiply and with speculum exam may be seen peeping through the cervical os. They are generally rather small, although they can become as thick as a little finger and may become so elongated that they can be seen protruding from the opening of the vagina.

When they are small they often don't cause symptoms; however, the larger ones, as a rule, usually do. The tip of the polyp may be subject to injury because of its exposed position and may therefore bleed on contact. Intercourse, douching, speculum examination, straining when going to the bathroom and the like may cause staining between periods or, in the case of larger polyps, prolonged and heavier bleeding.

Pain is not usually associated with cervical polyps. The polyp may crowd the cervical canal, blocking it off so that sperm cannot pass through, thereby causing an infertility problem. Polyps may also be associated with an increase in mucous discharge from the cervix, perhaps because of irritation to the glands, perhaps because of associated infection. This too may affect fertility.

Diagnosis

In the rare instances in which polyps grow from the surface of the vaginal portion of the cervix, they are usually associated with sores called cervical erosions, which are described above. Sometimes the bleeding symptoms will lead a woman to seek medical care, but at other times the polyps are discovered only in the course of a routine physical exam. The doctor may feel them

358

by manual exam or see them during speculum exam. The only real problem in diagnosis is that they may look like certain forms of cervical cancer and produce similar symptoms. A Pap smear and biopsy will determine the difference.

Treatment

The treatment of polyps is usually fairly easy and consists of removing them. Most of the time this can be done in a doctor's office under a local anesthetic. The doctor twists off the polyp at its stem and may touch the base with an electric cautery point. The removed polyp is examined microscopically to rule out the possibility of cancer.

It is particularly important to remove the polyp right down to the base. Only rarely does cervical cancer appear in a polyp, but on those rare occasions when it does the base is often involved. So the doctor must be sure that the polyp can be removed at the base before an office procedure is attempted.

Some polyps are too thick to remove in the office because of the danger of excessive bleeding. Likewise, if the polyps are multiple and the cervical canal is crowded, hospitalization might be necessary.

Polyps tend to recur, and if another polyp or significant bleeding occurs after initial treatment, the second attempt at treatment should be a dilation and curettage (D&C), done in a hospital. Decidual polyps, overgrowths of the decidua (which is part of the rich lining of the pregnant uterus), are usually not treated during pregnancy but are left alone because of the danger of excessive bleeding.

NABOTHIAN CYSTS

AKA: cysts on the cervix

Associated Terms: squamous metaplasia, epidermidalization

Nabothian cysts (Illustration 46) are cysts of the mucus-producing glands that are located in the cervical canal and on the surface of the cervix.

Causes

Most of the time the cysts are the result of natural healing processes known as squamous cell metaplasia or epidermidalization. As explained in the introduction of this section, the outside of the cervix is normally covered by squamous cell tissue, which is pink, and the inside of the cervical canal is lined with red, somewhat angry-looking tissue that contains mucus-producing

359

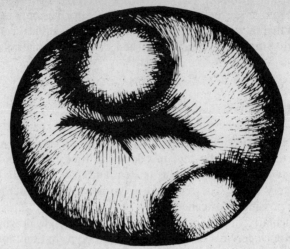

Illustration 46   *Nabothian Cysts*

glands and is known as columnar tissue. In most women these two tissues meet at the cervical os, the opening of the cervical canal. In cases of chronic cervicitis the squamous cell tissue attempts to grow over and cover up the raw, irritated areas of the infected cervix. In the process the squamous cell tissue may pinch off the mucus-producing glands either by growing beyond its normal limits and into the cervical canal or because the glandular tissue itself is located beyond its normal boundary at the os and is growing on the surface of the cervix (a condition known as cervical eversion). In either case, cysts may be formed.

Nabothian cysts are also found in older women, who are no longer producing much estrogen. With the decline in estrogen levels the tissue of the cervix thins and flattens. As a result the normal secretions, although more meager than those found in a younger woman, are trapped, again forming nabothian cysts.

Symptoms

The cysts may be single or multiple and range in size from as small as a pinhead to as large as a grape or even larger. They are usually filled with the clear mucus-type fluid that makes up the cervical secretions, but if the cervix is infected, the contents of the cyst may be somewhat cloudy and pus filled. The cysts generally do not cause any bothersome symptoms.

Treatment

The cysts do not become infected unless the entire cervix happens to become infected, as in cervicitis, so they do not usually require treatment. Nonetheless, some doctors will treat nabothian cysts by electric cautery or cryosurgery, which involves expense, healing time and possibly complications. But since nabothian cysts produce no symptoms, cause no problems and are in fact just the aftermath of a healing process or part of a natural aging process, we do not think that they need to be treated.

CERVICAL LACERATIONS

AKA: tears in or stretching of the cervix

Cervical lacerations are tears in the cervix that usually result from injuries during childbirth or abortion. They may be slight or deep and may be associated with relaxation of the muscles of the vaginal opening. Writers of medical textbooks, who seem to relish the creation of new categories, classify cervical lacerations as unilateral, bilateral and stellate. But as common sense will tell you, such tears may take all sorts of forms.

With improved medical care during childbirth and delivery, serious lacerations of this type are uncommon. Some amount of tearing during delivery is natural, and most of the tears that do occur do not require surgical repair. Cervical lacerations that result from abortions are more likely to need treatment. This is especially true of late abortions that are done by saline or prostaglandins. In such abortions the dead fetus is delivered through the cervix just as happens in normal deliveries, but because the normal process by which the cervix dilates and is prepared for delivery does not take place during such an abortion, tears in the unprepared cervix may occur as the fetus is expelled. Because these sorts of lacerations tend to be more severe and do not usually heal naturally, the doctor will often have to suture or sew them up.

It is an important but often ignored procedure to check for lacerations of the cervix after late abortions, so ask your doctor about this problem if you have this type of abortion.

Untreated lacerations of this type will often result in cervical stenosis, a closing up of the cervical canal. If the cervix is completely closed off, the menstrual debris cannot escape. There is a buildup of menstrual blood that can cause problems. Fistulas, abnormal connections between various genital organs—in this case, the cervical canal, vagina and uterus—can also result from such unrepaired lacerations. Cervical lacerations may also result in a condition known as cervical incompetence, which can cause miscarriages.

Lacerations are often associated with eversion, a condition in which the red glandular tissue that normally lies inside the cervical canal prolapses, or

361

falls, and pouts out of the cervical os onto the normally pink tissue that covers the surface of the cervix. Lacerations caused by late abortion may also be associated with cervical infections.

According to some authorities, lacerations caused by childbirth are similarly associated with infections of the cervix; however, there is some controversy here. Sometimes lacerations from childbirth heal up in such a way that they leave no sign except for long, fibrous scars. However, there is considerable debate about whether or not any given cervical laceration is healed or not. The traditional textbook explanation of events goes something like this: The tear or laceration occurs during delivery, and there is usually a subsequent infection. This is because the bacteria that are normally present in the vagina in limited numbers blossom in the pregnant vagina as a result of the hormones involved in pregnancy, which create an alkaline environment conducive to their growth. The laceration and the presence of the bacteria combine to produce cervical infection, so that the inflamed tissue must be treated with drugs; if this is unsuccessful, as it often is in cervical infections, the infected tissue must be cut, burned or frozen off.

In our experience, and that of many of our colleagues, it is uncommon for cervical lacerations from childbirth to become infected or for the symptoms of cervicitis—a bothersome discharge—to develop. In the rare cases where there is a discharge so heavy that it becomes an annoyance to the woman, we of course treat it. But in the majority of cases, cervical lacerations from childbirth don't require treatment and don't become infected. Part of the confusion here is caused by the nature of the tissue that makes up the cervix. It is soft, internal tissue, and what may look like an inflamed or irritated area is really just the way scar tissue manifests itself on this type of tissue. It is always possible to pick up some bacteria in the vagina. Thus this angry-looking scar tissue and the presence of bacteria may be interpreted as an infection, when it is not really a pathologic situation. Therefore, what a doctor who treats cervical lacerations with electric cautery or cryosurgery is really doing is simply removing scar tissue from the cervix, a bit of cosmetic surgery. No woman is vain enough to care whether the appearance of her cervix is flawed by scar tissue, so freezing, burning or cutting away such tissue is unnecessary—and may be uncomfortable and expensive as well.

INCOMPETENT CERVIX

AKA: premature dilation of the cervix during pregnancy

Some women have what is called an incompetent cervix, a condition that should probably be renamed, as the term sounds rather like a put-down of a woman with this condition. The cervix does not normally open up until a woman is in labor. Then it dilates until it is opened wide enough to permit the baby to pass through. In the case of an incompetent cervix the cervix opens up long before it should and the woman has a miscarriage. Typically, this occurs during the 18th to 32d week of pregnancy, even though there may *not* have been any prior problems, such as cramps or bleeding, during the pregnancy. The duration of each successive pregnancy is usually lessened. This sort of history will help the doctor make the diagnosis. Ultrasound techniques, methods of visualizing internal tissue by using high-frequency sound waves, may also help in diagnosis.

Causes

In some cases the woman with an incompetent cervix will have a history of therapeutic abortions or difficult childbirth that has resulted in tears or lacerations of the cervix. In other cases there is no such history, and the defect is thought to be congenital (that is, present since birth). There has recently been some evidence suggesting that women whose mothers took synthetic hormones, such as DES, during their pregnancies are more likely to have this congenital defect (*see* pp. 808–15).

Women with incompetent cervices used to be confined to bed for their entire pregnancies. Nowadays the Schirodkar procedure, whereby the cervix is tied closed, usually during the 12th to 16th week of pregnancy, permits such women to have normal pregnancies. Usually, the tie is cut before labor, and a vaginal delivery, rather than the riskier cesarean section, can take place.

Sometimes the cervix is tied off before the pregnancy takes place, a procedure called an internal trachelorrhaphy. There is some controversy about whether the cervix should be tied off before or after the pregnancy is established. The internal trachelorrhaphy will not prevent pregnancy, but some doctors are concerned because there is a 20 percent spontaneous abortion rate in all pregnancies and the uterus, if tied shut, will not be able to abort spontaneously. On the other hand, the process, no matter when it is done, is not always successful, and waiting to place the suture until the greatest risk of spontaneous abortion has passed—the 12th week—means cutting it pretty close to the wire, for some incompetent cervices will open up on or before the 12th week. Each case must be decided on its own merits, and a woman has a right to a full discussion with her doctor of the pros and cons of each method for her particular case.

CERVICAL STENOSIS

AKA: partial or total obstruction of the vaginal canal

Types: acquired stenosis
        congenital stenosis

Associated Terms: hematosalpinx, hydrometra

Cervical stenosis refers to a condition in which the cervical canal is partially or totally blocked.

Causes

Cervical stenosis may result from a variety of causes. In some cases the problem is congenital, that is, the blockage is present at birth. Owing to disturbances in embryonic development, the canal never opens properly, is absent altogether or is obstructed by a wall of tissue (see Congenital Abnormalities of the Uterus and Fallopian Tubes and Congenital Abnormalities of the Vagina, for a more complete discussion). Sometimes the closure of the canal results from a mechanical blockage. Thus abnormal growths, like cervical polyps, endometrial polyps and certain fibroid tumors of the uterus and cervix, may be the source of the obstruction. Scar tissue from conization or cauterization, especially in the hands of an unskilled, inexperienced doctor, can cause cervical stenosis as well. In fact, any surgical procedures involving the cervix—including biopsies and curettage, or scraping, of the cervical canal—can result in such a blockage. Infections in the cervix may result in adhesions, hardened bands of fibrous tissue produced by healthy tissue to wall off infections and prevent their spread, and these adhesions may cause blockage. Similar types of obstructing adhesions may occur after menopause and may also cause blockage.

Symptoms and Complications

A number of symptoms and complications can result from partial or total blockage of the cervix. First, there may be pain. Anything that obstructs the easy passage of menstrual blood may cause a bearing-down pain, painful uterine contractions and backache. If the obstruction is only partial, the menstrual blood will flow but is likely to be dark brown or almost black.

If the obstruction is total, passage of the menstrual blood is prevented altogether. In a young girl with a congenital blockage the problem may not be discovered until the expected time of menarche. She may seek help about her failure to menstruate. Sometimes such a girl will actually have started to menstruate and may have monthly menstrual symptoms but no external bleeding. The blood has backed up in her uterus, a condition known as hematometra that can cause abnormal swelling and pain, especially at the time of menstruation. If the process continues untreated for long enough, the fallopian tubes as well as the uterus may fill up with menstrual blood, a condition known as hematosalpinx. The blood may even back up through the tubes and spill out into the pelvic cavity. Because the lining of the pelvic cavity is sensitive to blood, this can cause a great deal of irritation and pain and the formation of pelvic adhesions. There may even be associated pelvic endometriosis, a condition in which bits of uterine lining tissue are found growing on the ovaries and other abnormal locations. The same thing can happen in a woman who has already begun to menstruate; however, they are less likely to go that far, because her failure to menstruate will usually prompt her to seek medical attention.

When the blockage occurs in a young girl or in a postmenopausal woman there may be a buildup of watery and mucous cervical secretions, a condition known as hydrometra. This buildup is less likely to happen in a postmenopausal woman, since her cervical secretions are diminished. If the blockage is associated with infection, there may be a backup of fluid and pus, a condition known as pyometra.

There may also be a fertility problem associated with the blockage, because it may be impossible for sperm to navigate the blocked canal. Even partial blockage may cause such problems.

Treatment

Treatment consists of removing the blockage surgically and may involve one or more follow-up dilations of the canal to prevent it from closing up again. This can be done in the doctor's office with a local anesthetic. If there has been a backup of fluids, they must be drained. Antibiotics are often given to prevent an infection from subsequently arising from the accumulated fluids, which, especially in the case of blood, tend to be a fertile breeding ground for bacteria.

CONGENITAL ABNORMALITIES OF THE CERVIX

AKA: cervical birth defects

Types: incompetent cervix
cervical stenosis
cervical eversion or ectropion
cervical agenesis
double cervix

>   septate cervix
>   transverse cervical ridges
>   hooded, rim, cockscomb, pseudopolypoid, or collar cervix

We have already discussed incompetent cervix, cervical stenosis and cervical eversion in this section. These conditions may be either congenital—present since birth—or acquired as the result of injury, infection or something else that has happened since birth. There are several additional congenital cervical abnormalities. These include a complete absence of the cervix, called cervical agenesis, and a double cervix, called a septate cervix, in which the cervix is divided down the center by a wall of tissue. These conditions are discussed under the heading Congenital Abnormalities of the Vagina and Congenital Abnormalities of the Uterus and Fallopian Tubes.

A special category of congenital cervical abnormalities includes transverse cervical ridges, which are ridges or ripples running across the surface of the cervix much as ridges of sand may form on a stretch of desert, and the hooded cervix, in which a flap of skin covers the top of the cervix. The terms "rim," "collar," "cockscomb" or "pseudopolypoid cervix" may also be used to describe the latter condition. The majority of birth defects in this category occur in women whose mothers took synthetic hormones, such as DES, during their pregnancies. These defects in and of themselves may not be serious; however, other more disturbing defects may occur along with these. This topic is discussed more fully under the heading DES.

LEUKOPLAKIA OF THE CERVIX

AKA: white patches on the cervix

Leukoplakia of the cervix is manifested as single or multiple white patches on the cervix that usually appear in women over age 40 and may be associated with vaginal discharge or bleeding. It is caused by an irregularity in cell growth and is thought by some to be precancerous.

Although it is certainly true that leukoplakia and cancer often coexist, it is not clear whether this is because malignant tissue is conducive to the development of leukoplakia or because leukoplakia is precancerous. A sort of which-came-first-the-chicken-or-the-egg situation exists. Certainly not all women with leukoplakia develop cancer. However, even though the answers are not yet in, the fact that it is possible for an area of leukoplakia to mask a cancer growing beneath it means that the usual treatment involves excision (cutting out) of the areas of leukoplakia.

The leukoplakia may be discovered because the woman has symptoms and seeks medical attention, or it may be discovered in the course of a routine gynecological exam with a speculum.

CERVICAL DYSPLASIA*

AKA: cervical intraepithelial neoplasia (CIN), grades I & II

Types: CIN grade I, basal cell hyperplasia, mild dysplasia, or moderate dysplasia
CIN grade II, or severe dysplasia

The term "dysplasia" means abnormal cell development; cervical dysplasia, then, is an abnormal condition of the cells of the cervix. It doesn't, as a rule, produce any obvious symptoms, nor in most cases can it be seen with the naked eye. The only way that most women know they have it is as a result of a routine Pap smear.

There is a good deal of controversy and confusion about dysplasia, especially about its relationship to cancer. Sometimes the cell abnormalities seen in cervical dysplasia become progressively more abnormal and the woman develops cervical cancer, but not all women with dysplasia do develop cervical cancer. Some 30 percent to 50 percent will, however, develop cervical cancer over a period of some years if the condition is not treated. Most authorities therefore consider dysplasia a precancerous condition.

Today there is a tendency to view dysplasia not as a separate entity but as the first step in a continuum of abnormal cell changes that progress in a few years to carcinoma in situ, which in turn progresses in about 5 to 10 years to invasive cancer. Thus the term "cervical intraepithelial neoplasia" (CIN) has been coined.

CIN is divided into three grades. Grade I includes mild and moderate dysplasia. In mild dysplasia, also known as basal cell hyperplasia, the cells in the bottom third or less of the tissue that covers the cervix (the cervical epithelium) are abnormal. Moderate dysplasia involves one-third to two-thirds of the cervical epithelium. Grade II is severe dysplasia, meaning that at least two-thirds but not the entire epithelial membrane is involved. Grade III, which is also known as carcinoma in situ, involves the full thickness of the cervical epithelium. Grades I and II are discussed here; Grade III is discussed under the heading Carcinoma in Situ.

Incidence and Cause

Cervical dysplasia is most frequently found in women aged 25 to 35 but can also occur in women in their teens or early 20s and in older women as well. The cause of cervical dysplasia, like the cause of any precancerous or cancerous condition is unknown; however, studies of the women that are at high risk for developing such conditions have indicated some possible causes. Risk factors and possible causes are discussed under the heading Cervical Cancer.

*Important background information is given in the section on the Pap smear.

Diagnosis

The first step is the Pap smear. If the Pap smear indicates mild, moderate or severe dysplasia, which may be referred to as a Class III smear, most doctors think that the next step should be a biopsy. The biopsy must be done to confirm the Pap smear, for Pap smears can be wrong. They may be falsely negative or falsely positive. Moreover, Pap smears are, not infrequently, "off" by one class. A woman whose Pap smear indicated dysplasia could, in reality, have carcinoma in situ. The Pap smear may even be off by more than one class, so that a woman with a smear indicating dysplasia could actually have invasive cancer. A biopsy, which involves taking a tissue sample, is more accurate. The Pap smear provides the pathologist only with isolated cells; the biopsy allows him or her to study the architecture of the cells' relationship to one another and thus to make a more accurate diagnosis.

Not all doctors perform a biopsy when a woman's Pap smear indicates that she has mild or moderate dysplasia, usually referred to as a Class III smear. Some doctors will merely tell her that her smear has indicated some abnormality and that another smear should be done in anywhere from 3 to 6 months. Their reasoning goes like this: Not all cases of dysplasia become cancer; some revert to normal on their own. Moreover, cancer of the cervix is usually a slowly progressing disease. Because the Pap smear indicates only the possibility of a precancerous condition, there is no great hurry. They maintain that, because these conditions progress so slowly, waiting will do no harm. Repeating the smear right away won't do any good, they say, because a lapse of at least a few months is necessary to give the condition enough time to progress, if indeed it is going to progress, to a more serious stage. Since the abnormal Pap smear may regress to normal by the time of the next smear, they argue that there is no need to subject a woman to a needless biopsy.

This wait-and-see approach should be taken only if the doctor cannot see or feel any irregularity on the cervix. If there is a visible abnormality, this approach should NEVER be used. A woman familiar with the appearance of her cervix can double-check her doctor on this. If the cervix looks different to her, she should insist on a biopsy, no matter what her doctor says. Likewise, the wait-and-see approach should be discontinued if the woman experiences any pain or bleeding between periods. In such cases a biopsy *must* be done.

If at the time of the second smear the dysplasia gets worse, or even if it has merely persisted, a biopsy should be done. The waiting should not be continued, for a smear that persists as positive is not likely to return to normal. Even if the second smear *is* negative, the woman must have follow-up smears every 3 to 6 months for the next 2 years. This is necessary because the follow-up smears may be incorrect. As pointed out earlier, it is not unusual for a smear to be one class more serious or one class less serious than the pathologist's report. Thus a follow-up smear with a report of no dysplasia does not guarantee that the dysplasia is gone, but merely that the cells collected in that particular smear and analyzed by that particular pathologist are not judged to be dysplastic.

Many women and many doctors question the wisdom of a wait-and-see approach. First of all, most authorities now feel that true dysplasia usually does not regress to normal.[1] They believe that those instances in which the Pap reverts to normal were actually misread in the first place (*see* pp. 783–87). Many women object to the mental anguish of waiting 3 to 6 months to find out if they have a precancerous or cancerous condition. There is also the risk of delaying treatment. Although it is true that cancer of the cervix is usually a slowly progressing condition, there are exceptions. An approach that delays a diagnosis could, then, be dangerous.

Most experts believe that there should be no delay in cases of severe dysplasia. No one knows for sure whether severe dysplasia always goes through a carcinoma in situ stage or whether some progress directly to invasive cancer, a much more serious condition. Moreover, because it is known that Pap smears are often inaccurate, the reported severe dysplasia may in reality already be carcinoma in situ or even invasive cancer.

It is our recommendation that women with dysplasia, regardless of the severity, insist on biopsies and not accept a wait-and-see approach, even if it means finding another doctor or traveling to another town for medical care.

The biopsy may be done in one of two ways. In the first approach the cervix is stained with a special solution, and biopsy specimens of any areas that do not take the stain are collected. The cervical canal must be also scraped, a procedure known as endocervical curettage, for the inside of the canal cannot be seen and yet that is where the cancerous or precancerous problem may lie. If the staining doesn't show any suspicious area or only a few such areas, biopsy specimens are taken from several locations on the cervix where studies have shown that these sorts of problems are most likely to occur. This is known as a blind biopsy.

The second way of doing the biopsy is to use a colposcope. The colposcope is a magnifying instrument, a sort of microscope on a stand. With a speculum in place, a beam of light from the colposcope is directed at the cervix. The doctor can often tell how serious the dysplasia is and can see suspicious areas not visible to the naked eye. In fact, the colposcope may detect suspicious areas even before cells that could be picked up on a Pap smear are shed. The interior of the canal still can't be seen, so it must be scraped. A special stain is also used in conjunction with the colposcope. The use of the colposcope means that numerous blind biopsies need not be taken.

The colposcope-directed biopsy is much more accurate. Even in the best of hands, the first method of biopsy is accurate in only 80 percent of the cases. The colposcope is more than 95 percent accurate. The problem is that not all doctors have colposcopes and not all are well trained in their use. If your doctor doesn't have a colposcope, ask to be referred to a clinic or doctor who does. Again, we recommend that women insist on cervical biopsies done with a colposcope, even if it means that they have to travel to another city or town.

Sometimes it is necessary to do a conization, a procedure whereby a cone of tissue is removed from the center of the cervix. Conization necessitates hospitalization and a general anesthetic. It may involve such complications as excessive bleeding, scar-tissue blockage of the cervical canal and infertility owing to destruction of the mucus-producing glands in the cervical canal. Because of this, a biopsy is preferred over conization. But if there is reason to suspect that the abnormality is in the cervical canal, a conization is necessary, for the scrapings from the cervical canal, like the Pap smear, provide only isolated cells. An actual biopsy of the canal—a conization—is necessary in the following instances:

☐ If the squamocolumnar junction (*see* pp. 350–51), the area where the squamous cells of the vaginal portion of the cervix and the columnar cells of the canal meet and where most cancers of the cervix originate, is not visible

☐ If the staining and colposcopic exam don't reveal any abnormalities on the surface of the cervix

☐ If the cells obtained by scraping the cervical canal are abnormal

☐ If the abnormal areas detected by staining or colposcopy lead into the canal

☐ If the Pap smear indicated severe dysplasia but the biopsy indicated only mild dysplasia, the colposcopic-directed biopsy should be repeated. If the inconsistency between the Pap and the biopsy persists, conizations should be done.

Women should not agree to conization unless a colposcopic exam has been done first, for it can discover abnormalities that a mere staining of the cervix may miss. If your doctor suggests conization, make sure you understand his or her reasoning. If you get one of those because-I'm-the-doctor-and-I-say-so replies or you are not satisfied with the explanation, seek a second opinion (*see* p. 238).

Treatment[2]

Treatment for dysplasia ranges from hysterectomy to conization to electric cautery or cryosurgery to merely following the condition closely, as described above.

Although hysterectomy is done for dysplasia, it is considered by most to be overtreatment, no matter what the woman's age. The risks and complications involved are too high a price to pay now that effective, less-radical treatment is available. If your doctor proposes to do a hysterectomy for dysplasia, read the section on hysterectomy carefully and get a second medical opinion before undergoing surgery.

If a conization has already been done as part of the diagnostic process, this may constitute treatment as well, as long as the cone was done properly and all suspicious areas seen by the colposcope were removed. However, a dysplasia will recur in 13 percent to 15 percent of the cases treated by conization. Because of this recurrence rate and because conization is a surgical procedure necessitating hospitalization and an anesthetic, and is known to have complications, it is not a good treatment choice, particularly for women who have future childbearing plans.

Either electrocautery (heat) or cryosurgery (freezing) can also be used to treat dysplasia. The dysplastic areas are destroyed, thereby allowing normal, unaffected tissue to grow back in its place. Most doctors favor cryosurgery because it goes deeper and destroys more possibly dysplastic tissue. Another big factor in favor of cryosurgery is that it is essentially painless. Moreover, such complications as closing of the cervical canal and infertility may be associated with electric cautery but not with cryosurgery. Women should insist on cryosurgery rather than electrocautery. Some doctors are now using laser surgery instead of cryosurgery, and this new form of therapy produces results as good as those from cryosurgery.

Follow-up is important, even when a hysterectomy has been done, for the vaginal tissue may develop cancer as well. Follow-up Pap smears and colposcopic exams are especially important in the less radical forms of treatment. (For more information on follow-up, *see* p. 390.)

Some doctors who treat dysplasia by the wait-and-see method are also recommending that the woman's sexual partner use a condom during the waiting period. Although we think it is a good idea for women who have been diagnosed as having a precancerous condition of the cervix or who are at high risk of developing such conditions to use condoms as their method of birth control (*see* pp. 375–78 for details), we are skeptical about its effectiveness as a *treatment* for dysplasia. Doctors who think the condom is effective in the treatment of dysplasia point to a study of 400 women with Class III Pap smears.[3] In this study, 139 of the women were not given treatment but were simply followed (as in the wait-and-see approached discussed above), and their sexual partners used condoms during the waiting period. In all but three of these women the dysplasia cleared up, a fact that the researcher inut three as showing a curative effect from condom use. However, the validity of this study has been questioned.[4] Critics point out that certain viruses, such as the condyloma virus, can cause changes on a Pap smear that mimic dysplasia and that such Pap smears are, therefore, frequently misdiagnosed as dysplasia and labeled as Class III. Condyloma will clear itself up without treatment in 30 percent to 40 percent of cases. These critics believe, as we do, that correctly

371

diagnosed Class III Pap smears showing dysplasia require effective treatment, not simply the use of condoms. Again, although condom use is not a bad idea, we do not recommend the wait-and-see approach.

CARCINOMA IN SITU*

AKA: intraepithelial carcinoma, preinvasive cancer, precancerous anaplasia, noninvasive carcinoma, Bowen's disease of the cervix, cervical intraepithelial neoplasia (CIN) grade III, Stage O of cervical cancer

Carcinoma in situ means "cancer that is in place," or cancer that has not invaded the surrounding tissue. It is a condition in which cells that have all the characteristics of cancer are found but only the top layers of the cervical tissues are involved, and there is no sign of the invasion of the surrounding tissue that characterizes true invasive cancer. Whether all carcinoma in situ of the cervix eventually progresses to invasive cancer is not known, largely because no one is willing to leave it untreated and risk the chance that it will become invasive.

At this time the generally accepted view is that carcinoma in situ arises from a background of severe dysplasia and is part of a continuum of disease that leads to invasive cancer. Working from this assumption, one expert has coined the term "cervical intraepithelial neoplasm" (CIN), or Stage O of cervical cancer. CIN is further divided into three types, or stages; grades I and II, which encompass the various degrees of dysplasia (see above), and grade III, which is carcinoma in situ, or Stage O of cervical cancer.

Carcinoma in situ most often arises in the area of the cervix known as the squamocolumnar junction. This is the point at which the pink, squamous tissue that covers the vagina and the vaginal portion of the cervix meets the red columnar tissue that lines the cervical canal. In the majority of women this junction lies just inside the cervical os (opening).

Incidence

Carcinoma in situ of the cervix is most frequently found in women in their 30s who have borne one or more children, as opposed to invasive cancer of the cervix, which is most often found in women in their 40s. Recently, however, carcinoma in situ is being found with increasing frequency in women in the 20- to 30-year-old age-group. For a discussion of the reasons for this increase in incidence in younger women, see the section on Cervical Cancer.

*See the general section on cancer, the previous section on dysplasia and the section on the Pap smear for background information.

Cause and Risk Factors

The cause of carcinoma in situ, like the cause of all cancers, is unknown. However, certain women seem more likely to develop this condition than others. For a discussion of causes and risk factors, see Cervical Cancer.

Symptoms

Carcinoma in situ of the cervix has no characteristic symptoms. Although it is true that 85 percent of the women with this condition will have some sort of abnormality in the appearance of the cervix, this is not surprising, because most of them have borne children. Cervical lacerations, erosions and eversions, which can cause abnormalities in the appearance of the cervix, are common among such women and are not necessarily related to cancer. In other words, although most women with carcinoma in situ have these conditions, that does not mean that most of the women who have them will develop cancer.

Bleeding between menstrual periods or after intercourse occurs in about a third of the women who are diagnosed as having cervical carcinoma in situ. However, although some women will show a history of such irregular bleeding and may even have cervices that bleed on the slightest contact, most women with this condition do not.

Cervical carcinoma in situ frequently occurs without any abnormality in the appearance of the cervix, particularly when it is located inside the cervical canal and when there is no bleeding. Luckily, even in the absence of symptoms or of abnormalities in the cervix, a routine Pap smear can detect carcinoma in situ.

Diagnosis

The Pap smear is the first step in diagnosis. If the smear shows carcinoma in situ, the next step is a biopsy, preferably a colposcopic biopsy, as described in the preceding section on cervical dysplasia. In certain cases a conization may be necessary. This too is described in the preceding section on dysplasia. A D&C may be done to rule out the possibility of invasive cancer.

Treatment[5]

Carcinoma in situ may be treated by hysterectomy, conization, electric cautery or cryosurgery (freezing). (*See* the preceding section on dysplasia.)

Hysterectomy offers a 100 percent cure and is usually recommended for postmenopausal women and premenopausal women who don't have future childbearing plans. In the past, women adamant about preserving their ability to bear children were sometimes treated by conization. Unfortunately, conization often has an effect on fertility. Only about 65 percent of women treated by conization are able to get pregnant, and of these, approximately 25 percent will have miscarriages. Today a new form of therapy, cryosurgery, which destroys the affected tissue by freezing, is available. Conization may still be done for women whose carcinoma in situ is located in the cervical canal, but for most women who want to preserve their childbearing capabilities, cryosurgery is the best choice.

Women who are treated by cryosurgery must commit themselves to a life-long follow-up program that includes Pap smears every 3 months, regular colposcopic exams and a yearly endocervical curettage, that is, a scraping of cells from the inside of the cervical canal. This follow-up program is essential, for in 7 percent to 11 percent of cases the cryosurgery will not be effective and the carcinoma in situ will recur. Without a careful follow-up program the recurrent carcinoma in situ might be missed and progress to frankly invasive cancer before being detected, which would greatly reduce a woman's chances of survival. If recurrent carcinoma in situ is discovered in follow-up, a second cryosurgery treatment or a hysterectomy may be done.

Most doctors feel that cryosurgery is an acceptable alternative to hysterectomy for women anxious to retain their ability to bear children. Even though they have no future childbearing plans, some women anxious to avoid the risk and expense of hysterectomy are choosing cryotherapy over hysterectomy.

Women who choose cryotherapy for carcinoma in situ are taking a certain risk. Theoretically, even if a woman were to report faithfully for her follow-up visits, there is a small chance that a recurrence could be missed. The cancer could recur high up inside the cervical canal, where it could not be seen with a colposcope. The Pap smear might fail to detect a recurrence. False negative rates (that is, failure to detect cancer that is actually there) of 1.4 percent to 30 percent have been reported in studies of Pap smears. The generally accepted false negative rate is 11 percent to 22 percent. It is highly unlikely that a woman who is having four Pap smears a year would be unlucky enough to have a false negative reading each time, but it is theoretically possible. It is also possible, although unlikely, that the yearly endocervical curettage could fail to detect a recurrence in the cervical canal. However, even if a recurrence were missed one year, it would probably be caught the next year, and because carcinoma in situ usually takes 7 years to progress to invasive cancer, missing it one year would not be too serious.

The other risk involves the problem of misdiagnosis. It is possible that the woman might really have invasive cancer, and not carcinoma in situ, but that a mistake was made in the diagnostic workup. If treated by hysterectomy, this misdiagnosis would probably not present a problem, for the cervix and uterus would have been removed. If, on the other hand, the woman is treated only with cryosurgery, she would not be cured of the invasive cancer.

Cryosurgery has not been used on a large enough group of women for a long enough period for anyone to say with *absolute certainty* that it is as safe as hysterectomy or to define precisely the magnitude of the risks involved. The studies done so far are very encouraging, however, and we personally feel comfortable with this form of treatment.

Cautery—destroying the tissues by burning—has also been used, but cautery involves more discomfort and complications that may affect fertility, so most doctors prefer cryosurgery. Recently, laser beam surgery has been used instead of cryosurgery, with good results.

CERVICAL CANCER

AKA: carcinoma of the cervix

Although the incidence of cervical cancer is on the rise, the death rate is declining. This is because the disease, thanks to widespread use of the Pap smear, is being detected in its earlier stages, when it is virtually 100 percent curable. The Pap smear, then, is an invaluable tool and should be part of every routine physical exam.

Incidence, Risk Factors and Cause

Cancer of the cervix is the third most common cancer occurring in women. The average age of the diagnosis of invasive cervical cancer is 48, but the disease may affect both younger and older women. The annual incidence rate in the United States is 14.9 cases per 100,000 women, but cases of cervical cancer are not randomly distributed throughout the population. In other words, not everyone is equally likely to get the disease; some women are definitely at higher risk of developing the disease than others. A number of factors come into play: Incidence rates vary according to ethnic group, for instance, with rates having been reported of 3.6 cases per 100,000 for Jewish women, 13.5 per 100,000 for non-Jewish white women, 47.8 per 100,000 for black women and a high of 97.6 per 100,000 for Puerto Rican women. It is also known that of the women with cervical cancer, 97 percent have had children. Women who marry at an early age and whose first child is born when they are still young also have higher incidence rates. Women with three or more husbands have higher rates, as do prostitutes. Numerous studies with results along these lines have been done.[6] It has not always been entirely clear what all this information means. At one time it was thought that having children at an early age or frequent sex put a woman at higher risk. At the present time, however,

375

most authorities feel that having sexual intercourse at an early age and multiple sex partners are the two factors most likely to increase a woman's chance of developing cervical cancer.[7] Some authorities question the accuracy of this. They point out that there are unproved assumptions behind the reasoning that earlier sex and multiple partners account for the high incidence among poor women. It has long been a popular piece of social folklore that the poor are more promiscuous, but there is no scientific evidence to substantiate this, and as one middle-class friend of ours says, "You couldn't prove it by me."

Still, there is other evidence to suggest that these two factors put a woman at higher risk of developing cervical cancer, carcinoma in situ or dysplasia. Women with these sexual patterns may want to have Pap smears more frequently.

The role of heredity is not considered to be important in cervical cancer. Cervical cancer does not seem to run in families, and the different incidence rates in various ethnic and economic groups is not thought to be the result of an inherited trait but of socioeconomic factors, since certain ethnic groups and women in low-income groups tend to marry earlier and have their children at an early age.

The fact that nuns never get cervical cancer, while prostitutes have high incidence rates, and that women who have sex at an early age or have multiple sex partners seem to be at greater risk, while women who use diaphragms[8] and condoms[9] for birth control (which presumably protect the cervix) are at lesser risk, first led to the suspicion that cervical cancer may be caused by some sort of agent—possibly a virus—passed during sexual intercourse. It is known that the cervical tissue is still maturing in a woman in her teens, and this maturation process may not be complete in some women until about age 20. It has been theorized, then, that the introduction of some sexually transmissible agent into the immature cervical tissue causes changes that only become apparent years later.

The evidence linking one agent known to be sexually transmitted, the herpes virus (*see* p. 569), to cervical cancer is strong. Over the past 10 years there has been a growing body of evidence suggesting a relationship between herpes virus and cervical cancer.[10] Studies that showed that herpes is found much more frequently in women with cervical cancer than in women without the disease were the first indication that herpes might be a factor in cervical cancer. A number of other studies further advance the case for a connection between herpes and cervical cancer.

A which-came-first-the-chicken-or-the-egg sort of question comes up in evaluating the relationship between herpes and cancer. Does herpes infection cause, or at least predispose a woman to, cancer, or does herpes just happen to find cancerous or precancerous tissue a more conducive environment in which to grow? Perhaps the cancerous or precancerous changes in the cervix make it more susceptible to herpes infection. However, the fact that the mean age of women with herpes is 20, that with cervical dysplasia it's 25, that with carcinoma in situ it's 31, and that with invasive cancer it's 48, does suggest that herpes may be the first step in a series that leads over the years to the development of cervical cancer. Moreover, studies that have followed women with herpes over a period of years have shown that such women are up to eight times more likely to subsequently develop some form of cervical cancer. But that may be because of precancerous changes that occur in the cervix years before the actual cancer is diagnosed and that also happen to make the cervix more susceptible to herpes infection. These sorts of data do not finally answer the chicken/egg question.

Still there is other laboratory evidence that doesn't look good for women with herpes. Herpes virus has been implicated in the development of tumors in laboratory animals. More to the point, herpes-associated substances have been found in cervical cancer tumors in humans. The laboratory evidence is again not conclusive, but there are persuasive indications that herpes is either a cause or a factor in the sequence of causative factors that leads to cervical cancer. Although the link between herpes and cervical cancer isn't strong enough to be called conclusive in the strictest medical sense, it is firm enough to suggest that any woman with a history of herpes should have at least an annual, probably even biannual, Pap smear. Other organisms, such as *Chlamydia* and the condyloma virus, are also being investigated as possible causative factors.[11] If further research confirms that there is a relationship with cervical cancer, women with histories of these infections may need Paps done more frequently.

Another causative factor in cervical cancer may be DES-type hormones taken during pregnancy by the mothers of the women with these conditions. This topic is discussed in greater detail elsewhere in this text.

The results of some studies show that women who smoke have higher rates of cervical cancer, carcinoma in situ and cervical dysplasia.[12] It is unclear whether this is because smoking has some kind of effect on the cervix or whether women who smoke also tend to have sex at an early age and multiple sex partners. Studies are being done to clarify this possible risk factor. If these studies prove that it is the smoking and not some associated sexual patterns that causes increased incidence, smoking may be listed as a risk factor for these conditions.

Women who use the Pill may also be at increased risk of developing dysplasia, carcinoma in situ and cervical cancer. Early studies of Pill users did not show such connection, but later studies that followed women for longer periods have shown an increased risk for Pill users.[13] Using the Pill for longer than 2 years seems to increase the risk. Women who use the Pill should have Pap smears at least once a year and possibly twice a year.

Because of the negative effect of the Pill and because methods like the diaphragm and condom have a protective affect, women who have had dysplasia, carcinoma in situ or cervical cancer or who have other risk factors for these conditions would probably do better to use a diaphragm or condom as their method of birth control.

Symptoms

The symptoms of cervical cancer include vaginal bleeding, discharge and an abnormal appearance of the cervix. In the later states there may be pain, weight loss and possibly urinary and bowel problems. Not all these symptoms are always present. In fact, the disease is often asymptomatic in the early stages. Approximately 70 percent of the women with Stage IA, or microinvasive, cancer have no unusual bleeding, and in 60 percent, the cervix appears normal. Only 20 percent of these women will have both symptoms.

Because the menstrual cycle is not disturbed, bleeding, when it does occur, is of the intermenstrual, or between periods, type. Except in advanced cases of this disease the bleeding is rarely of the gushing type, and in most cases the bleeding is slight. Spotting may occur after intercourse or douching. A woman may notice a slight vaginal bleeding while straining to make a bowel movement or after exercise, intercourse or even riding in a car. The bleeding may be so slight that it doesn't even require a sanitary pad. It is not nesessarily constant and tends to come and go. Several days may go by with no bleeding. Unfortunately, invasive cancer of the cervix tends to appear in women around the time of menopause and therefore such bleeding irregularities are often attributed to the menopause.

Bleeding is much more likely to appear in more advanced cases and is apt to be more profuse. However, even in these cases it may never be excessive, especially in the postmenopausal woman. Still, bleeding is one of the causes of death in the terminal cases of cervical cancer.

In the earlier stages of the disease, vaginal discharge tends to be constant but of such a slight amount that it is rarely enough to alarm a woman. The discharge is usually odorless, thin and watery. Only rarely does the discharge precede the bleeding; sometimes the two symptoms coexist. The color of the discharge varies from yellow to brown, depending on the amount of associated bleeding. The vaginal discharge tends to become more profuse and to smell bad in the advanced cases.

Pain combined with discharge and bleeding is the most frequent combination of symptoms in women with advanced disease. The pain varies in severity. It is usually a vague lower-back pain that may spread to the hip and down the side. It is usually worse at night and is not relieved by lying down. If the bladder and rectum are involved, there is often pain when voiding or when moving the bowels. There may also be constipation or retention of the urine.

The appearance of the cervix in invasive cancer varies considerably. About one-third of the women with this disease will have cervices that appear normal. Others, in the early stages, will have what appear to be cervical erosions or even slighter abnormalities. For example, there may be an area of the cervix that merely seems a bit redder, darker or less shiny than another, a condition that has been described as a "tomato blush."

In the more advanced stages the appearance of the cervix is more apt to be abnormal. If the disease is on the surface of the cervix, or growing from the canal outward, there may be a large sore or a bulky cauliflower-type growth. If the tumor is in the canal or tends to grow inward, the entire cervix may be increased in bulk, and although its surface may appear normal, the cervix takes on a barrel shape and extends lower into the vagina.

Recurrent cancer, that is, cancer that occurs even after the initial treatment, doesn't produce much in the way of symptoms in its early stages either; approximately 10 percent of such women will have some vaginal bleeding. As the disease becomes more extensive, there is usually pain in the lower back, radiating down the thighs. There may be swelling of the legs. If the bladder or ureters (the tubes that conduct urine from the kidney to the bladder) are affected, the woman may have associated urinary and kidney problems.[14]

Diagnosis and Staging

The first step in diagnosing cervical cancer is the Pap smear. Sometimes a woman will come to the doctor complaining of one of the symptoms described earlier, and in the course of investigating the cause of the symptom a Pap smear will be done. Often, however, there are not symptoms, and the abnormalities are discovered only in the course of a routine Pap smear. It is important, then, that all women have a Pap smear once a year. Biannual Pap smears might be a good idea for those women who are at high risk because of a particular history of sexual activity (see above) or a history of herpes infections or exposure to DES-type drugs or who are in the 40-to-50 year old age-group and thus are more likely to develop such cancer.

However, the Pap smear is only a screening test. Although it is 95 percent accurate in detecting cancer, it is not always accurate in indicating the seriousness of the disease. It is possible that the smear will show carcinoma in situ or even less serious cervical dysplasia when in fact invasive cancer is present. It is important, then, that the Pap smear be followed by a cervical biopsy. The Pap smear contains only isolated cells, but the biopsy provides a tissue specimen, which allows the pathologist to study the architecture of the cells. By studying the cells in relation to one another, the pathologist can make a more accurate diagnosis.

Scrapings may also be taken from the cervical canal in order to help the doctor determine whether the disease has spread to this area. Certain cases will require conization, in which the central core of the cervix is removed, a process somewhat akin to removing the core from an apple. The reasons for doing a conization, as well as important information about cervical biopsies, are discussed under the heading Cervical Dysplasia. In addition, a conization is always done in cases where the biopsy has indicated that the woman has microinvasive cancer (see below). *No woman should accept a diagnosis or treatment of microinvasive cancer unless a surgical cone has been done.* A simple biopsy does not provide enough tissue to allow for an accurate diagnosis of microinvasion; tissue samples from the more extensive conization procedure are necessary, for only three-quarters of cases diagnosed as microinvasive on biopsy will turn out to be so when a surgical cone is done.[15]

Moreover, it is essential that a number of sections of the cone be examined, for studies have shown that in busy labs, where only one section was studied, errors have run as high as 17 percent. Women should make sure that a board-certified pathologist (*see* p. 711) has examined her tissue slides.

Once the diagnosis of invasive cervical cancer has been confirmed by biopsy or, if necessary, by conization, the next step is staging the disease.

Staging is made before surgery and is based on the doctor's estimate of how far the disease has spread. Table 10 outlines the most widely used staging scheme for cervical cancer. TNM classifications, as outlined in Table 11, have recently been used as well.[16]

The first step in staging is a careful palpation of the cervix, vagina, bladder, uterus, rectum, pelvic lymph nodes and abdomen. This helps the doctor determine the size and spread of the cancer. Knowing the size is important, because smaller cancers are much less likely to have spread beyond the cervix and therefore will require less aggressive treatment.

Obviously, the skill and experience of the doctor will affect the accuracy of the staging. But in some cases even the best doctors will not be able to make an accurate pretreatment estimate of the spread of the disease. Scar tissue from previous pelvic diseases may lead the doctor to believe that cancer is present in areas where, in fact, there is no malignant disease. Similarly, lymph nodes may be swollen as a result of infection, and this swelling may be mistaken for the presence of cancer. On the other hand, the cancer may have spread to the surrounding tissue but may be too small or too inaccessibly placed to be felt, or the lymph nodes may contain cancer cells without being noticeably swollen. Then, too, not all nodes may be involved, and those that are may be too deeply placed to be felt.

Certain tests can help the doctor in making his or her estimate. Routine blood and urine tests may be of help. Chest X-rays are also done to rule out the possibility that the disease has already spread to the lungs. X-ray studies may be done to assess kidney, bowel and liver function. Specialized viewing instruments may be used to examine the bladder, lower colon and rectum.

Table 10
Staging Scheme for Cervical Cancer

Stage O:	Carcinoma in situ, also called intraepithelial carcinoma grade III, in which the cancer is limited to the outer skin (epithelial) layer of cervical tissue
Stage I:	Cancer strictly limited to the cervix
	Stage IA: Microinvasion, also called early stromal invasion. The cancer has penetrated deeper than the epithelial level described in Stage O, but the penetration into the lower tissue is limited to a depth of not more than 5 mm (some authorities use 3 mm as the cutoff point).
	Stage IB: The cancer is still limited to the cervix, but the penetration is more than 5 mm.
Stage II:	The cancer has extended beyond the cervix but has not extended to the pelvic wall.
	Stage IIA: The cancer has extended down into the vagina and all or part of the upper third of the vagina is involved, although the parametrium, the connective tissue surrounding and supporting the cervix, is not.
	Stage IIB: Same as above, only the parametrial tissues are involved, but not all the way to the pelvic wall.
Stage III:	The disease has now invaded the side wall of the pelvis and/or the lower third of the vagina.
	Stage IIIA: The cancer has invaded the lower half of the vagina but has not reached the pelvic wall.
	Stage IIIB: The cancer has reached the pelvic wall.
Stage IV:	The cancer has extended beyond the pelvis and/or has involved the bladder or rectum.
	Stage IVA: The bladder and/or rectum are involved.
	Stage IVB: Distant metastases

Table 11
TNM Classifications for Cervical Cancer

T = Primary Tumor

T1S:	Carcinoma in situ
T1:	Tumor confined to the cervix
T1a:	Microinvasive tumor
T1b:	Tumor beyond microinvasion but still confined to the cervix

Table 11
TNM Classifications for Cervical Cancer (continued)

T2:   Tumor extending beyond the cervix but not reaching the pelvic wall, or cancer
         involving the vagina but not the lower third
         T2a: Tumor has not infiltrated the tissues adjacent to the uterus and cervix
         T2b: Tumor has infiltrated beyond just the tissues adjacent to the uterus and
                cervix

T3:   Tumor involving either the lower third of the vagina or reaching the pelvic wall

T4:   Tumor involving the bladder and/or rectum or extending beyond the pelvis
         T4a: Tumor involving the bladder and/or rectum
         T4b: Distant metastases

N =Lymph Nodes

NX: Not possible to examine the nodes
N0:   No clinically obvious nodal involvement
N1:   Nodes involved as shown by diagnostic tests
N2:   Nodes involved

M =Metastasis

M0:   No evidence of metastases
M1:   Distant metastases

Stage/TNM Correlations*

Stage O:	T1S		
Stage I-A:	T1a	NX	M0
Stage I-B:	T1b	NX	M0
Stage II-A:	T2a	NX	M0
Stage II-B:	T2b	NX	M0
Stage III:	T3	NX	M0
	T1b	N2	M0
	T2a	N2	M0
	T2b	N2	M0
Stage IV-A:	T4	NX	M0
	T4	N2	M0
Stage IV-B:	Any M1		

*N0 and N1 are not taken into account in Stage grouping.

All the information gained from the palpation and tests to detect metastases (*see* p. 714) is used to stage the disease and to decide on the correct treatment. Unfortunately, this preoperative diagnosis or staging process is frequently in error. Indeed, in some 30 percent of cases the estimate of disease spread is incorrect. Because of this high rate of error, researchers have long sought other, more accurate methods of staging.

One of these is lymphangiography, which involves injecting a substance into the lymph system that will show up on X-ray film. Unfortunately, studies have shown that the estimates of lymph node involvement based on the lymphangiogram are wrong in more than 50 percent of cases. Too many times the lymphangiograph completely missed the cancer. The process is, nonetheless, of some value. When correlated with the results of palpation it may provide important clues. Moreover, a dye added to the injected substance will stain the nodes, and if surgery is the treatment of choice, this will make it easier for the surgeon to locate the nodes and remove them. The lymphangiogram can also act as a map for the radiotherapist if irradiation is the treatment of choice.

Another pretreatment method used by many doctors is an exploratory operation called a staging laparotomy. The doctor makes an incision in the abdomen that allows for direct inspection of all the pelvic organs and the lymph nodes for signs of disease. Biopsy specimens of suspicious lymph nodes are collected and examined. The staging laparotomy can help in making a more accurate estimate of disease spread and allows for removal of lymph nodes that may be too large to be cured by radiation therapy. The staging laparotomy also allows for biopsy of certain lymph nodes, known as the para-aortic nodes, that are located higher in the body, roughly at the level of the belly button. These nodes are not necessarily included in the field of radiation when treatment is given. Thus if cancer is present in these nodes, it will not be destroyed by the usual therapy. Anywhere from 30 percent to 50 percent of women with Stage III and Stage IV disease may have cancer in these para-aortic lymph nodes.[17] Unfortunately, the biopsy of the para-aortic nodes may not always indicate the cancer. The staging laparotomy is not, then, 100 percent accurate. And it's much more useful at the later stages of cancer. For instance, in Stage IB only 7 percent of the women show positive nodes; 93 percent do not.[18] For the majority of these women, then, the operation would not be beneficial. Moreover, the complications, which include death, may outweigh the benefits. Some lives have definitely been saved by prestaging laparotomy, but because of the risks, it is presently a controversial procedure. Most experts agree that if it is done, it should be done only on patients thought to have at least Stage IIB disease who are otherwise in good health and are therefore good operative risks.[19] This issue should be thoroughly discussed before surgery by the woman and her doctor.

Treatment

The treatment of cancer is always a complex subject. In some ways the treatment of cervical cancer, which usually involves either surgery or radiation therapy, or, in some cases, a combination of the two, is especially complex, because there is such a variety of treatment programs. Indeed, there are more than 10 surgical procedures that may be used in the treatment of this form of cancer. In another sense the treatment of cervical cancer is a fairly simple, straightforward subject, for although there are many treatment options, the decision as to which form of treatment should be given is fairly well defined—or at least more so than with other forms of cancer. In contrast to breast cancer, where the same woman might be treated in radically different ways, depending on the personal philosophy of the doctor doing the treatment, a woman with cervical cancer is apt to get pretty much the same treatment regardless of whom she sees. One surgeon or radiation therapist may be better or more skilled than another, but the same basic treatment approach will be used. There are exceptions to this generalization, however, especially in Stage IA, where there is some controversy, and, to a lesser degree, in Stage IB and Stage IIA, where there is a choice between radiation and surgery. Moreover, although Stage IV cases are generally treated by radiation, certain Stage IVA cases may be treated surgically.

In Stage IB and Stage IIA, where there is a choice between surgery and radiation, it is especially important that a woman with cervical cancer have opinions from both a radiologist and a surgeon. Human nature being what it is, specialists tend to think that if a choice of treatments exists, their specialty should be that choice. Thus, as a general rule, surgeons will recommend surgery and radiologists will favor radiation therapy. At larger cancer centers a team approach, involving experts from each specialty in the treatment decision-making process, is standard. At other places these routine consultations among experts may not automatically take place and a woman should then ask for second opinions or consultations (*see* p. 238) with board-certified doctors from each specialty. In cases where there is a difference of opinion as to the type of surgery, as there is in Stage IA, women should seek second opinions or consultations from various surgeons.

The basic aim of treatment, whether it's surgical or radiation therapy, is to destroy the cancer that is in the cervix, the adjacent tissues to which it may have spread and, in most cases, the lymph nodes in the area. The type of treatment chosen will depend largely on the extent of the disease and the age and general health of the woman.

Radiation Therapy

Radiation therapy is given in one of two ways:

External Beam Therapy: This type of radiation is delivered from outside the body by means of a beam of radiation generated by a machine and directed at an area of the body. With cervical cancer the beam of radiation is directed at the pelvic area and is designed to destroy cancer both in the tissues adjacent to the cervix and uterus and in the pelvic lymph nodes. In some cases the area radiated is more extensive and includes the para-aortic lymph nodes, which are located at about the level of the navel. In advanced cases, Stage III and Stage IV, some doctors routinely radiate this area in all their patients receiving curative radiation therapy; however, radiation to this area involves a significantly greater number of complications, some of which may be fatal.[20] Some doctors do the prestaging laparotomy discussed earlier and make the decision about radiation to the para-aortic nodes on this basis. The question of how to treat the para-aortic nodes is controversial. Women should discuss this issue as it applies to their cases with their doctors.

Often external beam therapy is given first because it will shrink the tumor, making it more susceptible to radiation implants. At other times implants are used before external beam therapy. In cases where the woman is in such poor health that she cannot withstand the anesthesia required for implants, external beam therapy is used alone, but the chances of a cure are usually reduced if the two methods of delivering radiation cannot be combined.

Intracavity Implants: This form of therapy is designed to destroy the cancer in the cervix, as well as any cancer in the uterus and vagina. Special containers are inserted into the vagina and the uterus, loaded with a radioactive material, and left in place until the specified dose of radiation has been achieved. In certain cases, hollow tubes or needles inserted into the tumor are used.

In some cases internal implants cannot be used. If, for instance, the woman has had previous pelvic surgery or pelvic inflammatory disease, there may be too much scar tissue in the pelvis. Older women whose vaginas and uteri are smaller, inelastic and distorted may be poor candidates for internal implants, because their anatomies will not permit the insertion of containers large enough to deliver an evenly spread dose of sufficient quantity to destroy the cancer.

Surgery

As mentioned earlier, there are a number of different surgical procedures used to treat cervical cancer. The most commonly used forms are described below:

Radical Hysterectomy and Pelvic Lymphadenectomy: This operation involves removal of the uterus, tubes, the tissues immediately adjacent to the uterus and cervix and the upper third of the vagina. The ovaries are usually removed as well, although in younger women the ovaries may be preserved in order to avoid a premature menopause. The pelvic lymph nodes are also removed.

Pelvic Exenteration: This operation removes all the pelvic organs, including the uterus, tubes, ovaries, adjacent pelvic tissues, the vagina, the bladder and/or the rectum. In some cases a partial exenteration procedure in which either the bladder or the rectum is preserved may be done. If the bladder is removed but the rectum is preserved, the urinary tract may be diverted to the bowels. If the rectum and/or the bladder are removed, new openings must be created on the outside of the body and waste products collected in plastic bags.

Stage-by-Stage Treatment Programs

Many factors will affect the choice of treatment. Stage-by-stage treatment programs are outlined below. Treatment of cervical cancer is not standardized but is highly individualized, and each case must be considered on its own merits. If the treatment recommended by your doctor differs from the treatment outlined below, this certainly does not mean that your doctor's recommendations are wrong; however, every woman has the right to know which type of therapy is planned and why. The following information is intended to provide a *general* understanding of the types of therapy available and the reasons for their use, so that you will have enough information to know the right questions to ask and to be able to evaluate your doctor's treatment recommendations.

Stage IA

The treatment of Stage IA, or microinvasive, cancer is somewhat controversial.[21] There is general agreement that it should be treated by some form of surgery (unless, of course, the woman is in such poor health that surgery is out of the question; such women are treated by radiation).

There is considerable disagreement, however, as to how extensive the surgery should be. A few doctors believe that a simple conization will suffice. Other doctors think that a radical hysterectomy and pelvic lymphadenectomy is necessary. Between these two extremes are the doctors who recommend either simple hysterectomy (removal of just the uterus and cervix); the somewhat more extensive radical hysterectomy, without the pelvic lymphadenectomy; or the Schauta procedure (also called the radical vaginal hysterectomy), which is rarely done anymore.

One reason that there is such disagreement about the extent of the surgery needed to treat microinvasive cancer is that no one is sure how this form of cancer behaves. We know that in more extensive cancer, like Stage IB, even though the cancer appears to be confined to the cervix, there is a significant chance that cancer cells are lurking in the supportive tissues immediately adjacent to the cervix and uterus or in the pelvic lymph nodes, so that these areas must be dealt with in planning treatment for Stage IB. Obviously, those who favor the radical hysterectomy and pelvic lymphadenectomy for Stage IA feel that there is a chance, although a small one, that the adjacent tissues and pelvic lymph nodes are harboring unsuspected cancer despite the microinvasive diagnosis. Those who favor the Schauta procedure or radical abdominal hysterectomy believe that Stage IA cancers may be accompanied by unsuspected cancer in the supportive tissues adjacent to the cervix, although not in the lymph nodes. Those who favor a simple hysterectomy think that neither the adjacent tissues nor the pelvic lymph nodes are harboring cancer cells and that removal of these tissues is therefore not necessary.

Even though they don't sound much different on paper, the radical hysterectomy and the pelvic lymphadenectomy involve significantly higher complication rates and mortality than the simple hysterectomy. For one thing, the ureters, the tubes that conduct urine from the kidneys to the bladder, may be damaged and a fistula, a hole, may be created. If this happens, the woman may have to have an operation whereby a new opening for urinary wastes is made and the urine then collected in a plastic bag attached to the outside of the body. Then, too, there is a higher death rate for radical operations than for a simple hysterectomy. All this must be balanced against the chances that doing less than a radical hysterectomy will leave microscopic areas of cancer behind.

A few doctors will argue that conization is sufficient, but most doctors believe that this form of surgery is inadequate for Stage IA cases. Even if the tissue removed by conization encompasses the entire microinvasive area, they think that the chances are too great that cancerous or precancerous cells may be lurking in the remaining portions of the cervix. Because some areas of the cervix have already ''gone bad''—have developed invasive cancer—they believe that there may be some basic fault in the cervical tissue that will eventually produce more cancer, which, if not detected in time, could become truly invasive cancer. If this happened, the woman's chances of surviving would be significantly reduced. Therefore, the majority of doctors do not advocate conization for Stage IA. Women whose doctors do suggest that conization is adequate treatment would be wise to seek a second opinion.

One reason that no one is sure how microinvasive cancer behaves, that is, whether or not the tissues adjacent to the cervix and the pelvic lymph nodes are ever involved, is that definitions of microinvasion differ. Basically, microinvasive cancer is a carcinoma cancer that is ''in place,'' that has begun to invade, but the invasion is in its very early stages. In fact, the invasion is microscopic. Some authorities are very conservative and define microinvasion as penetration of 3 mm or less; others use 5 mm as the cutoff. Still others think that it is the total volume of the cancer that is significant. Most doctors believe that evidence of invasion of the blood or lymph vessels excludes a diagnosis of microinvasion.

Because the definitions of microinvasion differ, it is difficult to compare the results of studies that attempt to find out whether microinvasion does or does not involve these adjacent tissues and lymph nodes. Studies in which radical hysterectomies and pelvic lymphadenectomies were done on women diagnosed as having microinvasive cancer and in which the removed lymph nodes were examined microscopically have reported between 0 percent and 5 percent incidence of lymph node involvement.[22] The trouble is that the authors of these studies have used different definitions of microinvasion. However, it seems fairly certain that microinvasive cases in which the penetration is less than 3 mm and the width less than 2.5 cm, and in which there is no sign of blood or lymph vessel penetration, don't involve the pelvic lymph nodes or adjacent tissue. A simple hysterectomy will therefore suffice in these cases.[23] Women with microinvasive cancer should discuss the various treatment options as they relate to their particular cases and should seek second opinions before deciding on a course of treatment.

Stages IB and IIA[24]

In Stage IB and Stage IIA it is necessary to treat the cervix, uterus, upper third of the vagina and the pelvic lymph nodes, for even when there is no obvious sign of involvement of these areas, there is a high likelihood that they are involved in the disease process.

Two forms of treatment, surgery and radiation therapy, are used to treat Stage IB and Stage IIA. In certain instances they may be used in combination. Both forms of treatment have been shown to be about equally effective in terms of survival rates. Generally speaking, if the woman is in good health, a radical hysterectomy and pelvic lymphadenectomy will be done, for this allows for better vaginal function. Radiation therapy causes a narrowing of the vaginal canal, a condition known as vaginal stenosis, which can make intercourse painful or downright impossible. Even though the upper portion of the vagina is removed surgically, and the vaginal canal is therefore shortened, intercourse is usually still possible.

Moreover, radiation destroys the ovaries, whereas surgery can sometimes allow for preservation of the ovaries. This is important in younger women, for destruction of the ovaries can cause premature menopause, which is apt to be more severe than a natural menopause. Even if the ovaries must be removed surgically, the operation is preferable to radiation, for there is some evidence that radiation-induced menopause puts a woman at higher risk for hypertension than a surgical or natural menopause.

Moreover, it is known that radiation can cause as well as cure cancer. By having surgical treatment the woman can avoid exposure to dangerous radiation. For older women this may not be as important a consideration as it is for younger women, since it may take 15 to 20 years for the radiation-induced cancer to develop.

If, after microscopic examination of the tissues removed surgically, cancer is found in the lymph nodes or at the outermost edges of the removed tissue, external beam therapy is given postoperatively. Postoperative radiation is also given if the cancer turns out to be more advanced than was originally thought, if there is any sign of ovarian involvement or if the tumor turns out to be too widespread for complete surgical removal. Radiation therapy is also used in cases where the woman's health will not permit surgery. External beam therapy is generally given first, before internal radiation. This shrinks the tumor and makes it easier to insert the containers for the radioactive implants. One advantage that radiation has over surgery in these cases is that should the woman treated with surgery require postoperative radiation, her complication rates are much higher. If she had been treated with radiation in the first place, she would have had fewer problems. Of course, the assumption in these Stage IB and Stage IIA cases is that the woman will not require postoperative radiation, but as explained above, pretreatment estimates of the disease are frequently wrong. On operation the disease may turn out to be more serious, requiring postoperative radiation.

In certain instances external beam therapy may be followed by surgery in the form of a hysterectomy. This is done when the woman has a tumor that is large and has caused the cervix to assume a bulky, barrel shape and protrude into the vagina. Such tumors are difficult to treat with radiation implants because of their size and because they distort the anatomy so much that the proper containers can't be inserted.

Stages IIB and IIIA and B[24]

The treatment choice in these cases is limited, for the disease has spread so widely that surgical removal is not feasible. The complication and fatality rates would simply be too high, so radiation is the treatment of choice. Generally, external beam therapy is given first, followed by radiation implants. In certain cases interstitial radiation, which involves inserting needles directly into the tumor, may be used.

Stage IV[24]

Most cases are treated with radiation therapy; however, in certain instances Stage IV surgery may be the treatment of choice. For example, if a woman has Stage IVA disease, in which the bladder and/or rectum is involved, but there is no evidence that the tissues adjacent to the uterus are involved, partial or total pelvic exenteration may be done, for the bladder and rectum are extremely sensitive to radiation and doses sufficient to kill the tumor would destroy these organs. In other Stage IV cases radiation therapy may be used. Sometimes, when the disease has spread to distant points in the body, lower doses of radiation may be given in hopes of providing relief of symptoms even if it is not possible to cure the disease.

389

Follow-Up and Recurrent Cancer[24]

Women who have been treated for cervical cancer will need lifelong follow-up. The nature of the follow-up program depends on the extent of the initial disease. Many cases of recurrent cancer are asymptomatic and may be discovered only when a Pap smear is made. If a woman has been treated by radiation therapy, however, there may be problems in diagnosing recurrent cancer, for radiation can alter the character of the cells and the Pap smear may be hard to read. Needle biopsies or conization may then be necessary.

Although many cases of recurrent cancer are asymptomatic, there is a classic triad of symptoms that is often present, which includes swelling of the legs, pain in the lower back and urinary problems.

Treatment of recurrent cancer will depend on what type of therapy was used initially. If radiation was used to treat the original cancer, surgery must be used to treat the recurrent cancer, for, assuming that the woman was treated properly in the first place, the tissues in the area will already have had the maximum dose of radiation they can tolerate.

If the recurrent cancer is limited to the cervix, a radical hysterectomy and pelvic lymphadenectomy may suffice. But most recurrent cancer has already spread beyond the cervix and will require a partial or total pelvic exenteration. Not all women with recurrent cancer are in good enough health to allow for this radical form of surgery. For those who are, there is a 20 percent to 30 percent 5-year survival rate following pelvic exenteration,[25] so the operation may well be worth the risks. Several factors affect a woman's chances of surviving after radical surgery for recurrent cancer, including the presence or absence of obvious symptoms, the location and extent of the recurrence, the time between the primary treatment and the diagnosis of recurrent cancer and the results of special X-ray studies known as intravenous pyelograms. Each woman should discuss the exenteration procedure and survival rates as they apply to her case before deciding about this procedure.

If the woman was initially treated by surgery, the recurrent cancer is generally treated by radiation therapy. But in cases where the initial surgery was minimal, it may be possible to do more extensive surgery for recurrent cancer.

Survival Rates

Survival rates for cervical cancer are generally given in terms of 5 years. Table 12 reflects typical survival rates.

Table 12
Five-Year Survival Rates for Cervical Cancer*

Stage	Percent
I	79.2
II	58.1
III	32.5
IV	8.2

*SOURCE: Juan A. del Regado and Harlan J. Spjot, *Cancer,* 5th ed.
(St. Louis: C.V. Mosby Co., 1977), p. 789.

The Uterus and the Fallopian Tubes

The anatomy of the uterus and the fallopian tubes is described and illustrated in Chapter Two. The uterus has two parts, the body, or fundus, and the neck, or cervix. In this section we are concerned only with diseases that affect the fallopian tubes and the body of the uterus; cervical diseases are discussed in a separate section.

In some cases the uterus and tubes are just the focal point for more widespread pelvic diseases. For instance, the first disease in this section, pelvic inflammatory disease, may involve only the fallopian tubes or, less frequently, only the endometrial lining of the uterus; however, the infection in the tubes may spill out into the pelvic cavity, causing a more generalized infection. In a similar vein, endometriosis, described under the second heading in this section, is a condition that can affect the entire pelvic cavity. In endometriosis the endometrial tissue, which is normally found only on the inside of the uterus, grows on the ovaries or other organs in the abdominal cavity. Adenomyosis, the third condition discussed in this section, is basically the same as endometriosis, the only differences being that adenomyosis is usually diagnosed in older women and that the misplaced endometrial tissue is not spread throughout the pelvic cavity but is confined to the muscular tissue of the uterine walls.

Another set of problems that may involve the uterus and tubes are conditions that cause distortions of the normal anatomy. A woman may have congenital abnormalities and may be born with a uterus or tubes that are malformed or absent altogether. The uterus may not lie in the usual anatomical location. It may be tipped forward or backward. It may fall, or prolapse, to a lower position than normal. The anatomy of the uterus may also be disturbed by a condition known as Asherman's syndrome, in which the walls of the endometrial cavity are partially or totally stuck together.

Abnormal growths may be found in the uterus and/or the fallopian tubes. These may be noncancerous, like fibroid tumors, endometrial polyps and benign tumors of the tube, or they may be malignant, as in cancer of the uterus or cancer of the fallopian tube. Sometimes the endometrial lining of the uterus grows too thick, a condition known as hyperplasia, which, in some instances, may be the first step on the road to cancer.

Many of the conditions described in this chapter will cause abnormal uterine bleeding or irregular menstrual periods; however, a separate section, Menstrual Problems, is devoted to these topics.

PELVIC INFLAMMATORY DISEASE
AKA: PID

Types: subacute pelvic inflammatory disease
acute pelvic inflammatory disease
chronic pelvic inflammatory disease

Associated Terms: endometritis; endoparametritis; paraendometritis; salpingitis; oophoritis; peritonitis; pelvic cellulitis; tubal occlusion; tubal, tubo-ovarian, or pelvic abscess; tubo-ovarian cyst; pyosalpinx, hydrosalpinx, or pyohydrosalpinx; thrombophlebitis; blood poisoning or septicemia, actinomyces, chlamydia

Pelvic inflammatory disease (PID) is a catch-all phrase that refers to infections of the pelvic organs. PID has become increasingly common, affecting 500,000 women each year, and the disease can have serious, even fatal, consequences.[1] The disease may be subacute, acute or chronic. Subacute is the least severe and most common type. It is slow in its onset, and mild or moderate symptoms may persist for some time before a woman seeks treatment. Acute PID refers to an infection that is more sudden in its onset and more severe. The woman is apt to experience a sudden onset of pain, weakness and fever or chills. Chronic PID is a low-grade infection that may persist for a week or months, and in some women it never seems to go away completely. There may be constant mild, moderate or even severe pain, or the chronic infection may flare up occasionally, causing acute attacks.

Spread of PID

PID starts when germs from the vagina make their way through the cervical canal (the opening that leads from the vagina into the uterus) into the sterile (germ-free) uterus. Most of the time the cervical canal forms a natural barrier to prevent germs that normally live in the vagina or germs that have been introduced into the vagina by sexual intercourse or other means from getting into the uterus. However, at certain times the cervical canal is more dilated (opened up). For example, it is slightly dilated during your period to allow for the passage of menstrual blood. The cervical canal is also more dilated after childbirth, miscarriage, abortion, insertion of an intrauterine device (IUD) and certain gynecological operations, such as a D&C. At such times germs from the vagina can penetrate the natural barrier of the cervix and move into the uterus. The strings of the IUD may also serve as a ladder, allowing germs from the vagina to migrate up into the uterus.

Once in the uterus these germs may infect the blood-rich lining of the uterus (the endometrial lining, which thickens and is shed each month during the menstrual period). The term endometritis is used to refer to infections of the endometrial lining. Unfortunately, PID is rarely confined to the lining of the uterus. The blood in the lining provides a perfect breeding ground for germs, so the infection spreads rapidly. If the uterine wall also becomes infected, the terms endoparametritis and paraendometritis may be used. Frequently, the infection spreads to the fallopian tubes. If the tubes are infected, the term salpingitis is used. The infection may then spread along the length of the tubes and spill out the ends of the tubes, infecting the ovaries. Infections of the ovaries are called oophoritis. The infection may also spill into the pelvic cavity, causing an infection of the peritoneum, the layer of tissue that coats the inside of the pelvic cavity. This condition is called peritonitis. (The term "peritonitis" is not exclusively associated with PID, for a number of conditions, including a burst appendix or a ruptured ovarian cyst, can cause peritonitis.) If the infection spreads through the lymph or blood system, causing a generalized pelvic infection, the term "pelvic cellulitis" may be used.

The body typically attempts to defend itself from the spreading infection. Infection-fighting blood cells attempt to combat the infection, which can result in a good deal of pus that may distend the tubes. Cells surrounding the inflamed, infected areas of the tube secrete fibrous material that solidifies and forms bands of scar tissue or adhesions within the tube to block off the infected area. The ends of the tube may seal themselves off, either partially or totally, with adhesions in an attempt to halt the spread of the infection. In this manner, tubal occlusions (blockages), tubal abscess (collections of sealed-off infection and pus) or a hydrosalpinx (a watery collection of pus) may be formed. If the ovary is involved in the abscess, the term "tubo-ovarian abscess" or "tubo-ovarian inflammatory cyst" may be used to describe the condition. If the infection spills into the pelvic cavity, adhesions and abscesses, called pelvic abscesses, may be formed. Any of these abscesses may rupture (break open), leading to even more extensive infection and adhesions.

The adhesions may bind the tubes or other pelvic organs to the pelvic walls or to each other.

If the disease spreads through the blood system, infections in the veins may cause the formation of blood clots or cause blood poisoning (septicemia).

Complications

PID can be fatal if the infection becomes overwhelming, especially if septicemia or blood clots occur. Fortunately, most women with PID can be treated successfully before the disease progresses that far. In addition to death, PID carries other serious complications. The disease may become chronic, causing constant pain or intermittent flare-ups and necessitating hysterectomy, or it may cause infertility or sterility (inability to get pregnant) and ectopic pregnancy (a pregnancy in which the fertilized egg implants in the tube or some other abnormal location rather than in the uterus). Some of these complications may not become apparent until years after the PID has occurred, and they may occur even in women who have had only mild cases.

Ectopic Pregnancy

Between 1971 and 1977, as PID has become increasingly widespread, the incidence of ectopic pregnancies has doubled.[2] Half the cases are related to PID.[3]

Normally, the ovum (female egg) is fertilized by the sperm in the fallopian tube and travels to the uterus, where it implants in the uterine lining and grows into a baby. In women who have had PID and who have developed tubal adhesions or blockages, the sperm and ovum may be able to make their way past these barriers, so fertilization can still occur. But the fertilized egg may not be able to make it past these tubal barriers into the uterus, or pelvic adhesions from the PID may have impinged on the tube, inhibiting the normal contracting motion of the tube so that it cannot move the fertilized egg down the tube into the uterus. In such instances the fertilized egg implants in the tube rather than in the uterus, a situation known as an ectopic pregnancy. Because the tube cannot accommodate the developing pregnancy, it may burst, causing internal bleeding and necessitating immediate surgery. If too much blood is lost, the woman may die. The affected tube and ovary may need to be removed, and the remaining tube and ovary may be so damaged that the woman is rendered sterile. (See the section on ectopic pregnancy for details.)

Infertility and Sterility

In order to cure PID, removal of a woman's uterus, tubes and ovaries is sometimes necessary. In such cases the woman is sterile, unable to have children. As explained above, ectopic pregnancy can also result in sterility. In addition, PID can cause such severe tubal blockage, can restrict movement of the tube so completely that the woman cannot get pregnant. Sometimes a PID-related case of infertility can be cured by surgically removing the adhesions and unblocking the tube, but this is not always possible. Of the 500,000 women each year who develop PID, 34,000 to 92,000 will become sterile.[4] Others will be unable to get pregnant without surgical treatment.

Even a mild case can result in infertility or sterility. After a single episode of PID an estimated 9.4 percent of women aged 15 to 24 and 19.2 percent of women aged 25 to 34 (an average of 11.4 percent for all ages) will be infertile.[5] After two episodes of PID an average of 23.1 percent of women of all ages will become infertile (20.9 percent of women aged 15 to 24 and 31 percent of women aged 24 to 34). After three episodes of PID about 54.4 percent of women of all ages will become infertile (51.6 percent aged 15 to 24 and 60 percent aged 25 to 34).

Cause

As explained above, PID is caused by germs from the vagina ascending into the uterus, which is more apt to happen when the cervix is dilated. The strings of the IUD can also act as a ladder, allowing germs to travel along the strings into the uterus. It was thought that this problem occurred only with such IUDs as the Dalkon Shield, whose strings were twined together like a candlewick (*see* p. 119), but it is now thought that this can occur with any type of IUD. In fact, IUD users have a three- to fivefold increased risk of developing PID (see the section on the IUD).

Apparently, a number of organisms can cause PID. In the past, most cases of PID were attributed to *Gonococcus,* the organism that causes the sexually transmissible infection gonorrhea. Nowadays 80 percent of PID cases are nongonococcal.[6] Other organisms, some of which are sexually transmissible and some of which are normal inhabitants of the vagina or other areas of the body, are now implicated in PID, including *Chlamydia, Escherichia coli, Hemophilus, Actinomyces* and organisms called anaerobes (to mention a few). As it turns out, nongonococcal PID (i.e., PID caused by organisms other than *Gonococcus*) is generally more serious. Chronic PID and infertility occur more often in women who have nongonococcal PID.[7]

More than one organism may be at fault. Some doctors believe that the gonococcus initiates the pelvic infection and that this allows other organisms, such as *E. coli, Chlamydia* and anaerobes to further complicate the problem.[8] Still others believe that a combination of disease-causing organisms, which may or may not include *Gonococcus,* are involved in any given case of PID.

Symptoms

The kinds of symptoms produced by PID and their severity will depend on the type of germ causing the infection, the strength of the particular strain of bacteria, the organs that are affected as the disease spreads and the woman's own resistance to disease.

The symptoms, which may be mild, moderate or severe, may develop gradually or come on suddenly. Any of the following symptoms may occur with acute PID: abdominal pain or tenderness, low-back pain, pain during or after intercourse, persistent cramps, fever, chills, abnormal vaginal discharge, abnormal menstrual periods, bleeding between periods or after intercourse, urinary frequency and urgency, abdominal pain with bowel movements or urination, fatigue or weakness, cramping or rigidity of the abdominal muscles, swelling of the lymph nodes, nausea, vomiting or a rapid pulse.

Chronic PID may cause some of the same symptoms. The pain in chronic PID may range from a mild, bearing-down discomfort to a nagging discomfort in the lower abdomen to severe, sharp pains. The pain may be constant or may come and go. Characteristically, the pain symptoms are worse just before or during the menstrual period.

Diagnosis

Sometimes diagnosing PID is a fairly straightforward matter. A history of recent gonorrheal infection, childbirth, abortion, IUD insertion or other situations causing cervical dilation, plus the symptoms mentioned above, will make the doctor suspicious. Bimanual exam, which may be quite painful, may reveal tubal enlargement and the presence of tubal, tubo-ovarian or pelvic abscesses, which may feel hot and be extremely tender. Speculum exam may show pus dripping from the cervix, and the doctor will take a sample of the discharge and run a culture and sensitivity (C&S) test. This may indicate what type of organism is causing the disease and help the doctor to select an appropriate antibiotic. Unfortunately, C&S tests are not always accurate in determining the cause of PID. Even when pus is coming out of the uterus the

397

C&S test may be inaccurate, for a different organism may be at work in the tubes and ovaries than in the uterus.

The diagnosis of PID is not always an easy task. Both chronic and acute PID may be mistaken for a number of conditions, including appendicitis, ovarian cysts and tumors, ectopic pregnancy, fibroid tumors of the uterus or endometriosis. Sometimes the only way to make a definite diagnosis is through laparoscopic or culdoscopic examinations, in which specialized viewing instruments are inserted into the pelvic cavity through surgical incisions. In certain cases ultrasound or X-ray exams may be used in diagnosis.

Diagnosis can be a real problem in mild cases with subtle symptoms. One of the insidious things about PID is that a subtle, smoldering infection can cause infertility and lead to recurrent attacks of severe pain in the future. So if you have one of the symptoms described above, especially if you have recently given birth, had a miscarriage, abortion or surgery or have an IUD, be sure to consult a doctor.

Treatment

The treatment of PID, which involves some form of antibiotics, is a matter of some controversy. Not only is there some question as to which antibiotics should be used, but there is also debate as to *where* a woman should be treated. Some experts believe that *all* women with PID should be hospitalized; others think that many cases can be treated on an outpatient basis. Those who argue for hospitalization point out that the woman can be followed more closely in the hospital and that intravenous (IV) antibiotics can be used. Administering antibiotics directly into a vein allows for higher, more effective doses than can be absorbed through the stomach, when the drugs are given orally. Because the disease can become chronic if it is not eradicated successfully, and because it can lead to ectopic pregnancy and sterility, some experts believe that hospitalization and IV antibiotics are necessary, even in mild cases. Othere are of the opinion that mild cases can be treated on an outpatient basis.

All doctors agree that in certain instances the woman should be hospitalized; these instances include (1) a woman in whom the diagnosis is uncertain; (2) a woman who has or may have a tubal or pelvic abscess; (3) a woman with severe symptoms; (4) a pregnant woman; (5) a woman who has failed to improve after 48 to 72 hours of oral antibiotic therapy on an outpatient basis.

Regardless of whether they are administered orally or intravenously, antibiotics are given as soon as the diagnosis is made. It used to be that some doctors would wait until the results of a C&S were available before giving an antibiotic. But C&S tests take time and are not always accurate, so treatment is now begun immediately with a broad-spectrum antibiotic, such as tetracycline or doxycycline, that is effective against a wide variety of organisms. Although additional drugs may be given once the C&S results are known, a woman should not wait for C&S test results but should insist on immediate antibiotic therapy.

In the past, ampicillin was widely used in the initial treatment of PID, but tetracycline is now preferred, because it is more effective against *Chlamydia,* an organism frequently involved in PID (*see* p. 579).[9] In cases where the woman has an abscess or is an IUD user, IV metronidazole (*see* p. 309), which has recently been approved for this use by the Food and Drug Administration, may also be given.

Our knowledge of the organisms that cause PID and the specific drugs that are most effective against the disease is constantly being refined, so treatment recommendations change all the time. Not all doctors stay up-to-date with the latest research, so if you develop PID, you should ask your doctor what the Centers for Disease Control are currently recommending for PID. If your doctor does not know, you might consider getting a second opinion.

Even if you have been hospitalized and treated with IV antibiotics, you will need to take oral antibiotics for at least 10 days after you have completed the IV treatment. If you are being treated on an outpatient basis, you must return to the doctor within 2 to 3 days after you begin treatment, for evaluation of your progress. You must also return within 4 to 7 days after you have completed the oral medication, to make sure you are cured.

Many women are justifiably hesitant about taking antibiotics; however, PID is one of the instances in which antibiotics are vitally important. Attempting home remedies can be dangerous in treating acute or subacute PID. It is important to treat the disease as early and as effectively as possible in order to prevent adhesions and abscesses, which can lead to infertility, sterility, chronic pain, surgical removal of the pelvic organs or, in extreme cases, death. All the prescribed medications should be taken, even if the symptoms have subsided, for an incomplete course of medication can lead to recurrences.

In addition to antibiotics, bed rest and plenty of fluids to flush out the body are *vitally* important. Bed rest will prevent jarring of the uterus and tubes, which might aggravate the inflammation and slow down the healing process. Ideally, the woman should stay in bed until the pain is gone and her temperature has returned to normal, getting up only to use the bathroom and to eat. Vaginal or anal intercourse, which can move the pelvic organs, should be avoided because it could spread pus from one part of the tube to the other or even cause pus to spill out into the pelvic cavity.

Heat is helpful in treating PID, for the blood flow to the tubes may be severely restricted and heat will increase the blood flow to the area. It will also help in relieving the pain. Hot sitz baths three or four times a day will bring

399

heat to the pelvic area. Hot-water bottles and heating pads are less efficient but still effective.

Another controversy in the treatment of PID centers around how to deal with a woman who has an IUD and develops PID. Most doctors believe that the IUD should be removed *immediately,* because its presence can aggravate the situation and hinder treatment. However, some doctors will wait 48 to 72 hours before removing the IUD to see if the woman will improve. We think immediate removal is generally preferable. Women with PID should discuss this with their doctors, and any woman whose PID has not improved after 48 to 72 hours should *insist* on removal.

There is one instance in which insisting on removal may present a problem—at least for some women. If the woman is in the middle of the menstrual cycle* and has had intercourse since her last period, there is a chance that removing the IUD may result in pregnancy. The IUD works by making it impossible for the fertilized egg to implant in the uterus or by dislodging it soon after it implants. With the IUD removed at midcycle the woman could, then, get pregnant. Many doctors argue that PID *overrides* other considerations and that the IUD should be removed, even in midcycle. They point out that such women could be treated with the morning-after pill or that the lining of the uterus could be suctioned out when the IUD is removed, to prevent pregnancy. Or the woman could "wait and see" and have an abortion if necessary. But women who have moral objections to abortion or who think that even the morning-after pill or suctioning out the lining of the uterus is morally wrong may be faced with a dilemma. We encourage such women to have the IUD removed because of the risks involved in leaving it in place. But the final decision in such cases rests, of course, with the woman herself.

It should be noted that a rare form of PID, caused by an organism known as *Actinomyces,* may deserve special treatment. This is discussed more fully in the section on IUD.

Sometimes the disease will become chronic. Tissues may have been so damaged by the infection that they never heal properly, making a woman vulnerable to repeated infection, or the bacteria may become walled off by adhesions or become buried in pelvic abscesses, where antibiotics cannot reach them. Thus the woman may have a low-grade infection and chronic pain that may flare up in acute attacks of PID from time to time.

There are a number of treatment options with chronic PID. If oral antibiotics have failed, IV antibiotic treatment, as outlined above, may be tried. If,

*The middle of the cycle would be from Day 12 to Day 16 of the cycle in a woman with a 28-day cycle. For information about how to determine if you are in the middle, most fertile portion of your cycle, *see* pp. 65–67).

however, there are pelvic abscesses, even IV antibiotics may not work. In such cases it is sometimes possible to operate and drain the abscesses.

If a woman has tubo-ovarian abscesses, it may be necessary to operate to make sure that the ovarian enlargement is not caused by a benign or malignant ovarian tumor. Moreover, the abscesses could rupture and cause acute peritonitis or blood poisoning. In some cases it is possible to drain these abscesses.

Sometimes a hysterectomy is the only way for a woman to get relief from chronic pain; however, women should ask their doctors if IV antibiotics or drainage can be attempted before consenting to a hysterectomy. If the PID is not too severe, some women choose to live with their symptoms or to explore alternative therapies, like acupuncture, rather than having a hysterectomy. In certain cases it is possible to remove the uterus and obtain relief from chronic PID and yet spare at least one ovary, thereby preventing premature menopause. Women who are anxious to obtain relief but who are reluctant to have a premature menopause should investigate this possibility with their doctors.

Prevention

Women can minimize their chances of getting PID by being careful anytime the cervix becomes dilated. For 2 to 3 weeks after having an abortion, a D&C or a miscarriage nothing should be put into the vagina. This means no intercourse, tampons, fingers or douche nozzles. Nor should they take a bath, swim or douche. (Showers or sponge baths are all right.) After childbirth the same precautions should apply, but for a period of 6 weeks.

If a woman wants to minimize her chances of getting PID or has a history of pelvic infections, she should probably not use an IUD. IUD users have a three- to fivefold increased risk of developing PID as compared with nonusers.[10] Women who use barrier methods of birth control, such as the diaphragm and condom, are less likely to get PID.[11] Women who use the Pill have even a lower risk than women who use the barrier methods, probably because the Pill reduces the amount of menstrual blood.[12]

Avoiding intercourse during the menstrual period, especially for women who have a history of PID or who have multiple sex partners (and are therefore subject to more sexually transmitted infections), may also help prevent PID.

Wiping from front to back after a bowel movement will help prevent rectal bacteria from entering the vagina. Prompt treatment of vaginal infections may also help to prevent PID. Routine gonorrhea cultures are also an important part of PID prevention.

ENDOMETRIOSIS

Associated Terms: chocolate cysts

The uterus is lined with a special type of tissue, the endometrium, which, in response to stimulation by the female hormones, swells and thickens each month in preparation for the possibility of pregnancy. If there is no pregnancy, this blood-rich lining is no longer needed. It then breaks down, begins to shed and the menstrual flow starts. Normally, this type of hormone-responsive tissue is found only inside the uterus; hence the name, endometrial —*endo* ("inside") and *metrial* ("uterus") tissue.

With endometriosis it's a case of the right thing in the wrong place, for endometriosis is a condition in which the endometrial tissue is found growing outside the uterus. It may, for instance, be found on the ovaries or on the peritoneum, the layer of tissue that coats the surfaces of the organs and the interior walls of the pelvic cavity. In some rare cases it has even been found in such remote locations as the forearm and the lungs. Even though the endometrial tissue has wound up in some abnormal location, it continues to thicken, break down and shed each month, which, as we shall see, can cause pain and other problems.

Incidence

Because the condition is related to hormone production, it is not surprising that it is most commonly reported in women whose hormones are active, that is, women between the ages of puberty and menopause. Seventy-five percent of cases are reported in women aged 25 to 45. It has, however, been found both in adolescents and in older women who have passed menopause and are no longer menstruating. Some doctors think that pregnancy has a preventive or curative effect on endometriosis.

Cause

No one is certain what causes this condition. There are basically three theories, all of which may be correct. One theory is that tiny shreds of endometrial tissue find their way into the pelvic cavity through the fallopian tubes during menstruation. In other words, it's a sort of backup problem (please excuse the plumbing analogy). Instead of being shed through the cervical os into the vagina and onto a sanitary napkin or tampon, some bits of menstrual tissue and blood may float up through the tubes, spill out the ends and float around the pelvic cavity until they attach themselves to the ovaries or to one of the other organs in the area.*

Another theory is based on the fact that, for the most part, the tissue that makes up the organs in the female pelvis is the same basic tissue with various modifications. It all develops from the same fetal tissue. As the fetus grows, this tissue is modified. The simplest modifications of this basic tissue form one kind of organ; with a few more modifications there is another variety of tissue that becomes another sort of organ, and so on, until a very fancy material, the endometrial tissue, develops that can do all sorts of wonderful tricks and is complete with such options as the ability to respond to hormonal messages by growing rich and thick or breaking down and to feed the developing fetus in the case of pregnancy. In a sense, the other pelvic tissues are just endometrial tissues that didn't continue developing and get all these extra options. With all this unrealized growth potential in these other tissues it's not surprising, according to this theory, that here and there are nests of tissue that, perhaps in response to hormone stimulation, haven't stopped modifying. Thus this tissue goes on to get the extra options, even though they aren't necessary for the job it's supposed to be doing.

The third theory suggests that endometriosis may be spread through the blood or lymph systems, which would explain the presence, although rare, of endometriosis in some bizarre locations, such as the lungs, underarms and thighs.

Symptoms

Endometriosis can occur almost anywhere in the pelvic cavity. It will look and behave somewhat differently, depending on where the endometrial tissue is located.

On the ovaries, which are involved in about 60 percent of cases, there may be single or multiple areas of endometriosis. The areas may be as small as a pinhead and are rarely larger than an orange. The smaller ones look like blood blisters and may be blue, dusty red or brownish black, depending on how much fresh or old blood is present. Typically, both ovaries are affected.

The ovarian tissue may protect itself from this foreign endometrial tissue by growing a sort of lid of tissue over the implant, forming what is called an endometrial cyst. Since the misplaced endometrial tissue can respond to hormones just as the normal tissue within the uterus does, it may bleed cyclically, at the time of menstruation. Thus the cysts swell with menstrual blood. Over time this blood takes on a thick, tarry texture and turns dark brown;

*Vaginal tampons cannot *cause* the menstrual flow to back up. In fact, tampons actually act as a wick to draw the blood out of the uterus.

403

hence the term "chocolate cysts" that is sometimes used in reference to endometriosis.

The periodic swelling may cause the cyst to rupture, usually just before or immediately after menstruation. When the cyst breaks the contents are spilled into the pelvic cavity. This is one way in which bits of endometrial tissue may be spread to other parts of the pelvic cavity.

This swelling and rupture also explain much of the pain that is associated with endometriosis. The old blood from the cyst is highly irritating to the lining of the pelvic cavity and causes inflammation and pain. In some cases the pain may be so severe that emergency surgery is necessary.

In response to this inflammation the cells in the rest of the area secrete bands of fibrous material that solidify and, typically, seal over the ruptured cyst. These fibrous adhesions can literally plaster the ovary to the broad ligament, the wall of supportive tissue that extends from the side of the uterus to the wall of the pelvic cavity. Repeated spillage from ruptured cysts can produce adhesions that bind the organs together, so that the pelvic organs become one large, immovable mass. Then the pelvis can no longer yield to pressure. Movement of the cervix as a result of intercourse or a doctor's exam or any sort of pressure on this unyielding pelvis can produce severe pain and backache.

Endometriosis may also be present in other locations in the body, either in conjunction with endometriosis on the ovary or independently. If endometriosis is present on the lining of the pelvic cavity or on the supportive tissues that hold the uterus in place, it may look and behave somewhat differently. In most cases it appears as a varying number of small, blueberrylike spots. These may group together to form solid, knobby bumps. These areas of endometriosis may also menstruate at first, but as the disease progresses so much scar tissue is formed that the endometrial tissue is compressed and can no longer menstruate. Thus there will often be puckered, clawlike areas of endometriosis that are no longer active. The damage may be considerable before this inactive stage is reached, for the scarring draws more tissue to adjacent organs inward as it progresses. The endometrial tissue, even though it is no longer menstruating, may continue to swell somewhat each month. Since the scar tissue is firm and unyielding, this can result in a considerable amount of pain.

Endometriosis can also affect the large and small intestines. On the large intestine it may look just like cancer, but unlike cancer, endometriosis, except in rare instances, will not cause bleeding from the rectum. In the rare case where such bleeding is associated with endometriosis, it occurs only at the time of menstruation. In both the large and small intestines the endometrial implants can cause obstruction. In the large bowel this may cause increasing constipation, which worsens at the time of menstruation and is often accompanied by a sharp cramp and the urgent need to go to the bathroom even though little urine or feces is eliminated. In the small intestine this endometrial blockage may be associated with lower-abdominal pain, abdominal swelling and vomiting. These symptoms may also be aggravated at the time of menstruation but not as noticeably as in the large intestine.

If the endometriosis is extensive, it may involve the rectum, vagina and vulva. In the vagina it can be seen on speculum examination as firm, blue, domelike bulges. These may cause considerable pain on intercourse if located near the top of the vagina. Less often, these blue bulges may be seen on the vulva. If the rectum is involved, there may be severe intestinal cramps and pain when moving the bowels, especially at the time of the menstrual period.

Infrequently, endometriosis affects the bladder and the urethra, the tube that runs from the bladder to the urinary opening. When this does happen it can cause pain on urination, urinary retention, urinary frequency, very occasionally blood in the urine (particularly on or at the time of menstruation) and pain in the flanks radiating toward the groin.

Single nodules of endometrial tissue, called endometriomas, may be found in scars from operations and childbirth. Although such growths have appeared as long as 16 years later, most appear in less than 2 years. Similarly, these endometriomas may appear in the region of the belly button even if there has not been an operation. They may appear as blue bulges and occasionally will break through the skin and cause bleeding. In rare cases endometriomas have even been found in lungs, thighs, forearms and underarms. Endometriomas are firm, even hard, vary considerably in size and are painful and tender to the touch, especially when they swell as menstruation approaches.

In general, pelvic pain associated with the menstrual cycle is the earliest and most common symptom associated with endometriosis. The pain is usually one of two types. The first type of pain, associated with the menstrual period, typically occurs in women who have previously had relatively pain-free periods. It is usually steady and dull as opposed to cramplike and becomes progressively worse with each subsequent menstrual period. In contrast to this type of pain, the second type is a lower-abdominal pain that begins just before the period. It varies according to the location and extent of the endometriosis. In certain locations there is no pain. In fact, about 25 percent of women afflicted have no pain. In the early stages there is usually less pain, but it gets progressively worse.

One curious thing is that women with relatively little endometriosis may have a lot more pain than women who have fairly widespread implants. It is not entirely clear why this happens, but it is probably related to the amount of scar tissue, where it occurs and how often the cysts rupture. For example, women with large ovarian cysts may not ovulate, whereas those who have endometriosis only on the lining of the pelvic cavity often do. Absence of ovulation seems to cause the disease to regress and thereby minimizes pain.

Women who have endometriosis frequently have abnormal menstrual bleeding. About one-half to two-thirds of all patients with endometriosis have such problems. However, it is not clear that the irregular bleeding is caused by the endometriosis. The disease is often accompanied by associated problems, such as fibroids and uterine polyps. The bleeding may actually be caused by these associated diseases. If women with associated fibroids and/or polyps are eliminated, only about 20 percent of women with endometriosis will complain of menstrual irregularities.

Infertility is also common to women who have endometriosis; however, about 20 percent of the women involved already have one or more children. Often such women will be unable to add other children to their families no matter how hard they try. No one is sure just why such women are infertile. Perhaps the adhesions around the ovary and fallopian tube interfere with the normal process of ovulation. The pain associated with intercourse may have some relationship to the low fertility rate as well.

Diagnosis

At times the diagnosis of endometriosis is a simple matter, but at other times it can be tricky, especially when the endometriosis is minimal. The symptoms may alert the doctor to the possibility, but 25 percent of women with endometriosis will be asymptomatic. Moreover, many times the symptoms that are present could be caused by a number of diseases. Sometimes a careful bimanual exam will help the doctor make the diagnosis. If, for instance, the doctor can feel knobby endometrial growths in certain areas, it may clear up the confusion that often exists between endometriosis and chronic pelvic inflammatory disease. But sometimes the areas of endometriosis are too small to be felt or too inaccessibly placed to be reached by the examining doctor's fingers. Sometimes the doctor's palpation (feeling) will identify swollen areas that might be endometriosis but could also be other things. For instance, chocolate cysts on the ovaries may be large enough to be felt, but it may not be clear whether these are ovarian tumors or endometrial tissue.

It is often impossible, then, to make a definite diagnosis of endometriosis without actually taking a look at the pelvic organs by means of a laparoscopic examination, which involves making a small incision in the abdomen and inserting a lighted viewing instrument into the abdominal cavity. Sometimes a culdoscopic examination, which involves inserting a similar viewing instrument into the pelvic cavity through an incision in the upper vagina, will be useful.

Because a definite diagnosis can be obtained only by laparoscopic or culdoscopic examination, both of which involve the risks of surgery, in certain cases a woman might decide to try hormone therapy (described below) even though her doctor cannot be sure that she actually has endometriosis without these examinations. (This choice, however, cannot be made if the woman has ovarian enlargement, for reasons explained under Treatment.) However, since diagnosis made without benefit of laparoscopic or culdoscopic evaluation are wrong in more than 40 percent of cases, accepting treatment on the basis of a presumptive rather than a definite diagnosis may very likely mean that the woman is subjecting herself to unnecessary treatment. If a woman decides to accept treatment on the basis of the presumptive diagnosis, she should be convinced that the risks and expense of laparoscopy outweigh the risks and expense of undergoing possibly unnecessary hormone therapy.

Treatment[13]

Treatment of endometriosis is a complex subject. The type of treatment suggested will depend on many factors, including the age of the woman, the severity of the symptoms, the location and extent of the endometriosis and future childbearing plans. In certain cases there is general agreement among doctors about treatment of the condition, but in other cases there is considerable debate. Since there is such controversy, women with endometriosis should familiarize themselves with the various treatments available.

If the symptoms are not severe and the endometriosis is not widespread, a wait-and-see approach may be appropriate. Women nearing menopause may decide to avoid the risks and expense of treatment and to use painkillers or live with their symptoms, since, with the diminished output of ovarian hormones at menopause, the condition often regresses. Younger women with mild symptoms may make the same sort of decision, especially if they don't have an associated infertility problem or future childbearing plans. Even women in their 20s who *do* plan to have children in the future will sometimes decide to forego treatment, at least temporarily, for a number of women with endometriosis do achieve pregnancy without treatment. Indeed, spontaneous cures of endometriosis sometimes occur. But many doctors recommend that women with endometriosis begin their childbearing earlier than they may have otherwise intended because the disease generally becomes progressively worse and may impair fertility. Delaying pregnancy may make it difficult or even impossible for such women to get pregnant.

In cases where there are large areas of endometriosis on the ovaries a wait-and-see approach is not appropriate, even if the symptoms are minimal. This is true for a number of reasons. First, the enlargement of the ovaries may be caused by cancerous or noncancerous ovarian growths. Since this possibility exists, any persistent ovarian enlargement deserves investigation. Second, the possibility also exists that the ovarian endometrial cyst will rupture, necessitating emergency surgery. Rupture could also spread disease to other areas of the pelvic cavity, causing more severe symptoms and necessitating more radical surgery later on. Moreover, the endometrial cyst may continue to grow larger, progressively displacing the ovarian tissue and impairing ovarian function, which could bring on premature menopause or result in infertility.

When there are large areas of ovarian endometriosis, severe symptoms or an infertility problem that cannot be traced to another cause and that the woman is anxious to overcome, the wait-and-see approach must be abandoned. Two types of treatment are then available: hormone therapy and surgery.

Hormone Therapy

The idea of using hormones to treat endometriosis stemmed from the observations of early researchers that pregnancy, a time of high hormonal levels and suppression of ovulation, often resulted in cures, or at least 9 symptom-free months. Some researchers have since disputed this observation, claiming that as many cases of endometriosis progressed as regressed during pregnancy. The traditional recommendation that a woman have her first child at an early age and space her children every few years in order to prevent or cure endometriosis is therefore losing credibility, perhaps because women decided the "cure" (that is, having a large family) was more limiting than the disease. At any rate, aside from the question of whether or not the original observations about pregnancy and regression of endometriosis were valid, the fact remains that hormone therapy has worked for many women.

Over the years a variety of different hormone therapies have been used. All these treatments have one thing in common: They stop a woman from having her period. Stopping the process during which the thickened endometrial lining inside the uterus breaks down and is shed means that the misplaced endometrial lining won't thicken or shed either, and that the symptoms of endometriosis, which are aggravated by this thickening and shedding process, are therefore relieved. Sometimes stopping menstruation for a while also seems to "dry up" existing disease, resulting in a cure. In the past, male-type androgen hormones in the form of methyltestosterone, sold under such brand names as Metandren and Oreton, were used, but these often caused masculinizing side effects, like male hair-growth patterns, decrease in breast size, clitoral enlargement and deepening of the voice, some of which were not reversible once drug use was discontinued. Moreover, since this type of hormone therapy did not always suppress ovulation, there was a chance that the woman might get pregnant, and if so, there was the very real risk that the child would have abnormalities. Thus this type of therapy is rarely used today, and any woman whose doctor suggests it should question the reasoning behind this type of therapy. She should also seek a second opinion (*see* p. 238) before accepting such treatment.

High doses of estrogen were also used in the past; this therapy also produced a high rate of side effects of the type associated with any overabundance of estrogen (nausea, breast tenderness and weight gain). Moreover, the use of estrogen, particularly in high doses, has been associated with serious, even fatal, complications, so that it too has fallen out of favor.

Today a new drug, danazol, sold under the brand name Danocrine, is the preferred medical treatment for moderate and severe cases of endometriosis. It stops ovulation, preventing the egg from bursting out of its follicular sac. Without a burst follicle, no progesterone can be produced. Thus there is no shedding of endometrial tissue, which in turn means relief from symptoms. In addition, danazol seems to work directly on the endometriosis, "drying" it up. It also works faster than the other types of hormone treatments, often providing relief of pain during the first menstrual period after treatment is begun. Moreover, women taking danazol, unlike those taking progesterone-type drugs (see below), whose menstrual cycles may take many months or even years to return to normal after treatment is stopped, resume normal menstrual cycles within, at most, 3 months after the drug is discontinued. Thus the drug is particularly appropriate for women who have future childbearing plans. Then, too, while on the drug a woman reportedly cannot get pregnant, so the chances of hormone-induced birth defects are eliminated. Pregnant women should not, however, take danazol, for the possibility of birth defects does exist.

Danazol also has less severe side effects than many of the other hormone treatments. This is not to say that danazol doesn't have side effects; it does. It can cause weight gain, bloating, bleeding between periods, acne, growth of facial and chest hair, decrease in breast size, deepening of the voice, increased skin and hair oiliness, enlargement of the clitoris, and symptoms associated with diminished estrogen, such as hot flashes, postmenopausal vaginitis and postmenopausal vulvitis. The larger the dose, the greater the incidence of side effects. The original researchers testing danazol used 800-mg doses, but many doctors today believe that 600 or 400 mg will work as well. These lower doses significantly reduce side effects. Women taking danazol should discuss dosage levels with their doctors, for some of the masculinizing kinds of side effects may not be reversible once the drug is stopped.

Another advantage that danazol enthusiasts point out is that unlike other hormone treatments, danazol does not lead to a softening of ovarian endometrial growths, which has led to rupture of these growths in some women on other hormone therapies. However, other doctors have reported that this problem does exist in patients on danazol, so this point is still being debated.

Despite all its advantages in comparison with other hormone therapies, danazol is not the only type of hormone therapy recommended by experts, for

409

it has a big drawback in terms of cost. Danazol is expensive. Each 200-mg pill costs anywhere from $1 to $1.50. Treatment, depending on the dosage prescribed, costs anywhere from $2 to $6 a day! Minimally, the treatment takes 3 to 4 months and, in a number of cases, requires 9 months. Treatment, then, could cost anywhere from $180 to $1,600, and this figure includes only the cost of the drug. Office visits for checkups during the treatment period would, of course, add to the cost of treatment. Some insurance companies, realizing that use of danazol may preclude the necessity of even more costly surgery, will cover this expense; others will not. Medicaid programs may not cover the cost of danazol either; however, if the doctor is willing to write a letter explaining the need for this drug, payment can often be authorized.

Some women—those with certain heart and kidney conditions, those who are pregnant or breast-feeding, or those in whom side effects are too pronounced—cannot use danazol. If, for whatever reasons, danazol cannot be used, the second choice for hormonal treatment of moderate or severe endometriosis is a progesterone-type drug. Continual progesterone stimulation will stop the menstrual period. The progesterone drug used by many doctors is Provera. Its generic name is medroxy-progesterone. Provera is less expensive than danazol, sold under the brand name Danocrin, but also less effective. It carries the same risks and may cause the same side effects as the progesterone used in birth control pills, as well as estrogen-deprivation symptoms. It may soften ovarian endometrial implants, which could result in rupture and the spillage of the irritating contents into the pelvic cavity, causing pain, scar tissue (which could cause infertility) and further spread of the disease. Moreover, although it is unlikely, women on Provera can become pregnant. Pregnancy while on such hormones may result in birth defects.

The biggest problem with Provera is that it disrupts normal hormonal processes so thoroughly that it may take some time before normal menstrual cycles are resumed. Women who are using the injectable form of the drug, Depo-Provera (*see* p. 796), may become permanently infertile. Even with oral forms, subsequent pregnancy rates are low and disease-recurrence rates are high. The drug, then, to put it mildly, has serious drawbacks for a woman with future childbearing plans.

In mild cases of endometriosis it may not be necessary to use either danazol or Provera. Such cases may respond to treatment by low-dose oral contraceptives. Some doctors will merely put women with this problem on birth control pills. Preventing ovulation in this fashion, even though there may be withdrawal bleeding, can be effective in relieving symptoms in mild cases. More often it will be necessary to use the birth control pills continuously, rather than in the usual off/on cyclical dosage pattern followed when the pills are used for contraception. However, after a while, in order to prevent breakthrough bleeding, it may become necessary to take four to eight birth control pills a day, and the side effects from taking this many pills may be so severe that the woman has to discontinue treatment. Some doctors will stop the treatment for a week once dosage gets this high and then start again. The problems of softening and possible rupture also exist. This type of treatment is generally considered to control rather than cure the condition and is often followed by a recurrence of the endometriosis. It also prevents conception for the treatment period, which may be as long as 1½ years, and defeats the purpose of a woman who is seeking prompt treatment for endometriosis-related infertility. Many doctors have abandoned this form of treatment.

It should be noted that most doctors don't like to prescribe hormone therapy without first confirming the diagnosis of endometriosis by laparoscopy. As noted earlier, diagnoses made on the basis of physical exam are frequently wrong. Thus there is good possibility that the woman may have a condition that won't benefit from hormone therapy. It may even worsen. Moreover, the laparoscopic exam will reveal whether or not adhesions, which could be causing infertility, are present. If such adhesions are present, hormone therapy will not solve the infertility problem. Some doctors are strongly against giving hormone therapy without laparoscopic confirmation. They believe that before beginning treatment of this magnitude they want a laparoscopic exam to be sure the diagnosis is correct.

Other doctors are willing to try the less drastic forms of hormone therapy first, especially if they are fairly confident of their diagnosis. They point out that even laparoscopy done under a local anesthetic carries risk. Five out of every 1,000 women will have complications; about half those complications will be serious ones.[14] If a general anesthetic is used, the risk as well as the cost is increased.

Certain characteristic signs may make the doctor more sure that s/he is actually dealing with endometriosis. If the doctor feels nodules or thickenings on the uterosacral ligaments, the bands of supporting tissue that hold the uterus in place, or in the cul-de-sac, the area behind the uterus and in between it and the bowels, this increases the likelihood that the woman has endometriosis. If these signs are present and the woman has the classic symptoms of endometriosis, coupled with a family history of the disease, she may feel more comfortable about the doctor's diagnosis and thus may be willing to forego laparoscopy. But this is one of those areas in which there are no clear-cut medical answers, and each woman must, with the aid of the medical opinions she gathers, make her own decisions.

No type of hormone treatment is 100 percent effective. Approximately 30 percent to 40 percent of women using the most effective treatment, danazol, will have a recurrence of the disease within 3 years.[15] The treatment can, however, be repeated. No hormone therapy is effective in cases where there is marked ovarian enlargement. Still, most doctors think that hormone therapy, in the absence of marked ovarian enlargement, should be tried before resorting to surgery. There is some debate about the wisdom of trying hormone therapy before attempting surgery in women in their late 20s and early 30s who are anxious to have children, but before unraveling that issue the types of surgery used to treat endometriosis will be reviewed.

Surgery

The surgery may range from conservative—removal of the areas of endometriosis—to radical—removal of the uterus, ovaries and tubes.

In conservative surgery, which usually requires a general anesthetic, the doctor will remove as much of the endometriosis as possible by cutting, laser beam therapy, or burning with electric cautery, depending on where the endometriosis is located. If there are cysts on the ovary, these will be removed, leaving as much normal tissue as possible. Even if only a small nub of normal tissue is left, the ovary can often still function normally.

Some doctors will also do procedures known as presacral and uterosacral neurectomy, in which the nerves that transmit pain to the brain are cut. Even if the woman has not had pain as a symptom, some doctors will do this in order to prevent pain should the endometriosis recur. This procedure will also prevent involuntary contractions or spasms of the uterus thought by some doctors to be a factor in the backup through the tubes of endometrial tissues that causes the condition in the first place. Other doctors are less inclined to do this procedure, fearing that it will cause scar tissue reactions that could reduce fertility, one of the problems that they are often trying to avoid. It is important for women who have this procedure done to know that they may not have any pain in the first stages of labor and thus may not head toward the hospital until the middle of giving birth. (The woman occasionally may not make it to the hospital.) Women who have future childbearing plans and whose doctors suggest this procedure should seek a second opinion before making a decision.

If there are adhesions around the fallopian tubes or binding the pelvic organs together, these will also be cut. If the uterus has been pulled back toward the spine by adhesions, these adhesions are also cut. The doctor will then perform a uterine suspension, a procedure that tightens the uterine supports and lifts the uterus.

The problem with conservative surgery is that it doesn't always work. In a fair number of cases the disease will recur, requiring further surgery. A younger woman with hopes of future pregnancy may decide that the time she buys by conservative surgery is worth the risk of needing a second surgery, for she has a fair chance of achieving pregnancy. A woman who doesn't have future childbearing plans may decide that something more extensive than the conservative surgery described above is preferable. More radical surgery may be necessary when the disease is so extensive that there is no choice but to remove the uterus, ovaries and tubes, regardless of the woman's desire to have children. However, in some women the question of preserving the ovaries comes up. This is probably not a serious question when the woman is approaching or has passed menopause, but with younger women, removing the ovaries as well as the uterus will cause premature menopause, which may result in distressing problems and possibly increase her risk of certain serious diseases. Some doctors will simply do a hysterectomy in younger women with extensive disease in whom ovarian preservation is possible. They remove all the visible endometrial implants as well as the uterus. They point out that even though the ovaries are still there to produce the hormones that aggravate the disease, removing the uterus eliminates the menstrual pain and bleeding problems, much of the abdominal pain and pain on intercourse and "quiets the pelvis down." Although the recurrence rate is somewhat higher in women whose ovaries remain and continue to put out estrogen, which of course could aggravate any remaining disease, premature menopause is avoided. Other doctors, less concerned about ovarian preservation, point out that leaving the ovaries in means that the disease will not be cured. They also point out that the recurrence rate is higher when the ovaries remain. Here again, women have to balance the risks and problems of premature menopause against the likelihood of recurrence of the disease, which might then require a second surgery.

Hormones vs. Surgery

One of the great debates in gynecology is whether to treat endometriosis in those women in their late 20s and 30s who are anxious to get pregnant with hormones or with surgery. A woman's fertility declines significantly after age 30. Since hormone therapy often suppresses the menstrual period for 6 to 9 months or more, and on top of that, it often takes some time for the menstrual cycle to resume its normal rhythm after the therapy, sometimes as long as a year depending on the type of hormones administered, a woman on hormone therapy may thereby lose a year or two of fertility. If she is over 30, her statistical chances of achieving pregnancy are all the while declining. Some doctors believe that such a woman has a better chance of achieving pregnancy if her endometriosis is treated by surgery instead of hormone treatments. A woman in this situation owes it to herself to get opinions from doctors on both sides of this debate.

Endometriosis can recur after any form of therapy but is most likely to happen with the hormone treatments. Recurrence rates after conservative surgery vary, depending on whether the woman got pregnant after surgery. In about 4 percent of those who get pregnant after conservative surgery, there will be a recurrence, but the figure may be as high as 40 percent in those who don't become pregnant.[16]

The recurrence rates after hysterectomy, regardless of whether or not the ovaries are removed, is low. If there is a recurrence, it is generally treated with danazol; however, at times a second or even third conservative operation may be done, and removal of the ovaries may eventually be necessary in some rare cases.

Sometimes, after surgical treatment in cases where there have been widely scattered small implants, danazol may be given to clear up any endometriosis that was missed. In the past, hormones were given before surgery to soften up the pelvis, making surgery easier, and to enlarge the endometriosis so the surgeon will be less likely to miss it. However, this approach has now been discredited and any doctor who suggests it may be a bit behind the times.

Radiation Therapy and New Drugs

X-ray treatment is never appropriate for endometriosis, the exception being cases of ovarian endometriosis in which the surgeon wasn't able to remove all the fragments of ovarian tissue. Low doses of radiation therapy may be used, but this would be a rare case.

Because of the side effects involved in danazol therapy, researchers are experimenting with new drugs. In the future, then, alternatives to danazol may be available.

ADENOMYOSIS

AKA: internal endometriosis, endometriosis interna

Adenomyosis is a condition in which the endometrial tissue that lines the inside of the uterus (and which is shed each month during the period) is found growing into the muscle wall of the uterus. It is thought that the endometrial lining grows down into the muscle owing to some weakness in the muscle wall. Sometimes the surrounding muscle tissue will "pinch off" the invading endometrial tissue, creating islands of endometrial tissue within the muscle. At other times the invading tissue is still connected to the normal endometrial lining inside the uterine cavity. In still other cases the endometrial tissue will grow all the way through the muscle wall to the outer surface of the uterus.

At one time this condition was called internal endometriosis, since both adenomyosis and endometriosis, the condition described above, involve endometrial tissue in abnormal locations. In adenomyosis the endometrial tissue is confined to the muscle wall, whereas in endometriosis it is found growing on the ovaries and other pelvic organs entirely separate from the uterus. Moreover, adenomyosis is usually diagnosed in women who are in their 40s and 50s and who have borne children, whereas endometriosis is most commonly found in younger women who have not borne children.

According to some authorities, the two conditions frequently coexist; others say this is true in only a minority of cases. It is now thought that the two conditions are separate and distinct, so the term "internal endometriosis" (or "endometriosis interna") is no longer used.

Incidence and Cause

There is some debate about how frequently adenomyosis occurs. Many women, even though they have a considerable amount of disease, are symptomless. The disease may not, then, be discovered until the uterus is removed for some other reason and examined microscopically. These reported incidence rates range from 10 percent to 60 percent. The wide variation is owing to different definitions of exactly what constitutes adenomyosis, that is, experts do not agree on how much endometrial tissue, how far down in the muscle tissue it should be and which type of cells have to be present before adenomyosis is diagnosed. The method of sampling (single samples or multiple samples) also has an effect on incidence rates, because adenomyosis may exist in one tissue sample whereas another sample from another location may be disease-free.

As mentioned, most women treated for adenomyosis are in their late 40s or 50s and have had one or two children. It is uncommon to find the disease in much younger women or in women who have never borne children. This lends credence to the theory that adenomyosis results from bits of endometrial tissue getting more or less "caught" in the muscle tissue in a process known as involution, during which the uterus returns to its normal size after pregnancy. Some doctors think of adenomyosis as a sort of endometrial hernia that has poked through the weak spots in the muscle wall—weak spots that were perhaps the result of repeated pregnancies. There are, however, other (somewhat less plausible) theories, and the actual mechanism by which the endometrial tissue invades the muscle wall is not clear.

Symptoms

The two chief symptoms of adenomyosis are abnormal menstrual bleeding and menstrual pain, although for some unknown reason, about 25 percent of those with the disease are free of symptoms. Adenomyosis is characterized by profuse or prolonged periods. This occurs in about two-thirds of the cases. Frequently, the bleeding is so excessive that the woman is actually hemorrhaging. The severity of the bleeding seems to be related more to how widespread the condition is within the uterus than to how deep the penetrations are. This abnormal bleeding suggests a hormonal imbalance. It is suspected that adenomyosis may also be related to excessive hormone production.

About a third of the women treated for adenomyosis will have severe, sometimes incapacitating pain with their menstrual periods. One explanation for the pain is that the ingrown endometrial tissue continues to develop and swell each month in response to the monthly ebb and flow of hormones. Since the muscle walls of the uterus are unyielding and do not permit expansion, pain results. However, there is some question about whether or not the ingrown tissue always continues to respond to hormones. Another explanation is that the increase in the blood vessels in the area that usually accompanies this disease causes the walls of the uterus to become swollen with blood. This swelling, along with the scarring within the walls where the endometrial tissue has invaded, interferes with the normal contractibility of the muscle walls, causing pain. In any case the degree of pain seems to be related to the depth of penetration into the muscle wall. It is interesting that although bleeding and pain are the two common symptoms, they occur together in only 20 percent of women with adenomyosis.

Diagnosis

On physical examination the doctor will usually find a uterus that is rather firm and diffusely enlarged, but the enlargement rarely exceeds three times its normal size. This, in addition to the symptoms mentioned above, may make the doctor suspect adenomyosis, but a definite diagnosis is difficult because there are many diseases that coexist with adenomyosis. Often the diagnosis is impossible short of an actual operation and dissection of the uterus.

Moreover, sometimes it is hard to distinguish between adenomyosis and certain other diseases. Some types of uterine fibroids, for example, produce excessive bleeding, although in adenomyosis there is less tendency toward the gushing-type flow associated with these fibroids. Certain fibroids also produce a symmetrical enlargement of the uterus, but generally a uterus with adenomyosis feels firmer. The chief point of difference between these types of fibroids and adenomyosis is pain. The fibroids, although they may produce pain, are less likely to do so than adenomyosis. Adenomyosis will be suspected in a woman who has borne children when there is a diffusely enlarged uterus with symptoms of cramplike uterine pain that persists through the entire period, becoming worse as menopause approaches. During the rest of the cycle the adenomyosis is relatively pain-free, which distinguishes it from endometriosis.

Treatment

When adenomyosis is accompanied by only moderate degrees of uterine enlargement the woman is frequently treated for dysfunctional bleeding with hormones or by dilation and curettage (D&C), a scraping of the uterine cavity, neither of which will be successful. Indeed, the hormones may make the situation worse.

Because the disease is related to estrogen and its chief symptoms—menstrual pain and excessive menstrual bleeding—diminish once menopause occurs, a woman near menopausal age with only minimal symptoms can just be given treatment to relieve or minimize the symptoms. Such women should, however, have a D&C to rule out uterine cancer, which could also produce these symptoms.

If, however, the symptoms are extreme, surgery—in the form of a hysterectomy, removal of the uterus and possibly the tubes and ovaries—may be necessary. If a hysterectomy is performed, the fate of the ovaries will be decided on the basis of such factors as the personal judgment of the surgeon, the age of the patient and the presence or absence of associated diseases. Any woman whose doctor suggests a hysterectomy for adenomyosis should carefully weigh the decision. Are the symptoms that severe? Is menopause—and relief—just around the corner? The risks of hysterectomy must be weighed against the severity of the adenomyosis.

CONGENITAL ABNORMALITIES OF THE UTERUS AND FALLOPIAN TUBES*

Types: congenital absence of the uterus
unicornuate, unicornous, or unicorn uterus
rudimentary uterine horn, uterus bicornis unicollis or blind uterine horn
double uterus, double symmetrical uterus, uterus didelphys, uterus duplex, uterus bicornis bicollis, bicornuate uterus
septate uterus, subseptate uterus, uterine partitioning
arcuate uterus
immature, or undeveloped uterus
T-shaped uterus

Back when we were all developing embryos in our mothers' wombs, certain masses of tissue with specific functions began to develop and differentiate themselves from the surrounding tissue. In females, two tubelike embryonic structures known as müllerian ducts fuse together to form what will become the uterus, the fallopian tubes and the middle and upper portions of the vagina, at some time before the 8th week. Sometimes this normal process of development and fusion is disturbed, causing a wide variety of congenital abnormalities (Illustration 47).

---

*The position of the uterus within the pelvic cavity may also be unusual, and sometimes this results from congenital problems; however, these are discussed separately under the headings Tipped Uterus and Prolapse of the Uterus, Vagina and Cervix.

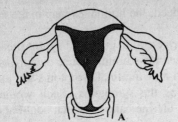
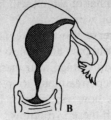
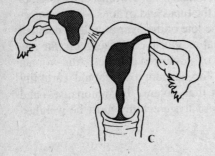
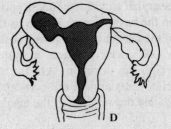
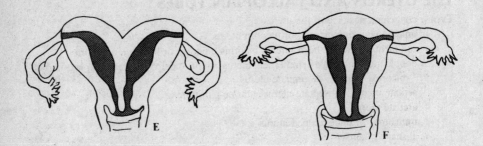
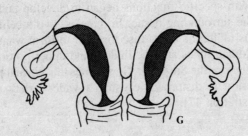

Illustration 47 *Congenital Abnormalities of the Uterus: (A) Normal, (B) Unicornus, (C) Rudimentary Uterine Horn, (D) Rudimentary Uterine Horn (with cavities connecting), (E) Bicornuate, (F) Septate and (G) Didelphys.*

Types

Different doctors use different categories to classify and describe the various types of congenital abnormalities of the uterus and tubes. We have found the following ones useful:

Congenital Absence of the Uterus

Sometimes there are no müllerian ducts, so there is a total failure of development. Or both ducts fail to develop properly and cannot fuse. Such women, then, have no uterus. This absence is almost always accompanied by absence of the vagina. Absence of the uterus may also be associated with certain congenital abnormalities of the ovary.

Unicorn Uterus

If only one of the müllerian ducts fails to develop, the uterus and the fallopian tube may be formed from the other duct. This condition may cause fewer problems than the other uterine abnormalities. It is known also as unicornuate uterus, or unicornous uterus.

Rudimentary Uterine Horn

When the development of one müllerian duct is normal but the other is abnormal or underdeveloped, varying degrees of what is called a rudimentary uterine horn will result. The term ''uterus bicornis unicollis'' is used to describe certain types of rudimentary horns. In some instances of rudimentary horns there is some fusion between the underdeveloped duct and the normal uterus that has developed from the other duct. In such cases the rudimentary horn and the uterus are said to ''communicate,'' meaning that there is a passageway between them. If so, pregnancy can occur in the underdeveloped portion, which, as we shall see, can cause problems. More often the underdeveloped duct does not communicate but is merely attached to the uterus by a band of connecting tissue. In some of these attached horns the endometrial lining, which normally covers the inside of the uterus and bleeds, or menstruates, each month, is not functional. But in other cases the lining of the horn behaves just like normal uterine lining, swelling and shedding blood each month. However, since the horn is closed off, there is no place for the menstrual debris to go, which can lead to problems.

Blind Uterine Horn

If the two embryonic müllerian ducts develop about equally well but one fails to ''communicate'' with the other or with the cervix, a condition referred to as a blind uterine horn results. It differs from the rudimentary horn in that it is fully or almost fully developed. But, like some types of rudimentary horns, it has no passageway to the other, normally developed uterus or to the cervix. Since the blind horn is sufficiently developed to menstruate but has no outlet for the menstrual debris, once again there are apt to be problems.

Double Uterus

When the two müllerian ducts develop fully, so that there are two uterine cavities, two tubes, two cervices and two vaginas, but there is no passageway or communication between them, this is referred to as a double, or double symmetrical, uterus, or uterus didelphys. There are a number of variations. A single vagina with all other structures duplicated is a uterus duplex, or a uterus bicornis bicollis. If both the vagina and cervix are single, the term for this is ''uterus bicornis unicollis,'' or ''bicornuate uterus.''

Septate Uterus

Sometimes the double uterus does not consist of two totally separate systems. On the outside it may feel like a single uterus. There may just be a septum, or wall of tissue, inside the uterus that separates it into two cavities. If this wall of tissue runs from the top to the bottom of the interior cavity, it is called a septate uterus, and if the wall of tissue is only partial, it is known as a subseptate uterus.

Arcuate Uterus

Sometimes there is a single vagina, a single cervix and two fallopian tubes, and the uterine cavity is almost normal, except for a slight depression at the top of the uterus caused by an incomplete fusion. This results in a sort of heart-shaped interior cavity and is referred to as an arcuate uterus.

Underdeveloped Uterus

Some doctors recognize yet another type of uterine abnormality, which they call an underdeveloped, or immature, uterus. Such uteri are smaller than average. Many times these sorts of uteri are associated with other abnormalities, such as hermaphroditism or polycystic ovarian disease. Sometimes these so-called underdeveloped uteri will cause difficulties in getting pregnant, in carrying a baby to term or in delivery, but this is usually only in association with other conditions. Some doctors attempt to stimulate the growth of an underdeveloped uterus with hormones, but it is usually not successful nor is it necessary. Unless a woman actually has some underlying disease there is no reason to do anything about a small uterus. We don't worry whether a woman is 6 feet 2 inches or 4 feet 9 inches tall when she has a baby, and it is our experience that the size of the uterus is equally irrelevant.

T-Shaped Uterus

Another type of uterine abnormality, called a T-shaped uterus, has recently been discovered in some of the daughters of the mothers who took the synthetic hormone DES during their pregnancies. For more information, see the section on DES.

Incidence and Cause

No one knows what causes these abnormalities or how frequently they occur. Many of these defects don't cause any symptoms and don't interfere with fertility or pregnancy, so they are not discovered unless there is an autopsy at death or they are found in the course of another operation.

Symptoms, Complications and Diagnosis

Many women have no symptoms. For those who do, pain is a common complaint. Women with certain of these abnormalities may experience severe pain with their menstrual periods. There may also be irregularities in the menstrual bleeding pattern. The bleeding is apt to be very heavy and may last for many days, especially in double uterus, where there is more endometrial tissue and hence more bleeding. The periods are likely to be delayed. If there is a double vagina or if one of the horns of the uterus is in an inappropriate position, there may be pain associated with intercourse.

Infertility is often associated with uterine abnormalities. In cases where there is a complete absence of the uterus or vagina the reason for this infertility is obvious. However, with other types of uterine abnormalities the cause of difficulty in achieving pregnancy is unclear. Perhaps there is a problem in implantation owing to lack of space in the malformed uterus. The consensus of opinion is that uterine abnormalities are not usually the cause, per se, of a woman's inability to get pregnant, although abnormalities that are related may be. The presence of uterine abnormalities does not mean that a woman

421

cannot get pregnant, for many women—probably the majority—do, but it certainly doesn't increase the chances. However, once a woman with a congenital abnormality of the uterus does become pregnant, she is apt to have problems. Miscarriage is not uncommon.

Many times these uterine abnormalities are not diagnosed until a woman comes to the doctor because she is unable to get pregnant or because she has some of the symptoms described above. Careful examination with a speculum will reveal the abnormality if it is one that involves a double vagina or cervix. Or the doctor may be able to feel an abnormality in shape when a bimanual exam is done.

A history of repeated miscarriages will also help the doctor in diagnosis, for if a woman with a congenital abnormality of the uterus does conceive, there are likely to be problems. Such women generally have only about a 50 percent chance of carrying the pregnancy for a full 9 months, as compared with the normal rate of 85 percent. This is probably owing to lack of sufficient space to allow the fetus to develop properly. Certain types of abnormalities are especially likely to result in spontaneous abortions. For instance, approximately 33 percent of all pregnancies occurring in a septate uterus will result in miscarriage in the 3d or 6th month of pregnancy.

Pregnancy in one horn of a double uterus may proceed to term, where it produces its own particular problem, but miscarriages are also frequent. If a woman with a double uterus becomes pregnant, she may continue to bleed cyclically from the other, nonpregnant uterus. Pregnancy in a rudimentary horn can be difficult to recognize and is often mistaken for a fibroid tumor. Of course, the rudimentary horn is too underdeveloped to sustain a pregnancy. Such a pregnancy involves the same dangers as an ectopic pregnancy. As the fetus grows, the rudimentary horn ruptures, or bursts open, and this can result in the death of the fetus and the mother.

Even when a woman with uterine abnormalities does manage to get pregnant and carry her baby to term, there are likely to be problems. If the woman has a unicorn uterus, there may not be so many problems, but most abnormalities result in difficult deliveries and a much-reduced chance of having a normal baby; 93 percent of babies born from normal uteri are healthy, as compared with 64 percent born from abnormal uteri. It depends somewhat on the extent of the malformation, but even the only slightly abnormal arcuate uterus results in a high number of complications, including premature or postmature delivery, prolonged labor, sudden fetal death and breech or transverse presentations, in which the baby is born feet first or sideways.

Another serious complication of uterine abnormalities involves the buildup of menstrual blood. If a woman has a blind uterine horn or a rudimentary horn that does not communicate with the normal uterus but does bleed, there is no place for the menstrual blood to go. It builds up over time and forms a collection of blood known as a hematometra. This can cause abdominal swelling, especially at the time of the menstrual period, and pain. If there is a fallopian tube, this too may fill up with blood (hematosalpinx). These conditions are discussed more fully in relation to a condition known as imperforate hymen. Pelvic endometriosis, a condition in which menstrual debris backs up through the fallopian tubes, spills into the pelvic cavity and starts growing on the ovaries or in other abnormal locations, where it can cause serious problems, is also associated with these types of uterine abnormalities. In addition to these complications, women with uterine abnormalities often have associated abnormalities of the urinary system, for the tissues from which these two structures evolve are closely related.

Treatment

Generally, a doctor will not operate to correct a uterine abnormality unless a woman has a history of repeated miscarriages, long and complicated labors or infertility in which all other causes have been ruled out. Then the partition between the double uterus or the abnormal portions of the uterus may be removed. Obviously, if there is no uterus, it is impossible to create one; however, it is possible to use plastic surgery procedures to create a vagina, if necessary.

In some cases where delivery could be particularly dangerous to the mother, the doctor may suggest sterilization, but although the fetal death rate is nearly 10 times higher in the malformed uterus, the maternal death rate is approximately normal, so only in rare cases is sterilization an appropriate option.

TIPPED UTERUS

AKA: displaced uterus

Types: anteflexed uterus
retroflexed uterus
retroverted uterus

Associated Terms: pelvic passive congestion syndrome, Masters-Allen syndrome

A woman's uterus may be located in an unusual position in the pelvis (Illustration 48). Basically, the uterus can be located forward (ante) or backward (retro). (It may also be lower; lowered uteri are discussed separately under the heading Prolapse of the Uterus, Vagina and Cervix.) The terminology used to describe the various forward and backward positions may be slightly confusing.

In most women the uterus is tilted forward, almost forming a right angle to

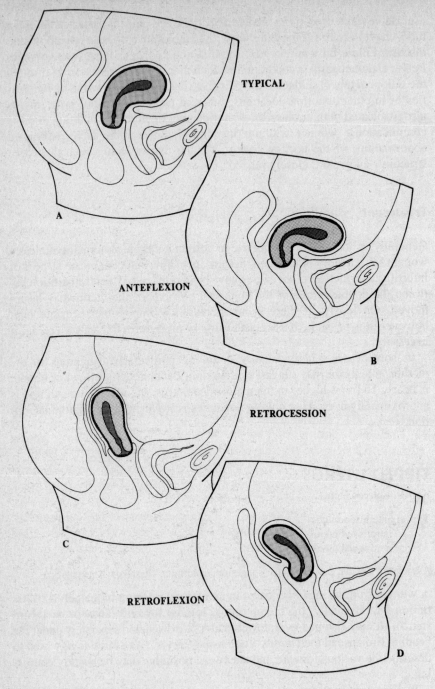

TYPICAL

A

ANTEFLEXION

B

RETROCESSION

C

RETROFLEXION

D

Illustration 48 *Tipped Uterus*

the vagina and resting on the bladder. In some women the cervix and the body of the uterus are at a more acute angle than usual, that is, the uterus is bent at the neck. The term anteflexion'' is used to describe such uteri. About 20 percent to 25 percent of all women have a uterus that is retrodisplaced, that is, one that is tipped backward, away from the bladder. The term ''retroflexion'' is used to describe this situation. If the uterus is tipped backward and is bent at the neck, the term ''retrocession'' may be used. The term ''tipped uteri'' is a general one, used to refer to anteflexion, retroflexion and retrocession.

Cause

A woman's uterus may become tipped in one of three ways. First, the problem may be congenital. As mentioned, 20 percent to 25 percent of all women are born with retrodisplaced uteri. Second, the uterus may become retrodisplaced if the ligaments that normally hold it in a forward position become stretched as a result of childbirth. And third, such diseases as pelvic inflammatory disease and endometriosis may cause adhesions—bands of scar tissue—that may fix the uterus in an abnormal position. A large ovarian tumor or fibroid tumor may push the uterus out of its normal position.

Symptoms

The majority of women who are either born with a tipped uterus or develop one after childbirth don't have any symptoms. Occasionally, a severely tipped uterus that is lying right next to the end of the vagina will cause pain on intercourse, but this is not generally the case.

A uterus that is fixed or forced into retrodisplacement because of some pelvic disease may produce symptoms. If, in such cases, the uterus is immovable and cannot yield to pressure, there may be pain on intercourse or a constant dull pain in the pelvis and lower back. Menstrual bleeding may be irregular, and there may be pain associated with it. These symptoms, however, are not owing to the position of the uterus but to the fact that it is fixed in place.

In the past, gynecologists attributed a multitude of symptoms to the tipped uterus. Because the tipped uterus and backache were such common everyday conditions, putting the two together gave doctors a seemingly logical explanation for the pain (and also a quick and lucrative method of treating it). However, more discerning gynecologists began to realize that the majority of women with tipped uteri did not have any symtpoms and that treatment didn't usually relieve the backache. Indeed, it is now realized that less than 1 percent of all backache is related to uterine problems.

Still, misunderstanding about the tipped uterus persists among both women and doctors. There are some women who have chronic pelvic pain, and the term "chronic pelvic passive congestion syndrome" is sometimes used to describe the condition. It is usually associated with a retrodisplaced uterus that is congested with blood. There is some question as to whether this condition really exists or not. Another similarly vague condition is the Masters-Allen syndrome. In this condition the broad ligaments that help support the uterus have tears or holes—thought to be the result of trauma during delivery—and therefore are not able to hold the uterus firmly in place.

Diagnosis

The diagnosis is made by bimanual pelvic exam. Some doctors will not mention the fact that the woman's uterus is displaced unless it's causing problems because they don't want to alarm her or because they think that she might invent symptoms once she knows she has this condition. We, of course, believe that a woman has a right to any information a doctor may have about her body.

Treatment

At one time it was quite the fashion to treat a tipped uterus by inserting a pessary, a ringlike support device, to hold the uterus in the usual position or by performing an operation known as a uterine suspension, in which an incision is made in the abdomen and the ligaments that hold the uterus forward are shortened, which pulls the uterus back into position. But the majority of women with tipped uteri do not require treatment of any kind.

It is fortunate that the use of the pessary has fallen out of favor, for it almost invariably causes infections and sores. Besides, if the pessary can push the uterus forward easily, there is no need for one, and if there are adhesions present, there is no pessary in the world that can move the uterus. It has been jokingly said that some gynecologists have gotten wealthy inserting pessaries and that others have gotten wealthy removing them. (This is funny?) A woman whose doctor proposes the use of a pessary for her tipped uterus should pass on this "joke" and seek a second opinion (*see* p. 238).

Sometimes a woman will seek medical help because she is unable to get pregnant, but the doctor won't be able to discover any reason for her infertility. If such a woman has a displaced uterus, the doctor may suspect that uterine displacement and the resulting displacement of the cervix is the problem. The cervix may be at such a weird angle that it does not lie in the pool of seminal fluid, and thus the sperm cannot easily move up the cervical os into the uterus. Some doctors will treat this problem surgically, with a uterine suspension operation, resuspending the uterus and sewing it back into its so-called proper place. In our opinion this is unnecessary, a case of overtreatment somewhat akin to using an elephant gun to kill a chicken. In the rare case where infertility is related to uterine displacement, there are much simpler solutions. First, during and for half an hour or so after intercourse the woman should lie on her back, with her hips elevated. Or she may lie on her stomach and the man enters from the rear. In extreme cases a vaginal pessary may be used on a temporary basis; however, women whose doctors suggest a uterine suspension for infertility should seek a second opinion.

The doctor may also suggest a uterine suspension for the relief of chronic backache; however, this too is of questionable value. Any woman whose doctor proposes the use of a pessary, uterine suspension operation or, heaven forbid, a hysterectomy for the relief of back pain should realize that such treatment is not likely to relieve the pain. She should, by all means, seek a second opinion.

PROLAPSE OF THE UTERUS, VAGINA AND CERVIX

AKA: descensus uteri, uterine descent or fallen uterus, fallen vagina or cervix.

Types: first-degree prolapse
  second-degree prolapse
  third-degree prolapse, complete prolapse or procidentia uteri

Prolapse of the uterus (Illustration 49) refers to a condition in which the uterus "falls," or is displaced, from its normal position. Prolapses are classified in three categories, depending on the degree of the displacement. In first-degree prolapse the uterus has fallen into the vaginal cavity but does not protrude through the vaginal opening. In such cases the uterus has usually fallen or flopped backward so that it is not in its normal position, resting on the bladder, but instead lies closer to the rectum. This is called retrodisplacement. This position usually prevents further prolapse. In second-degree prolapse the uterus has fallen so far that all or part of the cervix protrudes through the vaginal opening. In such cases part of the vaginal vault may also have fallen or collapsed in on itself. In third-degree prolapse there is a complete descent of the entire uterus, with inversion of the entire vaginal canal. Third-degree prolapse is also called complete prolapse, or procidentia.

Prolapse of the uterus is usually associated with prolapse of other organs, such as the bladder (cystocele), the urethra (urethrocele) and the rectum (rectocele).

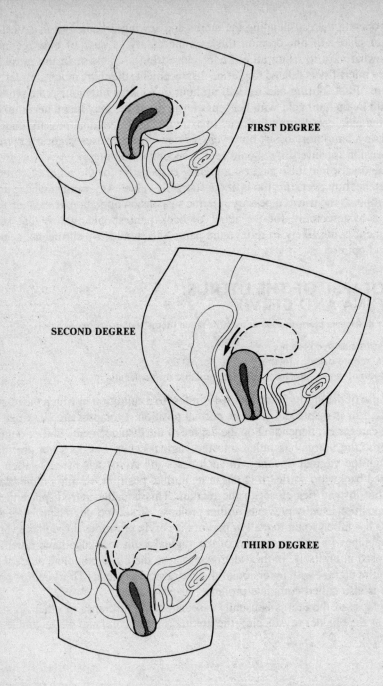

FIRST DEGREE

SECOND DEGREE

THIRD DEGREE

Illustration 49   *Prolapse of the Uterus*

Cause

The underlying cause of prolapse is some sort of injury to the support tissues, usually during childbirth. However, since many women have traumatic deliveries and never have prolapse, and since in some cases women who have never had children have prolapse, it is thought that some sort of congenital or inherent weakness in the support structures is also a factor. Although the initial injury may occur during childbirth, it usually takes years for the signs and symptoms of uterine prolapse to develop, and it appears most often in women over age 40.

In some rare cases there may be prolapse of the vagina after the surgical removal of the uterus, and this may be difficult to repair if a functioning vagina is to be preserved.

Symptoms

A minimal degree of prolapse may not cause any symptoms. But as the uterus falls lower, many women have a heavy, bearing-down sensation in the vagina. Others, particularly when they stand, may have a feeling that something is falling out of their vaginas. These symptoms are apt to be worse if the woman has been standing on her feet all day. If the cervix or the entire uterus is protruding from the vagina, sores and other irritants may develop, because of its exposed position.

Diagnosis

The diagnosis of uterine prolapse is fairly easy, although when a woman is lying down it may not be as obvious. The doctor may ask the woman to bear down, may pull at the cervix gently with an instrument or may ask her to stand up in order to make a diagnosis. The doctor should be careful to make sure that it is not a case of an elongated or swollen cervix owing to cervicitis or cervical cancer and that the uterus is actually descended. If there have been associated urinary tract infections, a tube may be inserted and urine extracted and examined microscopically for signs of infection.

Treatment

Treatment of uterine prolapse will depend on the age of the woman, whether or not she desires to have children, the severity of the symptoms and the extent of the prolapse. If a woman has only first-degree prolapse with no bothersome symptoms, it is usually not treated and is examined on a yearly basis. When the discomfort is intense and the prolapse is severe, the treatment of choice in women who have completed their families is a hysterectomy. Prolapse is often accompanied by a cystocele, urethrocele or rectocele, and these can be repaired at the same time that the hysterectomy is done.

If the prolapse is severe or if a woman is having symptoms but wishes to avoid a hysterectomy or is unable to have surgery because of health problems or advanced age, the doctor may prescribe a device known as a vaginal pessary to help alleviate the symptoms. The pessary comes in various shapes and sizes and is made of rubber. It fits up around the cervix at the top of the vaginal vault and helps prop up the prolapsed organs. Although a pessary won't cure the prolapse, it will prevent it from worsening. There are, however, problems with the pessary. It has to be removed (by either a doctor or the woman), cleaned and replaced each month. Sometimes, despite daily douches, the rubber sets up an irritation that produces an annoying vaginal discharge. This may even cause open sores or ulcers to develop, perhaps with bleeding, making it necessary to remove the pessary. If the pessary is too large, it may press against the urethra, the tube through which urine is eliminated, causing urinary retention. If it is too small, it may cause sores or slip out. Sometimes a woman's particular anatomy precludes a correct fit with any of the standard pessaries available. Then, too, over the years the pessary may lose its effectiveness.

ASHERMAN'S SYNDROME

AKA: Asherman's disease, uterine synechia, sclerosis of the uterus

Asherman's syndrome is a condition in which the walls of the uterus are partially stuck together by bridges of scar tissue (synechiae) or in which the front and back walls of the uterus are totally adherent.

Cause

The condition is caused by too vigorous a scraping of the uterine walls during a D&C or, more rarely, by genital tuberculosis. Sometimes a suction curettage can also result in Asherman's syndrome.

Symptoms

One symptom associated with Asherman's syndrome is infrequent menstrual periods. If the scarring is too great, the endometrial layer may be too thin to build up enough thickness to allow any menstruation. There is also infertility, because the fertilized egg cannot implant in the uterine wall or because the embryo cannot develop properly in the constricted uterus. Only about 33 percent of women with Asherman's syndrome will be able to get pregnant, and to carry full term is even less likely.

Diagnosis

A history of curettage for gynecological problems, along with the symptoms mentioned above, will suggest the possibility of Asherman's syndrome. The doctor may explore the uterine cavity with a curette and collect a biopsy specimen of any obstruction encountered. A hysteroscope, an instrument used to view the inside of the uterus, or special X-ray studies of the uterus, called hysterograms, may also be used to diagnose Asherman's syndrome.

Treatment

Sometimes the insertion of an IUD will succeed in separating the uterine walls enough so that the endometrial lining is restored. Sometimes hormone treatment will also succeed in building up the endometrial lining so that menstrual bleeding can be resumed.

UTERINE FIBROIDS

AKA: leiomyoma uteri, fibroleiomyoma or fibromyoma of the uterus, myomas, leiomyomas, fibroid tumors of the uterus

Types: intramural, or interstitial, fibroids
subserous, or subperitoneal, fibroids
submucous fibroids
cervical fibroids

Associated Terms: fibroid polyp

Uterine fibroids (Illustration 50) are noncancerous tumors of the uterus. They grow in the thick muscular wall of the uterus and vary greatly in size from microscopic to mammoth. Although freak tumors of immense proportions are lavishly illustrated in grotesque detail in gynecological textbooks, such tumors are uncommon. Most women seek treatment before the tumors get that large.

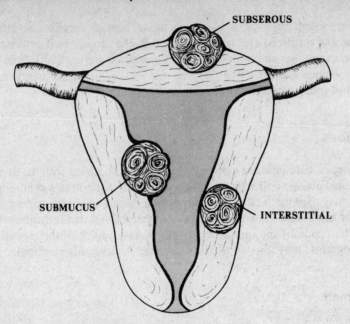

Illustration 50   *Uterine Fibroids*

Incidence

No one knows how common fibroids are because many of these tumors produce no bothersome symptoms and are too small or too inaccessibly placed to be felt by the doctor. An estimated 1 out of every 5 women over age 30 has a fibroid. Next to pregnancy, it is the most common cause of an enlarged uterus.

Fibroids are rarely seen before puberty and don't usually develop or grow larger after menopause. They are most frequently found in women who are in their middle and late menstrual years. In black women, who, for unknown reasons, seem to be particularly susceptible, the peak incidence occurs slightly earlier.

Cause

The cause of uterine fibroids is unknown, but it appears that they are related to the production of the hormone estrogen. They are prevalent in women who are in their reproductive years and producing a monthly ebb and flow of estrogen. In pregnant women and women on birth control pills, both of whom have higher estrogen levels, the normally slow growth rate of fibroids is acceler-

432

ated. Moreover, fibroids rarely develop, and indeed often shrink, after menopause, when the level of estrogen is diminished.

Symptoms

Not all fibroids cause bothersome symptoms. A woman may have small single or multiple tumors, or even a fairly large one, without troublesome symptoms. She may not even be aware of the fibroid until her doctor happens to discover it in the course of a routine pelvic examination. A fibroid tumor may also be present for many years before it begins to produce symptoms.

If there are symptoms, their nature will depend in great part on exactly where in the uterus the fibroid is located. The tumors usually begin as small seedlings in the thick muscle wall of the uterus. They are well separated from the surrounding tissue by a capsule and may be single or multiple. Most fibroids stay confined within the muscle wall, and these are referred to as intramural, or interstitial, fibroids. They may grow large and expand in the direction of the outer surface of the uterus, in which case they are called subserous, or subperitoneal, fibroids. Less often they may grow toward the interior uterine cavity, in which case they are called submucous fibroids. In some rare cases fibroids may appear in the lower, cervical portion of the uterus and these are called cervical fibroids.

Frequently, there are small multiple tumors scattered throughout the muscular wall of the uterus, and the uterus is symmetrically enlarged owing to the presence of the tumors and the swelling they produce in the surrounding tissue. If the tumors grow in the direction of the outer surface of the uterus, the fibroids may be felt as irregular bumps, or nodules, on the surface of the uterus. They may continue to grow larger and in an outward direction. Then they may become pedunculated, which means that they grow a stalk or stem, called a pedicle, by which they are attached to the uterus. In this instance they are more mobile and may move to various locations within the pelvis. The pedicle may be broad and provide an adequate blood supply to nourish further growth or it may become very thin. A large tumor supported by a thin pedicle is subject to twisting of the stem, an event which in medical circles is known as "torsion of the pedicle." If this happens, there may be a good deal of pain. Also, the blood supply to the tumor may be cut off, which results in necrosis, or death, of all or part of the tissue that makes up the fibroid. If necrosis occurs, the dying tissues may swell up, causing pressure on the outer capsule of the fibroid and pain. If the tumor grows out toward the bladder or becomes pedunculated and moves into a position that causes pressure on the bladder, it may cause pain and disturbances in urination. A cervical fibroid growing out toward the bladder can also cause these sorts of disturbances. Sometimes the cervical fibroid will remain within the wall of the cervix and cause distortion and elongation of the cervix, pushing it down into the vaginal cavity. In extreme cases the fibroid may even protrude through the vaginal opening.

Less frequently a fibroid will grow in the direction of the interior cavity of the uterus. These are most often single tumors and may fill the entire uterine cavity, which becomes increasingly larger as the fibroid grows. Usually, the uterus enlarges symmetrically, and the tumor cannot be felt as a separate growth. The uterus does not tolerate this submucous type of fibroid and reacts, as it does to any foreign body, by contracting in an effort to expel it with each menstrual period. Severe menstrual pain that continues throughout the menstrual flow is common in women with submucous fibroids. As a result of the continued uterine contractions, these tumors may also become pedunculated. They may even dilate the cervix and protrude into the vagina, in which case they are called fibroid polyps. Then the blood supply to the tumor may be affected, resulting in necrosis of some of the tissue. If the fibroid protrudes through the cervix, it is subject to injury and infection.

Submucous fibroids may bleed as a result of the tissue death, injury and/or infection. They also tend to produce excessive menstrual bleeding of the gushing or flooding type, probably because they distort the endometrial lining of the uterine cavity and because they interfere with the normal contractions of the uterine muscle that aid in slowing down blood loss during menstruation. Even small submucous fibroids can produce excessive bleeding. Other types of fibroids may interfere with these normal contractions. If they grow large enough, they too can distort the endometrial lining and produce menstrual irregularities. But it is usually only the submucous fibroids that are responsible for heavy, prolonged menstruation and for the shortening of intervals between periods that sometimes occurs.

Sometimes submucous fibroids produce a vaginal discharge, which, if present, is usually mucuslike. If the fibroid becomes infected, the discharge may also include pus and may be tinged with blood. If portions of the tissue that makes up the tumor die, the discharge may become thin, watery and brown and have a bad odor.

Pain, as we have said, may accompany the fibroid. The exact nature of this pain will depend on the location of the fibroid. Intramural (within the wall) fibroids are apt to produce a pain that comes on suddenly over a localized area in the lower abdomen. The initial pain may be severe, gradually subsiding into a dull, pelvic "toothache." A pedunculated tumor that has twisted on its stem may produce pain that is apt to be sudden, colicky and severe.

If inflammation is associated with the fibroid, adhesions (thick banks of fibrous tissue formed by the surrounding tissues to protect themselves) may be created. The adhesions may cement the organs in the area together, causing a constant back or lower-abdominal pain that may worsen at menstruation. Submucous fibroids may produce a cramplike uterine pain that may become almost as intense as labor pains as the uterus tries to expel the fibroid through the cervix. Subserous tumors, because they may have veins stretched over their surface, can produce pain if an abdominal injury results in rupture of the veins, causing bleeding into the pelvic cavity, which is very sensitive to blood. However, this rarely occurs.

The fibroids may also produce discomfort through pressure on nearby organs or tissue. Such pain is usually felt in the back, the lower portion of the abdomen or the thighs. Prolonged standing, particularly at the time of the period, exaggerates the discomfort. A large tumor may produce pressure on the stomach or diaphragm, causing gastric or respiratory disturbances. Similarly, pressure on the veins may result in swollen, distended veins in the legs, a condition known as varicose veins, or in hemorrhoids.

The bladder or ureter (the tube that leads from kidney to bladder) may be compressed, producing pain in the flank and kidney area on the affected side, as well as urinary symptoms. There may be urinary retention, which may be chronic and partial or sudden and total, requiring catheterization (insertion of a tube through the urinary opening to the bladder). This sudden blockage is most likely to occur at the time of menstruation when the pelvis is congested with blood, which results in swelling of the fibroid. If the bladder is constantly distended, incontinence (lack of control of urine flow) may result, as the urine in the bladder spills over. Such overdistention and retention of urine lead to infection, since stagnant urine is a perfect breeding ground for bacteria. The infection may in turn cause pain on urination.

Infertility is often associated with fibroids, although sometimes the fibroid itself is not to blame. For instance, the infertility may actually be owing to endometriosis, a condition in which uterine tissue grows outside the uterus, or salpingitis, an infection of the fallopian tubes, either of which frequently co-exists with uterine fibroids. However, in other cases the fibroid itself may be the culprit. If the normally blood-rich lining of the womb is thinned out over a protruding fibroid, the implanted egg will have difficulty surviving, owing to the faulty blood supply. Miscarriage may also be a problem for women with fibroids; however, many women get pregnant and have no trouble with their pregnancies despite the presence of fibroids.

Diagnosis

Fibroids are diagnosed by abdominal palpation (feeling) and bimanual pelvic exam. They are usually felt as one or more firm, nontender bumps on the uterus. Sometimes it is easy to make a diagnosis of fibroids—but not always. If the fibroid is growing from the side of the uterus, it may be difficult to distinguish it from a solid ovarian tumor. If portions of the fibroid have broken down and become liquefied, so that the tumor takes on a soft feel, it may then be hard to distinguish from an ovarian cyst. Ultrasound, a method of visualizing the internal organs by means of sound waves, may be reliable in distinguishing between fibroids and ovarian growths.

Another problem in diagnosis is the confusion between a soft, enlarged uterus caused by a fibroid, particularly one that has undergone cystic degeneration, and one caused by pregnancy. A pregnancy test will clear up the confusion.

A submucous fibroid may not cause uterine enlargement or irregularities that can be felt by physical exam, and yet it may produce troublesome bleeding. These fibroids are usually diagnosed by a dilation and curettage (D&C), a procedure in which the cervix is dilated and the uterine lining is scraped. During the D&C the doctor feels inside the uterus with an instrument known as a curette. If the doctor feels a lump that is too firm to be removed, s/he knows that it is probably a submucous fibroid rather than a uterine polyp.

A special X-ray examination, known as a hysterosalpingogram, in which a special fluid that will show up on X-ray film is injected into the uterus, will sometimes reveal the presence of a submucous fibroid.

Treatment

Not all fibroids will require treatment. A wait-and-see approach, in which the woman is carefully followed at regular intervals, may suffice, particularly if the woman is near menopause, after which fibroids tend to regress. If, however, the tumor grows larger, treatment becomes necessary, for the possibility exists that this is not a fibroid but uterine cancer.

A fibroid tumor that is larger than a 12-to-14-week pregnancy also requires treatment, even if it isn't producing symptoms, for large tumors can create serious surgical problems. Large tumors are also subject to necrosis, cystic degeneration and other complications. Moroeever, in all likelihood they will begin to produce symptoms sooner or later. It is best to remove them before they grow large or complications occur and they begin to produce symptoms.

The wait-and-see approach may have to be abandoned if the fibroid arises in or near the cervix, for such fibroids frequently cause urinary problems. Moreover, they may also cause infertility or create problems during childbirth.

In the face of severe symptoms the wait-and-see approach doesn't make sense, particularly if there is bleeding with severe blood loss. Some doctors will try to control such bleeding with hormone therapy by giving birth control pills. This treatment is not usually successful, but it may be worth a try, particularly in a woman approaching menopause for whom it may thus be possible to avoid surgery.

If surgical treatment is necessary, it may be possible on rare occasions to remove a pedunculated submucous fibrois with a D&C. A cervical or submucous fibroid that protrudes from the uterine wall can occasionally be removed during a D&C as well. However, most fibroids require at least a myomectomy (Illustration 51). A myomectomy involves simply removing the fibroids and leaving the uterus intact. In some cases myomectomy is a simple operation. If the fibroid is attached to the outside of the uterus by a pedicle, removal might be easy, but if the fibroids are multiple and scattered through the uterus, the operation is hard or sometimes impossible. The myomectomy has a slightly higher mortality and a much higher complication rate than the hysterectomy. The uterus is a very muscular organ, with a rich blood supply. Thus shelling out the tumors can lead to bleeding complications. It may also leave scars and cause adhesions, or hardened bands of connective tissue, that could bind the uterus to other pelvic organs. This could lead to pain on intercourse, backaches and abnormal uterine bleeding. Moreover, in about 10 percent of cases the fibroids will recur, for some of the seedlings within the uterine wall may have been missed and the basic underlying cause of the fibroids won't have been dealt with. Usually, only women who are particularly anxious to have children should have a myomectomy. Although the uterine wall is weakened by myomectomy, women in whom the operation can be done have about a 50 percent chance of subsequently getting pregnant. Even

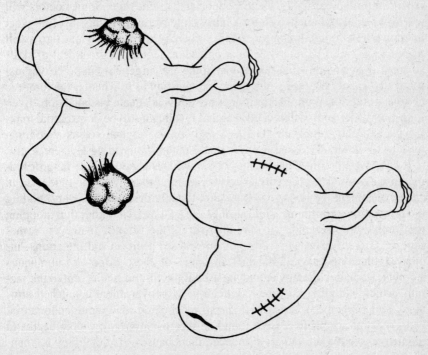

Illustration 51   *Myomectomy: Sometimes fibroids on the surface of the uterus can be removed by an operation known as myomectomy.*

some women who have had more than one myomectomy have been able to have a normal pregnancy.

Before surgery, there is usually no way of telling for sure whether or not a myomectomy is possible. Women who are particularly anxious for pregnancy should make the doctor aware of their desires. Because myomectomies are done only rarely, it is hard to find an experienced doctor, but experience is important, for it cuts down on complications. Don't hesitate to question your doctor about his or her experience in doing myomectomies and to seek out another doctor with more experience if necessary.

Because of the high estrogen levels in pregnancy, some asymptomatic fibroids will flare up at that time, growing larger and creating such severe symptoms that myomectomy is required. Unfortunately, many times a myomectomy in a pregnant woman will result in a miscarriage, so it should not be attempted unless absolutely necessary.

In women whose condition precludes myomectomy, who do not wish to have children or who are older, a hysterectomy is done. The hysterectomy can be done by a vaginal or abdominal approach. If the tumor is small, the vaginal approach is often used. The vaginal approach is a less serious operation, requires a substantially shorter recovery time and allows for any vaginal repair for prolapse or cystocele to be done at the same time. Some doctors will use the vaginal approach even for a fairly large fibroid, but this involves what is known as a morcellation procedure, whereby the tumor is cut into small pieces before vaginal removal. This procedure requires a great deal of skill, so most doctors prefer an abdominal route for large fibroids. The vaginal route also cannot be used when there is a question as to whether the tumor is ovarian or uterine in origin, for it does not allow adequate visualization. Even if an abdominal approach is used, vaginal repair can still be done before making the abdominal incision. The pros and cons of vaginal versus abdominal hysterectomy are discussed in more detail under the heading Hysterectomy.

If surgery is not possible because a woman has serious heart, lung or kidney disease and is a poor surgical risk, radiation therapy of the type used in cancer treatment may be used. Radiation therapy destroys the ovary, ending the production of hormones, and shrinks the endometrial lining, thus stopping the troublesome bleeding. It may also shrink the fibroid. However, sometimes it fails to shrink large fibroids and causes necrosis and infections; increased bleeding may then result in some of these large or submucous fibroids. Radiation therapy cannot be used if the fibroid is adherent to the rectum, which is highly sensitive to radiation. Moreover, there is much controversy about whether a radiation-induced menopause may incite endometrial cancer. Some researchers have found an increase in pelvic cancer deaths in women who have had radiation-induced menopauses. Radiotherapy is, then, only rarely used to treat fibroids.

Although some doctors will prescribe birth control pills, women with fibroids should probably not use them because there is a risk of increasing the size of the fibroid and thus perhaps necessitating a hysterectomy. If a woman with fibroids does take the Pill, she should be monitored closely and examined every 3 to 4 months to make sure the fibroids are not growing larger.

ENDOMETRIAL POLYPS

AKA: uterine polyps

An endometrial polyp is a soft outgrowth of the endometrial lining. The term "polyp" is used to describe any growth that is attached by means of a stem, or pedicle. Endometrial polyps are generally small, although they may grow large enough to fill the entire uterine cavity. They may be single or multiple.

Incidence and Cause

Endometrial polyps can affect any age-group but are most commonly found in women who are at the age of menopause. Since hormone levels fluctuate in women in this age-group, this suggests that polyps may be caused by some sort of hormonal imbalance. The exact incidence, however, is hard to determine, for polyps may be removed piecemeal during a D&C, a procedure in which the cervix is dilated and the uterine lining removed, and may therefore be unrecognizable.

Symptoms

Sometimes the polyp doesn't produce any symptoms and is discovered only in the course of an operation done for some other reason.

The most common symptom is abnormal bleeding. This may take the form of bleeding in between periods of premenopausal women. The bleeding is not usually profuse, although on occasion a polyp may cause heavy bleeding.

At times the polyp may protrude through the cervical opening. It may cause some cramping as it dilates the cervical opening. The polyp may even grow such a long stem that it actually protrudes through the vaginal opening. These protruding polyps may become injured because of their exposed position. Large ones may outgrow their blood supply, causing portions of the tissue to die. Similarly, the polyp may become twisted on its stem, causing disruption of the blood supply and tissue death. If any of these things occur, the polyp may become infected. There may be a foul-smelling vaginal discharge. Occasionally, a woman's infertility problem can be traced to an endometrial polyp.

Diagnosis

Polyps that protrude through the cervical or vaginal opening are readily diagnosed, although in such cases they may be confused with a cervical polyp. More commonly they don't protrude and are discovered only during the course of a D&C, although, as mentioned before, they may be unrecognizable. Occasionally, a polyp will be located high up inside the uterus and may be missed during a D&C.

Treatment

Treatment of a protruding polyp is removal by D&C. If the polyp's presence has been discovered during a D&C, cure has already been effected. Infrequently, a hysterectomy, or removal of the uterus, may be in order. The polyp is, by and large, a benign condition. Cancerous polyps are extremely rare, and those that occur are usually found in women in their 60s. A hysterectomy would be in order only if the polyp found showed cancerous or precancerous changes. If, for instance, the polyp showed changes resembling those found in adenomatous hyperplasia, treatment similar to the one used for that condition would be in order.

BENIGN TUMORS OF THE FALLOPIAN TUBES

AKA: fibroid tumors
   paraovarian cysts
   tubo-ovarian inflammatory cysts
   endometrial cysts
   noncancerous tumors of the tubes

Types: adenomatoid tumors
   salpingitis isthmica nodosa

"Tumor," in the broadest medical sense of the term, means simply a "swelling." "Benign," of course, means "noncancerous." A number of benign tumors can affect the fallopian tubes as well as the broad ligaments and uterosacral ligaments (the bands of tissue that support the uterus and other pelvic organs).

These tumors are generally small and don't cause any symptoms, although occasionally they are thought to play a role in causing infertility or ectopic pregnancy. If they become large, they may lead to torsion, or twisting, of the fallopian tube, which can cause a great deal of pain, not unlike that associated with an ovarian tumor that has undergone torsion. Since they are generally small and don't cause symptoms they are usually not discovered unless surgery is done for some other reason.

Types

Many of these benign tumors of the tubes have been discussed in more detail elsewhere in this book. For instance, fibroid tumors of the type found in the uterus can affect the tubes and the ligaments, but fibroids are less common in these areas than in the uterus. Paraovarian cysts and tubo-ovarian inflammatory cysts, which are discussed under the section on the ovary, are all associated with the tubes as well. Endometriosis can also affect the tubes and ligaments.

Although they are relatively rare, the two most common types of tumors of the tube are adenomatoid tumors and salpingitis isthmica nodosa. The adenomatoid tumors are frequently associated with salpingitis, inflammation of the fallopian tubes and are sometimes mistaken for cancer.

Salpingitis isthmica nodosa are tumors that are also associated with salpingitis. The condition has a number of names, including diverticulosis of the tube, adenosalpingitis and adenomyosis of the tube. These tumors may occur at any age. They tend to be small and rather firm; their presence may stimulate the formation of scar tissue and adhesions.

Treatment

Most of these benign tumors don't require treatment unless they produce pain or there is an associated fertility problem. If fertility is a problem, it is sometimes possible to remove the affected section of the tube and to rejoin the remaining healthy portion of the tube to the uterus.

ENDOMETRIAL HYPERPLASIA

Types: cystic hyperplasia
adenomatous hyperplasia
carcinoma in situ or Stage O uterine cancer

Endometrial hyperplasia is an abnormal condition in which the endometrial lining has grown too thick. The term "hyperplasia" means "overgrowth." "Endometrial" refers to the endometrium, the specialized tissue that lines the inside of the uterus, thickening each month in preparation for pregnancy and breaking down and shedding during menstruation if pregnancy does not occur. The endometrium is normally rather thin, and about half its thickness is lost each month during menstruation.

Most of the time, hyperplasia is not too serious. It is usually a benign disease that may not even require treatment in a young girl. At other times it may be the first step on the road to endometrial cancer.

Types

Basically, there are two types of hyperplasia: cystic hyperplasia and adenomatous hyperplasia. The only way to tell the difference between the two is to examine the endometrial tissue under a microscope. It is possible for both types to exist in the same woman, and either type may coexist with endometrial cancer.

The majority of cases of hyperplasia do not lead to cancer. Cystic hyperplasia is less likely to lead to cancer than adenomatous hyperplasia. The age at which the hyperplasia occurs is an important factor. Hyperplasia in the young girl is less serious than hyperplasia in the older woman. Some studies have indicated that as many as 30 percent of postmenopausal women with adenomatous hyperplasia will develop endometrial cancer, usually within 3 to 6 years.[17] Because of the precancerous nature of adenomatous hyperplasia, some doctors use the term "carcinoma in situ" or "Stage O endometrial carcinoma" to describe this condition.

Cause

Hyperplasia is caused by continual estrogen stimulation of the uterine lining without the counterbalancing effect of progesterone. During the first half of the menstrual cycle, the hormone estrogen stimulates the endometrial lining of the uterus, causing it to thicken and grow. After the ripe egg bursts from its follicle on the surface of the ovary, the hormone progesterone, which is produced by the remnants of the burst follicle, further stimulates the uterine lining, so that it will be able to nourish a fertilized egg. If the egg is not fertilized, the endometrial lining is no longer needed. Progesterone plays a role in the breakdown and shedding of the endometrial lining. If, for a variety of possible reasons, the egg does not burst from the surface of the ovary, no progesterone is produced. The estrogen continues to stimulate the lining, which grows thicker and thicker without the progesterone to help it break down and shed.

In postmenopausal women, estrogen replacement therapy may cause hyperplasia. However, hyperplasia may also occur in postmenopausal women who are not taking estrogen as well as in women with functioning ovarian tumors or polycystic ovaries.

Incidence

Hyperplasia usually occurs at the beginning and end of menstrual life, just after puberty or during the menopausal years, when irregularities in ovulation are most common, as the monthly cycle gears up or slows down.

Symptoms

Hyperplasia causes irregular menstrual bleeding. At first there may be a period of amenorrhea (absence of menstruation), as the estrogen continually stimulates the endometrial lining. Eventually, the estrogen cannot support the overgrowth it has stimulated, and portions of it break down and shed. This may start as minimal spotting but may progress to profuse and prolonged periods.

Diagnosis and Treatment

Endometrial hyperplasia may be diagnosed by a D&C, a procedure in which the endometrial lining is removed. The lining is then examined microscopically to rule out the possibility of cancer and to determine which type of hyperplasia is present. Endometrial biopsies may also reveal the presence of hyperplasia, but they may not indicate which type of hyperplasia is present or whether cancer is also present.

The treatment of hyperplasia will depend on the age of the woman, the severity of her symptoms and her childbearing plans, as well as on the microscopic analysis of the tissue. Sometimes a D&C will cure the problem. Hormone therapy may be used, but sometimes a hysterectomy is necessary.

If the woman is in her teens, it is often wise to try to avoid a D&C. There is little point in subjecting her to this procedure, for the problem often corrects itself with time. Using birth control pills for a few months may "prime" her ovaries and bring on regular ovulation, eliminating the hyperplasia problem.

In women who are past their teens, however, the D&C is important. First, it will rule out the possibility of cancer and allow the doctor to determine the type of hyperplasia. Second, unlike teenagers, women in the older age-group are not likely to experience a spontaneous cure. Moreover, a D&C often provides a cure for the hyperplasia.

If the pathologist's microscopic examination of the tissue removed by

D&C indicates *cystic* hyperplasia, further treatment may not be necessary, for, as noted, the D&C often cures the problem. If symptoms do persist, a second or even a third D&C may be done. If the woman is premenopausal, some form of progesterone, perhaps oral Provera, may be given instead of a repeat D&C. Within 2 weeks of stopping the drug, all the progesterone is excreted from the body. The drop in the body's level of progesterone causes the endometrial lining to break down and shed, thus eliminating the hyperplasia and the irregular bleeding. The therapy may be continued for several months and then discontinued to allow the woman's body to resume its natural functioning.

If the microscopic examination of the tissue removed by D&C indicates *adenomatous* hyperplasia, more drastic treatment is necessary because of the relationship between adenomatous hyperplasia and endometrial cancer. The treatment of choice is a hysterectomy, removal of the uterus. Depending on age and other factors, the hysterectomy may be accompanied by removal of the ovaries and tubes, a procedure known as bilateral oophorectomy or salpingo-oophorectomy. An alternative form of treatment uses progesterone therapy. Although this type of therapy is often used for cystic hyperplasia, its use in adenomatous hyperplasia is controversial. It has been used with apparent success, but there have been no long-term studies of its effectiveness. The progesterone can apparently cause the abnormal condition of the endometrium to regress to normal. But even if a woman's symptoms subside, she should have a repeat D&C in 3 to 4 months to check for cancer. She must then continue the progesterone therapy and must be followed regularly with endometrial biopsies. The problem is that endometrial biopsies sample only a small portion of the endometrial tissue. Cancer could be lurking in another part of the uterine lining. The woman could conceivably be followed up with D&C's on a regular basis, which would rule out the possibility that cancer was present elsewhere in the lining. But the effect on a woman's body and uterus of frequent D&C's, not to mention the expense and risk involved in such frequent surgery, makes this impractical.

Even if a woman with adenomatous hyperplasia who is treated with progesterone is followed carefully, there is still the possibility that cancer could develop between follow-ups or be missed by the endometrial biopsy. If the cancer should become invasive before being discovered, it might require more extensive surgery and/or radiation therapy, and the woman's chance of survival would be significantly affected. Perhaps in the future, more data will be available on this alternative form of therapy, but until then, women with adenomatous hyperplasia who are anxious to retain their childbearing capacity or to avoid hysterectomy and who elect to try this therapy should realize that they are taking a calculated risk. No one should attempt this form of therapy unless they are willing to commit themselves to a lifelong follow-up program including frequent endometrial biopsies (which, not incidentally, can be quite painful).

Another important issue in endometrial hyperplasia involves the use of terminology. Different doctors use different terminology. Some will call a precancerous growth pattern ''adenomatous hyperplasia,'' whereas others will use the term ''atypical hyperplasia'' to refer to the same growth pattern. Some doctors will refer to both cystic hyperplasia and adenomatous hyperplasia as ''benign'' unless the condition is definitely cancerous.

Over the years there has been some confusion and controversy about endometrial hyperplasia. Some doctors thought it was basically a benign condition; others thought it represented the early stage of cancer. Perhaps this confusion was owing to the lack of standardized terminology and a failure to distinguish between the different types of hyperplasia. Today most gynecologists think of adenomatous hyperplasia as the first step on the road to uterine cancer, even though not all cases will necessarily progress to cancer.

This confusion about hyperplasia has filtered down to general surgeons and family doctors, who may not understand the seriousness of adenomatous hyperplasia. Postmenopausal women will require a hysterectomy, and younger women who are treated with progesterone will need a repeat D&C, even in the absence of symptoms.

After the D&C is performed, the family doctor or general surgeon may get back a pathology report that indicates the presence of ''endometrial hyperplasia'' or merely ''hyperplasia'' and will then assure the woman that there was no sign of cancer and that everything is fine. Women should be sure to ask the doctor which type of hyperplasia is present—cystic or adenomatous. If a woman's D&C was done by a family doctor or general surgeon, she would be wise to seek a second opinion (*see* p. 238). Second pathology opinions (*see* p. 711) are also a good idea, especially for women who have been operated on in small, rural hospitals where only one pathologist is available.

UTERINE CANCER

AKA: carcinoma of the uterine corpus

Types: endometrial cancer
        sarcoma of the uterus

The uterus is made up of the body, or corpus, and the cervix, or neck. Cancer of the cervix is discussed elsewhere. Here we are concerned only with cancers that affect the corpus.

Most cancers of the uterus involve the endometrium, the uterine lining. There are, however, other forms of uterine cancer. Sarcomas, tumors that arise from connective and muscle tissue, may develop in the uterus, but these account for less than 1 percent of uterine malignancies and are mentioned briefly at the end of this section.

Incidence

The incidence of endometrial cancer appears to be increasing.[18] For reasons that are not clear, white women seem to develop the disease more frequently than do black women. The incidence rates for endometrial cancer in white woman are 21.6 per 100,000, whereas for black women the incidence rate is 12.2 per 100,000.[19]

Cause

The cause of endometrial cancer, like the cause of all cancer, is unknown; however, there is strong, if not conclusive, evidence indicating a link between endometrial cancer and the hormone estrogen.

Women whose bodies are subject to a certain type of estrogen influence known as unopposed estrogen are more likely to get endometrial cancer. Women with a history of menstrual irregularities who ovulate infrequently and therefore don't get the relief from constant estrogen stimulation normally provided by the hormone progesterone (which is produced after ovulation) are subject to unopposed estrogen. Overweight women who produce higher levels of estrogen in their excess fat tissue are also at higher risk, as are women who have a late menopause and therefore have more years of estrogen stimulation.[20]

Unopposed estrogen in certain birth control pills has also been associated with increased rates of endometrial cancer. Sequential birth control pills, which relied on unopposed estrogen, where withdrawn from the market for this reason.[21] The use of estrogen replacement therapy, frequently given to menopausal women for relief of menopausal problems, has been associated with an increased risk of endometrial cancer.[22] But combined birth control pills, which contain both estrogen and progesterone, may protect against uterine cancer (*see* pp. 85–6 for details).

Risk Factors

Certain women are more likely to develop endometrial cancer than others. The following risk factors have been identified.[23]

Obesity

Extreme obesity is a strong risk factor, especially in the postmenopausal years. About one-half the women with endometrial cancer are extremely overweight.

Childlessness

Women who have never borne children have an incidence rate about twice as high as those who have children and three times as high as those with five or more children. About one-half of women with this form of cancer have not borne children.

Late Menopause

The average age at menopause for women with the disease is higher. The risk of developing endometrial cancer is approximately two times greater for women whose menopause occurs after age 50 than for those whose menopause occurs before age 49.

Diabetes Mellitus

It is thought that women with diabetes, a disease of the pancreas, are at increased risk. Some authorities have placed the relative risk at slightly better than twofold for the development of endometrial cancer in a woman with a history of diabetes.

Hypertension

Hypertension, a condition characterized by high blood pressure, has not been as consistent a characteristic as the other factors listed here. It is not surprising to find high blood pressure in overweight women of this age-group with diabetes. So, although many women with endometrial cancer have this condition, it is not clear that high blood pressure is in and of itself a risk factor.

Ovarian Disorders

Both Stein-Leventhal syndrome and granulosa cell tumors of the ovary have been associated with increased risk of endometrial cancer.

Cancer of Other Sites

There are increased rates of endometrial cancer in women with breast and ovarian cancer. This may be because all these cancers have some common

447

cause or that women with these cancers have some common factor in their makeup or background that makes them susceptible to all three diseases. Cancer of the bowel has also been associated with increased risk.

Radiation Exposure

Exposure to radiation therapy, used to control postmenopausal bleeding (a form of treatment that has been discontinued), is associated with increased risk of developing this form of cancer. Some researchers think this is one of the best-documented examples of radiation-induced cancer; others suspect that the woman who is treated in this manner and subsequently develops cancer may actually have had cancer at the time of the radiation treatment.

Use of Estrogen Replacement Therapy

In several studies the use of estrogens has been observed to be associated with a four- to sevenfold (or greater) increase in the risk of endometrial cancer. This is discussed in detail under the heading Estrogen Replacement Therapy and in Chapter Five under the heading The Long-Term Effects.

Menstrual Irregularities

Almost 80 percent of women with endometrial cancer have a history of menstrual irregularities. One of the major symptoms of the disease is irregular menstrual bleeding owing to the disease itself; however, for many of these women the abnormal bleeding patterns date back as far as menarche, the first menstrual period. It is not entirely clear whether menstrual irregularities in and of themselves are risk factors or whether the women have menstrual irregularities because they have certain other risk factors, such as diabetes and ovarian problems, that are associated with menstrual irregularities.

Inherited Characteristics

Somewhere between 12 percent and 20 percent of women with endometrial cancer will have a family history of the disease. Here again, it is not entirely clear whether there is an inherited tendency to develop the disease itself or merely an inherited tendency to develop diabetes, obesity, polycystic ovaries, menstrual irregularities and other risk factors.

Women who are at high risk should discuss their medical situations with their doctors. In some instances it may be wise for women at high risk to have routine endometrial biopsies so that any cancer that might develop could be detected while still in its early stages.

Symptoms

The most common symptom is vaginal bleeding, which appears in more than 90 percent of cases. In premenopausal women the bleeding may take the form of a prolonged menstrual period, a sudden flow of blood between periods or a slight staining between periods or after going to the bathroom. In rare cases this type of bleeding may occur after douching or intercourse. These types of abnormal uterine bleeding may result from many other causes. Vaginal bleeding in premenopausal women is more likely the result of some other factor, but continued abnormal bleeding should be brought to the attention of a doctor.

In the menopausal woman, skipping menstrual periods and gradually "tapering off" is not uncommon, so abnormal vaginal bleeding owing to uterine cancer may be misinterpreted as normal menopausal bleeding. If the menstrual periods stop for 6 months to a year and then start up again, however, this should be investigated (see below).

Of the postmenopausal women who experience vaginal bleeding, about one-third will have cancer, one-third will be bleeding because of some benign condition and one-third will be bleeding for unknown reasons. The bleeding may be nothing more than intermittent spotting; however, it may be constant and may even be heavy. Any postmenopausal bleeding deserves investigation. Too often women taking estrogen replacement therapy (ERT) for menopausal symptoms and their doctors are apt to blame the bleeding on the drug, but we know that women on ERT are at increased risk for endometrial hyperplasia and uterine cancer, so it is particularly important that their bleeding symptoms be investigated.

Vaginal discharge is another symptom of uterine cancer, but here again, this symptom may be caused by a number of factors. The discharge may precede the bleeding. A clear, watery discharge is particularly significant, especially when it comes in bursts after heavy exertion or after straining while going to the bathroom. If the cervical canal is partially closed, as it often is in older women, there may be cramplike pain as the uterus tries to expel the discharge through a blocked cervical canal. This is particularly true if there is an associated pyometra, a condition in which a collection of pus and fluid is built up inside the uterus, either because of the cancer or some benign condition. The discharge may then become brown or blood tinged. If portions of the tumor begin to break down, the discharge may begin to smell bad.

Pain is sometimes present, but the significance of the pain is hard to evaluate. Pain in women with cancer is often a sign of advanced or incurable disease, but this is not always true with this form of cancer. Fibroids, endometrial polyps, pyometra and other benign conditions frequently coexist with endometrial cancer and may be the source of the pain.

Diagnosis

There is no simple, painless, screening test like the Pap smear, used to screen for cervical cancer, available for uterine cancer. Nor is the Pap smear reliable in detecting uterine cancer. It fails to detect the cancer too many times. For high-risk women an office procedure known as an endometrial biopsy may be done. This is a painful procedure and is not entirely accurate, so it is not a practical solution for mass screening.

Abnormal bleeding is a critical symptom, since it may be the only one. Once a woman comes to the doctor with abnormal bleeding, she may be given either an endometrial biopsy or a more involved hospital procedure known as a dilation and curettage (D&C), a procedure in which the cervix is opened and the lining of the endometrial cavity is removed. If the woman is menopausal or postmenopausal, an endometrial biopsy is usually done first. If the biopsy indicates that cancer is present, the doctor can proceed to treat the woman without subjecting her to the additional expense and risk of a D&C. If the biopsy is negative, a D&C must still be done, because the endometrial biopsy is not 100 percent accurate.

If, however, the woman is still in her menstrual years, it is much more likely that her abnormal uterine bleeding is caused by some less serious problem. Many of these more common causes of abnormal bleeding will be cured by the D&C. So in this age-group, the D&C, which will rule out cancer and may also be curative, rather than an endometrial biopsy, is generally done.

If the D&C is done, tissue samples from the cervix are taken separately to rule out the possibility that the disease has spread to the cervix. If a D&C is not done, cervical samples may be done at the time of surgery. The uterus is always measured, either during the D&C or on operation. This is an important step, for an enlarged uterus is generally a sign that a larger volume of cancer is present, which will require more aggressive treatment.

The tissue samples are sent to the pathology laboratory for analysis. The pathologist's report will indicate whether or not cancer is present. It will also reveal which grade (*see* p. 714) of cancer the woman has. The grade of the cancer is particularly important, for if the cancer is a low-grade one, this means that the cells are less abnormal and that the cancer is a less serious one. This will affect the treatment that is given.

Any of the standard preoperative tests to detect metastasis (*see* p. 714) may also be done as part of the diagnostic workup. Once the doctor actually operates, the abdominal cavity is carefully inspected for signs of cancer. The lymph nodes are carefully examined. Tissue samples from various locations within the abdominal cavity and, in particular, from certain lymph nodes may be taken in order to help the doctor detect microscopic spread of the disease.

Staging

The results of the pathologist's analysis of the cell and tissue samples and the doctor's measurement of the uterus and careful inspection of the abdominal cavity, along with the results of tests to detect metastasis, will be used to estimate the spread of the disease, that is, to stage the disease.

Table 13 outlines the official staging scheme for uterine cancer.[24] The grade of the tumor cell is of particular importance in Stage I. The grade refers to how well differentiated or mature the cells are. The less mature the cells, the higher the grade, and the higher the grade, the more serious the disease. Grade, as we shall see, can influence decisions about treatment.

Although it is not included in the official treatment scheme, the depth to which the cancer has penetrated the uterine wall will also affect treatment. The length of the uterus is also important, for experience has proved that the larger the uterus, the more likely it is that microscopic cancer has already spread to the adjacent tissues and lymph nodes.

Once the cancer has spread to the cervix (Stage II), the likelihood of involvement of the surrounding tissues and lymph network again increases and treatment must include the areas adjacent to the cervix as well. Once the cancer has spread outside the uterus itself, the situation becomes more serious. In Stage III this spread has begun and the adjacent tissues are obviously involved. Stage IV involves the bladder or rectum and/or spread to distant organs, frequently the lungs.

Table 13
Classification and Staging of Uterine Cancer

Stage I:	The cancer is confined to the body of the uterus
	Stage IA: The length of the uterine cavity is 8 cm or less
	Stage IB: The length of the uterine cavity is more than 8 cm
	Stage IA and Stage IB cases are subgrouped according to grade:
	GI: Highly differentiated
	G2: Highly differentiated with undifferentiated areas
	G3: Predominantly or entirely undifferentiated
Stage II:	The cancer has involved the body of the uterus and the cervix but has not extended outside the uterus
Stage III:	The cancer has extended outside the uterus to the adjacent tissues
Stage IV:	The cancer has involved the bladder or rectum
	Stage IVA: Direct spread to adjacent organs
	Stage IVB: Spread to distant organs

Treatment

Most of the time the treatment of endometrial cancer involves surgery and some form of radiation therapy. In certain cases one or the other form of treatment may be used alone, but the combination of the two generally offers the best chance for a cure.

Surgical Procedures

A variety of surgical procedures may be used in treatment of uterine cancer.

Hysterectomy: At a minimum the surgery will include removal of the uterus. A vaginal cuff, a small portion of the upper vagina that adjoins the cervix, is also removed.

Bilateral Salpingo-Oophorectomy: In this procedure the tubes and ovaries are removed as well.

Lymphadenectomy: This operation involves removing the lymph nodes in the area. There are a number of lymph passageways to which the cancer might spread. Cancer located high in the uterus might spread to one set, whereas cancer near the cervix typically spreads to other lymph nodes. The location of the cancer will be a factor in determining which nodes are removed. At the time of operation, biopsy specimens of certain key nodes may be collected and examined, using frozen section, to help determine which nodes should be treated.

Radical Hysterectomy: Sometimes this more extensive type of hysterectomy, in which the uterus, tubes, ovaries, upper one-third of the vagina and the connective tissues adjacent to the uterus and cervix are removed, is done.

Pelvic Exenteration: In a few cases this very radical form of surgery is used. It involves removal of the uterus, tubes, ovaries, vagina, bladder, connective tissues, urethra and rectum. In certain instances a partial exenteration, in which either the rectum or the bladder and urethra are preserved, can be done. If the bladder and/or rectum are removed, the urinary and bowel tracts must be diverted and new openings created on the outside of the body so that waste products can be collected in plastic bags.

Radiation Therapy

Two types of radiation therapy are commonly used to treat uterine cancer: radioactive implants and external beam therapy.

Radioactive Implants: This type of therapy involves inserting containers, or holders, into the woman's uterus and/or vagina. Once the containers are in the correct position, they are loaded with a radioactive material and left in place until the specified dose of radiation has been achieved. The implants will kill or disable the tumor cells in the uterus or vagina.

External Beam Therapy: This type of radiation is administered from outside the body by directing a beam from an X-ray machine at the cancerous area. It is used to treat cancer that has spread to the adjacent tissues and lymph nodes.

Radiation therapy is generally given before surgery for several reasons. First, it is thought that the radiation will alter the cancer cells in a manner that makes it impossible for the cells to implant elsewhere. Second, radiation causes scarring of the blood vessels and lymph nodes in the area. Thus by giving radiation before surgical treatment, the chances of spreading tumor cells to other areas of the body during surgery are supposedly reduced.[25]

Radiation is not always used preoperatively. In cases where a radical hysterectomy and lymphadenectomy are done, some experts believe that preop radiation is not as important, for a large area of tissue is removed, pretty much in one piece; thus, they argue, the danger of spilling cancer cells onto adjacent tissues or into the lymph system is not as great a problem.[26] Moreover, preoperative radiation delays surgery for anywhere from 1 to 6 weeks (depending on how much radiation is given), makes subsequent surgery more difficult, complicates healing owing to the radiation damage and makes it difficult—sometimes impossible—to tell how deeply the cancer has invaded the uterine wall. The depth of invasion is sometimes a critical factor. In certain cases where the cancer has not invaded the uterine wall or the invasion is limited to the upper one-third of the wall, radiation may not be required.[27] Avoiding preop radiation in these cases allows for a more accurate analysis of depth of invasion and makes it possible to avoid unnecessary radiation in some cases. There are, then, instances when radiation is not given preoperatively or is not used at all.

Similarly, surgery is not used in some cases or is done in only a limited fashion. The extent of the surgery that is done will depend on many factors. The stage of the disease and the grade of the cancer cells are important factors. The low-grade cancers are less likely to spread to the adjacent tissues and lymph system and will require less-radical treatment.

Many times the extent of the surgery is limited by the woman's general health. Since many of these women are obese and have associated medical problems, like high blood pressure, they are often poor surgical risks. The more extensive the surgery, the longer the anesthesia time required and the greater the potential for complications. Sometimes only a simple hysterectomy can be done, because the longer anesthesia time required for a radical hysterectomy or a pelvic examination procedure would pose too great a risk to the woman's life. Sometimes surgery cannot be done at all. Although the survival rates are lower when only radiation therapy is used, sometimes radiation therapy alone is used. Even radioactive implants require some form of anesthetic. Occasionally, a woman is in such poor health that only external beam therapy is used.

The woman's general health, the location and extent of the disease and the grade of the tumor cells will all influence the type of treatment given. The same woman might be treated differently by different doctors. A doctor may advocate a particular therapy program over another simply because s/he was trained that way or because in his or her experience that particular mode of therapy seems to yield superior results.

Although there are differences among doctors regarding treatment of endometrial cancer, there is not the sort of controversy that surrounds treatment of breast cancer. There are studies being conducted that should yield more precise information as to optimum treatment, but medical professionals don't expect these studies to reveal dramatic differences in survival rates.

Although, from the medical point of view, the results of these studies won't be all that significant, they may well be from the woman's point of view. If two plans of treatment are shown to be equally effective, but one causes the woman subsequent pain and difficulty with sexual relations, or makes sex altogether impossible, and the other one doesn't, many women would consider this a rather significant difference. Doctors tend to measure things more in terms of cure rates. Moreover, many women with endometrial cancer are in the older age-group. Despite obvious and unrefuted evidence to the contrary, many doctors persist in thinking that older women don't have sex lives and that, therefore, preservation of, say, vaginal function need not be a major concern. It is true that for some women, having a functioning vagina may not be of great importance in their sex lives. The clitoris is generally of more physiologic importance in sexual pleasure. But for other women, retaining a functioning vagina may be very important. Since the doctor may not consider these issues when planning treatment, it is important that women bring these subjects up and discuss their personal attitudes and priorities with their doctors.

Treatment Plans According to Stage and Grade

The treatment of uterine cancer, like the treatment of any form of cancer, is complex. Descriptions of what is done and explanations of why it is done in the treatment of various stages and grades are outlined below, but these are only generalizations. Treatment is individualized according to the particulars of a woman's case. If your doctor recommends a treatment plan different from the one outlined here, this certainly does not mean that the recommendation is wrong. The information given here is intended to provide basic information, so that women will understand the issues and know enough to ask the right questions. Remember, every woman has the right to a full explanation

454

of what the doctor plans to do and why. Second opinions (*see* p. 238) are, of course, always in order, and they are especially important in cancer.

Stage IA, Grade 1

These cases are usually treated by surgical removal of the uterus, tubes, ovaries and vaginal cuff. The uterus is then examined by the pathologist. If the cancer is indeed Stage IA, Grade 1, and has not penetrated beyond the first third of the uterine wall, some doctors do not recommend any further treatment.[28] If, however, there is deeper penetration, postoperative radiation may be given, for there is a greater likelihood that the cancer has spread to the adjacent tissues and lymph nodes.

There are some doctors who use preoperative radiation in these cases.[29] There are also some who use postoperative radiation regardless of the depth of penetration.[30] Those who advocate preoperative radiation point out that there is a chance, albeit a small one, of recurrence of cancer in the top of the vagina that can be prevented by preoperative radiation. Those who oppose it think that the risks and complications of radiation outweigh the benefits. In fact, some doctors don't think that radiation has any effect on survival in these cases.[31] Also, radiation therapy usually makes for poor vaginal function, so that intercourse becomes painful or sometimes impossible. Rather than treating everyone, some doctors prefer to follow these women carefully and to treat only those who do have recurrences. If a woman is conscientious about follow-up, vaginal recurrences are easy to detect.

Those who use postoperative radiation regardless of the depth of the invasion also do so in order to prevent vaginal recurrences. They point out that postoperative radiation is more comfortable and does not delay surgery. No one knows for certain which type of therapy is best, so decisions are based on the particulars of a woman's case and the doctor's personal experience and treatment preferences. Women with Stage IA, Grade 1 endometrial cancer, particularly those who are concerned about preserving vaginal function, will want to discuss these issues with their doctors and should certainly get multiple opinions before deciding on therapy.

Stage IA, Grades 2 and 3; Stage IB; Stage II[32]

These cases may be treated in a number of ways. Generally, radiation is given preoperatively. Implants may be given, followed in a week or two by hysterectomy and bilateral salpingo-oophorectomy, or in some cases a radical hysterectomy may be done. Depending on the pathologist's estimate of the depth of invasion, subsequent external beam therapy may then be used. Sometimes both implants and external beam therapy are used, followed by hysterectomy and bilateral salpingo-oophorectomy in 4 to 6 weeks (greater doses of preop

455

radiation mean a longer delay to allow for healing of radiation damage before surgery). Sometimes a radical hysterectomy and lymphadenectomy will be done first. This "surgery-first" treatment plan allows for a good pathological evaluation of the depth of penetration of the uterine wall and of the lymph nodes. In some cases no further treatment may be required. In other cases, where there is deep invasion in certain areas, subsequent external beam therapy may have to include the para-aortic as well as the pelvic nodes.

These cases represent one of those instances in which each of the available treatments has its advantages and drawbacks. For example, if radical surgery is done first, it may be possible in some cases to avoid subsequent radiation. Even though the upper one-third of the vagina is removed surgically, this usually permits better vaginal function than radiation therapy, which causes such severe vaginal scarring that intercourse may be painful or even impossible. However, doing surgery first means a delay in administering radiation therapy in those women who require it. If only implants rather than implants *and* external beam therapy are used, better vaginal function is possible.

Sometimes the particulars of a woman's case will dictate the choice of treatment plan. For example, a woman may be too poor a surgical risk for radical surgery and a pelvic lymphadenectomy to be done, so radiation followed by less-radical surgery may be the treatment of choice for her. Or, if a woman has a high-grade tumor or a Stage II tumor, which means the cancer is more likely to have spread to adjacent tissues and lymph nodes, the doctor may use both implants and external beam radiation before surgery to increase the chances of disabling these more lethal high-grade cells so that they won't implant, should they be spilled during surgery.

These again are instances in which the decision about which treatment plan to use is not clear-cut. Although studies are being done to compare these options, it may be years before the results are available. Some doctors are reluctant to use the surgery-first type of treatment because, based on their personal experience, they believe it to be less effective or simply because they have been trained to give preoperative radiation. Here again, women, particularly those who are concerned about preservation of vaginal function, should discuss the pros and cons of the various treatment options with their doctors and seek second opinions from doctors who are advocates of the various treatment plans that are possible options in their cases.

Stages III and IV [33]

Treatment of Stage III and Stage IV cases is highly individualized and will depend on the extent of the disease spread, its location and the general health of the woman. External beam therapy and implants are generally used. Surgery may also be done, and if it is done, it generally includes removal of the uterus, tubes and ovaries. More extensive surgery is done in some cases, but this is generally not possible because of the extent of the spread and the generally poor health of these women. In a few cases surgery as radical as pelvic exenteration may be done. In one study involving 33 women with Stage IV disease who were given pelvic exenteration, 6 survived longer than 5 years. Such surgery can, then, be worthwhile in certain cases.

Chemotherapy and hormone therapy may also be used in the treatment of these advanced cases. Generally, some form of the hormone progesterone is used. This is particularly valuable in Stage IVB cases, where there is metastasis to the lung. The progesterone will be effective in about one-third of these cases. It is also effective in treating metastases in other locations as well as local spread in the pelvis. Currently, there are a number of studies evaluating other forms of chemotherapy for advanced and recurrent uterine cancer. Having a doctor who is up-to-date on the latest developments is of prime importance.

Recurrent Cancer[34]

The treatment program for recurrent cancer will depend on the location and size of the tumor and what type of therapy was used in the treatment of the initial cancer. If it recurs locally, for instance in the vagina or nearby tissues, this may be treated by external beam therapy if only radioactive implants were used in the initial treatment; however, if both external beam therapy and implants were used initially, further radiation therapy cannot be given, for the maximum dose of radiation will have been given during the initial therapy. Further radiation would damage the healthy tissue so much that the woman would die. If the maximum radiation has already been given, in some cases pelvic exenteration may be done. Although this has been effective, it is rarely done, for the woman's health usually won't permit such radical surgery. If the disease recurs in some distant location and/or locally, chemotherapy of the type described above may be used.

Follow-Up[35]

Follow-up is important if recurrences are to be detected early. In the first year the woman will see the doctor at least every 3 months. Most recurrences happen within the first 2 or 3 years after treatment. By the 5th year, women are generally seen only once a year, unless problems occur.

The extent of the follow-up will depend on the extent of the disease. More advanced cancers are more likely to recur and therefore require more elaborate follow-up. At a minimum the doctor will do a Pap smear, bimanual examination, a thorough visual exam with a speculum, a careful palpation of the abdomen and liver and a complete physical. The abdomen may be measured and tapped to check for any accumulations of fluid. Symptoms like a cough or chest pain are important. Chest X-rays are often done routinely even if no symptoms are present since the lungs are a frequent site of recurrence. The bones may also be a site of metastasis, so any pain in the bones calls for a bone scan. The liver is another frequent site of recurrent endometrial cancer. So, in advanced cases, liver scans as well as intravenous pyelograms may be done. The exact nature of the follow-up program will depend on the seriousness of the original disease.

Sometimes women who have been treated for endometrial cancer don't visit the doctor for follow-up. If they had low-grade, Stage I cancer, they may think their problems are over, but recurrences happen even in the best of circumstances. Follow-up of women with early stages is especially important, for they have the best chance of cure should the cancer recur. Some women get lax about follow-up as the years go by. Although it is true that most recurrences are detected within the first 3 years after treatment, some don't appear for many years. Still, many women neglect follow-up because they have been so drained by the recovery from surgery or the side effects of radiation therapy that, in one woman's words, "It just took the fight out of me." Or they may feel that there is no hope for them should the cancer recur. Although it is true that those women whose disease was less serious in the first place, and hence required less extensive and physically draining therapy, have a better chance of survival if there is a recurrence, even women with late-stage cancers have been cured by subsequent therapy. Even though the cure rate for recurrent cancer is only 10 percent, treatment may succeed in prolonging life and in making the remaining time more comfortable.

Follow-up is important for all women. A woman's best chance of being the 1 in 10 who will survive recurrent cancer depends on early detection of the recurrence.

Sarcomas

Sarcomas, another form of uterine cancer, are often not detected until the cancer is in a fairly advanced stage. Treatment usually includes a hysterectomy and bilateral salpingo-oophorectomy. For certain types of sarcomas, treatment may involve radical hysterectomy and lymphadenectomy. In some cases radiation therapy may prove helpful. Chemotherapy is frequently used. Overall survival rates are around 20 percent to 30 percent but in early stages may run as high as 80 percent.

Survival

The survival rates for endometrial cancer vary with the stage of the disease, the grade of the tumor cells and other factors including whether or not the woman's health was good enough to allow for optimum treatment. Table 14 lists survival rates by stage and also breaks down survival rates for Stage I according to grade.

Table 14
Five-Year Survival Rates for Endometrial Cancer by Stage

Stage	Percent
IA	80
IB	65
II	41
III	17
IV	2

Five-Year Survival Rates for Stage I Endometrial Cancer by Grade

Grade	Percent
1	91
2	74
3	48

SOURCE: Adapted from John, Boutselis, "Endometrial Carcinoma," *Surgical Clinics of North America*, Vol. 58, No. 1, February 1978.

CANCER OF THE FALLOPIAN TUBES*

AKA: carcinoma of the fallopian tubes

Associated Terms: hematosalpinx, or hydrosalpinx; torsion of the tube, hydrops tubae profluens, or hemohydrops tubae perfluens

Cancer of the fallopian tube very rarely occurs. The disease may be primary, that is, it may originate in the tubes, or secondary, the result of direct extension of cancer of the uterus or the ovary or of distant metastasis. It is sometimes difficult to tell whether the disease is primary or secondary.

Cause and Incidence

The cause of cancer of the fallopian tube is unknown. It is extremely rare, accounting for somewhere between .3 percent and 1.1 percent of all gynecolog-

*See also the general discussion of cancer.

ical cancers.[36] Even those cancer specialists who treat only patients referred to them by other doctors are unlikely to see more than one patient a year with cancer of the fallopian tube.

Symptoms[37]

More than 90 percent of women with this disease will have symptoms. But the symptoms are often inconsistent, that is, they vary from case to case, are nonspecific (can be caused by many other diseases) and are so slight, at least in the early stages, that the symptoms are often ignored or misinterpreted.

Abnormal vaginal bleeding, spasmlike pain, heavy vaginal discharge that tends to be watery and mucus-filled or tinged with blood and abdominal distention are all possible symptoms of fallopian tube cancer.

Diagnosis

Most of the time this disease is found unexpectedly in the course of exploratory surgery or surgery done for some other reason. Less than 5 percent of cases are diagnosed preoperatively.

Spread and Staging

Decisions about how far the disease has spread are usually made at the time of the operation. Cancer of the fallopian tube most often spreads by direct invasion of the cancer into the surrounding organs. The disease may also be spread by the lymph system or blood system. Since the disease is so rare, no official staging scheme has been developed. The staging schemes used are similar to the ones used for ovarian cancer.

Treatment

The same principles that apply to the treatment of ovarian cancer apply to this disease. The treatment is primarily surgical and consists of total hysterectomy, that is, the removal of the tubes, uterus and ovaries.

Postoperative radiation in the form of external beam therapy may be given, although there is some debate about the effectiveness of such radiation.[38] Recently, chemotherapy has proved to be of some limited value. Despite the lack of spectacular results, chemotherapy is frequently used in the treatment of this disease.

Survival Rates

The overall 5-year survival rate for this disease is 38 percent.[39] The stage of the disease is, of course, a significant factor in the survival rates. Five-year survival rates as high as 60 percent have been reported for Stage I.[40] Most deaths occur in the first 2 years after diagnosis.

The Ovaries

The anatomy and function of the ovary, which is illustrated in Chapter Two and is discussed in Chapter Four, may be disrupted by a variety of disease processes. Basically, there are four kinds of things that can go wrong with the ovary.

Ovarian Infections

First, the ovary can become infected. Infections of the ovary alone, which are known in medical circles as oophoritis, are rare. When the ovary is infected it is usually a part of a more widespread infection involving the fallopian tubes and other pelvic organs. When these widespread infections occur, collections of pus, known as tubo-ovarian abscesses or cysts, may be formed. These infectious processes are discussed elsewhere in this book under the heading Pelvic Inflammatory Disease.

Birth Defects

Second, the ovary can be abnormal as a result of congenital problems, that is, owing to birth defects. For instance, a woman may be born without any ovaries or with extra ones. Her ovaries may not have the proper amount of eggs, causing her to have a premature menopause. A woman may have both ovaries and the male counterpart, testes, or may have testes instead of ovaries. Fortunately, these sorts of problems are uncommon and are discussed briefly under the first heading in this section, Congenital Abnormalities of the Ovary.

Ovulation Problems

There may be disturbances in the process by which an egg is matured and released from the ovary each month. The follicular sac, inside of which the ripening egg develops, may not behave properly and may swell up, creating a follicular cyst. The corpus luteum, which is formed from the remnants of the follicle after it has burst open and released its egg, may also function improperly, creating a luteum cyst. These are called physiologic cysts. Another type of ovarian problem associated with abnormal ovulation is a condition known as polycystic (meaning "many cyst") disease.

Ovarian Tumors

The fourth group of problems that can affect the ovary are ovarian tumors. The word "tumor" is a scary one that conjures up associations with cancer for most of us. But in the widest medical sense of the word the term "tumor" merely means a "swelling." A pimple, for instance, would be a tumor in medical jargon. The luteum and follicular cysts mentioned above are also considered tumors in the medical sense of the term, but they are generally not serious problems. Indeed, physiologic cysts usually do not even require treatment, for they generally disappear all by themselves. These physiologic cysts, the cysts associated with polycystic disease and the tubo-ovarian cysts mentioned above, as well as another type of ovarian cyst known as an endometrial cyst, are all nonneoplastic tumors, which means that they are *not* ("non") *new* ("neo") *growths* ("plastic").

All the other tumors of the ovary are neoplastic, or new growths. There are quite a few types of neoplastic tumors that can occur in the ovary, for the ovary is a complex organ containing many types of tissue. Moreoover, the ovary contains the ova, the female egg cells, which have the potential, if fertilized, to produce hair, skin, bone—indeed, all the types of tissue present in the adult human. Therefore, it is not surprising that a wide variety of tumors, including some rather bizarre ones that contain hair, teeth and bits of bone, can arise from the ovary.

These new growths may be cystic (fluid-filled), solid, semisolid or semicystic. They may be unilateral, affecting only one ovary, or bilateral, involving both ovaries. Most important, they may be either benign or malignant. Certain types of tumors are always benign, like the ovarian fibroma; others, like the cystadenocarcinomas, are, by definition, cancerous. Oftentimes,

463

there is not a clear dividing line between cancerous and noncancerous ovarian tumors, and these are called borderline tumors.

The new growths of the ovary are divided into two major groups: the benign tumors and the cancerous ones. We have also included a third group, known as the functioning ovarian tumors. They are referred to as functioning tumors because they are capable of producing hormones. Some produce male hormones, causing the woman to grow chest hair and a beard and to develop other masculine characteristics. Some produce the female hormone estrogen and can cause irregular bleeding. Some of these functioning tumors are benign and some are borderline or clearly cancerous.

Unfortunately, there is usually no way to tell whether an ovarian tumor is benign or malignant short of actually operating, removing the tumor and examining it under a microscope. The woman's age and the feel and location of the tumor may give the doctor some clues as to whether an ovarian tumor is benign or malignant. Solid tumors, for instance, are more likely to be malignant, as are bilateral tumors. If the woman is in her reproductive years, she probably has a benign tumor. If the woman is past menopause, the situation is more serious, for 50 percent of the ovarian tumors in these women will be cancerous.[1] If the doctor can feel a suspicious enlargement in the pelvis of a young girl, the situation is less serious than it would be in the postmenopausal woman. But it is more serious than in a woman who is in her reproductive years, for although ovarian cancer is rare in young girls, any type of ovarian enlargement in young girls is rare. Statistically, chances are that the young girl's suspicious enlargement is the result of some benign condition. Perhaps it is not even an ovarian enlargement, for it is sometimes hard for the doctor to determine by simply feeling a young girl's pelvis exactly where the enlargement is located. However, the doctor will always suspect cancer in a young girl who has a pelvic mass.

Exploratory Surgery for Ovarian Masses

But these signs are only clues. Cancer can occur in any age-group, regardless of whether the tumor is unilateral or bilateral, cystic or solid; therefore, any time the doctor feels a suspicious mass that might be ovarian in origin, prompt exploratory surgery is in order. This may be hard for some of us to accept, especially if the mass is small and not causing any symptoms. Such surgery may seem needless—why have an operation when it's not causing any problems?

The answer is twofold. First, there is the chance that it might be a cancerous tumor. Second, the tumor, even if it is benign, will continue to grow larger, eventually producing symptoms and possibly causing serious complications. Moreover, in women who have future childbearing plans or who are anxious to preserve their ovaries in order to avoid premature menopause and all its attendant problems, it is necessary to remove the tumor before it destroys the rest of the ovary.

There is one important exception to this prompt-surgery-for-ovarian-tumors rule. If a woman is in her reproductive years, is not using birth control pills and has a small, soft mass, chances are that she has a luteum or follicular cyst. Since these usually disappear spontaneously within one or two menstrual cycles, waiting for a few weeks before doing surgery will often allow a woman to avoid unnecessary surgery. If you fall into this category, don't allow yourself to be rushed into surgery, as too often happens. If your doctor suggests immediate surgery, discuss this issue with him or her and consider getting a second opinion (*see* p. 238) before consenting to surgery.

If you are scheduled for surgery for a possible ovarian tumor, you should read the sections on physiologic cysts, benign ovarian tumors, and ovarian cancer. There are many considerations. If the tumor turns out to be benign, do you want the doctor to remove your ovaries or try to conserve as much ovarian tissue as possible? Some doctors will routinely remove both ovaries in women over age 35 who have completed their families. Others will go to great lengths to save the ovaries, even if the woman is 45. A woman who has a family history of ovarian cancer might decide to have her ovaries removed regardless of her age. Another woman who is at high risk for developing hypertension, a condition characterized by high blood pressure that can have serious, even fatal, consequences, might decide to try and save her ovaries if possible, for premature menopause might increase her risk of developing hypertension. There are many factors involved, and each woman must make the decision for herself. Unfortunately, many doctors won't even present these alternatives to their patients or will present them in a biased fashion, pushing their own points of view.

Other questions are to be considered as well. If your tumor is benign and only one ovary needs to be removed, do you want the doctor to remove your uterus as well? If it turns out to be a certain type of cancer, there may be different treatment options and decisions you may want to have a voice in making. There are also certain things you should check out before operation. Is the pathologist top-notch? Will there be more than one pathologist reviewing your slides? These questions and other information that you, as a consumer of medical services, have a need to know are discussed in the following pages. Read and study them carefully, and then, armed with enough knowledge to enable you to ask the right questions, discuss these issues with your doctor, seeking second opinions wherever you feel the need.

CONGENITAL ABNORMALITIES OF THE OVARY

AKA: birth defects involving the ovary

Types: testicular feminization syndrome
true hermaphroditism
female hermaphroditism, pseudohermaphroditism, congenital adrenal hyperplasia
and adrenogenital syndrome
Turner's syndrome, gonadal dysgenesis, or gonadal agenesis
accessory ovaries
supernumerary ovaries
congenital absence of one ovary and fallopian tube

Many, but not all, of the congenital abnormalities (birth defects) of the ovary are caused by abnormalities in the chromosomes, which are microscopic substances in the center of a cell that govern the cell's behavior. These are called developmental abnormalities. There may also be associated congenital abnormalities of the vulva. These conditions vary in their severity. One of the relatively less serious ones, testicular feminization syndrome, is a condition in which a woman, normal in every other way, is born without a uterus and with organs that more closely resemble testes than ovaries. This is not as bizarre as it sounds, for testes and ovaries are actually rather similar and develop from the same fetal tissue. Such women have normal breast development and female secondary sex characteristics and function as normal women except that they do not have ovaries or a uterus and cannot, therefore, have children. The condition is generally diagnosed because the girl fails to start menstruating. It is difficult to distinguish between this syndrome and congenital absence of the uterus, but it is important to do so since the abnormal ovarian/testicular tissue must be removed, as it is subject to the development of cancer. The diagnosis and treatment of this syndrome is discussed under the heading Amenorrhea. Interestingly, women with this syndrome are often quite striking. They tend to be tall, with long graceful arms and legs.

True hermaphroditism is another developmental abnormality. It is a condition in which the person has male and female organs, both internally and externally. There may be both an ovary and testis on each side or an ovary on one side and a testis on the other. The condition is again owing to a defect in the chromosomes and is often associated with mental retardation. The external genital organs may appear normal, although usually they are also deformed. At puberty the development may be along male or female lines, depending on whether ovarian or testicular tissue predominates. Treatment may include hormone therapy and plastic surgery.

Female pseudohermaphroditism, congenital adrenal hyperplasia and adrenogenital syndrome are conditions in which masculine traits appear in a genetic female. These conditions may be detected at birth if the external genitals are abnormal. The clitoris may, for instance, be enlarged and may look more like a penis than a clitoris. Otherwise, they may not become apparent until puberty, when the child has rapid growth; a muscular, male body-type; early development of male hair patterns on the face and chest; acne and failure to have menstrual periods. These conditions are caused by an overproduction of hormones by the adrenal glands. In pseudohermaphroditism this overproduction results from a chromosomal abnormality. Adrenogenital syndrome, on the other hand, may not be a birth defect but may be caused by a tumor of the adrenal gland. The symptoms may be obvious or subtle. In some cases these conditions are diagnosed only because the girl fails to menstruate at the normal age. Diagnosis, which is made by certain laboratory tests, is discussed more fully under the heading Amenorrhea. Treatment may include surgery to correct abnormalities of the genitals, and hormone therapy to stimulate secondary sex characteristics. Other forms of pseudohermaphroditism, both male and female, can occur and require similar treatment.

Another type of developmental abnormality is Turner's syndrome, also called gonadal dysgenesis or gonadal agenesis. It is caused by abnormalities in the chromosomes of the genes. Since the ovaries are undeveloped or absent altogether, the hormones that stimulate growth and sexual development are also absent. The condition varies in its severity. It may be diagnosed at birth or may not become obvious until puberty or later. Children with this syndrome may have a webbed neck, a certain bone condition known as osteoporosis, widely spaced nipples, a low hairline, small jaw and short stature. The genitals do not develop properly, nor do the breasts. Such women have minimal sexual hair or sometimes none, do not menstruate and are infertile. The ovaries are absent or underdeveloped. The physical appearance and other symptoms will suggest the diagnosis, and it can be confirmed by special tests. Treatment may involve estrogen therapy to stimulate secondary sex characteristics, but such therapy carries certain risks. These are discussed under the heading Estrogen Replacement Therapy. Plastic surgery may be done to create a normal vagina and external genital organs. Turner's syndrome is used to refer to a specific type of chromosomal abnormality. There are other, similar conditions whose symptoms may vary slightly. For instance, the woman may be tall rather than short, but similar treatment is used.

Some congenital abnormalities of the ovary are thought to be the result of faulty development in the ovary rather than chromosomal abnormalities. These include an extremely rare condition known as accessory ovaries, in which excess ovarian tissue is found, usually located near or attached to the normal ovary; supernumerary ovaries, in which three or more ovaries are present; and the absence of one ovary and fallopian tube, which may be associated with certain congenital abnormalities of the uterus. These conditions are, fortunately, rather rare.

467

PHYSIOLOGIC CYSTS

AKA: ovarian cysts, functional cysts*

Types: follicle, or follicular, cysts
      luteum cysts

Associated Terms: corpus luteum hematoma, follicular hematoma

There are basically two types of physiologic cysts: luteum and follicle. Follicle cysts occur quite frequently, for they are really exaggerations of a normal process that occurs cyclically in the mature female. Each month a number of ova (eggs) resting inside sacs, called follicles, deep within the ovary are stimulated by hormones to develop and move toward the surface of the ovary. As they develop, specialized cells that line the interior cavity of the follicular sac secrete fluids that nourish the developing ovum, and these fluids cause the follicle to swell. Normally, only one of these swelling follicles is chosen to mature fully, reach the surface and release its egg at ovulation. Countless others don't develop fully and disintegrate into microscopic specks of scar tissue.

Sometimes this normal process goes awry. Either the chosen follicle fails to release its egg and continues to grow larger or one or more of the competing follicles doesn't disintegrate and continues to swell with fluid. If either of these things happens, one or more cysts, that is, encapsulated collections of fluid, known as follicular cysts, are formed.

Just as follicle cysts are the result of a distortion of the process of ovulation, so luteum cysts are an irregularity in the normal course of events. After the follicle bursts, releasing its egg at ovulation, the remnants of the burst follicle become the corpus luteum, which starts producing the hormone progesterone. This hormone helps the uterus get ready for a possible pregnancy by stimulating the uterine lining to grow rich and thick, so that the egg, if fertilized, will be well nourished. If a fertilized egg does not implant in the lining of the uterus, the corpus luteum normally stops producing progesterone and disintegrates. Without the progesterone to support its growth, the rich lining begins to disintegrate and is shed during the monthly period. In the case of a luteum cyst the corpus luteum does not disintegrate as it should but swells with fluid and persists on the surface of the ovary as a cyst. There is normally a small amount of bleeding into the corpus luteum after the follicle bursts. Sometimes this can become excessive, and the cyst fills with blood. This is called a corpus luteum hematoma. Similarly, blood may fill a follicular cyst in which case the name follicular hematoma is used.

*These cysts are sometimes called functional cysts because they develop from normal ovarian process or functions. This is not to be confused with the term "functioning cysts."

Symptoms

Physiologic cysts are generally rather small, for the pressure of the fluid on the cyst wall prevents the further production of fluid and greater enlargement.

They may produce the same symptoms as any other ovarian cyst (*see* p. 476); however, since they are usually small, they are less likely to produce severe symptoms. If, however, they grow large, there may be a dull ache on the affected side.

They may affect the menstrual cycle. The luteum cyst, which affects progesterone production, is more apt to alter the menstrual cycle. The continued stimulation of the uterine lining by the progesterone may delay the period. When menstrual flow does start, the bleeding may be rather scant since much of the lining may be retained because of the effect of the progesterone.

Physiologic cysts generally don't become pedunculated, that is, they don't grow stems, or pedicles, as so many other ovarian tumors do. If, however, they grow large, they may develop pedicles, in which case they are subject to the same complications and may produce the same symptoms as any other pedunculated ovarian cyst.

These cysts may rupture spontaneously or as a result of some physical exertion. If a follicle cyst ruptures, there is generally little pain, for the fluid that spills into the pelvic cavity is not irritating. If blood has seeped into the follicle cyst and the cyst then ruptures, there may be some discomfort but this usually passes and rarely reaches the emergency proportions that rupture of other types of ovarian cysts can cause.

The luteum cyst is less prone to rupture; however, should it rupture, it is more likely to cause pain since it is more apt to contain larger amounts of blood, and blood is highly irritating to the pelvic cavity. A ruptured corpus luteum cyst can produce symptoms similar to those of a ruptured ectopic pregnancy. Laparoscopic exam may be the only way to distinguish between the two.

Diagnosis

These cysts are often diagnosed when bothersome symptoms of pelvic pressure or pain bring the woman to the doctor, or they may be discovered in the course of a routine pelvic exam. The diagnostic procedures are the same as those used for any other type of ovarian tumor (*see* p. 480).

Treatment

As explained in the introduction to this section, ovarian cysts generally require prompt surgery because of the possibility that they may be cancerous, but younger women with small cystic masses should not allow themselves to be rushed into surgery, as too often happens. In all likelihood such a woman will have a follicular or luteum cyst that will rupture spontaneously or be reabsorbed by the body within one or two menstrual cycles. Waiting a few weeks can prevent unnecessary surgery. We generally wait one menstrual cycle in these cases. Some doctors will wait for two cycles, since some of these physiologic cysts take that long to disappear. This is certainly acceptable medical practice; however, we are a bit more conservative about this and will recommend an operation if a cyst persists for more than one cycle because of the possibility that this could be ovarian cancer, a very serious disease. Although this is our personal philosophy, many doctors believe that waiting for two cycles is justified.

If, however, the woman is past menopause or is using birth control pills, she is probably not ovulating and therefore probably does not have a physiologic cyst. In such women, surgery should not be delayed. Chances are that these women will have benign cysts, but follicular and luteum cysts are the only cysts that will disappear spontaneously, so there is nothing to be gained by delaying surgery in such women. Also, if a woman's cyst is larger than 5 cm, surgery should generally not be delayed, for cysts of that size rarely regress on their own.

If an operation is done and a follicular cyst is discovered, the ovary should not be removed, as is sometimes done. The contents of a smaller cyst can be aspirated with a needle, which will cause the cyst to collapse. The larger ones can be shelled out, leaving much of the normal ovary intact. If a luteum cyst is discovered, it is usually not removed or aspirated unless it is large or leaking blood into the pelvic cavity. The corpus luteum normally continues to function in the early stages of pregnancy to support the developing embryo. The woman might have an undiagnosed pregnancy and removing the corpus luteum could terminate the pregnancy.

A new treatment, known as ovarian cyst fenestration, may be recommended to women suspected of having physiologic cysts. However, as explained elsewhere (see p. 484), we think this procedure is too risky and do not recommend it.

Women who are troubled by recurrent physiologic cysts, especially those who have undergone repeat surgery for what turned out to be simple physiologic cysts, may want to consider using the birth control pill (unless, of course, they have contraindications to use of the Pill; see pp. 115–16). For such women the Pill may be a good idea, because the Pill inhibits ovulation. Since physiologic cysts result from disturbances in normal ovulation and because Pill users do not usually ovulate, physiologic cysts are uncommon among Pill users.* In fact, the incidence of such cysts in Pill users aged 20 to

---

*The Pill has not been shown to have the same protective effect against other benign cysts. The incidence of other noncancerous cysts is the same in Pill users and nonusers.

44 is only 3 cases per 100,000 women per year, as compared with 38 cases per 100,000 in women who do not use the Pill.[2] Although we are hardly Pill "fans," we *do* believe that the Pill might be a wise idea for women who are troubled with recurrent physiologic cysts.

Some doctors recommend that women who have *suspected* ovarian cysts, but no history of recurrent physiologic cysts, also go on the Pill, at least temporarily. We are not as comfortable with this advice. Doctors who recommend this course of action believe that the Pill will aid in the regression of the cyst—if it is a physiologic cyst—thus helping to avoid unnecessary surgery. Such doctors may point to the fact that physiologic cysts are less common among Pill users, or to studies like the one that involved 286 women with ovarian cysts who were put on the Pill as soon as their cysts were discovered.[3] In all but 81 of these women the cyst had regressed after 6 weeks on the Pill. The 81 women whose cysts had not regressed were subsequently operated on. Some had cancerous cysts and some had benign cysts, but none of the women had physiologic cysts. Some doctors have taken this to mean that the Pill aids in the regression of physiologic cysts. But we are a bit skeptical. Although it seems clear that the Pill can prevent physiologic cysts from developing in the first place, it is not clear how it would help get rid of a cyst that is already there. Moreover, it is already known that the majority of physiologic cysts will go away by themselves after 4 weeks, so it is not particularly surprising that the physiologic cysts in the women in this study had disappeared by 6 weeks. In fact, it seems altogether possible that the cysts would have gone away by themselves, Pill or no Pill. Until we get more convincing evidence that the Pill aids in regression of ovarian cysts, we will be reluctant to prescribe it for this purpose.

Not only is it unclear to us whether or not the Pill would help in making the cyst go away, we are also concerned about prescribing the Pill to a woman who may need surgery within a few weeks. The risk of post-surgical blood clots is increased in women on the Pill (see the section on the Pill). Doctors are urged, whenever possible, to take women off the Pill for at least a month before any anticipated surgery. If a woman with a cyst were given the Pill and her cyst persisted, necessitating surgery, she would add to the risks of surgery by having used the Pill.

POLYCYSTIC OVARIES

AKA: polycystic disease, or syndrome; Stein-Leventhal disease, or syndrome

Polycystic ovaries are another type of disturbance of ovulation. In the normal monthly course of events, follicles deep within the ovaries that contain unripe eggs are stimulated to grow, develop and move toward the surface of the ovary, where one of these follicles matures, bursts open and releases its egg. This process of stimulating eggs and their follicles is governed by hormones

471

from the pituitary gland. After the egg is released at ovulation the remnants of the burst follicle become the corpus luteum, which produces the hormone progesterone. The primary effect of this hormone is to stimulate the lining of the uterus to grow rich and thick in case it needs to support a fertilized egg. The rising levels of progesterone also affect the pituitary, which has been busily sending out its hormones to stimulate the eggs to develop. In effect the progesterone tells the pituitary, "Stop stimulating eggs; ovulation has occurred."

In patients with polycystic disease this normal progression of events doesn't take place. The follicles with the unripe eggs never get to the surface of the ovary. Instead, they just sit there, literally stuck beneath the surface of the ovary. Since there is no egg, there is no burst follicle. Therefore, no corpus luteum is formed and there are no rising levels of progesterone, which means that no "turn-off" message is sent to the pituitary. The pituitary therefore continues to send out its hormones, which stimulate more and more follicles.

These follicles continue to get trapped just below the surface of the ovary. After a while both ovaries become studded with multiple small cysts just below the surface. Even though these individual cysts may measure only a fraction of an inch, all together they can cause the ovary to enlarge to as much as two to three times its normal size. There is a sort of thickened capsule surrounding the ovary. It is unclear whether this thickened capsule is a result of the presence of many follicle cysts or perhaps the cause of them. Occasionally, some women with polycystic disease have a successful ovulation, but most of the time no ripened eggs are released.

Polycystic disease is also called Stein-Leventhal syndrome after Dr. Irving Stein, who defined the characteristic group of associated symptoms. Not all patients with polycystic ovaries have all the symptoms Dr. Stein identified. Some doctors don't use the term Stein-Leventhal in such cases, but most doctors use the two terms interchangeably.

Incidence and Cause

This disease is usually found in women between ages 17 and 30. The cause of the disease is unknown, but heredity seems to be a factor.

Symptoms

Symptoms include irregular or absent menstrual periods, infertility (owing to lack of ovulation), pain, abnormal hair growth and excessive weight gain.

The most outstanding symptom is irregularity or absence of menstrual bleeding. This symptom usually occurs shortly after a young woman begins to menstruate for the first time, but it can also occur in women who have been menstruating normally for quite some time. At first there may be heavy, erratic bleeding, interspersed with fairly regular periods. After a while the bleeding becomes scantier, less frequent and stops altogether. Because these women do not ovulate they are, of course, infertile.

Because of the thickened capsule surrounding the ovary, the follicles cannot develop normally, so that women with polycystic disease may have lower-abdominal pain owing to pressure as the follicles push against the capsule. About 40 percent of women with Stein-Leventhal syndrome are overweight. Approximately 70 percent of women with polycystic ovaries have a condition known as hirsutism, which means that they grow extra facial and body hair. This is probably because polycystic ovaries produce more androgens than normal ovaries do. The body converts androgens into testosterone, the so-called male hormone (so-called because all normal women have some testosterone in their bodies). Although there may be male-type body hair patterns, most women with this disease don't have the more drastic masculinization effects, such as decrease in breast size or balding. Some women do, however, have some enlargement of the clitoris, owing to an excess of male hormones. Polycystic ovaries are not the only cause of hirsutism. Unless the appearance of this excess hair is sudden, it is more likely that excessive body hair results from racial and individual genetic heritage.

Diagnosis

In addition to these symptoms the doctor will probably be able to feel an enlargement of the ovaries. Usually both ovaries are equally enlarged, although in some rare cases, in the very early stages of the disease, one ovary may be enlarged slightly more than the other. The uterus in Stein-Leventhal women is sometimes smaller than normal. It may in fact be about the same size as the enlarged ovaries, so that on bimanual exam the doctor feels three masses of about the same size.

These symptoms and signs are not enough to allow for a definite diagnosis of Stein-Leventhal syndrome. The doctor can also make certain hormone tests, since patients with polycystic disease generally have certain characteristic differences in their hormone levels. These tests are described more fully under the heading Amenorrhea. Diagnosis may include some form of visual examination of the ovaries either by culdoscopy or laparoscopy, procedures in which a special viewing instrument is inserted into the body through a small incision either in the vagina or the abdomen. The characteristic appearance of the ovaries and the absence of any corpus luteum (although, as mentioned before, in some cases there may be evidence of occasional ovulation) will help to establish the diagnosis.

Treatment

Once the diagnosis has been established, precise treatment can be given. The ultimate aim of treatment is to establish regular menstrual cycles, for if the lining of the uterus doesn't build up and shed in the usual cyclical fashion, precancerous conditions like endometrial hyperplasia or actual cancer of the uterine lining may occur. Some studies indicate that the rate of uterine cancer is high in Stein-Leventhal patients, although Stein himself reported very few cases, probably because he was careful to establish regular menstrual cycles in his patients.

Hormonal therapy is generally used for treatment. If a woman wants to become pregnant, fertility drugs or surgery may be used.

In women not concerned with pregnancy a progesterone compound, such as Provera, taken orally, is given once a month, usually for about 5 days. Within 24 hours this drug will cause the lining to thicken and swell, and once the drug is eliminated from the body the endometrial lining, deprived of the progesterone, will break down and shed. It may not be necessary to use progesterone each month. Most doctors think that every 2 or 3 months is sufficient to prevent hyperplasia or endometrial cancer.

Some doctors will prescribe birth control pills instead of progesterone therapy for women with polycystic disease. The progesterone in the Pill suppresses the pituitary hormones that keep stimulating all those follicles, thus stopping the continual cystic enlargement of the ovaries. Using the Pill cyclically, 3 weeks on and 1 week off, will allow the uterine lining to be shed. The Pill will also cut down on the amount of testosterone being produced and may solve hirsutism problems. In most cases Pill therapy won't make the excess hair growth that has already taken place disappear. However, a drug known as spironolactone (Aldectazide) has been shown to be effective, even against hair that is already there, but has not been approved by the Food and Drug Administration for this purpose.[4]

We prefer to use progesterone therapy rather than birth control pills in treating polycystic disease. The Pill also contains estrogen, which can have serious side effects and complications. Although progesterones can also cause problems, these are not thought to be as serious as estrogen's side effects and complications.

Even though progesterone treatment will cause menstrual bleeding, it won't cause a woman to ovulate. If a woman wishes to get pregnant, she must, of course, ovulate. In order to stimulate ovulation, fertility drugs, like Clomid, may be used. Some doctors will use Clomid to treat a woman with polycystic disease even if she doesn't want to become pregnant; however, the

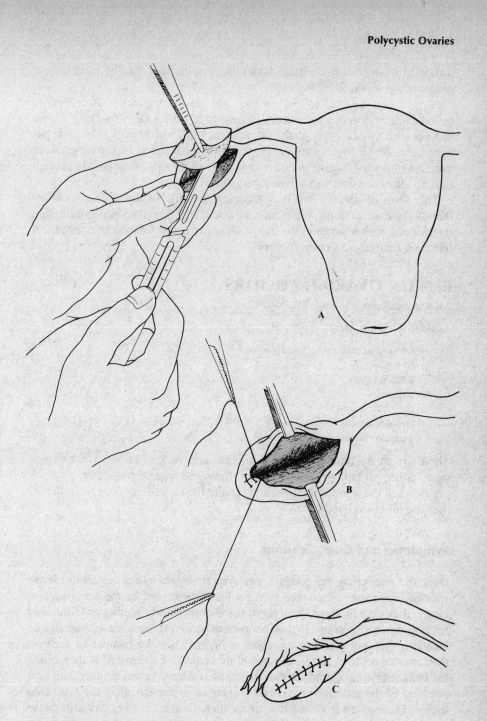

Illustration 52 *Wedge Resection: A wedge-shaped portion of the ovary is removed (A). The edges of the ovary are sutured (B), and the ovary is closed up (C).*

use of Clomid involves certain risks and we think it should be used only if pregnancy is desired.

Surgery may be used to treat women who desire pregnancy. A procedure called a bilateral wedge resection (Illustration 52) cures menstrual irregularity in 85 percent of cases and produces pregnancy in 75 percent of polycystic patients who desire it. Unfortunately, the beneficial effects of the surgery are usually temporary, lasting only a couple of years. But this is generally enough time to allow a woman to achieve pregnancy.

This form of surgery involves reducing the bulk of the ovaries, and although there are a couple of theories, no one is sure how it works. If ovulation doesn't occur after surgery, the use of Clomid may prove effective, even if it has been ineffective before surgery.

BENIGN OVARIAN TUMORS

AKA: noncancerous tumors of the ovary

Associated Terms: Meigs' syndrome

Types: serous and mucinous cystadenomas
       fibromas
       dermoid cysts
       teratomas
       paraovarian cysts
       Brenner tumors
       germinal inclusion cysts

There are many types of ovarian tumors, and no one knows what causes them. Since all benign tumors require the same type of treatment, produce pretty much the same symptoms and require the same diagnostic procedures, they are all considered here.

Symptoms and Complications

Ovarian tumors may not produce any symptoms when they are small. Some women, however, experience pain on intercourse, and as the tumors grow larger, they may produce swelling of the abdomen and a feeling of fullness or bearing-down discomfort in the abdomen or pelvis. If, because of their size or location, they put pressure on adjacent organs, like the bladder or rectum, they may cause irregularities in bowel movement or urination. If they block the blood or lymph channels, they can cause varicose veins, hemorrhoids and swelling of the legs or vulva. If they grow large enough, they may displace the uterus, moving it to one side or another. Ovarian tumors can also cause irregularities in the menstrual cycle or, in postmenopausal or prepubertal women, abnormal uterine bleeding. Certain ovarian tumors are capable of producing male or female hormones. These tumors often create menstrual problems as well as other symptoms related to hormonal imbalance, such as excessive facial hair, deepening of the voice, flattening of the breasts, and premature breast development and other symptoms of precocious puberty, depending on whether male or female hormones are produced by the tumor. These symptoms most often occur with these tumors, called functioning ovarian tumors, but can occur with other types of ovarian tumors as well.

There is generally little pain from the tumor itself, but these tumors, especially the cystic ones, are subject to certain complications that can produce pain. Some of these complications arise from the fact that these tumors may be pedunculated, which means that they are attached to the ovary by means of a stem or stalk, called a pedicle, through which the blood and lymph supply to the tumor circulates.

If the tumor is not blocked by scar tissue from previous pelvic infections and is light enough, and the pedicle is long enough, the tumor may rise upward in the pelvic cavity, floating like a helium balloon attached to a string and moving freely to different locations. It is then subject to twisting of the stem, an event known as torsion of the pedicle. This, of course, is much more likely to happen with the lighter, fluid-filled cystic tumors than with the heavier, solid ones.

Once the pedicle is twisted a number of things may happen, producing a variety of symptoms. The severity of the symptoms will depend on how much twisting there is and how rapidly the twisting takes place. If the twisting is only partial, there may be little in the way of symptoms. Even if the twisting is complete, the symptoms may not be too severe, provided that the twisting has occurred slowly. In fact, the cyst may untwist itself. On rare occasions it may twist itself completely off.

The pain associated with torsion of the pedicle may be sharp and persistent, or it may be only moderately severe and transitory. Not infrequently, however, it is sudden and excruciating. There may be nausea, vomiting, an accelerated pulse and a rise in temperature. If the ovary on the right side is affected, the doctor may think the woman has appendicitis. Severe symptoms like these may require emergency surgery.

If the twisting is only partial, the arteries that provide the blood supply to the ovary are not usually affected, but the veins that carry the blood away from the tumor may then become enlarged and swollen. They may break and cause bleeding into the tumor, which in turn causes the tumor to swell, producing pain owing to pressure on the walls of the tumor.

The blood supply to the tumor may be cut off if this swelling becomes too severe or if the pedicle is completely twisted. Without the nourishment provided by the blood flowing into the tumor, portions of it may die. Tumors that grow too large for their blood supply also tend to break down in their centers. This dying tissue can also cause the tumor to swell and may also produce pain owing to pressure on the tumor walls. These dying areas of the tumor are a perfect breeding ground for infection, again causing swelling and pain. Secondary infection of an ovarian cyst may produce symptoms similar to those produced by acute pelvic inflammatory disease.

On rare occasions the bleeding, tissue death or infection produces so much swelling that the tumor breaks open and the irritating contents of the tumor either leak or spill into the abdominal cavity.

Spontaneous rupture of cystic tumors can occur even though the stem is not twisted and the tumor has an adequate blood supply. Cysts have been known to rupture after intercourse, a fall, a direct blow to the abdomen or childbirth, or when they are being removed surgically. The symptoms produced by a ruptured cyst will depend on how irritating its contents are. There is bound to be some pain, but certain cysts contain fluids that produce a minimal amount of irritation in the abdominal cavity, whereas others contain much more irritating contents. However, as long as the contents are not infected, the reaction is usually not overwhelming. The contents tend to collect in certain areas. In defense, the neighboring tissue produces a fibrous substance that hardens into bands of tissue called adhesions, which wall off the irritating contents. These collections of cyst contents are usually tender to the touch and may cause pain on exertion or intercourse.

If, however, the rupture is accompanied by bleeding into the pelvic cavity, the symptoms of pain, nausea, vomiting and faintness may be severe. If a blood vessel has been broken, the bleeding may even be fatal. Such extreme bleeding is rare, however, for in the majority of cases cysts are made up of little separate compartments and only one is involved in the rupture. The initial pain and other symptoms may therefore subside after a few hours, although for a few days there may be tenderness and rigidity in the lower abdomen, with moderate fever. This may be confused with a ruptured ectopic pregnancy.

Sometimes ovarian tumors will be accompanied by the production of ascites, that is, they will leak fluid into the abdominal cavity. Ascites is more likely to occur with malignant tumors than with benign ones; however, it does happen even with benign tumors. Sometimes the fluid produced by the tumor will affect the area around the lungs as well. When an ovarian tumor is accompanied by ascites and this type of lung cavity involvement, the term Meigs' syndrome is used. Again, this can happen with either benign or malignant tumors.

Types

There are many types of benign ovarian tumors. Some of the more common ones are discussed below.

478

Serous and Mucinous Cystadenomas

Serous and mucinous cystadenomas are the most common of the cystic tumors of the ovary. They may be filled with a thin, watery serous fluid or a thick, sticky mucinous fluid. They are noted for their unusually large size. Sometimes they reach incredible proportions, weighing many pounds and completely filling the abdominal cavity. The mucinous varieties tend to be larger than the serous types. Doctors apparently love to take pictures of them, and no medical textbook is considered complete without at least a couple of photos of a 200-pounder.

They are often pedunculated and are subject to the types of problems that can occur with any pedunculated ovarian tumor, including rupture. If they do break down and spill their contents into the pelvic cavity, the mucinous cysts are more likely to cause pain and adhesions than are the serous ones, for the gluelike contents of the mucinous cysts are highly irritating to the lining of the pelvic cavity.

Fibromas

Fibromas are the most common of the solid benign ovarian tumors. These tumors are composed of fibrous connective tissue. Sometimes there are other types of tissue, such as bone or cartilage, in the tumor as well. They are usually solid, although they may contain one large or several small, soft, fluid-filled cystic areas. Certain varieties sometimes produce estrogen, just like the functioning ovarian tumors, and thus may cause some of the same symptoms associated with these tumors.

Dermoid Cyst

The dermoid cyst, one of the more bizarre types of ovarian cysts, is filled with an oily fluid and may contain hair and even teeth, bits of bone and cartilage. The dermoid belongs to a class of tumors that arise from the germ cells of the ovary, the cells that produce the egg, or ovum. Despite the fact that it has not been fertilized, the egg tissue can start to develop in an unstructured way and produce a dermoid tumor.

Dermoid cysts are the most common ovarian tumor in women younger than 20 and also the most common ovarian tumor occurring in pregnant women. They vary in size but are rarely large and tend to be unilateral (affecting only one ovary), although in 25 percent of the cases they are bilateral. They are often attached to the ovary by a stem, or pedicle, and are thus subject to the usual complications. They rarely rupture; however, if they do spill their contents into the pelvic cavity, they may cause extremely acute symptoms, for the contents of these tumors are highly irritating to the pelvic cavity.

Paraovarian Cysts

Paraovarian cysts are soft, fluid-filled benign tumors that take their name from the location in which they are found, the paraovarium, an area adjacent to the main body of the ovary. They are usually unilateral and are relatively common in women in their 30s and 40s. Most of the time they are small and don't produce symptoms, so they are generally found only in the course of an operation done for some other reason. They can, however, grow rather large, but even then they rarely reach the size of the cysts that affect the main body of the ovary. They don't have stems, or pedicles, so they are not subject to the complications that can occur with other ovarian cysts; however, if they are large, they may push the uterus to one side.

Brenner Tumors of the Ovary

Brenner tumors of the ovary are usually benign; however, in the past 10 years a small number of malignant Brenner tumors have been reported. They too are generally unilateral and small, but on occasion, tumors of considerable size, weighing many pounds, have been reported. They are mostly found in postmenopausal women but can occur in any age-group; however, they are only rarely seen in women under age 30. Sometimes these tumors produce excessive menstrual flow.

Germinal Inclusion Cysts

These cysts are microscopic in size, cause no symptoms, are entirely benign, require no treatment and, therefore, deserve only brief mention. They are found in both middle-aged and older women and are part of the normal aging process. They may be mentioned in a pathology report if the ovary has been biopsied or removed for some other reason. We only mention them since a woman reading the pathology report may be concerned about their significance (none, relax!).

Diagnosis and Treatment

An ovarian tumor may be discovered because bothersome symptoms bring the woman to the doctor or because a mass is found in the course of a routine pelvic exam.

One problem in diagnosing ovarian tumors is determining whether the

480

mass is actually on the ovary or on some other pelvic organ. Sometimes it will be obvious that the suspicious mass is ovarian in origin; at other times it is not so easy to determine the origin. For instance, it is sometimes difficult to distinguish between a pedunculated fibroid tumor of the uterus and an ovarian tumor. In a woman in her 30s it is often hard to tell the difference between endometriosis, pelvic inflammatory disease and an ovarian tumor. Indeed, there is a wide variety of diseases, from various bowel diseases to congenital abnormalities of the uterus to ectopic pregnancy, that can be confused with ovarian tumors. Even a full bladder may be confused with a pelvic mass—possibly an ovarian tumor—so the pelvic examination should be done only after the bladder is emptied. It is important not to ignore this step, for women have been operated on, only to have it found that the suspicious mass was merely a swollen bladder.

If the doctor is not certain whether or not a mass is ovarian in origin, s/he may perform certain diagnostic tests. Sonograms, pictures of internal organs taken by means of high-frequency sound waves, may be done; or laparoscopic or culdoscopic exams, procedures in which the ovaries are examined by means of special viewing instruments, may be done.

Another problem in diagnosing ovarian tumors centers around determining whether the tumor is benign or malignant. Generally, this cannot be done short of actually operating on the woman, removing the tumor and examining it microscopically. On rare occasions a cancerous ovarian tumor will be detected by a Pap smear, but the Pap smear is not reliable in detecting ovarian cancer.

Definite diagnosis requires an operation. Special X-ray tests, including possibly an intravenous pyelogram or a barium enema, may be done preoperatively. In addition, special viewing instruments, the cystoscope and the proctosigmoidoscope, may be used to examine the bladder and the small bowel.

Once the doctor has made the surgical incision, s/he removes all the tumor, or at least as much as possible. In some cases it may be necessary to remove the entire tube and ovary. If the tumor is a fluid-filled cyst, great care must be taken to remove it without spilling its contents, for if the cyst is cancerous, spillage of its contents could spread the cancer to other parts of the abdominal cavity. The tumor or the portions of it that have been removed are then sent to the pathology lab for analysis by frozen section.

It is particularly important that the pathologist be top-notch and up-to-date. New information has necessitated frequent changes in the terminology used to describe various types of ovarian tumors, but it takes time for these changes to percolate through the ranks of pathologists. Those pathologists who have not kept up with these changes may be providing out-of-date diagnoses to surgeons. It is also important that the surgeon and the pathologist have good communication so that they are sure they are both using the same terms to

481

mean the same thing. Mistakes do happen. Consider the case of a 19-year-old woman who was operated on for an ovarian tumor.[5] The pathologist reported that the woman had a cancerous tumor, on the basis of her frozen section. The permanent section, according to this pathologist, confirmed the diagnosis of cancer. Luckily for this woman, because of some technical problems at the time of operation, the surgeon removed only the ovary and referred her to an ovarian cancer specialist. A review of the pathology of her tumor revealed that she did not have cancer at all. She had what is known as a papillary serous cystadenoma, a benign tumor. Thus her other ovary and her childbearing capacity were preserved. The mistake was made because this woman's tumor had small papillary (nipple-shaped) protrusions. Although it is true that most papillary serous growths are malignant, this is not always the case.

A woman should find out ahead of time whether or not the pathologist is board-certified (*see* p. 235) and how many pathologists will be available to review her slides. The importance of having a high-caliber pathologist is discussed in greater detail in the section on cancer, along with more information about how to investigate the pathology situation before the operation.

While the surgeon carefully examines the rest of the pelvic organs, the pathologist examines the tissue and sends back a report to the surgeon. If the report indicates that the tumor is malignant or borderline, appropriate therapy, as described under the heading Ovarian Cancer, is done.

If the pathologist's report indicates that the tumor is benign, it nonetheless needs to be removed. Not only will it continue to grow larger, possibly creating the complications described above and destroying the healthy ovarian tissue, but with certain types of tumors there is the danger of malignant degeneration—of the tumor's becoming cancerous.

Sometimes it is possible to remove the tumor and to save the rest of the ovary (Illustration 53). Even a small nubbin of ovarian tissue may be capable of functioning normally, and women with such an ovary not only continue to produce ovarian hormones but are also, surprisingly, fertile. At other times the tumor will have destroyed so much ovarian tissue that the entire ovary must be removed. If there are tumors on both ovaries, sometimes both or at least one of the ovaries or some portion of ovarian tissue can be saved. In some cases it may be necessary to remove both ovaries.

In young women desirous of having children the doctor will make every effort to save all or some portion of the ovary. Even if the younger woman has completed her family, an effort is usually made to conserve the ovaries, for this will usually prevent premature menopause, which carries certain risks, including increased risk of developing hypertension or having a fatal heart attack, as well as other problems.

In older women the question of whether or not to conserve the ovary becomes more controversial. Some doctors advocate removal of both ovaries and the uterus as well in all women over age 35; others use 40 or 45 as the

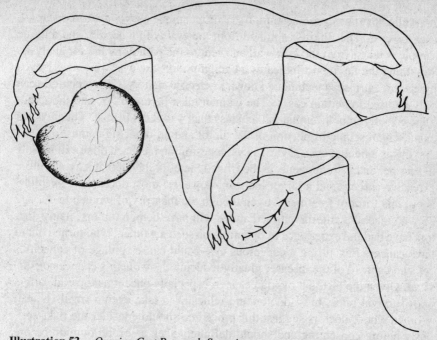

Illustration 53 *Ovarian Cyst Removal: Sometimes a cyst or tumor on the ovary can simply be removed and the wound sutured back together.*

cutoff. The pros and cons of removing the ovaries and uterus are discussed in more detail under the heading Hysterectomy.

Another controversy revolves around the treatment of the woman who, although she has no future childbearing plans, wants to preserve her ovarian tissue if possible. If such a woman needs to have only one ovary removed, the question of what to do with her uterus arises. Some doctors think it should be removed since the woman does not want to have children. Other doctors (and we lean toward this viewpoint) believe that since hysterectomy is a major surgical procedure, it should not be done unless necessary. We are reluctant to remove a healthy uterus. If birth control is a concern for the woman, we would recommend one of the barrier methods or, if she is adamant about sterilization, tubal ligation. The decision, of course, rests with the individual woman.

Women faced with ovarian tumor surgery should read the appropriate sections indicated in the text and discuss these issues in detail with their doctors before operation, seeking a second opinion (*see* p. 238) when necessary. It's better to find out that your doctor is from the ovaries-out-at-age-35 school of thought before the operation rather than afterward.

A new approach to treating ovarian tumors is being done in some hospitals.

It is called ovarian cyst fenestration.[6] This technique uses a laparoscope to locate the cyst. The fluid is aspirated from the cyst with a needle, and a tissue sample is taken from the cyst wall and sent to the pathology lab for analysis. Assuming the lab report indicates a benign tumor, the cyst wall is destroyed by electric current, a technique known as electric cautery. This technique can only be used in certain cases: The woman must be under 35, and the tumor must be soft, smooth, unilateral and less than 4 to 8 cm in size. The physical exam, laparoscopic inspection of the tumor and all other signs must indicate that this is a benign cyst. Ovarian cyst fenestration has been done extensively in Europe, and its proponents in the United States point out that it avoids more extensive surgery and a larger incision; however, most doctors are skeptical about this form of treatment. Even though the majority of women under age 35 who meet the criteria outlined above will have benign tumors, many doctors have had the experience of operating on such a woman, who turned out to have cancer. Puncturing a cancerous cyst could cause spillage of cancerous cells and spread of the disease, greatly reducing the woman's chances of survival. Given the fact that ovarian cancer, especially once it has spread, offers poor survival rates, most doctors are reluctant to take even a small chance. Women whose doctors suggest this procedure should consider the risks seriously before consenting and should definitely seek a second opinion before undergoing the procedure.

Having just spent the last several pages explaining the necessity for surgery in women with ovarian enlargements, we are now going to say something that may seem like a contradiction. As explained in the introduction to this section, a younger woman with a small (less than 5 cm), soft, unilateral, smooth tumor should not allow herself to be rushed into surgery, as often happens. The odds are that she has only a luteum or follicular cyst, which tends to disappear by itself. Waiting for one menstrual cycle (some doctors will wait for two or even three, but we think that that is taking too much of a chance) can prevent unnecessary surgery.

If, however, the younger woman is on birth control pills, waiting is riskier, for women on the Pill are unlikely to have physiologic cysts. If the cyst is larger than 5 cm, waiting is not recommended, for even if she has a physiologic cyst, a cyst of that size is unlikely to go away by itself, is displacing normal ovarian tissue and needs to be removed. Moreover, if the cyst is solid or grows larger during the waiting period, prompt surgery will be required, for even though it is still likely that she has a benign and not a cancerous growth, there is no way of telling for sure, short of operation.

FUNCTIONING OVARIAN TUMORS

AKA: hormone-producing tumors

Types: masculinizing tumors
      feminizing tumors
        granulosa cell tumors
        theca cell tumors
        dysgerminomas

Functioning ovarian tumors are tumors that are capable of producing hormones. There are many types of functioning ovarian tumors, but they all have this hormone-producing ability in common. This is not to say that they always *do* so, but some of them do, and when this occurs there are apt to be hormone-related symptoms.

Functioning ovarian tumors may be broken down into two subgroups: the masculinizing tumors and the more common feminizing tumors. They are considered here separately.

Masculinizing Ovarian Tumors

These tumors occur only rarely. They are usually small to moderate in size, although occasionally they grow quite large. They are usually unilateral and occur most frequently in women in their early 20s and 30s. Masculinizing tumors are capable of producing male hormones, which can produce such symptoms as absence of the menstrual period, decrease in the size of breasts, loss of the rounded contours of the female figure, change to male body-type, facial and chest hair, an enlarged clitoris and a deepening of the voice. All these symptoms, except for the change in the voice, generally disappear once the tumor is removed. Occasionally, for reasons that are not clear, these tumors will produce the type of symptoms usually associated with female hormones, such as excessive menstrual bleeding, and if this happens, there may be associated endometrial hyperplasia or endometrial cancer of the uterus.

If these tumors are hormonally active, the masculinizing symptoms they produce will help in the diagnosis; however, if the tumor is too small to be felt, there may be some question about diagnosis, for other conditions can cause these symptoms. The doctor will do certain laboratory tests and X-ray examinations to rule out other possibilities. The same sorts of diagnostic procedures used with other ovarian tumors and the same considerations involved in the treatment of benign ovarian tumors (see above) apply to benign masculinizing tumors. Treatment of malignant tumors is considered in the discussion of ovarian cancer.

Feminizing Ovarian Tumors

There are a number of types of feminizing tumors. The most common are the granulosa cell and theca cell tumors. Occasionally, these tumors may leak fluid (ascites), and the fluid may even involve the area around the lungs, a condition known as Meigs' syndrome. They vary considerably in size from very small to very large, averaging 5 to 10 cm in diameter. There seems to be little direct correlation between the size of the tumor and the hormone output, for very small tumors can produce excessive amounts of hormone whereas very large tumors may be hormonally inactive.

The symptoms that these tumors can cause are the same as those of any ovarian tumor (*see* p. 476). The larger tumors are prone to break down, and if this occurs, there is often blood in the fluid of the cystic areas. If such cysts rupture, their contents are apt to be highly irritating. In addition to the usual symptoms, tumors that are hormonally active can produce symptoms related to excessive hormone production. In young girls they may cause precocious puberty, a condition characterized by the early onset of menstruation and the early development of breasts, body hair and other secondary sexual characteristics. Although such symptoms as breast enlargement do not occur in women who are past the age of puberty, the menstrual cycle can be reactivated in postmenopausal women.

Abnormal uterine bleeding is the most distinctive hormone-related symptom. In some cases there may be an absence of menstruation, sometimes lasting for quite some time, followed by excessive vaginal bleeding. In other cases there may be irregularly spaced, excessively profuse periods.

Women with these tumors may still ovulate and get pregnant. The uterus may be enlarged to as much as twice its normal size. Part of this enlargement is owing to excessive hormonal stimulation but some of it can be explained by the fact that women with these tumors often have associated benign fibroid tumors of the uterus. The continuous estrogen stimulation may also account for the fact that 15 percent to 25 percent of women with feminizing ovarian tumors also have cancer of the uterus, for such cancer is related to the overproduction of estrogen. The older a woman with a feminizing tumor, the greater the chances that she will have associated uterine cancer. Since younger women are less likely to have uterine cancer anyhow (it is a disease that generally affects older women), it is not surprising that they are less likely to have uterine cancer along with their feminizing tumors. Nonetheless, the possibility does exist. As many as 70 percent to 80 percent of women with feminizing tumors may have endometrial hyperplasia, a condition that can, in some cases, lead to uterine cancer.

The distinctive, hormonal-induced symptoms of these tumors in prepubertal girls and postmenopausal women, coupled with the presence of a solid ovarian mass, may lead the doctor to strongly suspect the presence of some type of feminizing ovarian tumor. However, at times the tumor may be too small to be felt. Diagnosis and treatment involve the same problems and procedures as with other ovarian tumors (*see* p. 480). However, if the tumors are malignant, they may require special therapy (see the section on ovarian cancer).

Dysgerminomas are another type of functioning tumor. They aren't feminizing tumors in the usual sense of the word, for they produce hormones associated with pregnancy rather than female hormones. They are often hormonally inactive, although on occasion they are active and may produce a positive pregnancy test. They may be associated with an enlarged uterus and an absence of menstrual periods. They are often malignant and may require special treatment (see the section on ovarian cancer below).

OVARIAN CANCER

Types: epithelial cell tumors
        serous cystadenocarcinoma
        mucinous cystadenocarcinoma
        endometroid carcinoma
        clear cell, or mesonephroid, carcinoma
        Brenner tumors
        mixed tumors
        other metastatic or rare tumors
   germ cell tumors
        dysgerminoma
        embryonal tumors
        endodermal sinus tumors
        choriocarcinomas
        immature teratomas
        cancer arising inside a benign dermoid cyst
        mixed tumors
        other rare tumors
    sex cord stromal tumors
        granulosa cell tumors
        other functioning ovarian tumors
        other rare tumors

Ovarian cancer is a relatively rare form of cancer, accounting for about 5 percent of all gynecological cancers, but it is the fourth leading cause of cancer deaths in American women.[7] Nearly three-quarters of the women who get the disease die from it. The ovary is not an accessible organ in the way that the vulva, vagina and cervix are. Since it is not possible to get at the ovary easily in order to take cell samples or perform other screening tests to detect cancer early, ovarian cancer is generally not detected until it is in a fairly advanced stage.

Incidence and Risk Factors

There are approximately 14 new cases of ovarian cancer each year per 100,000 women of all ages.[8] The disease occurs most often in postmenopausal women, but beyond this, risk factors that could tell us which women are more likely to develop ovarian cancer have not yet been clearly defined. We do know that for women who have breast cancer, the risk of developing ovarian cancer increases twofold and vice versa.[9] Women who have an initial cancer of the intestine or rectum are also at increased risk. Women who use the birth control pill may be less apt to develop ovarian cancer than other women (*see* Chapter Five).

Types

As explained in the introduction to this section, a wide variety of tumors are found in the ovary. About 85 percent of ovarian cancers are epithelial tumors, which means that they arise from the epithelial tissue, a type of tissue that lines the cavities and passageways of the body and that covers the organs—in this case the ovary. The most common of the epithelial tumors is the serous cystadenocarcinoma, which is the cancerous form of the benign serous cystadenoma. The second most common is the mucinous cystadenocarcinoma, which is the cancerous form of a benign mucinous cystadenoma. These tumors may develop within a benign tumor or may arise initially in their cancerous form. Endometroid tumors, clear cell tumors, Brenner tumors and mixed tumors are some of the other types of epithelial tumors that may arise in the ovary and may be malignant.

Certain functioning ovarian tumors called sex cord stromal tumors may also be cancerous. There are a number of other less common types of ovarian cancer. These other tumors are also classified according to the type of tissue from which they arise. In addition, the ovary may be the site of a metastasized tumor that had its origin elsewhere in the body. Identifying the particular tissue type of the tumor is important in terms of selecting proper treatment and predicting chances of survival.

Grade

The grade (*see* p. 715) of the tumor, that is, whether the tumor cells are mature, well differentiated and low grade or immature, undifferentiated and high grade, is of particular importance in ovarian cancer, especially in the early stages of the disease. Low-grade tumors are referred to as borderline tumors or tumors of low malignant potential. They are less serious, generally result in better survival rates than the high-grade, undifferentiated ones and may require less aggressive treatment.

The concept of borderline tumors has been of great importance in the treatment of ovarian cancer. Until ovarian tumors were divided into three groups—benign, borderline and malignant—it was difficult to make sense of survival statistics and to compare the different methods of treatment used by different institutions. Survival rates for Stage I serous cystadenocarcinomas, for instance, ranged from around 60 percent to as high as 98 percent; however, once the concept of the borderline cancer was developed the survival rates became more uniform and there was no longer such a wide variance in the statistics (see below).

Symptoms

The symptoms that may appear in ovarian cancer are the same as those that may be associated with any type of ovarian tumor (*see* p. 476). In the early stages there may be no symptoms. The most common symptom is abdominal pain. The next most frequent symptom is abdominal swelling. A change in weight, usually weight loss, may be noted and may be owing to loss of appetite, intermittent nausea or occasional vomiting. As the tumor grows larger there may be symptoms of pelvic pressure, abnormal bleeding, a change in the menstrual cycle or postmenopausal bleeding, cramps, constipation or a frequent need to urinate. However, approximately one-third of women with ovarian cancer are asymptomatic at the time of diagnosis.

Diagnosis

Sometimes ovarian tumors can produce symptoms even when it is not possible for the doctor to feel a pelvic mass. Such women may have symptoms mimicking gastrointestinal tract diseases, such as gallbladder disease or spastic colon, and may be referred to an internist for treatment. If the gastrointestinal workup is negative, the possibility of an ovarian tumor must be considered and a laparoscopic exam should be done. Sometimes women who have tumors too small to be felt but have symptoms of persistent or recurrent pelvic pain do not receive the treatment they need. If they are young, they may be treated for salpingitis, an infection of the fallopian tube. If they are postmenopausal, they may be given a prescription for tranquilizers—in other words, the old it's-all-in-your-head-dearie diagnosis.[10] Unfortunately, some of these women actually have ovarian tumors. Women should insist on proper and complete diagnostic procedures for their symptoms.

If a woman has suspicious symptoms, the doctor should do a pelvic exam. If a suspicious mass is felt, an operation will be necessary. However, as we have seen, women with ovarian cancer may not have symptoms until the disease is fairly advanced. Many ovarian tumors are discovered in the course of a routine physical.

Occasionally, a Pap smear will pick up a case of ovarian cancer, but in order to show up in the Pap smear the cancerous cells would have had to travel down the fallopian tubes, through the uterus, out through the opening of the cervix and into the vagina. The Pap smear, then, is of little value in detecting ovarian cancer.

Many times the doctor will feel a suspicious mass in the pelvis but won't be able to tell, without specialized testing (*see* p. 480), whether the mass is growing on the ovary or on some other pelvic organ. If the mass is definitely an ovarian one, it is necessary to operate, for even if the tumor is not cancerous, it must be removed, as discussed under Benign Tumors of the Ovary. Much of the information there is pertinent to diagnosis of ovarian cancer and the reader should refer to that section before continuing here.

The consistency of the tumor, whether it is bilateral or unilateral and the age of the woman may make the doctor suspicious of cancer. If there is evidence of cancer in other sites in the pelvic cavity, the doctor may suspect that the woman has advanced ovarian cancer. If cancer is suspected, some of the diagnostic steps described in the general section on cancer should be done.

Most of the time, however, there is no way to find out for sure whether or not an ovarian tumor is cancerous short of operating on the woman and removing all or part of the tumor for microscopic evaluation. Whenever possible, the entire tumor will be removed. Great care must be taken with fluid-filled, cystic tumors so that the tumor capsule is not broken and the contents spilled, for if the tumor is cancerous, this could spread the disease. Sometimes, despite the surgeon's skill, the tumor will rupture and this may decrease the woman's chance of survival.

Sometimes it is not possible to remove all the tumor, and in such cases only a portion will be removed and sent to the lab for analysis. Even though it may be obvious from the appearance of the tumor that the woman has cancer, this analysis is necessary to determine the tissue-type of the tumor and the grade so that appropriate treatment can be planned. The possibility that the cancer has metastasized from some other site must be ruled out as well. And even if the appearance of the tumor convinces the doctor that it is benign, this analysis should still be done, for cancer can and does arise inside benign ovarian tumors.

The tissue removed at operation is sent to the pathology lab for analysis by frozen section. It is important that the pathologist examine all suspicious areas of the tumor and make multiple sections, for it is not uncommon for cancerous and noncancerous or borderline areas to exist in the same tumor. The pathologist makes the diagnosis on the basis of multiple frozen sections; however, permanent sections are also done.

Samples of any fluid in the area should be suctioned out and also sent to the lab for analysis. The presence of malignant cells in such fluid is an indication that the cancer has spread and will influence staging and treatment. Unfortunately, this vital step is sometimes ignored. A woman diagnosed as having Stage I cancer should ask if samples of fluid were taken. If the answer is no, she should seek a second opinion from a cancer specialist.

If the appearance of the tumor or the abdominal cavity suggests cancer, the surgeon will proceed to explore the abdominal cavity and take other tissue samples and cell specimens while waiting for the frozen-section analysis. Even if the surgeon is not certain, s/he may still explore the abdominal cavity while waiting for the tissue analysis from the pathology lab. If the pathologist sends back a report of cancer, a thorough exploration of the abdominal cavity is mandatory.

Unless the doctor had suspected cancer before the operation (because of the age of the woman, her symptoms, the feel and consistency of the tumor or the results of preoperative tests), the original incision for the operation may have been what is known as a Pfannenstiel incision (Illustration 54). However, if the frozen-section analysis reveals cancer, the doctor should make another muscle-cutting incision in order to do an adequate exploration of the abdominal cavity. Some doctors think that a Pfannenstiel incision does not allow for

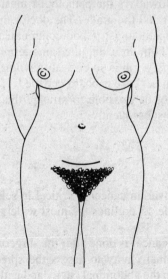

Illustration 54   *Pfannenstiel Incision*

an adequate inspection.[11] Any woman with ovarian cancer whose doctor has done only a Pfannenstiel incision should discuss this with her doctor. She may want to seek a second opinion.

If the doctor's exploration reveals other tumor areas, these must also be removed, if possible. If there is no other sign of tumor (in medical terms, "no gross tumor"), the doctor must take cell samples and tissue biopsies from various locations. If conservative surgery (see below) is a possibility, in addition to these tests, the opposite ovary must be examined, using a procedure known as a wedge biopsy. This must be done even if the other ovary appears normal, for cancer could be lurking inside the ovary.[12]

It is important that the surgeon be aware of the necessity for these other procedures in addition to the biopsy of the tumor itself. These tests will help to stage the disease and to indicate the need for further surgery or chemotherapy. They are not always done. Any woman being operated on for an ovarian mass should discuss the possibility of ovarian cancer and the need for the above-described tests with her doctor. If possible, she should have a board-certified doctor doing her surgery. If a woman who is diagnosed as having ovarian cancer has not had an opportunity before her operation to assure that adequate exploratory cell samples and biopsies were taken, she should investigate this afterward. If these tests have not been done, a "second look" operation (see below) by a cancer specialist should take place.

The skill and experience of the pathologist are of critical importance, as explained in detail in the general section on cancer (*see* p. 710). In the past, all the pathologist was expected to do was to report whether the tumor was benign or malignant. Nowadays the pathologist must also tell the surgeon the cell type of the tumor and the grade. The doctor must have a good working relationship with the pathologist. Good communication between them is essential to ensure that both are using the same terminology in the same way. Because the pathologist's job is so critical, a woman will want to make sure that the pathologist on her case is board-certified. If the operation is an emergency one, it may not be possible to arrange this ahead of time, but here again, it can be done subsequently.

Staging

Accurate staging of ovarian cancer is critical in selecting treatment and predicting survival. Table 15 outlines the most widely used staging scheme for ovarian cancer.[13]

Staging of ovarian cancer is done after the surgeon has removed the tumor, inspected the abdominal cavity to assess the spread of the disease, taken samples of the fluid in the abdominal cavity and gathered tissue samples from the ovary and/or other locations, to detect possible microscopic spread. Depending on the surgeon's findings, the pathologist's report and other standard tests to determine metastasis (*see* p. 714), the proper stage is assigned.

Treatment

Treatment of ovarian cancer usually involves surgery, followed by some form of chemotherapy. In the past, radiation therapy was also used, but chemotherapy has pretty much replaced radiation. If your doctor recommends radiation instead of chemotherapy, be sure you understand why. Second opinions are, of course, always a good idea.

The stage-by-stage treatments outlined below are general ones, and the specific treatment recommended by a woman's doctor may differ according to the particulars of her case. In some cases there is not yet uniform agreement among experts as to what is the best treatment in a given situation. The treatment program outlined here is not prescriptive but is intended to provide enough information to enable women to understand the issues, to ask intelligent questions, to begin to evaluate their doctors' recommendations and to recognize those instances in which they might be wise to seek a second opinion.

Table 15
Stages of Ovarian Cancer

Stage I:	Growth limited to the ovaries
	Stage IA: Growth limited to one ovary; no ascites*
	1. Tumor capsule unruptured and no tumor growth on the external surface of the tumor
	2. Tumor capsule ruptured and/or tumor growth on external surface of the tumor
	Stage IB: Growth limited to both ovaries; no ascites*
	1. Capsule unruptured and no tumor growth on the external surface of the tumor
	2. Capsule ruptured and/or tumor growth on external surface of the tumor
	Stage IC: Growth limited to one or both ovaries; ascites with malignant cells
Stage II:	Growth involving one or both ovaries with pelvic extension
	Stage IIA: Extension and/or metastasis to uterus and tubes only
	Stage IIB: Extension/metastasis to other pelvic tissues
	Stage IIC: Either IIA or IIB, with ascites present
Stage III:	Growth involving one or both ovaries, with widespread metastasis in the abdominal cavity
Stage IV:	Growth involving one or both ovaries, with distant metastasis outside the abdominal cavity

*Some amount of fluid is normal; the surgeon must judge whether the fluid exceeds normal amounts

Stage I

Most Stage I cases are treated by removal of the ovaries, tubes and uterus in operations known as bilateral salpingo-oophorectomies and hysterectomies. Part of the omentum, a fold of fat tissue that hangs from the bowels, should be removed as well. Sometimes the appendix is also removed.

In certain Stage I cases it may be possible to do less-radical surgery, removing only the affected ovary and leaving the other ovary and the uterus intact.[14] This can be done only in certain carefully selected cases and only if the woman is particularly anxious to retain her ability to bear children. Not all doctors have precisely the same criteria for selecting cases to be treated conservatively. Most doctors would restrict this conservative surgery to Stage IA(1) cancers. In this stage the tumor is confined to one ovary, there is no tumor growth on the outside of the tumor capsule, the tumor has not ruptured and there is no ascites. Further, the ovary must be nonadherent, which means that it must not be stuck to other pelvic organs. The cancer must be growing inside a cystic tumor. The pathologist's report must indicate that the tumor is a low-grade, borderline, well-differentiated type of tumor. Before this type of treatment is given the surgeon must have removed the tumor, taken samples of any fluid in the cavity, taken biopsies from various key areas, such as the omentum, and samples from various areas, such as the liver. In addition, the pathologist's report on the fluid samples and biopsy specimens must be negative. A wedge biopsy of the opposite ovary must also be done. Since this important procedure is not always done, a woman who may be a candidate for conservative surgery should discuss the wedge biopsy with her doctor before surgery.

Some doctors might extend the criteria for conservative surgery, but performing conservative surgery in other cases is controversial. Women should discuss their doctors' criteria for conservative surgery beforehand and seek a second opinion if necessary.

The other Stage I cases—Stage IA(2), IB, IC, those Stage IA(1) cases in which the tumor was not a well-differentiated low-grade borderline tumor and those Stage IA(1) cases in which the woman does not have future childbearing plans—will usually be treated by the more radical form of surgery outlined above.

Stage I cases may also be treated with adjuvant therapy—preventive treatment to destroy any microscopic cancer that may remain after surgery. It is sometimes difficult to determine the desirability of using adjuvant therapy or to decide on the optimum type. When adjuvant therapy is given, chemotherapy in the form of alkylating agents is used. There are several alkylating agents available, but the one most widely used for these cases is melphalan (Alkeran), which is well tolerated by most women. The drug is given for 12 to

18 months after surgery in an effort to eradicate any microscopic residual cancer. However, the use of melphalan in Stage I cancers has been seriously questioned. A study published in a major medical journal assessed the risks of acute leukemia after treatment of ovarian cancer by alkylating agents and found that the risk was greatly increased.[15] Although there were a number of problems with the study, and it could hardly be called "conclusive," it did raise serious questions about the advisability of using chemotherapy in Stage IA(1) cases.[16] The problem is that only about 35 percent of women with Stage IA(1) cases actually have unrecognized microscopic cancer after surgery; 65 percent do not. Only 35 percent would benefit from chemotherapy. According to this study, about 10 percent could be expected to develop leukemia from the chemotherapy. Because of these findings some doctors have discontinued chemotherapy in these cases.[17]* Generally, however, doctors will use chemotherapy if there are any cancer cells in the washings of the area that are done at the time of the operation. This is referred to as positive cytology. If the cytology is negative, most doctors don't give chemotherapy.

Women should discuss this issue with their doctors and should request an update on the most recent developments. If your doctor recommends chemotherapy for Stage IA or IB, be sure you understand why. Doctors are more inclined to give chemotherapy in Stage IC, but even here, you may want to seek a second opinion.

Stage II

Stage II cases are treated by removing the ovaries, tubes, uterus, omentum, appendix and as much of the tumor as possible. In some Stage II cases all the tumor can be removed, but in others this is not possible without causing damage to vital organs.

Further therapy is needed for Stage II cases. Even if the doctor has removed all the tumor, there is a high likelihood that microscopic cancer may remain. If some cancer remains after operation, chemotherapy is used (see below).[18]

Stages III and IV

The aim of surgery in Stage III and Stage IV is to remove as much of the tumor as possible without endangering the woman's life or producing excessive complications. Sometimes complete removal is possible. At the very least the ovaries and omentum should be removed, for relief of discomfort. Surgery in these cases calls for experienced judgment and great skill on the part of the

*See note 16 in the Ovary footnotes at the end of the book for more details about chemotherapy in Stage I disease.

surgeon. If all areas of tumor greater than 1.5 cm in diameter can be removed, the survival chances are significantly better, but if the tumor cannot be reduced this much, radical surgery won't significantly improve the woman's chance of survival.[19] In some cases, radical surgery, such as partial or total pelvic exenteration, which involves removing all the pelvic organs, including the bladder and/or rectum, may be done. But this is done only if one of two possibilities exist: (1) The radical surgery would result in such complete removal of the tumor that no single area of tumor larger than 1.5 cm in diameter would remain after surgery; or (2) areas larger than 1.5 cm remained, but in the surgeon's opinion, subsequent chemotherapy could reduce the tumor to the point where the doctor could, in a second operation, reduce all the remaining areas of tumor to less than 1.5 cm in diameter.

Obviously, having a skilled surgeon who is experienced and knowledgeable about chemotherapy and the ability of chemotherapy to reduce tumor bulk in various circumstances is of utmost importance. A less knowledgeable surgeon may be overwhelmed by the discovery of extensive tumor on operation. The woman might then be given only minimal surgery, be closed back up and given some form of chemotherapy, whereas another, more qualified surgeon might have been able to reduce the tumor to the point where chemotherapy would have a better chance of success. A woman should discuss her surgeon's qualifications before surgery and find out whether or not the doctor is qualified and experienced enough to do radical pelvic surgery, or if another doctor who is qualified can be called in, should the need for consultation arise. If she has not had the benefit of consultation with or surgery by a cancer specialist—either a surgical or gynecological oncologist—before diagnosis, *she should insist* that a second opinion be obtained before beginning chemotherapy.

Stages III and IV will always require further therapy. Chemotherapy is the treatment of choice. In the past a single agent, melphalan, was given; however, studies have shown that combinations of drugs are more effective than a single agent.[20] Any combination that includes the drug cisplatin may be used. Studies are now underway to investigate giving the chemotherapy by means of a method known as interperitoneal washings, in which the drugs are inserted into the pelvic cavity through a catheter (hollow tube).[21] Changes in chemotherapy for advanced ovarian cancer are taking place all the time, which is why it is important to have a doctor who is up-to-date on the latest developments in research and to seek second chemotherapy opinions.

Special Treatment Cases

The treatment program discussed so far holds true for the majority of ovarian cancers; however, less-common types may require different treatment. Dysgerminomas often present as Stage IA(1) and can be treated conservatively; however, biopsy of the other ovary is essential, for in 15 percent of cases the other, seemingly normal ovary will be involved. All other stages will require further therapy, which may be given by external beam radiation, since these tumors are very responsive to radiation.[22]

Granulosa cell tumors can also be treated conservatively in many cases. However, if the uterus is not removed, a D&C must be done, since these tumors are often associated with endometrial cancer. (If the D&C indicates cancer, the uterus must, of course, be removed.) It is important to note that women are frequently diagnosed as having this tumor when, in fact, their tumor is of another cell type.[23] Since granulosa cell tumors are treated differently, accurate diagnosis is important. Women who are told they have granulosa cella tumors should, therefore, confirm the diagnosis with second opinions from pathologists at cancer centers (see appendix).

Malignant embryonal tumors, endodermal sinus tumors and choriocarcinomas can never be treated conservatively because of their aggressive nature. They always require further therapy after surgery.

Follow-Up

Follow-up care is extremely important in ovarian cancer, in order to detect recurrent or persistent cancer and to monitor the success of chemotherapy so that the therapy can be changed if necessary or discontinued if it has been successful. Because of the associated leukemia risk, therapy should be discontinued as soon as it has proved successful.

Careful questioning about possible symptoms and a thorough pelvic exam are the foundation of follow-up care. Breast exam by the doctor and self-exam by the woman are also of vital importance, since women with ovarian cancer are at higher risk of developing breast cancer. The woman's weight, appetite and general well-being should be given careful attention. Nutrition is particularly important for women with ovarian cancer. Persistent ascites and abdominal swelling, signs of intestinal obstruction, nausea, vomiting and pain are important symptoms.

A "second-look" operation may be done in certain cases.[24] If the woman had only a biopsy of the tumor and did not have samples of ascites and the appropriate tissue biopsies or optimum surgery to remove the bulk of the tumor, she is a candidate for a second operation. Those women in whom it was not possible to remove all the tumor and who are receiving chemotherapy are also candidates for a second-look operation. The chemotherapy may have reduced the tumor to a point where it can all be removed surgically or where the remaining tumor could at least be reduced to less than 1.5 cm in diameter by further surgery. The presence or absence of tumor will be a guide to determining further chemotherapy.

Women who have had all gross tumor removed, who have no signs or symptoms of recurrence and who receive chemotherapy may also be candidates for a second-look operation, which might allow the doctor to discontinue the adjuvant therapy and thereby cut the risks involved in such therapy. Nowadays it is common practice to treat a woman with chemotherapy for 6 to 10 months and then do a second-look operation. If no cancer is found, chemotherapy is discontinued. If there is cancer, the doctor will attempt to reduce it to less than 1.5 cm and the chemotherapy is continued.

If a woman's tumor is known to be growing larger, however, there is no point in a second operation, for by the time a recurrence is large enough to be felt, the tumor is growing out of control and chemotherapy cannot control it. A second operation, which poses risks in and of itself, will do no good in these cases.

There is not total agreement among doctors as to which women are candidates for these operations or precisely when they should be done. Women should discuss this issue with their doctors, again seeking second opinions if necessary.

Sometimes laparoscopy rather than a second major operation may be possible. This second-look procedure will involve the same sorts of abdominal investigations, cell specimens and tissue biopsies as done in the original diagnostic procedure.

Culdocentesis, a method of extracting fluid by way of a needle inserted into the abdominal cavity, may be useful in following some cases. Chest and abdominal X-rays, intravenous pyelogram, liver scans and ultrasound examinations may all be used in follow-up. Certain rare forms of ovarian cancer may be followed up with special blood tests that allow the doctor to detect recurrences before the recurrent tumor has grown large enough to be felt and, hence, too large to control.

Survival Rates

The overall 5-year survival rate for ovarian cancer is about 30 percent to 35 percent; however, many factors will influence the survival rates.[25] Table 16 breaks down survival rates by stage and cell type. The grade of the tumor will also influence survival rates. For instance, survival rates better than 95 percent have been reported for Stage I borderline serous and mucinous tumors at some institutions.[26] In the more advanced cases, whether or not all or most of the tumor was removed during surgery will affect survival rates. A woman's doctor should be able to quote survival statistics for her particular situation.

Table 16
Five-Year Survival Rates for Various Stage and Cell-Type Ovarian Cancers

Type	Percent
Stage I	
Serous	70
Mucinous	84
Endometroid	73
Solid	58
Stage II	
Serous	39
Mucinous	68
Endometroid	79
Solid	24
Stage III	
Serous	6
Mucinous	17
Endometroid	28
Solid	2

SOURCE: Adapted from D.G. Decker, "The Diagnosis and Management of Ovarian Cancer," *South Me. J.* 66:369–374, 1973.

Survival rates vary, sometimes considerably, from one institution to another. This may be because borderline tumors are sometimes included along with frankly cancerous ones. It has also been suggested that high cure rates may result from misdiagnosis, where borderline or even benign tumors were incorrectly identified as cancerous, thus artificially raising the 5-year survival rates.

Table 17
Five-Year Survival Rate by Stage

Stage	Percent
Stage 1	61 (overall)
IA	65
1B	52
1C	52
Stage 2	40 (overall)
2A	60
2B	38
Stage 3	5
Stage 4	3

SOURCE: Adapted from S.S. Tobias, "Ovarian Cancer," *New England Journal of Medicine* 294 (1976):818–823.

The Breast

The anatomy and function of the breast are discussed in Chapter Three. In this section we are concerned with diseases of the breast, which may be either benign or malignant. These cancerous and noncancerous breast diseases can produce identical symptoms, so that it is generally impossible to distinguish between them on the basis of the symptoms alone.

Symptoms

The following symptoms, also listed in the symptoms index at the end of Chapter Six, may be associated with either benign or malignant breast diseases.

- ☐ A lump or thickening in the breast
- ☐ A depressed or bulging area in the skin or any change in the shape or symmetry of the breast
- ☐ A thickening on the skin of the breast that may feel warm to the touch
- ☐ Dilated veins in the breast. Some women normally have visible blue veins in their breasts; however, the appearance of such veins in a woman who has not had them previously or a change in the appearance of such veins in a woman who has previously had them calls for medical attention.
- ☐ A change in the texture or color of the skin of the breast. The appear-

ance of areas of skin with the texture of an orange peel, a condition known as peau d'orange, is particularly important.

☐ Any change in the condition of the nipple or the areola. Changes in the size, shape, skin texture or direction in which the nipple points; retraction of the nipple; cracks in the nipple or scaling of the skin around the nipple are important.

☐ Discharge from the nipple

☐ A lump in the axilla (armpit)

☐ A sore on the breast or nipple that does not heal

☐ A hot, swollen or sore breast

☐ Unusual ache or pain that persists and is not associated with cyclical changes and tenderness

A woman may have only one of these symptoms or any combination of them. If you have any of these symptoms, you should see a doctor, but many of us don't do so because we are afraid of what we might find. Our fear is that we will discover that we have cancer and that we will lose our breast or even our lives. Feeling upset and afraid is quite natural, but try to remember that the majority of women who discover these symptoms do not have cancer. Eight out of every ten lumps biopsied are benign.[1] Although 7 percent of women do develop cancer, the other 93 percent of them don't.[2] The odds are on your side.

Moreover, if it is cancer, you may save both your breast and your life by seeking prompt medical attention. Studies have shown that the earlier a cancer is detected, the greater the chances of survival.[3] Delaying treatment could cost you your life. There is nothing to be gained by waiting.

Having breast cancer does not necessarily mean that you will lose your breast. Today there are less radical therapies that hardly alter the appearance of the breast. Although these less radical therapies are still experimental, there has been enough evidence suggesting their effectiveness to have brought about large-scale studies at the nation's top cancer centers. No responsible investigator would treat a woman with these forms of therapy unless there was good, strong evidence to suggest their effectiveness. But women are eligible for these less disfiguring therapies only if their cancer has been discovered while it is still in the early stages. Here again, there is nothing to be gained by waiting, and everything, including your life and your breast, to be lost by delaying.

Breast Self-Exam

Every woman should practice monthly breast self-exam. If she discovers anything suspicious, she should consult her doctor. Even nonsymptoms, like a bruise that doesn't fade or a vague, indefinite feeling of thickening, deserve prompt attention.

Diagnostic Workup

If you have found a suspicious symptom, the doctor may do one of a number of things, starting with a careful palpation (feeling) of the breast. A needle biopsy may be done. This involves applying a local anesthetic to the breast and inserting a needle into the suspicious area. X-ray studies of the breast, known as mammograms, may be done. It may be necessary to do a surgical biopsy, in which all or part of the lump is removed and examined microscopically.

The many things that you as a consumer should know about the procedures involved in diagnosing breast cancer are discussed in detail in the section on breast cancer.

There is a great deal of information in the following pages. If you are reading this section because you have a suspicious symptom and are in the process of having a diagnostic workup, you may be feeling apprehensive, which, of course, makes it difficult to absorb so much new information. Ask a friend or relative to help you. It may be easier for your friend to absorb the information and think clearly than it is for you right now. Both of you should take notes and make lists of questions. Remember, you have the right to take someone else along with you on your doctor visits and to ask questions and receive answers to your questions.

The Pill and Breast Disease

The Pill apparently reduces a woman's chances of developing benign breast diseases. Because having a benign breast disease increases your chances of developing breast cancer, it is hoped that the Pill would decrease a woman's chances of developing breast cancer. Thus far there is no evidence to indicate that the Pill protects against breast cancer. Some researchers have worried that Pill use might *increase* a woman's chances of developing breast cancer because of the estrogen in the Pill. Although one study suggested that use of estrogen in menopausal women might increase the risk of breast cancer, no studies have shown an increase in breast cancer in Pill users. There is, however, one recent study that suggests that high-progesterone pills may increase the risk of breast cancer in certain women. For details, see the discussion of long-term effects of the Pill in Chapter Five.

CYSTIC DISEASE OF THE BREAST

AKA: adenofibrosis, fibroadenomatosis, fibrocystic disease, mastodynia, mammary dysplasia, chronic cystic mastitis, blunt duct adenosis, apocrine metaplasia, sclerosing adenosis, or ductal dysplasia

Cystic disease, often called fibrocystic disease, or mammary dysplasia, is a group of disorders that are an exaggeration of the normal changes that take place in the breast each month during a woman's reproductive years. Just as the lining of the uterus, in response to hormonal stimulation, thickens and prepares itself for the possibility of pregnancy each month, so the breast tissues respond to hormones and begin to prepare themselves for milk production each month.

In the first half of the menstrual cycle, when the hormone estrogen predominates, the cells of the milk-secreting glands, the ducts that carry the milk and the supporting fibrous tissue multiply. Once ovulation has occurred, progesterone levels rise and this triggers the first steps of the secreting process in the milk-gland cells. If pregnancy does not occur, the secretory process stops and the newly grown gland, duct and fibrous tissue breaks down, just as the thick, rich lining of the uterus breaks down and is shed in the form of menstrual blood. In the breast, however, there is no place for the debris to go, so it must be reabsorbed by the breast tissues. In the case of fibrocystic disease the process of growing the new cells and starting the secretory process goes too far and/or the process of breaking down and reabsorbing does not function correctly. Hence, small pockets of cellular debris and trapped secretions (cysts) are formed. These may coalesce together to form larger cysts.

Incidence

Since cystic conditions are related to hormone production, it is not surprising that they are most often found in women in their reproductive years. They can occur at any time between the first menstruation and menopause. After menopause, when the influence of hormones diminishes, the condition usually, but not always, subsides. A woman may develop cystic disease only to find that it disappears after a few menstrual cycles, or she may be bothered by it continually. Sometimes it disappears only to reappear years later.

Cystic disease is the most common benign condition of the breast. About 50 percent of female bodies autopsied will show some degree of cystic disease.[4]

Causes

The cause of cystic disease is not known; however, there is some indication that the tendency to develop the disease is hereditary. Pregnancy, birth con-

503

trol pills and menopause, because of their hormonal effects, usually cause the disease to regress. The disease may also regress spontaneously.

It seems clear that cystic disease is related to hormone levels. Fibrocystic changes are apt to become more exaggerated if the menstrual cycle becomes irregular because of some other problem. According to some authorities, irregularities in menstruation in normal women happen most often in late August and September for women in the northern hemisphere, especially when they are approaching menopause.[5] Also, in the months from December to May the ovaries are at their peak production for women living in the northern hemisphere. Women who usually have some tenderness and swelling are likely to notice fibrocystic lumps more often during these months.

There is also some evidence to indicate that fibrocystic disease may be related to diet (see below).

Cystic Disease and Cancer

One of the biggest concerns about fibrocystic disease is its relationship to cancer. Women with fibrocystic diseases are four times more likely to develop breast cancer than women who do not have these conditions.[6] It now looks as if certain forms of cystic disease may be more significantly related to cancer than others. Some doctors believe that the age at which a woman first develops cystic disease is a particularly important factor, and that women who develop it before age 20 are at higher risk than those who develop it later on.[7]

A mammogram, an X-ray study of the breast, is often done as part of the diagnostic workup for cystic disease. Mammograms can be classified into one of four categories: N_1, P_1, P_2 and DY. These are known as Wolfe's classifications. According to some experts, women whose mammograms fall into either the N_1 or P_1 classification are at low risk for developing cancer, whereas those whose mammograms fall into either the P_2 or DY classification seem to be at high risk.[8] This does not mean that all women who have P_2 or DY mammograms will develop cancer or that women with N_1 or P_1 mammograms will never develop the disease. Moreover, scientists are not in complete agreement about the significance of these mammogram patterns. Still, women who fall into one of these high-risk classifications may want to be followed closely.

Research is now being done to help pinpoint the particular forms of cystic disease that are related to cancer and to refine our estimates of increased risk for women with early versus late cystic disease. Until then, any woman with cystic disease, particularly those with early onset and high-risk mammogram patterns, should consider themselves at increased risk and, like all women, should carefully examine their breasts each month. Moreover, such women should have their breasts examined every six months by a doctor who is well informed about breast disease.

Symptoms

In the early stages of cystic disease a woman may feel nothing more than a general thickening about the size and shape of a thick pancake or a mass with indefinite borders, the edges of which seem to blend into the surrounding breast tissue. As her period approaches, her breast may become tender, or painful or swollen. These symptoms tend to disappear with the onset of the menstrual flow.

There seem to be two distinct types of cystic disease as far as symptoms go. One type is more diffuse and is characterized by lumpiness and tenderness, usually in both breasts, which is most pronounced in the week before the onset of the period. After menstruation there is usually less lumpiness and pain. The second type tends to occur in one breast, although it may occur in both, and is manifested by one, two or even three larger, rounded lumps that are usually quite distinct and freely movable within the breast tissue. If the larger cyst is actually a collection of smaller cysts, it may not be clearly separate from the rest of the breast tissue but may tend to shade off into the surrounding tissue and not be movable. This type of cystic disease is also likely to be more tender or painful in the week preceding menstruation and may also regress once the period starts, although usually not as much as the more diffuse type does. A single cyst may be relatively soft to firm or hard, depending on how much fluid it contains and the phase of the menstrual cycle in which it is noted. When it is full of compressed fluid or if the cyst is of long standing, it may feel quite hard.

The severity of the symptoms depends largely on how many of these cysts a woman has, their size and their location and how rapidly they enlarge. A woman with widely dispersed small cysts may not even be aware of them or may just feel small, nodular lumps throughout her breasts. On the other hand, an accumulation of relatively small cysts in the upper outer quarter of the breast, near the armpit, may cause considerable discomfort or pain in the days preceding the onset of the menstrual cycle, when hormone levels are fluctuating. A large cyst, responding to the same hormone stimulation, may become exceedingly painful as the fluids within the cyst press against the cyst walls. It too may shrink, or regress, as the period begins, but this tends not to be as noticeable with the large cysts. The off-again-on-again nature of the symptoms is characteristic of cystic disease and distinguishes benign cystic lumps from cancerous ones.

For some women the pain associated with fibrocystic disease can last as long as 3 weeks and may be excruciating. With large cysts, removal of them

505

will alleviate pain, but pain is often associated with the more diffuse, generalized form of cystic disease as well. Removal of these multiple, small cysts is often impractical. Some women find that wearing a good bra helps. Some studies suggest diet may be important. Avoiding excess salt, sugar, coffee, tea, alcohol and refined sugar will help relieve the symptoms.[9] Using oral contraceptives may help alleviate the pain. Some doctors prescribe Depo-Provera for relief of pain in cystic disease, but many others question the wisdom of using the drug in this way. For severe forms some doctors have been experimenting with a new drug called bromocriptine (Parlodel),[10] but this drug has numerous side effects and its use in this manner is also questioned by many. Another drug, danazol (*see* pp. 409–11), has also recently been used with some success, but it too carries certain risks and should be used only in extreme cases.

Diagnosis

The main aim of diagnosis is to distinguish cystic disease from cancer. The elements that help in the diagnosis are the mobility of the lumps, the absence of any suggestion of skin retraction, the feelings of tenderness and the typical waxing and waning of symptoms according to the phases of the menstrual cycle. These factors indicate that the cyst is more apt to be benign than cancerous; however, there are many forms of cystic disease, and the way in which symptoms manifest themselves may vary from woman to woman. Not all these symptoms will be present in each case. For instance, the waxing and waning during the menstrual cycle may not be evident.

The first step in diagnosis is a needle aspiration, a simple office procedure whereby a fine needle is inserted into the suspicious area and fluid or cells are drawn out. This may cause the cyst to collapse entirely, although it may refill later. The fluid or any other material extracted is then sent to the lab for analysis, to see if it contains any cancerous cells. If the cyst has collapsed, the lab report comes back negative (indicating that no cancer cells are present) and the symptoms indicate cystic disease, the doctor may decide that further tests and treatment are unnecessary. A "wait-and-see" policy is adopted, and the woman's breasts are examined in a month or two and then every 6 months. However, even if the lab report indicates that the cyst is benign, this does not guarantee that cancer is not present—just that there were no cancer cells in the fluid extracted. If there is any reason to be suspicious, the doctor may do further tests.

If no fluid is extracted, this may indicate that the tumor is a more serious one; however, many times fluid cannot be extracted in cystic disease. In this case the doctor may try another procedure, using a wider needle to remove a sample of tissue from the breast. Not all doctors are well versed in this procedure or have access to laboratories with pathologists who are trained to interpret such tissue samples. Even if the needle aspiration or needle biopsy indicated benign disease, a mammogram, which is an X-ray examination of the breast, is usually done. Sometimes the lump must actually be removed and examined microscopically to rule out the possibility of cancer. Breast biopsies are discussed in greater detail under the heading Breast Cancer.

MASTITIS

AKA: infections of the breast

Associated Terms: breast abscesses

Infections of the breast are rather rare in women who are not nursing a child but are not uncommon among those who are. The source of the infection is usually bacteria that enter through a crack, or fissure, in the nipple. Because the breast has a great deal of fatty tissue and a rather widely dispersed blood supply, the infection does not spread rapidly but tends to remain localized in an area of the breast.

Symptoms

The symptoms include swelling, redness, a sensation of heat in the infected area and pain or tenderness. The overlying skin may be red, and if the process continues for a long time, the infected area may become hardened. The infection may be mild, producing only an area of tenderness and a slight redness in the overlying skin, or it may be more severe, triggering a defense mechanism in the surrounding tissue. In such cases special cells in the neighboring tissue pour out secretions that harden and wall off the infected area, thus protecting the healthy tissue. This walled-off area, full of pus and infection, is called an abscess.

Diagnosis

Diagnosis is usually a fairly simple matter, at least in the woman who is, or has recently been, breast-feeding. However, the symptoms—pain, heat, redness, nipple discharge and a feeling of hardness—may be produced by certain forms of cancer as well, so there may be some difficulty in diagnosis, especially in the nonnursing woman.

If the woman has been breast-feeding, treatment is usually given for 1 week. In women who fail to respond to treatment or who don't have a recent history of breast-feeding, a needle aspiration may be done. The fluid aspirated by needle biopsy is examined microscopically and will usually reveal signs of infection indicating that this is a breast abscess and not a cancerous process. A mammogram or an excisional biopsy may be necessary in doubtful cases.

Treatment

In most cases it is not necessary to stop breast-feeding. The infection won't affect the baby, and nursing may help to clear it up. Minor infections may not require more than bed rest; the more severe cases may call for antibiotics. However, because the breast is made up of separate compartments of fatty tissue, it is sometimes difficult for antibiotics to reach the infection site. Thus antibiotic therapy is often ineffective, especially when the infection has progressed to the point of abscess.

In such cases the doctor must cut into the breast and drain the infected area. Here again the architecture of the breast, with all its little compartments of fatty tissue, can make treatment difficult. The cutting and draining must be extensive enough to include all the compartments where infection may be present. Treatment of small abscesses in the area of the areola are particularly tricky, since they tend to recur. This happens because the sinus tracts in the area, which are the drainage channels for blood and lymph, tend to become overgrown with cells as a result of defensive scar-tissue response on the part of the body. Antibiotics are frequently ineffective in this situation, as are incision and drainage. Small pockets of pus may remain in the sinus tracts and give rise to repeated abscesses. If this happens, the sinus tracts may have to be removed, but this procedure is not too damaging and heals with minimal scarring.

FAT NECROSIS OF THE BREAST

The breast has a good deal of fat tissue. Any blow or injury to this fat tissue can cause fat necrosis or death of the fat tissue, either because the blow has destroyed the tissue by crushing it or because it has damaged the blood vessels, which restricts the flow of blood to the fat tissue and causes it to die. The condition can occur in any age-group.

Symptoms

Fat necrosis tends to form a stony hard mass, or tumor, owing to a process of calcification that may take place in fat tissue. In response to the breakdown and decay of the fat tissue, the surrounding tissue exudes a fibrous substance that hardens and attempts to wall off the area of fat necrosis from the neighboring healthy tissue. This is called fibrotic response, and it tends to fix the mass of fat necrosis in place. If the fibrotic reaction is taking place just below the skin, it can cause retraction, or dimpling, of the skin.

These symptoms—a firm, fixed mass with skin retraction—may also suggest breast cancer. Furthermore, after injury an area of fat necrosis may enlarge gradually in much the same manner as certain forms of cancer. Moreover, areas of fat necrosis may break down and decay, setting up an inflammatory process and producing increased heat, tenderness and redness of the overlying skin; unfortunately, cancer may behave in this manner as well, so it is not easy to distinguish between fat necrosis and breast cancer.

Diagnosis and Treatment

If there is no bruise from the original blow, or if the bruise has subsided by the time the doctor feels the mass, s/he is apt to strongly suspect cancer. The diagnostic steps, described in the section on breast cancer, may be done, but since this condition can produce the same symptoms and even mimic cancer on a mammogram, an excisional biopsy, which is also curative, may be necessary.

FIBROADENOMAS

Types: adenofibromas
fibromas
adenomas

Fibroadenomas are benign tumors of the breast that are usually composed of fibrous (*fibro*) and gland (*adeno*) tissue. Other terms, such as "adenofibromas," "fibromas" and "adenomas," may also be used, depending on which type of tissue predominates.

Incidence

Fibroadenomas usually occur during a woman's menstruating years, most often in women aged 20 to 40. They are also the most common breast tumor found among adolescent girls (among whom breast tumors are uncommon).

Signs and Symptoms

Fibroadenomas are usually felt as firm, rounded tumors with a somewhat rubbery texture. They are usually sharply delineated from the surrounding breast

509

tissue, are freely movable and are not attached to the skin. They usually occur singly, but in about 15 percent of cases they are multiple. They are generally found around the nipple or in the upper sides of the breasts and tend to be small (1 to 5 cm), not to be tender and to produce no other symptoms.

There is a less common (7 percent of cases) so-called juvenile type of fibroadenoma that affects teenage girls. This juvenile type behaves quite differently from the so-called adult type (which, despite its name, also appears in young girls). Unlike the adult type, it tends to have dilated veins covering its surface. The skin over the tumor may be tense, but the tumor is not fixed to it. Because the juvenile tumor is generally larger and grows much faster, this is the type that is most often mistaken for cancer, but it is a benign condition.

On rare occasions a single fibroadenoma growing among a group of small tumors may take on an exaggerated growth pattern and produce what is called a massive fibroadenoma. The size varies, but they have been reported to reach 10 to 19 cm (see Cystosarcoma Phyllodes below).

The fibroadenoma is not significantly related to cancer. In adolescents there are few other conditions it may be confused with; however, in older women it may be confused with other, possibly precancerous conditions, such as fibrocystic disease. Certain types of cancer that occur almost exclusively in older women can also mimic the appearance of a fibroadenoma.

Treatment

It is sometimes best to delay treatment in young girls, since surgery may interfere with the development of the breast that is taking place at this stage of life. Although these tumors usually grow slowly in young women, they can take on an accelerated growth rate, especially during pregnancy. If this happens, it is usually wise to remove the tumor, along with a margin of normal tissue.

In older women the doctor will want to do the usual diagnostic tests for evaluating any breast lump (see the section on breast cancer) to eliminate the possibility of cancer. Treatment of this benign condition in older women consists of the removal of the tumor, along with a wide margin of surrounding tissue, for even though the condition is benign in the overwhelming majority of cases, there have been a few cases where cancer has arisen in adjacent tissues.

CYSTOSARCOMA PHYLLODES

AKA: giant or massive fibroadenoma

To anyone familiar with medical terminology, "cystosarcoma phyllodes" has an ominous ring, since the term "sarcoma" usually implies cancer. The name is misleading, however, for only about 10 percent of these growths are cancerous.

Cystosarcoma phyllodes is a variant of the fibroadenoma, and some authorities consider it merely an overgrown, or giant, fibroadenoma. These tumors are most often found in the breasts of postmenopausal women, although some cases have been reported in younger women and even in teenagers.

Signs and Symptoms

These growths are generally large, 15 cm or more, although some may be only 2 to 3 cm. The small ones, however, tend to grow rapidly in size. They are usually firm and freely movable within the breast. In some cases they become so large and the overlying skin so tightly stretched that it ulcerates (forms sores).

Diagnosis

The problem in diagnosis is, of course, to eliminate the possibility of cancer, particularly in postmenopausal women, so the usual diagnostic steps (described in the section on breast cancer) must be taken.

Treatment

Medical opinion on the type of treatment for a benign cystosarcoma phyllodes is somewhat divided. Some doctors, perhaps because of the ominous-sounding term "sarcoma," will treat the condition with a radical mastectomy. Most experts consider this overtreatment. They generally recommend simple removal of the tumor, along with a wide margin of the surrounding healthy tissue. This wide margin will help prevent recurrences. Even if the tumor recurs, more radical surgery may not be necessary as long as the second tumor is similar to the first one and doesn't show any suspicious, cancer-type changes. In some cases the tumor may be too extensive for local excision, so that mastectomy, amputation of the breast, may be necessary.

511

LIPOMAS AND OTHER SOFT TUMORS OF THE BREAST

Types: adenolipomas
      leiomyomas
      myoblastomas
      rhabdomyomas

Lipomas are noncancerous tumors of fat tissue. They are relatively uncommon but may occur in any age-group. On rare occasions they may include glandular elements (adenolipomas). Other benign tumors may occur in the smooth muscle of the erective tissue of the nipple area (leiomyomas) or may involve certain other types of muscle tissue (myoblastoma or rhabdomyoma).

Symptoms

These tumors usually occur singly and are firm, but soft rather than hard. Their size depends on how long they have been present. They are freely movable and do not produce skin retraction. They are well encapsulated, but at times their outline is not distinct, because they may blend into the surrounding fatty tissue of the breast.

Diagnosis and Treatment

Once they are discovered, the doctor may do any of the diagnostic tests used to rule out cancer (see the section on breast cancer).

Once the true nature of the lump is determined, it is not always necessary to remove it; however, it is frequently removed as part of the diagnostic workup.

INTRADUCTAL PAPILLOMAS

Types: simple papillomas
      duct papillomatosis

Intraductal papillomas are overgrowths of the lining of the duct system of the breast. Simple papillomas are entirely benign. Duct papillomatosis, however, is a form of cystic disease and is considered by many experts to be a precancerous condition.

Symptoms

The chief symptom is a bloody discharge from the nipple; however, this symptom is not always present. Lumps or thickenings in the breast may also appear.

Diagnosis and Treatment

Diagnosis may involve any of the procedures used in the diagnosis of breast lumps (see the section on breast cancer). If a definite mass can be felt, treatment of simple papillomas is surgical removal. In older women with duct papillomatosis and other risk factors for breast cancer, a subcutaneous mastectomy may be recommended. If no lump can be felt, the doctor may recommend careful follow-up, including biannual mammograms.

MAMMARY DUCT ECTASIA

AKA: plasma cell mastitis

Mammary duct ectasia is a condition in which the tissue that lines the milk duct breaks down. It usually occurs in postmenopausal women and is one of the few noncancerous conditions that can cause a firm mass in women of this age-group.

Symptoms

The process starts in the collecting ducts just beneath the nipple and areola. The lining of the ducts starts to break down and the stagnant duct contents begin to irritate the walls of the ducts. There is a fibrotic response to this irritation, which means that cells in the area secrete a fibrous substance that hardens and attempts to wall off the inflamed tissue, separating it from the surrounding healthy tissue. This fibrotic response and the resultant thickening of the ducts may shorten the ducts and cause nipple retraction. There may also be a nipple discharge as a result of the infection.

The process continues slowly and may take years. Eventually, the ducts themselves "spring a leak," and the irritation spreads to the surrounding tissue. As the duct contents continue to leak, a chronic inflammation is set up, along with an accompanying attempt by the body to defend itself by the fibrotic reaction described above. A firm, hard, fixed mass of fibrous tissue is formed. As it grows larger it grows downward into the breast. There may be pain and discomfort. The tumor has a tendency to break down. Portions of it begin to die, and there may then be redness, tenderness and warmth of the overlying skin. In extreme cases the whole breast and even the axillary lymph nodes may be involved.

Diagnosis and Treatment

The diagnostic steps used to evaluate any suspicious breast lump (see the section on breast cancer) are taken. Most of the time a definite diagnosis cannot be made short of an actual biopsy, for the symptoms mimic those of cancer. Treatment consists of removal of the lump.

GALACTORRHEA

AKA: abnormal production of breast milk

Associated Terms: Forbes-Albright syndrome, Chiari-Frommel syndrome, hypothyroidism, acromegaly, chromophore adenoma, idiopathic galactorrhea

Galactorrhea is defined as abnormal secretion of breast milk. Galactorrhea is a symptom of a number of problems that may have nothing to do with the breast per se. However, since the symptom involves the breast and the presence of this symptom often brings a woman to the doctor, we have chosen to consider it here along with breast diseases.

Symptoms

The thin, milky-white, watery discharge may be constant or intermittent; it may be present for a short time or for years; it may flow spontaneously or may be noticeable only when the breast is expressed, or "milked." It can occur both in women who have borne children, whether they breast-fed them or not, and in women who have never borne children.

Many times the menstrual period is also disturbed. There may be abnormal uterine bleeding, absence of menstrual bleeding or only occasional menstrual periods. Depending on the nature of the underlying cause, there may be additional symptoms, as described below.

Occasionally, a woman with normal menstrual periods will have a slight nipple discharge at certain points in her menstrual cycle. If this is her only symptom and there are no other abnormalities, such a woman does not usually require the complete diagnostic workup or the treatment described below. Such a woman would be wise, however, to discuss this symptom with her doctor, because galactorrhea can be an indication of serious problems. Similarly, women with post-Pill amenorrhea, that is, women who fail to resume their menstrual periods after discontinuing the use of birth control pills, may also experience galactorrhea. This may not be serious, but women who have both an absence of menstrual periods *and* galactorrhea must have the diagnostic workup described here to rule out more serious possibilities, whether they

514

have been on the Pill or not. We have come across women who have had both these symptoms whose doctors have told them not to worry about it unless they want to become pregnant. One such woman whom we saw recently turned out to have a brain tumor. Luckily, she did not heed her doctor's "not-to-worry" advice and sought a second opinion. The combination of these two symptoms *always* demands a complete diagnostic workup.

Causes

Galactorrhea may be caused by a number of factors. Many times, but not always, the galactorrhea is associated with abnormal levels of the hormone prolactin. Prolactin is manufactured in the pituitary gland and causes the breast to produce milk. Overproduction of prolactin may result from problems in the pituitary itself, from abnormal levels of certain other hormones, which alter the delicate interrelationships of hormones that stimulate or inhibit prolactin production, or from other substances that affect the chemical process through which brain messages are transmitted.

Hypothyroidism, a condition in which the thyroid gland produces insufficient amounts of thyroid, can produce galactorrhea as well as other distinctive symptoms, which are detailed elsewhere in this book. Injury to the chest or the use of certain tranquilizers can also cause galactorrhea.

Tumors in the pituitary glands sometimes, but not always, produce galactorrhea. There may be headaches and visual disturbances as well, although these may appear only after the tumor has grown rather large. A slow-growing tumor might be present for years before these sorts of symptoms appear. The term "Forbes-Albright syndrome" is used to describe a certain type of pituitary tumor known as a chromophore adenoma if the tumor is also associated with galactorrhea. Women with this rare syndrome tend to be somewhat overweight and don't usually have menstrual periods. If the tumor is successfully treated, the galactorrhea will disappear, and after a course of hormone therapy the menstrual cycle will return to normal. Other pituitary tumors may cause galactorrhea as well.

A condition known as Chiari-Frommel syndrome is also associated with galactorrhea. This rare syndrome follows childbirth. The woman fails to resume her normal menstrual periods and has persistent galactorrhea whether she has nursed her child or not. She may also have abdominal pain, backache and depression or other emotional upsets. The problem is thought to lie in the hypothalamus, the brain center that controls hormone production. Such women may also show signs of acromegaly, another condition associated with galactorrhea, in which the hands, feet, nose and lower jaw grow excessively large owing to a disturbance in growth hormones.

Sometimes it is not possible to identify a specific cause for the galactorrhea, in which case we call it idiopathic galactorrhea. Generally, this kind of diagnosis is good news, for it means that more serious causes have been ruled out. However, the fact that a woman has a diagnosis of idiopathic galactorrhea today does not mean that the cause of her galactorrhea will always be a mystery. It may be that she has a pituitary tumor too small to be detected even by our most sophisticated X-ray techniques or a thyroid problem that has not yet advanced to the point where it could be detected by our present methods of measuring thyroid levels. Thus the diagnosis of idiopathic galactorrhea may be changed in a year or two to a pituitary tumor or hypothyroidism. Women with idiopathic galactorrhea, then, need to be followed closely.

Diagnosis and Treatment

The first step in diagnosing galactorrhea involves expressing some of the discharge from the breast and examining it microscopically to make sure that it is actually breast milk and not discharge associated with a breast abscess or breast cancer. It is important that the doctor express, that is, "milk," the breast, for a simple breast palpation (feeling) that is normally done to detect tumors may not produce the discharge.

Once the doctor is sure that the discharge is breast milk, the next step is to get a test for hypothyroidism. If this test (a good one is the serum thyroid stimulating hormone, or TSH) shows an abnormal level of thyroid, the woman is started on thyroid therapy and followed up with regular serum TSH tests and tests to assess the level of prolactin. If prolactin production returns to normal during thyroid therapy, the diagnosis of hypothyroidism is confirmed and treatment for hypothyroidism is continued.

If the woman's TSH level is normal, the next step is to do a blood test to measure the prolactin level in her body. If it's high (above 200 nanograms, or ng, per milliliter), 90 percent of such women will have a pituitary tumor.[11] If moderately high (the 100-to-200-ng range), about two-thirds of the women will have pituitary tumors. If close to normal (20-to-100-ng range), about one-third of these women will have pituitary tumors. Pituitary tumors are, however, rather rare.

If the woman's prolactin level is normal, some doctors believe she still should have X-rays to rule out the possibility of a tumor. Although it is highly unlikely that such a woman would have a tumor, they think that the X-rays should be taken just to be safe. Still other doctors will order tomograms—a special type of X-ray study—but simpler X-rays, referred to as A/P laterals and cone-down views, which involve only about one-ninth as much radiation as a tomogram and only a quarter of the cost, are all that is necessary.[12] Only rarely will tomograms be necessary.

If the X-rays are normal, the woman has idiopathic galactorrhea, which needs to be followed. Some doctors will do prolactin tests every 6 months and A/P laterals and cone-down views every 2 years. (this may change to every 3 to 4 years, pending the results of studies now being done) just in case a tumor is present but is too small to be picked up by X-ray.[13] Other doctors don't believe this is necessary.

If the X-rays show some abnormality, the woman is referred to a specialist, who may do tomograms or sophisticated X-ray tests known as CAT scans. Treatment for a pituitary tumor is generally brain surgery to remove the tumor, although if the tumor is very small, a drug called bromocriptine, sold under the brand name Parlodel, may be used to destroy the tumor.[14]

If the prolactin levels are high, the woman will also need A/P laterals and cone-down views. Here again, the tomogram is not necessary. If the X-rays show some abnormality, the woman needs to be referred to a specialist, as described above. If the X-rays are normal, this is one case in which your doctor would be justified in ordering a tomogram. If the tomogram is abnormal, the woman should be referred to the specialist. If the tomogram is normal in these women with elevated prolactin, some doctors will treat the woman with the drug described above. However, because this drug has so many side effects, some doctors do not give it to women such as these, who have no demonstrable abnormalities.

Table 18 summarizes the diagnostic steps and treatment of women with galactorrhea.

BREAST CANCER
AKA: carcinoma of the breast

Breast cancer is one of the most controversial subjects in medicine today, and for this reason it is especially important that women understand the issues and become informed patients.

Breast cancer is a complex topic. It would take a book many times this size to thoroughly cover the subject. In the following pages the major issues are discussed. Vital information about symptoms, diagnosis and treatment is covered. Other important information about the emotional impact of the disease, recovering from the operation, dealing with having lost a breast, being fitted for an artificial breast and so forth is not covered in this section, for these topics have been dealt with in other books. In addition, refer to the introduction to this section, to Chapter Three, which discusses the anatomy of the breast and breast self-exam, and to the general background information on cancer, all of which will help to make the information in the following pages more comprehensible.

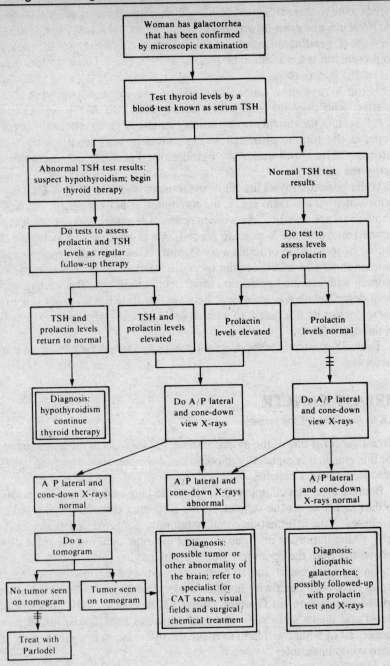

Woman has galactorrhea that has been confirmed by microscopic examination

Test thyroid levels by a blood test known as serum TSH

Abnormal TSH test results: suspect hypothyroidism; begin thyroid therapy

Normal TSH test results

Do tests to assess prolactin and TSH levels as regular follow-up therapy

Do test to assess levels of prolactin

TSH and prolactin levels return to normal

TSH and prolactin levels elevated

Prolactin levels elevated

Prolactin levels normal

Diagnosis: hypothyroidism continue thyroid therapy

Do A/P lateral and cone-down view X-rays

Do A/P lateral and cone-down view X-rays

A/P lateral and cone-down X-rays normal

A/P lateral and cone-down X-rays abnormal

A/P lateral and cone-down X-rays normal

Do a tomogram

Diagnosis: possible tumor or other abnormality of the brain; refer to specialist for CAT scans, visual fields and surgical/chemical treatment

Diagnosis: idiopathic galactorrhea; possibly followed-up with prolactin test and X-rays

No tumor seen on tomogram

Tumor seen on tomogram

Treat with Parlodel

⊧ indicates that this step is controversial.
⊧ See accompanying text for details.

518

Incidence

Of the women in the United States, 7 percent, or about 1 out of every 14, will develop breast cancer at some time in their lives. There are approximately 90,000 new cases each year.[15] It is the leading cause of cancer deaths in women and the leading cause of death from any cause in women aged 40 to 44.[16] Every 17 minutes another woman in the United States dies of this disease.[17] According to some authorities, the incidence rates are rising; others disagree with this and attribute the apparent rise to changes in the methods of collecting statistics.[18]

Risk Factors

Some women are more likely to get breast cancer than others. Risk factors have not been precisely defined, but the following conditions seem to be associated with increased risk:[19]

Previous Breast Cancer

The risk is highest for women who have previously had cancer in the other breast.

Other Forms of Cancer

Women with uterine cancer have about a twofold increase in risk of developing breast cancer and vice versa. Similarly, having ovarian cancer increases a woman's risk of developing breast cancer and vice versa. It is not known whether this is because having the other form of cancer increases risk per se or because these diseases have some common risk factors that would predispose a woman to all of them.

Women who have had cancer of the colon seem to be at increased risk of developing breast cancer; however, the opposite is not true. Women who have cancer in a major salivary gland are thought to have a risk about four times greater than that of the general population.

Family History

A family history (mother, sister, paternal or maternal aunts and grandmothers) of breast cancer puts a woman at a two- to threefold increased risk. There is some indication that the age at which a woman's mother or sister developed

519

breast cancer is significant. It seems that if the mother or sister developed breast cancer after the age of menopause, the risk is less than if she developed it earlier. If the mother or sister developed the cancer in her 30s, the risk could be severe. At any rate it does seem that the woman with a family history is likely to develop her cancer at a younger age than her relative did and that the cancer is apt to be more virulent.

Childbearing

Breast cancer risk increases with the age at which a woman bears her first child. Women who have their first child before age 18 have about one-third the breast cancer risk of those whose first delivery is delayed until age 35 or older. To be protective, a pregnancy must occur before age 30. In fact, a woman who has her first child after age 30 is at higher risk than a woman who has never had children. The protective effect of pregnancy is apparently limited to the first birth. Subsequent births convey little or no added protection. Only full-term pregnancy affords protection. An aborted pregnancy does not decrease risk.

Breast-feeding

The information about breast-feeding as a risk factor is contradictory. In the past it was thought that it was a protective factor. Several studies done in the past decade have failed to show any correlation between breast-feeding and lower cancer rates, but most of these studies were done in countries that generally had high rates of breast cancer. One study done in Japan, a country with low rates, indicated that there was a correlation. This may be because American women breast-feed for only relatively short periods, whereas Japanese women breast-feed for considerably longer periods, thus perhaps giving any protective influence a chance to manifest itself. No one is quite certain, then, about the significance of breast-feeding, but it is thought that if breast-feeding is indeed protective, the effect is probably not dramatic.

Menstrual History

Women who begin to menstruate at an earlier age are more likely to develop breast cancer. If a woman experiences menopause, either naturally or artificially, at a younger age, she is less likely to develop breast cancer. Women who go through menopause after age 55 are twice as likely to get breast cancer as those who experience menopause before age 45.

Fibrocystic Disease

Most studies show that women with a history of fibrocystic disease are four times more likely to develop breast cancer. Critics of these studies point out that many of the women studied were lost in the follow-up, and that the ones who are lost are probably the ones who never developed cancer, whereas the ones who do develop cancer are more likely to be the ones who stay in contact with the doctor and stay in the follow-up; hence the results of these studies may be heavily weighted on the side of a positive association between breast cancer and fibrocystic breast disease.

There is some indication that only certain types of cystic disease are precancerous, but not enough is known to refine the odds about which types are precancerous. One clue may be the age of onset. Cystic disease that is diagnosed before age 20 is considered by some experts to be particularly related to subsequent cancer.[20]

Diagnosing benign disease usually involves a special type of X-ray known as a mammogram. The pictures taken by mammography can be divided into categories according to their common characteristics. These categories, known as Wolfe's classifications, are N_1, P_1, P_2 and DY. Classifications P_2 and DY may be associated with a higher risk of developing breast cancer (*see* p. 504).[21]

Ethnic Background, Socioeconomic Class, Geography

These three factors play a role in increased risk, but since they are often cross-related, sorting them out is sometimes difficult. Affluent white women in northern climates have the highest rates. Women in Japan have considerably lower rates than do any women in the United States.

Incidence rates are higher in colder climates than in warmer ones, with the exception of Israel, which has high rates. These geographic variations may be owing to differences in childbearing practices in various climates, but this is hard to substantiate.

Heredity suggests itself as an explanation for ethnic and racial differences; however, the fact that women from low-risk racial or ethnic backgrounds increase their risk when they move to a high-risk country indicates that environmental factors, rather than inherited ones, are at work.

Diet

There has recently been a good deal of speculation that diet may be the factor that accounts for the racial, geographic and economic variables. A diet high in animal fats seems to be associated with increased risk. This could account

521

for the fact that people who live in warmer climates have lower rates, for these people consume less animal fat. Moreover, women in Japan have lower rates and less animal fat in their diets. Overweight women, who seem to be at higher risk, often have diets higher in animal fat. The fact that low-risk women increase their risk when they move to a country where the diets are high in animal fat also supports the idea that diet and nutrition are crucial factors.

An affluent Jewish woman over age 40 with a history of breast cancer either in herself or in her family, a history of benign breast disease with suspicious mammogram patterns, early menstruation, no children or a child born after age 35, late menopause, a history of long-term use of estrogens (see below) and a diet high in animal fats and proteins would be at highest risk. A low-income Asian woman with no family history of cancer, no prior breast disease, late menstruation, a child born before age 18, a surgical menopause before age 35 and a diet low in animal fats would be at lowest risk. Most authorities consider a personal or family history of cancer to be the most important risk factor.

Causes

The cause of breast cancer is not known. For one thing, breast cancer is not one disease, but perhaps 15 or more diseases. However, epidemiological studies have helped to identify risk factors and studies of laboratory animals have suggested some causes.

The discovery of a virus in the milk of mice with breast cancer that seems to be associated with tumor growth in mice suggested that there might be a viral factor transmitted by breast milk in humans. The identification of a virus in human milk of breast cancer patients that was similar, structurally, to the mouse-milk virus further strengthened the theory; however, the virus was found with equal frequency in women with a family history of breast cancer and in those without. Moreover, women who were breast-fed do not have a higher rate of breast cancer. Then, too, it is difficult to apply animal studies to humans, especially in cancer, which is an extremely species-specific disease, that is, it behaves differently in different animals. Breast cancer in mice does not usually metastasize and is generally not responsive to hormones, and the effect of pregnancy is to increase rather than decrease incidence rates. Breast cancer in rats, however, seems to mimic human breast cancer more closely. There is not persuasive evidence for a breast-milk–transmitted, cancer-causing virus in rats. Although the idea that cancer is caused by a virus transmitted through breast milk cannot be ruled out, the evidence is not strong.

The evidence that hormones play a role in breast cancer is suggestive but

522

often contradictory. The fact that women who have their first menstrual period late and their menopause early are at lower risk suggests that the ovarian hormones, estrogen and progesterone, may be a factor. The fact that overweight women, who produce higher levels of estrogen, are at high risk is also suggestive. We also know that the growth rate of some human breast cancer is affected by estrogen. Estrogen has been used to induce breast cancer in rats. However, if estrogen is a causal factor, it is hard to understand why only the first pregnancy seems to offer any protective effect and why breast-feeding, which also alters estrogen levels, doesn't necessarily have a protective effect. Moreover, estrogen in birth control pills has not been shown to increase breast cancer incidence. However, as critics of the Pill point out, the Pill has not yet been in use for a long enough period for all the effects to have manifested themselves. Then, too, there is some evidence that women who have taken estrogen replacement therapy for menopausal symptoms are at increased risk.[22] (For more information on the Pill and breast cancer, see the discussion of long-term effects in Chapter Five.)

Just to make things more confusing, it has also been demonstrated that women with low levels of certain hormones from the adrenal glands that are related to the body's production of estrogen have higher rates of breast cancer. Since these women with low levels of adrenal hormones are thought to have low levels of estrogen as well, this would suggest that low levels of estrogen increase the risk of breast cancer—which runs contrary to the other data we have. There has recently been some indication that the ratio of certain types of estrogen to certain other types is the critical factor. These particular ratios have been found to occur more commonly in Asian women, who have lower incidence rates, than in American women, who have higher rates.

Other hormones have also been implicated. Prolactin, the hormone that stimulates the production of breast milk, has been related to the development of breast cancer. Here again, the evidence is contradictory. In some instances low prolactin seems to bear a relationship to low rates of breast cancer. At other times high rates of prolactin are associated with low incidence.

Progesterone, the hormone produced during the second half of the menstrual cycle, has also been studied. Women who do not ovulate regularly and hence do not produce progesterone regularly have higher rates of breast cancer, and progesterone has been used to induce breast tumors in some species of laboratory animals. Progesterone receptors, which make a tumor sensitive to the hormone, have been found in some breast tumors. Human pregnancy, which is accompanied by very high levels of progesterone, is usually associated with lower disease rates. Here again, there is contradictory information. Findings of a recent study have suggested that birth control pills that are high in progesterone may be associated with increased risk for breast cancer in certain women. This study is discussed more fully in Chapter Five.

It seems clear that hormone levels have some sort of relationship to breast cancer, but the relationship is not a straightforward one. Many doctors are therefore concerned about the widespread use of hormones in the form of birth control pills and estrogen replacement therapy used to treat menopausal problems. There is no evidence that women on birth control pills have higher rates of breast cancer, but the Pill has been widely used for only about 10 years and breast cancers may take 15 to 20 years to develop. Moreover, even though evidence for hormones as a causative factor is controversial, we do know that estrogen, if not a seed, is at least a fertilizer, causing some existing cancers to accelerate their growth rate. For this reason many doctors are hesitant about prescribing oral contraceptives for women who are at high risk. Certainly women with personal or family histories of breast cancer should avoid use of any hormone medications unless specifically prescribed as part of their cancer treatment (see Treatment below).

Another, more clearly understood causative factor is exposure to radiation. Women who are treated for tuberculosis with radiation therapy are known to be at increased risk. Female survivors of the atom bomb exploded at Hiroshima in World War II also had increased incidence rates. Radiation has been used to induce breast cancer in laboratory animals. Although it is clear that radiation can increase breast cancer incidence in exposed women, the doses of radiation received have been large, far greater than those to which most women are exposed, so most authorities believe that only a fraction of human breast cancers are related to radiation exposure. This topic has been hotly debated and is discussed in greater detail below (see Mammography).

Symptoms

Breast cancer may be present for quite some time before it produces any symptoms. In about 80 percent of cases the disease will already have spread beyond the breast before the diagnosis is made.[23] Any of the symptoms listed in the introduction to this section may be associated with breast cancer; however, having one of these symptoms does not necessarily mean that a woman has breast cancer. These symptoms could also be caused by benign diseases of the breast. In fact, 8 out of every 10 lumps that are biopsied will be benign; only 2 will be cancerous. Nevertheless, any suspicious symptom deserves prompt medical attention.

Diagnosis

There are a number of important issues in the diagnosis of breast abnormalities that every woman should know about, including:

☐ The importance of monthly breast self-exam
☐ What constitutes a good breast exam, so that you know whether or not an exam is adequate
☐ The risks and benefits of mammography, an X-ray procedure used to detect breast cancer, and how to minimize risks
☐ The unnecessary expense and risk involved in certain types of breast biopsies
☐ The controversy about whether certain types of breast abnormalities are malignant or benign and the importance of getting multiple pathology opinions
☐ The fact that certain tests, known as hormone receptor assays, which could be of critical importance in planning treatment, are not done routinely at all hospitals and may have to be specially requested

These issues are discussed in more detail in the following pages.

Physical Exam

Most breast cancers are discovered by the woman herself, which is why breast self-exam, described in Chapter Three, is so important. Studies have shown that tumors discovered by self-exam tend to be diagnosed in an earlier stage than tumors that are discovered by accident.[24] Every woman should examine herself once a month, and women at high risk need to be especially conscientious about breast exam. Women should enlist their doctors' help in learning breast self-exam and should also have their breasts examined every 6 months by an experienced doctor.

Most women have their breasts examined by a gynecologist. Unfortunately, many gynecologists give only the most cursory of breast exams, just a few quick pats. The exam should be thorough. The doctor should examine the woman while she is sitting up with her arms resting at her sides to judge the symmetry of the breasts and to note any differences in the direction in which her nipples point or any irregularities in the contours of the breasts. The arms should then be raised over the head and the breasts carefully examined for the same things. Next, the woman should lay on her back, and the breasts and armpits should be palpated in the manner described in Chapter Three. It has been suggested that a woman at high risk should make a point of having a breast exam by a specialist at least once in her life, even if it means traveling to a breast-cancer care facility (see the appendix), so that she will know what a really thorough exam is like.

Any woman who discovers a suspicious symptom should consult a doctor right away. There is nothing to be gained by waiting. Sometimes we may be hesitant about consulting the doctor about a lump in our breasts, especially if we aren't sure whether the lump is actually there. We may be particularly reluctant to bother the doctor about certain symptoms, such as a vague pain or a bruise that doesn't go away. We may also fear losing our breasts. But breast cancer is a serious disease; no abnormality should be ignored. Early detection can literally save a woman's life—and in certain instances, her breast.

Any woman whose doctor dismisses her symptoms without a thorough investigation should look for another doctor. Studies have shown that doctors are sometimes responsible for significant delays in the diagnosis of suspicious breast symptoms, delays that affect a woman's chances of survival.

Mammography

Another important part of the diagnostic workup is the mammogram. Mammography is a special type of X-ray procedure that can detect abnormal tissue because such tissue absorbs radiation differently from normal tissue, and this shows up as a contrast on the X-ray film. There are two types of mammography: low-dose film mammography and xeromammography, or xerography, which produces a paper, Xerox-type print as opposed to the film print produced by the low-dose film mammography.

There has been considerable debate about which type of mammography is best. When xerography first became available it was considered superior by many radiologists because it took less time and produced a picture that had greater contrast and accuracy. Since that time, film mammography techniques have been greatly improved. Studies comparing the accuracy of the two methods are now underway. Thus far the accuracy of one method over the other seems to be related to the skill, experience and training of the person "reading" the mammogram.[25]

But even in the best of hands, mammography is plagued by a 6 percent false negative rate (in 6 percent of cases it fails to detect a cancer that is actually there) and an 11 percent false positive rate (in 11 percent of cases it notes a cancer that *isn't* there).[26] And that's in the best of hands; its accuracy can be considerably lower. We've heard reports of accuracy rates as low as 50 percent when used by supposedly well-trained radiologists.[27] Women should make sure that their mammograms are read by board-certified (*see* p. 235) radiologists.

Where the mammography is done is as important as who reads the mammogram. The amount of radiation received during the mammographic exam will depend on the type of X-ray machine and equipment used, how carefully the machine is monitored, the manner in which the film is processed and the skill of the technician running the machine. The amount of radiation received is of crucial importance, for as outlined earlier, and discussed in more detail below, mammography involves exposure to radiation, which itself is known to increase the incidence of breast cancer.

The amount of radiation exposure a woman receives can vary considerably.

526

Not all centers have the new types of low-dose mammography machines. One survey indicated that 10 percent of the radiologists were still using the older Egan machines, which expose women to unacceptably high levels of radiation.[28] Women should make sure that their mammograms are done on the new, low-dose machines.

Even if the machine is one of the low-dose types, a woman may still receive an unacceptably high dose of radiation. If the machine is not maintained and adjusted correctly, or if proper techniques are not used to process the film, the dose may be too high. Indeed, the very same machine may give higher exposures at one center than at another.[29] Sometimes higher doses of radiation are needed to get a more accurate picture of thick, glandular breasts, but some centers do not have their machines adjusted for the lowest possible dose.

The amount of radiation emitted from a machine is measured in units called roentgens, but the really critical factor is the number of rads. A rad is a unit of absorbed radiation. Skin dose refers to the number of rads absorbed on the surface of the skin. Midbreast dose refers to the number of rads absorbed in the midbreast area. The density and size of the breast will affect the number of rads received at the midbreast. It is not possible for anyone to tell how many rads will be received at midbreast, but it is estimated that the breast absorbs about 25 percent of the roentgens emitted by a machine. According to the guidelines issued by the National Cancer Institute (NCI), the total number of roentgens per mammographic exam (usually two breasts, three exposures per breast) should not exceed the number that will give a woman a maximum of 1 rad. A woman having mammograms should ask about the estimated dose of rads she will be receiving. If the answer is more than 1, she should look for another machine. The best place to find a well-calibrated, low-dose machine is at one of the major cancer-care facilities (see appendix).

Because the mammogram has a significant false negative rate, no woman should rely solely on a negative mammogram report if she has a suspicious symptom. A negative mammogram does not entirely rule out the possibility that a woman does not have cancer, for as noted above, mammography has a significant false negative rate. In certain cases a doctor may rely on the negative mammogram and decide to follow the woman carefully. This might be done if (1) the tumor looks and feels benign to the doctor (that is, it is soft, freely movable and there is no skin retraction) and (2) the woman is young (and therefore unlikely to have cancer) and (3) the negative mammogram is not one of the high-risk types (see above). Otherwise, further tests are necessary. Similarly, a positive mammogram doesn't always mean that the woman has cancer, for there is a significant false positive rate. But a positive mammogram definitely calls for further tests (see below).

Despite the fact that mammography is not 100 percent accurate, it is still a valuable tool. It can detect cancers that are too small to be felt by the doctor or the woman herself. Other, coexisting lumps may be discovered. It can indicate suspicious areas and help the doctor to decide which areas to biopsy. Moreover, the mammogram can be used as a record for the doctor to use in future comparisons.

Diagnostic mammography, as discussed above, is done on a woman who has a suspicious symptom—a lump, discharge, thickening of the skin and so forth—to help the doctor decide whether or not a lump is cancerous and where the biopsy should be done, or as part of the follow-up program for women who have been treated for breast cancer. In such cases the benefits of mammography clearly outweigh the possible radiation risks. However, when mammography is used as a screening device, that is, when regular, periodic mammograms are done on women who have no suspicious symptoms, in hopes of detecting cancer early, the question of risks versus benefits comes up. Do the potential benefits of screening—early detection and higher survival rates—outweigh the risks—radiation-induced cancer?

We know very little about how radiation affects the human body. Most of our information on this subject comes from women who have been exposed to large amounts of radiation, for example, survivors of the atom bomb dropped at Hiroshima. We know that these women have a higher incidence of breast cancer than those who did not receive such radiation. We also know that the effects of radiation are cumulative—they add up. In other words, it is thought that repeated exposure to small amounts of radiation over many years may be just as bad as exposure to a lot of radiation at any one time. Thus for some time there was concern that mammography might cause as many cancers as it detected;[30] however, new lower-dose machines have been developed. It is now generally agreed that the benefits of mammography exceed any risks that might be involved, at least for certain women. Clearly, in diagnostic mammography, the benefits outweigh the risks. Also, as a routine screening device for women over age 50 the benefits outweigh the risks. The NCI now recommends mammography as a routine screening device for:

1. All women age 50 or older
2. Women aged 44 to 49 only if they have a personal history of breast cancer or a mother or sister who has had breast cancer
3. Women aged 35 to 39 only if they have a personal history of breast cancer

A baseline mammogram at age 35 or 40 is also recommended. Then, after 50, yearly mammograms are recommended. Studies are now underway to determine whether a mammogram is necessary every year or whether less frequent mammograms, which would mean less exposure, would be as effective in detecting the cancer early. Recommendations for mammography may change again in the future, pending the results of the new studies.

The NCI guidelines for safe use of mammography apply only to machines that deliver exposure of 1 rad or less. The use of such mammography in asymptomatic women over age 50 is considered worthwhile because, by virtue of their age alone, they have fewer years left in which to develop radiation-induced cancer. Higher doses may not be safe for any woman, regardless of her age.

Women should realize that the NCI guidelines are just that—guidelines, not laws. Individual doctors may use mammography more or less liberally. Although we generally feel comfortable about the latest NCI guidelines, we do wonder about the value of mammograms in asymptomatic women over age 50 who are at extremely low risk, as, for instance, the hypothetical low-risk woman described earlier. Moreover, there are some instances in which we might recommend mammography more liberally than the guidelines suggest.

We have already discussed the fact that women with histories of benign breast disease who have certain characteristic mammogram patterns (*see* p. 504) seem to be at higher risk. The NCI reports have alluded to these high-risk mammogram patterns, but the NCI didn't consider them in making their guidelines, since they do not collect data on them. Whether or not such women should have regular mammograms and, if so, at what age they should have them and how frequently, is a matter of debate. All we can tell you is that one of the authors of this book has a history of benign breast disease of the high-risk type and has been having yearly mammograms since age 35.

Thermography, Ultrasound, GST and Other Diagnostic Tools

Thermography is another method of visualizing the interior of the breast. It relies on differences in heat patterns between normal and abnormal tissues. Initially, researchers were enthusiastic about the potential of thermography, which, unlike mammography, involves no radiation exposure and little risk. Studies have shown, however, that thermography is not very accurate; it has a 30 percent to 35 percent false negative rate.[31] Indeed, it is only slightly more accurate than choosing women at random and flipping a coin to determine if they have breast cancer. Although some experimental work is still being done, most centers have abandoned thermography. A woman should never rely on thermography alone as a screening or diagnostic technique.

Ultrasound, a method of visualizing internal tissues by means of high-frequency sound, is now being used experimentally. Although the technique is not yet reliable or practical enough for wide-scale use, it may play a role in the future.

GST (graphic stress telethermometry), another experimental diagnostic tool, also involves heat patterns in the breast tissue. The test can detect and distinguish between benign and cancerous breast tumors and does not involve radiation. This diagnostic tool is currently being tested, and if it proves effec-

529

tive, it may become the ideal method for mass screening of asymptomatic women. New, more precise X-ray procedures that involve similar or lower-dose radiation exposure also look promising. Experiments now underway may also yield simple blood tests that could be useful in diagnosing breast cancer.

Biopsy

The only way to tell for sure whether or not a lump is cancerous is to do a biopsy. There are several types of biopsies. Needle biopsy, or needle aspiration, is one type. This simple office procedure involves injecting a local anesthetic into the breast, inserting a needle into the lump and attempting to aspirate fluid. The fluid is then sent to the laboratory for analysis. If the laboratory report is negative and the lump collapses, a more extensive biopsy may not be necessary. If the pathology report is positive, cancer treatment can be planned. If, as sometimes happens, no fluid can be extracted, a more extensive biopsy is necessary. Similarly, if the pathology report is negative but the lump has not collapsed, a more extensive biopsy must be done, for the needle aspiration is not 100 percent accurate and the remaining lump may contain cancerous cells.

Another type of needle biopsy, known as a tru-cut, or wide-bore, biopsy, involves inserting a hollow needle into the lump and extracting a core of tissue. If the report from the lab is negative, a more extensive surgical biopsy is still necessary, for this type of biopsy also is not 100 percent accurate. Although there may not have been any cancer in the tissue sample, cancer might be lurking elsewhere in the lump. But if the lab report is positive, no further biopsy need be done, for the diagnosis has been made and treatment can be planned.

Another type of surgical biopsy, done in the operating room, is the incisional biopsy, in which part of the tumor is removed. Whenever possible, an excisional biopsy, in which the entire lump is removed, is done. The tissue is then sent to the lab for analysis.

One-Step Biopsies vs. Two-Step Biopsies

In the past, most breast biopsies were done in the hospital, using a general anesthetic. The woman was admitted to the hospital as a patient, prepared for surgery, wheeled into the operating room and given an anesthetic. The surgeon then performed the excisional or incisional biopsy and sent the tissue to the pathology lab for analysis. While the surgeon waited in the operating room, the pathologist examined the tissue in a quick procedure known as frozen-section analysis. Before the operation the woman had signed a consent form authorizing the doctor to remove the breast, a procedure known as mas-

530

tectomy (see below), should the lump prove cancerous. If the report from the pathologist came back positive, the surgeon removed the woman's breast.

This one-step biopsy/operation has come under a lot of criticism in the past few years. Many doctors are now doing a two-step procedure. The biopsy is done on an outpatient basis, using a local anesthetic. The woman comes into the office or hospital in the morning and is home again the same day.

This has several advantages. First, it is less expensive. A biopsy in which the woman is admitted to the hospital as a patient and in which a general anesthetic is used costs about seven times more than a biopsy done on an outpatient basis using a local anesthetic.[32] Moreover, only about 2 out of every 10 lumps that are biopsied will be cancerous. When one-step biopsies are done, 8 of these 10 women are paying unnecessary hospital and doctor costs. Since there is no postoperative hospital recovery time, the woman doesn't lose as much time from work.

Cost is not the only advantage to the two-step procedure. There is also less risk involved. Any time a general anesthetic is used there are risks and possible complications, sometimes fatal ones. One out of every 1,600 people requiring a general anesthetic will die just from the anesthetic.[33] Use of a local anesthetic involves less risk. The argument is sometimes made that by using a one-step biopsy the doctor can avoid subjecting the woman to two anesthetics—one for the biopsy and one for the mastectomy—but this argument is a fallacious one. First, a local rather than a general can be used. Second, only 2 out of every 10 women will need the second anesthetic, for the other 8 will not have cancer. With the two-step procedure, then, only those women who need it will be subjected to the risks of a general anesthetic.

In addition to lowering costs and reducing risk the two-step biopsy has other advantages. Instead of relying on the frozen-section analysis, which is done while the woman lies on the operating table, the pathologist can do a more accurate, but more time-consuming, permanent-section analysis. The frozen-section method sometimes distorts the cells, making it difficult for the pathologist to "read" the biopsy specimen. Admittedly, however, even if the one-step procedure and frozen-section analysis are done, it is unlikely that the pathologist would misread the slide and make an incorrect positive report to the surgeon, for if there is any doubt, the pathologist will await the permanent section. Only on extremely rare occasions will an unnecessary mastectomy be done because of a misreading of a frozen section. Still, mistakes can happen, and the permanent section is therefore preferable.

More important, use of a two-step biopsy means that the woman has time to seek a second pathology opinion before operation. Often this is done as a matter of routine. In small hospitals, however, this may not always be the case, and as explained in the general discussion of cancer, second pathology reports are always a good idea. Moreover, as explained below, in certain cases of breast cancer there is considerable debate even among experts about whether or not certain abnormalities are benign or malignant. Women who fall into this category will want to get second, third and perhaps even more pathology opinions from the very best experts in the field before deciding on a course of treatment. If they have a one-step biopsy, this will not be possible.

Another important advantage to the two-step procedure is the fact that it allows the doctor to do proper tests to detect metastasis before treatment. If a two-step procedure is done and the lump is malignant, the doctor will do chest X-rays, liver function tests and bone scans before beginning the cancer treatment. Many doctors think that if these tests indicate metastasis, there is no point in doing a mastectomy, for it won't enhance survival rates. Simple removal of the lump will suffice.

If a one-step biopsy is done, the doctor has two choices: S/he may either do the tests after the biopsy/mastectomy, although, as explained above, this might mean that a needless mastectomy was done, or s/he could do the tests before biopsy, although this might mean that if the woman turns out to have a benign lump, she will have been subjected to the needless expense and radiation risks involved in these tests. Only by doing a two-step procedure can these problems be avoided.

Perhaps the most important advantage to the two-step procedure is that it allows time for the woman to consider the various treatments available and make an informed decision about which type of therapy she wants, for, as discussed in more detail below, different doctors favor different types of therapy, some much less mutilating than others. It also allows the woman time to shop around for the doctor she wants to perform the therapy she chooses. A general surgeon might be competent to perform a biopsy, but if a woman elects to have a mastectomy, she should have her surgery done by a skilled and experienced surgeon who specializes in this type of operation, not by a doctor who performs only a few mastectomies a year. Moreover, for those women who are considering breast reconstruction (see below), the two-step procedure allows for consultation with a plastic surgeon before the operation.

The two-step procedure has so many obvious advantages that it is hard to understand why the one-step procedure is done. In the past the arguments were made that the cancer might be spread by disturbing the tumor during surgical removal and that the delay between biopsy and treatment would be dangerous; however, studies have shown this not to be true.[34] Delays of up to 2 weeks have been shown not to have any negative effect on survival rates. However, some very large lumps might be technically difficult to remove without discomfort to the woman if she has only a local anesthetic. And some tumors are so small that they cannot be felt and are detectable only by mammography. These cases might necessitate a general anesthetic. A one-step procedure might be done in these cases, but they are a minority. The majority of women can and should have two-step biopsies. In fact, a special committee set up by the NCI has now endorsed the two-step procedure.[35]

Given that it is rarely necessary to do a one-step biopsy, it seems obvious that the motivation for a one-step is largely financial. The one-step procedure is more lucrative for the anesthesiologist. If two-step procedures were done routinely, the anesthesiologist would do a major procedure only on the two women who actually had cancer, thereby losing the income from the other eight women in whom the less lucrative outpatient biopsy revealed benign disease. Hospital costs are also reduced when a two-step procedure is done.

Every woman should ask her doctor whether a one-step biopsy or two-step biopsy is planned and why. If the doctor is adamant about doing a one-step procedure, the woman should, by all means, seek a second opinion.

Biopsy Incision

Women should also ask about the type of incision the doctor plans to make in order to do the biopsy. In some cases the location of the tumor will dictate the type of incision that is made. Many times, however, it is possible to make the incision along the outer edge of the areola, which makes for a superior cosmetic result. In most cases such incisions are practically invisible once they have healed.

Pathology

Another important issue that women having breast biopsies should consider is the skill of the pathologist. As explained in the general section on cancer, the accuracy of the pathology report is a critical factor. This is especially important in breast cancer. Today, with the use of mammography, breast abnormalities of only 5 mm or less are being discovered. These small abnormalities are often noninvasive, that is, the cells are cancerous but there is no sign that they have invaded the neighboring healthy tissues. These are sometimes referred to as carcinomas in situ, cancers that are "in place." Some pathologists believe that these growths will eventually become invasive. Other pathologists have questioned this interpretation. They point to the fact that microscopic examinations of the breasts of women over age 70 revealed evidence of these types of minimal cancers at a rate 19 times higher than the reported incidence of breast cancer.[36] It may well be that not all these minimal abnormalities will become invasive cancer. Obviously, this has important implications for treatment: Is it necessary to remove these minimal abnormalities, let alone remove the entire breast? This issue is discussed in greater detail under Treatment, below. It also has implications for pathology: How should these abnormalities be classified, as benign or malignant?

Some diagnoses in pathology are difficult to make. Evidence of this fact comes from a pathology review of BCDDP findings in which a board of pathologists analyzed the minimal cancers discovered in the various BCDDP centers.[37] A total of 1,810 breast cancers had been discovered in the BCDDPs at the time of the review, of which 592 had been found to meet the definition of minimal cancer, that is, an abnormality that is either noninfiltrating (in situ) or infiltrating less than 1 cm. Of these, 506 were reviewed by the board, all top-notch pathologists. In 83 percent of cases reviewed the pathologists agreed that the abnormalities found were indeed cancerous. In 66 cases, or 13 percent of cases reviewed, the board found that the original diagnosis of cancer was incorrect and that the abnormalities were, after all, benign. In 22 cases, or 4 percent of cases reviewed, even the experts were unable to agree.* The review board thus found that 3.5 percent to 5 percent of the 1,810 cancers found in the BCDDPs were initially misdiagnosed.

How does all this sort out and what implications does it have? Well, first, it underscores the need for second opinions. Women who are diagnosed as having noninfiltrating cancers—in situ cancers—or infiltrating cancers less than 1 cm in size should, without exception, have two, three or even more pathology opinions before accepting treatment. Moreover, these second opinions should come from top-notch pathologists, the heads of departments of pathology at major university teaching hospitals or cancer-care facilities (see appendix). It is not necessary for women to travel to these locations to get second opinions. The woman or her doctor can arrange to have her slides sent to the pathologist for review.

Although second pathology opinions are always a good idea, studies have not shown these kinds of discrepancies in diagnosis when larger, infiltrating cancers have been reviewed by teams of pathologists.[39] Every woman should ask her doctor to explain the pathology report. Terms such as "noninvasive," "in situ," "noninfiltrating," "minimal" or "early" may all be used to describe the types of cases for which we think multiple pathology opinions are essential. Women should ask their doctors specifically, "Is my cancer an in situ cancer or an infiltrating cancer that is less than 1 cm?" If the answer is yes, multiple opinions from top-notch pathologists are in order.

Hormone Receptor Assays

The last but certainly not the least tests that should be considered by any woman having a breast biopsy are the hormone receptor assays. The results of these tests, which are also called steroid receptor assays, are of vital importance in planning further therapy. Unfortunately, they are not yet done routinely at all hospitals, so you may have to request it specially.

At the time of the biopsy a small segment of the tumor is removed. The segment is then analyzed to determine how sensitive the tumor is to hormones.

*Women who had minimal cancers diagnosed at BCDDP centers should read the important information given in note 38. More detailed and precise information about the number of cases misdiagnosed is also given there.

We have known for many years that estrogen can stimulate the growth of certain breast tumors. We know that progesterone also plays a role.

After careful research and investigation it was discovered that the presence of a certain number of estrogen or progesterone "receptors," which seem to sensitize the tumor to hormones, could be used to predict which treatment would reduce a woman's tumor. The tests are not always 100 percent accurate in their prediction, but they are a valuable tool that can help the doctor in planning therapy.

The test should be done at the time of the biopsy or, if a one-step procedure is done, at the time of mastectomy. If it is not done and the woman needs chemotherapy (see below) or cancer should recur in some inaccessible place, for instance in the bones, there is no way to biopsy the cancer and do a hormone receptor assay. Since the assay is not done routinely, a woman should check with her doctor before biopsy. If the doctor has not made arrangements to have the assay done, the woman should ask him or her to do so. If the hospital is not equipped to perform the assay, there are a number of commercial labs across the country that can do so. But advance arrangements are necessary, because the malignant tissue must be frozen for testing within 15 minutes. *All* women having biopsies should make sure that this assay will be done if the biopsy shows malignancy. It should be noted, however, that the test depends on having 1 gram of malignant tissue, so the test may not be possible for women who are fortunate enough to have very small tumors.

Staging

A number of staging schemes are used for breast cancer. Table 19 outlines one widely used classification scheme.[40] TNM classifications like those described in Table 20 are now more commonly used.[41]

One extremely important factor in staging, regardless of what classification scheme is used, is the size of the tumor. Generally, the larger the tumor, the greater the chance that disease has spread beyond the breast. This is not

Table 19
Staging Scheme for Breast Cancer

Stage I:	Tumor less than 2 cm in diameter; nodes clinically negative; no distant metastasis
Stage II:	Tumor less than 5 cm in diameter; nodes, if palpable, not fixed; no distant metastasis
Stage III:	Tumor greater than 5 cm, any size tumor that is fixed in place or evidences invasion of the skin or any tumor that is accompanied by nodes other than the axillary nodes that are clinically positive; no distant metastasis
Stage IV:	Tumor of any size accompanied by distant metastasis

Table 20
TNM Classifications for Breast Cancer

T = Tumor size

T1S:	Preinvasive cancer, carcinoma in situ, noninfiltrating intraductal carcinoma or Paget's disease of the nipple with no obvious tumor
TO:	No tumor can be felt
T1:*	Tumor 2 cm or less
	T1a: Tumor not fixed to underlying pectoral muscles
	T1b: Tumor fixed to underlying pectoral muscles
T2:*	Tumor more than 2 cm but less than 5 cm
	T2a/T2b: Same as above
T3:*	Tumor more than 5 cm
	T3a/T3b: Same as above
T4:	Tumor of any size with direct extension to the skin or ribs or underlying muscles other than the pectoral muscles
	T4a: Tumor fixed
	T4b: Swelling, sores or cancerous nodules on the skin of the breast, peau d'orange
	T4c: Both of the above

N = axillary lymph nodes

NO:	No palpable nodes
N1:	Palpable but freely movable nodes
	N1a: Nodes not considered to contain cancer
	N1b: Nodes considered to contain cancer
N2:	Nodes that are considered to contain growths and that are fixed
N3:	Nodes other than axillary nodes considered to contain growths or swelling of the arm

M = distant metastasis

MO:	No evidence of distant metastasis
M1:	Distant metastasis (including skin involvement beyond the breast area)

---

*Dimpling of the skin, nipple retraction or other skin changes except those noted in T4b may occur in T1, T2 or T3 without changing the classification.

always the case, for some cancers apparently grow relatively large within the breast before they spread.

The condition of the lymph nodes is also important. After careful palpation (feeling) of the nodes the doctor will decide whether the nodes are "clinically negative" (thought not to contain cancer) or "clinically positive" (thought to contain cancer). Clinical estimates of nodal status are incorrect in about a third of cases,[42] for nodes may be swollen without containing cancer or may feel normal even though cancer is present. The only way to tell for sure whether or not there is cancer in the lymph nodes is to remove them and examine them microscopically.

If the tumor is fixed in place and not freely movable, this is a serious sign. Open sores on the breast, swelling of the breast tissue, peau d'orange or cancerous nodules on the skin also indicate that the disease is more advanced.

Treatment

The treatment of breast cancer is one of the most controversial subjects in medicine today. At times the particulars of a woman's case, especially the stage of her disease, will dictate a specific form of treatment, but at other times, particularly during Stage I and Stage II, the form of treatment recommended may depend on the doctor's philosophy and personal preference. Most doctors recommend some form of mastectomy (Illustration 55), or removal of the breast, but treatments may range from a segmental mastectomy, or simple removal of the lump and surrounding tissue, to removal of one or both breasts as well as the axillary lymph nodes and the major and minor pectorals (the muscles of the upper chest). Sometimes hormone therapy, chemotherapy and radiation therapy are used.

Perhaps a bit of the history of breast cancer treatment is in order.[43] The first major breakthrough came with the development of the radical mastectomy, also called the Halsted mastectomy, after the doctor who pioneered this form of therapy. This operation involved removal of the breast, the lymph nodes in the axillary area and the major and minor pectorals, which are the muscles of the upper chest. Proponents of this form of treatment believed that the entire breast, rather than just the tumor, must be removed, for breast cancer is multicentric—has many points of origin. Merely removing the tumor would, they believed, be taking too great a risk, for the microscopic residual cancer left behind could metastasize before it was detected. The lymph nodes were removed because the cancer frequently spreads to this area. Even if the lymph nodes did not appear to be enlarged, microscopic cancer could be lurking in the nodes. (The only way to tell is to remove the nodes and examine them microscopically. If positive nodes are found, chemotherapy [see below] is given.)

The rationale for removing the pectorals was threefold. First, proponents of the radical mastectomy argued that it is difficult to remove all the lymph nodes without removing the pectorals. Second, they argued that removing the pectorals through which the lymph passes assured that any lymph vessels

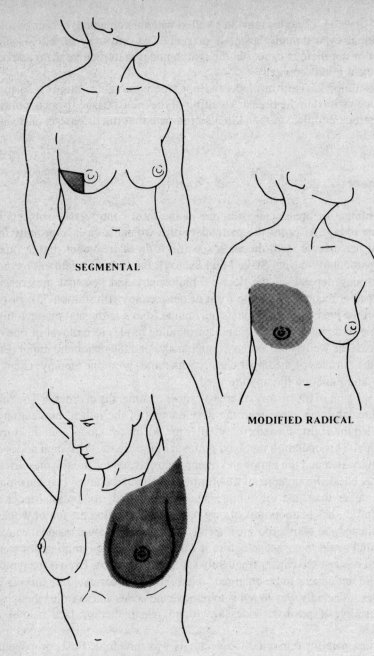

SEGMENTAL

MODIFIED RADICAL

RADICAL

Illustration 55 *Types of Mastectomies*

538

embedded in the muscle tissue that might contain cancer cells would also be removed. Lastly, removal of the pectorals allowed for what is known in medical circles as en bloc dissection. This means that all the tissue was removed in one piece, which supposedly lessened the chance of spilling tumor cells into adjacent tissue or into the lymph and blood systems during surgery.

This operation is, to say the least, disfiguring. Not only is the breast itself removed but also the chest muscles, which creates a hollow in the upper part of the chest. The scar is a long one and is hard to cover over with anything but high-necked dresses and tops. Sometimes skin grafts—layers of skin transplanted from another area of the body to the wound area—must be done in order to close the wound. The destruction of the lymph network can cause a condition known as lymphedema, in which the lymph fluid that normally travels from the arm through the axillary area becomes trapped, causing the arm to swell. Also known as milk arm, this condition can grossly distort the arm and cause grinding pain. In addition, the axillary muscles have to take over for the pectorals, and some women never regain use of the arm completely.

Because of these complications, changing notions about the spread of the disease and the fact that women seemed to be dying, not from local recurrences in the breast/chest/axillary area, but from distant metastasis, there was increasing interest in an operation known as the modified radical mastectomy. This operation involves removal of the breast and the lymph nodes, but the pectoral muscles are left intact. Although on paper it doesn't sound much different from the radical, the modified is a much less disfiguring operation. It has a much lower complication rate and has much better cosmetic results.[44] The incision is transverse rather than horizontal and is much easier to cover with clothing. The chances for breast reconstruction (see below) are much better. Lymphedema and muscle disability are reduced. Skin grafts are not usually necessary and recuperation is much more rapid.

Most cancer specialists now prefer the modified radical instead of the radical for Stage I and Stage II. Studies have shown that it is possible to remove just as many lymph nodes with a modified radical as with a radical mastectomy.[45] The fact that most women who die of breast cancer don't die of local recurrences but of disease that has already spread through the body first suggested that removal of the pectorals—at least in Stage I and Stage II—might not be necessary. Moreover, small-scale studies that gathered data about women who had had one or the other operation in the past indicated that in these cases there was no advantage in terms of survival, whether a modified or a radical was done.[46] Many doctors therefore believed that the modified was an acceptable alternative.

Many other doctors were hesitant to accept the superiority of the modified radical to the radical on the basis of the studies that had been done. Their hesitancy had to do with problems concerning statistical methods and the experimental design of the studies comparing the two methods of treatment. However, new studies, with better designs, have been done. The results of these studies shows that there is no advantage to having a radical instead of a modified radical.[47] A special consensus panel of the NCI has even agreed that the modified radical does just as well as the radical in Stage I and Stage II. Still, many doctors continue to do radicals. If your doctor suggests a radical mastectomy for Stage I or Stage II, *be sure to seek a second opinion.*

In the past, some doctors advocated total mastectomy and radiation therapy as a treatment for breast cancer. The total mastectomy, also called a simple mastectomy, involves removal of only the breast itself. The chest muscles and lymph nodes are not removed. Surgery can then be followed by radiation to the axillary area that destroys the cancer in the lymph nodes and axillary area. But this treatment doesn't produce better results than the modified radical[48] and doesn't involve actually removing the lymph nodes and examining them microscopically for signs of cancer. This has become increasingly important in recent years, for we now have chemotherapy that can provide better survival rates in cases where the disease has spread beyond the breast. However, as explained below, chemotherapy involves certain risks and should be given only to women who actually need it. The only way to tell whether the woman needs it is to remove the lymph nodes and examine them microscopically for signs of cancer. (Remember, although palpation of the nodes yields a finding of "clinically" positive or negative, it is not totally accurate; only the microscopic examination can tell for certain whether cancer is present in the nodes.) Thus, we now know that the total mastectomy plus radiation therapy, which doesn't allow for microscopic examination of the lymph nodes, is not the best treatment for Stage I and Stage II. If your doctor suggests total mastectomy plus radiation to the axillary areas, be sure to get a second opinion.

Once it became clear that the less disfiguring modified radical was preferable to the radical, doctors began to wonder if another form of therapy, known as segmental mastectomy, might prove to be as effective as the modified. Another term for segmental mastectomy is "partial mastectomy."* Basically, this form of therapy involves removal of the lump itself, along with a generous portion of breast tissue, with or withour subsequent chemotherapy. If you are considering a segmental, there are several things you should know. First, the lymph nodes in the armpit should also be removed. Some doctors will perform segmental mastectomy without axillary dissection, a procedure in which the lymph nodes in the armpit are removed. We strongly urge women to insist on an axillary dissection, for without actually removing the lymph nodes and examining them microscopically, there is no way of knowing whether or not

---

*The terms "tylectomy" and "lumpectomy" are not synonymous with segmental mastectomy although some doctors use them in that way.

cancer is present in them. Clinical estimates of whether or not the nodes are involved are too often inaccurate. Accurate decisions about the use of chemotherapy cannot be made unless the lymph nodes are examined microscopically. There are also some doctors who will perform a segmental mastectomy without a complete axillary dissection: They may remove only the lower lymph nodes. We think this is unwise. Removal of all the lymph nodes doesn't distract significantly from the cosmetic effects. Moreover, we know that cancer can "skip" lymph nodes; if the lower nodes are negative, this does not necessarily mean that the higher ones are not positive. Women should insist on an axillary dissection, and the axillary dissection should be a complete one.

You should also know that there is still some question as to whether the segmental will be as effective as the modified radical. In the past, doing a segmental mastectomy was considered too risky because it has long been known that cancer is a multicentric disease.[49] Multiple microscopic cancerous areas have been found in breasts removed by mastectomy. Doctors were afraid that if these small cancerous areas were left behind, they would continue to develop and might metastasize before they became large enough to be discovered. However, new developments in the field of breast cancer have led to a rethinking of this issue. Autopsies of women who have died have shown the presence of microscopic breast cancers even though the women never had breast cancer during their lifetimes. Autopsies of the breasts of women over age 70 who have died of other causes have revealed the presence of microscopic cancerous areas at a rate 19 times higher than the actual rate of breast cancer in this age-group.[50] This suggests that some of the multicentric cancers doctors have worried about will never become truly invasive cancers but will remain localized within the breast. The question then arises, Do we really need to remove the entire breast in all cases?

We also now know that a large percentage of women with breast cancer will have cancer in their lymph nodes at the time of diagnosis. Once the cancer has reached the lymph nodes, the chances are greater that it has spread to other parts of the body. Since chemotherapy is needed to treat metastasized disease, is the removal of the entire breast worthwhile? Will it prolong life or increase survival rates? Or will a segmental mastectomy suffice? Studies of women who have refused mastectomy or who were for health reasons unable to have this surgery, along with the development of effective chemotherapy, stimulated interest in the possibility that for certain women segmental mastectomy could be an acceptable alternative to the modified radical mastectomy.[51]

A number of doctors have been using the segmental mastectomy, either alone or in combination with chemotherapy or radiation therapy, in the past decade. The results, at least in Stage I and sometimes in Stage II, seem to be on a par with the modified radical mastectomy; however, these studies had certain technical problems, so no one could rely on them.

541

The indications were strong enough, however, to justify experiments. Thus experiments like those being done by the NSABP, under the direction of Dr. Bernard Fisher, have been set up to study the possibility that less extensive surgery might be as effective as the modified radical.[52] In order to be eligible, women must have tumors smaller than 4 cm. The nodes may be clinically positive or negative, but they cannot be fixed to the chest wall. There cannot be any ulceration (open sores) or any peau d'orange (skin textured like an orange peel). There can be no signs of distant metastasis. Basically, this means Stage I and Stage II. Also, the cancer cannot be located near the nipple, for tumors in this location are more likely to have metastasized and may have done so even though the chest X-rays and liver and bone scans give negative reports.

Women who are eligible are randomly assigned to different treatment programs, called arms, by computer to prevent bias on the part of the doctor giving the treatment. There are three treatment arms: (1) total mastectomy and axillary dissection (in other words, modified radical mastectomy), (2) segmental mastectomy plus axillary dissection and (3) segmental mastectomy plus axillary dissection plus radiation to the breast. In categories (2) and (3) any women who subsequently develop tumors in the remaining breast tissue will receive a total mastectomy. All women who are found to have positive nodes will receive chemotherapy. The treatment protocol is outlined in Table 21.

The above NSABP study shows segmental mastectomy to be equivalent to the modified radical masectomy. Furthermore, preliminary results from another well-designed study sponsored by NCI in Italy that compared less extensive therapies have indicated that segmental-type therapy is as effective as other, more extensive forms of surgery.[53] What are women with Stage I or Stage II breast cancer to do? Well, the women who want to play it safest should have a modified radical mastectomy. We know how that will work. The less extensive therapies will at best give equivalent survival rates. The only point of having one of the less extensive therapies is to preserve the breast, that is, to obtain better cosmetic results. Having a modified eliminates the problem of what will happen to the multicentric areas of breast cancer, for the entire breast is removed.

However, now that the preliminary results of the NSABP study and the Italian study are in there is, more than ever, good reason to suspect that a segmental will do just as well. Longer-term results may not be as encouraging. Thus, at this point in time, having a segmental is not as safe a bet as having a modified. We would encourage all women—those desiring modifieds, those who are undecided and those who are interested in these less extensive therapies—to seek treatment consultation from a doctor participating in an NSABP study. A list of participating doctors and hospitals is included in the appendix. For one thing, you'll be assured of being treated by doctors

NSABP Protocol B-6

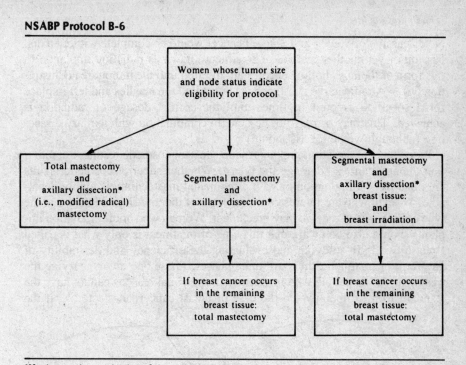

*If microscopic examination of the nodes indicates the presence of cancer, the woman is treated with chemotherapy.

who are up-to-date on the latest developments. Also, only by participating in these studies will we ever be able to answer the questions that now exist about breast cancer. Although the results may not help those of us who have breast cancer at this time, they will help our sisters and our daughters who may develop it in the future.

Women making the decision between a segmental mastectomy with axillary node dissection and a segmental and node dissection with radiation to the breast should know, if they have positive nodes and will therefore require chemotherapy, that some doctors believe that the radiation therapy will limit the effectiveness of chemotherapy. Others think that radiation therapy will cause the development of breast cancers in the future.* Here again, these issues cannot be resolved at the present time.

*The issue of radiation-induced breast cancer has been discussed earlier under the heading Mammography (*see* p. 525). Radiation therapy involves much, much more exposure to radiation than mammography, but the magnitude of the risk is not known.

Radiation Implants

No discussion of Stage I and Stage II cancer would be complete without a discussion of yet another method of treatment known as radiation implants. In this form of therapy, hollow needles are inserted into the tumor area (Illustration 56).[54] A radioactive substance is loaded into the needles and left in place for a specified amount of time, until the correct dosage of radiation is achieved. This may or may not be done in combination with axillary dissection (although we believe it should).

Proponents of radiation implants claim superior cosmetic results, but radiation therapy can also damage the breast. Whether superior cosmetic results are obtained with radiation or with a segmental mastectomy is highly debatable. Women who are interested in this form of therapy should know that the type of biopsy they receive may preclude it. Women who opt for radiation implants should also be aware that this type of treatment is only what is called ''phase two.'' In studying and evaluating the efficiency and desirability of any form of treatment, there are three phases. Phase one involves trying the treatment out on people who for medical or personal reasons cannot have the standard form of therapy—in the case of breast cancer, mastectomy. If the

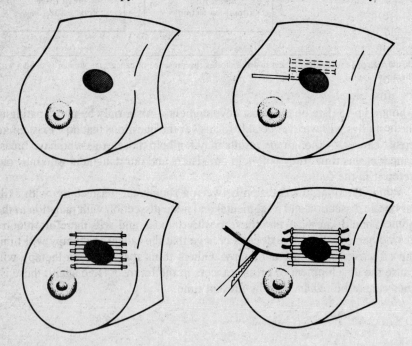

Illustration 56 *Radiation Implants: Hollow needles are inserted into the breast in the tumor area. Radioactive material is inserted into the tubes and left in place for a specified amount of time.*

results seem promising, a phase-two study is done. In phase two a number of subjects are given the treatment, and the results are compared with the results achieved in the past by giving the standard form of therapy to a comparable group. Phase-two studies are retrospective studies. If these results seem promising, phase-three studies are done. The NSABP studies are examples of phase-three studies—large-scale, randomized, prospective, carefully controlled studies. Perhaps in the future radiation implants will prove to be as valuable as the modified radical or the other types of treatment for Stage I and Stage II now being studied. But many doctors point out that this form of therapy, which does not always offer superior cosmetic results to those obtained with segmental mastectomy, also involved exposure to high amounts of radiation, which can cause cancer as well as cure it. Furthermore, future study results are needed before we can determine whether or not radiation therapy will have a negative effect on chemotherapy in women who will require such treatment.

Carcinoma in Situ

Before discussing the treatment of more advanced cancer, a word or two should be said about the treatment of carcinoma in situ of the breast. Carcinoma in situ, as you recall, means cancer that has not invaded the surrounding tissue. We have discussed the problems in the pathology diagnosis of this form of cancer elsewhere. Carcinoma in situ is highly controversial: in terms of defining the condition, determining whether or not it even exists and predicting whether it will develop into cancer. It is also not clear how to decide on the best treatment. With the improvement of mammography, cancer is being detected at earlier and earlier stages and more minimal cancers are being found. It is only recently that we have been able to detect cancers in this stage, for they are generally too small to be felt. It has not yet been determined which is the best form of treatment for this type of cancer. As a result, the type of treatment recommended varies widely, from modified radical to segmental mastectomy. Many doctors recommend an operation known as a subcutaneous mastectomy, an operation whereby most of the internal breast tissue (about 85 percent) is scooped out but enough skin and tissue is left to accommodate a silicone implant, which may be inserted at the time the subcutaneous mastectomy is done or during a second operation later on.[55]

A woman with in situ cancer of the breast has a difficult choice to make. First, as outlined above, she should have multiple pathology opinions before accepting any form of treatment. Like the woman with Stage I or Stage II disease, she could opt to be on the safe side and have a modified radical. Having this operation assures the woman that even if her pathology diagnosis were incorrect, and even if the multicentric areas that are quite possibly present in other areas of her breast were to become full-blown cancers, she would not have a problem, for the breast has been removed.

On the other hand, the fact that lesser surgeries are being done for Stage I and Stage II (NSABP studies outlined in Table 21, for example) certainly suggests that lesser therapies may be appropriate for carcinoma in situ. Both a subcutaneous and a segmental mastectomy are viable alternatives. The subcutaneous mastectomy removes 85 percent of the breast, and if multicentricity turns out to be a problem, this form of treatment has the advantage of having removed more tissue than the segmental mastectomy. However, some doctors argue that the silicone implants will make it harder to feel recurrences in the small amount of breast tissue that remains or may create confusing shadows on mammography.

The NSABP trials discussed above will shed some light on the behavior of the multicentric areas of cancer in the breast that may have implications for the treatment of carcinoma in situ as well. Until that time there is not much information on which to base treatment decisions.

Prophylactic Subcutaneous Mastectomy

A prophylactic (preventive) subcutaneous mastectomy may be recommended for women who don't actually have breast cancer but who are at high risk of developing it. When we first heard about this practice we were, quite frankly, horrified at the idea of removing perfectly normal tissue just to prevent the possible development of breast cancer. Although we're all for preventive medicine, this seemed, to say the least, a bit radical. Since that time we have changed our thinking somewhat. We realized that the average woman has about a 1 in 14 chance of developing breast cancer. As explained under the heading Risk Factors, for a woman who has a mother or sister with the disease, the chances are increased two- to threefold and perhaps even more if her mother or sister developed breast cancer before menopause. Moreover, women with certain types of benign breast disease are at greater risk as well. Reports of a fourfold and even higher increase in risk have been noted. Unfortunately, we have not yet been able to define risk factors precisely enough to say exactly how much having a combination of factors will affect a woman's chances of developing the disease, but women with family histories of breast cancer and histories of benign breast disease may have a better-than-50-50 chance of getting the disease. Certainly, a high-risk woman who has undergone the trauma of repeated breast biopsies for suspicious lumps might want to consider the possibility of having a subcutaneous mastectomy. At this time, however, the value of this procedure is highly debatable. Although 85 percent to 90 percent of the breast tissue is removed, the 10 percent to 15 percent of tissue that remains is still at high risk. Some doctors also believe that the implants make it difficult to detect cancer in the remaining tissue. Women interested in this procedure should have multiple opinions from experts at cancer-care centers.

Stages III and IV

Anyone who has read this far will not be surprised to discover that the treatment of advanced breast cancer is also controversial. Radical and modified radical mastectomies, radiation and even less extensive therapies may be used. In certain Stage IV cancers many doctors think that the mastectomy is useless and that simply removing the lump and using some form of adjuvant therapy will suffice.[56] In Stage III there are some cases in which the particulars of a woman's case will dictate the form of treatment. Radiation therapy is sometimes used. Chemotherapy is always used in these advanced cases. Hormone therapy and immunotherapy may also be used (see below). Because there is so much controversy and so many unanswered questions about the proper method of treatment in these cases, and because opinions are needed from surgeons, radiologists, chemotherapists and experts in immunology, we think that it is especially important for women with advanced disease to have the benefit of consultation by a team of experts, which is best obtained at a cancer-care facility or approved cancer hospital (see appendix).

Chemotherapy

Chemotherapy, the treatment of cancer by the use of drugs, has been one of the most promising developments in recent years. In the past, chemotherapy was given only to women whose pretreatment diagnostic tests to detect metastasis showed that the cancer had already spread beyond the breast or who had suffered a recurrence after the original treatment. The drugs were effective in relieving pain and shrinking tumors, but they could not totally eradicate the cancer.

As a result of studies on laboratory animals, it became evident that the smaller the tumor, the better the chances that the chemotherapy will be able to eliminate it. If, then, women could be given the chemotherapy before the metastatic cancer was large enough to be detected, it was thought that the chances of the chemotherapy's being effective might be much greater. Thus chemotherapy began to be used on less drastic cases.

We know that in about 80 percent of women diagnosed as having breast cancer the disease has already spread beyond the breast; however, in 20 percent, the disease has not spread. These 20 percent will not need chemotherapy. If it weren't for the fact that chemotherapy can have serious side effects, including the development of other forms of cancer in future years, it might make sense to give all women with breast cancer chemotherapy. As yet, however, there is no "safe" form of chemotherapy. We can't always tell for sure which women have disease confined to the breast and which have systemic disease. Therefore, only certain women are given chemotherapy.

Most women whose lymph nodes are examined microscopically and found to contain cancer (Stage II) will have a recurrence of the disease within 10 years,[57] so chemotherapy is given to these women. Women with the minimal or early cancers discussed above have a 90 percent survival rate, so most chemotherapists feel that chemotherapy should not be given to these women.[58] Women with Stage I disease and nodes judged negative on the basis of microscopic examination have about a 65 percent survival rate,[59] so chemotherapy is generally not given to these women. There are, however, exceptions to this rule. For example, a woman with Stage I disease, that is, a woman with negative nodes, *and* a negative estrogen receptor assay actually has a lower survival chance than a woman with Stage II disease, that is, a woman with positive nodes, and a positive estrogen test. Women with Stage I disease and negative estrogen assays are often given chemotherapy.

In the past a single agent chemotherapy was used. Recent NSABP studies have shown that combinations of two drugs can give superior results.[60] NSABP studies have been done comparing two-drug combinations with three-drug combinations.[61] Women in this protocol are given either a combination of L-phenylalanine (L-Pam) and 5-fluorouracil (5-FU) or L-Pam, 5-FU and methotrexate (MTX). Enthusiasm for a three-drug combination was originally generated by results from a study sponsored by the National Cancer Institute and conducted by Dr. G. Bonadonna in Milan, Italy, in which a three-drug combination known as CMF was used.[62] The initial results were positive not only for premenopausal women but also for postmenopausal women, who have, in the past, not done as well on chemotherapy. But the NSABP studies comparing two-drug and three-drug therapy have not shown any benefit from the addition of the third drug. In fact, when the results of the NSABP study using two drugs, the Italian study using three drugs and a study conducted by the Southwestern Oncology Group using five drugs.

Chemotherapy in combination with hormone therapy and immunotherapy is also being studied by the NSABP. These experiments are described below.[63] Again, we urge women who need chemotherapy to consult with one of the doctors participating in these NSABP studies. The only way we will ever answer these important questions is if women participate in carefully designed studies like those being done by the NSABP. Women who have had radicals and modified radicals and positive nodes are eligible, regardless of whether their original surgery was done by an NSABP doctor. Being part of an NSABP protocol also assures the woman that she is getting treatment from a doctor who is knowledgeable and up-to-date on the most recent developments in the field of chemotherapy.

Radiation Therapy

We have already discussed the NSABP protocol in which segmental mastectomy is followed by irradiation designed to destroy any residual cancer in the remaining breast tissue. We have also discussed the experimental use of radium implants and the use of radiation to the axillary area after a simple, or total, mastectomy. As explained above, this last form of therapy has fallen out of favor because of chemotherapy and the need to examine the nodes microscopically.

Another use of radiation in the treatment of breast cancer that has fallen out of favor is the so-called prophylactic, or preventive, radiation to the armpit after radical or modified radical mastectomy for Stage I or Stage II disease. At one time radiation was given in these cases to ''dry up'' any remaining cancer cells. However, carefully controlled studies have failed to show any benefit.[64] In fact, prophylactic radiation may even be harmful, in that the remaining healthy tissue can be damaged by radiation. Then too there is the danger of the development of radiation-induced cancer in 10 or 20 years.* Moreover, radiation therapy may hinder the effectiveness of chemotherapy. Today most, if not all, experts are opposed to radiation to the axillary area after modified or radical mastectomy or any form of therapy that involves removal of the lymph nodes. Unfortunately, the word has not yet percolated down through the ranks, and some doctors still use radiation in Stage I and Stage II disease after axillary dissection. Women who are Stage I or Stage II whose doctors recommend axillary radiation should seek a second opinion (see p. 238).

Some Stage III cases may require radiation. In Stage IV cases where the cancer has spread to the bone, some doctors use radiation therapy to treat the areas of bony metastasis; however, many doctors think that by the time the disease has gotten to the point where metastasis can be detected in the bone, there is no point in radiation, for the disease has already spread throughout the system.[65] Radiation, like surgery, is only a local form of therapy. Only chemotherapy can hope to control the disease once it has involved the whole system.

Because radiation may inhibit the effectiveness of chemotherapy, these doctors prefer to go right to chemotherapy without wasting time on radiation. Many of these doctors will, however, use radiation if the cancer is in a weight-bearing bone like the leg, since the cancer could weaken the bone and cause it to break. At the present time the question as to whether small areas of bony metastasis should be treated by chemotherapy or radiation has not been answered.[66]

A similar question comes up with regard to cancers that occur near the mid-

*Radiation risks are discussed under the heading Mammography.

dle of the chest. This area is drained by a group of lymph nodes known as the internal mammary chain, which runs along the breast bones, under the ribs. Some doctors favor radiation to destroy these nodes, but there is no way of telling whether or not the nodes are involved, so the use of radiation in these cases is controversial. Others favor chemotherapy because they reason that by the time the internal mammary chain nodes are involved, the disease, in all likelihood, has spread throughout the body and chemotherapy should be done.

Radiation is also used in advanced disease for palliation, or relief of symptoms. If, for instance, the cancer has metastasized to the brain or the bones, radiation may be given to shrink the tumor and provide relief.

Hormone Therapy

It has long been known that some breast cancer tumors are sensitive to hormones. At one time it was standard practice to remove the ovaries of all women who had breast cancer; however, the results of this type of therapy were rather unpredictable.[67] Some women seemed to benefit; others did not. Today we have the hormone assay receptor tests described above to help us predict whether or not a woman will respond to hormone therapy.

In the past, hormone therapy was only used to treat recurrent cancer and advanced disease; however, experiments are now being done that combine hormone therapy with chemotherapy in women with positive nodes. The preliminary results of these studies have been very encouraging, at least in certain instances. Chemotherapy alone has made a marked improvement in premenopausal women with one to three positive nodes and has had some effect in premenopausal women with four or more positive nodes. It has even made some improvement in postmenopausal women with four or more positive nodes, but there hasn't been any benefit for postmenopausal women with one to three positive nodes. However, the addition of hormone therapy, in the form of a drug called Tamoxifen, to the chemotherapy of postmenopausal women with positive hormone assays has made a marked improvement in the treatment of such women, both those with one to three positive nodes and those with four or more positive nodes.[68] This is one of the most exciting developments in breast cancer today. Unfortunately, Tamoxifen has not had the same effect in premenopausal women. No benefit has yet been shown for younger women.

Because of the positive results of Tamoxifen, there are now NSABP studies being conducted in which certain women with Stage I disease are being given Tamoxifen. It will be some time, however, before the results of these studies are available.

In addition to hormone therapy in the form of drugs to suppress hormone production, there are also surgical hormone therapies, which are used in the treatment of recurrent disease. The ovaries of a woman with recurrent cancer

550

may be removed, a procedure known as oophorectomy, or the ovaries may be destroyed by radiation. This is generally only done for premenopausal women.

Two other forms of surgery designed to curtail hormone production are sometimes done in advanced disease. The adrenal glands—two small glands located near the kidneys that produce essential hormones, including cortisone (which helps the body metabolize sugar), and are apparently able to produce some estrogen as well—may be removed. This operation, known as an adrenalectomy, may be done after oophorectomy in premenopausal women with recurrent cancer. It may also be done in postmenopausal women whose tumors are thought to be estrogen-sensitive, in an effort to remove a potential source of estrogen. The operation is a difficult one. Today, other drugs can be used to suppress the action of the adrenal glands. Although adrenalectomies are still done in some cases, drug therapy has pretty much replaced adrenalectomy.

Another surgical procedure used in the treatment of recurrent breast cancer is hypophysectomy, which involves removal of the anterior pituitary gland in the brain. The pituitary produces hormones that in turn stimulate the ovaries and the adrenal glands. By removing the anterior pituitary, the functioning of the ovaries and adrenals falls to a low level, almost as low as if the woman had had an oophorectomy and adrenalectomy. In addition, destruction of the pituitary effectively stops the production of growth hormone and of prolactin (the hormone responsible for milk production), both of which have been implicated in the stimulation of breast tumors. However, this operation requires major brain surgery and some risk. Even though the pituitary can now be destroyed by radiation instead of surgery, the procedure is not often done, for it is now known that estrogen can be produced in fatty tissues of the body, so even this extensive a procedure may not succeed in removing all the estrogen from a woman's body.

In the treatment of recurrent cancer—in addition to surgery, radiation or drugs used to destroy or suppress the body's production of hormones—sometimes large doses of hormones are given. For example, some women respond well to massive doese of estrogen. It seems that a change in the hormone climate of the woman's body—oophorectomy if she is premenopausal or, in certain cases, large doses of hormones if she is postmenopausal—will sometimes be helpful in relieving symptoms or slowing the growth of the tumor. The tumor will return eventually, however.

Breast Reconstruction[69]

Breast reconstruction is a procedure made possible by some of the same techniques plastic surgeons first devised for cosmetic reshaping of the breast. In the past, less than 1 percent of all women who had mastectomies had breast reconstruction. The techniques have improved greatly, however, and since many insurance companies now provide partial or total coverage for the procedure, more and more women are choosing to have it done.

The procedure and the outcome vary considerably. Sometimes the reconstruction can be done at the time of surgery. Most of the time a waiting period of at least 3 months is necessary. Reconstruction may also be done many years after surgery. In fact, successful reconstructions have been done as long as 20 years after mastectomy.

The reconstruction may require more than one operation, especially if the woman had a radical mastectomy, which leaves a hollow in the chest wall. Tissue from other parts of the body may be transplanted to fill in the hollow. More than one operation is sometimes needed if the nipple is also reconstructed. A new nipple can sometimes be constructed using tissue from the vulval lips or other areas of the body. Depending on the size of the other breast and the amount of muscle and skin remaining after mastectomy, it may be necessary to reduce the size of the other breast to restore symmetry. Sometimes this procedure, known as reductive mammoplasty, can be done at the same time as the reconstruction; at other times a separate operation must be done.

Basically, reconstruction involves inserting a plastic bag of silicone gel under the skin or muscle. The silicone gel implant, unlike silicone injections, which are now banned in most states, is not thought to be harmful to the body in any way. Some doctors do worry that the presence of the silicone implant might make it difficult to feel recurrent cancer on the chest wall under the implant or might create confusing shadows on a mammogram.

The results of reconstruction vary considerably. In some cases a very satisfactory result is obtained, but in others the results are disappointing. Women should not expect the breast to look the same as it did before mastectomy. The reconstructed breast is intended to look good under a bra, but in the nude its appearance may be marred by scarring and other imperfections. The woman's doctor should be able to give her an idea of how the reconstructed breast will look. Most good doctors will have "before and after" photos of other women. Women may wish to ask the surgeon if it's possible to talk with some of his or her previous patients, if any have given the doctor permission to offer their names to prospective patients. There is also an organization, AFTER (Ask a Friend to Explain Reconstruction), 99 Park Avenue, New York, New York 10016, that puts women in touch with other women who've had reconstructive surgery. The organization also publishes a pamphlet on the subject.

Reconstruction is a fairly new technique, so it is important to find a doctor who is skilled and experienced in this procedure. Ideally, the doctor should be a board-certified plastic surgeon who is experienced in performing the operation. A woman should shop around before making a decision, asking how many operations the doctor has done, talking with former patients and viewing before and after shots. The surgeon who is doing the mastectomy may be able to provide referrals. Cancer hot lines or medical-school–related hospitals may also provide names. Women can also contact the American Society of Plastic and Reconstructive Surgeons, 29 East Madison Street, Suite 807, Chicago, Illinois 60602, for a list of surgeons in their area. The Society also publishes an informative pamphlet on the subject. If possible, the plastic surgeon should consult with the doctor performing the cancer surgery before the operation. Although the cancer operation should never be compromised for the sake of better reconstruction, sometimes it is possible to perform the cancer operation in such a way that the plastic surgeon's job will be easier.

Not all women can have breast reconstruction. Sometimes the skin is too tight to allow for successful reconstruction. If radiation therapy has been used, the remaining tissue may be too badly damaged to allow for reconstruction. Many doctors discourage reconstruction in cases where the cancer has recurred or metastasized. Women on chemotherapy may have to wait until the chemotherapy is discontinued, for the drugs may suppress the white blood cell count, making surgery inadvisable.

Breast reconstruction can be costly, especially if more than one operation is required. A number of insurance companies now cover these costs, but some do not, so it is important to discuss finances before surgery.

Breast reconstruction, like any form of surgery, carries risks. There may be bleeding, infection and extensive scar formation. Occasionally, the blood supply of the skin may be inadequate and there may be partial skin loss. The implant may be rejected by the body. There may be distortion in shape or hardening of the areas around the implant, or the implant may fall. In these instances further surgery may be needed. However, many women have been pleased with reconstruction results.

Breast Prosthesis

Women who have had mastectomies are usually fitted for artificial breasts, called prostheses. This is done both for appearance and for medical reasons. The prosthesis will counterbalance the weight of the remaining breast, eliminating back strain, which can be caused by uneven weight distribution. The American Cancer Society sponsors a program, Reach to Recovery, run by volunteers who have had mastectomies themselves. These women can provide important information on fitting prostheses and can also offer invaluable assistance to women who've had mastectomies. Your doctor can put you in touch with this group. It should also be mentioned that a growing number of women are deciding to forego prosthesis and reconstruction, adopting the at-

553

titude that "This is how my body looks now and I don't see any reason to pretend otherwise."

Survival Rates

Survival rates for most forms of cancer are given in terms of 5 years because most of those who are alive at 5 years will be disease-free at 10 years. With breast cancer, 5-year survival rates do not mean as much, for a significant number of women will have recurrences 10 or even 20 years later. Table 22 lists survival rates according to both stage and nodal involvement. But it takes a number of years for the improvements that chemotherapy and hormone therapy have wrought to show up in the national statistics, so if you are having these forms of treatment, your survival statistics may be higher than those reflected in Table 22.

Table 22
Survival Rates for Breast Cancer by Stage

Stage	Five-Year Survival Rate (%) by Stage
I	82—94
II	47—74
III	7—8
IV	—

Survival Rates for Breast Cancer by Nodal Status

Condition of Nodes	Five-Year Survival Rates (%)	Ten-Year Survival Rates (%)
Negative axillary lymph nodes	78.1	64.9
Positive axillary lymph nodes	46.5	24.9
1–3 positive nodes	62.2	37.5
More than 4 positive nodes	32.0	13.4

SOURCE: Adapted from Craig Henderson, M.D., and George P. Canellos, M.D., "Cancer of the Breast: The Past Decade," *New England Journal of Medicine* 302:1 (Jan 3, 1980), pp. 17–30.

Follow-up

Women with breast cancer will need careful follow-up for the rest of their lives. Follow-up has three objectives:

1. The detection of metastasis
2. The detection of a possible second cancer in the opposite breast or in the remainin breast tissue if a segmental mastectomy has been done
3. The detection of other forms of cancer.

Metastasis usually occurs first in the lungs and soft tissues, such as the liver. Metastasis frequently occurs in the bones. Women who have had breast cancer are at higher risk of developing other forms of cancer, especially endometrial and ovarian cancer. Follow-up will then pay special attention to the remaining breast, the soft tissues, the skeletal system and the uterus and ovaries.

Many women we have spoken with in the course of writing this book have received less-than-adequate follow-up. Table 23 outlines a widely recommended follow-up program. The tests listed in this table are those

Table 23
Follow-Up Program for Breast Cancer Patients

I	Monthly breast self-exam
II	First year
	• Complete physical exam at 3-month intervals, with special attention to inspection and palpation of mastectomy area, remaining breast and lymph nodes and abdomen, liver, chest, pelvic and rectal areas, oral cavity, skin, chest and bones
	• CBC blood exam at 6-month intervals
	• SMA12 blood chemistry at 6-month intervals
	• X-ray of chest at 6-month intervals
	• Mammogram once a year
	• Liver, bone and brain scans as indicated
III	Second Year
	• All tests and examinations listed above should be performed twice a year, except for mammography, which should be done once a year
IV	Third and subsequent years
	• All tests and examinations listed above should be performed on an annual basis

recommended routinely in the absence of symptoms or signs. If symptoms appear, further tests will be needed. Significant symptoms include bone or chest pain, persistent cough, appetite or weight loss, weakness, headaches, falls, seizures and changes in behavior or psychological changes.

Sexually Transmissible Infections

Imagine what would happen if we were having an epidemic of a group of diseases that were transmitted by shaking hands, diseases that could, if not treated in time, lead to serious complications, including birth defects, infertility, arthritis, blindness, heart failure, mental retardation, insanity and even death. To complicate matters, suppose that some people didn't have symptoms in the early stages of these diseases and therefore didn't have any way of knowing they had been infected unless the person who had infected them passed the word on. Not only that, but what if the diseases were so widespread that only colds were more common. Indeed, what if every 15 seconds another person came down with one of these diseases. Suppose that just caring for the psychiatric and blinded victims cost taxpayers $50 million each year.

Well, for starters, a lot of people would wear gloves. Health officials would be passing out free pairs at clinics across the country. A massive education program would be launched to educate people about these diseases. The signs and symptoms of the diseases and how to recognize and prevent them would be the most important items in the curriculum of public-school health classes. Conscientious doctors would report each case to the state health department, and social workers would diligently track down the infected persons' contacts, warning them of the dangers and helping to stop the spread of the diseases. The government would pour vast sums of money into medical research projects in an effort to develop a vaccine. In a few short years, immunizations would be available, and the "shaking hands" disease would join the ranks of smallpox, polio, diphtheria, whooping cough and other conquered diseases.

You can stop imagining now, for as it turns out, we do have an epidemic of a group of diseases that can have the serious complications outlined above. But there aren't any massive education programs. The topic is ignored in most public schools. Doctors, despite legal requirements, aren't reporting the cases they treat to state health officials. Infectors aren't passing the word along to infectees. Methods of prevention are a well-kept secret. A mere pittance is spent on research; there is no vaccine.

Why not? Because you don't get these diseases by shaking hands; you get them by having sex with an infected person. They're called venereal disease (VD) or, if you prefer (as we do) the more direct term, sexually transmissible infections (STI).

Because these diseases are transmitted sexually the whole issue has been clouded by fear, guilt, moralizing and sexual hypocrisy. Since early childhood most of us have been taught to think of our genital organs as something unclean and of sex as something to be ashamed of, something "nice girls" don't do—don't even like to do. Getting VD, like getting pregnant, is an obvious indication that you've been "doin' it." Because most of us have at least some difficulty in talking about sex and in confronting our sexuality, dealing with VD, with all its sleazy connotations, is especially difficult. On both a personal and social level we've tended to ignore the VD problem, shoving it back into some dark, guilty corner, hoping it will go away.

But it won't go away. Indeed, VD is on the rise. In 1978 there were an estimated 468.3 cases of gonorrhea per 100,000 people, a rise from 466.8 per 100,000 in 1977.[1] Incidence rates for syphilis have risen too, and it's anybody's guess how many cases of herpes there are, since it is not a disease that must be reported, but clinics and private doctors are now seeing it more frequently than gonorrhea.

Apparently, "nice girls" *do* like to do it; either that or else there are an awful lot of "not-nice" girls around. A popular bit of folklore holds that nice people, meaning upper- and middle-class people, don't get VD, that it's a disease of the poor and of prostitutes. Not true. The disease occurs in the suburbs as well as the ghettos. The organisms that cause these diseases don't make moral judgments, aren't social snobs and make no distinctions as to race, color or creed. They'll attack anybody. Unfortunately, many in the medical profession don't seem to know this, so a lot of people who need testing don't get it, because their doctors have decided that they are "nice, middle-class people" who don't get such diseases. Conversely, many poor people can't get any kind of medical treatment without first being tested for VD.

Although most of these diseases are readily cured in their early stages, they can have serious, even fatal, complications. The symptoms may disappear, sometimes for years, but most of these diseases don't go away by themselves.

557

It is often possible to infect someone else even when you don't have symptoms.

Prevention

There are ways of protecting yourself—and your partners—against STIs, although these methods aren't receiving the public attention they deserve. Perhaps this stems from the old sex-is-bad-and-VD-is-a-punishment-for-your-sins school of thought. Moreover, these methods are not 100 percent effective, so many public information services, including some VD hotlines, don't tell people about them. They fear that people will think that these methods offer absolute protection and will therefore go ahead and have sex, even though they know they (or their partners) have one of these diseases. We don't think people are that dumb, however, and believe that it's important for them to know about any possible forms of protection. Even if these protective measures were only 25 percent effective, they'd make a big dent in the current epidemic.

At any rate we'll say it again: There are ways of protecting yourself and your partners, but these methods don't offer 100 percent protection. If you know for sure that you—or someone else—has the disease, you'd be a fool to rely on one of these protective devices and go ahead and have sex.

One of the best ways to protect yourself is to have your partners use condoms. Condoms, also called rubbers, have been shown to cut down on your chances of getting most STIs.[2] Widespread promotion and use of condoms in Sweden has cut the rate of STIs dramatically.[3] Condoms may not be as effective in preventing viral diseases, like herpes, however, because viruses are smaller than bacteria and can more easily penetrate the rubber. The condoms also don't protect your outer genitals. Still, they do afford some protection against herpes.

Certain foaming spermicides and various creams and jellies used with diaphragms, such as Delfen Foam, Emko Foam, Ortho-Cream, Perceptin Gel, Ortho-Gynol Jelly and Koromex A-II Vaginal Jelly, have been shown in laboratory studies to be effective against some of the organisms that cause STIs.[4] Whether or not they will be as effective in actual use has not yet been determined.*

You should also know that if you use the birth control pill, you are much more susceptible to certain STIs. This is because the Pill alters the acid/alkaline balance, or pH level, of your vagina, making it more conducive to

---

*We do not recommend these jellies and creams for birth control unless they are used with a diaphragm. Using a condom along with one of the foams will offer both better protection against STIs *and* better birth control.

the growth of some of the organisms that cause STIs. For instance, if you have sex with someone who has gonorrhea, you normally have about a 40 percent to 50 percent chance of catching it, but if you're on the Pill, you have nearly a 100 percent chance.[5] (However, you are less likely to have your gonorrhea progress to pelvic inflammatory disease if you're a Pill user; see the section on pelvic inflammatory disease for details.)

Urinating and washing the genitals with soap and water before and after sex will help, for the urine will help flush out germs and soap and water will kill some of them; however, although these sorts of precautions are of value, they are not highly reliable.

Another way of protecting yourself is to inspect your partner's sex organs for signs and symptoms of disease before having sex, which may require a bit of finesse. Look for sores, reddened areas and/or warts on the penis, scrotum (balls), anus and buttocks. If the man is not circumcised, pull back the foreskin, the flap of skin that covers the tip of the penis, and check there. Obviously, if your sex partner has any sores or symptoms, you should not have sex with him or her, and since some people can have the disease without obvious symptoms, you should use a condom and spermicide in heterosexual sex unless you have good reason to believe your partner is not infected.

Now, all this doesn't sound terribly romantic. If you don't feel comfortable saying, ''Hey, I want to check you for VD before we have sex,'' you can be a bit more subtle about it. Incorporate a quick check into your foreplay (men like foreplay too, you know). This is very important for those of us who have sex with a number of partners, especially if the partners are not people we know well whom we could count on to contact us if they were to discover later that they had one of these diseases.

In the case of herpes you'd be wise to ask your partners specifically if they have a history of herpes. You can figure out a way to bring it up in conversation if you don't want to ask point-blank. Many people don't realize that they can pass herpes on to others even though they don't have active symptoms.[6] This disease can be particularly devastating, for there is no cure, and having herpes may increase your chances of developing cervical cancer. Those planning to have children in the future should know that it has been implicated in birth defects, miscarriages and premature labor.[7]

Getting Treatment

It's important to learn the signs and symptoms of these diseases and not to ignore them if they do develop. In some of these diseases the early signs and symptoms may go away but the disease is still in your body. It is important too that you familiarize yourself with the tests available, because some tests are not reliable for women or won't detect the disease until it has been in your body for a certain time. If you are sexually active and have more than one sex partner (or if your sex partner does), you should have regular tests every 3 to 6 months. For lesbians who have sex only with other lesbians (not bisexuals), this precaution may not apply, as lesbians rarely get syphilis or gonorrhea. If you are married or fall into the class that some doctors vaguely define as "nice" people, you may have to insist that your doctor do the test. The doctor may pooh-pooh the idea, saying something like, "Oh, you couldn't possibly . . . ," but you should insist on the test or seek treatment elsewhere. If you have oral or anal sex, you may specifically have to ask your doctor to take cultures from these areas.

If you think you have an STI or have had sexual contact with someone who has, you should get medical help right away. Do not take any medications or douche before being tested, as this could lead to false negative test results. "Waiting to see" if you develop symptoms is dangerous. Eighty percent of women who get gonorrhea and 90 percent who get syphilis have no early symptoms. The diseases are readily cured in their early stages, but waiting could lead to serious complications.

Getting treatment for STIs is not always easy. First, a disease—any disease—is not a pleasant thing. If we feel uncomfortable with our sexuality and with talking about sexuality, asking for tests and treatment for STIs may not be easy. To make matters worse, many doctors have a moralistic or judgmental attitude about sexuality and about STIs. Finding a doctor or clinic that can provide, at a price you can afford, good medical care, accurate information and nonjudgmental support isn't always easy, but it can be done.

One place to try is a community "free clinic." These may be listed in the telephone book, or the information operator may be able to help you find the number. Local hotlines, help hotlines, rape hotlines, gay counseling centers, crisis intervention hotlines and so forth may be able to refer you to a free clinic or to a VD hotline, which in turn can refer you for testing and treatment. There is a national VD hotline that can answer questions and help you find treatment. You don't have to give your name to get information, and the numbers are toll-free. In California call 800-982-5883; in the rest of the country call 800-227-8922. The lines are open from 8:30 A.M. to 10:30 P.M., Pacific time, 7 days a week. Most state or county public health departments have a VD control or infectious disease section. They may be able to provide answers to the questions you have. They can usually refer you to a clinic, where you can at least get adequate testing and treatment at little or no cost. In some areas Planned Parenthood clinics, which provide birth control counseling, also provide testing and/or treatment for STIs or can refer you if they do not. They usually have sensitive, supportive, nonjudgmental staffs. If you prefer to be tested and treated by a private doctor, see Finding a Doctor in Chapter Six.

Minors

In most states minors can be treated confidentially. In California, for instance, the law says that doctors can treat anyone over age 12 for VD without a parent's consent. Puerto Rico and Wisconsin don't yet have such laws, but it is hoped that they will in the future. The specific age used to define a minor may vary from state to state, and the laws simply say the doctor doesn't have to notify the parents, not that they *can't* notify the parents. So if you are a minor and don't want your parents to know, you can do one of two things. First, once you have a list of community free clinics or county health departments clinics, call and ask what their policy is regarding minors. Second, remember that you don't have to give your parents' address or telephone number in order to get treatment.

Reporting

The law requires that a doctor treating you for syphilis or gonorrhea report your name to the state health department. This is done so that a special public health investigator can contact you and ask for your help in contacting the people you may have gotten the disease from or who may have given it to you. You are not required by law to provide any names. However, reporting the disease is important. Consider, for instance, a group of 10 people, each of whom has gonorrhea. If they each give it to one other person, that's a total of 20 people, and if each of the 10 newly infected people in turn pass it on to one other person, that's a total of 30 people, then 40, then 50 and so on. If that first group of 10 people were all reported and their 10 contacts tracked down, the next 10, 20, 30, 40 people wouldn't have gotten the disease.

Despite the law, not all doctors report the names of the people they treat for gonorrhea and syphilis. The failure of physicians to report these diseases has contributed to our inability to control VD. If you are being treated by a doctor who does not report your name, s/he is, in a sense, responsible for your having the disease, for if physicians were conscientious about this, others who have the disease would thus also get treatment and we wouldn't have an epidemic. You might want to point this out to your doctor.

The reporting of the diseases to the state health department may cause special problems for some people. If you have had sexual contact with a person who is a minor living with parents or with someone who is married or living with another sexual partner, this can be a bit sticky. You might then want to assume the burden of informing your sex partner yourself, in the most discreet way possible. You can't count on the public health investigator's discretion, which varies considerably from state to state and even from case to case. In the very best of circumstances, investigators will try to visit the person. They are usually quite discreet about this. The information you give them will help them to be discreet, and they aren't beyond telling white lies. In the case of a minor, for instance, the contact might be made through the school nurse, or a female investigator might call the home, saying that the school nurse, or a female investigator might call the home, saying that the school nurse needs to do "a routine eye test" or "bring the immunization records" up to date. Not all investigators are so discreet, and in the wake of cut-back state budgets there simply aren't funds available for this sort of fancy footwork. As a result, in some cases a postcard (which, of course, anyone can read) telling the person to contact the public health service may be sent to the home of your sexual contact. You have a right to know what kind of notification will be made and to meet the person making the contact before you provide names. But remember that we are dealing with diseases that can, for you, for your contacts or for someone else down the line, have serious, even fatal, complications.

Herpes is not a disease that must be reported, although there are efforts being made to change this. It is especially important that anyone with herpes inform everyone he or she sleeps with, for there is no cure for herpes. Once you have it, you always have it, and some authorities consider it the most serious of all venereal diseases.

In the following pages the most common STIs—gonorrhea, herpes, chlamydial infections, crabs, syphilis and venereal warts—are discussed, along with the less common chancroid, granuloma inguinale, and lymphogranuloma venereum. A special section, Other Sexually Transmissible Infections, includes information on diseases that may be transmitted sexually but are commonly transmitted in other ways, and on a group of little-understood diseases that are suspected of being sexually transmissible. Other diseases that can be transmitted sexually, such as trich, yeast infections, hemophilus and nonspecific vaginitis, are discussed in detail under the section on the vagina. In addition, there is a growing body of evidence suggesting that invasive cervical cancer and the early forms of cervical cancer, such as carcinoma in situ and dysplasia, may also be caused by a sexually transmissible agent. This topic is discussed in more detail under the heading Cervical Cancer.

GONORRHEA

AKA: dose, clap

Gonorrhea is an extremely widespread disease that, if untreated, may have serious consequences. Information on how to prevent this disease and where to seek treatment—which may be of particular interest to minors—is discussed in the general introduction to this section.

Incidence

Gonorrhea has the dubious distinction of having the highest incidence rate of any venereal disease in the United States.[8] It is epidemic and, if not treated correctly, can be a serious disease.

Cause and Transmission

The disease is caused by a very delicate, very discriminating germ, the *Neisseria gonorrhoeae,* or gonococcus, which can live only in the mucous membranes of the human body where there is both warmth and moisture—places such as the inside of the cheek, the throat, the genital organs, the rectum, the urethra and, occasionally, the eye. Air, sunlight, soap, water and a variation of only 3° in temperature supposedly destroy the gonococcus. Thus it is virtually impossible to get it other than through vaginal, oral-genital or anal sex with an infected person, the only exceptions being babies, who may get it from their mothers, and young girls, who may receive it from the hands of an adult and then unknowingly transfer it to their vulvar tissues. Gonorrheal eye infections can also be spread as a result of hands touching an infected area and then rubbing the eyes.

Gonorrhea is usually transmitted by sexual contact, when the mucous membranes of two people are in contact. A man need not ejaculate in order to infect a partner. Not every contact with an infected sex partner results in the other person's contracting the disease. Women, who are more likely to get it, have about a 50 percent chance of contracting it from one infected contact, unless they use birth control pills, in which case they have nearly a 100 percent likelihood of getting it.* Men run about a 20 percent to 40 percent chance.

Symptoms and Complications

Part of the problem with gonorrhea is that somewhere between 70 percent and 80 percent of the women who have the disease are asymptomatic. Some women don't have any noticeable symptoms or signs until weeks or even months after first contracting the disease. Men generally have obvious enough symptoms so that the majority seek treatment within 1 to 2 weeks.

*Although Pill users may be more susceptible, their gonorrhea is less likely to develop into pelvic inflammatory disease.

Only about 10 percent of males with gonorrhea are thought to be asymptomatic.

In women the disease most commonly affects the cervix, the urinary opening, Skene's duct, Bartholin's gland and the anus. The gonococci enter through minute cracks in the skin in these areas. Because the openings to the vagina, urinary tract, ducts and rectum are so close together, menstrual blood, vaginal discharges, sanitary napkins and/or careless wiping may spread the infection to one or more of these openings. Anal or oral-genital sex may spread the infection to the rectum or throat.

In women the first signs, if there are any, appear within 3 to 11 (usually 3 to 5) days after infection. The chief early symptoms, which may be so slight as to be unnoticeable, are pain or burning on urination, urinary frequency and an increase in vaginal discharge.

On speculum exam the cervix may appear red and swollen. The vagina is not usually the seat of gonorrheal infection, although in young children, pregnant women and older women the vagina itself is sometimes infected. The tissues of the normal adult vagina seem to provide protection against the penetrating power of the gonococci. In the young, the old and in pregnant women, however, this normal tissue either has not yet developed or has changed with age or with shifting hormone levels and does not afford the same protection. If the vaginal canal does appear to be red and swollen, this most often is because the cervix is infected and the vagina is subsequently irritated. In those cases where the vagina itself is actually infected, there may be a good deal of pain, and pus may cover literally every crevice of the vaginal walls.

The vulva, which is subject to discharges from all these openings, may become red and swollen. The lips may become so swollen that they fuse together and voiding may become painful. Occasionally, the vulva is so irritated that genital warts caused by a symbiotic virus appear. If the rectum is involved, there may be painful and bloody stools and a mucous discharge from the anus. If the Skene's and Bartholin's glands are infected, it may be possible to milk pus from the opening of the glands and they may become quite swollen (see Skeneitis and Bartholinitis).

Although any of the symptoms described here may appear in women in the early stages of the disease, most of the time they are not present or are so slight that they go unnoticed.

Unlike women, most men have obvious early symptoms that are usually recognized and treated early, so that the more serious complications and the chronic form of the disease do not affect them as often.

If the gonorrhea is not recognized and treated in its early stages, it can spread upward, beyond the cervix, and infect the uterus and tubes. This is known as pelvic inflammatory disease (PID).

The gonoccocci may even spill out through the tubes into the pelvic cavity.

Symptoms like pain on one or both sides of the lower abdomen, vomiting, fever and irregularities in the menstrual period may occur. The time interval from the initial contact until the appearance of symptoms of pelvic infection is quite variable and unpredictable. It may take months or years. Most of the time the upward spread of the gonococci takes place during the first menstrual period after infection, because the cervix opens up at this time and because the menstrual debris is a rich environment on which gonococci feed and thrive. When the disease does spread above the cervix, serious complications may result. If the fallopian tubes are infected, they may become permanently blocked. In some cases a hysterectomy may be necessary, and the disease may even be fatal. Even if the disease can be treated with drugs, the damage done may be permanent, and infertility and chronic pelvic pain are not uncommon. The symptoms and complications of gonorrhea that has spread beyond the cervix are discussed in more detail under the heading Pelvic Inflammatory Disease.

In addition to PID, gonorrhea may have other serious complications. The organisms may get into the bloodstream, and septicemia, or blood poisoning, may develop. The gonococci circulating in the blood can attack any organ in the body. Gonorrheal arthritis can occur if the circulating gonococci settle in the joints—the wrists, knees, knuckles and so on—causing them to fill with pus. The surrounding tissue becomes inflamed and swollen. The elastic cartilage tissue of the joints may be destroyed, causing the adjacent bones to atrophy. The joints may stiffen permanently. Symptoms vary; sometimes there is excruciating pain and marked swelling of the joints, and at other times there are intermittent attacks that recur over time. Carditis, an inflammation of the lining of the heart, and meningitis, an inflammation that causes destruction of the membrane covering the brain and spinal cord, may also be associated with gonorrhea. With the use of modern antibiotics, these complications are rare; however, they do exist and may be fatal.

Nonsexual Transmission

Adults with germs on their hands can pass gonorrhea on to female children, which is one of the few instances of the nonsexual spread of the disease. The immature tissue of the child's vulva makes the child more susceptible to what is called gonorrheal vulvitis, or vulvovaginitis. Fortunately, this infection is usually confined to the vulva and lower two-thirds of the vagina and does not progress beyond the cervix. There may be a vaginal discharge, but quite extensive infection may be present with little discharge or pain.

A pregnant woman who contracts gonorrhea is usually protected from the spread of the disease through her fallopian tubes and out into the pelvic cavity by the fact that the tubes normally close up shortly after pregnancy. Although there is short-term protection for the mother, this is not so for the child. The gonorrhea doesn't affect the baby until delivery, when its eyes come in contact with the infected membranes of the mother. The gonococci eat away at the delicate lining of the eyes. Before antibiotics this was a major cause of blindness, but now the law requires that all newborns be treated with silver nitrate drops or penicillin. Gonorrheal eye infections also occur in older children and adults as a result of rubbing the eyes after touching an infected area. When this disease does occur the damage ranges from a slight scarring of the cornea to such serious infection of one or both eyeballs that surgical removal is required.

Diagnosis

There are two methods of diagnosing gonorrhea: the smear and the culture. The smear involves using a swab to obtain discharges from various areas that are then wiped on a glass slide, stained with a special dye and examined under a microscope for the presence of the coffee-bean–shaped gonococci. The culture involves obtaining discharges with a swab and placing them in a special container with a culture medium that stimulates the growth of the gonococci. Because the gonococci are so easily destroyed by air and heat, it was not until the mid-1960s that a suitable culture medium was developed that would keep the gonococci alive and yet would not be conducive to the growth of other organisms that might mask the gonococci. Now that such a medium is available, the gonococci can be put in culture dishes, mailed to a laboratory, incubated for 16 to 24 hours and then examined to determine whether or not gonococci are present.

The smear is 99 percent accurate in diagnosing symptomatic men but is practically worthless in both asymptomatic men and in all women unless pus can be squeezed from the woman's urinary opening or gland ducts or is dripping from the cervix. The culture is 88 percent to 93 percent accurate in these women if a swab is taken from the cervix alone. If swabs are taken from both the cervix and the anus, the culture is 92 percent to 94 percent accurate. Most doctors do not take a swab from the anus if they are doing just a routine culture, for extra cultures cost more money. However, people who practice anal intercourse should have a swab taken from the anus even in a routine smear. They will probably have to ask for it specifically, because many doctors are too embarrassed to ask their patients if they practice anal intercourse. Similarly, people who practice oral-genital sex should have throat cultures taken. People who have symptoms or who have reason to think they've been exposed should *always* have both cervical and anal discharges cultured.

There are a number of reasons why the culture test is not 100 percent accurate: The woman may have douched before the doctor's visit (don't!) or may have tried to treat herself by taking a few antibiotic pills (again, don't!). The organisms may have already spread above the cervix, leaving only a few organisms at the original infection site. The disease may have retreated deep into the glands of the cervix or vulva. The discharge on the swab may have contained only dead gonococci, so that there were none that could grow in the culture. The culture might not have been processed correctly.

Given that undiagnosed gonorrhea can cause such serious problems, that the tests are unreliable and that women, especially those on the Pill, are highly susceptible, any woman who knows or even suspects that she has been exposed should not be satisfied until she has had negative test findings from *two consecutive sets of cultures* taken during her menstrual flow.

Treatment[9]

The best time to treat gonorrhea is early, before it spreads. One of the most common treatments is penicillin given by injection into the buttocks, usually in a single treatment. About an hour before the penicillin injection, a drug called probenecid (Benemid) is given orally to inhibit excretion (so that the penicillin is not eliminated from the body) and increase sensitivity to penicillin.

If a person is allergic to probenecid or penicillin, another antibiotic, tetracycline, is given orally four times a day for 7 days, or doxycycline is given twice a day for 7 days. Some doctors now prefer this treatment even for patients who are not allergic to penicillin, because, unlike penicillin therapy, it is also effective against chlamydial infections. As many as 45 percent of people with gonorrhea also have chlamydial infections, so this makes good sense. But unless you can be religious about taking the medication for the required week, this is not the form of treatment for you. If you do not take all the medication correctly for the required time, the infection can return and will be even stronger and harder to eradicate. This form of treatment, however, is ineffective against anal/rectal gonorrheal infections in men.

Another form of treatment that can be used by pregnant women and others who cannot use tetracycline is probenecid and ampicillin or amoxicillin, either orally or by injection. Like penicillin, this treatment can be given in a single dose, so you do not have to remember to take pills for an entire week. But it is not effective against *Chlamydia* and does not work against anal/rectal or mouth/throat gonorrheal infections.

Some doctors are combining the single-dose treatment of penicillin or ampicillin with the tetracycline treatment. This single dose ensures that the gonorrhea will be adequately treated, even if the person does not take all the tetracycline. By prescribing tetracycline also, such doctors hope to eradicate any coexisting chlamydia. However, the Centers for Disease Control is still

567

studying the effectiveness and side effects (if any) of such combined treatment and has not yet included it in their officially approved treatment guidelines.

Spectinomycin hydrochloride (Trobicin) has been developed for use against strains of gonococci that may have become resistant to tetracycline and penicillin. It seems to have little in the way of side effects, but it is more expensive, is not effective against *Chlamydia* and for some unexplained reason, is not effective against gonorrhea in the throat. It can be used by people who are allergic to both penicillin and tetracycline, however, and is also prescribed when other forms of treatment have failed.

If a person has a throat infection that has failed to respond to treatment because it is a penicillin-resistant strain, a single oral dose of nine tablets of trimethoprim/sulfamethoxazole is used.

The treatment of gonorrhea has come a long way from the old days, when a single shot of penicillin did the trick for everyone. The form of treatment you receive will depend on where in your body the infection is located, any drug sensitivities you may have, the possibility of a coexisting chlamydial infection, whether or not you can be religious about taking medication and whether or not you have a drug-resistant strain of gonorrhea. You should read the section on chlamydial infections, discuss these issues with your doctor and make sure you understand why s/he is recommending a particular form of treatment. Not all doctors stay up-to-date on the latest developments; indeed, some still prescribe oral penicillin, such as penicillin G benzathine, for gonorrhea. Such penicillins are not effective against gonorrhea; you want penicillin G procaine.

If you are worried that your doctor is not prescribing the correct medication, you can call the VD hotline (*see* p. 560) or your state or county health department and ask about the most current treatment recommendations.

Treatment of gonorrhea may change in the future, for although the drugs that are now available can cure the disease, it is taking increasing amounts of them to be effective against some of the particularly virulent strains.

Follow-up is essential, since cures are not always effective. The dosage may not have been high enough to combat a resistant strain, or the person's particular body chemistry may have affected the absorption and retention of the medicine. If single-dose oral therapy is given, the cure rate is lower. An incorrect choice of antibiotic and the problems that arise when the gonococci are present in more than one location both contribute to treatment failures. Because 1 out of every 10 people will require further treatment, it is essential to return 1 week after medication to have another culture taken. Then, in 1 more week, another culture should be taken.

There is no immunity to gonorrhea. A person could be treated and get reinfected immediately. *No one should have intercourse until they have had two consecutive negative cultures.* Even if you have no symptoms and your partner is also undergoing treatment, you face a real risk of reinfection if you have intercourse before you both have had two negative cultures.

HERPES

AKA: herpes simplex virus disease, herpes simplex, herpes virus hominis, herpes genitalis, herpes vaginitis

Types: herpes simplex type I, or HSV-1
herpes simplex type II, or HSV-2

Associated Terms: herpes zoster, herpes labialis, cold sores, fever blisters

Herpes is a viral infection that causes painful sores and that can have serious complications if proper precautions are not taken.

It is often said that there is no cure for herpes. This is true in the sense that once a person has been infected with the herpes simplex virus, the virus remains in the body forever. As yet, we do not have a medication that will eradicate the virus from the body, as certain antibiotics, for example, will eradicate the organism that causes gonorrhea. But saying that there is no cure does not mean that a person will have herpes sores forever. The sores are what doctors call "self-limiting," meaning that the sores will go away by themselves, without medication, usually within a few weeks. For many herpes sufferers the virus simply causes one initial attack of sores and, although it stays in the body, it becomes dormant, so the person cannot pass the virus on to someone else and is not troubled by recurrences of the sores. Other herpes sufferers are not as fortunate; for these people the virus is reactivated from time to time, causing a recurrence of the sores. Once the sores appear (and sometimes for a period before their appearance and after their disappearance) the person is infectious and can pass the virus to someone else (*see* Cause and Transmission below for details).

Herpes has been the source of a great deal of confusion and misunderstanding, and people who are suffering from the disease may have trouble getting accurate information. Part of the problem is the terminology. When doctors speak of herpes disease they may be referring to any one of a number of diseases caused by a special family of herpes known as herpesviruses. Chicken pox, shingles (also known as herpes zoster) and mononucleosis, for example, are all caused by herpesviruses.

When laypeople refer to herpes they are usually talking about herpes genitalis, a herpesvirus infection that affects the sexual organs and the genital area. Herpes genitalis should not be confused with herpes labialis, a herpesvirus infection that is more commonly known as a cold sore or fever blister. People confuse the two because both are caused by a herpesvirus known as herpes simplex virus (HSV). There are two types of HSV: herpes simplex type I (HSV-1), which is the causative agent in most cases of herpes

569

labialis, and herpes simplex type II (HSV-2), which is the causative agent for most cases of herpes genitalis. In the past, virtually all cases of herpes labialis were caused by HSV-1 and virtually all cases of herpes genitalis were caused by HSV-2. Recently, however, researchers have begun to find that about 10 percent of herpes genitalis cases are caused by HSV-1 and a similar percentage of herpes labialis cases are caused by HSV-2. Doctors theorize that more people are having oral-genital sex and that this explains why we are seeing some HSV-1 infections on the genitals and some HSV-2 infections on the lips. In the following pages, unless otherwise noted, we are referring to herpes infection affecting the sex organs and genital area.

Incidence

Despite the fact that herpes is a widespread disease with serious implications for its sufferers' health and sexuality, it is not a disease that must be reported, so there are no accurate figures as to how prevalent it is. Based on samplings from clinics, some researchers have estimated that there are 500,000 new cases of herpes in the United States each year and that about 20 million people have the disease.[10]

Symptoms

The symptoms of herpes are generally the same for both initial, or primary, attacks and recurrent attacks, but recurrent herpes is usually less severe and of a shorter duration than a primary attack.

The primary attack of herpes normally occurs within 2 to 20 days after the person has come in contact with the virus. Occasionally, a person will suffer what seems to be a primary attack even though they are sure they have not come in contact with an infected person in the past 20 days. There are several possible explanations for this: (1) Some people may be carriers of the disease, that is, they can transmit the disease but have never had an attack themselves (this is probably uncommon). (2) In some people the disease apparently takes longer than 20 days to manifest itself (again, this is unusual but possible). (3) In a small number of people the initial attack is so mild that it goes unnoticed. A recurrent attack could, then, be mistaken for a primary attack.

For many people the first sign of a herpes attack is tingling, a pins-and-needles sensation, burning or itching in the area where the sores will appear. This first sign, called the prodrome, usually lasts for hours but may last for a day or two. The prodrome is more apt to be noticed by recurrent sufferers, perhaps because they learn to recognize the feeling. But not all herpes sufferers are able to notice a prodrome.

570

For other people the first sign is the appearance of small red marks, usually less than ¼ inch in diameter, that may be single or multiple and look like a measles rash. For still others the first sign is a headache, mild fever, a general sick-all-over, achy feeling and/or a swelling of the lymph glands in the groin. For yet others the first sign is the actual sores themselves.

The red marks that are sometimes the initial symptom usually develop within a few hours into blisterlike, fluid-filled sores that may have red edges and gray centers. There may be a single sore or area of sores, or there may be multiple sores or areas. The sores are likely to be painful and/or itchy. They are generally more painful in women than in men and more bothersome during primary attacks than during recurrent attacks. The surrounding area may be painful, swollen, red and inflamed. If the sores are on the outer lips of the vulva, the lips may swell to as much as two times their normal size. The sores may appear anywhere on the genital area in both men and women and up inside the vagina in women. The anus, thighs and buttocks may also be affected. Women may have a vaginal discharge and men may have a watery discharge from the penis. There may be considerable difficulty or pain with urination.

Within 2 to 3 days the blisterlike sores usually break open and leak, or "weep," a fluid or pus. Scabs may form over these open sores. Once the scab forms, the swelling, pain, inflammation, headache and flu-like symptoms have usually begun to subside. With primary herpes, most people begin to feel better by the end of the 2nd week, but in some cases the sores persist for 3 to 6 weeks.

Sexual intercourse is painful and should not be attempted, because it may spread the disease (*see* Cause and Transmission below). In about 35 percent of herpes cases there is another venereal disease present at the same time, so symptoms of these diseases may appear as well.[11]

Although many people have only a primary attack and are never troubled with recurrences, more than 50 percent will have a recurrence within 6 months.[12] Some people have recurrences within a few days of the primary attack; others will go months or even years before they have recurrences. Some women experience monthly recurrences, often around the time of their menstrual periods.

Generally, these recurrent attacks are progressively less severe and heal more quickly. But for a small number of people the body never seems to develop much of an immunity, and their recurrences continue to be frequent and severe. Most people, however, notice that these attacks occur with less frequency after 6 to 10 recurrences. There is no way to predict when recurrences will happen, and no one knows what causes them. Stress seems to be a factor. The hormonal changes of pregnancy and menstruation seem to trigger attacks for some women. Some people report that sexual stimulation will trigger an attack.

571

Cause and Transmission

The viruses that cause colds and flu can be spread through airborne droplets, and other viruses can be spread through insects or animals, but most authorities believe that herpes simplex virus can be spread only through direct skin-to-skin contact with an infected person (by kissing, by intimate sexual contact—including oral/genital activity or sexual intercourse—and by fingers, which spread the virus from the mouth to the genital organs). Some people think that, theoretically, it is possible to become infected with herpes by using a washcloth that a person with active sores has just used or by sitting on a toilet seat just after a person with "weeping" sores. But the herpes simplex virus decomposes shortly after leaving the body, so these methods of transmission, although possible, are highly unlikely. The majority of herpes cases are transmitted by direct contact.

One of the big questions about herpes revolves around transmission. A person can transmit herpes whenever he or she is doing what scientists call "shedding active viruses." When a person is *not* shedding active virus, the virus retreats along nerve pathways into the body, where it assumes its dormant stage. During this dormant stage the disease cannot be transmitted, and the person has no active sores or other symptoms.

A person may shed active viruses at three separate times. First, when a person has actual sores he or she is shedding active viruses and can easily transmit the infection to anyone who comes in contact with the sore or the surrounding area. Second, when a person is about to have an attack, that is, during the prodrome (which many people learn to recognize), they can also shed active viruses and may therefore be infectious. Richard Hamilton, author of *The Herpes Book,* makes this misleading statement on page 9 of his book: "And, of course, when the sores aren't present, the disease can't be transmitted at all." This is not necessarily true, and Dr. Hamilton admits as much on page 89 of the same book, when he says, "Why should we care about the prodrome? Simply because that early, tingling, itchy feeling is not only the first warning sign of an impending recurrence of the virus but may also be an infectious state itself." Every authority we have consulted agrees that the disease may be transmitted during the prodrome, even before active sores are present.

The third time when a person may be shedding active viruses is after the healing of the sores. In one study a woman was still shedding active viruses 132 days after her last sore had healed.[13] However, it is thought that most people will have stopped shedding active viruses within 10 days after a primary attack and within 4 days after a recurrent attack.[14]

There is another way in which the disease can be transmitted even though the person does not seem to have an actual sore. Occasionally, a woman will have a sore only up inside her vagina or on her cervix, where there are few nerve endings, so that she is unaware of the sore's presence.

For information on how to reduce the chances of transmitting herpes, see Living with Herpes below.

Diagnosis

The appearance of the sores and the medical history usually provide enough information to make the diagnosis. Because other venereal diseases often occur at the same time, tests should be done for these diseases. In questionable cases or in cases involving pregnant women, where it is important to confirm the diagnosis, laboratory tests can be done.

A Pap smear is 90 percent accurate in diagnosing herpes if sores are present. Viral cultures can be grown that are also highly accurate, if they are done when the sores first appear, for that is when the concentration of virus is highest. A blood test known as an antibody titer can be used to rule out herpes. In most people the body will produce antibodies in an attempt to fight the herpes. But the antibodies may not show up in the test until several months after the first infection.

Complications

In the past decade there has been growing evidence linking herpes infection to cervical cancer.[15] Women with histories of herpes infection are eight times more likely to develop cervical cancer than women who have not had herpes. Herpes-type viral material has been found in malignant cervical tumors. The evidence suggesting that herpes is a causative factor (or one factor in a string of causes that eventually leads to cervical cancer in some women) is not conclusive, but any woman with a history of herpes should have Pap smears at least once and possibly twice a year. The association between herpes and cervical cancer is discussed in more detail under the heading Cervical Cancer.

The other serious complications that herpes may cause involve pregnancy and childbirth. Women with herpes have a rate of miscarriages that may be three times higher than normal.[16] Herpes infection increases the risk of premature delivery. Herpes simplex virus can also cause severe disease in infected infants. It is not common for babies to be infected, but when it does occur it is apt to be serious. The closer to term, the more dangerous the infection is for the infant, for the fetus has not yet had time to develop its own protective antibodies. The risk of infection is greater if the infant is exposed to an active infection in the mother's birth canal during delivery. In such a case the baby has a 40 percent to 50 percent chance of being infected.[17] The mortality from herpes in infected babies may be as high as 50 percent.[18] Even if the infection is not fatal, there may be birth defects, including blindness and diseases of the central nervous system. Because of the risk of infection during normal delivery, many doctors and women believe that cesarean delivery, that is, cutting open the abdomen to deliver rather than allowing the baby to move through the birth canal, should be done. Others think that this may not be necessary in some cases.[19] Some doctors will isolate the newborn and keep the baby in the hospital for a week or two after delivery to avoid transmission of the disease and in case the baby might be sick. Other doctors have found that transmission can be controlled by careful handwashing and other precautions. A pregnant woman with a history of herpes should try to find a doctor who is experienced in herpes deliveries; this may not be easy. Another alternative is for the woman or her doctor to contact a large university teaching hopsital, where up-to-date information may be available.

Stanford University Medical Center in Palo Alto, California, Division of Pediatric Infectious Diseases, has a Perinatal Herpes Simplex Program, headed by Dr. Anne S. Yeager, where new procedures for testing HSV are being investigated. By assessing risk to the infant late in pregnancy on the basis of antibody levels, indications of virus shedding and the timing of active lesions, they have been able to avoid cesarean deliveries in certain cases. They have also developed a protocol (treatment procedure) that minimizes the risk of infection during birth and avoids separating the mother and infant. Another way to get up-to-date information about herpes and pregnancy is through a program known as HELP (for more information, see Treatment below).

Treatment

There is at present no cure for herpes, because it is caused by a virus and we have very little in the way of antiviral medications. Nor are there any proven measures for preventing recurrences. However, there are ways to relieve the symptoms, and there are some things that may possibly speed up the healing process.

The problem in finding a cure for herpes is that after the sores heal, the inactive virus retreats into the nerve cells, where it may remain dormant or flare up again periodically. It is thought that this retreat to the nerve cells prevents the body's immune system from dealing effectively with the virus. Although some drugs can work against the active virus in the sores, these drugs work on the viruses only when they are reproducing, or replicating, themselves and thus are powerless against the dormant virus.

A number of treatments have been suggested for herpes in the past few years, among them smallpox vaccine, metronidazole, flu vaccine and a process called photodynamic activation, which involves painting the open sores with a special dye. The virus absorbs the dye and is then inactivated by exposure to a light source; however, this treatment is no longer used, for it has not proved effective and may cause cancerous changes in normal cells.[20] Many times the initial reports of these sorts of cures have been quite good; however, subsequent, more careful studies have always yielded disappointing results. A number of proposed cures are now in the experimental stage at various centers across the country, but until one or more are proven effective and become available in the marketplace, treatment must generally consist of alleviating the symptoms and speeding up the healing process.

Acyclovir, a drug sold under the brand name Zovirax, has been used in the treatment of primary herpes.[21] The cream, which must be applied with rubber gloves, comes in a 15-g tube that sells for about $20. The drug limits viral shedding time, reduces healing time if treatment is begun within 6 days of onset of symptoms and, in some people, decreases pain. It does not cure herpes or help prevent recurrences. It is *not* effective in limiting viral shedding or reducing healing time in recurrent attacks and should be used only for primary attacks.

Some doctors and other health-care workers we spoke with were not impressed by Zovirax's performance and thought the drug was overpriced. But apparently it is helpful for many people, at least during the primary attack.

You can also take other measures to promote healing of the sores and to make yourself more comfortable during attack. When you are having an attack be sure that the clothing you wear is clean, loose and absorbent. This means no tight pants or pantyhose. Cotton underwear is best. When possible, avoid clothing altogether and expose the sores to air. Washing the affected area with mild soap and running water two or three times daily and patting it dry with tissue afterward may also help. Some people find that drying the area with a hairdryer set on the *cool* setting several times a day is useful. Sitz baths (sitting in a tub of warm water and Epsom salts for 10 to 15 minutes) once or twice a day may ease discomfort and promote healing. (Any washcloths and towels that are used should be clean and should not be used by you again without laundering or by others if they have come in contact with the affected area.)

If you have pain on urination, try pouring water over the infected area while urinating or even voiding in a tub of water. Drink six to eight glasses of water a day to dilute the urine and reduce burning. Avoid coffee, tea, alcohol and carbonated beverages.

It is generally best to avoid creams and lotions. To ease the pain of urination, some people coat the sores with K-Y jelly first. But it must be washed off afterward, because any ointment on the sores may prolong healing. In fact, do not put anything other than medication prescribed by the doctor on the sores (this includes, for example, lipstick, makeup or Blistex on oral sores, that is, cold sores or fever blisters).

Aspirin may be taken to relieve the pain and flu-like symptoms. If necessary, pain relievers may be prescribed. If ulcers have formed and a secondary infection ensues, the doctor may prescribe antibiotics to fight the secondary infection, although antibiotics have no effect on the herpes virus.

Although the reason for its effectiveness is not clear, some reports have advocated the use of aspirin—one or two tablets every 4 hours, 5 days before the menstrual period—to prevent recurrences. Proper nutrition and avoidance of stress and direct sunlight are also thought to be factors in preventing recurrences. Taking a zinc pill three to four times a day is helpful for some people.

Living with Herpes

People with herpes need to be concerned about two problems: spreading the infection to others and spreading the infection to other parts of their own bodies, a process known as autoinoculation.

Autoinoculation can occur anytime you are shedding active viruses, that is, during the time you have sores and for a period before the sores appear and after the sores are healed. Frequent handwashing is important at these times, especially after touching the affected areas and before touching your eyes, mouth and genital areas, which are all more vulnerable to herpes than other parts of the body. Sight-threatening complications can result from herpes infections in the eyes. In fact, try not to touch the affected areas at all. If you tend to touch or scratch the sores in your sleep, wear loose cotton pajamas and wash your hands as soon as you wake up.

Contact lens wearers must wash their hands before removing or inserting their lenses. If you have oral herpes, never use saliva to wet your lenses, regardless of whether or not you have an active sore. If, despite your best efforts, eye symptoms develop (feels like sand in your eye, looks like "pinkeye"), do not panic, but see your doctor at once. Fortunately, herpes in the eye can be treated, but the sooner, the better.

Most people are worried about spreading the infection to others. Although there is no 100 percent guarantee of prevention, the following practices are just about the best anyone can do to reduce the risk to minimal. Avoid allowing others to come in direct contact with the affected areas when prodromal symptoms (tingling, a pins-and-needles sensation, itching, burning) or sores are present. When oral or facial sores are present this means *no kissing or oral sex.* When genital sores are present this means *no sex,* including any activity that would involve direct contact of another with the infected area.

These precautions apply for a time after the sore is healed. (Healing is deined as intact pink skin, although some redness may remain. Crusts or scabs

576

are not considered healed.) As noted above, viral shedding has been known to continue for as long as 132 days after the last active sore; however, most people will stop shedding viruses 10 days after healing of a primary attack and 4 days after healing of a recurrent attack. A person who has a primary attack should have a second culture taken 10 days after the sores heal. If the culture is negative, sexual activity may be resumed. After recurrent attacks a person could also have cultures taken before resuming sex, but for those who are troubled with frequent recurrences this may not be practical. Wait *at least* 4 days after *complete healing* in the case of recurrent attacks before resuming sex.

Using condoms and vaginal spermicides may help cut down on your chances of spreading the infection when you may be shedding active sores without realizing it. But *do not rely* on condoms or spermicides for protection during the prodromal, when you have active sores or for the time after healing (see above).

Newborns have no immunity to herpes and can become seriously ill if infected. If you are shedding active viruses, avoid contact with newborns, just as you would if you had a cold or the flu. If this is impossible, take *special care to wash hands well and avoid the affected areas*.

The measures described above will minimize your chances of spreading herpes to another person, but they do not absolutely, 100 percent guarantee that you will not pass the infection on to another person. For this reason many think it is only fair that you inform all potential sex partners that you have herpes. This is not always easy to do. The following tips, adapted from a list developed by herpes sufferers, may make it easier to handle the situation:[22]

☐ Never use the word "incurable" when explaining herpes to another person. The body does cure the sores, even without medication. Herpes is only incurable in the sense that it cannot be eradicated from the body. The term "incurable" conjures up a fatal, incapacitating disease in most people's minds. A better way to explain herpes might be to say it is an intermittent, self-limiting condition that comes and goes more or less on its own.

☐ Never preface your remarks to another person with something like "Better sit down, I've got something heavy to tell." Your attitude makes a big difference.

☐ Never tell an untruth about herpes. Stick to the facts as you know them. You risk your credibility and compromise your ability to be a helpful source of information to another person if you allow even one "white lie" to slip in.

☐ Assume that the person you are telling knows nothing about the infection. You will be right more often than you are wrong. Besides, what the person already "knows" about herpes is likely to be wrong.

☐ Follow the dictates of your own sense of what is right in deciding when to bring the subject up. If you would have liked to have known about herpes before becoming infected, use this as a guide in making your decision. The overwhelming opinion is that people have the right to know what is going on before they get into it.

☐ Open the subject up at a convenient time, when you can talk without interruptions.

☐ Use unprejudiced and neutral terminology in explaining what herpes is. You might start by asking the person if they know what a cold sore is. This is much better than launching into a complicated explanation of DNA, RNA and the various types of herpesviruses that are around.

☐ Don't forget to emphasize how preventable herpes is, particularly when people are well informed, motivated and sincere about not wanting to spread the infection. If you are going to mention infectiousness, you must also mention preventability. Ditto for the cervical cancer risks, the problems with babies and autoinoculation.

☐ Don't feel you have to be a walking encyclopedia about the disease. You can get more knowledgeable friends or a doctor to help you explain the disease to someone. Or, HELP, the organization described below, can help you answer any questions you or the person you are informing may have.

☐ Don't be surprised to learn that the person you are anxious about telling also has herpes and has been worrying about telling you. As many as a quarter of the people you meet may have herpes.

☐ Herpes is only one small part of who and what you are (that is, you are not a virus). As a whole person, it is reasonable to expect that people will relate to you, accept you and sometimes reject you on the basis of the blend of elements and attributes that makes you unique. Rarely will you be evaluated in terms of anything as one-dimensional as herpes, particularly if you don't see yourself in that way. If someone that you tell attempts to focus on this one element to the exclusion of all else, set him or her straight or walk away. It is his or her problem, not yours.

It is hoped that in the not-too-distant future there will be a cure for herpes. One way to keep abreast of the latest developments in herpes research is through an organization called HELP, which puts out an informative newsletter for its members every 12 weeks. Subscriptions cost $8 a year. (Pregnant women should get their special report, ''Herpes and Pregnancy,'' Vol. 1, No. 2.) For information, write to HELP, Box 100, Palo Alto, California 94302. PLEASE, PLEASE send a stamped, self-addressed No. 10 (business-size) envelope along with your request.

CHLAMYDIAL INFECTIONS

AKA: chlamydia, *Chlamydia trachomatis, C. trachomatis*

Associated Terms: nongonoccocal urethritis, NGU

Chlamydial infections are caused by *Chlamydia,* an unusual group of bacteria that have many of the characteristics of viruses. Until recently, chlamydial infections received much more attention in men than in women. In men, chlamydiae are responsible for perhaps as many as 60 percent of cases of nongonococcal urethritis (NGU), an infection of the urethra, the tube in men that runs down the inside of the penis and through which urine is eliminated.[23] NGU, like gonorrheal urethritis, is common in men.

The sexual partners of men with NGU sometimes have symptoms of cervical or urethral infection, but most of the time they are asymptomatic (without symptoms). Even women who have chlamydiae in cultures grown from their cervical secretions may be without symptoms. Because the organisms often do not cause symptoms in women, many doctors (present company included) did not treat women unless they had symptoms. Now, however, it is recognized that chlamydiae may play a role in pelvic inflammatory disease (*see* pp. 393–401) and may cause problems in pregnancy and in infants born to women with the infection. Moreover, untreated women may pass the disease along to another sexual partner. Therefore, chlamydial infections in women are now receiving more attention.

One type of chlamydia is responsible for an eye infection in adults that is a major cause of blindness in underdeveloped parts of the world but is rare in the United States. Another type of chlamydia causes lymphogranuloma venereum (*see* pp. 594–95). Here, we are concerned mainly with the type of chlamydia that causes genital infections in men and women.

Incidence

Chlamydial infections are rapidly becoming epidemic, and in many clinics they are seen more frequently than is herpes or gonorrhea. These infections are not reportable diseases (*see* pp. 561–62), but it is estimated that there are 3 million new cases each year.[24]

Transmission

In adults the organism is sexually transmitted, in much the same way that gonococci are transmitted (*see* p. 563). The organism may be transmitted to

579

the infant of an infected woman during delivery, as the infant passes through the birth canal.

Symptoms

Women with chlamydial infections are often asymptomatic. Some women, however, do develop symptoms. If the urethra is involved, there may be pain, difficulty or burning on urination. If the cervix is affected, there may be pain, especially on intercourse, and a discharge. In some women the cervix becomes extremely swollen and characerically has a beefy red appearance. There may be bleeding from the cervix.

In men, chlamydial NGU may cause pain, a discharge and difficulty, pain or burning on urination. One or all of these symptoms may be present. A small percentage of men are asymptomatic.

The symptoms of chlamydial infections generally appear within 7 to 14 days after the person comes in contact with the organism. But there have been cases in which symptoms appeared in as few as 4 days,[25] and some authorities believe that the organism can be present for years before symptoms appear.[26] The symptoms may disappear, even without treatment, but the person remains infected and is still capable of passing the organism along to others.

In infants, chlamydiae can cause an eye infection known as conjunctivitis, as well as pneumonia.[27] The eye infection is characterized by swelling of the eyelids, redness of the eyes and a discharge. It generally starts about 5 days after birth, and if treated promptly and correctly, does not affect the infant's vision. Chlamydia-induced pneumonia in infants is characterized by a repetitive, staccato cough and loss of appetite. There may be an accompanying fever, but often there is none. The pneumonia generally develops within the first 6 months after birth, usually within a month or two.

Complications

In women, chlamydiae can cause pelvic inflammatory disease (PID), a disease that can have serious complications, including infertility and death. In the past there was some question as to whether or not chlamydiae alone could cause PID. However, recent studies in which only chlamydiae could be found in women with PID have indicated that the organisms can indeed cause PID.[28]

One preliminary study has indicated that women who have chlamydial infections during pregnancy are at greater risk of having a premature birth, a stillborn infant or a infant who dies shortly after birth.[29] At the present time this study has not been confirmed by other studies, so the connection between chlamydiae and these problems is considered tentative. Other studies are now being conducted. If the results of this preliminary study are confirmed, this finding could become a key issue. Other studies have shown that between 4 percent and 13 percent of pregnant women have chlamydiae in their cervices.[30] We also know that as many as 70 percent of infants born to women with chlamydial infections will likewise be infected.[31] Some doctors are therefore recommending that all pregnant women have a chlamydial culture (see below) done shortly before they are about to deliver. And if their cultures are positive, these doctors recommend that the women be treated so the infants will not be infected. If further studies confirm that there is a connection between premature delivery, stillbirth or infant death and chlamydiae, many doctors may also recommend doing cultures in early pregnancy so that infected women can be treated promptly and, it is hoped, avoid such problems.

There is also some evidence that chlamydial may cause infertility in some women. Any woman whose chlamydial infection develops into PID may become infertile (*see* pp. 396). But even women whose chlamydial infections do not progress to PID and those who have mild or asymptomatic cases may have infertility problems.[32] Treating the infection will usually alleviate the infertility.

Men may also develop complications. Proctitis, an inflammation that involves the anus and rectum and that may make it difficult to have bowel movements, may occur. Epididymitis, an inflammation of the tubes that store sperm in the testes, may also be a problem.

Diagnosis

Unfortunately, we do not have a quick, inexpensive, readily available way of diagnosing chlamydial infections. Chlamydiae can be grown in a culture taken from the cervix or the urethra, but such cultures are expensive and few laboratories are equipped to do them. As a result, most doctors make what is known as a presumptive diagnosis. For example, a man who has symptoms of urethritis (discharge, pain, difficulty with urination) is tested for gonorrhea. If the test is positive, he is treated for gonorrhea; but if it is negative, he is presumed to have NGU and is treated accordingly (see below). If a woman presents symptoms of cervicitis or urethritis and the simple tests available to test for other organisms are negative, the doctor may make a presumptive diagnosis, especially if the woman's cervix has the characteristic beefy red appearance or if her sexual partner has been diagnosed as having NGU. In fact, if her partner has NGU, there is a 70 percent chance that she will have an infection, even if she does not have symptoms.[33] Rather than going to the expense of having a culture done, which can cost as much as $50 to $80, many doctors will make a presumptive diagnosis on the basis of the fact that her sexual partner has NGU symptoms and will go ahead and treat her. A presumptive diagnosis is also made for men who are asymptomatic but whose sexual partners have given birth to chlamydiae-infected infants as well as for the mothers of such infants.

Treatment

Infants and adults are treated with antibiotics. In adults the usual form of treatment is oral tetracycline taken four times a day for 7 days. If gonorrhea is also present, as is often the case, the tetracycline will also be active against the chlamydiae. But if only gonorrhea is diagnosed and penicillin is used to treat it, the chlamydial infection will persist, for penicillin is not effective against chlamydiae.

Anyone with symptoms in whom gonorrhea has been ruled out should be treated. To cut down on further spread of the disease and the possibility of PID, women whose sexual partners have NGU should be treated, even if they are asymptomatic. Asymptomatic men whose partners have chlamydial infections or whose partners have given birth to infected infants should be treated, as should the mothers of infants born with an infection.

Because pregnant women should not take tetracycline, erythromycin is used instead. Anyone taking medication for a chlamydial infection should be sure to take all the medication prescribed, even if the symptoms have cleared up.

SYPHILIS

AKA: Lues, bad blood

Many people think that syphilis is a thing of the past, but this is not true. Although the disease is readily cured in the early stages, it may not be detected, especially in women, until later, when it may be harder to cure. Information about prevention and how minors can get treatment without their parents being notified is discussed in the introduction to this section.

Incidence

Syphilis, like almost all venereal diseases, is on the rise. In 1977, 66,625 cases were reported, and it is estimated that another 500,000 cases either went undetected or unreported.[34]

Cause and Transmission

The disease is usually transmitted through sexual contact. It is caused by a strain of bacteria called *Treponema pallidum,* which dies rapidly without warmth and moisture, so that it is virtually impossible to get syphilis from toilet seats or infected clothing or towels. However, it is possible to get the disease by kissing someone with an open sore or by touching the infected sore. Anal-genital, oral-genital or genital-genital sexual contact can spread the disease. Although the disease is prevalent in the male homosexual population, lesbians (with no bisexual involvement) rarely get it. It may also be spread during pregnancy or during delivery to an infant by an infected mother. Although it is uncommon, a man who is in the tertiary stage (see below) of the disease can transmit it to a woman, but *only* if his sperm impregnates her ovum. Then the blood of both the mother and her infant become contaminated. This type of infection initially produces only a mild form of the disease, which may, therefore, go untreated for years.

Symptoms

The first symptoms of syphilis may appear anywhere from 10 to 90 days after the initial contact, the average being around 21 days. The disease is divided into stages. The first stage, called early, or primary, syphilis, is usually marked by the appearance of a small, reddish brown spot that may range from the size of a pinprick to the size of a dime and may look like a pimple, sore or blister. This sore, or chancre, as it is called, is located at the exact spot where the germs entered the body and is a by-product of the attempt of the body's white cells to fight the infection. It may grow to about the size of a marble and ulcerate, producing a round or oval sore with hard, raised edges and a depression in the center. The sore is generally painless, does not itch and usually lasts for 6 to 10 weeks, although it may disappear more quickly. It may leave a scar or disappear without a trace. In most cases it eventually goes away by itself, even if not treated. While the sore is present, as well as for some time preceding and following it, the person is contagious and can pass the disease along to others. The sore usually appears on the vulva or penis but can appear inside the vagina or on the cervix, anus, lips, mouth, fingers or breast. There may be an associated swelling of the lymph glands in the area around the groin.

Because the sore is painless, often very small and disappears quickly, it may not be noticed, particularly in women. A woman who practices self-exam on a regular basis has a much better chance of detecting it early, but about 90 percent of women with syphilis don't remember ever having seen the primary symptoms. Men are more apt (40 percent to 60 percent) to notice the primary symptoms. People who do notice primary symptoms should seek treatment immediately, for even though the symptoms go away, the disease is still there. All sexual contacts in the previous 6 weeks should be notified.

The second, or secondary, stage of syphilis may occur anywhere from 1 to 6 months after the initial contact. The symptoms vary from person to person, but generally they begin as slightly raised blotches—a skin rash about the color of raw ham that may change to copper red. The rash may resemble measles, chicken pox, scarlet fever or other infectious diseases. It is generally not painful, nor does it itch. It may appear on dry areas, like the palms or the soles, or may even cover the entire body. In moist areas, especially on black people, it may appear as slightly raised, round or oval sores with flat, gray surfaces that ooze a clear liquid. This liquid is full of germs, and the sores are highly contagious. The lymph glands in the groin, armpit, neck or elsewhere in the body may swell and feel tender. There may be a mild fever, headache, sore throat, hoarseness, loss of appetite, a dull ache in the joints and bones and a general feeling of illness. In some people the rash may cover the head and scalp and cause patches of hair to fall out. The untreated symptoms may last for 3 to 6 months and can even come and go for years. Most people, however, notice the symptoms and seek treatment at this point.

Next, during the latent phase, there is an apparent remission of the disease. The rash is gone and the infected person may look and feel fine. There is no limit as to how long this phase may last. It may even last a lifetime. During the first year or so after the symptoms disappear, a person may still pass the disease along to someone else; but after that time, with the exception of during pregnancy (when the fetus can be infected), they are generally no longer able to infect others.

No one knows what causes the disease to become active and flare up again during the third stage, which is also referred to as tertiary, or late, syphilis. About 25 percent of those with untreated syphilis will go on to the third stage.

When the disease does flare up it can attack with an incredible virulence. It may attack the skin, muscles, eyes, lungs, digestive system, liver, endocrine glands or the walls of the blood vessels. An internal, chancrelike sore called a gumma attacks the organs and eats away at them. The progress of the disease may be halted at this stage, but the damage that is already done is permanent.

The effects of syphilis in this stage can be devastating. Cardiovascular syphilis will affect the heart and blood vessels and may be fatal. Neurosyphilis destroys the fragile sensory nerves, so that the person is unable to sense what his or her legs are doing without looking at them. Walking becomes difficult, and the person may develop a peculiar gait. If untreated, neurosyphilis can cause lightning pain, feelings of pins and needles being stuck into the skin all over the body and severe pains and spasms in the throat. Syphilis can also cause a condition known as general paresis, which involves the cranial nerves and affects the facial muscles. Paresis can cause total personality changes, insanity or death. People with paresis may pass through a series of very pleasant and/or extremely unpleasant hallucinations until they are finally cut off totally from outside sensory impressions and are the sole occupants of a disease-induced fantasy world. Luckily, there are now treatments that can prevent the disease from progressing this far, provided that it is diagnosed and treated early enough.

Syphilis and Pregnancy

It is important to know that a pregnant woman with syphilis, regardless of which stage of the disease she is in, may pass the disease on to her unborn infant (in which case it is called congenital syphilis). Both the primary chancre and the secondary rash are generally mild in pregnant women and may pass by unnoticed. Syphilis in pregnant women may, therefore, go untreated for a longer period. The mother may pass the syphilis through the placenta to the fetus, or the infant may contract the disease if a secondary rash is present on the vagina or vulva during delivery. If the mother is treated before the 4th month, the child usually won't develop any symptoms. The fetus is cured as the mother is cured. However, if untreated, the placenta may be damaged, resulting in miscarriage or stillbirth or in the child's being born with the disease. Because the baby has received the syphilis bacteria directly into the bloodstream, there may be no primary or early secondary stages. The child may be born with latent syphilis that remains latent for anywhere from 2 years until the time of puberty. In some children there are birth defects and symptoms or problems that develop soon after birth, including distorted bones, misformed teeth, inflamed and clouded eyes, deafness, blindness and mental retardation. Every pregnant woman should be tested for syphilis at least twice during her pregnancy, once at the initial visit and again just before delivery.

Diagnosis

All people who develop a sore on the genitals should be tested for syphilis. The diagnosis of syphilis is made in a couple of ways. The doctor can examine scrapings of the chancre, or sore, under a special dark-field microscope that makes the spirochetes show up brightly. If you practice anal or oral-genital sex and have sores in these areas, make sure the doctor tests them as well. Since the *T. pallidum* may be confused with other organisms, it is important that this test be done by a highly skilled person. If such a microscope is available in the doctor's office or clinic, test results may be ready in a few minutes; otherwise, the sample can be sealed and sent to a laboratory for testing. The testing is done free of charge by the Public Health Service. It is important not to put any cream or lotion on the sore before seeing the doctor, as this may kill germs on the surface and upset test results.

All men and women believed to have syphilis are given a blood test, no matter what the results of a dark-field examination. All blood tests for syphilis rely on detecting the antibodies that the person's body has produced in reaction to the invading syphilis germs. The most widely used test is one called the VDRL, but it cannot detect syphilis until it has been in the body long enough to form antibodies, or for about 4 to 6 weeks. Even then, it is only about 76 percent accurate in detecting primary syphilis. It can give both false positive and false negative results. The FTA-ABS is a more accurate test that requires more expensive equipment and is more difficult to perform. It can detect syphilis earlier than the VDRL and is about 86 percent accurate in detecting primary syphilis. If you have been exposed to syphilis less than 4 weeks previously, request that an FTA-ABS be done rather than a VDRL. If you have had intercourse with an infected person, or with someone you suspect may be infected, and yet your test results indicate that you do not have syphilis, you should have the tests repeated in 6 weeks and again in 90 days. There is a third test, the TPI, that is used in special, confusing cases and is expensive and difficult to perform. In latent syphilis this test may be necessary to make sure that the disease is not continuing quietly in the central nervous system. In the TPI a needle is inserted between the bones of the spine and a sample of the spinal fluid that surrounds the spine is withdrawn for testing.

Treatment

The usual treatment for syphilis is penicillin, injected into the buttocks. Two injections, one in each buttock each time, must be given. Patients who are allergic to penicillin are treated with oral tetracycline. For pregnant women and others who cannot use tetracycline, another drug, erythromycin stearate (Erythromycin), is given by mouth for a couple of weeks, but because Erythromycin does not cross the placenta very easily, two new drugs that show promise, cephaloridine and, less often, doxycycline, may be used instead.

The introduction of the antibiotic will kill large numbers of the germs suddenly, and in dying the organisms break open and release their contents into the bloodstream. This release can cause a fever of 101° to 102°F, and if a chancre is present, it may become swollen and enlarged, but the reaction usually lasts only a few hours.

Everyone treated for syphilis needs several follow-up exams to make sure the disease is completely cleared up. If it is a case of primary or secondary syphilis, a follow-up blood test should be done 1 month later and then once every 3 months for 1 year. People with latent or late syphilis must be seen more often.

CRABS

AKA: pubic lice, cooties, pediculosis pubis, *Phthirus pubis*

Pubic lice are tiny, wingless insects that attach themselves to pubic hairs by means of their crablike claws. They insert their sucking-type mouths into the hair follicle and feed on the tiny blood vessels in the area. These perfectly loathsome creatures, which look like props from a grade B monster film, are about the size of a pinhead and are a nondescript white/yellow/gray that makes them difficult to see on light-skinned people. They appear to be a small scab or flake of skin until you look closely and see movement of the legs. They may be a bit easier to see after they have just finished a "meal," when they are gorged with blood and are consequently rather rust colored. Although they prefer pubic hair, they may also exist in any hairy part of the body, including eyelashes, underarms, eyebrows and hairy parts of the chest.

The lice cannot survive for longer than 24 hours unless they are attached to a human body. They have a life span of about 30 days and apparently have no knowledge of birth control—they put rabbits to shame, mating frequently and laying three eggs a day. The eggs, called nits, are oval, white, hard and glistening. The female cements the eggs to the side of a pubic hair, usually near the junction of the hair and skin. The eggs hatch in 7 to 9 days. By the time they are 17 days old the newly hatched lice can reproduce.

Transmission

Pubic lice are usually transmitted during sexual contact; however, a mere hug while nude will suffice. It is even possible to pick up crabs from articles of clothing, bed linen, mattresses, toilet seats—or anything that has been infested with the lice or their eggs.

Symptoms

The telltale symptom is an intolerable itching, often worse in the middle of the night. It is believed that the itching is caused by an allergic reaction to the saliva that the crabs secrete while feeding. Not all people develop this allergic reaction, so it is possible to have crabs without any symptoms. The itching causes scratching, which gives no relief and only intensifies the sensation. In some people the bites cause a mild rash of small, blue dots, which are the result of hemorrhage (bleeding) in the tiny blood vessels just below the surface of the skin.

Diagnosis

No special tests are required to diagnose crabs, for they are large enough to be seen with the naked eye; however, because the initial infestation involves only six to eight of these tiny creatures, they may be difficult to locate at first. Sometimes it is easier to see the glistening tiny eggs (nits) glued to the pubic hairs.

Treatment

Treatment involves killing the lice and their eggs on the body and sterilizing any clothing, bed linen, towels, mattresses, washcloths, toilet seats and such that may harbor the lice or their eggs. Your doctor, who can prescribe a product called Kwell that kills both the lice and their eggs. It comes in a shampoo or a cream lotion. There are also certain over-the-counter preparations that can be purchased in drugstores or pharmacies without a doctor's prescription. They are usually not as effective as Kwell; however, a new product, Rid, which can be purchased without a prescription, compared favorably with Kwell in a recent study.[35] Home remedies, such as kerosene and shaving the pubic hair, are rather extreme and can cause irritation of the genital skin. They also may not be as effective as Kwell.

Kwell lotion is used by applying a thin coating to the hair and skin of the pubic area, thighs, trunk and underarms. It is rubbed into the hair and skin, left in place for 12 hours and followed by a thorough washing. The Kwell shampoo is a bit easier to use. First, apply enough shampoo to wet the hair and skin of the hairy areas of the body. Once thoroughly wetted, add water a bit at a time to work up a good lather. Then, shampoo for 4 minutes. Rinse well and towel-dry briskly. A second treatment is sometimes necessary. Check yourself again in 7 days and repeat treatment if necessary. The dead nits can sometimes be removed with a fine-tooth comb. If they cannot, you may have to resort to the ancient art of nit picking.

Avoid getting Kwell on mucous membranes, the area between the lips of the vulva, the penis and the eyes, as it may irritate them. Kwell should be used with caution on children and by pregnant women, because the active ingredient can penetrate the skin and could potentialy poison the central nervous system. Crabs in the eyelashes may be treated with mercuric oxide ointment, available in pharmacies without a prescription.

Because the crabs can live briefly on clothing, bed linen and mattresses and can also lay their eggs in such places, it will be necessary to treat these things as well. This can be quite a hassle. Dry-cleaning or washing the items in boiling water will kill the lice and their eggs; however, if you can't afford to dry-clean your underwear and haven't got a kettle big enough to boil all the clothing, sheets and towels you've used in the past couple of weeks (not to mention your mattress), you can simply leave everything undisturbed and away from human contact for 2 weeks. The hatched crabs will die within 24 hours. The eggs take a week to 10 days to hatch and without a human host won't survive longer than 24 hours once they've hatched. If you treat yourself and any sexual partners or other contacts who might have crabs, scrub your toilet seat and stay away from everything for 2 weeks, your life will once again be crab-free.

GENITAL WARTS

AKA: condyloma acuminatum; verruca acuminata; verrucous lesions; pointed condyloma; papilloma acuminatum; papilloma venereum; fig, moist, wet, pointed or venereal warts

Despite the string of rather complicated medical terms by which it is known, the condyloma acuminatum is just a wart that grows in the genital area or, occasionally, in or around the mouth. It is sometimes confused with molluscum contagiosum or the condyloma latum which is associated with secondary syphilis.

Transmission

Genital warts are usually transmitted through vaginal, anal or oral sex, but it is possible to pick them up through others types of contact. The warts are more contagious in their early stages than when they have been present for a long time. About 50 percent to 70 percent of people who have intercourse with an infected partner will develop warts.[36]

Incidence

Like all venereal diseases, it is especially prevalent among the sexually active, and the incidence is on the rise. It is more common in women who have other sexually transmissible infections or one of the common vaginal infections, use birth control pills or are pregnant, and in uncircumcised men. In all

589

these instances a damp, moist environment is provided that is ideal for genital warts.

Symptoms

The warts usually appear within 1 to 2 months after the initial contact with an infected person, but as many as 9 months may go by before they appear.[37] They may grow near the vaginal opening or on the labia, the vulva, the vaginal walls, the cervix, the anus or elsewhere in the genital area. On men they usually grow on the tip or shaft of the penis or on the scrotum. If the warts grow on dry skin, like that on the outer vulva or the shaft of the penis, they look similar to the warts that grow on other parts of the body. If they grow on the moist areas, they may appear as small, dark pink bumps about the size of a grain of rice. They may grow singly or there may be several. In the moist areas they tend to grow together, forming clumps that look like small cauliflowers. There may be a foul-smelling discharge and itching. But their growth is stimulated by pregnancy, and in extreme cases they may block the vaginal opening, bleed during delivery or even necessitate a cesarean delivery.

Diagnosis and Treatment

Genital warts can often be diagnosed simply by their appearance, but in women, diagnosis should also include a Pap smear. Genital warts, at least those that affect the cervix, have been associated with the development of cervical cancer.[38] This does not mean that all women with genital warts will develop cervical cancer. But the incidence of cervical cancer *is* higher among women who have had genital warts on their cervices. Moreover, the virus that causes genital warts is a member of the herpes family, and herpes has been strongly associated with an increased risk for cervical cancer (*see* pp. 375–78). Women who develop genital warts should, therefore, have Pap smears done at the time the warts are diagnosed and at least once a year thereafter.[39]

Although the warts occasionally will disappear by themselves, they should be treated promptly, because they often increase rapidly in size and number. Because the warts can be sexually transmitted, sexual partners should be notified and treated if they too develop warts. Theoretically, a condom should cut down on transmission, but this has not yet been proved. Moreover, the warts often exist on areas other than the penis itself or the inside of the vagina. The condom will not, therefore, provide protection against transmission of warts on areas of the outer genitals that may come in contact during intercourse. Thus people affected by warts have to forego intercourse until they are cured.

Treating vaginal warts can be a bit tricky in women who have another vaginal infection that is causing a lot of moisture and discharge. The first step will be to dry up the area by treating any related infections. In some cases it may be necessary for a woman to temporarily stop using the birth control pill in order to get rid of the warts.

The specific treatment will depend on the size, number and location of the warts. Most people can be treated successfully with a solution of a substance called podophyllin. The solution is painted on the warts, left on for 4 hours and then washed off. In a few days the warts fall off; however, the treatment may have to be applied a few times in order to get rid of all the warts. If you don't get all the warts, the whole mess usually recurs.

Generally, the podophyllin is applied by a doctor or nurse, since the solution is irritating to the skin and care must be taken to apply it only to the wart itself. Four hours after treatment the area is washed thoroughly with soap and water. If a burning sensation develops, the area must be washed off right away. If there is pain, aspirin and/or hot sitz baths are suggested. If these measures don't relieve the pain, the doctor can prescribe a cream to soothe the area.

Podophyllin cannot be used by pregnant women, since it has been known to cause miscarriage and premature labor. It cannot be used to treat extensive cases, for if the warts are too large, only the outer layers of tissue will be killed, the wart will not disappear completely and the dying tissue will be particularly susceptible to infection. If the warts persist after more than 4 weeks of treatment, or if podophyllin cannot be used for some reason, the problem is treated in other ways.

In the past, extensive or stubborn warts were treated with chemical or electric burning (cautery); however, it is now possible to destroy them by freezing, a procedure known as cryosurgery, which is more effective and more comfortable for the woman. Laser beam therapy is also being used to treat stubborn cases, but this form of treatment is still experimental and not widely available at the present time. In extreme cases an operation known as a "skinning" vulvectomy, which removes the outer layers of the vulval skin, is sometimes done. But this is a rather extreme solution, and we would encourage anyone facing this sort of operation to investigate the possibility of laser therapy. (Contact the nearest medical school and ask to speak to the Sexually Transmitted Disease or Communicable Disease or Gynecology Department to find out where laser therapy is available in your area.)

Women who have warts on their cervices should not be treated with podophyllin. In fact, such women should not be treated at all until the results of their Pap smears are in, for treatment could obscure the results of the smear. If their Pap smears are abnormal (*see* the section on Pap smears), they should be treated the same way that any woman with an abnormal smear should be treated (*see* the section on cervical dysplasia).

GRANULOMA INGUINALE

AKA: granuloma pudendi, ulcerating granuloma of the pudenda

Granuloma inguinale is usually lumped in with venereal diseases because the disease is thought to be transmitted sexually; however, this has not been conclusively proven. Perhaps the only nice thing about this disease is that you are not likely to get it unless you live in a tropical climate. Only a few hundred cases are reported in the United States each year, mostly in the southern states.[40]

Symptoms

The symptoms may be quite delayed, appearing anywhere from 4 days to 12 weeks after infection. The first symptoms are small bumps or blisters, which may appear in the area of the vulva, anus or, occasionally, on the cervix. In the man they may be found on the tip of the penis, under the foreskin and in the area of the anus as well. The blisters rapidly turn into red, raw, oozing sores and may bleed or exude pus. Secondary infection is common, with painful, tender sores or bumps that emit a pungent odor. The spreading sores may affect the urinary and rectal openings, making elimination difficult. Contraction of the vaginal opening and tenderness in the area limit sexual activity. Indeed, even sitting or walking may be uncomfortable.

Diagnosis and Treatment

The diagnosis is made on the basis of the symptoms and microscopic examination that reveals the presence of the organism *Donovania granulomatis,* which causes the disease.

Treatment usually consists of tetracycline taken by mouth every 6 hours for 2 to 3 weeks. For pregnant women and others who cannot take tetracycline, another antibiotic, ampicillin, is given orally over a period of 3 to 12 weeks. Patients should be followed up every 3 to 4 months after they start treatment.

CHANCROID

AKA: soft chancre, ulcus molle

On a worldwide basis, chancroid is more common than syphilis; however, it is usually found only in tropical climates. Less than 1,000 cases are reported in the United States each year, and most of these occur in the southeastern states.[41]

Causes and Symptoms

The disease is caused by a tiny rod-shaped bacterium, the *Hemophilus ducreyi,* which usually enters the body through some preexisting cut, scrape or crack in the skin of the genital organs. In the United States the disease is usually transmitted through vaginal, anal or oral-genital sex. In other parts of the world, where it is more widespread, it is probably transmitted through other forms of contact as well.

It is possible to have the disease without having any symptoms. When symptoms do appear it is usually within 1 to 5 days after intercourse with the infected person; however, it can be as long as 10 days. The first symptom is the appearance of one or more small, raised bumps with a narrow red border that may be located on the vulva, vagina, cervix, anal opening or urethra. In men they may appear on the shaft of the penis, the foreskin or the anal opening. They may look like small pimples or blisters that soon rupture to form small, red, saucer-shaped sores. The sores may produce a great deal of foul-smelling pus. They are usually soft and painful or tender and may bleed easily when touched. They may spread to adjacent areas, like the groin, thighs, abdomen and stomach.

The lymph glands in the groin may also swell, and if untreated, the enlarged glands will gather into a large, red, painful swelling called a bubo. The bubo usually ruptures and pus may drain out, in which case a person is highly susceptible to secondary infection. There may be such acute pain that the person has difficulty even in walking.

Diagnosis and Treatment

The disease is difficult to diagnose. It is easily confused with syphilis and lymphogranuloma venereum. No one test is completely accurate, so the doctor will have to do several.

Different doctors will choose different methods of treating the disease, for there is no clear indication of which treatment is most effective. Most of the time, sulfa drugs or tetracycline are used.

Since there is no immunity to chancroid, reinfections are common. It is important to be examined every 2 to 3 months for 1 year after treatment.

LYMPHOGRANULOMA VENEREUM

AKA: LGV, lymphopathia, lymphopathia venereum

LGV is widespread throughout the world, especially in tropical areas, but until recently was fairly rare in the United States. There are only a few thousand cases reported each year; however, the incidence is increasing, possibly because servicemen brought the disease back from Southeast Asia.[42]

Cause and Transmission

The organism that causes LGV displays characteristics of both a virus and a bacterium and is not yet fully understood. The disease is usually spread by vaginal, anal or oral-genital sex, although in tropical climates it is probably spread by other forms of contact as well. It is not as contagious as syphilis or gonorrhea and is more common in men.

Symptoms

Symptoms may appear anywhere from 1 to 12 weeks after the infected contact but usually appear within 7 to 12 days. A small, painless sore or blister appears on the sex organs. In women it may appear on the cervix, vulva or interior walls of the vagina. In men it usually appears on the tip of the penis or in the urethra. Since the sore is painless, may be hidden from view and disappears rapidly, it often goes unnoticed. Within a few days the infection spreads to the lymph glands. If the sore appears on the external genitals, the lymph glands in the groin may become swollen and inflamed. If the initial sore is in the vagina, or in the rectum as the result of anal intercourse, the deeper pelvic lymph nodes may be affected.

The tender, enlarged glands may fuse together to form a hard, painful swelling called a bubo. The skin over the bubo may be bluish red. The lymph nodes may be destroyed. The buboes may break through the skin and drain pus. This bubo formation usually occurs anywhere from 10 to 30 days after the appearance of the first sore. If it involves the deep pelvic lymph nodes, it may go unnoticed. In both men and women there may be fever, chills, pain, an aching in the joints and loss of appetite.

The untreated disease can cause a number of complications that may appear in the first several months or as late as 20 years afterward. The swollen lymph vessels in the penis or vagina may block the normal flow of lymph. The fluids back up and cause an enormous swelling called genital elephantiasis. This occurs more often in women and can cause unbearable pain. It may require plastic surgery to restore the vulva to its normal size.

Complications involving the anus occur more frequently in women and homosexual men. Pain and bloody discharge are common symptoms. If the disease isn't treated, scar tissue may form, partially blocking the rectum and causing painful bowel movements. This may require surgery to correct.

Diagnosis and Treatment

The diagnosis of the disease cannot be based on symptoms alone, for they are easily confused with other STIs and other nonvenereal diseases as well. In the presence of swollen lymph glands, the doctor may want to test for all these possibilities. There are also special skin and blood tests for LGV.

LGV responds slowly to treatment. The treatment of first choice is tetracycline, given orally for a few weeks. Sulfa drugs may also be used.

LGV is a difficult disease to get out of the system and needs to be checked frequently. An LGV blood test should be taken every 3 months for the first year and then once a year for at least 2 years.

OTHER SEXUALLY TRANSMISSIBLE INFECTIONS

Types: mycoplasmas
        cytomegalovirus, or CMV
        hepatitis B
        scabies
        molluscum contagiosum

In addition to the common and not so common sexually transmitted diseases described in the preceding pages, there are a number of other diseases that may be associated with sexual intercourse. First there are the common vaginal infections, such as trich, hemophilus, nonspecific vaginitis and yeast infections, although the latter are more frequently caused by nonsexual means. There is also a growing body of evidence that dysplasia, carcinoma in situ and invasive cancer of the cervix may be caused by some sexually transmitted agent. In addition, there are certain diseases that are suspected of being transmitted sexually or are known to be sexually transmitted although they are more frequently passed in other ways. These diseases are discussed below.

Mycoplasmas

Mycoplasmas are unique organisms that, like chlamydiae, are now considered bacteria, although they also have characteristics of viruses. It is known that they can be passed through sexual intercourse, but their role in genital infections is unclear. Although they can be cultured from sex organs, it is not known whether they actually cause diseases.

Cytomegalovirus

Cytomegalovirus (CMV) belongs to the same group of viruses as the herpes simplex virus and, like herpes, may infect infants. In fact, CMV is one of the most common causes of such birth defects as mental retardation, blindness and deafness. There is increasing evidence that the disease may be sexually transmitted among adults; however, it causes few, if any, symptoms in adults. It is thought that the mother may in turn pass it on to the infant. At present there is no treatment. Further research is needed to determine how the disease is transmitted and to develop ways to treat and prevent these infections.

Hepatitis B

Hepatitis B, or serum hepatitis, is a form of viral hepatitis, an infection of the liver. It was once thought that this disease could be transmitted only through contaminated blood transfusions or through injections using a contaminated needle. It is now recognized that the disease can be transmitted in other ways, including sexual contact. Symptoms include fever, loss of appetite, weakness, nausea, hives and a yellowing of the skin. There is no specific medical treatment available. Although most cases clear up by themselves, some do not, and the disease may have serious, even fatal, complications. There is no way to prevent the disease except to avoid exposure to people known to have it.

Scabies

Scabies, which are caused by small parasitic mites (bugs), cannot technically be called a sexually transmissible infection, for the bugs are often passed through nonsexual contact. Scabies often occur in children and tend to affect warm, moist areas of skin around the wrists, between the fingers and on the elbows. However, scabies have recently become common on the external genitals. The symptoms include severe itching and the appearance of small, red bumps or lines caused by the female mite burrowing under the skin to lay her eggs. Diagnosis involves extracting the mite from the burrows and examining it microscopically. Treatment is the same as that used for crabs.

Molluscum Contagiosum

Molluscum contagiosum is a condition in which small, smooth, white, raised growths with depressed centers appear on the male or female genital organs. There may be as few as one or as many as 20 of these growths. They may fuse together to form larger growths. In the past the disease occurred mainly in children on other areas of the body, but recently it has been found with increasing frequency on the genital organs in adults, which has led many doctors to believe that it is sexually transmitted. However, the evidence is far from conclusive, for the sexual partners of people with molluscum contagiosum are frequently not affected. The disease is often confused with vulvar folliculitis, and definite diagnosis can be made only by microscopic examination. For some reason the disease seems to disappear spontaneously, but in extreme cases this may take as long as 2 to 4 years. It is generally not worthwhile to treat the growths unless they become infected, in which case treatment consists of removing them and painting the area with a special solution to prevent scarring.

Problems Related to the Menstrual Cycle

The conditions discussed in this section are not really diseases; rather they are symptoms of some underlying problem whose cause may or may not be understood. For instance, the first heading in this section, Premenstrual Syndrome, describes the changes that many women experience in the days preceding the menstrual flow. Although there are some theories to explain these changes, no one knows for sure what causes them. The same is true for menstrual cramps. In the case of the third condition in this section, amenorrhea, a term that refers to an absence of menstrual periods, it is sometimes possible to pinpoint a cause, but not always. Similarly, abnormal uterine bleeding, which includes any variation from the usual menstrual pattern as well as any other abnormal bleeding from the vagina, can sometimes, but not always, be traced to a specific cause.

The last three conditions in this section—precocious puberty, menopausal problems, and premature menopause—are related to the larger cycles of a woman's life stages rather than to the monthly cycle of menstruation. Here again, these conditions are symptoms rather than diseases, and the cause of these symptoms cannot always be identified.

Women seeking medical treatment for the conditions described in this section may not be taken seriously by their doctors. In part the doctor's response will depend on which of these conditions a woman has. If a girl is experiencing precocious puberty, her problem is not likely to be dismissed by her doctor. Likewise, a woman who has a premature menopause will probably receive serious consideration from her doctor, for there is usually a history of surgical or radiation damage to the ovaries to explain her condition. Even

598

when there isn't, there are tests the doctor can do to confirm the fact that her ovaries really have stopped functioning. Abnormal uterine bleeding is also likely to be viewed by doctors as a "real" problem, since there is an observable symptom—blood loss—and since medical science can often pinpoint the cause of the abnormal bleeding. Moreover, even if the doctors can't explain why a woman is bleeding, they can always "cure" her problem by removing her uterus.

If you have amenorrhea, you can also expect to have your condition considered in an objective, rational manner—at least initially. Again, you have an observable symptom—lack of menstrual flow—and the doctor has lots of tests s/he can perform to find out why. If, however, the doctor's tests fail to explain your condition, you, along with those women seeking treatment for premenstrual syndrome, menstrual cramps and menopausal problems, are apt to find yourself up against the old it's-all-in-your-head-dearie diagnosis or the I-can't-figure-out-what's-wrong-with-you-so-you-must-be-crazy syndrome.

Consider, for example, what the most recent edition of one of the most widely used gynecological textbooks in the United States has to say about the diagnosis of puzzling cases of amenorrhea.[1] After pointing out that even the most exhaustive tests administered by the most conscientious doctors will sometimes fail to pinpoint a cause for amenorrhea, the authors conclude, "It is undoubtedly incorrect to classify all such cases as of psychogenic origin, but such a practice is not uncommon and, until additional evidence is available, no more satisfactory solution can be suggested."

"Psychogenic" means "of emotional or mental origin"—in other words, it's all in your head. The authors of that widely read textbook, who apparently think that it's perfectly all right to diagnose a woman as neurotic just because they have failed to find out what's wrong with her, are obviously suffering from the I-can't-figure-out-what's-wrong-with-you-so-you-must-be-crazy syndrome. These women aren't even given the benefit of the traditional judicial principle, innocent till proven guilty; instead, they are to be judged as crazy (or to put it in politer medical terminology, as having problems of psychogenic origin) until "additional evidence" proves otherwise. The doctors who authored the text can't suggest a "more satisfactory solution" to their inability to diagnose the cause of a woman's amenorrhea, but we can. How about a simple, honest "I don't know"?

If this sort of thing happened only after doctors had performed exhaustive tests and given women the benefit of what medical science had to offer, it wouldn't be such a problem. Women could perhaps learn to recognize this as one of the peculiar foibles to which doctors are prone and take such a diagnosis with an appropriate grain of salt. But all too often these attitudes prevent doctors from giving their women patients proper medical care.

Menstrual cramps, which have traditionally received the psychogenic "diagnosis" are an excellent example of how this works. One woman we know had cramps and vomited each time she had her period. Her gynecologist (who had no psychiatric training) decided she was neurotic and referred her to a psychiatrist. After extensive and expensive therapy, in which her male therapist helped her explore "her rejection of her femininity" as symbolized by her menstrual problems, she finally consulted another gynecologist. This doctor did not assume her problems were psychogenic and performed a thorough diagnostic workup, including a laparoscopic exam. It was then discovered that this woman had a condition known as endometriosis that was affecting her bowels. We don't know whether she ever got around to accepting whatever it was she'd been rejecting, but once the endometriosis was treated she did stop vomiting and having pain each month. This is just one example of the ways in which doctors' prejudices and assumptions can negatively affect the health care a woman receives.

Women who suffer from cramps and other unpleasant symptoms before the onset of menstruation may have trouble in finding relief. The idea that these symptoms, which cannot be observed, measured or otherwise verified by the doctor, are imaginary, made up or psychosomatic has been so firmly ingrained in doctors' thinking that the medical profession has paid little attention to them. However, some recent research, including some fascinating studies about the levels of little-understood substances called prostaglandins, which are found in higher concentrations among women who suffer menstrual pain, is leading toward a tangible, physiological explanation for menstrual cramps. Perhaps now that doctors are beginning to understand the reasons for menstrual cramps, they will admit that they do exist and are not imaginary problems made up by hysterical women.

Women seeking treatment for these sorts of medical problems should insist on a complete and thorough investigation of their symptoms. The appropriate diagnostic steps are outlined in the following pages. (Reviewing the discussion of the menstrual cycle in Chapter Four, making notes on the terminology and referring to these notes may be helpful as you read through the information in this section.)

If, after a thorough diagnostic workup, your doctor cannot identify the source of your problem, don't allow yourself to be made to feel that you have psychological problems. In all likelihood the problem is that medical science hasn't advanced far enough yet to understand your condition.

PREMENSTRUAL SYNDROME

AKA: PMS, premenstrual tension or congestive dysmenorrhea

Premenstrual syndrome (PMS) is a physical condition that is characterized by a wide variety of symptoms that regularly recur during the same phase of the menstrual cycle, usually in the 7 to 10 days before the menstrual period starts.

The symptoms may be physical and/or emotional and may include tension, irritability, forgetfulness, depression, mood swings, muscle pains, cramps, cravings for certain foods or for alcohol, headaches and bowel or urinary symptoms, just to mention a few. They may be mild, moderate or severe.

Because a small number of women who suffer from severe PMS may experience dramatic psychological symptoms, such as crying jags, panic attacks, suicidal depressions and bouts of violent or abusive behavior, the popular press has dubbed PMS "the Jekyll-and-Hyde" syndrome.

Public attention was focused on PMS largely because of two celebrated criminal cases in England in which the women—one accused of murder and the other of attempted murder—had their sentences reduced because they were suffering from this condition.[2] PMS has subsequently become a hotly debated issue in feminist circles. On the one hand, some celebrate the fact that PMS has finally "come out of the closet." Although the syndrome has been described in the medical literature since the early thirties, many doctors have been reluctant to treat it or even to recognize its existence. As a result, women suffering from PMS symptoms have generally been given the it's-all-in-your-head-dearie diagnosis. Because the symptoms usually occur *before* rather than *during* the menstrual cycle, women themselves often fail to make the connection between the symptoms and their menstrual cycles. Women suffering from severe emotional PMS symptoms have been hospitalized—or even institutionalized—for emotional symptoms instead of receiving the treatment they need. Thus the growing recognition of the syndrome has been applauded by many feminists.

On the other hand, many women, feminist or not, are leery of the attention PMS has been receiving. They fear that PMS, which may affect as many as 40 percent of the women in the United States, will be used as proof that women are emotionally unstable creatures, subject to "raging homicidal imbalances" and therefore unfit to hold positions of leadership and responsibility. They are concerned that allowing women to plead some special kind of insanity because of physical reactions to their menstrual cycles will have a dangerous effect on the legal rights of women in general. As attorney Elizabeth Heltsman points out, "In custody cases, for instance, the husband could charge that his wife is too unreliable to take care of a child for several days out of the month because of her raging hormones. It could also be used as an excuse to discriminate against women in employment and promotions. After all, if those raging hormones make them too dangerous to control their emotions, do we really want to trust them with important decisions or, for that matter, with complicated machinery?"[3]

A number of people are unwilling to even recognize PMS for fear of the implications it may have for women's rights. On the surface, PMS does seem to confirm the old notion that women, or at least a large percentage of them, are periodically unstable, subject to physical and emotional menstrual symptoms that, to some degree, interfere with their normal functioning. But we think that there is a middle ground between those who would deny that PMS exists and those who see PMS as an affliction that somehow makes a large percentage of women, by virtue of the fact that they menstruate, less emotionally and physically able than men are. We believe that PMS is a real condition that causes problems for some women. Most women experience some of the PMS symptoms listed below sometime in their lives, and these symptoms are probably related to the monthly ebb and flow of hormones in a woman's body. But it seems a bit much to say that because women notice bodily changes in relation to their menstrual cycles they are unreliable or unfit emotionally for certain jobs. For one thing, many women undergo a sort of reverse PMS; they experience extra energy, drive or especially "high" or "fit" feelings before their menstrual cycles. Moreover, most of those who *do* have negative symptoms don't think that these symptoms affect their work.[4] Rather than deny the existence of PMS (and thereby deprive women of needed treatment) or see it as "proof" that women are unstable creatures subject to raging hormonal imbalances, we view PMS as a problem that affects many women to a mild degree and a small number to such a severe degree that steps need to be taken to alleviate the problem.

Incidence

Almost every woman experiences at least one PMS symptom at some time in her life. Estimates of incidence vary according to how the syndrome is defined. The commonly quoted incidence rate indicates that about 40 percent of women suffer some mild PMS symptoms on a fairly regular basis. About 5 percent to 10 percent of these women experience regular symptoms to a degree that leads them to seek medical assistance.

PMS is uncommon among adolescents, more common in women who are in their 20s and more apt to be serious in women who are in their mid-30s. Some adolescents have developed PMS, however, and the syndrome has even been found in postmenopausal women. PMS often affects women who have undergone major hormonal changes, such as those connected with childbirth, miscarriage, abortion, stopping birth control pills, tubal ligation or amenorrhea.

Symptoms

More than 150 symptoms have been associated with PMS, the following being some of the most common:

- ☐ Tension, anxiety, mood swings, crying jags, irritability, aggressive or violent behavior, lethargy, fatigue, depression, forgetfulness or mental confusion, panic attacks, insomnia
- ☐ Accident proneness, clumsiness
- ☐ Acne (cyclic), growth of facial hair, susceptibility to herpes outbreaks and cold sores, itching, rashes, bruising
- ☐ Headaches, migraines, backaches, cramps, joint or muscle pain
- ☐ Water retention (which may cause weight gain), breast swelling and tenderness, abdominal bloating and discomfort, swelling of joints, ankles, hands, feet, arms, legs or eyelids
- ☐ Sensitivity to light, mistiness of vision, burning pain or inflammation in the eyes, styes, flashes of light
- ☐ Constipation, diarrhea, urinary disorders, hemorrhoids
- ☐ Asthma, sinus disorders, sore throats
- ☐ Cravings for alcohol, sweets, carbohydrates or salty foods; increased general appetite; decreased appetite; digestive disorders

Some women have only one symptom, but most experience several. For most PMS sufferers the symptoms recur monthly during the 7 to 10 days preceding the onset of the menstrual flow; however, symptoms may occur at the time of ovulation or during another phase of the cycle. Some women have only one symptom-free week in each cycle. The pattern that seems to characterize PMS is a regularly recurring set of symptoms, followed by a symptom-free period.

PMS may be broken down into four different classes, depending on which symptoms predominate.[5] The following classification system is widely used:

PMT-A: Nervous tension, anxiety, irritability, mood swings

PMT-C: Increased appetite, craving for sweets (primarily chocolate; rarely for starch), headache, dizziness, heart pounding

PMT-H: Weight gain, swelling of the extremities, abdominal swelling and tenderness, breast congestion and tenderness

PMT-D: Depression, forgetfulness, crying easily, confusion, insomnia

A woman may have more than one type of PMS.

Cause

No one knows what causes PMS. The syndrome has been variously attributed to overproduction of estrogen, under- and overproduction of progesterone, a disturbance in the estrogen/progesterone balance, water retention, salt retention, a disturbance in the master gland that regulates hormone production, an insulin imbalance, a liver malfunction, stress and inadequate nutrition.

Cause is an important issue in PMS, for theories of causation have implications for treatment. For example, one prominent researcher, Guy Abrahams, believes that at least one type of PMS, PMT-C, is a stress-related condition.[6] This type is characterized by headache, dizziness, heart pounding, increased appetite and a craving for chocolate. The brain normally requires about 20 percent of total body energy, but under stress the percentage increases. The brain gets this energy from conversion of a substance called glucose. The body supplies the brain with glucose by the liver breakdown of the glycogen that is consumed. But in order to effectively break down glycogen into glucose the liver needs sufficient amounts of magnesium. According to Dr. Abrahams, women with PMT-C have a magnesium deficency that becomes apparent when they are under stress, hence the craving for magnesium-rich chocolate. But eating chocolate increases insulin levels, which can intensify other PMS symptoms. (Alas, eating Hershey Kisses is not a cure for PMS!) Dr. Abrahams claims that increased intake of magnesium-rich foods and supplements of vitamin B$_6$, which increases the body's ability to metabolize magnesium, is effective in treating PMS.

Another prominent researcher, Kathryn Dalton, believes that PMS is caused by an imbalance in the amount of progesterone and estrogen produced by the body.[7] (Neither this nor any other theory has been substantiated by controlled scientific experiments.) Therefore, Dr. Dalton prescribes the hormone progesterone (not progestin—see below) to treat PMS.

Diagnosis

Many of the PMS clinics that have sprung up in the United States (see below) "diagnose" PMS with a pelvic exam and an elaborate series of blood tests that may cost from $200 to $500.[8] Although a general physical and pelvic exam should be done to rule out other possible causes of the symptoms, elaborate laboratory tests are of questionable value. (Many clinics prescribe treatment before the test results are back from the lab.) Every expert we consulted agreed that the only way to diagnose the condition is to have the woman keep a careful record of her symptoms for at least 2 months.

If you think you may have PMS, and if your symptoms are severe enough that you are considering medical treatment, you can save some time and the cost of expensive office or clinic visits by arriving at the doctor's with your symptoms already recorded for at least 2 months. You can use a chart like the one shown in Table 24 to record your symptoms.

Begin the chart on Day 1 of your menstrual cycle, that is, on the 1st day you begin to bleed. Write the date your period starts under the column marked 1, on the date line. For example, if your period started on January 5, you would write 1/5 in the column numbered 1, on the horizontal line labeled "Date." Weigh yourself on that day and mark your weight on the chart. If you suspect that weight gain is one of your symptoms, weigh yourself carefully at the same time each day and note your weight on the chart in the spaces provided.

Mark the chart each day until your next period begins. Each evening read down the list of symptoms on the left-hand side of the chart. If you haven't experienced a symptom on that particular day, put a 0 in the box for that day. If the symptom was present but was mild and didn't interfere with your activities, put a 1 in the box. If the symptom was moderate, interfered in some way with your activities but wasn't disabling, put a 2 in the box for that day. If the symptom was severe and disabling, put a 3 in the box. For example, if on Day 23 of your cycle you experienced a mild headache, a mild craving for sweets and such severe dizziness that you had to lay down for awhile, you would put a 1 on the line marked "Headache" under column 23, a 1 on the line marked "Craving for sweets" under column 23 and a 3 on the dizziness or faintness line under column 23. If those were the only symptoms you experienced on that day, the rest of the boxes in column 23 would get a 0.

If you experience any other symptoms described in the section on symptoms but not listed on the chart, or if you experience any physical or emotional changes that you suspect may be related to PMS, record them in the space labeled "Other" at the bottom of the chart. Write the date and a short note about the symptom. For example, suppose you had a sore throat on Day 24 of your cycle; you would make a note in the space provided under "Other" that might say something like, "Day 24, awoke with a slight sore throat that persisted until early evening."

Mark your chart every day throughout your menstrual cycle. When you have your next period, consider the 1st day of bleeding as Day 1 of your next cycle, and start a new chart (photocopy the one provided here). By arriving at the doctor's office or the clinic with at least 2 months of charts, you'll have a head start on treatment.

Treatment

The treatment of PMS is *extremely* controversial. There are basically two schools of thought: (1) the progesterone approach and (2) the nutritional/life-style changes approach. We favor the second approach.

The first treatment approach, pioneered by Dr. Dalton, involves the use of progesterone, which is given by injection, by means of vaginal or rectal suppositories or in powder form, placed under the tongue. Although progester-

Table 24
PMS SYMPTOMS CHART

Name

Amount of Menstrual Bleeding (circle one): 0–none; 1–slight; 2–moderate; 3–heavy; 4–heavy with clots

Grading of Symptoms: 0–none; 1–mild (symptom present but does not interfere with activities); 2–moderate (symptom present and interferes with activities but not disabling); 3–symptom severe and/or disabling

DAY OF CYCLE	1	2	3	4	5	6	7	8	9	10	11	12	13	14	15	16	17	18	19	20	21	22	23	24	25	26	27	28	29	30	31	32	33	34	35	36	37	38
DATE																																						
WEIGHT																																						
Abdominal bloating																																						
Aches, pains																																						
Anxiety																																						
Appetite increase																																						
Backache																																						
Breast tenderness																																						
Chest pain																																						
Confusion																																						
Constipation																																						
Craving for alcohol																																						
Craving for sweets																																						
Cramps (abdominal)																																						
Crying spells																																						

Depression																														
Diarrhea																														
Dizziness/Faintness																														
Fatigue																														
Forgetfulness																														
Headache																														
Heart pounding																														
Hot flashes																														
Insomnia																														
Irritability																														
Itching																														
Moodswings																														
Nausea/vomiting																														
Nervous tension																														
Swelling of extremities																														
Urinary problems																														
Vision symptoms																														
Other																														

one has been approved by the Food and Drug Administration for use in treating certain forms of cancer, it has not been approved for PMS treatment. There haven't, as yet, been any controlled, scientific studies to determine whether progesterone helps, does nothing or makes PMS worse. Nevertheless, it is widely prescribed for PMS, and we have spoken with a number of women who had histories of severe depression, suicide attempts, repeated hospitalizations for mental problems and other dramatic PMS symptoms who claim their lives have been changed by progesterone treatment. We think that progesterone should be used only when all else has failed and only when the symptoms are severe enough to warrant the risks. There are undeniable risks associated with progesterone use. Researchers have found that large doses of progesterone can cause breast cancer in laboratory animals.[9] Moreover, the use of high-potency progesterone birth control pills has been associated with an increased risk of developing breast cancer in some women (see Chapter Five). Other potential side effects include early or late menstrual periods, spotting between periods, weight gain or loss, increased menstrual cramps, change in sex drive and euphoria or faintness. With rectal suppositories there may be diarrhea, abdominal cramps or rectal irritation. Medication given under the tongue may cause dizziness and sensitivity to alcohol. Hypotension, a sudden lowering of blood pressure, has also been reported when progesterone is administered in this way.

Progesterone has been found not to be safe in pregnancy and may be associated with increased risk of birth defects in the infants of women taking the drug during pregnancy.[10] Pregnant women *should not* use progesterone.

Women who accept progesterone treatment should be aware of the risks involved in its use. Also, Dr. Dalton cautions against the use of progestins (synthetic progesterones), which are sometimes prescribed for PMS; she believes that only natural progesterone, which cannot be taken orally, is effective in treating PMS.

Because of the risks associated with progesterone use and the lack of scientific evidence to document its effectiveness, many doctors think, as we do, that the nutritional/life-style changes approach is preferable.

Women should also be aware fact that, in the wake of the publicity surrounding PMS, clinics specializing in this disorder have sprung up all over the United States. Many PMS clinics are excellent; they are staffed by competent, well-trained people and offer a wide variety of treatment approaches. Unfortunately, some have been established by unscrupulous people who are out to make a quick buck and profiteer from women's misfortunes. Because PMS is so "new" and so many doctors are not well informed about it, being treated at a clinic that specializes in PMS makes sense, but you need to know how to tell the difference between a good clinic and an unscrupulous one. The following guidelines will help:

1. Ask how the clinic diagnoses PMS. If the clinic performs a lot of tests but doesn't require you to keep a chart of symptoms like the one described above, find another clinic.
2. Ask if progesterone is prescribed routinely on the first visit. A clinic that offers progesterone to patients on the basis of just one visit, without waiting for test results and without first trying the nutritional/life-style changes approach described below, is not likely to be a good one.
3. Ask what forms of treatment most patients at the clinic receive. If they all receive progesterone, or if most do, the clinic probably isn't top-notch. If progesterone therapy is the *only* form of treatment prescribed, find another clinic.

The second approach to treating PMS is by natural means, involving nutrition, dietary changes and exercise. Reducing the intake of calories, caffeine, sugar, salt, dairy products and white flour has proved helpful for some women. It is generally recommended that PMS sufferers eat smaller meals, more frequently (six times a day). Vitamin B_6 supplements (200 mg a day) have been shown to reduce symptoms. Calcium and magnesium supplements have also been used, as well as zinc, copper, vitamins A and E and various amino acids and enzymes. Good nutritional counseling is important if you are going to try the natural approach. You need to know, for example, that zinc and copper taken at the same time may not be effective and that some doctors believe that doses of vitamin B_6 greater than 200 mg a day may be toxic. Women who are interested in finding a doctor who uses the natural approach can contact the National PMS Society, P.O. Box 11467, Durham, North Carolina 27703 (919-489-6577); Premenstrual Syndrome Action, P.O. Box 9326, Madison, Wisconsin 53715 (608-274-6688) or the Premenstrual Syndrome Program, 40 Salem Street, Lynnfield, Massachusetts 01940. Two good books on the subject are *Self-Help for Premenstrual Syndrome,* by Dr. Michelle Harrison (Matrix Press, 1982), and *PMS: Premenstrual Syndrome,* by Dr. Neils Laversen and Eileen Stukane (Fireside, 1983).

Regular exercise is important. Some authorities think that milder forms of exercise, such as swimming, yoga, fast walking or bike riding, are preferable to aerobic exercise.[11]

MENSTRUAL CRAMPS

AKA: dysmenorrhea

Types: primary, or essential, dysmenorrhea
　　　secondary dysmenorrhea
　　　congestive dysmenorrhea, or premenstrual tension
　　　spasmodic dysmenorrhea

"Dysmenorrhea" is a fancy medical term for "menstrual cramps." Dysmenorrhea may be either secondary or primary. Secondary dysmenorrhea is men-

609

strual pain that is caused by some associated disease—pain that is secondary to some other illness. Primary dysmenorrhea is menstrual pain that is not associated with some other disease—in other words, menstrual cramps whose cause is unknown.

Incidence

Menstrual cramps are common. Indeed, it is rare to find a woman who has never experienced some degree of menstrual pain. Secondary dysmenorrhea typically appears for the first time in women who are in their 20s or 30s. Primary dysmenorrhea usually makes its appearance in the early teens and is usually less severe after about age 25 or after childbirth. Primary dysmenorrhea doesn't occur as often in women who are not ovulating, which explains why young girls during the first year or two after menarche don't have cramps, for they usually are not yet actually ovulating. It also explains why most women who use birth control pills, which suppresses ovulation, don't experience menstrual cramps. Dysmenorrhea can occur in women of any age, however, and may persist until menopause.

Symptoms

The pain may vary in severity and from month to month or year to year. Some doctors recognize two types of menstrual pain: congestive and spasmodic. Congestive dysmenorrhea is really a form of premenstrual syndrome and occurs just before the menstrual period begins. There may be a dull, achy feeling in the lower abdomen; painful swelling of the abdomen, breast, genitals, hands and/or feet; headache; backache; depression; fatigue; diarrhea or constipation, to mention just some of the symptoms.

Spasmodic dysmenorrhea, as the name implies, involves spasms of dull or acute pain in the lower abdomen. The pain is usually localized, involving only the lower abdomen and genitals, but may include the entire pelvic area, the inside of the thighs and the lower back. Normally, it begins on the 1st day of the menstrual cycle and is relieved by the 3d or 4th day but may affect some women for the entire period. Some women are plagued by this type of dysmenorrhea all their lives, but many gain relief after childbirth. Severity may vary from a vague sense of pelvic heaviness (which one friend aptly calls "lead vagina") to severe, incapacitating pain.

If the dysmenorrhea is secondary, the symptoms may have certain characteristics that are related to the underlying cause. For instance, if the dysmenorrhea is caused by a uterine fibroid tumor, there may be a gushing, flooding type of menstrual bleeding, followed by cramping. If endometriosis is the cause, there may be premenstrual staining as well as pain on intercourse, and the pain tends to worsen with each period. If pelvic inflammatory disease is the causative factor, the pain tends to be bilateral. If the pain is associated with adenomyosis, it may not abate after the first few days but may continue through the entire menstrual period.

Cause

Secondary dysmenorrhea may be caused by endometriosis, pelvic inflammatory disease, fibroid tumors, cervical polyps, adenomyosis, cervical stenosis or endometrial polyps.

The cause of primary dysmenorrhea is not well understood. There are a number of theories, each of which may partially explain primary dysmenorrhea. An old but popular theory holds that women with narrow cervical canals have cramps because the menstrual flow is obstructed. On the one hand, the fact that bearing children or having a D&C, a surgical procedure in which the lining of the uterus is removed—both of which stretch the cervical opening—often relieves menstrual cramps seems to support this theory. On the other hand, the fact that X-ray studies of women who experience menstrual pain have failed to correlate cramps with narrow cervical canals, as well as the fact that many women with cervical stenosis don't experience menstrual pain tend to discredit this theory.

Another theory holds that cramps occur because the uterus is excessively sensitive to progesterone. The uterus may have an allergic reaction to progesterone that causes it to contract sharply, leading to pain. This theory could account for the fact that primary dysmenorrhea often starts when ovulation first occurs, a year or two after the first menstrual period. This is when progesterone is first introduced into the body, and sensitivity would therefore be greatest at that time. It could also account for the fact that primary dysmenorrhea tends to become less severe as the woman grows older, for according to this theory, the uterus is desensitized to the progesterone over time and the allergic reaction is therefore less severe. Moreover, it could also account for the relief of pain that occurs in women who have borne children, for during pregnancy the body is flooded with progesterone, thus desensitizing the uterus and quelling the allergic reaction. This theory would, however, fail to account for the fact that cramps are experienced by some women who have borne children and by some women who use birth control pills and therefore don't ovulate or produce large amounts of progesterone. Another problem with this theory is that progesterone is thought to have a relaxing effect on the uterus.

Hormonal imbalances have long been blamed for menstrual cramps. Some researchers think that spasmodic dysmenorrhea occurs when there is too much progesterone in relation to estrogen. By giving the woman extra estrogen they claim to relieve such cases. But not all doctors have had equally good results with this type of treatment. The same researchers also argue that congestive dysmenorrhea, or premenstrual tension, results from too much estrogen in relation to progesterone (in which case birth control pills would make the cramps worse). They therefore use progesterone to treat this type of menstrual pain. Again, not all doctors report equally good results, casting doubts on the ability of this theory to explain all cases of menstrual pain.

A theory that has received a lot of publicity lately is that menstrual cramps are the result of overproduction of substances called prostaglandins. There are many types of prostaglandins in the body, and one type is apparently responsible for causing uterine contractions. Some studies have shown that women with menstrual cramps have higher levels of prostaglandins in their bodies, and antiprostaglandin medication has been effective in relieving pain in some, but not all, women with menstrual cramps.[12]

Despite the fact that so many women experience menstrual pain at some point in their lives, comparatively little research has been done in this area. Not surprisingly, the it's-all-in-your-head-dearie diagnosis has been widely used to explain menstrual cramps. Some doctors point out that women whose mothers have histories of menstrual discomfort are more likely to suffer themselves, suggesting that such women may "learn" to have menstrual cramps because their mothers "made such a fuss." This interpretation of facts ignores the possibility that there is indeed some physical cause for menstrual cramps that may be an inherited problem.

Although it is undoubtedly true that some women consciously or unconsciously create their own menstrual pain, it is hardly logical to explain a phenomenon as widespread as cramps as being psychological in origin. On some level it may be true that all disease has a psychological component; however, it is only in the field of gynecology, which deals with women's ailments, that medical science so readily accepts the notion that disease is psychosomatic and is so willing to ignore physical causes.

Diagnosis and Treatment

The first step in diagnosis is to obtain a thorough medical and menstrual history, including the type, severity and time of onset of pain and a description of any associated symptoms.

Next, the doctor should do a careful pelvic examination. If there are signs of endometriosis, fibroids, polyps, pelvic inflammatory disease or any of the other conditions that can cause secondary dysmenorrhea, the diagnostic procedures appropriate to those conditions should be done.

If these steps fail to turn up anything and the woman is over 25, making her a less likely candidate for primary dysmenorrhea, a more thorough investigation, including perhaps a D&C and/or laparoscopic examination, a method of examining the pelvic cavity by means of a lighted viewing instrument, may be in order to rule out the possibility that the cramps are owing to some disease or abnormality known to cause secondary dysmenorrhea. Too many times such women are merely dismissed as neurotic and are not given a thorough diagnostic workup. Women have a right to and should insist on a complete workup.

The treatment of secondary dysmenorrhea depends on the nature of the underlying cause. The various treatments are described under the appropriate headings elsewhere in this book.

The treatment of primary dysmenorrhea depends on the severity of the symptoms. A number of natural or home remedies have proved to be successful. Sometimes having an orgasm, either by masturbation or by having sex with another person, can help relieve menstrual pain, for it relaxes the uterus and draws blood to the cramped muscles. Heat methods, such as hot baths, applying heat to the area and massaging the area, will, like orgasm, promote blood flow to the muscles and relax spasms. Yoga, pelvic exercises, deep breathing, acupuncture, acupressure and herbal remedies have all been used successfully. (It should be noted, however, that herbal remedies are often powerful medicines and should be used only by people knowledgeable about herbs. For instance, pennyroyal, an herb used for menstrual cramps, can cause serious, even fatal, poisoning.) Some women have found that acupressure is effective in treating menstrual cramps. Personally, we have had some good results with a device called the "Point-H Band," a rubber stimulator strapped around the ankle so it comes in contact with the acupoint used in the Chinese medical treatment of urinary and genital problems. (For a Point-H Band and a booklet explaining how to locate the point, send $19.95 plus $1.50 for postage and handling to AcuTechnics, 1827 Haight Street, Suite 2, San Francisco, California 94117.)

Another approach to treating cramps is the use of analgesics. The most popular analgesic, aspirin, will relieve the pain for some women. Interestingly, aspirin, as well as being a pain reliever, is an antiprostaglandin agent. Nonaspirin pain relievers, such as Tylenol, are also effective for some women. A number of other over-the-counter drugs, such as Midol, Pamprin, Trendar, Femicin, and Humphrey's No. 11, work for some women. They usually contain aspirin, caffeine, an antispasmodic and, sometimes, a diuretic. Alcohol is sometimes helpful. Prescription painkillers, such as codeine compounds, work for some women. Darvon and other prescription painkillers are often ordered, although double-blind randomized studies have proved that Darvon is only slightly more effective than a sugar pill in relieving pain of any sort. In the past a drug called Edrisal, which contained aspirin and amphetamine, was available, but the Food and Drug Administration removed it from the market in an effort to control the prescription of amphetamines. Although amphetamines are dangerous drugs, their careful use may be justified in women who suffer from severe cramps and for whom other remedies are unsuccessful. A doctor can, of course, still write a prescription for the same amounts of amphetamine and other drugs that were contained in Edrisal, as long as the prescriptions are filed separately.

Birth control pills have been used to treat dysmenorrhea. They prevent ovulation and hence the production of progesterone, which may account for their effectiveness. But the safety of hormone therapy has been seriously questioned (*see* p. 104–5). Sometimes the hormones need only be prescribed for a few months, after which the woman's system may adjust itself. Short-term use of hormones may not involve as serious risks as prolonged use for purposes of birth control.

Recently, antiprostaglandin agents, such as indomethacin (Indocin), have been studied and seem to be effective.[13] However, this drug may have unpleasant side effects in some women. Other antiprostaglandin medications, such as naproxen (Naprosyn)[14] and mefenamic acid (Ponstel),[15] have been studied. These drugs seem to be effective in relieving pain but may not have any effect on the vomiting and diarrhea that some women experience. Doctors convinced of the efficacy of prostaglandin inhibitors also emphasize their safety and practicality relative to oral contraceptives. The prostaglandin inhibitors are needed only for 1 to 3 days and in low doses compared with oral contraceptives or hormones, which must be taken for 21 days.

Another new treatment for menstrual cramps now being investigated involves dilating the cervix with a slender, dry rod of sterile seaweed called a laminaria. The rod, which gradually expands as it absorbs water and dilates the cervix painlessly, is inserted in the doctor's office without an anesthetic and is left in place for about 6 hours.

A D&C, which may be done as part of the diagnostic workup for menstrual pain, may also provide relief for some women. Another surgical procedure, presacral neurectomy, in which the nerve passageways that transmit pain messages from the lower abdomen to the brain are severed, has been effective in preventing menstrual pain in 60 percent to 70 percent of cases in which it has been tried; however, the operation involves risk and complications.[16] As with any operation necessitating a general anesthetic, the possibility of fatal complications exists. Moreover, the surgery may result in damage to the sensory fibers of the bladder; a number of women gradually lose control of their bladders after the operation and experience problems in retaining urine that may last anywhere from a few weeks to a lifetime. Also, women who have had this procedure done may not feel any contractions in the early stages of labor. This operation should be done only by a surgeon who is experienced in this type of therapy and only after less drastic forms of treatment have failed. A new form of surgery, uterosacral ligament resection, has recently been used.[17] This procedure is thought by some doctors to have the same effect but without any interference, even temporarily, with bladder function. It has been effective in 75 percent to 80 percent of cases in which it has been tried, and in women who have borne children it can be done vaginally, without an abdominal incision.

Sometimes it is hard for a woman to receive adequate treatment for her menstrual cramps. In mild to moderate cases she may get nothing more than advice to "grin and bear it." If her pain is severe enough for her to persist in seeking treatment, she may wind up with a referral to a psychiatrist. All women, and particularly those over age 25, deserve a thorough gynecological investigation of their menstrual pain, for it may be the symptom of an underlying disease that needs treatment. Any woman whose doctor suggests psychiatric referral without first giving her an exhaustive diagnostic workup as outlined above should find herself another doctor.

AMENORRHEA

AKA: absence of menstrual periods

Types: primary amenorrhea, delayed menarche, or delayed puberty
      secondary amenorrhea
      physiologic amenorrhea

Associated Terms: cryptomenorrhea, galactorrhea, hirsutism

Amenorrhea means without (*a*) menstruation (*menorrhea*), or the absence of menstrual periods. Amenorrhea may be either primary or secondary. Primary amenorrhea, which is also called delayed puberty or delayed menarche, is defined as the failure to have a menstrual period by age 14, 16 or 18, depending on who's doing the defining. The majority of women will have had their first menstrual periods by age 14. Some women, although they are normal, won't have their periods until age 16, and a small number won't menstruate until age 18. There have been cases of normal women who didn't start menstruating until they were in their 20s, but generally, failure to menstruate by age 18 is an indication that something is wrong. It would be wise to at least consult a doctor if menstruation fails to occur by age 14.

Secondary amenorrhea is the absence of menstrual periods in a woman who has previously menstruated. It is not uncommon for a woman to miss an occasional menstrual period, or even two or more in a row. For this reason most doctors define secondary amenorrhea as the absence of menstruation for 6 months or longer. In our opinion any woman who goes to the trouble and expense of consulting a doctor because she is concerned about her failure to menstruate can legitimately consider herself as having amenorrhea. She deserves a complete physical exam and medical history and, if pregnancy is even a remote possibility, a pregnancy test. If the physical exam or medical history leads the doctor to suspect one of the specific causes outlined below, appropriate tests should be done. If no specific abnormalities suggest themselves, as is often the case, and the woman is not particularly anxious to get pregnant, we recommend that she wait until she has missed her period for at least 3 to 6 months before subjecting herself to the progesterone withdrawal test (described below), a standard part of the diagnostic workup. In most cases this waiting period will avoid unnecessary doctors' visits and unnecessary use of progesterone, which carries certain risks, since most women will resume their periods normally within 6 months.

Another type of amenorrhea is known as physiologic amenorrhea. One obvious example of this would be pregnancy, for pregnant women do not menstruate.* Menopausal women also experience physiologic amenorrhea as they go through the change of life. After childbirth the majority of women do not menstruate for anywhere from 6 weeks to 3 months. If a woman is breast-feeding, this period of physiologic amenorrhea may be even longer. Some women don't menstruate again until they stop breast-feeding.

Symptoms

Amenorrhea is not, in and of itself, a disease, but it may be a symptom of some underlying hormonal problem, often an imbalance, which may be serious or just a minor, temporary imbalance. Sometimes, depending on the underlying cause, other symptoms occur along with the amenorrhea. For instance, some women with amenorrhea also have galactorrhea—a milky-white, watery discharge that can be expressed or may flow spontaneously from the nipples. Hirsutism—male hair-growth patterns—may appear in certain women with amenorrhea. Other symptoms that may accompany amenorrhea are considered in detail in the following discussion of causes.

Causes

As indicated by Table 25, amenorrhea can be caused by a multitude of factors. Some of these underlying causes fall within the realm of gynecology, and since they are discussed elsewhere in the book, they are mentioned only briefly here. Amenorrhea can also be caused by diseases or conditions that are not strictly gynecological, and these are discussed in more detail. It may be helpful to review Chapter Four before reading the following pages.

*There is an occasional woman who has menstrual-type bleeding during the 1st month or 2 of pregnancy.

Table 25
Causes of Amenorrhea

Physiologic Causes
    Pregnancy
    Childbirth
    Breast-feeding
    Menopause

End Organ Problems
    Imperforate hymen
    Septate vagina
    Transverse vaginal septum
    Double vagina
    Congenital abnormalities of the uterus
    Cervical stenosis
    Vaginal stenosis
    Asherman's syndrome
    Congenital absence of the uterus

Ovarian Problems
    Congenital developmental defects
    Congenital abnormalities of the ovary
    Premature menopause
    Benign ovarian tumors
    Malignant ovarian tumors
    Tubo-ovarian abscesses
    Functioning ovarian tumors
    Polycystic ovarian disease

Hypothalamic Problems
    Emotional stress or shock
    Organic brain disease
    Idiopathic hypothalamic insufficiency
    Chiari-Frommel Syndrome
    Birth control pills
    Drugs
    Anorexia nervosa
    Psychiatric problems

Pituitarian Problems
    Simmonds' disease
    Sheehan's syndrome
    Pituitary tumors
    Hypogonadotropic eunuchoidism

Chronic Diseases
    Tuberculosis
    Hepatitis
    Cirrhosis of the liver
    Other chronic systemic diseases

Pancreatic Problems
    Diabetes (insufficiency in the
      pancreas)

Thyroid Problems
    Hyperthyroidism
    Hypothyroidism

Adrenal Problems
    Addison's disease
    Congenital adrenal hyperplasia
    Cushing's disease or syndrome

Other Causes
    Malnutrition
    Excessive weight gain
    Excessive weight loss
    Rigorous athletic training

End Organ Problems

A woman's amenorrhea may be caused by an end organ problem, that is, one involving the uterus, cervix or vagina, and it may be either an acquired problem or a congenital one (one that has been present since birth). A woman may have an imperforate hymen, a condition in which a thin sheet of tissue completely covers the vaginal opening, so that no blood can escape. Or she may have a septate vagina, a transverse vaginal septum, a double vagina or a complete absence of the vagina, any of which could result in amenorrhea. Likewise, she may have certain congenital abnormalities of the uterus or stenosis (blockage) of the cervix or of the vagina, which could also block the menstrual flow. In all the conditions mentioned thus far the woman may actually be menstruating and may notice cyclical signs of menstruation, such as weight gain, breast tenderness and mood swings, but no blood flow, owing to the blockage. This absence of blood flow is called cryptomenorrhea. The diagnosis can usually be made by physical examination, although certain types of uterine abnormalities may necessitate more extensive diagnostic procedures.

Another type of end organ problem that can cause amenorrhea is a condition known as Asherman's syndrome, in which the endometrial lining has been so badly damaged that it can no longer respond to hormonal stimulation. A history of certain types of surgery, coupled with a careful physical examination, will lead to a diagnosis of Asherman's syndrome.

A woman may also miss her menstrual periods because she does not have a uterus. She may have been born without one, or she may have a condition known as testicular feminization syndrome. A careful physical examination will reveal the fact that the woman doesn't have a uterus but won't tell the doctor which of these two conditions she has. Diagnosis of such women is discussed in more detail below.

Ovarian Problems

Amenorrhea may also be caused by problems involving the ovaries. If the ovaries are not working properly and thus are not producing the proper amounts of estrogen and progesterone, the woman may have amenorrhea. Women with congenital developmental defects, such as Turner's syndrome, hermaphroditism or the testicular feminization syndrome mentioned above, will have primary amenorrhea. Other congenital abnormalities of the ovary can also produce amenorrhea. In addition, a woman might have a premature menopause as a result of irradiation, surgery or other factors. The ovaries might be destroyed or impaired by benign or malignant ovarian tumors or a tubo-ovarian abscess. Certain ovarian tumors, called functioning ovarian tumors, can produce hormones and thus cause amenorrhea.

Hypothalamic Problems

If the ovary is not producing hormones, sometimes it's because the ovary is not receiving proper stimulation from the pituitary gland. In some cases the pituitary itself is the source of the problem. In other cases the pituitary per se may be normal but may function improperly because *it* is not receiving sufficient stimulation from the hypothalamus. For instance, polycystic ovarian disease, a condition associated with amenorrhea in which the follicles in the ovary never release their eggs, may be caused by a problem in the ovary itself or by a problem in the hypothalamus.

There are a number of reasons why the hypothalamus could fail to function properly, for it is a finely tuned organ that is sensitive to all sorts of outside events. Indeed, the hypothalamus is so sensitive that even the sound of a baby crying in the next room is sometimes enough to trigger substances within it that could, in turn, cause milk to flow from a nursing mother's breasts. In a similar fashion, stress, perhaps from the death of someone close or from problems at work or with love relationships, can cause a woman to miss one or more periods. This may be owing to some sort of protective mechanism cleverly designed by mother nature to prevent us from adding the demands of pregnancy to our bodies when we are stressed and therefore have lowered resistance to disease or other abnormalities. Less dramatic types of emotional stress may also cause amenorrhea, presumably because of the effect on the hypothalamus. Even after the initial stress has passed, the amenorrhea may persist, for the hypothalamus may not get back into synch by itself.

Hypothalamic amenorrhea is also associated with anorexia nervosa, a condition that most often occurs in adolescents and women in their early 20s. The woman develops a distaste or aversion for food and consequently eats nothing or next to nothing, losing a great deal of weight. Unlike the woman with Simmonds' disease (discussed below), a woman with anorexia nervosa is not usually lethargic and may have a considerable amount of energy. The loss of weight and extreme malnutrition may be the cause of the amenorrhea, but in most cases the amenorrhea precedes the dramatic loss in weight. In 10 percent to 20 percent of cases, anorexia nervosa results in irreversible, fatal malnutrition. If the woman can regain her normal weight, which sometimes necessitates hospitalization and intravenous feeding, menstruation may be restored.

Although anorexia nervosa is commonly held to result from a psychological disturbance, one wonders about the accuracy of this diagnosis. It is true that the hypothalamus is profoundly influenced by emotional states, and as we have seen, psychological stress or problems can and undoubtedly do disrupt its normal functioning. However, it may be that some supposedly psychologically caused conditions result from an as-yet-mysterious organic disruption of normal glandular process. Certainly, in this case the fact that the amenorrhea precedes the weight loss and that patients who are receiving cer-

619

tain forms of cancer treatment often experience anorexia nervosa, presumably because of drug or radiation upset to their systems, should alert us to the possibility that there may be a physical cause for this disease.

In general, women who are diagnosed as having psychogenic amenorrhea and who do not have a history of psychological stress should view this diagnosis with a good deal of skepticism. In the future, medical science may find, just as we have found with menstrual cramps, that so-called psychological problems have a physiological basis. Even removing the stigma of "psychological problem" from the diagnosis could provide a certain relief. In the case of anorexia nervosa, for instance, it might help relieve parental guilt and thus temper the parents' incessant and unsuccessful efforts to nag the patient into eating.

Hypothalamic amenorrhea can also be caused by prolonged use of certain drugs. Some women who have used birth control pills for long periods stop menstruating once the Pill is discontinued. There is some disagreement as to whether this post-Pill amenorrhea is caused by the birth control pill, since many of the women who experience it had irregular menstrual patterns before going on the Pill. At any rate, most of the women with post-Pill amenorrhea eventually resume menstruation. Some, however, do not, and such women may also experience premature menopause.

Certain drugs used to treat psychiatric problems, some tranquilizers and some of the drugs used to treat hypertension, a condition characterized by high blood pressure, may, if used for long periods, cause amenorrhea. Heroin addicts and women on methadone may also have amenorrhea. Most cases of drug- or medicine-related amenorrhea will revert to normal when the drug is discontinued.

A number of other factors can cause the hypothalamus to malfunction. Organic brain disease, which can be caused by encephalitis, a viral infection of the brain, as well as other related infections, head injuries, scars, tumors and exposure to poisonous substances all can interfere with hypothalamic function and hence produce amenorrhea. A history of such disease—along with such symptoms as unconsciousness; dizziness; headache; bleeding from the mouth, nose or ears; vomiting; drowsiness; confusion and/or fever—will help the doctor make the diagnosis. If the underlying problem can be treated, the menstrual cycle will usually return to normal. If portions of the brain have been damaged permanently, it may be necessary to give the woman some form of oral medication to take the place of the substances her body cannot produce (see below).

Some women are apparently born with hypothalamuses that don't secrete the usual amounts of hormone-releasing factors or that are particularly sensitive to the "turn-off" messages that are sent to it by means of ovarian hormones at certain points in the menstrual cycle. In medical jargon this condition is known as idiopathic hypothalamic insufficiency. Such women will have amenorrhea punctuated by an occasional menstrual period. There is often a family history of menstrual irregularities. Once the diagnosis has been clearly established (see below), there is usually no need to treat these women.

Another type of amenorrhea thought to be related to a problem in the hypothalamus is the Chiari-Frommel syndrome. It occurs in women after childbirth. Galactorrhea, in which there is a milky-white discharge from the nipples, accompanies the amenorrhea in these women. Such women are usually somewhat overweight and may have some excessive hair growth. The uterus and ovaries are small. It is thought that the factor in the hypothalamus that normally suppresses the pituitary hormone prolactin (which causes the breast to produce milk) is absent. Without this inhibiting factor from the hypothalamus the pituitary overproduces prolactin. This throws the rest of the hormonal balance out of whack, causing amenorrhea. Diagnosis is made by the symptoms, the history of childbirth and X-rays to rule out a pituitary tumor. The Chiari-Frommel syndrome is often resistant to treatment.

Pituitary Problems

The pituitary gland can also be the source of the problem, even if the hypothalamus is functioning normally. There may be an insufficiency of pituitary hormones as a result of either Simmonds' disease or Sheehan's syndrome. Simmonds' disease, which usually occurs after traumatic or infected childbirth but which occasionally may be caused in other ways, involves destruction of the pituitary gland. The woman with Simmonds' disease may have amenorrhea, a smaller uterus, postmenopausal vaginitis, a decline in breast size and other symptoms of menopause, owing to ovarian failure. Such failure results from insufficient stimulation of the ovary by the pituitary hormones. The thyroid gland also is insufficiently stimulated, and any of the symptoms of hypothyroidism (described below) may also appear. There may be a deterioration of connective and muscle tissue. Typically, the hair begins to fall out, first from the armpits and later from the scalp and pubic area. The woman may give the appearance of having aged prematurely and may be severely emaciated.

Sheehan's syndrome, which is also associated with blood loss and shock owing to childbirth or severe infection after childbirth, likewise results in damage to the pituitary gland, although usually not as extensive as in Simmonds' disease. However, the woman with Sheehan's syndrome is apt to maintain her body weight or to become overweight. It may take years for the symptoms of Sheehan's disease to become obvious. The classic symptoms include amenorrhea; inability to produce breast milk; menopausal-type changes in the vagina and uterus; loss of armpit and pubic hair; gradual thinning of the eyebrows; dry, pale skin that is sensitive to cold and does not perspire; loss of

621

appetite; vomiting; a tendency to spells of weakness and fainting and lethargy.

Diagnosis of Simmonds' disease and Sheehan's syndrome is suggested by the symptoms and a history of bleeding and infection associated with childbirth; it may be confirmed by laboratory tests. Treatment depends on the extent of the damage to the pituitary gland. Cortisone-type drugs to replace the missing pituitary hormones may be given. Estrogen replacement therapy may be given to make up for the lack of ovarian hormone. Progesterone-type drugs may be given as well. Thyroid may be given to make up for the lack of natural thyroid. Women with minimal Sheehan's syndrome may only need temporary replacement therapy, for after a rest the unimpaired portions of the pituitary gland may resume function and the woman may return to normal. For some women, however, cortisone, estrogen and thyroid therapy may have to be continued. Sometimes, although the estrogen, thyroid and cortisone therapy may relieve the symptoms, including the amenorrhea, a cure may not be possible, and in some cases death can occur.

Pituitary tumors can cause amenorrhea. Such women may have headaches and visual disturbances as well, although these may appear only in the late stages. A slow-growing tumor might be present for years before these two symptoms appeared. One type of pituitary tumor, called a chromophobe adenoma, produces amenorrhea, because it destroys so much of the pituitary gland. Sometimes these tumors produce the hormone prolactin and the woman may have a milky discharge from her breasts, in which case the term "Forbes-Albright syndrome" is used to describe the condition.

Another type of pituitary tumor, the acidophilic adenoma, is associated with amenorrhea. Women with this condition may also have a condition known as acromegaly, in which the hands, feet, nose and lower jaw grow excessively large owing to a disturbance of growth hormones. The tumors are radiosensitive and are often treated by radiation therapy. Menstrual periods generally resume after successful treatment, but if the pituitary has been destroyed, amenorrhea will persist.

Some women are born with pituitaries that are not capable of producing the correct amounts of hormones. This condition is referred to as hypogonadotropic eunuchoidism. Diagnosis involves a complete hormone workup by a specialist (see below).

Pancreatic Problems

Disturbances in the pancreas, the gland that produces substances to help the body convert the food we eat into a usable form, can also cause amenorrhea. Women who have diabetes mellitus, a disease in which the pancreas fails to produce the hormone insulin, so that the body is unable to metabolize nutriments—in particular, to utilize sugar properly—may have amenorrhea, although excessive menstrual bleeding is a more common symptom for such women. Other symptoms include excessive thirst, urination or hunger; weight loss; generalized weakness; skin disorders; yeast infections of the vagina; blurred vision; numbness; dry mouth and cramps in the legs. Diagnosis is made by blood tests. Mild forms of the disease may be controlled by proper diet and exercise. Medication, usually insulin by mouth or injection, may be necessary. Amenorrhea should disappear with successful treatment of the diabetes.

Thyroid Problems

Both excessive and inadequate production of thyroid, conditions known as hyperthyroidism and hypothyroidism respectively, may be associated with menstrual abnormalities, including amenorrhea.

Hyperthyroidism, whose cause is unknown, may produce the following symptoms: enlarged thyroid gland; nervousness; emotional outbursts; excessive sweating; intolerance to heat; hyperactivity; weight loss; weakness; tiredness; thin hair; diarrhea; warm, moist, smooth skin; rapid pulse; bulging eyes and vision disturbances. Diagnosis is based on the amenorrhea and other symptoms and confirmed by special tests designed to measure thyroid levels. Treatment may include surgical removal of part of the thyroid gland or radiation.

Hypothyroidism may be caused by a birth defect, and children who are so affected may have impaired mental and physical development. The disease may also be acquired later in life as a result of destruction of the thyroid gland through radiation or surgery, of too much or too little iodine in the diet or of certain drugs and foods; however, the cause is not always clear. Symptoms, which may be mild or severe, include apathy; sluggishness; increased sensitivity to cold; brittle hair; low, husky voice; dry, cool, rough skin; puffy hands, face and eyelids; discolored fingernails; weak muscles; slow pulse rate; weight gain; slow reflexes; constipation and anemia. Diagnosis is made by specific tests used to measure thyroid levels. Treatment consists of iodine supplements, which may succeed in some cases, but daily administration of thyroid tablets is usually necessary.

Adrenal Problems

Over- or underproduction of the adrenal glands may also cause amenorrhea. In the past, tuberculosis infections were responsible for most cases of Addison's disease, in which there is underactivity of the adrenal glands. Today, with tuberculosis under control, wasting of the glands from unknown causes, a tumor, infection or insufficient pituitary hormones are the main causes of Addison's disease. Symptoms include weakness, lethargy, nausea, vomiting, abdominal pain, drop in blood pressure, depression, anemia and irritability. The disease may develop slowly, and severe attacks may be brought on by stress, injury or infection. Diagnosis is made by the symptoms, which indicate to the doctor that tests measuring adrenal hormone levels in the blood and in urine should be done. Once the tests have confirmed the diagnosis, treatment involves daily doses of the adrenal hormones. Although women may have amenorrhea in the later stages of Addison's disease, it is not clear whether this is owing to the lack of adrenal hormones or to associated malnutrition.

Overproduction of the adrenal glands can also cause amenorrhea. One cause of such overproduction is a condition known as congenital adrenal hyperplasia. Women with this condition usually have deformities of the external genitals. For instance, the clitoris may be enlarged and may resemble the tip of a penis. The condition may be diagnosed at birth, or at puberty, when male hair-growth patterns develop and menstruation fails to occur. Milder forms may not be recognized until later in life, when whiskers, chest hair and other male hair-growth patterns appear in the woman. The breasts may get smaller, the clitoris may enlarge, baldness and acne may occur, the voice may deepen and a male-type body structure may develop. The menstrual cycle is altered until, finally, menstruation stops altogether. Treatment may include the removal of the tumor or one or both adrenal glands; in rare cases, radiation of the pituitary may be recommended.

Conditions known as Cushing's disease and Cushing's syndrome are also associated with amenorrhea. They may be caused by tumors in the pituitary or in the adrenal glands or by other problems in the pituitary or adrenals. Women with these conditions may bruise easily and have male hair-growth patterns, acne, a deepening of the voice, muscle weakness and smaller breasts, uterus and ovaries. These women are typically overweight and tend to have large abdomens, thin arms and legs and round "moon" faces. They may have pads of fat over their shoulders, a condition that has been described as "buffalo hump," and purplish lines or stretch marks, called striae, in certain areas of their bodies. Diagnosis is made by the physical appearance and confirmed by laboratory tests. Treatment depends on the site of the problem and may include surgical removal of the tumor, removal of one or more of the adrenal glands or, in rare cases, irradiation of the pituitary gland. Symptoms usually regress after treatment.

Chronic Disease

Chronic diseases may exert their influence on proper hormone interaction between the pituitary, hypothalamus and ovaries and thus be associated with amenorrhea. Tuberculosis, for instance, can cause amenorrhea through either a specific attack on the ovary or uterus, or its effects on the whole system.

Since hormones are eliminated from the body through urine, a chronic kidney disease called nephritis, which interferes with the normal elimination process, can alter the correct hormone balance and result in amenorrhea. In addition to amenorrhea, symptoms include puffiness of the face, eyelids and ankles; a swollen abdomen; high blood pressure, headache; insomnia; poor vision; excessive urination at night; anemia and shortness of breath. Diagnosis is confirmed by urine tests, which may show blood and certain proteins in the urine. Treatment includes bed rest; a high-vitamin, low-salt diet; sedatives and medication to control high blood pressure; iron compounds for anemia and, in extreme cases, blood transfusions. If the kidney is damaged severely, hemodialysis, in which the blood is circulated through an artificial kidney machine that washes it clean of wastes and poisons, may be necessary. If the disease itself can be treated, the amenorrhea will usually disappear.

Similarly, the liver plays a role in metabolizing estrogen. Disturbances in liver function, such as cirrhosis of the liver, a condition that is usually associated with alcoholism but is occasionally caused by B-virus hepatitis, can result in excessive menstrual bleeding, followed by periods of amenorrhea. Other symptoms include nausea, vomiting, gas, weight loss, liver enlargement, bad breath, puffiness of the feet and legs, reddened palms, enlarged blood vessels in the chest and shoulders, swollen abdomen, nosebleeds, hemorrhoids, vomiting of blood and blood in the feces. Treatment includes abstinence from alcohol, a diet rich in proteins and low in salt, and medications to help the body eliminate fluids. A woman who has such severe cirrhosis that she misses her menstrual periods may not resume menstruation.

Other Causes

Excessive and rapid weight loss, poor eating habits or malnutrition may cause amenorrhea. Women athletes who are involved in unusually strenuous conditioning programs sometimes experience amenorrhea, because they have altered the ratio of body fat and muscle in their bodies and a certain proportion of fat is apparently necessary for ovulation.

Diagnosis and Treatment

As we have seen, amenorrhea can be caused by a number of factors. Diagnosis, then, is pretty much a process of elimination and involves trying to identify the cause or at least to rule out the more grave possibilities. Once the cause has been identified, proper treatment—if indeed treatment is necessary—can be given.

A careful medical history, physical exam and bimanual pelvic exam are the first steps in diagnosis. A pregnancy test should also be done, to rule out that possibility. A careful medical history is important, but some doctors don't spend a sufficient amount of time on it. This is another instance in which nurse practitioners can be of great value, for they can afford the time to take thorough history. For instance, past psychological stress may have thrown the hypothalamus out of whack, and although the stress may have passed, the hypothalamus may never have gotten back in synch. Careful questioning in the course of a thorough medical history might reveal such a situation. Similarly, a history of diabetes in the family, an abortion, a D&C, difficulties in childbirth, rapid weight gain or loss, poor eating habits and other suggestive information that could point to a diagnosis may be discovered in the course of a thorough medical history. The age of the woman, a recent history of childbirth or breast-feeding may point to physiologic causes. A bimanual pelvic exam may rule out end organ problems or detect ovarian tumors or abscesses.

If a woman has been taking birth control pills, she may have post-Pill amenorrhea, so the doctor should ask the woman if she has had any nipple discharge and carefully examine the woman's breasts, trying to express any discharge. If there is or has been a discharge, further testing, which is described in the section on galactorrhea, is necessary. If the woman has no nipple discharge problem, the doctor will want to know how long ago she stopped taking the Pill. If she has been off the Pill for less than 6 months, the doctor will not usually do anything, for the majority of women who have troubles with amenorrhea after they stop using the Pill will resume menstruation by the time 6 months have passed. If a woman fails to resume menstruation after 6 months, she should return to the doctor at that time for further diagnostic workup, as described below.

Sometimes the physical exam will reveal the classic signs of pituitary, adrenal or thyroid problems, in which case the doctor will prescribe certain tests that can lead to a diagnosis. If a woman has the signs of Cushing's disease, for instance, the doctor should do a dexamethasone suppression test.[18] At 11 PM the woman takes 1 mg of a drug called dexamethasone by mouth. She may also be given a tranquilizer. Between 8 AM and 9 AM the next day she reports to the doctor and has a blood sample taken and analyzed. If the level of the substances measured in this test are low, she does not have Cushing's disease. If they are high, she may or may not have Cushing's and must be referred to a specialist known as a medical endocrinologist for a more complex and more expensive series of tests. Some doctors neglect to do the dexamethasone screening test and either refer the woman directly to a specialist or immediately order the more elaborate, expensive series of tests. Any woman with amenorrhea and symptoms suggestive of Cushing's syndrome whose doctor orders the extensive tests or refers her to a specialist without first doing the simpler test should discuss this with her doctor and should consider getting a second opinion (*see* p. 238) before undergoing more elaborate testing.

If the dexamethasone suppression test results show high levels, the woman, along with anyone who shows signs of specific pituitary or adrenal problems, will need a complete endocrinology workup, with elaborate urine and blood tests. Hospitalization, in order to draw blood from certain veins deep inside the body, may be necessary, but this is uncommon. Although in the past many women were subjected to these tests, most of the tests were unnecessary. Today a simple test known as a progesterone withdrawal or progesterone-challenge test, described below, is done instead.

If the physical exam, medical history or accompanying symptoms fail to indicate the cause of the amenorrhea, the woman will fall into one of three groups. The characteristics of each of these groups, along with the appropriate diagnostic steps, are outlined in Table 26 A, B and C explained in detail in the following text.

Here again, jotting down notes on the terminology and abbreviations used to describe the menstrual cycle and keeping the notes handy will help you to sort through the somewhat complex process of diagnosing amenorrhea.

Group One

In the first group are those women with primary amenorrhea (that is, they've never had a period) who have normal uteri and cervices but do not have the secondary sex characteristics, like breast development and pubic hair, that normally appear during puberty in response to rising levels of estrogen. The first step is to do a hormone test, known as a serum FSH, that measures levels of FSH, the follicle-stimulating hormone from the pituitary that stimulates the follicles inside the ovary to produce estrogen. A woman who doesn't have secondary sex characteristics is lacking in estrogen. The doctor wants to know whether this lack of estrogen results from a problem in the ovary or in the brain, either in the pituitary or in the hypothalamus.

If the FSH test results indicate high levels of FSH, the doctor knows that the pituitary and hypothalamus are both doing their part, for if they weren't, the FSH levels would be low. So it must be that the ovary is, for some reason, failing to produce estrogen. Unfortunately, not all doctors have a clear understanding of how hormones work in the female body. Some doctors will mistakenly refer women with high FSH levels to medical centers for elaborate testing, looking for tumors or other brain abnormalities, when the problem is in the ovary.* Women (or parents of these females, for they are often young

*There is no such thing as an FSH-producing brain tumor.

Diagnosing Amenorrhea

Physical Signs and Symptoms

Group One

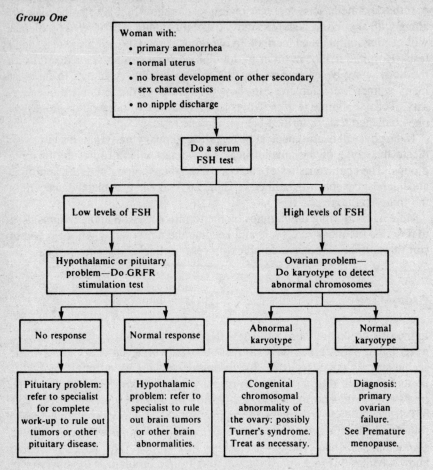

girls) who have primary amenorrhea, normal uteri, no secondary sex characteristics and high FSH levels should seek a second opinion if their doctors recommend X-ray studies.

If the FSH is high, the next step is to do a karyotype, which is a study of the
chromosomes. If the karyotype is abnormal, the doctor knows (depending on
the nature of the test results) that the woman has Turner's syndrome or one of
the other congenital developmental abnormalities of the ovary. If the karyotype is normal, the doctor will suspect primary ovarian failure. Treatment of
these conditions is discussed in detail elsewhere and may include some form
of estrogen replacement therapy to stimulate secondary sex characteristics.

628

Diagnosing Amenorrhea

Physical Signs and Symptoms

Group Two

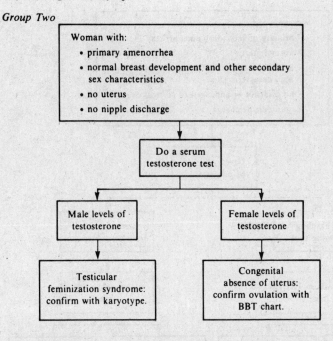

If the FSH is low, this indicates that the pituitary isn't producing enough FSH to stimulate the ovaries to make estrogen; hence there are no secondary sex characteristics. This may be caused by a malfunctioning pituitary that isn't producing enough hormone to stimulate the ovary. Or, it may be caused by a malfunctioning hypothalamus that isn't producing enough FSH releasing factor. Without the FSH releasing factor from the hypothalamus the pituitary can't produce FSH, which in turn means no estrogen from the ovaries and, again, no menstrual periods or secondary sex characteristics.

Some women may get back FSH test results that indicate FSH levels in the normal range. These levels are not actually normal, but what doctors call pseudonormal, for they are low for the particular woman's body.[19]

Further testing may be done to tell whether the problem is in the hypothalamus or the pituitary. The test is done by injecting some of the releasing factor substances normally made by the hypothalamus into the woman's body and then doing blood tests to measure the levels of pituitary hormones in her body. It is called a gonadotropin releasing factor response (GRFR) test. If there is no response to the test, the doctor will know that it is the pituitary gland that is not doing its job and will refer the woman to a specialist who will

629

Diagnosing Amenorrhea

Physical Signs and Symptoms

Group Three

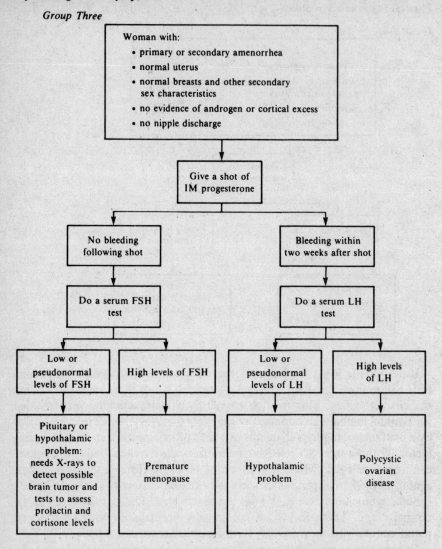

Woman with:
- primary or secondary amenorrhea
- normal uterus
- normal breasts and other secondary sex characteristics
- no evidence of androgen or cortical excess
- no nipple discharge

↓

Give a shot of IM progesterone

No bleeding following shot	Bleeding within two weeks after shot
Do a serum FSH test	Do a serum LH test

Low or pseudonormal levels of FSH	High levels of FSH	Low or pseudonormal levels of LH	High levels of LH
Pituitary or hypothalamic problem: needs X-rays to detect possible brain tumor and tests to assess prolactin and cortisone levels	Premature menopause	Hypothalamic problem	Polycystic ovarian disease

do X-rays and other tests to rule out the possibility of a brain tumor or other pituitary abnormalities. If the GRFR test results are normal, the doctor will know that the pituitary is capable of responding to these releasing factors. There must, then, be an insufficiency of releasing factors from the hypothalamus. Again, a specialist is needed to perform certain tests to rule out a brain tumor. Depending on the results of the test, the woman may be given replace-

630

ment therapy, that is, drugs to replace the substances her body is unable to produce.

Group Two

In the second group of women are those who have primary amenorrhea (that is, they have never had a period), who have normal breast development and other secondary sex characteristics but who on physical examination turn out to be missing their uteri. These women fall into one of two categories: those who were born without a uterus, a condition known as congenital absence of the uterus, and those with testicular feminization syndrome, a condition associated with chromosomal abnormalities in which a woman who is normal in other ways has male-type testicular tissue instead of ovaries. Women with the syndrome need to have this testicular-type tissue removed because it is subject to cancerous tumors, so it is important to distinguish between the two conditions. This is done by giving a blood test known as a serum testosterone test.

If the test shows that the woman has female levels of the hormone testosterone in her body, the doctor can be fairly sure that the woman has congenital absence of the uterus. Such women usually ovulate and don't need estrogen replacement therapy. Careful questioning may reveal that the woman has cyclical swelling of the breasts, weight gain, mood changes or other symptoms related to the menstrual cycle, which would indicate that the ovaries and other hormone-producing organs are functioning properly and that it is just the absence of the uterus that is causing the problem. A basal body temperature chart will confirm the diagnosis.

If the serum testosterone measurement is at a male level, the diagnosis of testicular feminization can be confirmed by a karyotype test, which will reveal the chromosomal abnormalities characteristic of women with this condition. The testicular-type tissue must be removed because of the potential of developing cancer. Again, the woman may be put on estrogen replacement therapy; however, estrogen involves certain risks, so it must be used with caution.

Group Three

In the third group are women with primary or secondary amenorrhea, normal uteri, normal breasts and other secondary sex characteristics, no signs of adrenal problems (for example, excessive hair growth) and no nipple discharge. This is by far the largest of the three groups. These women should have, as the first step in diagnosis, a progesterone withdrawal test. They should not allow themselves to be subjected to the expense, inconvenience and risk of a complete workup (which may include blood and urine tests and X-rays) unless this simple test has been done first. On the other hand, women with secondary amenorrhea (women who have menstruated previously) but no other symptoms should probably not have a progesterone withdrawal test done until they have missed at least three, or possibly six, periods, for the use of progesterone carries certain risks and the shot can be quite painful. Because of the possibility of birth defects caused by progesterone, no one should have this test unless pregnancy has been ruled out by the most sensitive tests (*see* p. 788).

The first thing the doctor wants to know is whether or not the woman is producing estrogen. That is why she is given the shot of progesterone. The progesterone will gradually be excreted by the body over a 2-week period. As the levels of progesterone fall, the endometrial lining, which you will recall from Chapter Four is built up by estrogen in the first place, will break down and be shed, causing bleeding from the uterus.

Bleeding After Progesterone Shot

If the woman does start bleeding (usually within 2 weeks), this will tell the doctor that the ovary is indeed producing estrogen, for if it weren't, there wouldn't be any endometrial lining to be shed and hence there wouldn't be any bleeding. If bleeding does occur, the doctor also knows that the pituitary gland is functioning normally, for without the proper follicle-stimulating hormone from the pituitary the follicles in the ovary wouldn't be stimulated to produce their estrogen and, again, there would be no endometrial lining and thus no bleeding after the progesterone shot.

Since the woman who bleeds after the progesterone withdrawal test isn't lacking estrogen, the doctor knows that her problem must be a lack of the other hormone that regulates the menstrual cycle, progesterone. The next step is to figure out *why* she is lacking progesterone. There are two possibilities. The first is that the woman has polycystic ovarian disease, a condition in which the egg follicles that produce estrogen never make it to the surface of the ovary to release their eggs at ovulation. Since the follicle never bursts open, the corpus luteum, which is formed from the remnants of the burst follicle after ovulation, never develops. The absence of the corpus luteum, whose job it is to produce progesterone in the second half of the cycle, accounts for the lack of this hormone in women with this condition. Although these women do produce enough estrogen to stimulate the growth of the endometrium and to trigger the surge of luteinizing hormone (LH) that would normally trigger ovulation, some other factor, perhaps something in the follicle

632

itself, prevents the LH from causing ovulation, so that there is no progesterone.

The second possible explanation for a woman's inability to produce progesterone is that the ovary is not getting enough LH, so that there is not enough stimulation to cause the follicle to burst open and release its egg. Again, without ovulation there is no corpus luteum and therefore no progesterone. Theoretically, the lack of LH could be caused by a problem in the pituitary or hypothalamus. However, since the woman has bled after the shot of progesterone, the doctor already knows the pituitary is functioning normally or, as outlined above, the woman would not have estrogen and would not have bled. Thus her problem must be in the hypothalamus.

In order to tell whether the problem is in the hypothalamus or in the ovary, the next step is to do a blood test to measure levels of LH. This test is called a serum LH. If the test indicates high levels of LH, the doctor knows the woman has polycystic ovarian disease. The explanation for the diagnosis is as follows: In polycystic ovarian disease the pituitary is constantly sending out FSH, which keeps stimulating more follicles to develop and thus creates high levels of estrogen (which is made in the follicle). The high levels of estrogen keep stimulating the pituitary to produce LH, so the woman has high levels of this hormone as well. Since there is no progesterone to tell the pituitary to "stop producing FSH," the pituitary continues to churn out both FSH and LH. This series of events is confirmed by the serum LH test. Once the diagnosis of polycystic ovarian disease is indicated by the high LH levels, treatment, which is described under the heading Polycystic Ovarian Disease, may be given.

The serum LH test may also indicate low levels of LH. Some women may get back test results that indicate the LH is in the normal range, but the LH is not really normal.[20] Here again, this result is what doctors call pseudonormal and the LH level is really low for that particular woman. Low or pseudonormal LH levels indicate a problem in the hypothalamus. There is some LH because there is estrogen that is stimulating the pituitary to put out a certain amount of LH. But there is not enough LH to trigger ovulation because the hypothalamus is not producing its luteinizing hormone releasing factor (LHRF), without which the pituitary is unable to produce the surge of LH that causes ovulation.

This woman does not, however, need a workup to detect a brain tumor or other such abnormalities, for the fact that the hypothalamus is producing follicle stimulating hormone releasing factors (as evidenced by the fact that the pituitary is indeed releasing FSH, which in turn is causing the ovary to produce estrogen, as demonstrated by the fact that the woman bled after the shot of progesterone) shows that a serious abnormality is not present. These are the cases in which the women have psychological stress problems, weight gains or losses or other problems that are not well understood. These women will often resume menstruation of their own accord. Generally, treatment involves inducing a menstrual period every 2 to 3 months by giving oral progesterone. This will prevent the uterine lining from growing too thick, a condition known as endometrial hyperplasia that is sometimes a precursor to cancer, and will also serve as a follow-up, a way of checking to see that the woman is indeed still producing estrogen.

Some women have long spells of amenorrhea punctuated by occasional menstrual periods. This can result from any one of the problems outlined earlier or it may be normal for that woman's body. Her hypothalamus may work differently. If serious problems have been ruled out and pregnancy is not a concern, these women don't need treatment.

Before discussing the woman who fails to bleed from the shot of progesterone, a word or two about the progesterone shot itself is in order.

As noted earlier, in the past, women were given a battery of fancy tests instead of the shot of progesterone. Some doctors still prescribe these tests, but in the majority of women with amenorrhea they are unnecessary; 50 cents' worth of progesterone will do the trick.

A particular type of progesterone, call I.M. progesterone, is used for this purpose. Depo-Provera, Delalutin and other, similar progesterones cannot be used for this purpose, because when they are given by injection they often cause long periods of amenorrhea.

The I.M. progesterone can be given mixed with either oil or water; however, progesterone mixed with water has caused abscesses in some women, so oil is preferred.[21] Usually, 100 mg of I.M. progesterone is injected into the buttocks. This should cause the woman to bleed within 2 weeks.

If the woman fails to bleed from a 100-mg injection, the doctor will give a second injection of 200 mg. Some doctors will give the 200-mg injection right away, but most women who are going to bleed will do so on 100 mg, and since the 200-mg shot can be rather painful, the doctor will usually try 100 mg first, unless the woman lives far away. Rubbing down the area where the shot is given for the first few hours afterward can help eliminate much of the subsequent discomfort.

Women who are given progesterone shots may bleed quite noticeably, or there may be only slight, brown staining. This slight, brown staining is also blood. It is brown because it is old blood, but it is still a sign that estrogen is being produced, so women should examine their underclothes carefully to make sure they don't miss this vital sign.

After being given the shot of progesterone, the woman is then asked to return to the doctor's office in 3 weeks. One of two things will have happened: Either the woman will have had bleeding, as we have discussed, or she will not have had any bleeding.

Failure to Bleed After Progesterone Shot

The woman who fails to bleed after the shot of progesterone has a somewhat more serious problem. The next test the doctor should do is a serum FSH. If the FSH level is high, this indicates (in the woman who has failed to bleed from a shot of progesterone) that the ovaries have failed, for there is plenty of FSH to stimulate the follicles and produce estrogen. The problem is in the ovary, and this woman has premature menopause.

If the woman fails to bleed after the shot of progesterone but the FSH levels are low or pseudonormal, this woman has a problem in either the pituitary, which is the source of FSH, or the hypothalamus, which is indirectly responsible for FSH production. She must be referred to a specialist for X-rays and other studies to rule out a tumor or other abnormality.

After a woman with amenorrhea has received a complete diagnostic workup, as described above, treatment may be given. In those cases where a brain tumor or disease has been ruled out but the woman remains amenorrheic, menstruation may be induced every few months as follow-up and to prevent hyperplasia. If the woman wants to get pregnant and is not ovulating because of a hormonal imbalance, it is sometimes possible to use fertility drugs to achieve pregnancy.

ABNORMAL UTERINE BLEEDING

Types: anatomical uterine bleeding
dysfunctional uterine bleeding

Associated Terms: hypomenorrhea, hypermenorrhea, oligomenorrhea, polymenorrhea, menorrhagia, intermenstrual bleeding, contact bleeding, metrorrhagia, postmenopausal bleeding, breakthrough bleeding, withdrawal bleeding

Abnormal uterine bleeding is not a disease but a symptom. It may result from a wide variety of factors, and sometimes its cause is not understood. The bleeding may vary from mild to severe and may take on a number of patterns. It may be indicative of a serious problem or may be only a temporary, minor problem. Any persistent abnormalities in the usual monthly bleeding pattern or unexpected vaginal bleeding should be brought to a doctor's attention.

Incidence

Abnormal bleeding is common in young women who have just begun to menstruate, for their cycles have not yet stabilized. It is also common during menopause, when the menstrual cycle is tapering off.

Types and Causes

Abnormal uterine bleeding may take many forms. The menstrual period may be disturbed. The flow may be scanty (hypomenorrhea) or it may be excessive, requiring more than six to eight napkins or tampons a day to control the flow (hypermenorrhea). The interval between periods (which may range from 20 to 36 or 40 days and still be considered normal) may be excessively long (oligomenorrhea) or too short (polymenorrhea). If the bleeding is profuse and the period is prolonged as well, the term "menorrhagia" is used.

The menstrual period may be late and the bleeding very heavy. This can happen with an ectopic pregnancy or a miscarriage. Women who don't ovulate for one reason or another may also have this sort of bleeding pattern.

The bleeding may occur at regular intervals, but it might be prolonged or heavy. Pelvic inflammatory disease, endometrial polyps, fibroid tumors, and adenomyosis are all examples of diseases or conditions that could cause this type of abnormal uterine bleeding. The use of an IUD may be a factor. Women who have certain blood disorders, such as severe anemia or leukemia, or whose blood doesn't clot properly because of medications they are taking or because they have a particular disease may also have long, heavy periods.

The bleeding may take the form of spotting in between periods or light bleeding that occurs at the time of ovulation. About 10 percent of women experience bleeding at ovulation, probably because of the drop in estrogen levels that occurs at that time. If a woman has this type of bleeding, which is harmless, her period should start almost exactly 14 days later.

Sometimes the bleeding will be irregular and unpredictable. In such cases the term "metrorrhagia" is used. The bleeding may be continuous or the woman may bleed for several days, stop for a few days, and then start again. The bleeding may be slight or it may be profuse. This type of bleeding may be caused by pelvic inflammatory disease, endometrial polyps, birth control pills, an IUD, thyroid deficiency, ectopic pregnancy, uterine or cervical cancer, endometrial hyperplasia or any disturbance in hormonal balance.

Abnormal bleeding that occurs in postmenopausal women may result from estrogen replacement therapy, postmenopausal vaginitis or endometrial hyperplasia, but it may also be caused by cervical or uterine cancer. Since women in this age-group are more likely to have cancer than are younger women, postmenopausal abnormal bleeding requires prompt attention.

Hormonal imbalances may be responsible for a variety of abnormal uterine bleeding patterns. Problems in the hypothalamus, the master gland that orchestrates the menstrual cycle, the pituitary gland or the ovaries can be responsible for abnormal bleeding. Sometimes the hormones are disturbed in such a way that ovulation fails to occur. This is called anovulatory bleeding. Sometimes the corpus luteum, the remnants of the follicle containing the ripe egg that bursts open at ovulation and that produces progesterone, functions improperly, producing too little or too much progesterone. If the thyroid gland isn't producing enough thyroid, this too may upset the delicate hormonal balance. Since the kidney is responsible for eliminating estrogen from the body, chronic kidney infections can interfere with the body's elimination, causing too high a level of estrogen in the body. In a similar fashion, chronic liver problems can lead to hormone imbalances.

Table 27 lists the many causes of abnormal uterine bleeding.

Diagnosis

The diagnosis of the cause of abnormal uterine bleeding is basically a process of elimination. A careful medical history, bimanual pelvic and speculum exams, pregnancy tests and a Pap smear may lead to the discovery of the cause of the abnormal bleeding. Blood tests may also pinpoint the cause of the disease. Thyroid tests may also be useful. X-ray studies of the uterus, called hysterosalpingograms, may be done. In some cases, laparoscopic or culdoscopic examination may be necessary.

A dilation and curettage (D&C), a process by which the cervix is dilated, the endometrial lining removed and the inside of the cervix carefully explored for abnormalities, may also be called for. In teenage girls the doctor will try to avoid the D&C. Abnormal uterine bleeding often occurs in this age-group

Table 27
Causes of Abnormal Uterine Bleeding

Pelvic inflammatory disease	Uterine cancer
Endometrial polyps	Estrogen replacement therapy
Endometrial hyperplasia	Chronic kidney or liver problems
Uterine fibroids	Benign ovarian tumors
Adenomyosis	Polycystic ovarian disease (onset)
Endometriosis	Physiologic cysts of the ovaries
Intrauterine devices	Functioning ovarian tumors
Severe anemia	Ovarian cancer
Blood disorders	Cancer of the fallopian tubes
Birth control pills	Tumors of the fallopian tubes
Ectopic pregnancy	Miscarriage
Thyroid deficiency	Hormonal imbalances
Cervical cancer	Trophoblastic disease
Cervical erosion	Ovulation
Cervical polyps	

when the menstrual cycle is just starting up and the system is not yet perfectly synchronized, and the cycle often stabilizes itself with the passage of time. In older women, particularly in postmenopausal women, a D&C must be done to rule out cancer and other causes.

One important diagnostic question is whether or not the woman is ovulating. Vaginal smears, endometrial biopsies, basal body temperature charts or urinary tests to detect progesterone may help the doctor decide whether or not the woman is ovulating. If a D&C is done, examination of the tissue removed will indicate whether or not the woman has been ovulating. If the woman is ovulating, the search for an organic or anatomical cause must be thorough, for dysfunctional bleeding occurs with ovulating cycles in only about 10 percent of cases. When such cases do occur it's usually because the corpus luteum, the source of progesterone, has failed to regress completely.

If the woman's cycles are anovulatory and no specific disease that could cause failure of ovulation is found, a complete hormone workup done by a specialist may be necessary.

Treatment

Treatment of abnormal uterine bleeding will depend on the severity of the bleeding, the suspected cause of the bleeding and the age of the patient.

If a D&C has been done as part of the diagnostic workup, further treatment may not be required, because for reasons that are not clear, the cleaning out of the uterus puts an end to the abnormal bleeding problems in 40 percent to 60 percent of such cases. Sometimes even if the first D&C has no effect, a repeat D&C may be successful. If the problem is a polyp, a submucous fibroid tumor, or a hormonal imbalance, the D&C cannot cure the problem.

Hormone therapy may be used to treat abnormal uterine bleeding. This type of therapy may be used in young girls in whom the doctor is trying to avoid a D&C, in women whose diagnostic tests have suggested a hormonal cause for the bleeding and in women whose first D&C proved unsuccessful.

The aim of hormonal therapy is usually twofold: to stop severe bleeding and, once that is accomplished, to restore normal menstrual cycles. Estrogen, progesterone and combinations of the two have been used, and all these will stop the bleeding. However, most authorities today believe it is best to use a drug that is predominately progesterone but that also has mild estrogen and androgen (male-type hormone) effects, such as norethindrone (Norlutin). This type of drug gives the most prompt relief from bleeding, is well tolerated by most women, isn't associated with the severe side effects caused by the other drugs and doesn't cause breakthrough bleeding. Provera may also be used. The drug is given continuously for various amounts of time, depending on how heavy the bleeding is. If the bleeding is severe, the woman may be kept on the drug for several weeks to allow her blood levels to return to normal. (Hormone therapy should not be started until pregnancy has been ruled out, since hormones have been associated with birth defects.)

Once the bleeding has been stopped for the appropriate amount of time, the medication is discontinued, which will usually cause the bleeding to begin again in a few days.

The bleeding occurs as a result of a process similar to that which takes place in a normal menstrual cycle: The constant progesterone stimulation of the medication causes the endometrial lining to thicken, just as it does in response to the progesterone normally produced by the body during the second half of the menstrual cycle. In the normal menstrual cycle if pregnancy does not occur, the levels of progesterone gradually diminish, causing the endometrial lining to break down and shed. Discontinuing the medication brings about the same result. The levels of progesterone in the body fall and the lining breaks down and is shed; hence bleeding resumes. In effect, the medication accomplishes the same thing as a D&C—removing the endometrial lining by a sort of "medical curettage."

After the bleeding has continued for 4 days the medication is given again from Day 5 to Day 25 of the menstrual cycle. This regimen is followed for a few months. The medication is then discontinued altogether, to allow the woman's body to resume normal menstrual function by itself. Many times this sort of hormonal therapy will have the effect of "priming the pump"; the boost of the hormone treatment will be enough to return the woman's cycles to normal.

Unfortunately, some doctors don't have a clear understanding of the underlying hormonal problems that can cause abnormal uterine bleeding or the effects of the various types of hormone medications available. According to authorities in the field, the four most common mistakes made in medical treatment are as follows:[22]

1. The doctor may choose a drug that has an estrogen/progesterone balance unfavorable to the prompt relief of bleeding
2. The doctor may not prescribe an adequate dose of the hormone, prescribing an amount sufficient for contraception but not sufficient for treatment of abnormal bleeding
3. The doctor may interpret the initial stoppage of bleeding as success of the treatment and discontinue the drug
4. The doctor may misinterpret the initial withdrawal bleeding after the drug is discontinued as failure of treatment and recurrence of the abnormal bleeding problem

These kinds of mistakes could lead to unnecessary D&C's or even to unnecessary hysterectomies.

The type of hormone therapy described here is just one of many possibilities. It has particular applications for abnormal uterine bleeding associated with anovulatory cycles. Other instances may require different therapies. For instance, Clomid, a drug that stimulates ovulation, may be effective in treating cases where the problem is related to persistent activity of the corpus luteum. In such cases, although the bleeding is not anovulatory, Clomid has proved to be effective. It is also effective in women who have anovulatory cycles and who wish to become pregnant. Women who have anovulatory cycles but who have recurrent bleeding after a D&C or hormone therapy, may be treated successfully with Clomid as well. Many doctors, however, don't like to use Clomid unless a woman is particularly desirous of pregnancy, since use of the drug carries certain risks.

It is impossible to describe all the varieties of hormone therapy, but since, as outlined above, mistakes are made by doctors, a woman whose doctor suggests another type of hormone therapy would do well to take this book with her and ask the doctor why s/he is suggesting a particular form of therapy. That way the woman will be sure that her doctor is acting from a legitimate medical basis rather than from ignorance.

A hysterectomy, a surgical removal of the uterus, is sometimes necessary. If the bleeding is associated with fibroid tumors, endometriosis or pelvic inflammatory disease, and if less drastic forms of treatment for these conditions are not successful—or if the cause of the bleeding cannot be identified and repeated D&C's and hormone therapy have not been successful—in all these cases a hysterectomy may be in order, depending on the severity of the bleeding.

PRECOCIOUS PUBERTY

Types: true, or constitutional, precocious puberty
      pseudoprecocious puberty

Definitions differ somewhat, but generally, if breast development, pubic hair and other signs of puberty appear before age 8, the girl is said to have precocious puberty.

Types and Causes

Basically, there are two types of precocious puberty: true, or constitutional, precocious puberty and pseudoprecocious puberty. In true precocious puberty the whole maturation process has for some reason been stepped up. Girls with this type of precocious puberty go through the normal sequence of developmental stages and ovulate and function as completely normal women; however, they do so abnormally early in life. Pseudoprecocious puberty, on the other hand, is not an acceleration of the normal maturation process. Instead,

640

some disease or abnormality has caused the body to produce estrogen. These girls are not really biologically mature, for they do not ovulate (produce a ripe egg from the ovary each month). They do, however, show signs of sexual development owing to the abnormal amounts of estrogen in their bodies.

Pseudoprecocious puberty may be caused by an ovarian tumor, hypothyroidism, a tumor of the adrenal glands, a brain tumor or some other form of brain disease.

Symptoms

The symptoms of both types of precocious puberty are pretty much the same and are the changes normally associated with puberty: development of breast buds, darkening of the skin around the nipple and the lips of the vulva, the growth of pubic and underarm hair and bleeding from the uterus. In true precocious puberty this bleeding is true menstrual bleeding: The estrogen stimulates the lining to grow thicker and thicker; a ripe egg bursts out of its follicular sac in the ovary; the remnants of this burst follicular sac then produce progesterone. If pregnancy does not occur, progesterone levels fall and the lining of the uterus, which has grown thick and rich in response to the progesterone and estrogen, breaks down and is shed, just as in normal females.

In pseudoprecocious puberty the girl may also bleed from the uterus on a fairly regular basis, but this is not true menstrual bleeding, and she doesn't ovulate or produce progesterone. However, the estrogen in her body stimulates the uterine lining to grow rich and thick, and finally, it gets so thick that pieces of it break away and are shed, mimicking menstrual bleeding.

Girls with precocious puberty differ from normal girls in several noteworthy respects: Although they are tall for their age when they first begin to develop symptoms, this growth spurt is not sustained, and such girls often end up being shorter than average by the time they reach their 20s. Moreover, their heads tend to be larger than normal and they tend to have a long trunk and short legs.

Diagnosis and Treatment

It is important to distinguish between true precocious puberty and pseudoprecocious puberty. In the former case the girl can get pregnant, and in the second case there is an underlying disease that requires treatment. Electroencephalograms, tests that measure brain waves, hormone tests and X-rays may be needed. Girls with true precocious puberty generally do not require treatment. Girls with pseudoprecocious puberty need to have surgery or other appropriate forms of treatment. Sometimes treatment is not possible, and such children may die. The cause of such deaths is not well understood, but luckily they are uncommon.

MENOPAUSAL CHANGES

AKA: change of life, menopause, climacteric

Associated Terms: menopausal syndrome, climacteric syndrome, hot flashes, hot flushes

When a woman reaches her late 40s or early to middle 50s she stops ovulating (producing a ripe egg) and menstruating each month. Thus the levels of the hormones estrogen and progesterone produced by her body are generally much lower than before menopause. The term "menopause" refers to the end of ovulation and menstruation. The broader term "climacteric" refers to the transition years between the reproductive and postreproductive years in a woman's life. Even though the two terms don't have precisely the same meaning, they are often used interchangeably.

We have included this section on menopausal changes here in the reference section on diseases because some women experience problems and symptoms during their menopause that lead them to seek medical care. However, by including menopausal changes in this reference section, we don't mean to imply that menopause is some kind of problem or disease. Most women don't have any more problems going through the climacteric, or the menopause, than they did going through puberty. This doesn't mean that they don't notice changes in their bodies. Just as we notice bodily changes during puberty, when the monthly menstrual cycle is first gearing up, so we notice changes during menopause, when the menstrual cycle and the monthly ebb and flow of hormones is slowing down. But for most women those changes don't cause any problems. According to a study done in England, about 90 percent of women go through menopause and carry on their normal activities without interruption.[23] Approximately 16 percent of the women in that study had no symptoms associated with their menopause. For about 62 percent of women the only symptoms or bodily changes they noticed were hot flashes (see below). Only about 10 percent of women experienced menopausal symptoms or bodily changes serious enough to lead them to seek medical help. Studies done in the United States confirm that only about 10 percent of menopausal women seek help for symptoms they associate with menopause.

Despite the fact that only 10 percent of women experience disturbing symptoms during menopause, the medical profession has tended to view menopause in all women as a disease of some sort. Because a woman stops ovulating, and consequently stops (usually) producing as much estrogen as she did when she was younger, doctors have thought of menopause as an estrogen-deficiency disease that they could "cure" by giving women daily doses of estrogen tablets. Beginning in the 1950s it became fashionable among gynecologists to prescribe estrogen for menopausal women to keep them "forever young" (as the advertising slogan went). Estrogen replacement therapy (ERT), that is, daily doses of prescribed estrogen, were supposed to keep women young, wrinkle-free, slim and trim and to prevent the depression and the decline in sexual interest that menopausal women were supposedly prone to.

We now know that taking estrogen will not keep you "forever young," and that the declining levels of estrogen in most menopausal women's bodies are in no way related to wrinkles, sexual desire, weight gain, depression or most of the symptoms for which ERT was once prescribed. Menopause is no longer considered—at least not among enlightened doctors—a disease. Moreover, it is now recognized that the only bodily changes occurring during menopause that are actually a result of the decreased levels of estrogen are hot flashes, the drying and thinning of urinary and vaginal tissues and osteoporosis, a condition associated with loss of bone density.

In this section we discuss the kinds of bodily changes menopausal women may experience, with particular emphasis on those changes that may cause problems in about 10 percent of menopausal women.

Incidence

The average age at menopause for American women is 51.4 years.[24] However, some women experience menopause as young as age 40 (see the next section on premature menopause), and others don't stop menstruating until their mid-50s. As noted above, only about 10 percent of women experience menopausal problems serious enough to lead them to consult their doctors.

Signs and Symptoms

The most obvious sign that tells a woman she is going through the climacteric is the cessation of menstruation. Some women menstruate fairly regularly until they come to an abrupt stop; they don't have a period 1 month and never have one again. Others gear down more slowly. Some experience a gradual tapering off; the amount of flow during the period may decrease over a number of months, becoming scantier until the flow stops altogether. Some experience progressively scantier flows and/or longer times between periods, perhaps alternating with regular periods and/or missed periods, until menstruation finally ceases altogether. Some women experience heavier and/or more frequent periods until they finally stop menstruating altogether. All these patterns of bleeding are considered normal. If the flow of menstrual blood is unusually heavy or gushing, if periods occur more frequently than every 21 days

643

or if bleeding starts again a year or more after the last period, you should consult your doctor. These bleeding patterns don't necessarily mean that something is wrong, but they should be checked out. We encourage women to trust their instincts in this matter. If you have any bleeding that doesn't "feel right" to you, we think it's a good idea to see your doctor.

One of the most common bodily changes related to the decrease in estrogen during menopause are hot flashes, or flushes. A hot flash, or flush, is a feeling of being heated from inside. Researchers are not sure what causes this feeling, but it does seem to be related to the lowered levels of hormones that usually follow menopause. A flash often begins as a feeling of heat in the chest that spreads to the neck and head; at times the whole body may be affected. The skin may become bright red. Some women perspire profusely and are chilled or experience a wet, clammy feeling afterward. The flash may last for a few seconds to several minutes. It takes a half hour or so for some women's bodies to return to normal. Flashes may be accompanied by dizziness, headaches, a tingling feeling and/or palpitations (rapid heartbeats).

Flashes may occur as the menstrual cycle begins to wane, or they may not appear until sometime after the periods have stopped. For some women they occur singly; for others they occur in a series of successive flashes over a period of hours. Flashes may occur several times a day or only once or twice a week or month. They are often worse at night. Some women experience such severe night sweats that their bedclothes are literally drenched with perspiration, and they may suffer from insomnia as a result of their night sweats.

Many women say that their flashes are more apt to occur when they are tense, nervous or excited. Some women report that flashes occur more frequently when they've eaten too fast; when they've had alcohol or hot drinks; when they've eaten heavy, hot or spicy foods; when they've exercised heavily or been "rushing around"; when they've engaged in vigorous lovemaking or when they've worn excessively heavy clothing and/or covered themselves with too many blankets. Flashes may continue off and on for a year or two, but some women have them for as long as 5 years after menopause.

Some women—most in fact—might have only mild flashes. Such women may notice only that they perspire more than usual or that they sometimes suddenly find the room they're in is "too hot." Others simply have a feeling that they have to catch their breath. Some women report that their flashes are an energizing feeling.

The important thing to remember is that hot flashes are harmless. Women who are unprepared for the experience are often frightened the first time it happens. A sudden hot flash, perspiration and dizziness or palpitations can be scary if you don't know that what's happening is completely normal. But flashes are normal and, although disconcerting, are not painful.

Women cope with hot flashes in different ways. Wearing "layers" of clothing so that you can remove a sweater or jacket when you're having a flash may be helpful. Loosening your belt, unbuttoning your blouse, taking off your shoes, sitting quietly and taking a few breaths, fanning yourself, taking a shower, drinking a cool drink all may be helpful. If you have severe and troublesome flashes, some of the treatments described below may be helpful.

Another bodily change occurring during the climacteric that is related to lower levels of estrogen produced by most menopausal women's bodies is the drying out and thinning of the vulvar, vaginal and urinary tissues. When ovulation ceases the body generally produces less estrogen, hence these tissues dry out and thin. Some medical textbooks make this normal process sound horrible. Terms like "atrophic" or "senile vaginitis" are used to describe this natural process and medical descriptions can make it sound as if you're going to dry up or decay. But these terms simply mean that the vaginal tissues become drier, and the vagina itself becomes narrower and smaller. (In fact, so do the cervix and uterus.) In some women this thinning and drying out causes problems. A woman may find that she is more susceptible to urinary tract, vulvar and/or vaginal infections (*see* Postmenopausal Vaginitis and Postmenopausal Vulvitis). In some women this thinning and drying out of the vaginal and urinary tissues is associated with a prolapse (falling down) of the urinary organs, the vagina or the uterus (*see* Cystocele and Urethrocele, Rectocele and Enterocele and Prolapse of the Uterus, Vagina and Cervix).

Vaginal lubrication that occurs as a woman becomes aroused sexually may also change. During adolescence and the 20s, lubrication occurs within 10 to 30 seconds of foreplay. As a woman approaches menopause 1 to 3 minutes may be required, and lubrication may not be as profuse as it was when she was younger. This change may affect a woman's sex life. Her mate may interpret this change in body response as some sort of rejection or disinterest in sex. An understanding of this menopausal change and a frank discussion between you and your sex partner may help alleviate such misunderstandings. Treatments for this condition are described below. Some women find that the change in vaginal size makes for a "tighter fit" and increased sexual pleasure. Also, some women enjoy the fact that more foreplay is involved before they become lubricated fully.

The myth that menopausal women lose interest in sex because of the lower levels of hormones in their bodies has persisted for a long time. This myth is not true. Estrogen doesn't affect libido (sexual energy). Androgens may affect libido, but androgen production is not affected by menopause. Of course, if a woman suffers from repeated bouts of postmenopausal vaginitis or has intercourse before she is lubricated fully, intercourse may be painful. Unless these conditions are dealt with she may well be less interested in sex. But Masters and Johnson found that in healthy women menopause did not decrease the capacity for orgasm or libido.[25] Men, however, do experience changes, such as a longer time to achieve an erection and longer time interval between erections. Women's supposed sexual problems during menopause are sometimes caused by men who are bewildered by the changes in their own sexual performance and attempt to shift the ''blame'' to their partners.

Some women feel less sexually desirable after menopause, and this may affect their sex lives. Given our society's preoccupation with youth, our rather restricted Madison Avenue notions of beauty and our cultural notion that a woman's femininity is connected with her ability to bear children, it's not surprising that they feel that way. But many women experience increased sexual responsiveness after menopause, once pregnancy and birth control are no longer concerns. Menopausal changes in sexual responsiveness, if they occur, are not related to menopause itself.

Such psychological symptoms as depression, irritability, nervousness and instability have long been associated with menopause. Actually, menopausal women have only about a 7 percent incidence of depression and emotional problems serious enough to require psychiatric care, as compared with a 6 percent incidence for other age-groups.[26] According to some studies, climacteric women report a slightly higher incidence of nervousness, irritability, headaches and ''feeling blue'' than other age-groups.[27] Other studies fail to confirm these feelings. Not surprisingly, women who experience severe hot flashes that disturb their sleep are more likely to experience psychological tension than are women who don't experience insomnia. This is not to discount the psychological upset some women experience during these years. In our culture, with its sexist stereotypes and limited roles for women, the menopausal woman who has been a homemaker may find that her children have left home and she feels as if she is suddenly unemployed. Like any person forced into retirement, she may feel useless and inadequate, but these feelings and the psychological problems they create have nothing to do with menopause per se.

Another condition that apparently *is* related to menopause per se is osteoporosis, a loss in bone density. Women begin to lose bone density beginning at about age 30. Once a woman goes through menopause she begins to lose bone more rapidly, a phenomenon that is apparently related to lower levels of the hormone estrogen. Other factors, such as nutrition, exercise, cigarette smoking, body build and heredity, also play a role in osteoporosis. The effects of osteoporosis may not show up until 10 or more years after menopause. Some women have extensive loss of bone density without ever having any problems, but others are troubled by backache and dowager's hump (a hump in the back caused by compression of the vertebrae). Still others are troubled by bone fractures. Hip fractures are particularly dangerous in elderly women, for complications related to the fractures, such as heart attacks, blood clots, and pneumonia from being bedridden, can be fatal. More than 120,000 hip fractures occur in elderly women each year, resulting in 50,000 deaths.[28] Estrogen replacement therapy (ERT) can apparently prevent bone loss and bone fractures resulting from osteoporosis.[29] For this reason some doctors believe that *all* postmenopausal women should take ERT at the onset of menopause and continue to take it throughout their lives. ERT carries certain risks, however, and cannot be used by everyone. Also, osteoporosis may be prevented in other ways, so many doctors are opposed to giving ERT to every postmenopausal woman. If you are going through menopause, be sure to read the section on ERT before deciding whether or not to take hormones.

Some menopausal women put on extra weight, but weight gain has nothing to do with menopause per se. Rather, women in this age-group tend to get less exercise and don't reduce their calorie intake. Decreased levels of hormones do not cause weight gain, and taking hormones will not result in weight loss.

Menopausal women may notice the effects of aging on their skin— wrinkles, age spots and so forth. Again, these skin changes are not caused by menopause per se, and taking hormones will not prevent them. In fact, there is some evidence that estrogen can cause drying and wrinkling of the skin.[30]

Menopausal women may notice many other changes in their bodies— various aches and pains, for example—but these changes are related to the general aging process, not to menopause and changes in hormone levels.

Treatment

Many doctors prescribe ERT for menopausal changes. Women who take ERT should know that the only menopausal changes for which such treatment is effective are hot flashes, osteoporosis and the drying and thinning of vaginal and urinary tissues, and that recent research indicates that they shouldn't take estrogen without also taking progesterone.[31] ERT will not cure depression, prevent wrinkles or keep you "forever young" (*see* pp. 797–807). Also, this therapy carries certain risks and cannot be used by all women. Any woman considering hormone therapy should read the section on ERT and carefully weigh the risks against the benefits before accepting this treatment.

Alternatives to ERT can be used to treat menopausal changes. Hot flashes have been treated with Bellergal tablets taken two to four times a day. The tablets contain phenobarbital, a barbiturate sedative; ergotamine tartrate, which inhibits the nervous system; and a belladonnalike substance that also inhibits nervous system activity.[32] Like any drug, it too carries risks and side effects and cannot be used by women who have peripheral vascular disease, liver or kidney problems or glaucoma or by women who are taking dopamine for Parkinson's disease.

Daily doses of Provera (10 mg) and megestrol acetate (20 mg) taken orally have also been used to control hot flashes, as have monthly 100-mg injections of Depo-Provera.[33] But progesterone preparations also carry risks and cannot be used by all women (*see* section on Depo-Provera for details). Clonidine, an antihypertensive (anti–high blood pressure) taken orally twice a day, has also been used, although it is generally less effective in controlling flashes.[34] Also, a high rate of side effects, including dry mouth, sedation, constipation, dizziness, headache and fatigue, have been noted in women who are not hypertensive. Many doctors believe this drug should be used to control hot flashes only in women who have high blood pressure anyway.

All these drug treatments can carry risks and side effects, so many women try nondrug approaches to hot flashes. Avoiding situations and conditions that bring on flashes (see above) and the coping mechanisms, such as "layering" clothes (see above), are enough to allow some women to deal with their flashes. An ice bag or a pitcher of ice water kept by the bed may be helpful for women with night sweats. Also, a drink of cold water will stave off a flash in some women. Many women have found relief through "natural" approaches. These "natural" approaches, which include dietary changes and supplements of various vitamins and minerals and herbs like ginseng, don't work for every woman, but they may be worth a try. Rosetta Reitz, author of *Menopause: A Positive Approach* (Chilton, 1977), suggests taking 2,000 to 3,000 mg of vitamin C at intervals throughout the day, 1,000 mg of calcium from dolomite or bone meal, also taken at intervals, and vitamin E. Barbara Seaman, in her book *Women and the Crisis in Sex Hormones* (Rawson, 1977), also recommends vitamins and the Chinese herb ginseng for treatment of hot flashes. Bioflavonoids and vitamin C, as well as vitamin E and kelp, are mentioned in Emirka Padus's book, *The Woman's Encyclopedia of Health and Natural Healing* (Rodale Press, 1981). Almost everyone who advocates natural approaches stresses exercise and good diet. For details, see the aforementioned books. These books also contain good information on skin care, weight gain and other changes that, although they are not related to menopause per se, may occur at this time in a woman's life.

If vaginal lubrication is a problem, lubricants like K-Y jelly, Transi-Lube, Personal Lubrication and Surgilube, which can be purchased without a doctor's prescription, may be helpful. Petroleum jellies, such as Vaseline, should not be used as vaginal lubricants, because the petroleum derivatives may irritate the vagina. (Besides, they don't wash off easily with soap and water.)

Perhaps the best "cure" for diminished vaginal lubrication is to have sex regularly. Masters and Johnson, the noted sex researchers, found that women who had intercourse twice weekly had fewer problems with vaginal lubrication than did women who had sexual activity less often.[35] They also found that menopausal women who were more sexually active had less reduction of their estrogen production after menopause. Although it has not been proved scientifically, it seems logical that having sex on a regular basis and its consequent higher levels of estrogen may well influence other menopausal symptoms related to lower levels of estrogen (for example, hot flashes, thinning and drying of urinary and vaginal tissues and their complications—postmenopausal vulvitis and vaginitis, cystocele, urethrocele and uterine/vaginal/cervical prolapse and, perhaps, even osteoporosis). At any rate the inescapable conclusion is that regular sexual activity after menopause is good for your health. For women who don't have regular sexual partners, masturbation, which is also a form of sexual activity, will undoubtedly have the same beneficial effects.

The treatment of postmenopausal vaginitis and vulvitis, cystoceles, rectoceles and prolapse of the uterus, vagina and cervix are discussed under the appropriate headings elsewhere in this book. The treatment of osteoporosis is discussed in the section on estrogen replacement therapy.

PREMATURE MENOPAUSE

AKA: early menopause

Types: artificial, or induced, menopause
       primary ovarian failure

Premature menopause is a condition in which a woman experiences menopause, the cessation of menstrual periods, before the usual age. A premature menopause may be artificial or induced. This occurs when both ovaries are destroyed by surgery, radiation therapy, disease or, in rare cases, the use of certain medications. Sometimes, even though a woman hasn't had an induced menopause, her ovaries cease to function normally. This condition is called primary ovarian failure.

Any induced menopause is a premature menopause. If a woman has primary ovarian failure and experiences menopause before age 40, most doctors would call this a premature menopause; others use age 35 and still others age 45 to define premature menopause.

Causes

As noted, artificial or induced menopause can be caused by radiation therapy, disease, the use of large doses of fertility drugs or, in rare instances, tubal ligation done for sterilization purposes.

The ovaries may be destroyed by ovarian tumors, pelvic inflammatory disease or cancer, and they are then removed in an operation known as bilateral oophorectomy. Sometimes, however, the ovaries are removed even though they are healthy. Some doctors remove the ovaries as well as the uterus in all women over age 35 who are having hysterectomies. Others remove the ovaries in their hysterectomy patients who are over age 40; still others use age 45 as a cutoff. The pros and cons of combining the removal of healthy ovaries in women having hysterectomies are discussed in greater detail under the heading Hysterectomy. Whether the ovaries removed are diseased or healthy, this

649

type of surgery generally results in premature menopause. Sometimes a hysterectomy will result in premature menopause even if the ovaries have not been removed. Tubal ligation (female sterilization) may also, on rare occasions, cause a premature menopause. In both cases the condition probably results from interruption of the blood supply to the ovaries or damage to the ovaries during surgery.

Although the causes of primary ovarian failure are not well understood, it is thought that some women are born with ovaries that have a fewer number of eggs and hence "run out" of eggs at an earlier age; or it may be that the ovaries have received too much stimulation from the pituitary gland, causing the ovary to exhaust its supply of eggs and thus bringing on a premature menopause.

Symptoms

The symptoms of premature menopause are the same as those of a natural menopause, only they are usually severer. In artificial menopause, instead of a gradual decline in hormone production, there is an abrupt cessation. Since the body isn't able to adjust gradually to lowered levels of hormones as it does in a natural menopause, the abrupt transition may be more difficult and the menopausal symptoms intensified.

In women who have primary ovarian failure the most obvious symptom will be the absence of menstruation. The diagnosis of women with primary ovarian failure is covered in more detail under the heading Amenorrhea.

Women who have a premature menopause may be at higher risk of developing heart disease; hypertension, a condition characterized by high blood pressure; and osteoporosis, a condition in which there is a loss of bone density, making the woman more susceptible to bone fractures. However, women who have a premature menopause may be at decreased risk of developing breast cancer.

Treatment

Premature menopause may not require any treatment. If, however, a woman has severe symptoms, these may be dealt with in the same manner as severe menopausal symptoms (see the previous section on Menopausal Changes).

There is disagreement among doctors as to whether or not women who experience menopause at a particularly early age, yet do not have symptoms, should be given estrogen replacement therapy. This is discussed more fully under the heading Estrogen Replacement Therapy.

TOXIC SHOCK SYNDROME[36]

AKA: TSS

Toxic shock syndrome (TSS) is not, strictly speaking, a menstrual problem. It is an overwhelming systemic infection that can begin in the vagina, but since the majority of women who get TSS get it during their menstrual periods, and since it seems to be related to the use of tampons, we have chosen to include it here.

TSS is a newly defined disease about which there are many unanswered questions. Some doctors believe that the disease has been around, although not defined as such, for more than 60 years. Others believe that TSS, at least the form of the disease that affects menstruating women, is a fairly recent phenomenon.

Incidence

TSS is supposedly a relatively uncommon disease. The incidence rate is 8.9 to 15 cases per 100,000 menstruating women.[37] Some researchers believe the actual incidence rate may be much higher.[38] They point out that milder cases may go unrecognized or unreported.

TSS usually affects menstruating women under age 30, but men and children as well as nonmenstruating and older women have been affected by what may be the same disease.

Cause

The disease is thought to be caused by *Staphylococcus aureus,* a bacterium that is often found in the nose and mouth, or by an associated virus.[39] Approximately 5 percent to 15 percent of women have this organism in their vaginas. The organisms produce a toxin. If a sufficient number of organisms are present and enough toxin is released into the bloodstream, the woman may develop an overwhelming infection that may have fatal consequences.

Tampons apparently play a role in the disease. The majority of women with the disease have been tampon users. One brand in particular, Rely tampons, has been associated with the disease, but other brands, contraceptive sponges and the natural sponges some women use to collect the menstrual flow have been associated with TSS. The syndrome was first identified about the time that Rely came on the market. Rely contained new superabsorbent fibers and quickly captured 20 percent of the market. Competitors followed suit and reconstituted their tampons, so that most of the tampons now on the market contain some sort of superabsorbent fiber.

651

No one is certain how tampon usage contributes to the disease. The most widely held theory is that tampons trap the blood and staph organisms, thereby providing a breeding ground for the staph. Because the superabsorbent tampons tend to be left in for longer periods, they may be giving the organisms more of a chance to produce their toxins. However, the disease has also occurred in women who have changed their tampons frequently. Another theory holds that the tampons absorb the normal vaginal secretions as well as the menstrual blood, thereby altering the acid/alkaline environment of the vagina and making it more conducive to the growth of the staph organisms (*see* p. 299).

Another possibility is that the staph can get into the bloodstream more easily because of microscopic lacerations or abrasions that these superabsorbent fibers can create on the vaginal wall. Still another possibility is that there is something about the makeup of the fibers themselves that aids the growth of the staph organism.

Symptoms

The disease is characterized by the sudden onset of fever, vomiting and diarrhea. Sometimes there is accompanying headache, sore throat and aching muscles. The women may feel dizzy and/or faint. Within about 48 hours there may be a dramatic drop in blood pressure. The woman may go into shock and become disoriented, and her kidneys may fail. At the same time a red rash that peels like sunburn may develop. The disease tends to recur, usually within the first few menstrual cycles, in about 30 percent of cases and may be fatal. In milder cases only some of these symptoms may be evident.

If you are menstruating and experience a sudden high fever (usually over 102°F), accompanied by vomiting and/or diarrhea, contact your doctor immediately. If you are wearing a tampon, remove it.

Treatment

Medication to stabilize the blood pressure and fluids may be given. Large doses of antibiotics are given to combat the infection. Antibiotics are important even in milder cases as they have been shown to cut down on recurrences. Treatment with a special type of antibiotic known as a beta lactamase–resistant antibiotic (ampicillin, streptomycin) has been shown to cut down on recurrence rates.[40]

Prevention

The best prevention is to stop using tampons, at least until more is known. If you continue to wear them, don't use the Rely brand (they've been withdrawn by manufacturers); use all-cotton tampons, like regular Tampax; change your tampons at least four times a day; alternate between tampons and pads (this is thought shown to reduce your chances of getting TSS); use the lowest possible absorbency tampon.

Some women are using natural sponges instead of tampons, but at least one case of TSS has been associated with natural sponge usage. Some researchers have found sand and other impurities in these sponges, so if their use becomes more widespread, we may see more cases of sponge-related TSS.

If you do develop TSS, do not use tampons even after the disease has cleared up because of the possibility of recurrence.

Complications

TSS may produce aneurysms—dilations of the blood vessels—that can lead to heart and vascular problems. Some researchers advise women who've had TSS to keep to a low-cholesterol diet and to have frequent checkups for cardiovascular irregularities.[41] About 5 percent of women who develop TSS die as a result of complications.[42]

Problems Related to Pregnancy and Fertility

The conditions described in this section are related to pregnancy and fertility. A complete survey of the medical considerations of pregnancy is beyond the scope of this book; however, we have chosen to include certain of these conditions because they occur in the early stages of pregnancy, in some cases before a woman is even aware that she is pregnant, and can produce symptoms, such as vaginal bleeding and lower abdominal pain, that may be associated with a number of gynecological problems in the nonpregnant woman.

All the conditions described here involve either the inability to get pregnant—infertility—or the involuntary termination of a pregnancy, either because of a miscarriage, an ectopic pregnancy, trophoblastic disease or repeated miscarriages. Women who don't have menstrual periods, a condition known as amenorrhea, will also have an infertility problem, but this is discussed in the section on menstrual problems.

Myths About Infertility

There are a number of myths surrounding infertility, some of which can make the emotionally difficult task of dealing with this problem even harder. One myth is that infertility is largely a psychological problem, that, deep down, infertile couples—or more specifically, infertile women—really don't want to become pregnant. This is simply not true; in 70 percent to 90 percent of cases, a specific medical explanation for the infertility can be found. This does not necessarily mean, in the remaining cases, for which no medical explanation can be discovered, that "psychological factors" are responsible; it merely means that medical science has not advanced enough to identify the problem.

Another myth is that infertile couples often conceive after having adopted children. Again, this is simply not true. About 5 percent of infertile couples will indeed conceive after adopting, but 5 percent of all infertile couples will experience a spontaneous cure of their problem whether they adopt or not.[1]

Yet another myth is that female factors are most often the cause of fertility problems—also not true. In about 35 percent to 40 percent of cases in which a specific cause for the problem can be found, female factors are responsible; in another 35 percent to 40 percent it's male factors. In the 20 percent to 30 percent that remain, it is either a shared problem or there is a cause that cannot be identified.

Emotional Stress and Infertility

A couple with an infertility problem is likely to encounter a lot of social pressure. Relatives are apt to come up with questions such as, "When are you going to give us the grandchild we're waiting for?" People who hardly know us are apt to question us about our childless state or our future childbearing plans. Because of all the myths and misinformation about infertility, people often interpret the anxiety, frustration and depression an infertile couple is likely to experience as the *cause* rather than the *result* of the problem. "Just relax, and you'll get pregnant" is a typical piece of advice. Such advice not only shows an ignorance of the medical realities of the situation but is also a huge put-down, implying that it is the couple's fault—their own uptightness—that is keeping them from conceiving.

Cultural expectations and assumptions about sexuality, femininity, masculinity and fertility add to the problem. Most of us, either consciously or unconsciously, think that a man's ability to father children is somehow tied up with his virility, with his worth as a man, and that a woman's ability to become pregnant is somehow a sign of her womanliness, an indication of her femininity. These old roles and notions are changing, but they still exert a strong influence on our emotional selves. Men and women with infertility problems are likely to have questions about their sexual selves. There may be terrible doubts about their adequacy and their worth as human beings.

Being diagnosed for an infertility problem can also put a strain on the infertile couple. Having to subject the details of their sex life to a doctor's scrutiny, scheduling lovemaking for optimum chances of conception and having to keep records and charts of sexual activity can have a bad effect on a couple's sex life. The importance that each act of lovemaking takes on—for after all, *this* could be *the* time—can be exciting but also stressful.

655

It is not unusual for such couples to experience impotence, a decrease in sex drive and inability to reach orgasm during this time. All aspects of their relationship may suffer, not just their sex life, especially if one partner wants the pregnancy more than the other, or if, as is often the case, it is seen as the woman's problem and responsibility—*her* charts, *her* sexual schedules, *her* doctor's appointments. Agreeing to take a vacation from sex for a time, sharing the responsibility for keeping charts and so on, as well as talking ahead of time about the kinds of feelings you are likely to experience, can be helpful.

Finding a doctor with whom you feel comfortable and who not only can answer your questions but also offer emotional support is vitally important. Finding a support group composed of other couples who are going through the same crisis can also be helpful, and your doctor or a staff member at an infertility clinic at a large medical center should be able to put you in touch with such groups. There is also a national organization called RESOLVE that is specifically designed to help people with infertility problems. A local chapter may be listed in your phone book, or you can contact the national headquarters (P.O. Box 474, Belmont, Massachusetts 02178, 617-484-2424) for information about RESOLVE chapters in your area.

If the fertility workup fails to disclose a specific cause for the fertility problem, or if treatment is not possible or is unsuccessful and the couple remains childless, there are apt to be feelings of intense disappointment and grief, mourning for all the children that will never be born. Anger and resentment are natural reactions as well. If the cause has been isolated and one partner or the other is the source of the infertility problem, the infertile partner is apt to feel that the fertile partner wants to leave the relationship and is concealing terrible, negative feelings about the infertile partner. It may be true that the fertile partner has feelings of disappointment and anger. It is better to talk out these feelings honestly rather than bottle them up, for they will eventually come out in other, less direct, less healthy ways. Finding a therapist to help you work through this emotional crisis can help. For many couples this difficult experience can actually bring them closer together, creating a new and special kind of caring and feeling for each other out of their shared disappointment.

Anywhere from 30 percent to 50 percent of couples being treated for infertility will become pregnant within the first 2 years of treatment. After that, there is still hope. Five percent of all such couples experience a spontaneous cure, sometimes after many years of childlessness. Then, too, new techniques are being developed all the time. But this glimmer of hope is only that—a glimmer—and for some couples this tiny chance may be more difficult to deal with than the absolute knowledge that they can never conceive.

656

Miscarriage

Miscarriages are also likely to result in emotional complications. Grief and sorrow, especially if the pregnancy was eagerly awaited, are, of course, the overwhelming reactions. There may also be feelings of guilt. Many couples think their sex life was too vigorous, causing the miscarriage (not true). A woman is apt to believe that something she did or didn't do was responsible for the spontaneous abortion or that there is something wrong with her. Fear that it will happen again is also a natural response. However, 80 percent of women who have a single miscarriage will have no problems with subsequent pregnancies.

All these emotions may be further compounded by the frustrations a couple experiences when they try to seek answers to their basic questions, "Why did this happen? Is there something wrong with me or with us? Will it happen again?"

Repeated Miscarriages

A couple or a woman who experiences a series of miscarriages, a condition known as habitual abortion, is likely to experience even more severe emotional trauma. One miscarriage is bad enough, but two, three, four or more can be totally wrenching. To make matters worse, the couple, in particular the woman, is likely to encounter a good deal of prejudice about her condition and a lot of sexist attitudes from the medical profession. Many, if not most, doctors have been trained to think of women who are habitual aborters as neurotic personality types and to attribute a habitual abortion problem for which they are unable to identify a specific medical cause to emotional factors, even though there is no scientific evidence to support this viewpoint. This myth is perhaps the cruelest of all, for it is believed by many doctors, the very people to whom the woman suffering from this problem must turn for help.

A look at how the topic of habitual abortion and psychological factors is treated in the most recent edition of one of the most widely used gynecological textbooks in the United States, reveals the incredible prejudice that clouds doctors' thinking on this subject.[2]

"There is mounting evidence that emotional factors play a role in etiology [cause] of repeated pregnancy loss," claim the authors. The "mounting evidence" subsequently cited in this text includes the opinion of two doctors who "have *always felt* [emphasis ours] that stress and emotional problems were responsible for many cases of habitual abortion." These two doctors claim an 80 percent success rate in treating habitual abortion through psychotherapy; but as the authors themselves point out, an 80 percent cure rate is about what one would expect from the treatment of infertility cases.

657

The authors further inform their medical-student readers that another team of two doctors has "noted two distinct types of personality among women who abort repeatedly: (a) basically immature women who are not ready to assume the full responsibility of being either a woman or a mother, or (b) they are frustrated women who have adjusted to a man's world and whose main aspirations are beyond what they believe to be their feminine limits." Moreover, the reader is told that "a few of these women have the instinct to destroy not only themselves but others." No mention is made of the type of psychological tests employed to determine who is "immature" or "frustrated," because obviously there are no valid psychological tests to measure such sexist perceptions. The evidence that women who are habitual aborters are neurotic personality types is merely the opinion of these male doctors.

The medical student reading these texts is then told that therapy is a good idea for such women and should "proceed along common sense lines . . ." The therapy, which apparently is administered not by a trained psychotherapist but by the gynecologist, is "time consuming" and requires "repetitive visits." No mention is made of how expensive these visits are for the "irresponsible" and "immature" habitual aborter who has to pay for them, nor of how profitable they are for the doctor who is going to charge her for them even though, by the authors' own admission, her chances of improving her habitual abortion problem will not be significantly improved.

The authors close with the following totally unscientific statement endorsing their commonsense therapy: "This type of therapy is far more effective than the older methods of pampering the mother by putting her to bed, applying heat, giving vitamins and hormones and telling her to avoid intercourse." We do not recommend the old therapy, especially in light of new evidence that estrogen or progesterone hormone therapy is not only ineffective but may also cause birth defects. Indeed, such estrogen therapy has clearly been shown to cause abnormalities, including a rare form of vaginal cancer in the teenage daughters of women who were given the hormone DES to prevent miscarriage.[3] However, the new therapy of "common sense" psychotherapy, administered by gynecologists steeped in sexist prejudices of the kind reflected in this text and untrained in psychotherapy, hardly seems much of an improvement.

If you are seeking help for an habitual abortion problem, you should remember that chances are your doctor used this very text (or, heaven forbid, an earlier edition) in medical school. Although the good doc may do a bang-up job of assaying your hormone levels, any nonmedical conclusions are likely to be just so much nonsense. If the source of your problem lies beyond the limits of present medical knowledge, and the doctor can't identify the cause or find a cure, it is possible that instead of frankly admitting ignorance the doctor will pull the old switcheroo: "I-can't-figure-out-what's-wrong-with-you-so-you-must-be-crazy."

A woman who has gone through the trauma of three or more miscarriages and suffered the loss of new and eagerly awaited life growing in her body, may quite naturally feel shaky emotionally. She may be having terrible feelings of inadequacy and is apt to be vulnerable. The last thing she needs is a doctor who tells her, directly or indirectly, that she is neurotic and that her emotional problems are the cause of her habitual abortion problem. Indeed, for doctors to inflict this sexist assumption, for which there is absolutely no scientific evidence, on such women is cruel and irresponsible.

If your doctor seems to be working from an "it's-all-in-your-head-dearie" diagnosis, don't buy it. Such prejudiced assumptions about your condition could stand in the way of your receiving the optimum medical care for your condition. Find another doctor.

INFERTILITY AND STERILITY

AKA: inability to get pregnant

Sterility is defined as the absolute inability to conceive. Infertility is defined as the inability to get pregnant after 1 year or more of regular sexual activity (without the use of contraception, of course) or the inability to carry a pregnancy to a live birth. The problems of miscarriage and habitual abortion are discussed elsewhere. Here we are concerned only with the inability to conceive. Some doctors define infertility in terms of 1 year; others use 2 years as the cutoff. The particular length of time used in the definition is based on studies that have shown that about 56 percent of fertile couples trying for pregnancy will do so within 1 month and about 77 percent within the first 6 months. An additional 5 percent to 10 percent will become pregnant within the following year. However, anyone has the right to seek medical help whenever they themselves believe that infertility is a problem. Women in their 30s who are having trouble getting pregnant may want to seek help after only 4 or 5 months, for their fertility is dropping and the chances of getting pregnant are declining with the passage of time. Moreover, after 35 the incidence of birth defects is much higher. Women who are not menstruating regularly may also want to seek treatment without waiting, since irregular menstrual cycles may mean that they are not ovulating. Such women are not likely to conceive without treatment. A woman who has a history of pelvic infections or a man who has a history of mumps might also forego the waiting period.

Most people seeking help for an infertility problem are couples; however, in some cases either the male partner refuses to seek medical help or the woman is single. If the husband refuses to participate in the diagnostic tests, this will obviously limit the scope of the diagnostic investigation.

Some doctors will refuse to treat a single woman. Indeed, some may even refuse to treat an unmarried couple. A single woman seeking help for an infer-

659

tility problem should read this section carefully so that she is familiar with the tests available; otherwise, she may be given only the most cursory of exams and told there is nothing wrong with her. A more extensive diagnostic workup might have uncovered the source of the problem.

Infertility is a fairly common problem; about 10 percent to 18 percent of the population, or about one out of every six couples, is infertile at any given time. Fertility in women declines markedly with age. A woman is at the height of her fertility in her mid-20s and this slowly tapers off to about age 30 and then begins to decline. A man's fertility decreases slowly until about age 40, and then there is a more rapid decline. The incidence of infertility is rising.

Causes and Treatment of Female Infertility

There are many possible explanations for infertility. Many people believe that infertility is usually the woman's problem, but this is not true; the problem may be traced to the female or the male, or the infertility may be a result of a factor involving both of them. Most of these causes and treatments of infertility are discussed in depth elsewhere in this book. Only a summary is included here.

Pelvic Scar Tissue and Adhesions

One of the leading causes of female infertility is scar tissue and adhesions in the uterus and fallopian tubes and around the ovary. The scar tissue may be formed as the result of such infections as gonorrhea and other types of pelvic inflammatory disease. Indeed, any major infection in the pelvic cavity, for instance, an inflammation set up by a ruptured appendix, can cause scar tissue. The treatment for these problems may be a dilation and curettage (D&C), which may remove the scar tissue. Endometrial polyps, which may also be the result of infection, can be cured by D&C as well. If extensive scarring is present, laparoscopy, hysteroscopy or even major pelvic surgery, laparotomy, may be necessary to cut the scar tissue. The ligaments that hold the uterus may be tightened, lifting the entire uterus. This closes the space behind the uterus and reduces the area where scar tissue, which could bind the tube, can occur. However, many doctors question the wisdom of this operation, both because its effectiveness is questionable and because the ureters, the tubes that conduct urine from the kidney to the bladder, are so close that they could easily be damaged.

Endometriosis, a condition in which the tissue that lines the inside of the

660

uterus is found growing in abnormal locations in the pelvic cavity—for instance, on the ovaries or tubes—can also cause scar tissue and adhesions. This abnormally placed tissue tends to behave just like the normal tissue in the uterus, bleeding in response to the monthly ebb and flow of hormones. The lining of the pelvis is very sensitive to blood, and so bleeding sets up a defensive reaction in the neighboring tissue that may result in extensive adhesions and cysts on the ovaries. Treatment may be by either surgery or drugs. There is some controversy as to which is the most effective method for treating infertility associated with endometriosis. This is discussed in more detail under the heading Endometriosis.

Cervical Problems

The cervix may be the seat of a woman's infertility problem. Mucus secreted by the cervical gland changes in character and consistency over the course of a woman's menstrual cycle. At the time of ovulation it is clear and thin. On a microscopic level, the molecules of the mucus form tunnels that facilitate the sperm on its journey into the uterus. At other times of the month it is thick and impassable. If a woman's cervical mucus is always thick and impassable, this can sometimes be corrected with low doses of the hormone estrogen; however, this may involve certain risks.* Chronic cervical infections can also cause a discharge that either slows the sperm down or makes it difficult for the sperm to pass through the cervix and up into the uterus. This condition, cervicitis, may be treated with antibiotics, and if this treatment is not successful, as is often the case, the infected tissue can be destroyed by heat or freezing. This is usually a simple office procedure. Sometimes a woman's cervical secretions are too acidic, and this may create an environment that is hostile to the sperm. These overly acidic secretions can sometimes be neutralized by using certain douches just before intercourse. If these methods of dealing with a cervical mucus problem are not successful, it is sometimes possible to mechanically inject some of the husband's sperm up into the uterus, a technique known as husband insemination. This too may involve certain risks. The fertilized egg may implant too low in the uterus or may implant poorly, causing death of the fetus and miscarriage.

Then, too, mechanical obstructions, such as cervical polyps or cervical fibroid tumors, may block the passage of the sperm. Removing polyps is usually a simple piece of surgery that can be done in the office. Removing a cervical fibroid tumor may be somewhat more difficult and less successful and is an operation that necessitates hospitalization.

*See the section on fertility drugs for details.

Hormonal Imbalances

In some women the second half of the menstrual cycle, from ovulation to menstruation, is abnormally short. This is known as corpus luteum insufficiency, or luteal phase defect. The corpus luteum, the source of the hormone progesterone in the second half of the menstrual cycle, begins to degenerate after only 4 or 5 days rather than after the normal 8 or 10 days. Without the hormone progesterone the lining of the uterus is not prepared adequately for implantation of the fertilized egg; hence the woman is unable to sustain a pregnancy or has continual miscarriages. Progesterone treatments have been used, but progesterone has been implicated in birth defects. However, in 30 years of treatment using this method at Johns Hopkins Hospital, where the treatment was developed, they have "been unable to document any adverse effects of progesterone suppository use."[4] But the progesterone must be given in suppository form. Under no circumstances should oral progesterone preparations, such as Provera or Norlutin, be used, for they may harm the fetus.[5] Low doses of certain fertility drugs, such as HCG and Clomid, have been used as well.

If a woman frequently has menstrual cycles in which she does not ovulate (called anovulatory cycles), she can't possibly get pregnant, since no ripened egg is being produced. She is likely to have menstrual irregularities as well. Failure to ovulate may be caused by a malfunction of any of the glands involved in regulating the menstrual cycle. Tests to check the function of these glands can be done, and sometimes treating the underlying imbalance will solve the infertility problem. This is discussed more fully under the heading Amenorrhea. Certain powerful fertility drugs, like Clomid and Pergonal, may be used to stimulate ovulation, but these involve certain risks.

Ovarian Problems

A condition like Stein-Leventhal disease, in which the ovary may be surrounded by a thick, fibrous capsule and in which the woman only rarely, if ever, ovulates, is also associated with infertility. This disease may be treated with drugs, such as Clomid, or by surgery. In some rare cases a woman is born without ovaries—a condition called Turner's syndrome—and such women are usually sterile and can't achieve pregnancy. Women with Turner's syndrome usually have other symptoms that are generally evident long before the infertility. However, in some cases these women may have rudimentary, or streak, gonads, and the symptoms of ovarian absence may not be as obvious. Occasionally, one of these women will have a small number of eggs in the streak gonad and will ovulate, and on rare occasions such women have become pregnant.

The ovaries may also fail to produce eggs because there has been extensive ovarian surgery, exposure to radiation or excessive stimulation from fertility drugs or because the blood supply to the ovaries has been cut off. This is known as primary ovarian failure, or premature menopause.

Uterine and Tubal Problems

Structural problems in the uterus, such as fibroid tumors and congenital abnormalities of the female organs, can affect a woman's ability to carry a pregnancy to term or her ability to conceive. Some of these abnormalities may result from certain hormones, such as DES, taken by the mothers of those women during pregnancy. Congenital abnormalities can often be corrected surgically. Many women have what is called a tipped uterus. Such women may have to use special techniques (see below), but they usually don't need surgery in order to become pregnant. Fibroids can sometimes be removed through surgery, a procedure known as myomectomy. This is not always possible, however, for if the tumors are extensive, requiring that a lot of tissue be removed, this might weaken the walls of the uterus so much that the entire uterus would have to be removed.

A new method of removing certain fibroids with the aid of a viewing instrument called a hysteroscope may be better than a myomectomy in some cases.[6]

The fallopian tubes may be blocked, causing infertility. Plastic surgery known as tuboplasty may be used to repair damage. This is a rather elaborate procedure in which microsurgery is performed. The success of any tubal surgery depends on exactly where in the tube the blockage is and whether one or both tubes is affected. After surgery there is an increased risk (5 percent to 10 percent) of ectopic pregnancy. If one tube is hopelessly blocked, some doctors will recommend that the ovary on that side be removed. Ovulation normally alternates, so that an egg is produced from the right ovary one month and from the left ovary the next. Removing the ovary on the side of the blocked tube forces the woman to ovulate from the remaining ovary, thus increasing her chances of fertility. But most doctors question this procedure and won't remove a healthy ovary in case something should ever happen to the remaining ovary.

Other

Any infection of the uterus can cause infertility, for if the uterine wall is too irritated, the egg cannot implant. Vaginal and cervical infections can also affect fertility. Any chronic disease, thyroid conditions, alcoholism or drug abuse can affect the sensitive hypothalamus, the control center in the brain that regulates the menstrual cycle, thereby causing infertility. Exposure to radiation and environmental pollutants has been implicated in fertility problems in women as well as men (see below).

Causes and Treatment of Male Infertility

So far we've been talking about female infertility, but male fertility may also be impaired. Basically, there are four ways in which a man's fertility can be affected: inadequate sperm production or sperm maturation, insufficient sperm motility (the sperm's ability to swim or move), a blockage or other problem somewhere in the sperm delivery system or inability to place the sperm properly in the vagina.

Sperm Count

The absence of sperm or a low sperm count can be caused by any infection associated with high fever that occurs after puberty. Mumps infections have long been associated with male infertility. If a male past the age of puberty gets the mumps, he may be rendered permanently sterile. In many cases, only one testis is affected. If both are affected, the situation is less hopeful; however, even in such cases a man may gradually recover his fertility, usually within a year. A number of other infections, notably the sexually transmissible infections, can temporarily depress sperm count and, if untreated, may render a man permanently sterile. Recovery of normal sperm production after a high-fever illness takes at least 3 months, for it takes the testes that long to produce mature sperm.

If the testes do not descend into the scrotum before puberty (undescended testes) this will also affect sperm production. Fertility is affected because the testes function at a slightly lower temperature than the rest of the body organs. They need to be within the scrotum to have their optimum temperature. A surgical cure for undescended testes is possible, but best results are achieved if the surgery is done before age 6. In some cases there may be abnormalities within the testis itself that affect sperm production, and these cannot be corrected surgically.

Other congenital factors, for instance, Klinefelter's syndrome (which is similar to Turner's syndrome in females), can also affect sperm production. A man with Klinefelter's syndrome tends to have small testes and an absence of sperm in his ejaculation.

The undescended testis is not the only condition that can cause too high a temperature in the scrotum and hence lower sperm count. A varicocele, which is a varicose or twisted vein of the testis, can also cause this problem. This condition can be corrected surgically, and in 80 percent of cases the sperm count improves. Higher than usual heat from frequent use of athletic supporters, the wearing of tight pants, hot tubs, sauna baths, long hot showers and so on can also temporarily slow down sperm maturation. Here again, the effect is usually reversible within 3 months.

Any abnormalities in the testes can affect sperm count; however, even if a man has only one testis, he can still be fertile. Injury to any of the reproductive organs from a serious accident may cut off the blood supply to the tissue, resulting in the death of that tissue. In rare cases this has also occurred as a result of a hernia operation or other type of surgery.

Radiation can render both men and women permanently sterile, although in some cases the effect on male fertility may be only temporary, for he is constantly producing new sperm, whereas a woman at birth already has all the eggs she will ever have. Once these eggs have been damaged, new, healthy ones cannot be produced.

If a man suffers from chronic illness, including alcoholism or drug addiction, fertility may also be impaired. Heavy and prolonged use of marijuana has been associated with lowered sperm counts. Certain medications, including some tranquilizers, antimalarial drugs and methotrexate, can affect sperm production. Stress, both physical and emotional, can likewise affect fertility. Hormonal imbalances, the result of diseases of the pituitary or hypothalamus, such as tumors, can also cause infertility. If these imbalances are treated successfully, fertility may be restored.

Toxic pesticides and herbicides and environmental pollutants also affect fertility.[7] Agent Orange, an herbicide used extensively in Vietnam to defoliate the jungles, has been implicated in sterility as well as miscarriage, birth defects, skin cancers and other problems. This same herbicide, 2-4-5-T, is used extensively by lumbering firms in the United States. In one area in Oregon where this chemical has been used the rate of birth defects is as high as 40 percent. Other toxic substances have also been implicated in infertility, miscarriage, birth defects and cancer. PCB, a chemical used in electric transformers, fluorescent bulbs, TV sets and even carbon paper has been found in almost all sperm tested for its presence. These and other contaminants may be responsible for the fact that the average sperm count in American men has fallen by as much as 30 percent in the past 30 years. Smoking and alcohol may also affect sperm quality.[8]

Sperm Motility

Many of the factors mentioned above will also cause inadequate sperm motility. Prostatitis, an infection of the prostate gland, which produces the milky fluid released with the sperm during ejaculation, or surgical removal of the gland will also affect sperm motility. Chronic illness or hormonal problems will likewise have an effect on the sperm's ability to swim. Curing the illness or infection, when possible, will usually improve fertility. Sometimes the female hormone estrogen may be given to improve a man's sperm production, but long-term use of estrogen may have feminizing effects. Some doctors use testosterone, a male hormone, to achieve a "rebound" effect from the feminization effects, but most doctors believe that this can cause the permanent suppression of sperm production. Drugs called corticosteroids are also used, but only rarely, for they have also been implicated as a cause of reduced sperm production. Human chorionic gonadotropin (HCG), another hormone, stimulates the production of testosterone, which improves sperm motility in some men. Clomid has also been used to stimulate sperm production and improve motility. In cases in which the man has a borderline sperm count and problems with motility, a technique known as split ejaculate, in which the man catches the first half of his ejaculate (the part that has the greatest number of live sperm) in a glass jar, may be used. The sperm is then used to artificially inseminate the wife. Artificial, or donor, insemination, in which an anonymous donor's sperm is injected into the uterus, is another possibility.

Sperm Delivery

Untreated sexually transmissible infections or other illnesses can cause a blockage in the sperm delivery system. Injury from surgery or an accident, a varicocele or a vasectomy can all cause such blockage as well. Sometimes surgical repair can correct these problems, but this is not always possible, especially in the case of a vasectomy. Another problem that can affect the sperm delivery system is a condition known as retrograde ejaculation, in which the sperm are deposited in the man's bladder instead of continuing out through the urethra. This condition may be permanent or temporary and may be caused by certain drugs, injury during surgery or damage to the nerve. Men with retrograde ejaculation have no visible sperm and their urine tends to look milky after sex. The condition can sometimes be treated by drugs. For a couple seriously intent on pregnancy it may be possible to recover sperm from the bladder and impregnate the woman, using the technique of husband insemination described earlier.

Impotence (the inability to achieve and maintain an erection), premature ejaculation ("coming" before the penis can be inserted in the vagina) and the inability to ejaculate can all cause infertility. Sometimes these forms of sexual dysfunction will have an organic, physical cause, but the problem may also be psychological. Sex therapy a la Masters and Johnson has been effective in treating these problems.

666

Sperm Antibodies

In some cases antibodies to sperm may be the source of the infertility problem. In a man, immunity to his own sperm may result from an injury or infection that allows the sperm to enter the surrounding tissue, where they may trigger his immune system and cause an antibody reaction. If the injury or infection can be treated, sometimes this will stop the production of antibodies. A woman may also have antibodies that attack the sperm. Such women are, in essence, allergic to sperm, and each time they have intercourse, more antibodies are produced. Sometimes this problem can be successfully treated by having the man use a condom (a rubber) during intercourse for a period of 3 to 6 months. During this time the level of a woman's antibodies are measured, and when they drop the couple can begin to have sex without a condom, but only at the time of optimum fertility, around ovulation.

A condition known as sperm agglutinization, in which the heads of the sperm clump together, may affect motility. This condition has been treated successfully with vitamin C.[9]

Sexual Practices That May Affect Fertility

Sometimes the couple's sexual practice may affect fertility. The use of lubricants like petroleum jelly or K-Y jelly must be discontinued, since these are known to weaken or in some cases even kill sperm. The position the couple uses during intercourse may also be affecting their ability to conceive. For most couples the best position is the missionary style, with the man on top and the woman's hips raised on a pillow. The man should penetrate as deeply as possible. If the woman draws her knees up to her chest, this facilitates deep penetration. The man should stop thrusting and hold his penis still when he experiences orgasm. The woman should hold her knees in this position for half an hour after intercourse. The exception to this rule is the woman who has a tipped uterus, for whom entry from behind may be best. The frequency of a couple's sexual activity is an important factor. The longer a man goes without ejaculating, the less sperm he generates. Having sex two or three times a week is considered optimum for conception. The timing of sexual activity is also important, and charting a woman's fertile period (see the section on natural family planning) will help the couple determine the optimum time for conception. Generally, a woman will ovulate 14 days, give or take 24 hours each way, before the beginning of her next period, so her best chances of conceiving are on the 13th, 14th and 15th day before the day on which her next period is expected to begin. During these 3 days the couple should have intercourse no more than once every 30 to 36 hours. This will avoid exhausting the man's sperm supply and will assure that active sperm are in the reproductive tract during the woman's fertile time. For best results the couple should have intercourse on each of the 2 days before this 3-day period so that the male's sperm production will be stimulated.

Diagnosis

Because so many factors can affect fertility and because more than one factor may be responsible, diagnosing the causes of infertility involves a number of tests. A couple may want to look for a doctor who specializes in fertility. The American Board of Obstetrics and Gynecology now certifies specialists in fertility, but there are few of them. Most are associated with medical schools. The American Fertility Society, 1608 13th Avenue S, Suite 101, Birmingham, Alabama 35205, has a listing of fertility centers and specialists across the country. A specialist may not be necessary for the preliminary steps, but if a test such as a laparoscopy or a procedure such as tubal surgery is needed, do seek referral to a specialist.

Nurse practitioners are assuming an important role in fertility workups. The doctor still supervises the tests and diagnostic workup, but much of the patient contact is done by the nurse practitioner. This can have advantages for everyone. The nurse practitioner is generally less pressed for time and is therefore able to spend the time needed to take a thorough medical history and to answer questions and explain procedures. Many times the nurse practitioner is better at explaining things in lay terms than the doctor is. Couples being treated for infertility who spend much of their time with the nurse practitioner should not feel as though they are being slighted or receiving less-than-adequate care. Although the nurse practitioner works closely with the doctor, the fee for his or her time is less than for the doctor's time, which can be a particularly important factor, since fertility workups can be expensive and many times insurance policies don't cover these costs. People with an infertility problem should discuss the financial aspects with the doctor and with their insurance companies.

If you are planning to see a doctor for a fertility workup, it is a good idea to start keeping a BBT chart (*see* pp. 174–79). The doctor will probably ask you to keep one anyhow, because it helps to determine whether or not the woman is ovulating, to time intercourse so the couple has sex when the chances of conceiving are optimum and to determine the best time to do certain tests. Arriving at the doctor's office with a chart on your first visit will speed up the testing process and may save a repeat office visit.

Step one is an initial interview that should, if at all possible, include the man and the woman. The doctor or nurse will take a detailed medical history from the man and the woman that will include information about how often they have sex, the positions used, past pregnancies (if any), the woman's menstrual history and medical problems, any sexually transmissible infections or any other diseases or conditions that might affect fertility. Sometimes the man or the woman may have certain information in his or her medical history, such as past abortions or a history of sexually transmissible infections, that he or she does not wish to discuss in front of the partner. For this reason we prefer to take the medical histories separately. If this is true for you, or if you suspect it may be true for your partner, you can ask that your medical histories be taken privately when you call to make your first appointment.

The first interview usually involves a complete physical exam of the woman, including a bimanual pelvic exam. Tests like a Pap smear, blood count, urinalysis and tests for such infections as gonorrhea and syphilis may be done. The man may also get a complete physical, or this may not be done until later if the results of the tests of his sperm are not normal.

If you are not already keeping a BBT chart, you will probably be asked to do so and to time intercourse in relation to the chart.

If your menstrual periods have not occurred regularly every 28 days, give or take 7 days each way, you may not be ovulating. This problem is discussed under the heading Amenorrhea.

Assuming everything looks normal after your first visit, you will begin on a fertility workup, which should take only 2 to 3 months. The standard fertility workup involves five tests—semen analysis, postcoital test, hysterosalpingography, endometrial biopsy and laparoscopy—which will pinpoint a cause for the infertility in 90 percent of cases, but in 10 percent of cases no specific cause will be found.

The semen analysis, or sperm count, allows the doctor to assess the quality and quantity of the man's sperm. The test involves the man's masturbating and ejaculating sperm into a clean glass container. This can be done in the office, but if the man has ejaculated in the previous 2 days, the sperm may be depleted. If the man *has* ejaculated in the previous 2 days or if he prefers, he may collect the sperm at home and bring it to the doctor or the lab for analysis within an hour of ejaculation. Catching all the ejaculate is particularly important, since most of the sperm are in the first half of the ejaculate. The sperm must be kept at room temperature. If for religious or other reasons a man cannot masturbate, a special type of condom may be used during intercourse to collect the sperm sample. If there is a religious objection to birth control, a small pinhole can be made at the top of the condom. Coitus interruptus, or withdrawal, as a method of collecting the semen is not as satisfactory because some of the early ejaculate may be lost.

If the sperm count is normal, tests on the woman will continue. A semen analysis must show at least 20 million sperm per ml, with at least 60 percent of the sperm having good mobility and normal shape and form. If the semen analysis does not meet the minimal standard, it may be repeated, depending on the type and extent of abnormality. Having one abnormal sperm count does not necessarily mean that something is wrong. A man's production of sperm varies markedly from time to time, so a second test may be done. If the sperm count is clearly abnormal, the man is usually referred to a urologist, who will do an extensive workup, looking for such problems as a history of DES exposure or a varicocele. A testicular biopsy, an office procedure that involves removing a tiny bit of tissue to be examined microscopically, may be done.

If the semen analysis is normal, investigation of the woman continues with the second test in the fertility workup, known as a postcoital, or Huhner, test, which requires that a woman arrive at the doctor's office within a few hours after intercourse without having washed or douched. A sample of her cervical mucus is studied to see if the sperm have been able to penetrate the mucus and survive in this environment.

Some authorities have suggested that the postcoital test precede the semen analysis, because this "avoids the stress associated with semen analysis."[10] (The "stress" is apparently embarrassment at masturbating into a jar.) Although this may be true, it does so at the expense of the woman, who has to undergo the "stress" of the postcoital exam.[11] All too often women are tested before their partners' sperm has been examined. Even the more painful and more invasive tests, such as hysterosalpingography, endometrial biopsy or laparoscopy, are sometimes done before the man's sperm has been tested. And as incredible as it seems, some women are put on fertility drugs and/or subjected to surgery without their partners' sperm having been tested. If your doctor recommends any of these tests or procedures before a semen analysis is done, be sure you understand why. You may want to seek a second opinion.

The postcoital test should be done immediately before ovulation. The BBT will help to determine the correct time for the test. The presence of white blood cells or bacteria in the mucus indicates an infection, which may be treated by taking a cervical culture and administering an appropriate antibiotic. The test may also show inadequate mucus, which may be corrected by taking low doses of estrogen. If no sperm are in the mucus, this may mean that the test was not done correctly, improper intercourse technique was used, a toxic factor exists in the cervix or vagina or there's an antibody/immunological problem. Repeat testing may be necessary, or the couple may have to be instructed in proper intercourse technique (see above). If on the basis of this test the doctor suspects an antibody problem, it may be treated by abstaining from sex for awhile, using a condom for 6 months or administering drugs called corticosteroids.

If neither the semen analysis nor the postcoital test reveals a problem, the third test, a hysterosalpingography, is done to investigate the possibility of uterine or tubal abnormalities. The hysterosalpingogram, or uterotubogram, is an X-ray that is taken after a dye that will show up on X-ray film is injected into the uterus through the cervix. Normally, the dye will fill the uterus and spill out through the fallopian tubes into the pelvis, where it will be absorbed. If the tubes are blocked, this test will reveal such tubal blockage and may be quite painful. (Women should plan to have someone else drive them home after the test.) In some cases this test may even be curative, because the fluid may flush out any slight blockage and the small (not harmful) amount of radiation in the special dye may stimulate the ovaries. The test should be done after the woman's period but before ovulation.

A tubal insufflation, or Rubin's test, may be done, in which a small amount of gas is blown into the uterus and, if the tubes are open, out into the pelvic cavity, where it is eventually absorbed. This test is a simple, harmless procedure that can be done in a doctor's office, but it doesn't tell whether one or both tubes are open or whether the gas has escaped in some other manner. Most specialists, therefore, no longer use it, relying on X-ray studies instead. Although tubal insufflation may be useful in some cases, a woman whose doctor suggests this test should question him/her carefully as to what s/he hopes to accomplish, for such a doctor may be a bit behind the times.

The fourth test, which may also be painful, is the endometrial biopsy, which is done to detect a possible luteal phase defect (see above). It is done 2 to 3 days before the woman expects her menstrual period to start. Other, less commonly used methods to detect a luteal defect include a plasma progesterone level test obtained 3, 8 and 11 days after ovulation or before the menstrual period.

If all these diagnostic tests are inconclusive, the doctor may want to do a fifth test, a laparoscopic exam, which must be done in the hospital. A viewing instrument is inserted through a small incision in the abdomen, allowing the doctor to inspect the tubes, ovaries, uterus and pelvic cavity directly. If laparoscopy is done because of suspected tubal adhesions, perhaps a specialist should be consulted, because if it turns out that microsurgery is needed to correct the problem, only specially trained doctors can perform this operation. If the doctor who does the exploratory laparoscopy is unable to perform the microsurgery, the surgery will have to be done by the specialist. Expert consultation may, then, require a repetition of the laparoscopy. It's better to have the laparoscopy done by the person whom you would have do any surgery that might be required.

Treatment

If a specific cause can be identified, the doctor may attempt the various treatments outlined above. Some doctors have recently been successful in treating unexplained infertility with a new drug, danazol (*see* p. 409).[12] If treatment of infertility is not possible or is unsuccessful, such techniques as husband insemination, in which some of the male partner's sperm is injected directly into the woman's uterus, may be possible. If the male partner's sperm is not satisfactory or, in the case of a single woman desiring artificial insemination, there is no male partner, artificial donor insemination is a possibility, although there may be a higher-than-usual rate of miscarriage associated with this procedure. Sperm donors, usually medical students who are paid a fee for their services, are screened and, in the case of couples, matched as closely as possible to the ethnic background, height and complexion of the male partner. There has recently been a great deal of interest in special "Nobel Prize Winner" sperm banks, which offer frozen sperm from men who are particularly bright or successful. Frozen sperm can be used, but the use of fresh sperm is more effective.

The process is strictly confidential. To ensure total anonymity, some doctors select two donors and use both sperm samples. Anonymity has become an issue because of questions that have been raised about the legal aspects of artificial insemination. Although it is hard to imagine a case in which a donor would sue for information about his artificially inseminated offspring, anything can happen. A doctor who had used two or more donors would not be able to testify as to whose sperm resulted in the pregnancy. Some doctors send their artificially inseminated couples to obstetricians who are unaware of the couple's history so that the man and woman will automatically be listed as mother and father on the birth certificate. Questions regarding inheritance, custody and child support in the event of divorce are other possible legal complications, and a couple may wish to discuss the legal aspects with a lawyer first.

Artificial insemination, especially when it involves a single woman, is a highly controversial topic. In recent years some gay women have chosen to be artificially inseminated. This, needless to say, is even more controversial, and such women may have a difficult time finding a doctor. They would probably do best to seek help from doctors who are gay and/or sympathetic to gays (see Chapter Six).

In any case, artificial insemination has legal, philosophical and emotional aspects that deserve careful consideration by anyone considering the procedure.

Equally controversial is the so-called test-tube baby, which is more correctly referred to as in vitro fertilization. In this procedure the sperm from the male and an egg taken from the female are brought together in the laboratory. The fertilized egg is then put into the mother's body and allowed to develop as in a normal pregnancy. A great deal of media attention has recently been focused on the first publicly acknowledged "test-tube baby," Louise Brown, born in England. The procedure is being done in the United States on a limited basis. The first publicly announced program, which has a long waiting list, is being run at the University of Virginia Medical School. Other universities have since begun programs, and private clinics have opened up recently in various parts of the country. Your doctor should be able to refer you to a university or private clinic in your area.

MISCARRIAGE

AKA: spontaneous abortion, fetal or pregnancy wastage

Types: threatened abortion
       inevitable, or incipient, abortion
       incomplete abortion
       missed abortion
       habitual abortion

Associated Terms: septic, or infected, abortion

Miscarriages, or spontaneous abortions, occur, as the name implies, spontaneously, in contrast to therapeutic, or induced, abortions, which are performed deliberately to terminate an unwanted pregnancy. There are several types or stages of spontaneous abortion (Illustration 57). The term "threatened abortion" is used to describe a condition characterized by bleeding and, sometimes, cramplike pain, which may or may not be followed by the expulsion of the fetus. Inevitable, or incipient, abortion refers to a threatened abortion that has progressed so far that there is no longer any question as to whether the pregnancy will continue. When a miscarriage does occur it may be complete, meaning that the uterus has expelled all the fetal and placental tissue, or it may be incomplete, meaning that some of the tissue is still inside the uterus. In some cases even though the fetus has died it is not immediately expelled. The dead tissue remains trapped inside the uterus, and this is known as a missed abortion.

Incidence

Miscarriages are said to occur in 10 percent to 15 percent of all pregnancies. The actual figure may be much higher than this, for some abortions undoubtedly occur without a woman's having realized she was pregnant. In such a case all that the woman might notice would be a slightly delayed, heavier-than-normal period with, perhaps, some unusually large blood clots.

Any given woman's chances of having a miscarriage depend on a couple of factors. For instance, the chances are about 1 in 400 if the woman is under 25, got pregnant within 3 months of trying and has no previous history of miscarriage. The chances are considerably higher—40 in 100—if the woman is over 35, took 6 months or more to get pregnant and/or has had previous miscarriages.[13]

Cause

It is not always possible to pinpoint the cause of a miscarriage. In the majority of cases some abnormality in either the sperm or the ovum results in the fail-

673

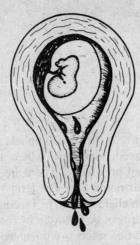

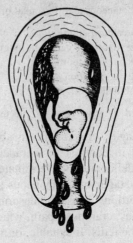

THREATENED ABORTION

INEVITABLE ABORTION

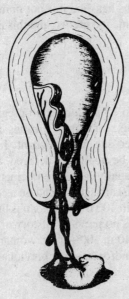

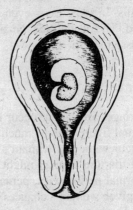

MISSED ABORTION

INCOMPLETE ABORTION

Illustration 57 *Types of Spontaneous Abortion (Miscarriage)*

ure of the fertilized egg to undergo its first important cell divisions properly; thus the embryo is incapable of growing or surviving beyond 10 or 12 weeks. The abnormal tissue dies and by the 2d or 3d month of pregnancy is expelled from the body.

The fact that a fetus is abnormal and is spontaneously aborted does not necessarily mean that there is something basically wrong with the mother's ova or the father's sperm. In the majority of cases it is thought that the deformity was just a chance event. Just because a woman has one miscarriage it does not follow that she will have trouble with her other pregnancies. In fact, normal delivery of a healthy infant occurs in about 80 percent of women who have had a previous miscarriage and in about 60 percent of cases where there have been two previous miscarriages. If, however, a woman has three or more spontaneous abortions, a condition known as habitual abortion, the chances of her having a normal subsequent pregnancy drop considerably.

Although in the past most of these single instances of miscarriage were attributed to chance, new information is accumulating to suggest possible causes. Cigarette smoking has been linked to a higher rate of miscarriage, as has poor nutrition.[14] Environmental pollutants have been linked to higher rates of miscarriage as well as birth defects, infertility, cancer and other abnormalities.[15] For instance, an herbicide known as 2-4-5-T, used widely in the Northwest by lumbering firms to retard the growth of underbrush in forests, has been implicated in higher rates of spontaneous abortion and birth defects. Women living in the area of Alsea, Oregon, where there has been intensive spraying of 2-4-5-T, have a 40 percent increase in the rate of birth defects or miscarriages. In one neighborhood in the Niagara Falls area, near Buffalo, the birth defect rate climbed to 56 percent and the miscarriage rate to 25 percent above normal when noxious chemicals started leaking from a dump site running right through a residential area.

Some studies indicate that women who have had two or more prior induced abortions are more likely to have miscarriages than women who haven't had induced abortions or have had only one.[16]

In addition to these sorts of problems, miscarriage may be caused by many other factors. These are described under the heading Repeated Miscarriage.

Symptoms

Most miscarriages—about 75 percent of them—occur in the first 3 months of pregnancy. In very early abortions a woman might not even be aware that she was pregnant.

The first indication that a miscarriage might occur is vaginal bleeding. The bleeding may appear for only 1 day and be quite heavy or it may continue for weeks as scanty spotting. Sometimes the blood is bright; at other times it is dark brown, indicating that the bleeding has been going on for some time. The longer the bleeding continues and the heavier it is, the more likely it is that an abortion will occur. The later in the pregnancy that the signs and symptoms appear, the greater the chances that the pregnancy will continue.

Pain may also be a sign that an abortion is in the offing, although in some threatened abortions there is little or no pain. If there is pain, it is usually preceded by bleeding in a woman who is going to have an early abortion. Occasionally, pain and bleeding occur together. In late abortions the pain usually precedes the bleeding. Pain may occur in normal pregnancy because of pressure from the growing fetus; however, women should not hesitate to consult their doctors if pain occurs.

After the initial symptoms of pain and/or bleeding, indicating a threatened abortion, the situation may develop in a number of ways. The symptoms may worsen, and on speculum exam it may be possible to see parts of the fetal tissue protruding through the cervix. Once this has happened, abortion is inevitable.

The symptoms progress until a complete abortion takes place and all the fetal and placental tissue are expelled from the womb. An early miscarriage may not feel any more uncomfortable than a heavy period. There may be one or more large clots in the blood. In a late first-trimester miscarriage—one that occurs in the 3d month of pregnancy—there may be cramping and bleeding on and off for days, until the uterus is completely emptied. If the miscarriage occurs after the 3d month of pregnancy, there are usually strong, regular uterine contractions as the cervix dilates, and for many women this may be associated with a good deal of pain. Once the fetus is expelled, the bleeding should stop within a few days.

A woman who has a miscarriage and is aware of passing the fetus and placenta should try and collect the tissue in a clean container. This may be a very difficult task emotionally, but by looking at the tissue the doctor may be able to tell whether the miscarriage was a chance event or was owing to some other problem that can be treated before the next pregnancy.

Another possible turn of events is an incomplete abortion, in which portions of the fetal or placental tissue remain in the uterus. In this case the cramping and bleeding do not stop and may get a good deal worse. Sometimes there is a gushing, flooding type of bleeding. This can be quite scary. Although this unusual amount of bleeding requires *immediate* medical attention, it is sometimes surprising how much blood a pregnant woman can pass without the loss being threatening to her life. Here again, fragments of recognizable fetal or placental tissue may be passed, and if possible, these should be saved.

Sometimes, even in the presence of severe symptoms, the threatened abortion never takes place. The symptoms subside. The pregnancy continues to term, and in most cases a normal baby is delivered, although there is a slight increase in the number of birth defects in such cases.

At other times, even though symptoms have subsided, the outcome is not as happy. The fetus has died, but the uterus has not expelled the dead tissue, a situation known as a missed abortion. The cervix closes up and the bleeding stops, although in some cases there may be light bleeding if the cervix does not close tightly. As the trapped tissue decays, such bleeding is apt to be brown and to smell bad. In women known to be pregnant, the failure of the uterus to grow larger after the bleeding episode is another sign of a missed abortion. In women who were not yet aware that they were pregnant, missed menstrual periods may be a sign of missed abortion.

Diagnosis

It is not always immediately possible to distinguish between a threatened abortion and an inevitable abortion. The amount of blood lost is often a clue. Keeping a count of how many sanitary napkins are used will help the doctor to estimate blood loss. Once portions of the fetal tissue are seen protruding through the cervix, the diagnosis is clear.

If the fetal tissue has been passed and the bleeding doesn't stop within a few days, this is an indication that there is something wrong. The woman may have had an incomplete rather than a complete abortion. If, however, a woman is not aware of having passed the fetus, the continued bleeding may sometimes be misinterpreted as a sign of a threatened abortion. A pregnancy test is not much help, for the test may remain positive for a while. Moreover, large blood clots in the uterus may be mistakenly interpreted to mean that the fetus is still inside the uterus. Bleeding tends to be rather profuse in an incomplete abortion, but this may not be so initially. The opening to the cervix tends to be dilated, but again, this may be less obvious if most of the tissue has been expelled. Thus a clear diagnosis cannot always be made right away.

Diagnosing these conditions may be particularly difficult in very early threatened abortions, when the characteristic signs of pregnancy—the enlarged uterus and softened cervix—may not yet be obvious. If a woman has irregular periods, doesn't have a clear idea of when her last period was or, as sometimes happens, has menstruated even though she is actually pregnant, her situation may be even more confusing. Her intermittent spotting or even heavier bleeding may be caused by a number of factors. A Pap smear, pregnancy test, endometrial biopsy or perhaps a D&C may be necessary. Even if a woman is aware of having missed a menstrual period and pregnancy is suspected—or has been confirmed—the diagnosis of the scant bleeding and cramps that accompany threatened abortion can be difficult. One of the most common errors in diagnosis is to mistake what is really a tubal pregnancy,

677

that is, a pregnancy that has implanted in the fallopian tube rather than in the uterus, for an early threatened abortion.

Consider Table 28. This neat list represents the clues a doctor uses in making this diagnosis. Unfortunately, real-life situations are rarely so clear-cut. For instance, pelvic pain is often reflected and generalized, so that it may be hard to tell exactly where the source of the pain is. A woman may not know exactly when she last menstruated, so clue No. 4, which is not a hard-and-fast rule anyway, is not always an aid in diagnosis. Sometimes anemia is not present in either case and, if it is present, may be owing to another condition. If the threatened abortion is very early, uterine enlargement and cervical softening may not yet be obvious. Likewise, the symptoms of fever, vomiting and fainting are not always present in tubal pregnancy. Moreover, should the threatened abortion become infected, some of these same symptoms might occur.

Since tubal pregnancy is a potentially life-threatening situation that requires immediate surgery once the diagnosis has been made, the doctor may have to use some specialized diagnostic tools to rule out the possibility if the symptoms are ambiguous. These diagnostic tools might include a culdoscope or a laparoscope, which are specialized viewing instruments that are inserted into the pelvic cavity, or culdocentesis, a procedure in which a needle is inserted through the vagina into the pelvic cavity in order to withdraw fluid from the pelvic cavity. The reasons for using these tools are discussed under the heading Ectopic Pregnancy.

Table 28
Symptoms of Tubal Pregnancy and Early Threatened Abortion

Tubal Pregnancy	*Early Threatened Abortion*
1. Scant vaginal bleeding	1. Scant vaginal bleeding
2. Enlargement on one side of the uterus owing to embryo in the tube	2. Possible enlargement on one side of the uterus owing to corpus luteum cyst of pregnancy
3. Sharp, cramplike pain on the affected side	3. Pain, if present, less severe; located in the middle rather than to the side
4. Time between the last menstrual period and the onset of bleeding is apt to be shorter, usually 6 to 8 weeks	4. Time between the last menstrual period and the onset of bleeding is apt to be longer, usually 8 to 10 weeks
5. Anemia, if present, out of proportion to observable blood loss from internal bleeding	5. Anemia not usually present, except if there is profuse bleeding, and then it is in line with observable blood loss
6. Uterus not enlarged, cervix not softened	6. Uterus enlarged, cervix softened
7. Nausea, vomiting, faintness	7. No nausea, vomiting, faintness

Diagnosis may be a bit easier in a woman with a previously established pregnancy who has a missed abortion. The stopping of the initial bleeding and the failure of the uterus to grow larger are telling clues. In later stages of pregnancy, absence of fetal heartbeat and movement are strong indications. If the formerly positive pregnancy test becomes negative, this pretty much cinches the diagnosis, but the possibility, although rare, does exist that the missed abortion is actually a form of trophoblastic disease, an abnormality of the developing embryo. Although sonography, a method of taking internal pictures by sound waves, may be helpful in differentiating between a missed abortion and trophoblastic disease, it is rarely possible to tell until the fetus has been expelled or removed.

Treatment

Once the process has begun there is not really much that can be done to prevent a threatened abortion from taking place. Generally, a wait-and-see approach is adopted. The woman is confined to her bed and intercourse is prohibited. If the bleeding stops of its own accord, she is usually confined to bed for another couple of days. She will be given a pregnancy test to make sure that her apparent recovery was not, in fact, a missed abortion.

In the past, hormone treatment was given to help prevent miscarriages. The now infamous DES, a synthetic estrogen, was given to millions of women in the years between 1947 and 1969 to help prevent miscarriages. When some of the teenage daughters of these women developed a rare form of cancer and other abnormalities, the dangers of this treatment became apparent (see the section on DES for details). Moreover, it is now known that DES was not even effective in preventing miscarriage.

Progesterone hormone therapy is sometimes given. There is some indication that this hormone too may cause abnormalities in the fetus.[17] It should certainly not be used without tests that demonstrate an actual deficiency, and even then, its lack of success and its possible dangers make it a highly questionable treatment.

Many threatened abortions eventually do abort. The fetus will usually be expelled within a short period of its death, but sometimes this doesn't happen for a few days. If there is no fever and the blood loss is minimal or sporadic, there is usually no medical need to go to the hospital to have the fetus removed, so the woman will be spared this expense. The tissue will be expelled by contractions of the uterus and the bleeding should stop within a few days. If the bleeding gets too heavy, the woman must be hospitalized, blood transfusions prepared and the uterus emptied by suction curettage, a vacuumlike method of emptying the uterus. The suction curettage is often followed by gentle scraping of the uterus with a blunt instrument called a curette. This has

679

several advantages. First, it rules out the possibility of a congenital abnormality of the uterus, a fibroid tumor or a polyp, any of which might have distorted the shape of the uterus and thereby caused the miscarriage. Certain tissue samples can be taken to help rule out the possibility that trophoblastic disease is present. Moreover, it assures that the uterus has indeed been completely emptied.

Although the tendency in treatment is to let nature take its course and to allow the uterus to expel the fetal tissue on its own, provided that the bleeding is not too severe, there are two factors that might suggest a more aggressive course of action. First, even though a missed abortion will eventually be expelled, this can take some time, perhaps a month or more. Carrying the dead fetus and not knowing when it will be expelled may be more of an emotional strain than a woman cares to deal with and so a suction curettage may be performed.

The second factor is infection. In an incomplete abortion the cervical os is dilated, leaving the uterus open for bacterial invasion. The dying or dead fetal tissue is fertile ground for breeding bacteria. At the first sign of infection, the uterus must be emptied. If infection does occur, it may be mild, moderate or severe, depending on whether or not the infection has spread beyond the uterus. Such an infection, which is called an infected, or septic, abortion, can cause high fever and chills. If the infection spreads, there may be serious complications, which are discussed under the heading Pelvic Inflammatory Disease. Given the possibility of infection, some doctors and women will decide, even when there is no heavy bleeding, to do a suction curettage as a preventive measure. Although this can be done with a local anesthetic in the doctor's office, this procedure is sometimes more painful than normal abortion procedures, so the woman may decide to have it done in the hospital with a general anesthetic, which, although more expensive and riskier, is also more comfortable.

Prevention

Because the cause of a single spontaneous abortion is not well understood and because about 80 percent of women who experience it do not have subsequent medical problems, prevention has not been emphasized. With new information about cigarette smoking, environmental pollutants, over-the-counter drugs and nutrition, many clinics are now emphasizing nutritional and genetic counseling in preparation for subsequent pregnancies, even for women who have had only one miscarriage.

REPEATED MISCARRIAGE

AKA: recurrent miscarriage, repeated spontaneous abortion, habitual abortion

In medicalese, repeated miscarriage is called habitual abortion. The term "habitual abortion" is generally used when a woman has three or more successive pregnancies that end in miscarriage. Some authorities apply the term to women who have had only two successive miscarriages. Still others use the term to apply to any woman who has a tendency to abort, regardless of whether the abortions occur sequentially or are interspersed with live births.

Causes and Treatment

It is thought that most miscarriages are the result of a "blighted ovum," that is, a fertilized egg or embryo that is too defective to survive. Such "blighted ova" are thought to be chance events, although recent research and discoveries have implicated various drugs, cigarette smoking, poor nutrition and environmental pollutants as factors in higher rates of miscarriage. Although it may be true that most spontaneous abortions can be attributed to such chance abnormalities, it is statistically unlikely that successive abortions could be traced to this cause. The odds of a random mutation happening twice, let alone three times, in the same woman are probably less than one in a million. If, on the other hand, rather than successive abortions, there were miscarriages interspersed with normal live births, a genetic factor might be suspected. Under these conditions an analysis of the mother's and father's chromosomes, a testing process known as karyotyping, might reveal the source of the problem; however, at this time there is no known treatment for such a genetic defect. Genetic counseling as to the possible risks involved in future pregnancies and odds for recurrence may be offered to such couples.

In some cases abnormalities in the father's sperm may be a factor in habitual abortion. Sperm analysis may therefore help to pinpoint the cause of a woman's habitual abortion. In some instances, although certainly not in all, the sperm abnormalities can be corrected. For details see the discussion of male factors under the heading Infertility and Sterility.

Abnormalities that distort the shape of the uterus can be a factor in habitual abortion. The abnormalities may be congenital (present since birth). For instance, a woman may have a uterus that is divided in half by a wall of tissue. Such abnormalities and their treatment are discussed in detail under the heading Congenital Abnormalities of the Uterus. Congenital abnormalities of the uterus and cervix that may affect fertility have recently been found in the daughters of women who took the synthetic hormone DES during their pregnancies.

Such distortions may also be acquired (the result of new disease or injury

681

that has happened since birth). For instance, a woman may have fibroid tumors of the uterus or uterine growths known as endometrial polyps. Any of these conditions may distort the uterine cavity and make it impossible for the fertilized egg to implant or the developing embryo to grow properly. These conditions may be diagnosed by the symptoms they produce, careful physical exam, a gentle scraping of the uterine lining by a process known as dilation and curettage or, in some cases, by hysterogram, an X-ray picture of the uterus taken after the injection of a contrast fluid that makes the uterus and tubes visible on the X-ray film. Treatment of these abnormalities is generally surgical and is not always successful.

An incompetent cervix, a condition in which the cervix opens up spontaneously, can cause repeated miscarriage. Incompetent cervix may result from injury or a congenital defect. DES daughters may have this problem. Abortions linked to cervical incompetence typically occur in the 18th to 32d week of pregnancy without any prior bleeding or symptoms of impending abortion, and the duration of each succeeding pregnancy is shorter. Diagnosis is made on the basis of a history of such abortions, evidence of prior injury to the cervix and, if necessary, by ultrasound, a method of visualizing the inside of the body using high-frequency sound waves. Treatment involves tying off the cervix to prevent premature dilation.

Hormonal imbalances of the type discussed under the heading Infertility and Sterility may also cause habitual abortion, although there is disagreement among the experts about whether such imbalances are a frequent or rare cause. In any case progesterone therapy, the treatment for these abnormalities, should not be given unless the various tests used to measure hormonal deficiencies indicate a definite lack. Some doctors, perhaps overcome by the logic of progesterone deficiency as an explanation for habitual abortion (and it does seem to fit right in), prescribe progesterone without the preliminary assays. This practice is questioned by many. A word of caution should be injected at this point. In the past, realizing that estrogen was important in maintaining pregnancy and that the levels of a specific type of estrogen were low in patients who aborted, doctors prescribed a treatment program using estrogen substitution in the form of the now-infamous synthetic estrogen DES for a large number of pregnant women to prevent miscarriage. An alarming number of abnormalities have begun to be found in the teenage daughters born to women who took DES during their pregnancies (see the section on DES for details). Recent reports suggesting that synthetic progesterone therapy may be responsible for malformations among the offspring of women wno took it may make the use of progesterone equally questionable.[18]

There is some evidence that certain incompatibilities in the mother's and father's blood may be a factor in miscarriage, but why or how is not known. Couples with a history that runs along these lines—one normal pregnancy, then perhaps a pregnancy resulting in a jaundiced baby and then recurrent abortions at earlier and earlier stages in the pregnancy—are thought by some authorities to be suffering from certain blood incompatibilities. At the present time there is no treatment for this condition. Women who have an Rh-negative blood type may have problems with miscarriage.

Certain bacterial and viral infections, such as herpes, have been implicated in recurrent miscarriages. Anemia, acute and chronic diseases, including alcoholism, and constitutional illness may play a role. Certainly, treatment of such problems should be attempted when possible. Nutritional factors may play a role. Cigarette smoking is also associated with a higher rate of miscarriage.[19]

In many cases no specific medical cause can be identified. Many doctors attribute cases of habitual abortion for which they are unable to find a cure to "psychological factors." It may be true that psychological factors play a role in all disease processes, but it has long been the habit of the medical establishment to blame women's diseases they have not been able to understand on women's supposed psychological problems. (Menstrual pain is an excellent case in point.) Any woman who is told that her problem is "all in her head," or is treated as if it were, should read the introduction to this section carefully and consider seeking another medical opinion.

Diagnosis and Treatment

Finding a doctor who is sensitive and skilled in treating these problems is important. For specific information on finding a fertility specialist, see the section on Infertility and Sterility. For general information on choosing a doctor, see Chapter Six.

Diagnosing a woman with a habitual abortion problem should be done with the help of laboratory tests on the aborted tissue whenever possible. Physical exams and certain tests similar to those described under the heading Infertility and Sterility may be done on both the mother and the father. Treatment for the particular problem, based on the outcome of these diagnostic tests, may then be undertaken. These treatments are discussed in detail under the specific diseases and conditions mentioned above.

ECTOPIC PREGNANCY

AKA: extrauterine pregnancy

Types: tubal, isthmic, ampullar, or infundibular, pregnancy
cornual, or interstitial, pregnancy
abdominal pregnancy
cervical pregnancy
ovarian pregnancy

Associated Terms: tubal abortion; tubal rupture; hematoma, or blood tumor; hematocele, or blood cyst

In a normal pregnancy the egg is fertilized by the sperm inside the fallopian tube. It then travels through the tube to the uterus, where it attaches itself to the lush uterine wall and begins to grow. In an ectopic pregnancy the fertilized egg doesn't attach to the uterine wall but instead attaches to some other inappropriate tissue. In most ectopic pregnancies the egg implants in the fallopian tube, but as indicated in Illustration 58, other locations are also possible.

Because only the uterus, with its rich lining and its ability to expand as the fetus grows, is equipped to nourish a fetus and to expand to accommodate a developing pregnancy, most ectopic pregnancies abort or rupture within 6 to 14 weeks. There have been cases of certain types of ectopic pregnancy in which the pregnancy was carried to term and a normal infant delivered by cesarean section, but the incidence of birth defects in such infants is considerably higher.

Incidence

The incidence of ectopic pregnancy is hard to determine, because many times the symptoms are vague and minimal and the embryo is reabsorbed by the

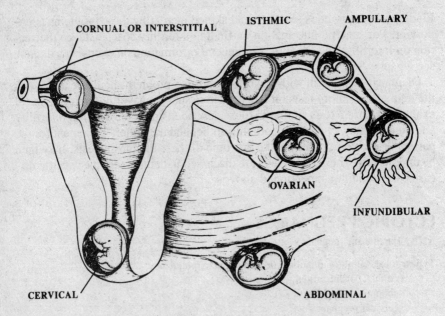

Illustration 58 *Sites of Ectopic Pregnancies*

body, without the woman's being aware there was an ectopic pregnancy. Also, an ectopic pregnancy may be confused with a miscarriage or other gynecological conditions.

The reported statistics in the United States range from 1 in 300 to 1 in 40 pregnancies. The incidence is related to socioeconomic status, with much higher rates being reported among poor, minority women, who are less likely to have the benefit of good medical care. Twice as many black women as white die as a result of ectopic pregnancies, which are estimated to be responsible for about 6.5 percent of all maternal deaths. There is good evidence that ectopic pregnancies are on the increase. Some doctors attribute this rise to the increase in the use of the IUD as a method of birth control. The increase in the incidence of pelvic inflammatory disease (PID) may also explain the rise in the number of ectopic pregnancies.

Cause

There are a number of theories to explain ectopic pregnancies, some of them rather far-fetched; however, in most cases the function of the fallopian tube is impaired in some way, which prevents the fertilized egg from making its usual journey through the tube and into the uterus. There may be an obstruction or a distortion in the shape of the tube that might have been caused by PID, endometriosis, scar tissue from previous tubal or pelvic surgery, congenital deformities of the uterus and tubes, tumors of the tube or by ovarian or fibroid tumors pressing on the tubes. In addition to obstructing the tube, these conditions may also cause problems with the normal muscle contractions and the action of the tiny, hairlike cilia that help move the fertile egg through the tube and into the uterus. It has also been suggested that bits of the normal uterine lining tissue may be found growing in the tubes. If this is the case, it is not surprising that the egg might incorrectly implant in such tissue.

Symptoms of Tubal Pregnancy

The fertilized egg implants in the wall of the tube, which develops an increased blood supply in response to the needs of the growing pregnancy and stretches to accommodate the enlarging embryo. But since the tube was not designed to support a pregnancy, sooner or later something has to happen. As the embryo burrows into and sometimes beyond the wall of the tube in its search for sustenance and the tube stretches, there is bound to be some bleeding. One of several things may then happen (Illustration 59).

If a woman is fortunate and the embryo has implanted near the end of the tube, the bleeding may separate the embryo from the wall of the tube and

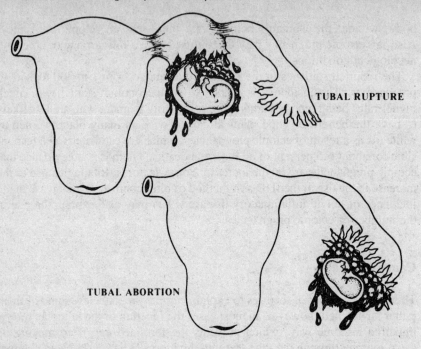

TUBAL RUPTURE

TUBAL ABORTION

Illustration 59   *Possible Outcomes of Ectopic Pregnancy*

force it backward through the tube and out into the pelvic cavity. This is called a tubal abortion. If this happens early on, the embryo may be reabsorbed by the body. As long as no major blood vessels have been injured, the bleeding stops. There may be only minimal symptoms, like a slight delay in the menstrual period and perhaps a dull, aching pain for a few days, but nothing serious enough to require medical attention. This sort of ectopic pregnancy may go unrecognized or be discovered years later when, in the course of another operation, the remnants of the tubal pregnancy are found.

If the embryo is still partially attached to the wall of the tube, the expulsion is more likely to take place gradually, over a period of 2 to 4 weeks. The bleeding is intermittent, only a portion of the embryo being detached each time. A hematoma (blood tumor) may form around the *end* of the tube, and it may grow larger with each bleeding eipsode, eventually causing the tube to rupture, usually between the 8th and 12th weeks. Tubal rupture may also occur if blood collects *in* the tube, a condition known as a hematosalpinx.

The tubal rupture may happen suddenly, as the tube literally bursts, or it may develop more slowly, a leaking process that takes place over a period of weeks. The bleeding may be slight or profuse; sometimes it is so excessive as to be fatal. The tubal rupture may be set off by intercourse or even by straining at the bowels.

686

Tubal ruptures and tubal abortions can cause external as well as internal bleeding. The first sign or symptom is apt to be a 7-to-14-day delay in menstruation, followed by slight bleeding, a red or brown vaginal discharge that persists. There is usually only a scant show of blood each day. Although this spotting type of bleeding is characteristic, the bleeding may be more profuse. In some cases the bleeding will occur before the expected time of menstruation, and in other cases the external bleeding may not occur until after two or more menstrual periods have been missed.

Pain is also an early symptom, although in some cases it is mild. At first there may be a vague soreness on the affected side or a sort of "stitch in the side" that precedes or accompanies the spotty bleeding. Later there may also be intermittent sharp, colicky pains. In either the complete tubal abortion or the tubal rupture the pain may be severe, and there may be faintness, nausea and vomiting. These symptoms result from the irritation of the lining of the pelvic cavity, which is particularly sensitive to blood. If the bleeding into the pelvic cavity is severe, there may be symptoms of shock: rapid, irregular pulse; pallor; cold, clammy skin; subnormal temperature and difficulty in breathing. Such a case, if not treated promptly, can be fatal. In cases of excessive internal bleeding there may be referred pain in the top of the shoulder if blood has collected beneath the diaphragm. More often the bleeding is slight and of an on-again, off-again nature. Then the pain may subside quickly, leaving only soreness in between more acute attacks.

Since the developing pregnancy, even if it implants ectopically, produces hormones, the hormone-induced changes that occur in a normal pregnancy may also occur in the uterus of an ectopic pregnancy. One of these changes is the formation of a decidual lining, which becomes part of the blood-rich placenta that helps nourish a fetus during pregnancy. Once the ectopic embryo dies, the hormone production stops and this decidual lining may be shed in fragments or even in one piece. Thus there may also be vaginal bleeding of this nature. If the lining is cast off in one piece, the woman and her doctor may mistakenly assume that the woman has had a spontaneous abortion. It is important for a woman to save any such tissue so the doctor can examine it. If there are no signs of embryonic tissue, this may suggest an ectopic pregnancy.

The usual symptoms of pregnancy—morning sickness, swelling of the breasts and so on—are not often seen because the embryo usually dies so early; but in cases where it does survive such symptoms may develop.

If the embryo develops to a large enough size, or if the tube is sufficiently swollen with blood, the doctor may be able to feel a tender swelling on one side or the other. The whole abdomen may be swollen, possibly so swollen that it's stretched as tight as a drum, as a result of the bleeding into the abdomen. The cervix may be softened and opened up, and the uterus may be enlarged even in early tubal pregnancy, although in most early cases this may not be noticeable. If the swelling of the tube is large enough, the doctor may be able to feel a uterus that has been pushed to one side.

There is generally little or no fever unless a hematocele (blood cyst) has formed in the pelvis and has become secondarily infected.

Diagnosis

The diagnosis of ectopic pregnancy may be difficult, for there are a number of other conditions that may be confused with ectopic pregnancy. A threatened or incomplete abortion, for instance, is often confused with ectopic pregnancy. Both can cause a delay in the onset of menstruation, although the length of time of the delay is longer with threatened or incomplete abortion. Moreover, the uterus is likely to be softer and larger, the pain less severe and located in the middle rather than the side and the bleeding more profuse in the case of incomplete abortion. In tubal pregnancy, where there is a great deal of internal bleeding, the anemia that results is out of proportion to the external blood loss, whereas in miscarriage any anemia is more or less in line with the observable blood loss.

PID can also behave like a tubal pregnancy and vice versa, the major difference being that in PID the infection of the tubes and their swelling is usually bilateral, whereas in ectopic pregnancy it is usually one-sided. It does happen, however, that the swelling in PID may be larger on one side than the other and thus appear to be unilateral. Also, IUD-related cases of PID are frequently unilateral. Although ectopic pregnancy usually produces scant, spotty bleeding, it may occasionally produce bursts of bleeding, like PID. Acute PID that affects the tubes usually produces high fever and a high white blood cell count that is not seen in ectopic pregnancy, but chronic PID may not produce these signs.

The sudden onset of pain with nausea and vomiting that may accompany tubal rupture or tubal abortion may also occur with an ovarian cyst that has become twisted on its stem, but there is usually no menstrual irregularity with the latter. It isn't too important to make the correct diagnosis in this particular situation, for both conditions constitute an emergency and surgery is done in either case.

Luteum and follicle cysts on the ovary may also cause a delay in menstruation, followed by persistent slight bleeding, just as a tubal pregnancy does. Moreover, the enlargement of the ovary produced by these cysts may be hard to distinguish from a tubal swelling in ectopic pregnancy, especially when it is near the end of the tube. In the rare case where the tubal pregnancy implants on the ovary, this may be especially difficult.

Sometimes the corpus luteum, which produces hormones in the early stages of a normal pregnancy, will bleed into the pelvic cavity. The bleeding may be so scant that it doesn't require surgery, but it may be the cause of the pain some women experience in the first 3 months of pregnancy. On occasion the bleeding may be extensive and may be difficult to distinguish from the shock symptoms produced by certain ectopic pregnancies, even though such symptoms as external bleeding and a tender pelvic mass are absent.

Diagnosis of an ectopic pregnancy, then, can be difficult and often it is not made until the tube has ruptured and the woman has had to be rushed to the hospital. Because ectopic pregnancy is a potentially life-threatening situation, it used to be that all women with suspected ectopics were operated on. Now there are specific tools that can help in the diagnosis. Culdocentesis, a procedure in which a needle is inserted into the pelvic cavity through the rear wall of the vagina, may be done. If unclotted blood is aspirated, this usually indicates an ectopic pregnancy. Culdoscopy, another procedure that can be done under a local anesthetic, allows the doctor to insert a viewing instrument into the pelvis and visually inspect the uterus, tubes and ovary. Laparoscopy, although it involves more risks and possible complications, may allow a better view and a more accurate diagnosis.

Treatment

Once a tubal pregnancy has been diagnosed, surgery must be performed. Even if a woman has little in the way of symptoms, surgery must not be delayed for too long because of the risk of fatal bleeding from a tubal abortion or rupture. In cases where the internal bleeding has been profuse, immediate surgery is necessary, and blood transfusions before or during surgery may be given.

In most cases involving younger women who have future childbearing plans, only the affected tube will be removed. There are, however, some important exceptions to this general rule in which either more or less extensive surgery may be done.

On the more extensive side there is the older woman who has long since completed her family. In her case the uterus, tubes and, if she is close to menopause, the ovaries as well may be removed. Pros and cons on the removal of the uterus and ovaries and the age at which this should or should not be done are discussed under the heading Hysterectomy. Sometimes, on operation, the doctor will discover that the other tube is also diseased. The same sort of scar tissue or disease that affected the first tube and caused the ectopic pregnancy may have affected the second tube. If the tube is hopelessly damaged, the doctor will remove it as well. Unless the ovaries are so diseased as to be nonfunctional or are so hopelessly matted together with the tube as to require removal, the doctor will try to leave the ovaries to prevent a premature menopause. If both tubes are taken, the majority of doctors think that the uterus should be removed as well.

On the less extensive side there are some cases in which it may be possible to avoid removing the affected tube. If the tube has not burst and the pregnancy is located near the open end of the tube, it may be possible to "milk" it out. Even if the pregnancy is not located at the end, as long as the tube has not yet burst, it may be possible to make an incision in the tube, remove the embryo and repair the tube. This is not always possible, and some surgeons are hesitant to try, even when one of these options seems feasible. Such doctors believe that the tube was probably defective in the first place—hence the ectopic pregnancy—or that the ectopic pregnancy has probably done irrevocable damage to it. They think that leaving the tube in would not increase the woman's chances of having a subsequent, successful pregnancy and might even increase her chances of having another ectopic pregnancy.

Other doctors point out that there have been many cases of women whose other tube had previously been removed who have had successful pregnancies after such operations. A woman, especially one who has only one tube and who very much wants to have a child, may decide to assume the risks. It is important that such a woman discuss her attitudes with the doctor before surgery and that she feel sure that the doctor is both willing to follow her wishes if possible and sufficiently competent and experienced in this special type of surgery to do it if the situation demands it.

A similar sort of dilemma may confront the woman even if her tube has already ruptured or is so damaged that there is no choice but to remove it. Often the other tube has been affected by the same underlying disease. In cases where it is feasible the surgeon may choose to repair the other tube at the same time. In emergency ectopics, where the woman has lost a good deal of blood, such a procedure cannot be considered, for prolonging the operation even by half an hour could risk the woman's life. In less severe situations this procedure may be possible. However, many women who have such operations are unable to get pregnant again, and for those who do, the rate of second ectopics is high. Only about 50 percent of such women will subsequently have successful pregnancies. Some women may decide that they are willing to assume the risks involved. Here again, women need to discuss their feelings on this matter with the surgeon before the operation. Women who want the chance to get pregnant again should know that most gynecologists are not skilled in the special type of tubal repair surgery, known as microtuboplasty, that in some cases may be necessary to save the tube. In order to avoid the risks and complications of another operation at a later date, as well as more loss of fertility time while the body readjusts after surgery (a factor that could be critical in women in their 30s), such women might decide to seek out a surgeon who is skilled in microtuboplasty before having an operation for what is deemed to be an ectopic pregnancy. This, of course, will not be possible in cases demanding emergency surgery.

Other Types of Ectopic Pregnancies

Thus far this discussion of ectopic pregnancy has centered around the more common tubal pregnancies. However, as noted in the illustration at the beginning of this section, there are other possible locations. The interstitial, or cornual, pregnancy is located where the fallopian tube joins the uterus. It is often mistaken for a soft uterine fibroid or an early miscarriage. The symptoms are similar to those of a tubal pregnancy, although the pain may not be as severe and the delay of menstruation may be a bit longer, since this location is more favorable and the embryo may survive longer. Should a rupture occur, the bleeding into the pelvic cavity may be heavy, producing the same sorts of symptoms and necessitating the same treatment as a heavily bleeding tubal abortion or rupture.

Most medical authorities believe that ovarian pregnancy is rare, probably because the egg given off by the ovary is not fully mature, a process that is usually completed during the egg's journey through the fallopian tube. Thus the immature egg cannot be fertilized and implant anywhere. Some doctors believe that the IUD may be a factor in ovarian pregnancies. Ovarian pregnancy may also be more common than is generally thought, many cases of what are assumed to be ruptured corpus luteum cysts being in reality early ectopic ovarian pregnancies.

It is also possible for an egg to be fertilized and travel into the pelvic cavity (instead of through the tube to the uterus). This is called abdominal pregnancy and can also result from tubal abortion or rupture in which the embryo and its partially detached placenta grow out from the tube and latch on to the lining of the abdominal cavity. In removing one of these the surgeon will leave the placenta in place, since detaching it may cause massive bleeding. Some doctors use a drug called methotrexate, which is sometimes used to treat cancer, to aid in the absorption of the placenta; others think that this highly toxic drug should not be used in this manner. Women should seek second opinions (*see* p. 238) before consenting to this type of therapy.

Although rare, the possibility of a cervical pregnancy does exist. This bizarre type of pregnancy produces profuse bleeding that may be fatal and usually necessitates hysterectomy. There have also been cases of tubal pregnancy accompanied by normal pregnancy, simultaneous pregnancy in both tubes and twin, and even triplet, pregnancy in one tube. There was even a case where a woman had intercourse the night before her hysterectomy, subsequently carried an abdominal pregnancy and delivered a normal baby.

Subsequent Pregnancies

Once a woman has had an ectopic pregnancy, she is at higher risk for having another one, so subsequent pregnancies should be monitored carefully. Providing that too much blood has not been lost and the woman is not anemic, pregnancy can be attempted after resumption of the first normal menstrual period.

TROPHOBLASTIC DISEASE*

AKA: gestational trophoblastic disease, TRD

Types: hydatidiform, or benign, mole
      nonmetastatic TRD, chorioadenoma destruens, or invasive mole
      metastatic TRD, choriocarcinoma, or chorioepithelioma

Trophoblastic disease (TRD) is a condition involving the trophoblast, the layer of specialized cells on the outside of the sac in which the fertilized egg develops. In normal pregnancies the embryo attaches itself to the uterus by means of this trophoblastic tissue. The trophoblast then invades the uterine wall and develops projections called chorionic villi through which the embryo receives nourishment from the mother's bloodstream.

TRD is usually a benign (noncancerous) disease, but in some cases it may degenerate into cancer. The benign form of TRD is known as hydatidiform mole (the term "mole" here means a swelling, not the kind of mole seen on the skin). Hydatidiform mole occurs when the fetus is stunted, has died or has never developed. If the fetus has died, it may be expelled in a spontaneous or induced abortion, or it may remain within the uterus, as in a missed abortion. In any case, even though the fetus is dead or absent altogether, the trophoblast continues to live and, temporarily, to grow. Since the fetus is dead and its circulatory system is no longer functioning, the fluid from the chorionic villi that would normally be absorbed by the fetus is not used. Thus the chorionic villi become swollen with fluid. The resultant mass of swollen villi has the appearance of a cluster of pale grapes. In some rare cases a few villi will develop in the same manner in the course of a normal pregnancy and a normal baby can be delivered in those cases. Also, parts of the placenta, the tissue through which the mother's blood reaches the infant, may be retained after childbirth and may develop a few of these similarly swollen villi.

Although TRD is most often a benign disease, it does on occasion become cancerous. The cancerous forms of TRD are metastatic and nonmetastatic TRD. They may occur after a hydatidiform mole or, in some cases, after a normal delivery, an abortion or, even more rarely, after an ectopic preg-

*Readers seeking information on cancerous forms of TRD should also read the general section on cancer.

nancy, but when they do occur it is always after a pregnancy, even though the pregnancy may have been of such a short duration that the woman was not even aware that she had been pregnant. Both metastatic and nonmetastatic TRD involve abnormalities of the process by which the trophoblast invades the rich uterine lining.

The nature of these abnormalities is not clear. Even in normal pregnancies the process by which the trophoblast implants is not well understood. The fetus and the trophoblast are actually foreign bodies to the mother's uterus, and why they are not rejected remains a mystery. It is thought that the mother's immune system, which normally attacks foreign bodies, is somehow switched off, thereby allowing the trophoblastic tissue to make its invasion without resistance. The trophoblast is allowed to go only so far and is stopped before it can grow into the lower levels of the uterine wall. It is thought that the mother's immune system somehow sets limits on this invasive process.

In all other instances in which one type of tissue invades another, we are talking about a malignant, or cancerous, growth pattern, the exception being the curious case of the trophoblast in a normal pregnancy. The trophoblast has another similarity to cancer. Just as cells from a cancerous tumor may travel to other parts of the body and set up new colonies of cancerous tissue—a process known as metastasis—so cells from the trophoblast may travel through the bloodstream from the mother's uterus to her lungs. In a normal pregnancy this metastasized trophoblastic tissue in the lung causes no harm. Here again, there is probably some mechanism in the mother's immune system that prevents trophoblastic metastasis from becoming a problem.

Sometimes this little-understood process of trophoblastic invasion, which as we have seen may also include metastasis, goes awry. The trophoblast may not stop growing, continuing to grow beyond the uterine wall and even through it into the pelvis or vagina, a process that produces an alarming and sometimes even fatal amount of bleeding. If this growth pattern, which is now considered a cancerous one, is accompanied by metastatic colonies of trophoblastic tissue invading the lung, the terms "metastatic trophoblastic disease," "choriocarcinoma" or "chorioepithelioma" are used. If there is no metastasis to the lung or other points in the body but there is growth into the uterine wall or beyond, the condition is considered nonmetastatic trophoblastic disease, which is also known as chorioadenoma destruens or, more simply, invasive mole.

Incidence

Fortunately, trophoblastic disease is rather rare in the United States, occurring in only about 1 in every 1,500 or 2,000 pregnancies.[20] It is more common at the extremes of reproductive life, that is, in women over age 40 or under age 20. Cancerous types of TRD are much less common than the benign hydatidiform mole. Two percent of women who have a hydatidiform mole pregnancy will have moles in subsequent pregnancies, which, although it is a low incidence, is 40 times the normal rate for women who have not had previous moles.

Symptoms

The chief symptom of hydatidiform mole is painless vaginal bleeding. The bleeding occurs after at least one or two menstrual periods have been missed. There is little to distinguish this bleeding from that of an early miscarriage, except that the hydatidiform mole generally occurs later, usually beyond the 10th week of pregnancy. In the case of a mole the bleeding usually does not stop once it has started. It continues until the uterus has been emptied of all abnormal tissue.

About half the women with hydatidiform mole will have enlarged uteri.[21] If a woman is known to be pregnant, the doctor may become suspicious when s/he feels a uterus that is larger than it should be for the stage of her pregnancy. An enlarged uterus in a pregnant woman with vaginal bleeding is going to make the doctor suspicious of several possibilities. However, not all women show this symptom, and some may even have uteri that are smaller than expected through the duration of the pregnancy.

Women with hydatidiform mole may show signs of toxemia, a condition that is characterized by swelling, headaches, vision disturbances (from swelling in the brain), high blood pressure, nausea and protein in the urine. About one-half of the women will have vomiting.[22] These symptoms are probably caused by the hormone HCG, human chorionic gonadotropin. During pregnancy this hormone is secreted by the placenta, the organ through which nutrients are filtered from mother to fetus and which develops in part from the trophoblast. In TRD the hormone is secreted in abnormally excessive amounts. There may be an excess of other hormones as well. In about 10 percent of cases of hydatidiform mole there will be evidence of an overactive thyroid gland.

A woman may pass pale, grapelike clusters of villi, or sometimes these may be seen on speculum exam as pale grapes protruding through the cervical os. There may be bleeding if the woman spontaneously aborts the mole. Although the vaginal bleeding discussed above is painless, the bleeding that accompanies the expulsion of the mole is usually associated with uterine cramps.

The ovaries may also be affected in TRD. Apparently, the excessive amount of the hormone HCG triggers the first steps in the process of ovulation. The stimulated eggs do not burst out of their capsules but remain on the surface of the ovary as cysts. These cysts may be small or large; in about a third of cases of TRD they are large enough to be felt by the doctor in the course of a bimanual pelvic exam.[23] However, these same sorts of cysts may be large enough to be felt in a normal pregnancy as well.

For some reason these cysts seem to grow rapidly after the mole has been expelled from the uterus. Another curious fact is that they sometimes disappear spontaneously as the disease progresses. Some experts have suggested that these cysts may provide protection against the subsequent development of choriocarcinoma. The large amount of estrogen produced by these cysts seems to act as a brake against excessive trophoblastic growth; thus a woman without ovarian enlargement may be more likely to have her hydatidiform mole undergo malignant transformation.

Diagnosis of the Hydatidiform Mole

Diagnosis of a hydatidiform mole is not always a simple process. The painless vaginal bleeding is likely to be interpreted as a sign of impending miscarriage, a more common occurrence than hydatidiform mole. A woman with such bleeding and a uterus that is overenlarged for the duration of her pregnancy should cause a doctor to be suspicious enough to run tests. Likewise, the onset of symptoms of toxemia before the 20th week of pregnancy in a woman without underlying disease to which the toxemia could be attributed should make the doctor suspicious. If the doctor can't hear fetal heart tones by the 12th week of pregnancy, or if there is no evidence of fetal movement by the 18th to 20th week, TRD should be suspected.

If all or some of these symptoms—bleeding, enlarged uterus, toxemia and absence of fetal heart tone and movement—are present, the doctor should be suspicious enough to run extensive laboratory tests. Laboratory evidence from the series of tests indicating higher-than-normal levels of HCG are extremely useful, although not conclusive, for HCG levels may vary in individuals. Moreover, a twin pregnancy could also yield high levels of HCG. When the high levels of HCG are accompanied by low levels of certain other hormones normally associated with pregnancy but not with TRD, the doctor will have an almost certain diagnosis.

The next step will probably be ultrasound examination, a method of visualizing the soft tissue inside the body by the use of high-frequency sound waves. If the ultrasound examination shows fetal parts, the diagnosis of hydatidiform mole is pretty much ruled out, since a developed fetus and a mole rarely coexist. One rare example might be a twin pregnancy in which one of the pregnancies is molar and the other one normal.

X-ray examination can also be used to determine whether or not a fetal skeleton is present, but because of the possible risks involved in radiating the

695

fetus, the X-ray examination is not used until the doctor is fairly certain that a viable fetus is not present.

Many times the diagnosis of hydatidiform mole is not made until the woman actually starts to pass the characteristic clusters of swollen, grapelike villi. Any woman who passes something unusual should save the tissue if at all possible, so that her doctor can examine it.

Treatment of the Hydatidiform Mole

Treatment of a hydatidiform mole is threefold. The first step is to determine the best method of removing the mole and then to do so. The next step is to rule out the possibility that the mole has undergone cancerous transformation. The third step is to plan and execute a careful follow-up program.

If the diagnosis of hydatidiform mole is not made until the woman is spontaneously aborting the mole, the woman is hospitalized and given a drug that aids the uterine contractions and helps in the expulsion of the mole.

In the absence of labor a decision must be made as to how to evacuate the mole. If the woman is over age 35 and has finished her family, a hysterectomy may be the treatment of choice, since there is a much higher incidence of malignant TRD in women over 35. If there is cancer and it is only a localized, nonmetastatic form of TRD, the hysterectomy will be curative. But the hysterectomy is more treatment than is really needed for 85 percent of women with TRD, since only 15 percent of TRD patients will have cancerous complications. Although in the past, hysterectomy was the only alternative, today, thanks to two developments—the sensitivity of tests to detect HCG and the development of drugs that can offer close to a 100 percent cure rate—not all women with a molar pregnancy need to have their uteri removed.

In most cases the uterus can be emptied by a D&C or a suction curettage, a vacuumlike procedure used to suck out the contents of the uterus. Once the evacuation has been accomplished, by whatever method, the tissue is studied carefully for signs of cancer. Unfortunately, such studies are not conclusive; therefore, a careful follow-up program, which involves measuring levels of HCG, must be instituted to rule out the possibility of cancer.

In 2 to 4 weeks most women's HCG levels will return to normal.[24] Even after the HCG levels drop a woman must be tested once a month for 6 months and then once every other month for 6 more months, since the trophoblastic tissue may still be present, either in the pelvic area or in some other location as a result of metastasis, and it might take this long for the remaining tissue to grow large enough to produce a quantity of HCG that could be measured even by the most sensitive of tests now available. A woman should not become pregnant during this time because pregnancy would create higher levels of HCG, which would confuse the picture.

Since metastasis, if it occurs, frequently affects the lungs, chest X-rays are done every 2 weeks until HCG levels return to normal and then every 3 months for a year. Bimanual pelvic exams to check that the uterus is returning to normal size and to allow the doctor to examine the vulva and vagina for masses of TRD are also done every 2 weeks until HCG levels return to normal and then every 3 months for a year.

Metastatic and Nonmetastatic Trophoblastic Disease

Invasive mole is the nonmetastatic form of TRD that occurs when the trophoblast of a hydatidiform mole takes on a cancerous growth pattern. There is apt to be bleeding beyond the normal 6 to 8 weeks after the mole has been expelled or removed from the uterus. If the uterus has been perforated by the invasive mole, there may be a great deal of bleeding, sometimes enough to be fatal. Also, if perforation has occurred, there may be infection, chills and fever. If the mole has spread beyond the uterus, it may be possible to feel masses in the pelvis or vagina. Choriocarcinoma is a metastatic form of TRD and can produce symptoms like those of invasive moles.

If vaginal bleeding continues for too long a time after a mole has been evacuated, this may indicate that the trophoblastic tissue is still present. If the HCG levels remain elevated for longer than 60 days, or if the HCG rises at any time during the follow-up, this is also taken as a sign that the trophoblastic tissue is still present and that it has taken on a cancerous growth pattern. Only about 40 percent of women whose HCG levels remain elevated after 60 days actually have metastatic or nonmetastatic TRD, but it is impossible at this point to tell whether any given woman is among the 60 percent who will progress to cancer or among the 40 percent who will not.[25] Chemotherapy, treatment of cancer by drugs, must be given to all such women, for the risks of withholding treatment are too great.

Chemotherapy is usually given orally or by injections for 5 days, followed by a resting stage of 1 week, while new tests of HCG levels are obtained. If HCG levels continue to decrease, subsequent chemotherapy is continued until the tests are negative. The tests are then repeated until they remain negative for 1 year. If during the therapy there is a rise in HCG or evidence of drug toxicity, another type of chemotherapy is used. Although a few experts recommend giving preventive drug therapy to all women with hydatidiform mole, this practice is questioned by most experts, since 85 percent of these women will not develop TRD and these drugs are highly toxic.[26] Any woman whose doctor suggests prophylactic, or preventive, chemotherapy just because she had a mole should seek a second opinion (see p. 238).

Cancer that starts out as a seemingly normal pregnancy and turns out to be a life-threatening, horrible disease is not a pleasant prospect for any woman.

However, the progress that has been made in treating what was formerly a highly lethal disease is encouraging. Cure rates of 80 percent to 100 percent for nonmetastatic TRD and 36 percent to 95 percent for metastatic TRD have been reported.[27] Because the disease is hardly a common one, many doctors are not equipped, trained or experienced enough to treat it correctly. A woman with TRD should consider contacting one of the trophoblastic-disease study centers around the country. Her doctor should be able to find out where the nearest center is located. If not, the nearest medical school should be able to answer this question.

The TRD study centers generally have some form of counseling available. Any woman, especially one who is childless, may need counseling in these circumstances. She is apt to feel that there is something monstrous about her. Both she and her partner or family may benefit from such counseling. Normal pregnancies can and do follow drug therapy. If the woman wants to get pregnant again, she must wait until follow-up therapy has been completed. She may also find special counseling and support during pregnancy valuable.

Cancer

Madison Avenue and public health agencies, in an effort to make us aware of the cancer problem and to encourage us to seek early treatment for suspicious symptoms, have in some ways oversold cancer to us, the American public. Most of us are terrified of the disease, although great strides have been made in treating it and some forms are now virtually 100 percent curable. Yet even those of us with curable forms of the disease are apt to find being diagnosed as having cancer, or even going through a diagnostic workup for a possible cancer, a frightening experience, for confronting cancer brings us face to face with the possibility of our own death.

Too many times our fear makes us act hastily, choosing a doctor or accepting a form of treatment before we understand our options; but these decisions are important ones, sometimes even matters of life and death, and they deserve our careful consideration. The treatment of cancer is one of the most controversial subjects in medicine. The type of treatment you receive will depend on many factors, including your age, menstrual status and the type and extent of your cancer. The quality of treatment as well as the kind of treatment you receive may also depend on the particular doctor you choose. The same woman may be treated differently by different doctors.

It's especially important to be an informed consumer if you have or may have cancer. But it isn't always easy to be a wise consumer when you're anxious and apprehensive, as anyone confronting cancer is apt to be. For this reason we suggest that you enlist the help of a friend or relative. The following pages provide general information about cancer and advice on how to assure yourself of getting optimum care. In addition, specific types of female can-

699

cers are discussed in greater detail in other sections of this book. Read these pages carefully, taking notes as necessary, and ask your friend or relative to do the same thing. Working together, make a list of the important issues and questions to be discussed with the doctor.

When you visit the doctor, take that person along with you. When we are upset we may not be thinking rationally and often misunderstand what is being said. Having someone else with you can therefore be invaluable. A good doctor will not object to your bringing someone else along. If your doctor refuses to allow you to include someone else in your consultations, find another doctor.

Do not allow yourself to be rushed into a decision about treatment. By the time a cancer is discovered, it has already been in your body for some time. Taking a few days or, with certain types of cancer, even a week or two to inform yourself fully and to seek consultations and second opinions won't hurt and may be a lifesaving step.

In the following pages we provide basic information about cancer and how it behaves. We also define basic terms and concepts used in connection with cancer. More specific information on the various types of cancer is discussed in the section on the particular organ involved—breast cancer, for instance, is covered in the section on the breast. The information on each of the specific types of cancer is broken down into various subheadings, such as Incidence, Risk Factors, Symptoms, Diagnosis, Stage, Treatment, Follow-Up and so forth. Basic information on these topics is also included here, and you will probably find it useful to review this more general information before you turn to the discussion of the specific type of cancer with which you are concerned.

What Is Cancer?

In order to be an informed consumer of the medical services available to cancer patients, it helps to have an understanding of what cancer is. Cancer is not a single disease but many diseases that may present a variety of symptoms, may have different causes and may require different forms of treatment. The nature of cancer is not understood, but the one thing that all cancers have in common is irregular growth of abnormal cells.

Our bodies are a collection of organs and tissues that are made up of trillions of cells, which are microscopic bits of Jell-O-like material. Each cell has a center, called a nucleus, and is surrounded by a special membrane that acts like a filter, permitting certain substances to enter or leave the cell. Throughout the cell are tiny "factories" that process the nutrients that have filtered through the cell membrane from the bloodstream. Each type of cell has its particular job to do. By interacting physically and chemically with one another the cells produce energy to support the function of the particular organ in which they are located. Cancerous cells can interfere with the function of the organ in which they are located because they don't do their job properly.

There are many types of cells, and each type has its own characteristics. Some are long and slender, others are round. The size of the nucleus also varies. Each type of cell also has its own particular architecture. Glandular cells, for instance, form circular patterns. Skin cells form flat sheets. Whatever the pattern, these cells build up, layer by layer, in a neat, orderly fashion.

Cells grow up and mature in the same sense that a person does. Young cells look different than fully mature cells. Normal cells at the same stage of growth in any given class of cells look pretty much the same. Cancerous cells sometimes look rather like the normal cells, but sometimes they look wildly different. They do not organize themselves into the same orderly architecture, although there is a tendency to mimic the normal growth patterns. Cancerous gland cells, for instance, often organize into circlelike patterns. Their circular architecture is not, however, as orderly as that of normal gland cells.

As normal cells mature and develop, so that they are able to perform their particular job, they are said to be differentiating. A fully mature cell, then, is one that is well differentiated. This term, "differentiated," is an important one in cancer, especially in certain types of cancer. If the cells of a cancerous tumor are undifferentiated, this means they are immature and look quite different than the normal, mature, differentiated cells, which generally means that the cancer is a more serious one. The term "grade" is used to refer to the degree of differentiation. Grade is discussed in more detail below.

Normal cells constantly wear out and die and are replaced by new ones. Most cells in our bodies reproduce by a process known as cell division, or mitosis. Inside the nucleus of each cell are strands called chromosomes, which are the bearers of substances called genes. Genes are made of the protein molecule DNA. These chromosomal strips, with their genes and DNA, are the cell's mastermind, a sort of computer headquarters that directs its behavior. When a cell is ready to reproduce itself it grows a duplicate set of chromosomes, a process known as twinning. Once there is a complete duplicate set, the two sets begin to move apart, migrating to opposite sides of the cell. Meanwhile, the outer membrane of the cell begins to indent and then quickly starts to cleave, pinching in until it divides into two separate cells, as shown in Illustration 60.

After resting awhile, the cells begin twinning and dividing again. Different types of cells have different resting times. Specific directions are "printed" in the DNA of the chromosome strip that let the cell know how long to rest and stay dormant until the tissue of which it is a part needs new cells to replace those that have died.

701

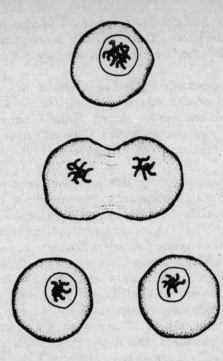

Illustration 60   *Twinning: The Reproductive Process of a Cell*

If everything goes well, the new twin strip of chromosomes is identical to the original strip and the new cell will then behave exactly like the original one in every detail, right down to the specific amount of resting time in between reproductive cycles. Sometimes, however, errors, or mutations, occur. The twinning process goes awry and the new cell is not an exact replica. If the mutation is severe, the cell may die. If the mutation is a minor one, it may merely affect one particular behavior of that cell. If, for instance, one of the cell's jobs is to absorb iron from the bloodstream and the new cell has an error in twinning that involves the gene that regulates iron absorption, that cell and its descendants will not absorb iron in the usual fashion. In most cases an error like this is not likely to affect the overall functioning of the organ. If, however, the error or mutation in the twinning process involves the gene that controls the length of time the cell spends resting in between reproduction, the result could be cancer.

Once the mutation has occurred it is repeated each time the cell reproduces. So the 1 mutated cell becomes 2. The 2 become 4; the 4 become 8, the 8, 16; the 16, 32 and so on, until after about 20 cell generations there are about 1 million cells, weighing about 1/1,000 of a gram. By 30 generations there will be about 1 billion cells weighing about 1 gram. A tumor of this size, depending on where it is located, may be large enough to be felt. The tumor grows 1,000 times larger in just half the time that it took to grow to the 1/1,000 gram weight. By the 31st generation it will increase to 2 grams, and by the 32d, it will weigh 4 grams.

This explains a phenomenon that people often find puzzling—the fact that although cancer is said to take years to develop, once a cancer is discovered it often seems to grow at a rapid-fire pace. Actually, the rate of growth is constant. This rate, the average time required for all the cells in the tumor to reproduce, is called the doubling time. The doubling time varies according to the type of tissue. If the normal cells in an organ grow slowly, generally the cancer in that tissue will have a relatively slow rate of growth. Liver cells, for instance, are slow-growing and so are cancerous liver cells. Some cancers grow more quickly. Breast cancer has a doubling time of anywhere from 6 to 540 days, depending on the particular kind of cells involved.

A tumor that had a 100-day doubling time would take 9 years to grow from a single cell to a 1-gram tumor that could be felt, but in only 15 more months it would weight 16 grams—about half an ounce—and in 15 more months it would weigh almost a pound! Thus, although the doubling rate is steady—100 days—the fact that every cell in the entire tumor doubles every 100 days—a geometric progression—explains the rapid acceleration in its size.

Meanwhile, the other cells of the organ are plodding away, reproducing at the preprogrammed rate designed to assure that the proper numbers of the right kinds of cells will be in the proper ratio to one another so that the organ will function as it should. But as we have seen, the cancer cells are not resting; they are reproducing at too fast a rate. Although the cancer cells, like normal cells, wear out and die, their birth rate far outstrips their death rate.

The invaded organ has no use for this overabundance of cells. Thus the cancerous cells may throw the organ out of whack by their sheer bulk; because they have not matured properly, are undifferentiated and unable to do their job; or by gobbling up the food that should nourish the other cells. Not only do they endanger the proper functioning of the organ by their overabundance within a particular area, but they also tend to invade other tissues as their exuberant growth continues. If one of these mutant cells gets into the blood or lymph system, it may be carried to another part of the body and start a new colony of aberrant tissue, a phenomenon known as metastasis.

Spread

Different types of cancer can spread from the tissues in which they originate in a number of ways. The cancerous tumor may simply keep growing in the same place (in which case it is said to be localized), getting bigger and bigger, until it invades and destroys the neighboring tissue. When this happens the terms "direct extension" and "invasion" are used. As noted above, sometimes the cancer spreads because the abnormal cells get into the bloodstream or the lymph system, which is an intricate network of interconnected passageways through which a fluid known as lymph is circulated. The lymph system is part of the body's defense system. The abnormal cells may then be carried to other parts of the body, where they start growing. The tumor is then said to have metastasized. Metastatic tumors, then, are colonies of new tumors composed of cells that have been transplanted. Once either direct invasion or metastasis (plural: metastases) has taken place, the malignant disease is said to be disseminated.

Particular types of cancer have a tendency to spread to particular organs. Breast cancer, for instance, generally metastasizes from the primary site in the breast to the liver, bones, lungs or brain. Even though a breast cancer has metastasized from the breast to the bones, it is still called breast cancer, for the cancer, although now located in the bones, is made of breast cancer cells, not bone cancer cells.

Sometimes it is easy to identify whether a cancer is primary (had its origin in the tissue in which it is found) or secondary (is the result of metastasis or direct invasion from some other site). But sometimes it isn't so easy. If, for instance, there is a widespread cancer involving the vulva, vagina and cervix, it may be impossible to say just where the cancer started or, indeed, if there were just one primary cancer. In the case of metastatic cancer in a distant organ, if the cancer cells are quite abnormal, it may be impossible to clearly identify the original source.

Some cancers metastasize early in the course of their development; others tend to grow relatively large or to invade directly before they metastasize. Thus it is sometimes possible for the secondary cancer to be discovered before the primary one.

Identifying a cancer as either primary or secondary is important for two reasons. First, if it's a secondary cancer, the primary one needs to be found and treated. Second, not all types of cancer are responsive to the same forms of treatment. A bone cancer that has metastasized from the breast will be treated most successfully by therapies effective against breast cancer cells, not by treatments designed to cure bone cancer.

Causes

Why these cell abnormalities and errors in twinning occur is not known—in other words, nobody knows what causes cancer. But with all the twinning that is constantly going on inside our bodies, it's not surprising that once in a while something will go wrong.

Chemicals or even natural substances that get into our tissues in one way or another are thought to play a role. Hormones, both natural and synthetic, are also thought to be factors. Vaginal clear cell adenocarcinoma is related to the use of the synthetic hormone DES.[1] Uterine cancer is linked to both naturally produced hormones[2] and the estrogens used to treat menopausal symptoms.[3] Viruses that can penetrate the cell membrane and alter the DNA have been implicated in cancer. Cervical cancer is strongly linked to the herpesvirus.[4] Radiation from the sun, X-rays and nuclear particles can also alter the microscopic DNA and cause cancer. Safe levels of radiation have not yet been determined, which is why there is so much controversy surrounding the use of X-rays in diagnosing various diseases and in treating anything less serious than cancer.

Many researchers believe that our bodies are probably producing mutant cells, some of them cancerous, all the time, but that our incredibly efficient immunological system is able to isolate and destroy these aberrant cells. People who have organ transplants and are given drugs to suppress the immunological system so that their bodies won't reject the transplants are particularly susceptible to cancer. Some scientists think that it is only when those errors in twinning occur *and* our immunological system is unable to cope that cancer occurs.

Cancer also seems to be related to aging. Although cancer can affect children and young adults, the overwhelming majority of cancer occurs in people over age 55. Some researchers attribute this to a decline in the efficiency of the immunological system with age.

You cannot catch cancer the way you can catch a cold, nor can you transmit cancer to someone else. (There is, however, some speculation that cervical cancer may be related to a sexually transmissible agent, perhaps the herpesvirus; see the section on cervical cancer for details.)

Types of Abnormal Cell Growth

Not all the irregularities in cell growth are so extreme as to be called cancerous, or malignant. Sometimes growth irregularities occur in which the cells, unlike cancerous cells, are not so abnormal, don't destroy the neighboring normal cells, don't grow as rapidly, don't spread into or invade the surrounding tissue and are not capable of metastasizing to other organs. These growths are called benign tumors, "benign" meaning "noncancerous" and "tumors" meaning simply "new growth." A wart or a uterine fibroid would be an example of a benign tumor.

Abnormal cells that do not or have not yet metastasized to other organs or invaded the surrounding tissue, yet do have the extreme abnormalities of cancer cells, are called carcinoma in situ ("carcinoma" being a medical term for a particular kind of cancer and "in situ" meaning "in place"). It is not

705

known whether carcinoma in situ always progresses to cancer. We know that some carcinoma in situ does become true invasive, and eventually metastatic, cancer, but it may be that some carcinoma in situ remains dormant.

There is, then, some controversy about the term "carcinoma in situ." Some doctors object to calling something cancerous that does not actually invade the surrounding tissue.

Certain other abnormal cell growth patterns are also possibly precancerous. These include dysplasia and hyperplasia. Sometimes they will progress to carcinoma in situ (or, possibly, directly to invasive cancer), but other times they will revert to normal.

In routine autopsies of people who have died of other causes these carcinomas in situ and other precancerous conditions are found in much higher numbers than are true cancers. In one series of autopsies of women over age 70 these sorts of precancerous conditions were found in the breast at a rate 19 times higher than the actual rate of cancer in this age-group.[5] Thus it is obvious that not all these precancerous conditions and carcinomas in situ do become true cancer. It is thought that the body's efficient immune system prevents this. This, as we shall see, raises some questions about the value of early detection and may have important implications for the treatment of cancer.

Another lesser form of cancer is microinvasive cancer. This is true cancer that is actually invading the neighboring tissue, but that has been diagnosed while the spread is still minimal. Precise definitions of what constitutes microinvasion have not been established, so different doctors will use different definitions.

Types of Cancer

There are many types of cancer, and cancers may be classified in a number of ways. They may be classified as to the organ in which they arise, which is how this book classifies them. They include:

- ☐ Preinvasive cancer of the vulva
- ☐ Vulvar cancer
- ☐ Clear cell adenocarcinoma of the vagina and cervix
- ☐ Vaginal cancer
- ☐ Cervical dysplasia
- ☐ Carcinoma in situ of the cervix
- ☐ Cervical cancer
- ☐ Endometrial hyperplasia
- ☐ Uterine cancer
- ☐ Cancer of the fallopian tube

☐ Cancer of the ovary
☐ Breast cancer
☐ Choriocarcinoma (cancer of fetal tissue)

Most of the cancers discussed in this book are carcinomas, cancers that arise from tissues that cover the surface or line the interior of internal organs and passageways of the body. A few sarcomas, cancers that arise from the connective or muscle tissue, are discussed, but in less detail, since carcinoma is far more common.

Cancers are also classified by the type of cell. This is known as histological classification. An adenocarcinoma would be composed of glandular (*adeno*) cells, whereas an epithelial carcinoma would be composed of epithelial, or skin, cells. These may be further broken down into subcategories. A squamous cell carcinoma would be one that arose from the particular type of epithelial tissue known as squamous cell epithelium that lines the vaginal cavity. Sometimes the histological type will greatly influence the choice of treatment, as well as the chances of surviving.

Cancerous tumors are generally solid, but they may become fluid-filled, either because the tumor itself secretes fluid or because it breaks down in its center. In either case they are referred to as cystic. A mucinous cystadenocarcinoma of the ovary, then, is a fluid-filled cancer of a specific type of epithelial gland tissue that produces a mucus-type secretion.

Incidence

Incidence rates are given in terms of the number of people per 100,000 who contract the disease each year. Most of the time incidence rates for cancer are age-adjusted so that people too young to develop the disease have been eliminated from the figuring. For many types of gynecological cancer the incidence rates are adjusted to include only women in their reproductive and postmenopausal years, since gynecological cancers are uncommon in prepubertal girls.

Incidence rates are valuable for two reasons. Differences in incidence rates among certain groups may help isolate causes related to difference in diet, behavior, environment or other factors. Incidence rates can also help us identify women who are at high risk. If a woman knows she is at high risk, she can take extra precautions and undergo more frequent routine tests, so that the disease, should she develop it, can be detected in its earlier stages. For example, women with histories of herpes have higher rates of cervical cancer, so such women might decide to have Pap smears more frequently.

Risk Factors

Being at "high risk" means that your chances of getting the disease are, statistically, greater than those of the general population. But this high risk does not necessarily mean that you will get the disease. Conversely, not having any of the high-risk characteristics doesn't mean that you won't develop the disease. Epidemiologists—scientists who study the kinds of people who get certain diseases—have been able to identify risk factors for some forms of cancer, but not for all.

Symptoms

The symptoms of cancer vary according to the organ in which the cancer arises and the stage of the cancer. The particular location within the organ may have an influence on the symptoms. Sometimes the particular cell type of the tumor will play a role in determining the symptoms.

The American Cancer Society lists these warning signs or symptoms:

- ☐ Unusual bleeding or discharge
- ☐ A lump that does not go away
- ☐ A sore that does not heal within 2 weeks
- ☐ Change in bowel or bladder habits
- ☐ Persistent hoarseness or cough
- ☐ Indigestion or difficulty in swallowing
- ☐ Change in a wart or mole

These symptoms can, of course, be produced by other, noncancerous conditions. Cancer is frequently asymptomatic until it is fairly advanced, although some cancers will produce symptoms fairly early. The specific symptoms associated with the female cancers are discussed under the appropriate headings.

Diagnosis

A suspicious symptom may be discovered by the woman herself or by her doctor in the course of a routine physical.

Screening Tests

For some forms of cancers there are tests that can detect cancer even before there are obvious symptoms. These tests may be used to screen asymptomatic women for cancer. For example, the Pap smear, which can detect cervical cancer in its earliest stages, has been used to screen large numbers of women. Mammograms, X-ray studies of the breast, can detect breast tumors before they are large enough to be felt, but X-rays carry some risk and there has been considerable controversy about the routine use of mammography to screen women for breast cancer. The endometrial biopsy can be used to screen women who are at high risk for uterine cancer, but since the endometrial biopsy is not a simple, painless, inexpensive procedure like the Pap smear—indeed, it can be quite painful—it is not used routinely on all women.

Biopsy

Screening tests and symptoms are not usually enough to confirm a diagnosis. A biopsy, which involves removing all or part of the suspicious tissue and examining sections of it microscopically, is the most reliable method of determining whether or not cancer is present. If only a portion of the tumor is removed, the term "incisional biopsy" is used. If the entire tumor is removed, the term "excisional biopsy" is used. Sometimes a needle is used to obtain a tissue sample, and this is termed a "needle biopsy."

One-Step and Two-Step Biopsies: Frozen and Permanent Sections

Different types of biopsies are done for different types of cancer. Sometimes a one-step procedure is done. In one-step procedures the woman is prepared for major surgery and given a general anesthetic. The surgeon then performs the biopsy and, while the woman remains on the operating table, the tissue sample is sent to a laboratory in the hospital, where it is examined by a pathologist, a specially trained doctor. The pathologist carefully cuts the tumor into sections. One or more of these tissue sections are then placed on a slide, quick-frozen and examined microscopically. The process, which is called a frozen section, takes about 10 to 15 minutes. The pathologist then reports back to the surgeon in the operating room. If the pathologist's diagnosis is "benign," the woman is "closed up" and taken to the recovery room. If a malignancy is diagnosed, the doctor will usually proceed with a cancer operation.

In the two-step procedure the biopsy and the treatment are done at separate times. The biopsy may be done in the doctor's office or on an outpatient basis at the hospital, depending on the type of cancer the woman is being tested for. Generally, only a local anesthetic is needed. The biopsy specimen is again sent to the pathologist, but in the two-step procedure the pathologist performs a permanent section, rather than a frozen section. It takes longer to get the results from a permanent section—generally a few days—but the results are easier to "read" than a frozen section, for the freezing process may distort the cells and make it more difficult to tell if the cells are normal.

Whenever possible a two-step procedure should be done. If the biopsy indicates cancer, the two-step procedure allows for further testing, second opinions and time for the woman to make important decisions before the cancer operation. The permanent section is also more accurate than the frozen section. However, as long as she is being treated at a good hospital with a good pathology department (see below), a woman need not be overly concerned about inaccuracy in frozen sections, for a good pathologist will realize when the frozen section is too distorted for conclusive diagnosis. If there is any doubt in the pathologist's mind, s/he will tell the surgeon that the case is borderline and that it is necessary to wait for the results of the permanent section. Even in one-step procedures, where surgical decisions are based on frozen sections, permanent sections are always done afterward as a double check.

Most biopsies can be done as two-step procedures; however, in certain types of cancer, when the suspicious mass is located deep inside the body, it may not be possible to do a two-step procedure. If, for example, a woman had a suspicious ovarian mass, a two-step procedure would not be done. Major surgery is already necessary in order to get at the ovary for the biopsy, and there would be no point in doing a two-step procedure and subjecting the woman who did turn out to have cancer to a second major surgery. In breast cancer, one-step procedures are sometimes done, even though it is generally possible to do two-step procedures. This is one of the important consumer issues that women with breast lumps should be aware of, and it is discussed more fully in the section on breast cancer.

Biopsies may also be done at the time of the cancer surgery to detect the possibility of microscopic spread to other organs, adjacent tissues and lymph nodes and are a common part of cancer treatment. These may be analyzed by frozen section so that more extensive surgery can be done right away. If the doctor plans to use radiation therapy to treat any further spread should the biopsies be positive, a permanent section will be done. Here again, even when frozen sections are done, permanent sections will also be done to double-check the results.

Pathology

Regardless of how or when the biopsy is done, its accuracy will depend on the skill and experience of the doctor doing the biopsy, the skill and experience of the pathologist, and good communication between the doctor and pathologist. Mistakes can happen and may have tragic consequences. A woman's reproductive organs or breast could be removed unnecessarily, or, conversely, necessary, lifesaving surgery could be neglected. No one knows for sure how frequently this happens. It is probably rather uncommon, but since on at least some occasions it does happen, a woman should be aware of the possibility and take proper precautions.

One type of mistake that could lead to misdiagnosis is insufficient medical history. If, for instance, a doctor sends the pathologist a tissue sample from a uterine tumor that is actually a benign fibroid but neglects to tell the pathologist that the woman is pregnant or taking some form of hormone treatment, the benign fibroid could be misinterpreted as a sarcoma, a cancerous condition. Such a woman could end up having her uterus removed or her pregnancy terminated unnecessarily. Similarly, a woman with genital warts who had been treated a few days before biopsy with a medication called podophyllin might get a pathology report of dysplasia or even carcinoma in situ if her doctor failed to tell the pathologist about the podophyllin treatment. One way that women can protect themselves from these sorts of problems is to make sure that the doctor doing the biopsy is board-certified. Although board-certification doesn't guarantee that mistakes won't happen, it is a valuable indicator of a doctor's competency.

Good communication between the doctor and the pathologist is of utmost importance. First, because the same terms can be used differently by different doctors, the woman's doctor and the pathologist must be aware of each other's use of terminology. It is a good idea, then, to find out whether or not the doctor has consulted personally with the pathologist on your case rather than merely having read the report and, if not, to request that s/he do so, because failures of communication are more likely to be detected in discussion between them than through a written report.

It is also a good idea for a woman to request a second pathology opinion. This may already have been done, for some doctors do it as a matter of routine. But not all doctors are this conscientious, so by all means, women should ask about this and should seek second opinions if necessary. If a one-step biopsy is done, or if further biopsies are done at the time of surgery, it isn't possible to get a second opinion before treatment. Obviously, an anesthetized woman flat out on an operating table cannot run down to the pathology lab and request a second opinion on her frozen section. There are, however, things she can do before surgery to assure an accurate diagnosis.

First, she can find out how many pathologists will be on duty. If only one pathologist will be on hand at the time of her operation, the woman might choose to have her surgery done at a time when more pathologists will be available or at another hospital with a larger pathology staff. Second, she can find out whether the pathologist in charge of her case is board-certified. Pathologists are certified by the American Board of Pathology. In order to be certified the pathologist must first complete basic medical training and then must complete 4 years of training in pathology in general and 3 years of specialized training in either clinical or anatomical pathology, or have 8 years of practical experience. In addition, the pathologist must pass certain oral and written examinations. Although many good pathologists are not board-certified, and although board-certification doesn't guarantee competency, it is nonetheless a reliable guide to judging the skill and experience of your pathologist.

Pathology is not a hard-and-fast science: Equally skilled, board-certified pathologists sometimes disagree. There are certain gray areas, where what one doctor calls benign, another may call malignant. This is most likely to happen in very early-stage cancers. In such cases more than two pathology opinions may be in order, and if necessary, they can be obtained long distance—the slides being mailed to expert pathologists for review. Some doctors do this as a matter of routine, especially if there is disagreement within their own pathology department. However, women should realize that they may not be informed about differences in opinion. Sometimes the doctor may say something along the lines of "You have a borderline case and we're not sure if you have a malignant or benign disease, so we'll have to follow this closely," which may be a completely accurate description of the situation. All the pathologists may have looked at your slide and been unable to determine whether it was benign or malignant.

On the other hand, this kind of statement may actually be a subtle variation on the truth of the matter. A "borderline case" in which the doctor is "not sure" may also be one in which three experts thought the slide revealed a malignancy and three others read it as benign. You should know the doctors' opinions so that you can, if you wish, play a part in choosing the treatment.

Suppose there was this sort of disagreement among the experts and that a woman possibly had breast cancer. One woman might decide to "play it safe" and have herself treated as if she did have breast cancer, for fear that the three experts who said "malignant" were right and that some tumor cells might break away and spread to other locations, thus greatly reducing her chances of surviving, before the follow-up program revealed that it actually was cancer; another woman might not want to take the chance of losing a breast unnecessarily and might decide to go with the pathologists who said the disease was benign, hoping that if they were wrong, the follow-up program would catch it before it metastasized. Still others might decide to have treatment but to have minimal surgery or radiation therapy, which is less likely to disfigure the breast but which has not proved to be as effective as surgical removal of the breast.

Such a decision would certainly be a tough one for a woman to make. Some doctors would hesitate to confront a woman with such a decision, perhaps for fear of overburdening her or perhaps because they believed their judgment was superior to hers (the old M.D.eity syndrome). Hospital politics may sometimes come into play too, especially at a large teaching hospital or cancer center, where a woman is being treated by a doctor who is on staff rather than by a private doctor. If the official diagnosis of the pathology department was benign disease, a doctor who operated on such a woman would be in serious trouble, indeed would risk his or her career if s/he went ahead and performed a mastectomy in the face of an official diagnosis of benign disease.

Regardless of the motivation that would lead a doctor to give a woman less-than-accurate information, we think it is wrong to withhold such information. The decision, no matter how difficult, is hers and hers alone. Women should be alert to the possibilities of conflicting pathology reports; they should ask the doctor whether there were any conflicting opinions or whether their cancer is one of the debatable types. If questioned directly, most doctors will have to answer frankly or risk a possible malpractice suit. Once again, it's all a matter of knowing the right questions to ask.

Staging

The stage of the cancer—Stage I, Stage II, Stage III and Stage IV—gives an indication of how far the disease has spread and how serious a particular case of cancer is. The stage will influence the type of treatment and the chances of survival. Staging is also helpful because it allows doctors to compare the results of various treatments in order to determine which is most effective.

The two basic types of staging are clinical staging and surgical staging. Clinical staging is done before treatment and is based on careful physical exam, symptoms and palpation (feeling) of the pelvic organs, breasts and lymph nodes. Certain X-ray studies and other laboratory tests may be used as well. Clinical staging is generally an estimate, the doctor's considered opinion as to how far the disease has spread. It is often inaccurate. Mistakes in clinical staging are not necessarily a reflection on the doctor's ability. Sometimes lymph nodes are enlarged, which leads the doctor to believe that the cancer has already spread to the lymph nodes and therefore to assign the case to a higher stage. But lymph nodes may become enlarged because of infection and there may not be any cancer in the nodes. On the other hand, lymph nodes may appear normal yet contain cancer.

Moreover, the spreading cancer may be located in an area that cannot be reached by the doctor's examining fingers. Or the metastasized cancer may be too small to be detected by even the most sensitive type of X-rays or tests.

Surgical staging is based on the doctor's inspection of the abdominal cavity during surgery and/or on the results of the pathologist's analysis of biopsies and tissue removed during surgery. In ovarian cancer, for example, the doctor carefully inspects the entire abdominal cavity for signs of spread. The ovarian tumor is removed. Cell samples and biopsies are also taken at the time of the operation. The removed tissue is examined by the pathologist. On the basis of this information, along with the results of tests to detect metastasis, the disease is assigned to a particular stage.

Tests to Detect Metastasis and Evaluate the Extent of the Spread of Disease

Doctors are often accused of ordering too many tests, but in the diagnosis of cancer such tests are generally necessary. If anything, there may be too few tests. The testing required will depend on the type of cancer and what the doctor finds from the physical exam and palpation. Women have a right to a full explanation of the tests that may be used, exactly what will be done and why it is necessary. Any of the procedures listed below may be used in the staging workup:

- ☐ Basic blood tests
- ☐ Urinalysis
- ☐ Liver function tests
- ☐ Chest X-rays
- ☐ Cystography
- ☐ Hysterography
- ☐ Lymphangiography
- ☐ Barium enema
- ☐ Intravenous pyelography
- ☐ Bone scans
- ☐ Liver scans
- ☐ Tomography
- ☐ CAT scans
- ☐ Ultrasound examinations
- ☐ Cystoscopy
- ☐ Hysteroscopy
- ☐ Colposcopy
- ☐ Culdoscopy
- ☐ Laparoscopy
- ☐ Proctosigmoidoscopy
- ☐ Colonoscopy

TNM Code

In addition to staging, doctors sometimes use a TNM code to classify a particular case of cancer. The *T* stands for *tumor*, *N* for *lymph nodes* and *M* for *metastasis*.

The T is accompanied by a number or letter. The number generally refers to the size of the tumor, T1 being a small tumor and T4, a larger one. In some cases—for example, in endometrial cancer—the number may indicate the depth of invasion of the tumor. The particular size or depth represented by the various numbers varies from cancer to cancer. A T1 designation in breast cancer, for instance, would mean a tumor that was 2 cm or less in diameter.

TIS means carcinoma in situ; TX means the size of the tumor cannot be determined or even estimated, and TO means that there is no evidence of the primary tumor. A TO classification might, for instance, be used for a cancer that obviously did not originate at the site in which it was found when either its cells were too abnormal to determine its original site or the tumor in the primary site was still too small to be detected.

The N, which designates lymph node involvement, may be accompanied by an O (NO), meaning no lymph node involvement, or an X (NX), meaning nodal involvement cannot, for some reason, be assessed. Numbers 1 to 4 may also be used to indicate the number of lymph nodes involved or the size of the involved nodes. The exact manner in which the numbers are used will vary from cancer to cancer.

In a similar vein, MO means no known metastases; MX means this has not been assessed; M+ indicates that evidence of metastasis is present. Numerals may be used to indicate the amount or extent of the spread and letters might be used to indicate the organ to which the disease has spread. A P, for instance, might indicate pulmonary metastasis, or spread to the lungs.

Grade

Confusion sometimes exists between the grade of the tumor, which depends on the individual cell characteristics, and the stage of the disease, which refers to how widely the disease has spread. Generally, the stage of the disease has more influence on the type of treatment selected and the chances of survival, but grade too may play a role, especially in certain forms of cancer, like cancer of the ovary or uterus.

Grade refers to how well differentiated the cells are, that is, the degree of immaturity or abnormality. High-grade cancers are those that are poorly differentiated, immature and quite abnormal. Low-grade cancers are well differentiated, less abnormal and generally less serious. Various grading schemes have been devised. One commonly used scheme uses three numerical grades, ranging from Grade 1 for low-grade, less serious tumors to Grade 3 for the more abnormal tumors.

Treatment

The type of treatment you receive will depend on many factors, including the type of cancer you have, the extent and location of the disease and your general physical condition. There are basically five types of treatment available: surgery, which involves cutting away the affected tissue; radiation, which involves destroying or disabling the cancer cells by the use of high-energy rays; chemotherapy, which involves the use of drugs that cripple or destroy cancer cells; hormones, which alter the growth of the cancer; and immunotherapy, which makes use of the body's immune system. Often different therapies are used in combination with one another.

The various specialists involved in cancer treatment are discussed in the following pages and in Chapter Seven. You may be referred to one of these specialists by your own doctor. Sometimes there is a choice of treatments. You should discuss this with your referring doctor and ask to be referred to doctors who are specialists in the various treatment options available to you. Second opinions and consultations (*see* p. 238) are always a good idea.

Where you are treated is important. The National Cancer Institute (NCI) has designated 20 comprehensive cancer-care centers across the country. These hospitals provide the finest and most up-to-date treatment. If you live near one of these centers, which are listed in the appendix of this book, you should by all means take advantage of it.

The NCI also supports programs known as nonclinical and clinical centers. The nonclinical centers conduct research, but the clinical centers treat patients and can offer most of the same services as a comprehensive care center. These are also listed in the appendix. In addition, there are cancer clinical cooperative groups sponsored by NCI. Each of these groups specializes in a particular type of cancer and conducts studies to determine the most effective forms of treatment. You or your doctor can call the Cancer Information Service Hotline for the names, locations and phone numbers of the national directors of each of the various clinical cooperative groups. It doesn't matter where the national directors are located, because they will be able to give you the names and phone numbers of those doctors in your area who are participating in these groups.

Being treated by cancer specialists at one of these special cancer-care facilities has several advantages. First, it assures you that a team approach will be used in your treatment. Doctors from all the various specialties will confer and consult on your case. Doctors who are part of these programs are more apt to be up to date on the latest treatment advances. Sometimes it takes a while for these developments to percolate through the rank and file of the medical profession. Some doctors are still using forms of treatment that have been abandoned by the experts, and you will want to make sure that you have the advantage of the latest knowledge and most effective treatments. Moreover, doctors at these major centers and those participating in these groups are likely to have more experience in the operations and other forms of therapy used in the treatment of cancer, for they receive referrals from many doctors.

If you can take advantage of one of the NCI-sponsored cancer programs, by all means do so. If you have an early-stage cancer, seeking treatment at one of these centers is not as critical. Still, you will want to make sure that your doctor and the hospital* in which you are treated are top-notch.

The American College of Surgeons' Commission on Cancer operates a voluntary surveillance program whereby hospitals are approved if they meet certain criteria that, if properly used, will promote a high level of care for the patient with cancer. The commission does not judge the actual care given to the patient. In order to be approved, the hospital must meet certain basic standards: It must have a cancer registry, a cancer committee, an educational program for doctors and a system for evaluating the quality of the care in that institution.

Approved cancer programs are listed in a directory entitled *Cancer Programs Approved by the Commission on Cancer of the American College of Surgeons*, which is updated twice yearly. Most medical libraries have one, or it can be obtained by writing to the Director, Cancer Department, American College of Surgeons, 55 East Erie Street, Chicago, Illinois 60611.

Surgery

Surgery is the most widely used form of therapy employed in the treatment of cancer. The nature of the surgery will depend on the type of cancer and the extent of its spread. A number of surgical procedures may be used, and these are discussed in detail in the sections on the specific types of cancer and in the section on operations, tests and procedures.

Extent of Surgery

Generally, the more extensive the cancer, the more radical the surgery. In conservative therapy the tumor itself and perhaps the organ in which it is located are removed. In more radical surgery the adjacent tissues and lymph nodes in the area may be removed as well. Sometimes this more extensive surgery is done because there is clear evidence that the cancer has spread to these areas, but at other times the tissue is removed even though cancer cells have not been detected, for experience has shown that there is a high likelihood that tumors too small to be detected, which could grow and metastasize before they *were* detected, may be lurking in these tissues.

Surgery is performed with the idea of removing all the obvious, visible cancer. A margin of surrounding, apparently healthy tissue may be removed as a safeguard. However, it is not always possible to remove all the cancer surgically. If it is obvious that the disease has already metastasized, there may be no point in performing surgery. Yet even in these cases, surgery may be performed, to relieve symptoms and to prolong life.

*Additional information on hospitals is included in Chapter Seven.

Sometimes surgery is used in combination with radiation therapy, or chemotherapy, which will shrink the tumor to the point where it can be removed by subsequent surgery.

Since it is not always possible to determine the extent of the disease before surgery, sometimes more extensive surgery than was originally planned will be necessary. There are also instances in which there is a choice between conservative and more radical surgery. Unfortunately, a number of doctors fail to discuss the options with their clients. Anyone considering cancer surgery should ask the questions listed in Chapter Seven before consenting to surgery.

Cancer Surgeons

Cancer surgery may be performed by a gynecologist, a general surgeon, a surgical oncologist or a gynecological oncologist. Any of these doctors may be qualified to perform surgery for early cancers, but for more advanced cancers you may want to seek out a surgical or gynecological oncologist, for these doctors have specialized training and concentrate on the treatment of cancer.

No matter which type of doctor you choose, you will want to check his or her credentials and, preferably, you will have a board-certified doctor perform your surgery. The board-certification process for gynecologists is discussed in Chapter Six and board-certification for general surgeons, in Chapter Seven. Gynecological oncology is a board-certifiable subspecialty of gynecology. Additional years of training in the treatment of cancer of the female reproductive organs is required for certification in this subspecialty. Rigorous written and oral examinations are also required. Unfortunately, surgical oncology is not yet a board-certifiable subspecialty of surgery, so it is a bit more difficult to check the credentials of a surgical oncologist. At a minimum the surgical oncologist should be a board-certified general surgeon. You might also ask where the surgical oncologist received special training in cancer surgery and whether s/he is a member of the Society of Surgical Oncologists. Be suspicious of any doctor who claims to be a surgical oncologist who is not a board-certified general surgeon.

It is sometimes difficult for a layperson to know when to seek out a specialist, and if your doctor is not a specialist, s/he may not readily refer you to one. If, for example, a general surgeon has performed your breast biopsy, s/he may want to also perform your mastectomy. Although many general surgeons do excellent mastectomies, our preference is to seek out an oncologist who has specialized in this field. S/he is much more likely to be skilled and experienced in the operation than a doctor who performs this surgery only a few times a year. It is always a good idea to have a second opinion before any type of surgery, and in the case of cancer, having a second opinion from a surgical oncologist or a gynecological oncologist is especially wise.

Radiation Therapy

Radiation is caused by electromagnetic waves similar to light and heat waves. Radiation therapy uses these high-energy rays to destroy cancer cells or to alter them in such a way that they can no longer reproduce. The rays destroy the malignant cells when they are most vulnerable, during their twinning phase, when the chromosome strips are replicating themselves. As the cells die they break down and are carried away in the bloodstream and excreted from the body, so the tumor shrinks in size.

These rays also destroy normal healthy cells, but since cancer cells are reproducing at a faster rate than normal cells, a greater number of cancer cells will be twinning at any given time. This is why radiation therapy can sometimes be effective against malignant cells without causing undue damage to normal cells.

Not all the cancer cells in a tumor are reproducing at the same time. Since only those in the process of twinning will be affected by the radiation, only a certain percentage of cells will be destroyed in a single therapy session. This is why radiation therapy involves either constant, low doses of radiation or a number of short, higher-intensity exposures spread out over a period of time.

Radiation therapy is used in a number of ways in the treatment of cancer. Sometimes it is used alone and can successfully destroy all the cancer cells. This is known as curative therapy.

Sometimes the cancer is so large that radiation cannot hope to destroy all the cancer cells without undue damage to the surrounding tissue. In these cases lower doses of radiation designed to shrink the tumor may be given, for shrinking the tumor may provide relief of symptoms. If, for example, the tumor is pressing on a vital organ, the radiation may succeed in shrinking the tumor, providing relief from the pressure effects of the tumor. Or if metastatic cancer is growing in a weight-bearing bone, radiation therapy may be used to shrink the tumor and prevent fractures. When radiation therapy is used in this manner the term ''palliative treatment'' is used.

At other times radiation therapy is used in combination with other forms of therapy. Sometimes radiation is given before surgery to shrink the tumor to the point where it is small enough to be removed surgically. Radiation may be used after surgery to ''dry up'' any microscopic areas of cancer that may have been left behind. This is known as adjuvant radiation therapy.

Radiation therapy is given in one of two ways: externally or internally.

External Radiation

External radiation involves a machine that produces a high-energy beam that is directed at the cancerous area. This is known as external beam therapy. External beam therapy makes use either of X-rays from a machine known as a linear accelerator or gamma rays from a cobalt machine. External beam therapy is sometimes used alone. For example, a woman too sick to undergo surgery or even to withstand the use of the local anesthetic that is sometimes used for internal radiation therapy may be treated by external therapy alone. However, external beam therapy generally is used in conjunction with surgery or internal radiation. A number of treatments may be required, for external beam therapy only kills a certain percentage of the cells at a single therapy session.

Internal Radiation

Internal radiation involves placing a radioactive substance, such as radium or cesium, inside the body as close to the tumor as possible. If the radioactive source is placed in special containers and inserted into a body cavity, the term "intracavity implant" is used. If special needles or hollow plastic tubes are inserted into the tumor area, the term "interstitial implant" or "needle implant" may be used. Sometimes a radioactive substance is mixed with a fluid and circulated through a body cavity, and this is called radioactive colloid therapy.

Internal radiation requires the use of either a local or general anesthetic so that the containers or needle can be inserted near the tumor. Since the containers are inserted into a hollow body cavity (the uterus or vagina) or the needles are inserted into the tumor area, a surgical incision is not required. X-rays are usually taken to assure that the containers are placed correctly. Then the radioactive substance is loaded into the needles or containers and is left in place until the specified dose of radiation is achieved. This may take a few hours or several days, and since certain of these substances put out rays that could be harmful to others, the woman may be isolated in a special room of the hospital. If the containers or needles create discomfort, painkillers may be used.

Since the radioactive substance is left in place for some time, many cancer cells will come into the twinning phase during treatment and will be destroyed. Internal radiation is limited and can only affect cancer fairly close to the source. The effect of the rays decreases dramatically as the distance from the source increases. It is often combined with external beam therapy, which can affect cancer cells that have spread beyond the initial tumors to the adjacent tissues or lymph nodes. More than one internal treatment session may be necessary, but once the radioactive source is removed from the body, the woman is no longer radioactive and can continue her normal routine.

Side Effects

There may be some side effects from radiation therapy. These side effects usually develop after 1 or 2 weeks. In some cases they may persist from 4 to 6 weeks after treatment. The intensity of the side effects depends on the location of the cancer, the intensity of the therapy, the woman's tolerance to radiation and her general health. Some women experience little or nothing in the way of side effects. For some the effects are severe.

Most women experience some degree of fatigue. Some women experience nausea and vomiting. If this happens, antinausea medication may be prescribed. There may be some hair loss in the area being treated, for instance, pubic or armpit hair may be lost, but unless the head is being treated, the woman should not experience hair loss there from the radiation therapy.

In addition, any of the following side effects may occur: dizziness, sore throat, diarrhea, constipation, skin irritation and difficulty in swallowing. Although most of these symptoms are not serious and are generally short-lived, they should be reported to the doctor, for they may be signs of something more serious.

Complications

Just as a surgical wound can heal incorrectly, causing an unsightly scar, so radiation can cause scarring. Different women's tissues react differently to radiation. For example, one woman's breast may be changed only slightly after radiation therapy, whereas another's breast may become misshapen and distorted. There is no way to predict how a woman will react.

Since the bowels, rectum, bladder and other parts of the urinary tract are especially sensitive to radiation, exposure to high doses of radiation can cause permanent damage to these tissues. Fistulas, which are abnormal holes connecting the bladder and the vagina, the vagina and rectum or other areas, may occur. The bowels, intestines or urinary tract may become obstructed, which can cause serious, even fatal problems.

A possible long-term complication is radiation-induced cancer. We know that exposure to radiation can increase a person's chance of developing cancer in future years, but we know little about how radiation affects the development of cancer in the human body. There has been a great deal of concern recently about radiation risks from diagnostic X-rays, which involve only a fraction of the exposure that radiation therapy does. It may be that women treated with radiation will develop radiation-induced cancer in 15 to 20 years, but this risk is considered worthwhile, because the radiation can cure the existing cancer.

721

Radiation Oncologist

A specially trained doctor called a radiation therapist, therapeutic radiologist, radiotherapist or radiation oncologist plans and administers radiation therapy. Women are usually referred to such specialists by their doctors, and since radiation oncologists have varying levels of skill, women should make sure that the one recommended is a good one. Often your doctor may make a recommendation based on location, not necessarily on quality. If you need radiation therapy, you may have to balance the convenience of being treated at a small nearby community hospital or private facility against the advantages associated with being treated at a major medical center or large hospital more likely to have the latest equipment and the most highly skilled doctors.

One way to evaluate the skill of your doctor is to find out whether s/he is board-certified. The American Board of Radiology certifies doctors in two radiation specialties: diagnostic radiology and therapeutic radiology. A diagnostic radiologist is skilled in interpreting X-rays taken to diagnose a disease. A therapeutic radiologist is skilled in treating disease with radiation and is the specialist that women being treated for cancer will want to be treated by. This separation of the two specialties by the American Board of Radiology is fairly recent. Before the mid-1960s the two fields were not separated, so doctors certified before that time may not have certificates saying "therapeutic radiology." Such a doctor may be as skilled in therapeutic radiology as a younger doctor who is certified as a therapeutic radiologist.

Being board-certified doesn't assure competence, and many good doctors are not board-certified. But board-certification is an indication that the doctor's colleagues have evaluated his or her training and skill and have found it to be of the highest quality.

For certain types of cancer there may be a choice between radiation therapy and surgery. If a woman is treated at a large hospital or a cancer center, consultations between surgeons and radiologists as to which method of treatment is best for her may be a matter of routine. But at smaller hospitals such consultations may not take place, and women would do well to seek consultations with specialists in both fields.

Chemotherapy

Chemotherapy involves the use of drugs to kill cancer cells. Most of these drugs work by interfering with the growth of the cancer cells or by preventing them from reproducing. Chemotherapy generally is used in combination with other forms of treatment.

Unlike surgery or radiation, which can be effective in dealing with local disease, chemotherapy, which enters the bloodstream, can be effective in treating disease that has spread throughout the body. It is used in the treatment of metastatic or recurrent cancer. It may also be used as preventive, or adjuvant, therapy in cases where there is a high likelihood that the undetected microscopic cancer has already spread to other parts of the body. For instance, women with breast cancer whose lymph nodes are found to have cancer are given adjuvant chemotherapy, since there is a significant chance that undetected cancer is already lurking elsewhere in the body.

Chemotherapy used to be a last resort, but great strides have been made in this field. When the first studies were done the drugs were used only on women with advanced incurable disease. Although these women were not cured, the drugs were sometimes effective in reducing the size of the tumor, prolonging life and relieving symptoms. Experiments with laboratory animals suggested that if the chemotherapy were administered earlier, before the cancer had grown too large, it might be able to provide a cure as well.

Like radiation, chemotherapy is most effective at certain points in a cell's life cycle. Only a certain portion of the tumor's cells will be in this vulnerable situation at any given time, so repeated courses of the drug are necessary. The drug may be given orally or by injection. The particular dosage, drug, schedule and length of treatment will vary according to the individual woman and her particular type of cancer. In some cases only one drug is given, but many times a combination of drugs is used, for this has been shown to be more effective in certain instances.

Not all types of cancer are responsive to chemotherapy and not all women are suitable candidates for this form of therapy, for it carries certain risks that may outweigh any anticipated benefits.

Side Effects and Complications

Chemotherapy has its problems. The drugs used are powerful cell poisons, which affect the normal cells as well as the cancerous ones.

The side effects may last from a few hours to several days. The type and severity of the side effects will vary according to the drugs used and the woman's personal body chemistry. Any of the following effects may be noted and, if so, should be reported to the doctor:

Nausea	Flulike symptoms
Vomiting	Fatigue
Diarrhea	Male hair-patterns
Constipation	Headaches
Hair loss	Darkening of fingernails
Pain	Cough
Loss of appetite	Fever
Weight gain	Chills
Fluid retention	Swelling of veins

723

Cramps

Absence of menstrual periods

Prolonged and excessive menstrual periods

Blood in urine or stools

Abscesses or pain at injection site

Mouth sores

Tingling and numbness in feet and hands

Pale skin

Dry skin

Tendency to feel cold

Mental depression

Skin rashes tending toward infections

Excessive bleeding from cuts

In some cases these symptoms can be controlled by medications. For example, antinausea medicines may be given for nausea and vomiting. It may be necessary to alter your diet. Most of these side effects are relieved once chemotherapy is discontinued. Lost hair grows back, appetite returns and so forth; however, sometimes chemotherapy causes permanent damage to the liver, kidneys, lungs, heart and other organs. Chemotherapy has not been in use long enough for us to say with certainty what all the long-term risks and complications will be; only time will tell. We do know that chemotherapy can cause as well as cure cancer. Women who have been on certain forms of chemotherapy have a higher incidence of leukemia, a cancer of the blood-forming cells.

The Chemotherapist

Chemotherapy involves the use of potent drugs that have many potential side effects and complications. They are too risky to be administered by a general physician and should be administered by a chemotherapist, who may also be called a hematologist (blood specialist) or medical oncologist. The chemotherapist is a doctor of internal medicine who has specialized in the administration of drugs used to treat cancer. As with other specialists, a chemotherapist may be board-certified, which indicates that s/he has received special training and has passed rigorous oral and written exams.

The field of chemotherapy is always changing. There are new developments all the time. Women will want to be treated by doctors who are knowledgeable about the latest and most effective drugs. If there is no chemotherapist in your community, make sure your doctor takes advantage of the consultations offered to doctors by cancer centers. That way, you will receive the most effective drugs in the correct dose and will be monitored properly for side effects.

Experimental Drugs

New drugs are being tested constantly. Many of these drugs are available only at large cancer centers, where careful studies are being done to test their effectiveness. Programs sponsored by the National Cancer Institute to encourage the development of new cancer drugs are carefully controlled. In order to become approved for use, a drug must first be shown to be effective against tumors in mice and rats and then in larger animals. If the drug looks promising, it is tested on people with many types of advanced cancer who have failed to respond to other forms of treatment. Side effects as well as tumor response are carefully noted. This is referred to as phase I. Phase II also involves people with advanced disease who are not responding to other drugs. Only those with types of cancers that have responded in phase I studies are tested. Again, side effects and effectiveness are carefully noted. Next, in phase III, the new drug is compared with the standard therapy to determine whether it can produce superior results.

Experimental or investigational drugs should be administered only by cancer specialists chosen to participate in these experiments. Supposedly, no woman can be treated with an experimental drug without her knowledge. Everyone receiving an experimental drug must sign an informed consent form, which indicates that what is known about the risks and benefits of this form of therapy has been thoroughly explained to the woman. Not everyone can receive these experimental drugs. In order to be eligible, certain specific criteria must be met. For patients with advanced disease, being treated at a major hospital where these studies are being done may be the only way to be included in such studies.

Hormone Therapy

Hormone therapy involves controlling the output of certain substances produced by your body—hormones—to treat cancer. Hormone therapy is rarely curative. Generally, it is given in hopes of relieving symptoms and temporarily stopping or slowing the growth of the cancer. Hormone therapy may require the introduction of additional amounts of hormones into your body or, alternatively, the reduction of the amounts of those hormones by way of surgical removal, radiation of hormone-producing glands or administration of a drug that blocks hormone production. Hormone therapy, regardless of whether it involves the introduction of hormones or hormone-blocking drugs or the destruction of hormone-producing glands, may produce side effects, including a permanent or temporary absence of menstrual periods, infertility, sterility, premature menopause, menopausal symptoms, male hair-growth patterns, a deepening of the voice and other masculinization symptoms.

Of the cancers described in this book, hormone therapy has its widest application in the treatment of recurrent breast cancer, carcinoma in situ of the uterus and advanced uterine cancer and is discussed in more detail under these headings.

Immunotherapy

Immunotherapy is one of the newest types of cancer treatment and is still largely experimental. It makes use of the body's own defense system to fight cancer. Any time a foreign invader or something abnormal is detected by our immune systems, special substances called antibodies are produced to defend the body. Some doctors believe that cancerous cells are being produced constantly by the body and normally are dealt with by this incredibly efficient immune system. Only when there are too many cancerous cells or when the immune system is too weak to handle these cells do we develop cancers. Other doctors think that cancer cells have some way of tricking the immune system or camouflaging their abnormalities so that they are not detected and destroyed.

The fact that some tumors undergo a partial or complete spontaneous regression—that is, they disappear on their own without treatment—has stimulated interest in immunotherapy. Less than 500 well-documented cases of complete spontaneous remission have been reported in worldwide medical literature; however, it is not uncommon for a tumor to get smaller and even to disappear for a while and then to grow larger or to reappear at a later time. Some scientists think that the body's immune system may be responsible for these temporary remissions.

Most of us are familiar with immunotherapy in the form of vaccines. Small amounts of a weakened strain of a disease-causing organism or an antibody-stimulating substance are injected into the body in order to trigger antibody production that will protect the person from the disease in the future. In cancer the aim of immunotherapy is to bolster the person's own immune system. Vaccines may be prepared from the person's own tumor or from another person's tumor, or deactivated cancer cells incapable of reproducing may be used to trigger antibody reactions. Another type of immunotherapy involves transferring immune factors from one person to another person. Yet another type involves the use of agents known to be strong stimulators of the immune system.

Immunotherapy is still in its infancy; however, it is being used experimentally to treat certain advanced cancers. For instance, one substance made from human blood, interferon, is being used on a small group of women with breast cancer. Initial results have not shown cures, but significant regressions have been noted. Immunotherapy is not without risks and complications, some of them fatal. There is still much work to be done, but in the future interferon and other immunotherapeutic agents may play a role in the treatment of cancer.

Laetrile and Other Alternative Therapies

Because of the high mortality for many kinds of cancer and the suspicion and distrust that many people feel for the medical establishment, alternative treatments for cancer have received a good deal of attention, at least in the popular press.

Laetrile is perhaps the most widely known of these alternative cancer treatments. It is derived from apricot pits and contains cyanide. Although there is little in the way of sound scientific data to support its effectiveness, Laetrile has many passionate supporters.

Proponents of Laetrile and other alternative therapies usually offer case histories of cancer victims who have been cured by the alternative as proof of the treatment's effectiveness. Anyone considering these forms of therapy should be skeptical of this type of proof. Many times the people who were treated never had cancer in the first place. Breast cancer is a particularly good example of this. We know that 80 percent of all breast lumps are benign. The only way to tell for certain whether a lump is benign or malignant is to remove it and examine it microscopically. We also know that many of these benign lumps will disappear without treatment. Sometimes proper diet and avoiding coffee, tea, colas, chocolate and cigarettes will cause these benign lumps to disappear.[6] If a woman has a breast lump and has not had a biopsy to prove that it is cancerous, any claim of cure must be disregarded, for in all probability the woman never had breast cancer. If you are investigating these alternative treatments and talking to or reading about people who have been "cured" by these methods, be sure to find out how the diagnosis of cancer was made. Were the proper diagnostic tests and biopsies done? Were the diagnostic procedures done by the person or the clinic offering the alternative form of treatment, or were they done elsewhere, by a member of the traditional medical establishment? Were there second opinions on the diagnostic tests from recognized, establishment doctors? Be skeptical if the tests and biopsies were done by the person offering the alternative treatment and if they were not confirmed in second opinions from doctors not affiliated with the clinic or person offering the alternative therapy.

As far as scientific proof for Laetrile's effectiveness, there is little. Since the 1950s more than 23 experiments with Laetrile have been done with laboratory animals. None of the tests demonstrated any antitumor effects; however, the early tests have been criticized by Laetrile supporters, who claim that the Laetrile used in the testing was impure, lacked certain essential enzymes and was not employed in sufficient quantity.

Despite the lack of laboratory evidence, the NCI has continued research in

Laetrile because of pressure from Laetrile proponents. The NCI launched a nationwide search for cancer patients who had benefited from Laetrile.[7] Letters were sent to more than 835,000 doctors. In addition, some 70,000 health groups and professionals who supported Laetrile were contacted and the research effort was publicized nationally.

It was hoped that some 200 to 300 cases would be collected for study, but only 90 such patients signed consent forms allowing NCI to study their medical records. One problem was that the major groups advocating Laetrile refused to participate, because they did not think this was a good way to determine the drug's effectiveness. Only 67 of these cases had enough information in their medical files to allow for a review. A panel of experts from NCI eliminated 11 cases that had insufficient data and 35 others that were "non-evaluable" (because, for instance, chemotherapy had been given as well). Of the remaining 22 cases, 7 showed progressive disease, 9 showed stable disease (no change), 4 showed shrinkage of tumor by 50 percent or more and 2 showed complete remission.

Those who supported Laetrile saw the results as a victory; those opposing it saw the results as evidence that the drug has no value, pointing out that it is not uncommon for tumors to go into remission, only to flare up later. Thus the study that it was hoped would resolve the long-standing Laetrile controversy only served to fuel it. Still, in the wake of this study the NCI Decision Network Committee voted (14 to 11) to recommend that sound, scientific studies of Laetrile effectiveness should be undertaken.[8] Results from these tests are not yet available.

Follow-Up, Cures and Survival Rates

All cancer patients must be followed for life. The extent and timing of the follow-up program will depend on the type and seriousness of the cancer.

Survival rates for cancer are usually given in terms of 5 years, for if the disease has not recurred in that period it is not likely to; however, for certain types of cancer, survival rates may be given in terms of 10 years, and certain cancers can recur many, many years later. It is difficult, then, to think of some cancers as ever being cured. A cancer may regress or get smaller, but it may eventually begin to grow again. A remission is a regression of the disease, which means that the symptoms have disappeared and the doctor can no longer discover any signs of the disease. A partial remission means that the symptoms and signs have partially disappeared. Cancer may be in remission for many years, but if there are still cancer cells in the body, it may flare up again at a later date.

Survival rates for the various cancers in this book are listed under the appropriate headings. The prognosis (outcome) of your case may depend on many factors, and your doctor may be able to give you more accurate survival rates for your case.

Services for Cancer Patients

Two major organizations provide services for cancer patients: the American Cancer Society (ACS) and the Cancer Information Service (CIS).

The American Cancer Society is a national organization of volunteers that sponsors research and education and provides patient service and rehabilitation programs. Local chapters throughout the country provide information about various forms of treatment, assistance in obtaining social security, medicare and other benefits and counseling in regard to the problems and concerns of cancer patients. They can provide transportation to and from medical treatments for people who cannot make other arrangements; dressings (bandages); bed jackets, gowns and other items; rental or loan of wheelchairs, hospital beds, commodes and other equipment; household assistance according to the physical and financial needs of the patient and emotional and physical rehabilitation, which may be especially helpful to women who have had breast cancer operations or pelvic exenterations. They also sponsor Reach to Recovery, a program designed to meet the physical, emotional and cosmetic needs of women who have had mastectomies. Their services are often free. They are usually listed in the phone book, or contact the national office, ACS, 777 Third Avenue, New York, New York 10017, for the name of the office nearest you.

The Cancer Information Service, sponsored by the National Cancer Institute, has a nationwide telephone hot line for both patients and doctors. They can provide information on the medical aspects of cancer, rehabilitation assistance, medical facilities, home-care assistance programs, financial aid, emotional counseling and referrals to cancer specialists in the area. They also provide written materials about various forms of cancer. The phone numbers of the CIS hot lines are listed in the appendix.

Gynecological Operations, Tests, Procedures and Drugs

This chapter deals with surgery, tests, procedures and drugs used in gynecological medicine.

Surgery

Anyone who is faced with the prospect of surgery is apt to feel somewhat nervous or anxious about it. This is normal. Many people find that a detailed understanding of what is wrong, why the surgery is necessary and what the operation entails helps to relieve their anxiety. Coping with clear-cut information about the risks and possible complications is often easier than dealing with vague, uninformed fears. Some doctors don't discuss operations with their patients ahead of time for fear of upsetting them, so you may have to press your doctor for details. Remember, it's your body and you have a right to know.

Unnecessary Surgery

U.S. doctors are often criticized for performing unnecessary surgery. Hysterectomies are one of the most flagrant examples of the unnecessary surgical procedures done in the United States each year. In fact, the operation is jokingly referred to as "hip-pocket surgery." In case you have trouble, as we did, getting this "joke," it's called hip-pocket surgery because that's where doctors keep their wallets. Since so many hysterectomies are done when there is no medical necessity, the motivation for doing them is presumably financial, for hysterectomies are lucrative, netting the surgeon anywhere from about $1,000 to $3,000 or more per operation.

Surgery in general is a lucrative business. In 1978 the average gross income for surgeons in the United States was about $75,000.[1] This average is undoubtedly distorted by the superspecialists, who earn from $500,000 to a million dollars a year. There is probably a sizable group of surgeons earning $30,000 to $50,000 a year to counterbalance the six-figure incomes. Still, $30,000 to $50,000 is hardly chicken feed. In order to keep all these higher earners gainfully employed, a fair amount of surgery must be done. Doctors who specialize in obstetrics and gynecology and are therefore qualified to perform certain types of surgery have been accused of drumming up business, often in the form of hysterectomies, to bolster the falling income from the obstetrics side of their practices, which, with the decreasing birth rate, has declined considerably.

There is some objective eivdence to support this. In 1977 approximately 794,000 hysterectomies were performed, and as many as 30 percent to 40 percent of them may have been unnecessary.[2] Women who have medical insurance are twice as likely to undergo hysterectomy as those who don't.[3] The rate of hysterectomies in countries with socialized medical-care systems is considerably lower. The U.S. rate of hysterectomies is twice that of England and four times that of many other European countries.[4]

Overly Extensive Surgery

U.S. surgeons have a reputation for being "knife-happy." Not only do they sometimes perform unnecessary surgery, but they also are said to perform more extensive surgery than necessary. For instance, healthy ovaries are removed routinely by some surgeons every time they do a hysterectomy. Radical mastectomies, operations that involve removal of the breast, the lymph nodes in the armpit area and the muscles of the chest wall, are still performed in many cases where this more extensive and disfiguring operation is not necessary.

How to Avoid Unnecessary or Overly Extensive Surgery

How does a woman protect herself from unnecessary or overly extensive surgery? Well, first, never consent to surgery unless it has been made clear to you, in plain and simple terms, what the doctor plans to remove and why. Don't allow yourself to be intimidated by medical terminology. Your doctor's explanation of what is planned may not be clear to you. If it's not, insist on clarification. The doctor may, for instance, tell you that it is necessary to remove the uterus, tubes, ovaries and parametrial tissues. Not even the most

731

educated woman could be expected to know what parametrial tissues are, and the sad truth of the matter is that a whole lot of us, well educated or not, may not have a clear understanding of what even the uterus, tubes and ovaries are. There is an overwhelming ignorance about our bodies imposed on women in this culture. Don't hesitate to ask questions about anything you don't understand.

When the doctor answers your questions it may be done with an of-course-you-know-about-*that* air. Doctors use medical terminology every day and often assume that women are familiar with it. And if the terms the doctor uses *are* over our heads, many of us are too embarrassed to let on that we don't understand. We may feel rather like a naive girl at a cocktail party full of sophisticates, who dumbly nods agreement when someone says, "Don't you just love . . ." (the latest novel that we haven't read, the work of a painter we've never heard of). Embarrassed by our ignorance, we may feign knowledge and understanding when in reality we haven't the faintest idea what's being said. Don't allow yourself to be intimidated. It's your body that's going to be cut, and you have the right to know what's happening. Ask the doctor to draw you a picture so that you are sure you understand the procedure.

You should also ask the doctor why this surgery is necessary. Other questions you should ask include:

- ☐ What are the chances of success?
- ☐ What are the possible side effects and complications?
- ☐ How great are the risks?
- ☐ What will happen if I don't have surgery?
- ☐ Can the surgery be delayed?
- ☐ What will be the effects of delaying surgery?
- ☐ Are there any possible benefits from delaying surgery?
- ☐ Are there any less extensive, less deforming, less painful or less risky operations that are ever done in the treatment of cases like mine?
- ☐ Are there forms of treatment other than surgery that are ever used in cases like mine?
- ☐ Do you consider the other form of treatment to be as effective?
- ☐ Are there other doctors who feel it is as effective?
- ☐ What are the risks of the other forms of therapy?
- ☐ How do they compare with the risks of the surgery you are suggesting?
- ☐ Why do you think the form of treatment you are recommending is best?
- ☐ What will this operation cost? Will my insurance cover the costs? How will I be billed?

We encourage women to seek second opinions (*see* p. 238) before submitting to any form of surgery. In the reference section on diseases we have tried to indicate those instances in which alternative forms of treatment are available. Try to get second opinions from doctors who are advocates of the other forms of therapy. If your doctor has recommended a hysterectomy to treat carcinoma in situ of the cervix, for example, call the Cancer Information Service (*see* appendix) for names of doctors who perform cryosurgery, that being an alternative form of treatment for carcinoma in situ.

Choosing a Surgeon

Once you've determined that the surgery planned is neither unnecessary nor too extensive and that surgery is, indeed, the best choice of treatment, the next important factor to consider is the skill of the doctor performing the surgery. In Chapter Six we discuss how to go about finding a good gynecologist, and much of that information applies here as well. But perhaps a word or two about surgeons is in order.

Gynecologists are qualified to perform certain types of surgery. (Those gynecologists who specialize in gynecological surgery used to treat cancer are called gynecological oncologists and are discussed in the section on cancer.) Other types of surgeons also perform "female surgery." A general surgeon is qualified to perform operations in the abdominal and chest cavities. (General surgeons who specialize in cancer treatment are called surgical oncologists and are also discussed in the section on cancer.) Although the general practitioner/surgeon—the family doctor who performs surgery—is a dying breed, some older doctors have been around so long that they've managed to establish certain operating privileges at the hospital with which they are associated. Don't have your operation performed by one of these general practitioners; seek out a specialist, a gynecologist or a general surgeon.

Regardless of whether your surgery is done by a gynecologist or general surgeon, make sure that your doctor is board-certified. Surgery is risky business; 1 out of every 1,600 patients operated on dies as a result of anesthesia complications.[5] Sloppy operating procedures can cost you your life or can have crippling consequences, so it is vital that you find both a good surgeon and a board-certified anesthesiologist.

Board-certification does not guarantee that a doctor is top-notch, but it does tell you that his or her qualifications and experience have been carefully reviewed by colleagues and been judged outstanding. Board-certification requirements for a gynecologist are discussed in Chapter Six. In order to be certified by the American Board of Surgery a doctor must first be a licensed M.D. and must have a minimum of 4 years of residency training in general surgery. Then s/he must successfully complete written and oral exams. In addition, general surgeons must be recertified periodically to assure that they are keeping up to date in their fields.

Another important credential to check for is membership in the American College of Surgeons. In order to become a member the surgeon must be board-certified and must have been in practice for 2 years. His or her performance is then evaluated, and if it is satisfactory, the surgeon is inducted into the college. If a doctor has the initials F.A.C.S. after his or her name, this indicates the doctor is a Fellow of the College and has received special training and been judged extremely competent by his peers.

Besides checking these criteria you can find out about your surgeon's qualifications by doing a bit of detective work. Try to find a scrub nurse, an anesthesiologist (a doctor who specializes in anesthesia), an anesthetist (a specially trained nurse who administers anesthesia) or any member of the nursing staff who assists in operations. These people have inside information and can provide the most valuable recommendations.

Another important factor to consider is the experience the surgeon has in performing the operation you need. A doctor who performs an operation once or twice a year is not going to be as skilled as one who performs it two or three times a week.

Yet another consideration is the hospital in which the surgery will be done. Just as there are good surgeons and poor surgeons, so there are good hospitals and poor hospitals. There are more than 7,000 hospitals in the United States and of these about 4,700 are accredited by the Joint Commission on Accreditation of Hospitals (JCAH). This organization evaluates a hospital's performance carefully before extending accreditation. One thing they will evaluate is the surgical tissue committee, which reviews the operations done in the hospital. In a good hospital a doctor must first submit a preoperative diagnosis; then the removed tissue is examined by the hospital's pathology laboratory. If the preoperative diagnosis doesn't line up with the pathology report, the doctor is called before the tissue committee. If, for instance, a surgeon removed a woman's uterus as a treatment for endometriosis and the pathology department found no evidence of endometriosis, the doctor would be called before the tissue committee. (Note: In the case of unnecessary hysterectomy the preoperative diagnosis could be nonspecific, indicating that the doctor is not removing the uterus for any specific medical reason. Thus even though the pathology department finds that a healthy uterus has been removed, there is no tissue committee review, for there is no discrepancy between the pre- and postoperative diagnosis.)

In addition to reviewing the workings of the tissue committee the JCAH considers many other factors. They audit the surgical charts and investigate patient care, record keeping, administration, staff qualifications, facilities and equipment. JCAH accreditation does not guarantee that every doctor who operates in that hospital is top-notch, but these hospitals do have a higher per-

734

centage of board-certified doctors on their staffs. Just as there are many excellent doctors who are not board-certified, so there are excellent hospitals that are not accredited, but JCAH accreditation is a valuable guideline in helping you assess the quality of a hospital. Women who are being treated for cancer should read the discussion of cancer-care hospitals in the general section on cancer. A list of JCAH-accredited hospitals in your area may be obtained by writing to JCAH, 645 North Michigan Avenue, Chicago, Illinois 60611.

Before Surgery

Before surgery you will be asked to sign a consent form giving the doctor permission to perform the required surgery. READ IT CAREFULLY! Do not sign any ''blanket permission'' forms or anything you don't understand. Ask to see a copy of the form before you go to the hospital so that you will be able to read it and ask questions and make changes before the day of surgery.

The doctor usually will order certain tests before surgery. The type of tests ordered will depend on the nature of the surgery and the type of anesthetic being used. At a minimum a blood count and urinalysis will be done. If a general anesthetic is being used, tests to determine blood-clotting time may be done as well as blood-typing and cross-matching tests in case blood transfusions are necessary. If you are over age 40 or have had previous medical problems, chest X-rays and/or cardiograms may be done.

It is important that you arrive at the hospital on time, since your doctor has scheduled use of the operating room for a certain time, and if you are late, there might not be time to perform all the necessary preoperative tests. Follow any preoperative instructions carefully. You will probably be asked not to eat or drink anything for about 12 hours before the operation, because food or liquids in your stomach could be regurgitated while you were under the anesthetic and cause choking. Even if only a local anesthetic is planned, this fasting is necessary, for if complications should develop, a general anesthetic might be required.

If you have forgotten your doctor's instructions and have had anything to eat or drink, tell the doctor before the operation. It might mean rescheduling the operation, but this would be preferable to taking the risk of having anesthesia problems.

In some cases you may be given a sleeping pill the night before the operation. An hour or two before the operation an injection generally is given so that you will be in a calm, semiconscious state. An injection of a drug designed to dry up secretions in the mouth and throat is sometimes given preoperatively.

Being ''prepped'' (prepared) for surgery may include having the skin shaved and the area around the incision site cleansed with an antiseptic solution. This is done to cut down on the chances of infection. An enema may be

735

given the night before major surgery. A tube called a catheter may be inserted through the urinary opening and into the bladder so that the bladder will be empty and there will be less danger of injuring it during the operation. This may be done in your hospital room or in the operating room. If it is done before you are anesthetized, you may experience a brief stinging feeling as the tube is inserted.

If you are wearing jewelry or false teeth, these must be removed. Fingernail polish must be removed so that the anesthesiologist will be able to see the skin beneath your nails and monitor you for signs of oxygen deprivation. You usually are required to wear a sterile surgical gown and cap. Then you are placed on a wheeled cot or bed and taken to the operating room.

In the Operating Room

Once you are in the operating room you will be transferred to the operating table. The position in which you are placed will depend on the type of surgery you are having. If, for instance, you are having vaginal surgery, your feet may be placed in stirrups similar to those used during a gynecological exam. A needle attached to a tube and to a hanging bottle called an I.V. (intravenous) may be inserted into your hand or arm. This may contain special medications or sugar water. The anesthetic may be administered through the I.V. You may feel a slight pinprick when the I.V. needle is inserted, but once it is in place you shouldn't feel any pain.

If you are having a general anesthetic, you will be unconscious within a few moments of the injection of the drug. If you are having a local anesthetic, you might feel a slight pinprick or a tingling or numbness when the anesthetic is injected, but this generally passes within a few moments.

You should discuss the operating room procedures and any questions you have with the doctor before surgery. Once you have been sedated and wheeled into the operating room, you may not be able to get clear answers to your questions. First, you are apt to be feeling a little fuzzy from the sedative. Second, your doctor may not be there yet, and the assistant doctors or nurses may not be willing or able to answer your questions.

After the Operation

After the operation you will go to the recovery room, where your temperature, pulse, respiration and blood pressure will be monitored carefully until you recover from the effects of the anesthetic. The amount of time you spend in the recovery room will depend on the nature and extent of your surgery and the type of anesthetic used. Then you will be returned to your hospital room.

If you have had minor surgery requiring only a local anesthetic, you may leave within an hour or two after surgery, but you should not try to get home by yourself, for reflexes and reaction time may be slow for 24 to 48 hours. If you have had a general anesthetic, you may still be able to leave the hospital the same day after most minor forms of surgery, but if complications develop, you may have to remain in the hospital overnight or longer.

After major surgery you will usually have to stay in the hospital for at least 5 or 6 days. Bed rest usually is required, although you will be encouraged to change position and move your arms and legs to stimulate your circulation and to get you to breathe deeply so you will not form blood clots or develop pneumonia. After most types of major surgery you will be made to get out of bed and walk a bit the next day. Getting out of bed as soon as possible speeds recovery time and cuts down on the possibility of complications.

You may be allowed some fluids within a few hours and a bland diet on the following day. Depending on the nature of your surgery, pain medications, antibiotics, I.V.s, enemas or blood transfusions may be ordered. Ask your doctor what to expect postoperatively so that you are not shocked by waking up and finding various tubes and needles stuck in you.

Nausea and vomiting are not unusual after operations. You may feel dizzy and rather weak. Expect some soreness around the incision, gas pains and other discomfort. You may be given injections of a narcotic immediately after surgery. Later on you may be switched to pain pills.

Any form of surgery involves risks. In addition to the risks involved in the use of anesthetics there may be bleeding problems, infection or injury to adjacent organs during surgery. Before you leave the hospital make you you have a *written* list of possible danger signs, an emergency phone number and careful postoperative instructions. The list of postoperative instructions should tell you when you can shower, bathe, use tampons and have intercourse. If you have specific questions about certain activities—for example, When can I drive a car? Go back to work? Play tennis?—be sure to ask the doctor. A follow-up appointment should be scheduled before you leave the hospital.

In the reference section following, the various types of surgery mentioned in other sections of this book are described in greater detail. Descriptions of various diagnostic tests and other routine procedures are also included.

Diagnostic Tests and Procedures

Doctors often are accused of practicing defensive medicine—of ordering too many tests to protect themselves from malpractice suits. To protect yourself from unnecessary or overly extensive tests, ask the following questions:

☐ What is the purpose of this test and what will the test results tell you about my condition?

☐ Are there other tests that could be done instead? If so, are these other tests less expensive, less risky, less time-consuming or less painful?

☐ What are the risks involved in this test?

☐ Do I need to be hospitalized? For how long? Could this test be done on an outpatient basis? Why not?

☐ What will happen to me during the test?

☐ How long will it take to get test results?

☐ What could the test results possibly indicate and what decisions might I be faced with if the test results are positive?

☐ What type of doctor will be performing the tests or analyzing the results of the test? Are these doctors board-certified?

☐ What will the test cost? Will my insurance cover the costs? How will I be billed?

Only by asking questions and insisting on complete answers and explanations can women assure themselves of getting top-notch medical care.

Routine Exams

Although it is true that many tests are done unnecessarily, it is also true that many women don't have physical exams and routine screening tests—many of them simple office procedures—that could detect diseases and abnormalities in their earliest stages. The following routine examinations and screening tests are important to your health:

General physical exam: These should be done at regular intervals, but there is considerable controversy as to how often they should be done on healthy people with no symptoms. Many authorities believe that a general physical should be done by an internist or family practitioner rather than by a gynecologist, since gynecologists are trained to deal with problems affecting the reproductive tract, not with the body as a whole.

Blood pressure (BP): Women under age 40 should have their BP checked once a year and, according to some doctors, those over 40, every 6 months. Hypertension (high blood pressure), which is a common problem for women, can have serious consequences and often can be detected only by a BP check. Women on birth control pills, who may be especially susceptible, may want to have their BP checked every 6 months regardless of their age.

Urine tests: According to some experts, urine tests to determine protein and urine levels should be done once a year; others recommend once every 3 to 5 years. These tests can detect kidney or bladder disease, diabetes and other medical problems.

Breast exam: Every woman should practice monthly breast self-exam. Women under 40 should have a doctor examine their breasts once a year; women over 40 may want to be examined every 6 months.

Mammography: A single mammogram at age 35 will serve as a baseline with which to compare results from subsequent testing, which should be done once a year after age 50. Younger women at high risk of developing breast cancer (*see* p. 518) may want to have mammograms and doctor exams more frequently.

Complete blood count (CBC): This blood test can detect anemia. Some experts think it should be done on a yearly basis, whereas others recommend every 3 to 5 years.

Stool analysis: This should be done once every year or two after age 40.

Pelvic and rectal exam: This should be done once a year from age 16 to 18, or before if sexual activity is begun, and twice a year after age 40.

Pap smear: Although there is some debate as to how frequently this simple screening test for cervical cancer should be done, we recommend it on a yearly basis. Women at high risk of developing cervical cancer (*see* p. 375) may want to have a Pap smear twice a year.

VD tests: Tests for venereal disease should be done on a yearly basis for sexually active, heterosexual women.

Mulitple blood screening tests: Tests to measure cholesterol, blood sugar and blood urea, nitrogen and calcium are done by some doctors on a yearly basis, but most believe once every 5 years is sufficient. Some think cholesterol levels should be done once a year after age 50.

Proctosigmoidoscopy: Some doctors recommend this on a yearly basis for all women over 60; others recommend every 3 years after age 40.

Endometrial biopsy: Some doctors recommend this test for postmenopausal women who are using estrogen replacement therapy or who are otherwise at high risk of developing endometrial cancer (*see* p. 446–47).

Skin test for tuberculosis: This should be done once every 5 years until age 35.

Screening for vision and hearing: This should be done every 5 years after age 60.

Tonometry: This test can detect glaucoma, an eye disease that can cause blindness, in its earliest stages. Women over age 40 should have this test every 2 or 3 years or annually if there is a family history of glaucoma.

Electrocardiogram (ECG): The "resting" ECG is not as accurate as the "exercise" ECG. A single ECG at age 35 will serve as a baseline with which to compare results from subsequent testing, which should be done once every 10 years.

Chest X-ray: In the absence of symptoms the chest X-ray is not valuable as a periodic screening test. Lung cancer is rarely detected by chest X-ray early enough to affect the eventual outcome.

Drugs

Some of the most heated controversies in medicine today revolve around drugs, in particular around the use of hormones. DES, a synthetic estrogen given to millions of pregnant women in the United States between 1940 and 1971, has caused cancer[6] and other serious problems[7] in the offspring of those women who took the drug and may increase the chances of developing cancer in the DES mothers.[8] Estrogen products used to treat menopausal symptoms have been implicated in an increased risk of developing cancer of the endometrial lining of the uterus[9] and may play a role in the development of breast cancer.[10] Estrogen and synthetic progesterone used in birth control pills have caused the deaths of some women, and more than 50 side effects and complications have now been attributed to Pill usage.

Hormones have a definite role in gynecological medicine, but they should be used with caution. Women who are considering the use of hormones should read the information on side effects and complications given in the section on birth control. These risks have been determined as the result of studies of women using birth control pills containing estrogen and progestin (synthetic progesterone). It is not known whether women using hormone preparations that contain only estrogen or only progestin face the same risks as those associated with Pill usage. For instance, women given progestin for the treatment of abnormal bleeding and other problems may not face the same risks as women who are using progestin in combination with estrogen, but until the risks are clearly delineated, women using progestin-only preparations should consider themselves at similar risk and should watch for the same danger signs.

We know a bit more about the risks associated with estrogen-only preparations, for these drugs have been widely used in the treatment of women with menopausal symptoms. These women have been studied, but not as extensively as Pill users. In some cases the use of estrogen in menopausal women (called estrogen replacement therapy, or ERT) has resulted in problems similar to those experienced by Pill users, but menopausal women have not been studied for all the Pill effects. Here again, until these risks have been more clearly identified, women using estrogen-only preparations should consider themselves at similar risk to women using estrogen in birth control pills and should watch for the same danger signs.

Getting Information About Drugs

In the reference section that accompanies this chapter we have provided detailed information on some of the more common and some of the more controversial drugs used in gynecological medicine. In addition, certain drugs used

740

to treat a specific condition are described in the section on that disease. You can locate information on these drugs by referring to the index.

Manufacturers of hormone preparations are required by law to include printed package inserts; be sure to read the inserts carefully. Another way to obtain information about a drug is to use a reference book called the *Physician's Desk Reference,* or the *PDR,* for short. Most medical libraries and hospitals have copies, and it can also be purchased at or ordered from large bookstores. Although only those drug manufacturers that pay a fee are included in this book, most companies do pay and so are in it. Products are listed by manufacturer, with cross-references by brand name, generic name and uses. The *PDR* also includes detailed information on dosage, ingredients, uses, side effects, complications and contraindications for the drugs listed, as well as pictures of many of them. Although the *PDR* is a valuable source of information, it is essentially an advertising tool for the drug industry and, not surprisingly, tends to downplay adverse effects of drugs. For example, the side effects and complications associated with hormones are presented in the most restrained way. The *PDR,* by law, must reveal that estrogen replacement therapy has been implicated in the development of breast cancer, but it tosses this fact off in one sentence:[11]

> At the present time there is no satisfactory evidence that estrogens given to postmenopausal women increase the risk of cancer of the breast, although recent long-term follow-up of a single physician's practice has raised this possibility.

The *PDR* does not tell you that this was the first and only long-term study of breast cancer risk and estrogen replacement therapy or that the single physician happened to be Dr. Robert Hoover of the National Cancer Institute or that the study was published in the *New England Journal of Medicine,* the foremost medical journal in this country.[12]

The point of all this is that even though the *PDR* is a valuable source of information, it will never be accused of muckraking or sensationalism. As mentioned, it tends to downplay negative aspects. If the *PDR* lists something as a possible negative effect of a manufacturer's product, you can be sure there is significant and respected scientific opinion to back it up.

General Considerations

All drugs involve some risk, so before a drug is prescribed or taken you should observe certain precautions. First, be sure that the doctor knows about any allergic reactions you have had to drugs or to foods in the past. It is especially important to let the doctor know if you are pregnant, are breast-feeding or have a history of kidney or liver disease or any other special medical condition, such as diabetes. Also tell the doctor if you are on a special diet or are taking vitamins or other over-the-counter or prescription drugs, including birth control pills or insulin. Ask your doctor what side effects are associated with the use of the drug and what to do if such side effects occur, and find out if there are any foods you should avoid while taking the drug. Some antibiotics, for instance, won't work if you drink milk or eat dairy products; other drugs should not be taken in combination with alcoholic beverages.

It should also be clear to you how the drug is to be taken. If you are told to take it "three times a day," does this mean morning, noon and night? Before or after meals? If it is to be taken "every 6 hours," does this mean only while you're awake or should you wake up to take the medicine? Should you take the medicine until it is all gone or just until you feel better? With some medications it is important to take all the medicine or the disease is apt to recur. You should always read labels carefully for storing instructions. Some drugs must be refrigerated or stored in special ways. Discard medicines that are outdated. If there are children around your home, ask for child-proof caps on medicines.

You should ask whether the drug being prescribed has been approved by the Food and Drug Administration (FDA) *for the specific condition that you have*. It is important to take this precaution, because doctors can and do prescribe drugs to treat conditions even though the FDA has not approved the drug for that particular condition. In order for a drug to become available for a doctor to prescribe, it must be tested for safety and effectiveness. But the FDA's job is to regulate the pharmaceutical industry, not the medical profession. Once a drug is approved, a doctor may prescribe it for any condition.

For example, consider the drug Depo-Provera. This drug has been associated with a number of serious side effects, including cancer in studies involving laboratory animals.[13] The FDA, however, approved it as a treatment for advanced uterine cancer, because in these cases it was felt that the proven benefits outweighed the possible risks.[14] Depo-Provera also works as a contraceptive, but since it is associated with cervical cancer in women[15] and with other serious complications, the FDA has not given its approval for use of the drug as a contraceptive.[16] This has not stopped doctors from prescribing it for that use. According to the Ralph Nader–affiliated Health Research Group, Depo-Provera was prescribed as a contraceptive for some 10,000 U.S. women in 1975.[17]

Be sure to ask whether the drug being prescribed has been clearly proven to be effective for the condition for which it is being prescribed. It was not until 1962 that the FDA required that effectiveness as well as safety be proved before a drug could be approved. Some doctors still prescribe drugs for conditions for which the drugs have not been proven effective. Consider, for example, sulfanilamide, sold under brand names like AVC Cream, Sufamal and Vagitrol. This drug is widely used to treat vaginitis, but a review of the drug by the National Academy of Science/National Research Council found that it was only "possibly" effective for the treatment of trich, candidiasis and hemophilus.[18]

If your doctor cannot assure you that the drug is approved for the condition you have or has been proven effective for that condition, your use of the drug is "investigational" or "experimental" and you should be given a consent form to sign that explains the possible risks and benefits. In some cases a woman may be acting wisely in her decision to take a drug on this basis. If, for example, you are being treated for breast cancer, it might be worthwhile to take an experimental drug. In other instances, where the disease is not a serious one, you may decide that you are not interested in the risks of experimentation.

One way to check on whether or not a drug is approved for and effective in treating your condition is to look it up in the *PDR;* however, it is possible for a drug to have been proven effective for a condition and not be so listed in the *PDR,* since some drugs (penicillin, for instance) are effective for so many conditions that it is impractical to list all the indications. You may also call your local FDA office (look in the phone book for the nearest major city under U.S. Government, Department of Health and Human Services, Food and Drug Administration). If you suspect you have been given a drug for an unapproved use, you can contact the Institute for the Study of Medical Ethics, P. O. Box 17307, Los Angeles, California 90017, (213) 413-4997.

Buying Drugs

The cost of the same drug may vary considerably from one pharmacy to another. Do a little comparison shopping by phone and you may find that you save yourself quite a bit of money. Also, ask your doctor if it is possible to prescribe the drug by a generic name rather than by a brand name. A generic name is the chemical name for a substance, whereas a brand name is the name used for this same substance by a particular company. For example, aspirin is the generic term for a product that may be sold under various brand names, such as Bayer or Bufferin. There is no difference in the painkilling quality of these drugs, for any drug that claims to be aspirin must meet the FDA standards set for that drug.

There may, however, be differences between products with the same generic name that are manufactured by different companies. To use aspirin as an example again, certain brands of aspirin may contain additional substances that aid in the breakdown and absorption of the aspirin so that it gets out of your stomach faster. With aspirin, which has detrimental effects on the lining of the stomach, these additional substances may make a crucial difference. In most instances, however, there is no difference between generic and brand name drugs. Indeed, many times the generic product is manufactured and sold by one company that also sells it in bulk to another company that then prints its own brand-name label and sells the identical product to you at a higher price. For example, consider ampicillin, a widely used antibiotic that is sold under 224 brand names but is made by only 24 manufacturers, or conjugated estrogens, sold under 219 names but made by only 45 manufacturers.

Many doctors are not aware that the differences in price between brand-name and generic drugs can be quite hefty. They are used to prescribing a particular brand or have been wooed by drug salesmen, who are liberally supplied with expense accounts for just this purpose, and so they don't consider writing prescriptions for the less expensive, generic drugs. In some states there are now laws that allow pharmacists, after informing patients, to substitute generic drugs for brand names when the substances are equivalent. This is not true in all states, so women should ask their doctors about the generic alternatives.

Reference Section:
Operations, Tests, Procedures and Drugs

VULVECTOMY

AKA: removal of the vulvar tissue

Types: "skinning" vulvectomy
simple, or total, vulvectomy
radical vulvectomy

A vulvectomy is an operation in which all or part of the vulva is removed. A "skinning" vulvectomy involves removal of the outer layers of the vulvar skin. It is used to treat certain deep-seated vulvar infections, in severe cases of condyloma acuminata and for precancerous vulvar conditions. It is sometimes used to treat vulvar dystrophies, but many experts believe it is ineffective in these cases and should not be used.

A simple, or total, vulvectomy involves the removal of the skin of the vulvar area, as well as the skin of the vaginal lips and the skin of the clitoris. It is more extensive than a skinning vulvectomy, but in both procedures new skin usually will grow back to replace the skin that has been removed.

A radical vulvectomy is used to treat invasive vulvar cancer. In this operation the vaginal lips, clitoris and the skin surrounding the vulva are removed. A pelvic lymphadenectomy—removal of the pelvic lymph nodes—usually is done at the same time. Skin grafts may be required to close the wound.

A general anesthetic is required, and the woman is usually confined to bed for at least 2 days. For a simple vulvectomy the hospital stay generally is 2

745

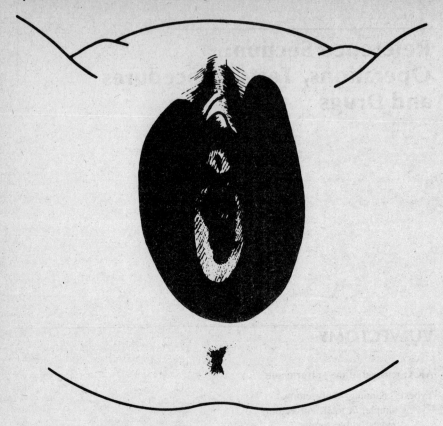

Illustration 61   *Simple Vulvectomy*

weeks or less. To cut down on infections and other complications, the wound is irrigated frequently with salt water. Heat lamps, whirlpool baths and hot sitz baths may be ordered. Honey may be applied to the wound to promote healing.

Women who have had vulvectomies can become pregnant, although it may be necessary to perform a cesarean rather than to use a vaginal delivery; however, most women who have vulvectomies are well past the childbearing years. Intercourse is still possible, but depending on the extensiveness of the vulvectomy, sexual responsiveness may be diminished. If a radical vulvectomy is done, the nerve endings of the clitoris may be so damaged that orgasm is not possible. Since vulvectomies are usually done in older women, doctors tend to ignore the importance of retaining the ability to experience orgasm, for they assume that this is not important to older women. If you need to have a vulvectomy, be sure to discuss this with your doctor. It may be possible to perform the operation in such a way that sexual functioning will not be impaired. If you don't discuss this issue with your doctor, s/he may rely on assumptions about older women and sexuality and perform a more extensive procedure as a matter of routine.

VAGINECTOMY

AKA: removal of all or part of the vagina

Types: partial vaginectomy
total vaginectomy

Vaginectomy is a removal of all or part of the vagina. This operation is used in the treatment of certain forms of cancer. It usually is part of another operative procedure, such as a radical hysterectomy or a pelvic exenteration. Vaginectomies have been used to treat women with vaginal adenosis, but the operation is no longer recommended for this purpose.

If the entire vagina is removed, it may be possible to reconstruct a new vagina using plastic surgery techniques. If only part of the vagina—generally the upper third—is removed, there may not be any problems; however, many women experience pain on intercourse or vaginal stenosis after such surgery. The risks and complications are similar to those of any major form of surgery.

HYSTERECTOMY

AKA: removal of the uterus

Types: subtotal hysterectomy
total, or simple, abdominal hysterectomy
total, or simple, abdominal hysterectomy with bilateral salpingo-oophorectomy, or complete hysterectomy
radical abdominal, or Wertheim's, hysterectomy
vaginal hysterectomy
radical vaginal hysterectomy, or Schauta procedure

In Chapter One we discussed the well-documented fact that many hysterectomies are performed unnecessarily. Of course, a woman's doctor does not say, "How would you like to have an unnecessary hysterectomy?" It's done with a good deal more subtlety than that. Consider, for example, what might happen to a woman who, although she has no symptoms, happens to have a small fibroid tumor in her uterus that is discovered by her doctor in the course of a

747

routine physical. The doctor could push all her panic buttons by telling her that she has a tumor in her uterus that might be cancer. S/he might further tell her that although in all probability the tumor is benign, there's always the chance that it's cancer, so "just to make sure," s/he recommends an operation. Another doctor, dealing with the same woman, might tell her that she has a tumor that in all probability is a benign one that may well get smaller after menopause, and although it should be watched carefully, unless it starts to grow larger or cause problems there is no need to subject her to the risk and expense of major surgery. Most of us are so frightened of cancer that had we seen the doctor who suggested the possibility of cancer, we might well have panicked and agreed to an unnecessary operation, without investigating the alternatives and seeking second opinions. This is just one of the many ways in which unnecessary hysterectomies are foisted on women.

Indications

The only times that a hysterectomy is absolutely necessary are:

- ☐ To remove cancer of the vagina, cervix, uterus, fallopian tubes or ovaries. In the early stages of these diseases it is sometimes possible to avoid hysterectomy.
- ☐ To stop severe, uncontrollable infection
- ☐ To stop severe, uncontrollable bleeding
- ☐ As part of surgery for life-threatening problems affecting other organs when it is technically impossible to treat the other problem without removing the uterus

Hysterectomy may be a wise choice in certain other cases as well, but if it is proposed, make sure you understand why. Read the section of this book that relates to your particular problem so that you will understand your options and alternatives. Get your doctor to answer the questions listed in Chapter Seven, and by all means get a second opinion (*see* p. 238) before consenting to surgery.

Risks and Complications

In many of the cases where hysterectomy is not an absolute medical necessity you will have to weigh the risks versus the benefits before making your decision.

Hysterectomy is a major surgical procedure requiring the use of a general anesthetic and can have serious complications, including death. The risks depend on your age, general health, the competence of the surgeon, the quality of the hospital and the specific type of hysterectomy you are having. For a relatively healthy woman under age 45, the mortality for hysterectomy is about 50 per 100,000 operations performed.[1] For a woman over 50 with high blood pressure the mortality is 15 times higher. The more extensive the type of hysterectomy, the greater the risks.

Although deaths from hysterectomies are relatively rare, complications are not. The most common complication is infection.[2] These infections are usually mild or moderate and can be controlled with oral antibiotics. Bleeding during the operation is also common, with about 15 percent of patients requiring blood transfusions.[3] Bleeding may also occur after the operation, although less than 1 percent of women having hysterectomies require transfusions or readmission to the hospital because of postsurgical bleeding complications.

Urinary tract problems are also rather common but usually are not serious. A portion of the women will have a bladder or kidney infection after the operation. However, damage to the bladder or tubes that carry urine from the kidneys occurs in about 1 out of every 200 operations. Bowel problems caused by damage to the intestines during surgery or scar tissue that prevents the intestines from contracting properly are relatively rare, but about 2 percent of all hysterectomy patients require a second surgery to remove scar tissue on the bowels. Blood clots occur in 1 percent of women having hysterectomies and may be fatal. Some women experience a loss of pelvic support and such problems as cystoceles and rectoceles after hysterectomy.

If the ovaries are also removed in a premenopausal woman, she will probably experience premature menopause. Even if the ovaries are spared, a woman may still experience a premature menopause, for at times the blood supply to the ovaries is disrupted and they gradually lose their ability to produce hormones. At other times the disruption to the ovaries during surgery leads to the subsequent formation of ovarian cysts that require a second operation and removal of the cysts and ovaries, again causing premature menopause. Loss of ovarian function after removal of the uterus alone is an uncommon complication, but it does happen.

Hysterectomy and Your Sex Life

One area that has received little attention is the effect of hysterectomy on a woman's sex life. For women who have had hysterectomies for conditions that were causing pain, their sex lives may be greatly improved. For some women, freedom from the fear of pregnancy and the hassles of birth control may have beneficial effects on their sex lives. For others the fact that they can no longer bear children may make sex less enjoyable. These are psychological effects and vary from woman to woman, depending on her own personal attitudes about sex and her role as a woman.

After certain types of hysterectomies the vagina may be shortened somewhat, which can make intercourse more difficult. Scar tissue may also form in the pelvis or at the top of the vagina after any type of hysterectomy, and this can cause painful intercourse.

The ability to achieve orgasm is not lost when your uterus and ovaries are removed. Many women don't notice any change in their orgasms at all, but some do. Some women find that their orgasms are less intense. Until recently, the observations of such women were dismissed as psychological. We now know from the pioneering work of well-known sex researchers Masters and Johnson that the uterus becomes congested with blood before orgasm and participates in the general release of congestion at the time of orgasm. This is yet another example of the discovery of a physiological basis for a phenomenon formerly considered to be of the "it's-all-in-your-head" variety. There has been little research done in this area, and doctors rarely mention it to their patients. Not all women have this reaction, but some do, and we feel that women should be made aware of this possibility.

Types

There are several types of hysterectomies (Illustration 62), including:

The subtotal hysterectomy: This operation involves removal of the body of the uterus but not the lower cervical portion. Since the cervix has no function once the uterus is removed, and since the cervix may be the site of cancer in the future, this operation is rarely done anymore. No surgeon does it deliberately. It is done only when circumstances force it, if, for instance, removal of the uterus has been difficult and time-consuming and taking extra time to remove the cervix would prolong the woman's time under anesthesia and subject her to undue risks.

The total, or simple, abdominal hysterectomy: Both the body of the uterus and the cervix are removed through an abdominal incision.

The complete hysterectomy (total, or simple, abdominal hysterectomy plus bilateral salpingo-oophorectomy): Same as the above except that the ovaries and tubes are also removed.

The radical abdominal, or Wertheim's, hysterectomy: Same as above except that the upper third of the vagina and the parametrial tissues (the tissues adjacent to the uterus and cervix) are also removed. This operation is used to treat certain types of cancer.

Vaginal hysterectomy: This operation involves removal of the entire uterus, the cervix and the body of the uterus through a vaginal incision. It is also possible to remove the ovaries and tubes through a vaginal incision—to

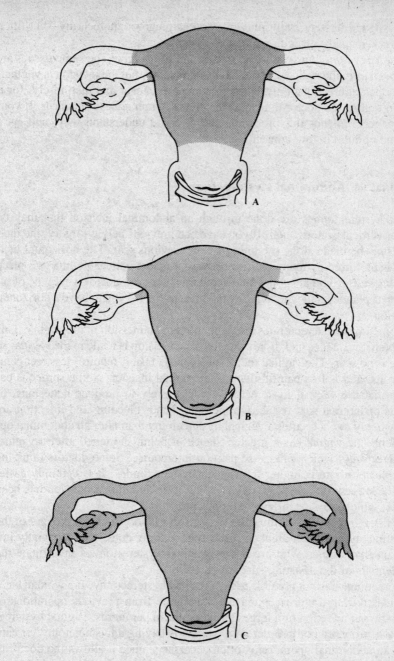

Illustration 62 *Subtotal Hysterectomy (A); Total, or Simple, Hysterectomy (B); and Total, or Simple, Hysterectomy with Bilateral Salpingo-Oophorectomy (C).*

do a vaginal hysterectomy plus bilateral salpingo-oophorectomy—but often this is technically difficult and usually is not done.

Radical vaginal hysterectomy, or Schauta procedure: The same tissues are removed as in the radical abdominal hysterectomy, but the incision is vaginal. This operation is done only in the treatment of cancer and then rarely, for it doesn't allow the doctor to inspect the pelvic lymph nodes for cancer. If your doctor recommends this procedure, be sure you understand why, and get a second opinion before consenting to it.

Vaginal vs. Abdominal Hysterectomy

Most hysterectomies are done through an abdominal incision that may be either vertical or horizontal. If you have had previous pelvic surgery, the incision may be made along the lines of your previous scar. The horizontal incision is preferred by many women because it is less noticeable in a two-piece bathing suit. If you are concerned about this, ask your doctor what type of incision is planned and whether it would be possible for you to have a horizontal incision.

Sometimes hysterectomies are done through an incision in the vagina. This has both advantages and disadvantages. The incision is made in the vagina, so there is no scar. The vaginal incision also heals faster, requires less recuperation time and is less painful than an abdominal incision. Some surgeons believe that the vaginal hysterectomy is less likely to produce adhesions, or bands of internal scar tissue. On the other hand, bleeding and infection are more likely to occur after a vaginal hysterectomy than after an abdominal operation. The vagina has a greater chance of being shortened after a vaginal hysterectomy, which can cause pain on intercourse. Some doctors think the complication rate is higher for vaginal hysterectomies. It is certainly easier for the surgeon to see what s/he is doing if an abdominal incision has been made, which may mean fewer complications.

The vaginal hysterectomy calls for a greater involvement on the part of the assisting surgeon than an abdominal hysterectomy does. It is especially important that women who are having vaginal hysterectomies investigate the credentials of the assisting surgeon carefully.

Sometimes it is not possible to do a vaginal hysterectomy. If a woman has a particularly large uterus, extensive scar tissue from previous operations or from pelvic infection or a large fibroid tumor in her uterus, vaginal hysterectomy is probably not in order. If a woman is having a hysterectomy for cancer, an abdominal operation is often necessary, since it allows the doctor to get a complete view of the abdominal cavity. Although it is possible to remove the ovaries as well as the uterus through a vaginal incision, it is more difficult to do so. The main indication for a vaginal hysterectomy is for prolapse of the uterus when there is associated prolapse of the other pelvic organs. The vaginal repair of the other prolapses can be done through the same approach.

You should ask your doctor which type of hysterectomy is planned and why. Women who are being operated on in teaching hospitals should realize that since vaginal hysterectomies are done less frequently, doctors may sometimes push this form of surgery so that students have a chance to learn how to do it. If your ovaries are being removed or you require a radical operation for cancer and your doctor recommends a vaginal hysterectomy, you would do well to question the reasoning behind this and to seek a second opinion.

Removal of the Ovaries

Sometimes the ovaries must be removed because of the nature of the disease, but at times doctors performing hysterectomies will remove healthy ovaries as well, even though this is not strictly necessary to cure the disease. Some doctors routinely remove the ovaries in all their women patients over age 35 who are having hysterectomies; others use 40 as the cut-off, and still others use 45. Most doctors will remove the ovaries in postmenopausal women having hysterectomies.

Those who argue for removal of the ovaries have three points to make. First, they argue that removing the ovaries precludes the development of ovarian cancer. Second, they point out that the hysterectomy interferes with the blood supply to the ovaries. In a small number of women this results in cystic ovaries and pelvic pain, requiring a second operation to remove the ovaries. Even though the number of women to whom this happens is small, these doctors consider it foolish to take the risk. Third, they point out that in a number of women—again, a small percentage—the ovaries cease functioning within a few years after the hysterectomy. Thus, they say, it is better to remove the ovaries and prevent possible cancer than to leave them in when they may function for only a few years anyway.

Those who prefer to leave the ovaries in point out that removing the ovaries usually will cause premature menopause. Premature menopause increases a woman's risk of developing hypertension, a disease characterized by high blood pressure, and osteoporosis, a disease associated with loss of bone density. Since both of these diseases can have serious, even fatal, consequences, they favor preserving the ovaries. Moreover, with removal of the ovaries there is an abrupt cessation of hormone production rather than the gradual tapering off that occurs in a natural menopause, so that menopausal symptoms are likely to be more severe. In the past those who favored removal of the ovaries countered these arguments by pointing out that a woman who has a surgical menopause can be given estrogen replacement therapy (ERT). The

753

fact that ERT can cause uterine cancer[4] would not be a problem for such a woman, since she no longer has her uterus. However, a recent study, while not conclusive, has indicated that women on ERT may be at increased risk of developing breast cancer.[5] Thus posthysterectomy women can no longer take ERT with complete assurance that it is safe to do so. (For details, see the section on ERT.)

A doctor's decision to remove or preserve the ovaries may depend on his or her personal experience. For instance, a surgeon who treats many ovarian cancer patients might be more apt to remove the ovaries in younger women than a doctor who doesn't deal with these sorts of cases. As one doctor put it, "Sometimes whether or not I remove the ovaries depends on what has happened to me in the last few weeks. If I've watched a patient die from cancer of the ovary, I often remove them. But if I've been free of this experience for a while, I'm more inclined to leave them in."[6]

Although this doctor's attitude is understandable, it is hardly scientific. Women should realize that doctors' decisions on this issue are often made on the basis of personal beliefs and attitudes rather than scientific facts. Moreover, women should realize that many doctors don't even discuss this issue with their patients. Women should take the initiative and ask their doctors the appropriate questions—does s/he plan to remove one or both ovaries or to leave one or both of them intact and why or why not?—before surgery. It is not always possible for the doctor to preserve the ovaries, although s/he may intend to. On operation the doctor may discover some unsuspected condition that requires that the ovaries be removed, but women should nonetheless discuss the doctor's intent before surgery.

Women should also make sure that they understand the doctor's terminology, for one doctor may use the term "total hysterectomy" to include removal of the ovaries, whereas another uses the term to refer to an operation in which the ovaries are not removed.

Our personal preference is to leave the ovaries intact in a younger woman, but different doctors can in good faith and for sound reasons disagree. Furthermore, although this is our recommendation, it is the patient's decision, and if she wants her ovaries removed, we will respect her wishes. In postmenopausal women we recommend removal of the ovaries, for there is nothing to be gained by leaving them in and there is a possibility of cancer developing later on. Even though there is some new evidence that the postmenopausal ovaries are not the functionless organs we once thought,[7] there is no evidence that the value of leaving them in outweighs the possible risks. We therefore would not perform a hysterectomy on a postmenopausal woman without removing her ovaries.

After Hysterectomy

The majority of women who have hysterectomies leave the hospital within 7 to 10 days. Recovery times vary greatly. Most women return to work in about 6 weeks, but some women take 9 weeks or longer, especially those over age 36. It is not uncommon for women to say that they didn't really feel back to normal for an entire year. Many women experience severe fatigue in the first few days at home, and some find they must spend an entire week in bed.

Women often have feelings of depression after hysterectomy. This is quite natural, and these feelings do not usually last for too long. Try to arrange with loved ones and friends for support so that you can have someone to talk to if you're feeling blue.

Many women experience hot flashes after hysterectomy even if their ovaries have not been removed. This may be owing to a disruption in the blood supply of the ovaries during surgery. For most women these are relatively short-lived.

You will probably have some vaginal bleeding that may be brown, but this should taper off in a few days. You are also likely to experience some pain and discomfort, for hysterectomy is a major operation.

Women are usually told not to have sex for 6 to 8 weeks because of the possibility of infection or of jarring the stitches. Most doctors recommend a 2- to 3-month wait before returning to active sports like tennis. You should use your common sense and consult with your doctor about postoperative activities.

If you have any of the following symptoms after surgery, call your doctor, for they might be signs of complication.

☐ Fever over 100.4°F
☐ Pain that is not relieved by the painkillers the doctor gave you
☐ More than 3 days without a normal bowel movement.
☐ Persistent pain in the bladder, burning sensation on urination, blood in the urine or an inability to urinate
☐ Pain, swelling, tenderness or redness in your leg
☐ Chest pain, cough, difficulty in breathing and coughing up blood
☐ Bright red vaginal bleeding that soaks two or more pads in an hour or forms large clots.

OOPHORECTOMY

AKA: removal of one or both ovaries, salpingo-oophorectomy, ovariectomy

Types: bilateral oophorectomy
unilateral oophorectomy

A bilateral oophorectomy (Illustration 63) is a procedure in which the ovaries are removed. The correct term for this operation is "bilateral salpingo-

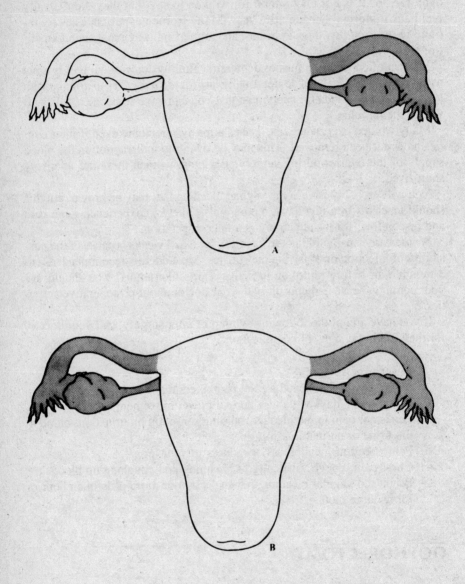

Illustration 63   *Unilateral Oophorectomy (A) and Bilateral Oophorectomy (B)*

756

oophorectomy,'' since the fallopian tubes (*salpingo*) as well as the ovaries (*oophoro*) are removed. A unilateral oophorectomy is the removal of one ovary or a portion of the ovary and may also be accompanied by salpingectomy, or removal of the fallopian tube. Bilateral salpingo-oophorectomy is generally accompanied by a hysterectomy, since without the ovaries, the uterus has no function and may be the site of future problems. Sometimes both ovaries are removed because of a problem in the ovaries themselves, but some doctors routinely remove healthy ovaries in women having hysterectomies. This is discussed in more detail under the heading Hysterectomy above.

Oophorectomies may be done to treat a number of conditions, including ectopic pregnancy, benign and malignant ovarian cysts and tumors and pelvic inflammatory disease.

A unilateral oophorectomy, in which only one ovary is removed, is sometimes possible. With a unilateral oophorectomy a woman is not subject to premature menopause and she preserves her ability to bear children, for even a small nub of ovarian tissue can continue to produce hormones. Women who have had a unilateral oophorectomy are still fertile.

Oophorectomy is a major operation and involves the same risks and potential complications as any form of major surgery. If both the ovaries are removed in a premenopausal woman, she will have a premature menopause. The doctor may recommend estrogen replacement therapy (ERT) in such cases; however, women should read the section on ERT and carefully weigh the risks and benefits before making a decision about ERT.

PELVIC EXENTERATION

AKA: removal of the pelvic organs

Types: total exenteration
     partial exenteration
       anterior exenteration
       posterior exenteration

Pelvic exenteration (Illustration 64) is an ultraradical form of surgery used in the treatment of cancer. A total exenteration involves removal of the uterus, tubes, ovaries, vagina, the tissues adjacent to these organs, the bladder, the urethra and the rectum. Sometimes a partial exenteration, either anterior or posterior, is done. An anterior exenteration involves removal of all the pelvic tissues except the rectum. A posterior exenteration spares the bladder and urethra.

If a total exenteration is done, urinary and fecal wastes are collected in plastic bags attached to the outside of the body. If an anterior exenteration is

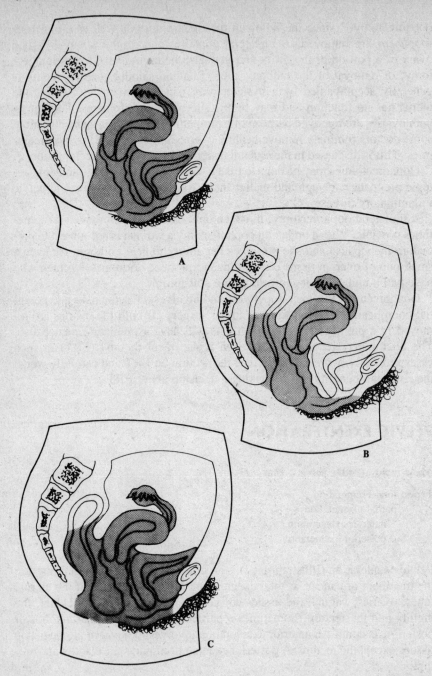

Illustration 64 *Anterior Pelvic Exenteration (A), Posterior Pelvic Exenteration (B) and Total Pelvic Exenteration (C)*

done, it may be possible to divert urinary wastes to the bowels and thereby avoid the external collection bag. If a posterior exeneration is done, the urinary tract may function normally, but fecal wastes must be collected in a bag.

Understandably, many women find the idea of having to empty the bags that collect the waste materials distasteful. Anyone who has grown up in this culture is apt to have intensely negative associations with the natural bodily processes of elimination. Yet many people who have this operation do learn to adjust. Moreover, the operation need not affect a woman's sexual responsiveness, and for women who desire it, plastic surgery techniques can be used to reconstruct the vagina. One way of finding out about the effects of this operation is by talking to people who have gone through it. The United Ostomy Association, at 1111 Wilshire Boulevard, Los Angeles, California 90017, telephone (213) 481-2811, is a support group for people who have had this type of surgery, and they can be helpful in answering questions and helping you to adjust.

The survival rates for women having this procedure are often high enough to justify the risks and complications involved. Women with advanced cancer who are candidates for this radical procedure (and not everyone is) are entitled to a frank discussion of risks and benefits with their doctors before making a decision.

CONIZATION

AKA: cold-knife conization, or cone; surgical conization, or cone; cone biopsy

Conization (Illustration 65) is a surgical procedure whereby a cone of tissue is removed from the center of the cervix, a process somewhat akin to paring out the core of an apple. It is considered a major surgical procedure and must be done in a hospital, using a general anesthetic. Although it sounds like a fairly simple procedure, it requires a good deal of skill. The tissue should be removed in one piece rather than whittled out in little bits, so that the pathologist can study the architecture of the cells.

Indications

Conization is used both as a diagnostic procedure for cervical cancer and as a form of treatment for cervical dysplasia and carcinoma in situ of the cervix. In the past, conization was used as a treatment for chronic cervicitis, but cryosurgery, which is less expensive and less risky, has pretty much replaced conization for this purpose.

759

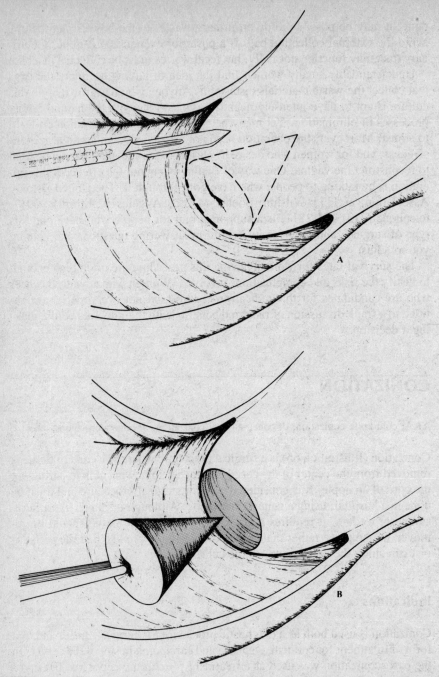

Illustration 65 *Conization: An incision is made in the cervix (A), and a cone-shaped wedge of tissue is removed (B).*

Before colposcopy was available, conization was used to do biopsies of the cervix. But since colposcopy is painless, has no complications, is less expensive and is less risky, it is now the preferred method in most cases. If, however, a woman has an abnormal Pap smear but the colposcopic examination fails to reveal any abnormalities on the surface of the cervix, if the abnormal area is quite large or if the abnormality that is seen leads into the cervical canal, conization must still be done. But whenever possible colposcopy should be done instead of conization. Not all doctors are skilled colposcopists, and some might be tempted to go ahead and do a conization rather than refer you to a doctor who is. If conization is recommended, always ask why conization, rather than colposcopy and biopsy, is being done.

Conization plays a vital role in establishing the diagnosis of microinvasive (Stage IA) cervical cancer. No woman should accept a diagnosis of microinvasive cancer unless a conization has been done.

Procedure

The woman is taken to the operating room and placed in stirrups as if she were having a routine gynecological exam. A speculum is placed in the vagina, and the cervix and vagina are washed with an antiseptic solution. A general anesthetic is given, and the doctor places sutures (stitches) on either side of the cervix to steady it and to diminish bleeding. A circular incision large enough to include the entire affected area is made on the surface of the cervix and is extended deep into the cervix, so that the lower part of the cervix that opens into the uterus is also removed. The cut edges of the cervix are then sutured together.

Complications

Heavy bleeding is a common complication and may occur immediately after surgery or about 10 days later, when the stitches are absorbed. One woman in ten requires transfusion, further surgery or readmission to the hospital because of bleeding problems. Infection and perforation of the uterus, although uncommon, are other complications that can result from conization.

Conization is apt to have a negative affect on fertility, depending on how much tissue has to be removed. If the cervical mucus glands, which produce the secretions that help the sperm swim up into the uterus, are destroyed, the woman may not be able to get pregnant. Cervical stenosis and incompetent cervix may also follow conization and affect fertility. About 25 percent of women who have conizations are not able to get pregnant. About 25 percent of those who do get pregnant will miscarry.

DILATION AND CURETTAGE

AKA: D&C, uterine scraping

The D&C (Illustration 66), a simple operation in which the endometrial lining of the uterus is surgically removed, is one of the most commonly performed surgical procedures and takes only about 10 to 15 minutes. It can be done using either a local or a general anesthetic. Most doctors prefer to use a general anesthetic. First, the local doesn't fully eliminate the pain. Second, often the point of doing a D&C is to allow the doctor to make a careful examination of the uterine cavity, and patient discomfort under a local might cause him or her to hurry, resulting in a less thorough procedure. It is possible, however, to use a local. Regardless of the anesthetic used, the D&C, a hospital procedure, usually can be done on an outpatient basis.

Procedure

The woman is taken to the operating room, given a general (or local) anesthetic and put on a table with stirrups in a position similar to that used in the routine gynecological examination. The vagina, vulva and cervix are carefully cleaned with an antiseptic solution. Although some doctors shave the pubic hair to reduce the chances of infection, most do not. The doctor does a careful bimanual pelvic exam. Under the anesthetic the muscles are completely relaxed and this allows the doctor to feel the pelvic organs more readily than is possible if the woman is not anesthetized. A speculum is inserted into the vagina. The cervix is gently grasped with a clamplike instrument called a tenaculum to hold it steady. If a local anesthetic is used, it is usually injected into the cervix and the ligaments that support the uterus at this point.

A thin metal rod called a uterine sound is used to measure the depth and position of the uterus. It resembles the device used to check the oil level in a car's engine and is introduced into the uterus through the cervical opening. Then a tapered rod is inserted into the cervical opening to widen (dilate) it. A series of graduated rods of varying widths are inserted until the cervix is dilated about a half inch. An instrument called a curette, a thin rod with a sharp, spoon-shaped tip, is inserted into the uterus, and the uterine lining is gently scraped out. A curette may be used to take samples of the tissue lining the cervical canal as well. The doctor will carefully explore the entire uterine cavity with the curette.

The tissue removed through curettage is collected carefully and sent to the lab for analysis. In 24 to 48 hours the pathologist will know whether or

762

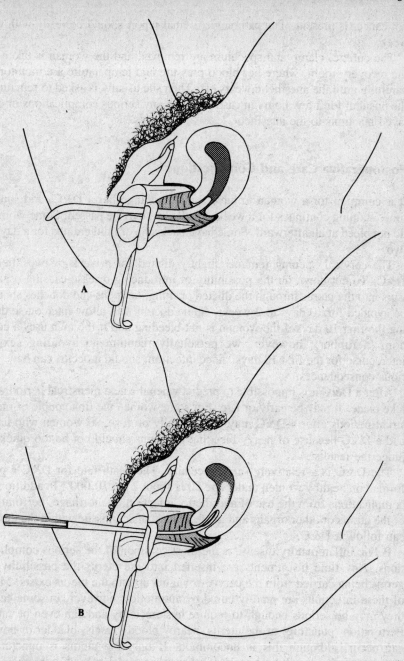

Illustration 66 *Dilation and Curettage: The cervix is dilated with a dilating rod (A), and the uterine lining is removed with a curette (B).*

763

not cancer is present. The pathologist's final report should be ready within a week.

The curette, clamp and speculum are removed and the woman is taken to the recovery room, where her blood pressure and temperature are monitored carefully until the anesthetic wears off. Then she usually is asked to remain at the hospital for a few hours in case there are any serious complications or delayed reactions to the anesthetic.

Postoperative Care and Complications

It is common for a woman to have some bleeding after a D&C, and sometimes staining continues for a week. Small clots may be passed. Some women do not bleed at all afterward. Some have backache or mild cramps for a day or two.

The cervical opening remains slightly dilated for a week or two after a D&C. To cut down on the possibility of introducing disease-causing organisms into the uterus through the dilated opening, tampons and douches should be avoided for 10 days to 2 weeks. Some doctors will allow intercourse during the first 10 days if the woman is not bleeding and if the man uses a condom (a rubber); however, we personally recommend avoiding sexual intercourse for the first 10 days, since infection, should it occur, can have serious consequences.

After a D&C it is impossible to predict when the next menstrual period will take place. It may be early or late. For some women the first couple of menstrual periods after a D&C may be unusually profuse, so women who have had a D&C because of heavy bleeding problems should not be too quick to judge the results.

The D&C is a relatively safe procedure. The death rate for D&C's performed on healthy women under age 50 is about 2 per 10,000.[8] In addition to complications from the use of anesthetic, infection, hemorrhage, perforation of the uterus or other organs and the formation of scar tissue within the uterus can follow a D&C.

Pelvic inflammatory disease is the most common of the serious complications. Any time instruments are inserted into the uterus the possibility of germs being carried from the cervix or vagina up into the uterus exists. Most of these infections are readily cured by antibiotics; however, in some cases they may be serious enough to require hysterectomy and can even be fatal. Perforation (puncture) of the uterus, nearby blood vessels, bladder or bowel can occur, although this is uncommon. If only the uterus is punctured, chances are that it will heal itself. If other organs are damaged, immediate reparative surgery may be necessary. If puncture is suspected, the woman is asked to remain in the hospital and laparoscopy may be recommended to assess the possible damage. Heavy bleeding may occur if the walls of the uterus or the cervix are injured or if a polyp or fibroid tumor is only partially removed, but in general, heavy bleeding is a rare complication, more likely to occur in women who have certain blood disorders. Another rare complication, known as Asherman's syndrome, a condition in which scar tissue forms in the uterus, causing an absence of menstrual periods and infertility, may also follow a D&C.

A checkup usually is done 2 weeks after the D&C. At that time the doctor will check for tenderness in the uterus and tubes, which could indicate infection, and to see that the cervix is normal. If any of the following signs or symptoms occur, the woman should contact her doctor *immediately:*

- ☐ A fever of 100.4°F or higher
- ☐ Persistent abdominal pain or cramps
- ☐ Faintness, weakness or dizziness
- ☐ A foul-smelling vaginal discharge
- ☐ Heavy bleeding (more than three pads soaked in 1 hour)

Indications

The D&C is a diagnostic tool and sometimes a cure for certain conditions. It is used to diagnose uterine cancer and is sometimes part of the diagnostic workup in cervical cancer. It may be used to diagnose abnormal uterine bleeding. Endometritis, which is an infection of the uterine lining that can cause abnormal bleeding, may be cured by a D&C if the infected lining is totally removed. Fibroid tumors that distort the endometrial cavity, causing abnormal bleeding, can be diagnosed by a D&C, for the doctor will feel a "bump" as the curette moves over the surface of the uterine cavity. On occasion, small, protruding fibroids can be removed during a D&C, but most of the time more extensive surgery is necessary. Endometrial polyps, another source of abnormal bleeding, can be diagnosed and treated by a D&C. Cervical polyps will at times necessitate a D&C. Endometrial hyperplasia, yet another source of abnormal bleeding, can also be diagnosed and cured by a D&C. It may also be used to treat Asherman's syndrome.

Sometimes a D&C will allow a woman nearing menopause who has been experiencing abnormal bleeding to avoid a hysterectomy. Sometimes the D&C itself can be avoided by the use of hormone treatment. This is discussed in more detail under the headings Abnormal Uterine Bleeding and Endometrial Hyperplasia. The D&C should be a last resort in young girls with abnormal bleeding problems, for in this age-group such problems often revert to normal by themselves or can be handled with hormone therapy. If a doctor suggests a D&C as the first step in the treatment of abnormal bleeding in this age-group, it would probably be wise to seek a second medical opinion (*see* p. 238).

A D&C is not a treatment for infertility or menstrual cramps. On occasion, the D&C may be part of the diagnostic workup for these conditions but not until other, less drastic diagnostic procedures, such as endometrial biopsy and certain X-ray or ultrasound techniques, have been used. Although the D&C was once used for abortions, the newer, safer suction methods are now preferred.

If the first D&C is not successful in controlling abnormal bleeding, a second or even a third D&C may be in order; however, after that a woman may begin to consider a hysterectomy as an alternative to repeated D&Cs. Factors like the number of years until menopause, whether or not the abnormal bleeding is getting progressively worse and whether or not the hyperplasia (if it exists) is getting progressively more serious in nature will influence this decision. Some women choose to undergo a number of D&C's rather than have a hysterectomy.

CAUTERY

AKA: electric or heat cautery, cauterization, burning

Cauterization (Illustration 67) involves destroying tissues by means of a controlled electric current. A pointed instrument is electrically heated until the tip becomes red-hot. The instrument is then applied to the affected area. The heat destroys the surface layers of tissue, allowing new and unaffected cell growth to replace the burned-off tissue. A scab forms as the tissue heals. The scab sloughs off in a week or two, leaving new, healthy tissue.

Indications

Cautery is used to treat such conditions as chronic cervicitis, dysplasia, carcinoma in situ and vaginal or vulvar warts. It may also be used to close off the tubes in certain sterilization procedures and to destroy areas of endometriosis.

Procedure

If, as is often the case, it is the cervix that is to be treated, a speculum is first inserted into the vagina. The vagina and cervix are cleaned and the cautery

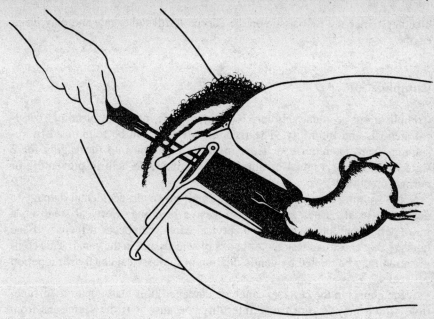

Illustration 67 *Cautery*

tip is applied to the affected area. A gray green scab forms and falls off in a week or two. Underneath the scab, new, healthy tissue will have formed. Complete healing usually takes 7 to 8 weeks, and some doctors prescribe antiseptic creams and jellies during this time to promote healing.

The procedure can usually be done in a doctor's office without an anesthetic although if the area to be treated is up inside the cervical canal, hospitalization and a general anesthetic may be necessary.

Because cauterization causes temporary swelling of the cervix and narrowing of the cervical canal, it usually is performed just after a woman's menstrual period so that the swelling and narrowing will have subsided by the next period and there won't be any blockage of the menstrual flow. The next menstrual period after treatment may, however, be heavier than usual.

There is apt to be a profuse discharge, sometimes with blood in it, for 2 to 3 weeks after treatment; this is normal. If the discharge turns yellow or develops a foul odor, this may be a sign of infection and your doctor should be notified.

Sanitary napkins may be used to catch the discharge, but tampons cannot be used. In fact, most doctors recommend that nothing be inserted in the vagina for 2 to 3 weeks, which means that intercourse and douching are also prohibited.

After the scab falls away the discharge subsides. There may still be some

767

bleeding, since the new tissue on the cervix is still rather raw and may bleed easily.

Complications

Complications are relatively rare but may include infection, bleeding, cervical stenosis and infertility. The risks of infection can be minimized by refraining from intercourse or from inserting anything into the vagina for 2 weeks. Antibiotic vaginal creams or jellies may also help in preventing or curing infection.

Some spotting or even bleeding is normal; however, accidental damage to deeper cervical tissues can cause excessive bleeding. Cervical stenosis, a more permanent narrowing of the cervical canal, can occur if there is tissue damage that causes adhesions, or bands of scar tissue, in the canal. This complication may be treated by gentle dilation of the cervical canal over a period of weeks.

If the glands in the cervical canal are damaged, this may impair their function, which may in turn cause infertility, because it is the secretions from these glands that help nourish the sperm and aid them on their journey into the uterus.

Some doctors fear that electric cautery may cause such scarring that subsequent Pap smears may be difficult to interpret. Certainly, the Pap smear will not be accurate until the healing process is complete.

Cautery vs. Cryosurgery

Cryosurgery (see below) can often be used instead of cautery. Cryosurgery has several advantages. First, it is less painful. Although the textbooks say that cautery causes only mild to moderate discomfort and point out that the treatment takes just a short time, many women we have talked to have found the treatment quite painful.

Moreover, the doctor is better able to control the depth of tissue destruction with cryosurgery, which accounts for the fact that cryosurgery has a lower complication rate than cautery. In certain instances cryosurgery is inappropriate and cautery must be used, but these are rare.

Unfortunately, many doctors do not have cryosurgery equipment in their offices. If you doctor suggests cautery, ask whether cryosurgery could be done instead. If so, request cryosurgery or referral to a cryosurgeon if your doctor does not have the necessary equipment.

CRYOSURGERY

AKA: freezing, cold cautery

Cryosurgery (Illustration 68) is a new technique that is replacing cautery (described above) in many instances. It involves the use of nitrogen or carbon dioxide to quick-freeze the affected areas, killing the abnormal tissue and allowing new, unaffected tissue to take its place. It can be used to treat the same conditions as cautery. Much of the information given in the above description of cautery applies to cryosurgery, so be sure to read that section as well.

Procedure

Cryosurgery is an office procedure and does not require an anesthetic. If the cervix is to be treated, a speculum is placed in the vagina. An instrument that looks like a miniature spear gun is attached to a tank of compressed gas. The gas is released into the gun and expands rapidly to produce intense cold. The

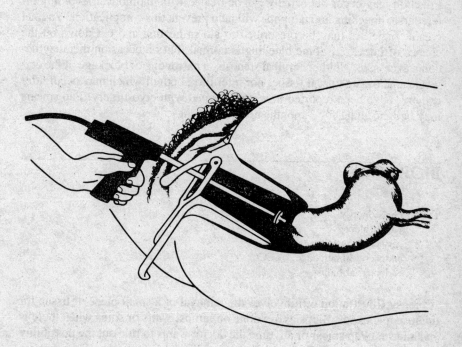

Illustration 68 *Cryosurgery*

tip of the gun is then applied to the area to be treated. The treatment takes about 2 minutes. You may experience a feeling of intense cold and a mild cramp. Because some women experience dizziness and light-headedness afterward, you will be asked to remain lying down for 15 minutes to a half hour after treatment.

Immediately after treatment the cervix is like a block of ice. Within 24 hours the cervix turns deep purple blue and is so swollen that it is impossible to distinguish the cervical os (opening).

Most women have a profuse discharge for a week or two after treatment. The discharge occasionally is bloody, and this is normal. The next period may be heavier than usual, and this is also normal. If the discharge becomes yellow or develops a foul odor, this may be a sign of infection and you should contact the doctor.

Douching, intercourse and the use of tampons are prohibited until the discharge subsides, in about 2 weeks.

Complications

Infection may occur but usually can be treated with antibiotics. Avoiding intercourse, douching and tampons will help prevent this complication. Vaginal creams or jellies may be prescribed to aid in healing and cut down on the chance of infection. Some bleeding is normal, but on occasion this may become excessive. Neither cervical stenosis, a narrowing or blockage of the cervical canal owing to scar tissue, nor infertility, both of which may occur after cautery, have been reported in women treated with cryosurgery. Pap smears may be inaccurate for 3 months after treatment.

BIOPSIES

Types: breast biopsy
vulvar biopsy
cervical biopsy
endocervical curettage, or ECC
endometrial biopsy

A biopsy (Illustration 69) involves the removal of a small piece of tissue for microscopic exam. Biopsies are done on lumps, warts or sores when there is an abnormal Pap smear or anytime the doctor wants to rule out the possibility that cancer is present. General information about biopsies is given in the section on cancer. Breast biopsies are discussed in the section on breast cancer

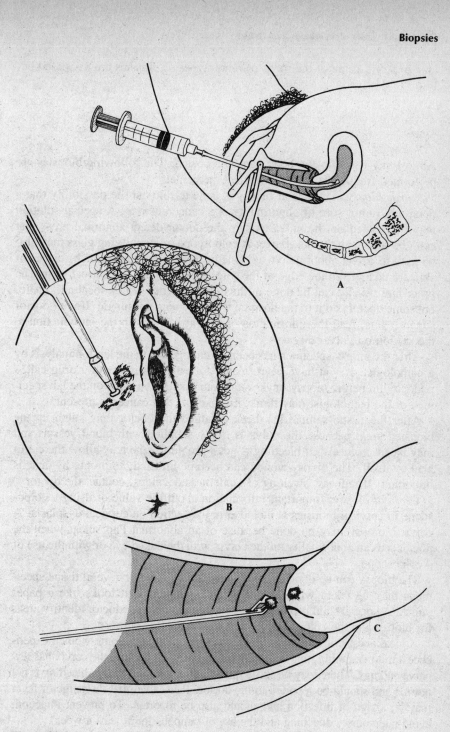

Illustration 69   *Endometrial Biopsy (A), Vulvar Biopsy (B) and Cervical Biopsy*

771

(*see* p. 529). Some of the more common types of biopsies are discussed below.

Types

Almost any tissue in the body can be biopsied. The following biopsies are performed frequently in gynecological medicine:

Vulvar biopsy: The vulvar biopsy is done to rule out the possibility that a persistent lump, sore or abnormality is a cancerous one. A special solution may be painted on the vulva to help the doctor detect abnormal areas that can't be seen with the naked eye. A colposcope or magnifying glass may also be used to detect abnormal areas. One or more tiny (quarter-inch) pieces of skin are taken from the edge of the sore, where it joins the normal skin. The procedure usually can be done in the doctor's office with a local anesthetic, but some doctors do it in the hospital with a general anesthetic. If your doctor suggests this, read the information on vulvar biopsies in the introduction to the section on vulvar diseases.

After the biopsy specimen has been taken it is sent to the lab for analysis by a pathologist. If you have been treated for vulvar warts with a drug called podophyllin before biopsy, make sure your doctor notes this on the lab specimen or the pathologist may think, mistakenly, that cancer is present.

After the tissue sample has been obtained the doctor may stitch up the biopsied area, because the vulva is richly supplied with blood vessels and may bleed profusely; if bleeding is not a problem, s/he may allow the cut to heal by itself. The biopsy wound can become infected, so proper hygiene is important. If redness, swelling or tenderness develops, contact the doctor.

Cervical biopsy: Important information about the value of using a colposcope in cervical biopsies is included in the section on cervical dysplasia. A cervical biopsy may be done because of an abnormal Pap smear when the doctor sees an abnormality on the cervix with the naked eye or with the use of a colposcope.

The biopsy can be done in the doctor's office. One or several tissue specimens may be taken with the aid of an instrument that looks like a paper punch. A special stain is painted on the cervix to help the doctor identify areas for biopsy and the colposcope is also useful for this purpose.

A local anesthetic is generally not necessary. Although some women experience a mild cramping, this is usually not too painful, because the cervix has few nerve endings. There may be some spotting afterward, but heavy bleeding is not normal and should be reported to the doctor. Pain, abnormal discharge or fever may be a sign of infection and should also be reported. To prevent infection, avoid intercourse, douching and the use of tampons for at least a week.

Endocervical curettage: Many times the cervical biopsy will include an endocervical curettage (ECC). A thin instrument with a spoon-shaped tip is used to scrape cells from the cervical canal. ECC is recommended when the abnormal area on the cervix extends into the canal and in the follow-up of women with dysplasia or carcinoma in situ who have been treated by cryosurgery. Like the cervical biopsy, ECC is an office procedure that doesn't usually require an anesthetic, although it may cause mild cramping and, on occasion, infection.

Endometrial biopsy: An endometrial biopsy involves the use of a small scraping instrument, a curette, which is inserted through the cervix into the uterine cavity. The spoon-shaped tip of the curette is used to obtain a tissue sample of the endometrial lining of the uterus. The biopsy can be done in the doctor's office. Most women experience moderate to strong cramping, and a local anesthetic may relieve the pain somewhat.

The endometrial biopsy is often used in fertility workups to tell whether or not the woman is ovulating. It can also detect uterine cancer in women who have abnormal bleeding. If the endometrial biopsy is negative, this does not rule out the possibility of cancer, for the cancer may exist in one area but not in another. A positive endometrial biopsy—one that shows cancerous cells—may eliminate the need for a diagnostic D&C, but a D&C is still necessary if the endometrial biopsy is negative.

Although the endometrial biopsy may fail to detect cancer that is present, it does have a high rate of accuracy (about 85 percent) and may be used to screen women who are at high risk of developing uterine cancer. In particular, many doctors recommend yearly endometrial biopsies for women who use estrogen replacement therapy.

ENDOSCOPY

Types: cystoscopy
        proctosigmoidoscopy
        laparoscopy
        culdoscopy
        colposcopy

Endoscopic examination involves using lighted, magnifying instruments called endoscopes to view the interior of a body cavity.

Types

There are a number of types of endoscopy, including:

Cystoscopy: Cystoscopy allows the doctor to inspect the interior of the bladder for fistulas, stones, tumors and other irregularities. It is often used in the diagnostic workup of gynecological cancer and in the investigation of persistent and puzzling urinary tract problems or blood in the urine. The bladder is first filled with air or fluid, and then the thin cystoscope is inserted through the urethra into the bladder. The cystoscope can collect cell samples and remove small tumors.

Proctosigmoidoscopy: This procedure, in which an instrument is inserted through the rectum, allows the doctor to inspect the lower portion of the gastrointestinal tract, usually without an anesthetic. It is often used to detect cancer of the rectum and colon. Its main application in gynecology is in the staging of certain gynecological cancers.

Hysteroscopy: The hysteroscope is a fairly recent innovation and is not yet widely used. It allows the doctor to view the inside of the uterus and can be used to look for lost IUDs, and to detect the presence of certain fibroid tumors and other benign and malignant uterine tumors. It is also being used in fertility workups. The hysteroscope looks like a diver's spear gun and has a flexible tip and an eyepiece to allow a full view of the uterus. The tube of the instrument is inserted into the vagina, through the cervix and into the uterine cavity. The procedure can usually be done on an outpatient basis, using a local anesthetic.

Laparoscopy: Laparoscopy is a surgical procedure in which a tubelike, lighted endoscope called a laparoscope is inserted into the pelvic cavity through a ½-to-1-inch incision just below the navel. The laparoscope works on the same principle as the periscope of a submarine and allows the doctor to look at the uterus, ovaries and tubes.

Although laparoscopy has been around for longer than 60 years, it is only in the past few years that the newly refined instrument has been used widely in the United States. It has proved to be a valuable diagnostic tool, enabling doctors to diagnose questionable cases without major exploratory surgery. In some instances it can be used to treat certain diseases by means of special instruments inserted through the tube that holds the laparoscope. It is also used in sterilization procedures.

Laparoscopic examinations are done in the hospital, using either local or general anesthetic, but unless complications occur it isn't necessary for the woman to stay overnight. Some doctors prefer a local anesthetic, which involves less risk, whereas others prefer a general anesthetic, both because it is pain-free and because, should complications arise and emergency surgery be necessary, there won't be any time lost while the patient is put under a general. The procedure is described in more detail under the heading Laparoscopic Tubal Ligation.

Culdoscopy: Culdoscopy (Illustration 70) is similar to laparoscopy except that the incision is made in the vagina and the culdoscope is inserted into the body through this incision. This allows the doctor to view the cul-de-sac, an

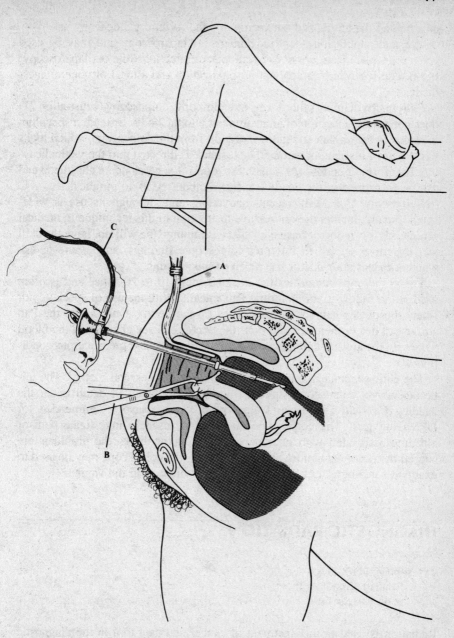

Illustration 70   *Culdoscopy: The woman is placed on the operating table in a knee-chest position. The vagina is held open by means of vaginal retractors (A). The cervix is held down with a tenaculum (B). The culdoscope (C) is inserted through an incision in the back of the vaginal wall.*

area behind the uterus and between it and the rectum. Culdoscopy has many of the same applications and advantages as laparoscopy and may be used when scar tissue from previous operations or infections rule out laparoscopy. It too requires at least outpatient hospitalization and a local or general anesthetic.

Colposcopy: Unlike other forms of endoscopy, colposcopy (Illustration 71) does not require insertion of an instrument into the body. Instead, a speculum is placed in the vagina and a beam of light from the colposcope, which looks like a pair of binoculars mounted on a stand, is directed into the vaginal cavity. This form of endoscopy is painless, doesn't necessitate an anesthetic and can be performed in the doctor's office in about 10 to 20 minutes.

Colposcopy is a fairly recent innovation, and although its use is widespread, many doctors did not receive instruction in this technique in medical school. Unless a doctor has taken special training s/he will not have the skill and expertise needed to interpret colposcopic findings, so be sure to ask whether or not your doctor has received this training.

The colposcope magnifies the doctor's view 10 to 20 times and is often used in the follow-up of abnormal Pap smears. With the use of special color filters the doctor can see abnormalities on the cervix even before the Pap smear can detect them. In addition, the doctor can see changes in the blood vessels in the area that are associated with cancerous and precancerous conditions.

The culposcope is also used to identify areas for cervical biopsy. The importance of a colposcopic-directed biopsy is discussed in detail under the heading Cervical Dysplasia. Colposcopic exam is also recommended for DES daughters. The colposcope may also be used to investigate pain or bleeding associated with intercourse if the doctor thinks the problems are caused by a cervical abnormality. In addition, the colposcope may be used to examine sores or other abnormalities on the vulva or in the vagina.

DIAGNOSTIC RADIATION

Types: plain film X-rays
      contrast X-rays
      radioactive scans

Radiation is used in the treatment of cancer and as a tool in the diagnostic workup of a wide variety of diseases and abnormalities, including many gynecological conditions. X-rays are the most widely used type of diagnostic radiation. They are taken by positioning the area of the body to be studied between an X-ray machine and a sheet of film. A short burst of rays is then

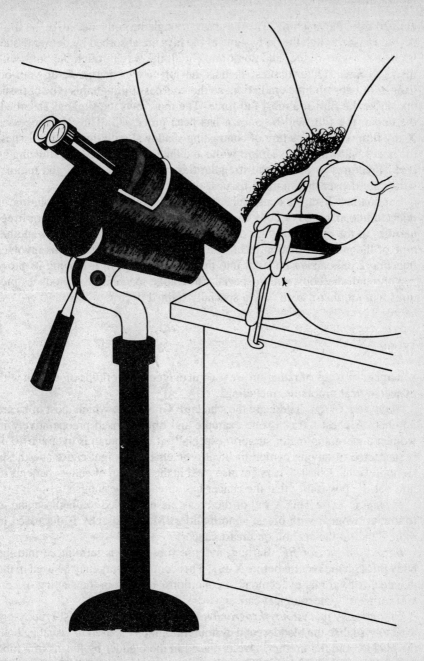

Illustration 71   *Colposcopy: A speculum is placed in the vagina. A beam of light from the colposcope is directed toward the cervix, and the doctor views the cervix and the interior of the vagina through the eyepiece of the colposcope.*

emitted from the machine. The rays pass through the body and strike the film. As they pass through the body some of the rays are absorbed by denser tissue, such as the bone tissue, and don't make it all the way through the body with their full force. Other tissues, such as the soft tissues that make up your organs, don't absorb much radiation, so the rays pass through this type of tissue and strike the film at almost full force. The more rays the film has absorbed, the darker the film will be once it has been processed. Thus the processed X-ray film will be a picture of contrasting shadows, with the densest tissues, the bones, showing up as almost white and the least dense tissues showing up dark. Fractures or other bone irregularities can be seen easily, and tumors, which are denser than normal tissues, often can be seen.

For contrast X-rays a dense substance called a dye, or contrast solution, is injected into an organ or body cavity before the X-ray so that tumors or irregularities in the outline of your organs can be seen more clearly. Yet another type of diagnostic radiation technique is the radioactive scan. This involves injecting a radioactive material into the bloodstream and following its progress through the body with a special cameralike machine that produces pictures that are then "read" by a specially trained doctor.

Types

A number of types of radiation are used in diagnostic workups of women with gynecological problems, including:

Plain film X-rays: These are the standard X-rays with which most of us are familiar. A chest X-ray is one example and often is used preoperatively in women undergoing major surgery, especially if the woman is over age 40 or is suspected of having certain medical problems that might cause anesthesia complications. Chest X-rays are also used in the workup of cancer patients to rule out the possibility that the cancer has spread to the lungs.

Mammography: This X-ray of the breast tissue is used to diagnose and to follow-up women with breast abnormalities. Mammography is discussed in more detail in the section on breast cancer.

Barium enema, or BE: Barium, a dense substance, is introduced into the body through the rectum before X-ray. This contrast X-ray may be used in the diagnosis of various gynecological conditions, notably in the staging of certain forms of gynecological cancer.

Cystography or cystourethrography: Cystography is a contrast-type X-ray used to visualize the bladder, and cystourethrography is used to visualize both the bladder and the urethra. Dye is placed in the bladder by means of a tube known as a urinary catheter. These X-rays are used in the workup of gynecological cancer and other gynecological and urinary diseases.

Hysterography, or hysterosalpingography: Again, this is a contrast-type

778

X-ray in which a dye is injected into the uterus through a small tube. It outlines the interior of the uterus and fallopian tubes. It is used frequently in the workup of fertility patients.

Intravenous pyelography (IVP): Yet another type of contrast X-ray, the IVP outlines the urinary tract, kidneys, ureters and bladder. The dye is injected into a vein in the arm. It often is used in the workup of cancer patients and before operations done to investigate or remove pelvic masses.

Lymphangiography: This contrast X-ray is used to visualize the lymph nodes. Dye is injected into the lymph system through an incision in the big toe. Because the lymph vessels are small, it usually takes a couple of hours before the dye is distributed fully and the X-rays can be taken. The procedure often is used in the staging workup of women with gynecological cancer. The procedure is not totally reliable, for even though the X-rays show some sort of obstruction to the flow of the dye, this may be owing to infection and does not necessarily indicate that cancer is present in the lymph system. Conversely, cancer too small to be detected by lymphangiography may be present. Still, lymphangiography techniques are being improved constantly and in many instances the lymphangiogram can be correlated with other findings to yield information valuable in diagnosing and staging cancer. Moreover, the dye usually is retained by the body for some time and may be useful in helping the surgeon locate and identify lymph nodes if surgical removal of the nodes is necessary.

Radioactive scans: Radioactive scans, which are more sensitive than standard X-rays, are used in the workup of cancer patients to determine whether or not the cancer has spread to other organs. They are also used in the follow-up of certain types of cancer. One type of scan that is used frequently in women with cancer, particularly those with breast cancer, is the bone scan. A liquid containing a mildly radioactive substance is injected into the bloodstream and carried to the bones. Cancerous areas in the bone usually will absorb more radiation than other areas. The pictures taken by the scanning machines will show denser concentrations in this area. These concentrations, or "hot spots," as they are called, can be caused by infections, injuries, arthritis and other abnormal conditions as well as by cancer, so having a hot spot does not necessarily mean that a woman has metastatic cancer.

Liver scans and brain scans, which work in similar fashion, may also be used in the diagnostic workup and the follow-up program of women with female cancers.

The Diagnostic Radiologist

Two types of doctors specialize in radiation: therapeutic radiologists, who are involved in using radiation to treat diseases, and diagnostic radiologists, who

779

interpret the results of diagnostic radiation exams. The use of radiation involves certain risks (see below), and because accurate interpretation requires experience, judgment and skill, you might want to insist on a board-certified radiologist. In order to be board-certified as a diagnostic radiologist, a doctor must be a graduate of an approved medical school, have completed 4 years of postgraduate training in a department of radiology and have passed written and oral examinations administered by the board. Although many good radiologists are not board-certified and certification is not an absolute assurance that a radiologist is competent, it does indicate that their training, skill and performance have been evaluated by their peers and judged to be of the highest quality.

Radiation Risks*

Radiation can cause as well as cure cancer. When radioactive rays pass through the body they damage the cells of our bodies. Radiation can destroy these cells outright or can damage them so that they are unable to reproduce. Sometimes the cells are damaged but are still able to reproduce. However, the reproduced cells may be abnormal. As you may recall from the section on cancer, cancer results when damaged cells that do not have the proper "brakes" to tell them when to stop reproducing continue doing so at a wild pace. Even subtle damage to a single cell could increase the risk of cancer in a susceptible individual, although it may take many years for the damage to manifest itself. Of course, not everyone who is exposed to radiation will develop cancer. In most people the damaged cells will die or the body's immune system will destroy the abnormal cells. But in some people, exposure to radiation can cause cancer.

Most of our knowledge of radiation-induced cancer comes from studies of people exposed to large amounts of radiation—more than 100 rads. Radiation doses are measured in rems and rads. A rem, or roentgen, is a unit of measurement of the amount *emitted* by the X-ray machine or source of radiation. A rad is a unit of measurement of radiation *absorbed* by the body. Terms like "millirem" (mrem) or "millirad" (mrad) are used to denote one-thousandth of a rem (.001 rem) or of a rad (.001 rad). We are all subject to a certain amount of natural radiation from the earth and the sun, about 130 millirems a year. It is not known whether or not this "natural" radiation is harmful.

We do know that people who are exposed to large amounts of radiation, for instance, survivors of the atom bomb dropped in World War II, have higher rates of cancer than would normally be expected. Until recently, it was thought that exposure to lower levels of radiation associated with medical di-

*For more details, see the section on Mammography.

agnostic X-rays or on-the-job exposure would not be harmful. But now most experts believe that radiation risks are cumulative—they add up. Exposure to low levels over a period of time may be just as bad as exposure to a large amount in a single dose.

Part of the controversy about low-level radiation risks comes from the few studies that have been done. One study begun in 1964 involved workers in Hanford, Washington, who were exposed to very low doses, .5 rem a year, over a number of years.[9] A 6 percent to 7 percent increase in cancer was found in this group. These and other, similar studies have been sharply criticized. The Hanford study involved 35,000 workers, but many experts point out that in order to be statistically valid, such a study would have to include millions of people; otherwise the 6 percent to 7 percent increase could be a mere statistical fluke.

To those unfamiliar with statistics, 35,000 seems like a substantial enough number from which to draw conclusions, but it is not. Radiation-induced cancers are but a small fraction of the cancers expected to occur normally. In a group of 400,000 people we would expect 65,000 of them to die of cancer in any event. If such a group were exposed to low-level radiation and 50 cancers more than the 65,000 expected cancers were found, could we attribute this to radiation exposure or could it be a mere statistical fluke?

These questions are unanswered at this time. But the fact that this study and others have suggested that low-level radiation over a period of years may be harmful should make us cautious about the use of X-rays.[10] Because as many as 30 percent of the medical X-rays ordered in the United States each year may be unnecessary,[11] you should take precautions.

- ☐ Never submit to an X-ray without understanding why.
- ☐ Always ask if other tests, for instance, ultrasound (see below), could be done instead.
- ☐ Give careful consideration to a decision to visit a hospital emergency room for a bump on the head or a superficial wound. Fear of malpractice may lead the doctor to recommend an X-ray that may not be strictly necessary.
- ☐ Avoid repetitions by telling the doctor about similar X-rays you have had. If you have a chronic condition or are getting a second opinion, you can ask to have a second copy of your X-ray made for your own files for a nominal fee.
- ☐ Make sure that the X-ray machine is well calibrated and is giving the lowest exposure possible. Ask which agency inspects the machine and how often. Have your X-rays done in a hospital or radiologist's office. These machines usually give less exposure than those taken in a doctor's office or a mobile X-ray unit.

781

☐ Never submit to an X-ray if you think you might be pregnant unless it is *absolutely* necessary.

ULTRASOUND

AKA: sonograms, sonography, B-Scans

Ultrasound is a method of visualizing the interior of the body by means of high-frequency sound waves. Unlike X-rays, sonograms do not involve radiation and are therefore thought to be less risky. But sonography is a relatively new technique, and we do not yet know if there are any long-term effects. Many health-care activists are therefore questioning the routine use of sonography on pregnant women. Although there may be a legitimate need in certain high-risk pregnancies and although ultrasound is probably preferable to X-rays in such instances, sonography may not be necessary in routine pregnancies.

Uses

Sonography is used to detect structural defects in pregnancy, to determine the size of the uterus, to estimate the length of the pregnancy, to monitor the fetal heartbeat and the strength and frequency of contractions during labor, to confirm the presence of twins and to determine the position of the fetus. It also may be used to locate a lost IUD or to detect an ectopic pregnancy and often is useful in evaluating ovarian enlargements and pelvic masses and in planning radiation therapy for cancer.

Procedure

Ultrasound is painless. You will be asked to drink a glass of water about an hour before the examination so that your bladder will be full and will serve as a reference point for the technician performing the examination. Sound waves are directed toward your body by means of a microphone-type instrument that is passed over it. The sound waves bounce back to the microphone receiver, and these "echo patterns" are translated into a picture.

You may be required to lie still and to hold your breath for part of the exam. The whole exam takes about half an hour and usually is done at a hospital or at a radiologist's office.

PAP SMEAR

AKA: Papanicolaou smear, Pap test, vaginal smear, cervical smear

The Pap smear is a simple, painless office procedure that is used primarily to screen for cervical cancer and precancerous conditions of the cervix. The doctor inserts a speculum into the vagina. The surface of the cervix is then gently scraped with a wooden spatula. The cells thus collected are smeared onto a slide that is then labeled and sent to a pathology laboratory for analysis.

How the Pap Smear Works

In order to understand how a Pap smear works it is necessary to know a bit about the cellular makeup of the cervix. The cervix is covered by layers of tissue known as epithelial (skin) tissue, which grows from the bottom layer, known as the basal cell layer, outward toward the surface. The tissue regenerates itself constantly. New cells on the bottom layer are very active, dividing, growing and multiplying constantly. As they grow they force the more mature cells upward, toward the surface layers.

As the cells mature and move upward they change character. At the bottom level, where they are active and reproducing constantly, the cells have large nuclei, or centers. At the middle level the cells themselves are larger, the nuclei are smaller, and they show less activity. They're getting older. By the time they get to the surface they are flattened out, less active and nearly dead, about to be shed.

On our outer skin we recognize such cells as flaky scales or dandruff. The same continual process of shedding takes place in the skin tissue of the cervix, and it is these sloughed-off cells that are picked up in a Pap smear.

As long as the cells picked up in the Pap smear are all mature, flattened-out inactive cells, the smear is normal. But if immature cells that are still active and dividing constantly are seen on the surface, this abnormality may mean that a cancerous or precancerous change is taking place, for, as explained in the section on cancer, cancer is a disease that involves irregularities in the growth patterns of cells.

Classifying Pap Smear Results

If the pathologist looks at the slide and sees only mature, flattened-out, near dead cells, the smear will be labeled "normal," "benign" or "Class I."

783

Sometimes a woman will have an infection that has irritated the surface layers of the cervical tissue. In such cases inflammatory cells, disease-fighting white blood cells and perhaps infectious bacteria may be present as well. Because the surface layer of the cervical epithelium has been disturbed, immature cells may reach the surface and may be picked up in the Pap smear. These are referred to as atypical cells. The pathologist may use such terms as "inflammatory," "atypical," "atypical metaplasia" or "Class II" to describe this type of smear. Although the smear is abnormal, it does not indicate that a cancerous or precancerous condition exists. It is a benign smear, and the cells can be expected to revert to normal once the infection has healed. Some women routinely have unexplained inflammatory cells in their Pap smears. Although this is not serious, it's inconvenient, for such women must have Pap smears frequently.

If the pathologist looks at a slide and sees immature and abnormal cells, s/he will classify the Pap as abnormal. If the degree of abnormality is relatively mild, s/he will use such terms as "mild or moderate cervical intraepithelial neoplasia," "mild or moderate CIN," "mild or moderate dysplasia" or "Class III" to describe the smear. These changes are considered precancerous, meaning that a large portion of *untreated* cases would, eventually, progress to cervical cancer. However, these conditions are 100 percent curable. Diagnosis and treatment of these conditions is discussed in the section on the cervix under the heading Cervical Dysplasia.

If the pathologist looks at a smear and sees more severe abnormalities and a greater proportion of immature cells, s/he may use such terms as "cervical intraepithelial neoplasia, grade three," "carcinoma in situ" or "Class IV." Again, this is a precancerous condition that, if not treated, has a high likelihood of progressing to cervical cancer but with treatment is virtually 100 percent curable. Diagnostic steps and treatment are discussed in the section on the cervix under the heading Carcinoma in Situ.

If the pathologist looks at the slide and sees extremely abnormal, immature, cancerous cells, s/he will use such terms as "malignant," "invasive" or "Class V." This means that the pathologist thinks there is evidence of cervical cancer, and that further tests and treatment, which are discussed under the heading Cervical Cancer, will be needed. Table 29 summarizes Pap smear classifications. Some laboratories use a slightly different classification scheme, so if your smear is anything other than Class I, be sure to ask what terms the laboratory has used to describe your condition as well as the class number.

Table 29
Pap Smear Results

Class	Terms Used to Describe
I	Normal, negative, benign
II	Benign, inflammatory, atypical, atypical metaplasia
III	Mild or moderate cervical intraepithelial neoplasia (CIN), mild or moderate dysplasia, CIN, grades I and II
IV	Severe cervical intraepithelial neoplasia (CIN), severe dysplasia, CIN, grade III, carcinoma in situ
V	Malignant, invasive cancer

Accuracy

The Pap smear is not 100 percent accurate. Sometimes it fails to detect cancer that is actually there. At other times it may suggest a cancerous or precancerous condition when in fact everything is normal. The smear may be inaccurate for a number of reasons. Faulty technique in collecting the cells from the cervix or improper preparation or handling of the slides can cause inaccurate results, but many times no one is at fault. For example, precancerous cells may be present but may not be among those picked when the cervix is scraped. Still, the Pap smear is about 95 percent accurate in detecting cancerous and precancerous cell changes. The fact that it is sometimes inaccurate is not too disturbing, for cervical cancer is usually a slowly progressing disease. It generally takes at least about 5 years for dysplasia to progress to invasive cancer, so even if the cancerous or precancerous cells are missed one time, they probably will be picked up on the next smear.

Although the Pap smear is 95 percent accurate in determining whether or not abnormal cancerous or precancerous cells are present, it is less accurate in detecting the degree of abnormality. It is not uncommon for Pap smears to be "off" by one or more steps. Thus a smear that indicates carcinoma in situ may, in reality, be invasive cancer, or a smear that indicates moderate dysplasia may actually be carcinoma in situ.

Pathology is not a hard-and-fast science. Classifying a Pap smear is a matter of judgment. One pathologist may look at a slide and call it dysplasia, whereas another might classify it as carcinoma in situ. Then too the smear may only have picked up dysplastic cells when, in reality, the more abnormal carcinoma in situ cells were present but just didn't happen to be picked up. Other, noncancerous conditions, such as condyloma, may fool the pathologist into thinking cancerous cells are present when they are not.

Because of this lack of accuracy, cancerous and precancerous smears must be followed up with cervical biopsies, preferably biopsies done with the aid of a colposcope. This is discussed in detail under the heading Cervical Dysplasia.

785

Frequency

Once a young woman begins sexual activity or reaches age 16 or 18, she should have periodic Pap smears. Until recently, it was recommended that women have a Pap smear once a year unless they were at high risk of developing cervical cancer (*see* pp. 375–78), had abnormal Pap results in the past, had a history of herpes or were DES daughters, in which case more frequent Pap smears might be called for. However, the American Cancer Society changed this recently and now recommends that all women age 20 and over and those under 20 who are sexually active have a Pap smear annually for two negative examinations and then one at least every 3 years until age 65. There is some controversy about the new recommendation, and many doctors still recommend annual Pap smears.*

Those who favor the once-every-3-years schedule argue that cervical cancer is a slowly progressing disease that usually takes at least 5 to 7 years to become invasive cancer, so once every 3 years should be sufficient to detect it. Those who favor the once-a-year schedule argue that even though the precancerous conditions usually take several years to develop into cancer, this may not always be the case. Moreover, because the Pap smear is not 100 percent accurate, getting a Pap smear yearly can minimize the risk of inaccurate results, as it would be rare to get a false negative 2 or 3 years in a row. Otherwise a false negative that wasn't corrected for 3 years could mean that invasive cervical cancer was allowed to develop in the interim. Invasive cervical cancer, unlike carcinoma in situ, is not 100 percent curable and may require more drastic treatment. Although the number of women who would be adversely affected by the once-every-3-years schedule is small, to be on the safe side we recommend once-a-year Pap smears.

Another reason we favor the once-a-year schedule is that it's easier to remember. Many of us would have a hard time recalling whether 2 or 3 years had gone by since our last smears. It would be too easy to let 3 years slide into 4 or even 5. The Pap smear is a safe, simple, painless, relatively inexpensive, lifesaving test, but one that too many women still ignore; there is no reason *not* to have it every year. If money is a problem, family-planning clinics or Planned Parenthood clinics usually offer Pap smears and are considerably less expensive than private clinics.

Other Uses

The Pap smear will sometimes pick up cancer of the uterus, fallopian tubes or ovaries. In order for this to occur the cancerous cells from the other organs

*Some doctors would suggest annual or biannual Pap smears for Pill users, because there is some evidence to suggest that Pill users may be at increased risk of developing cervical cancer. See Chapter Five for details.

would have to have made their way through the cervical canal and onto the slide. If this happened, it would be a lucky coincidence, for the Pap smear is not a reliable screening method for any of these other forms of cancer.

Theoretically, a Pap smear could be used to screen for vaginal cancer, but this would involve scraping all the vaginal walls, which would be impractical, since the surface area of the vagina is much greater than that of the cervix. Scrapings are taken of the vaginal wall when there is an abnormality on the vagina that can be seen with the naked eye or with a colposcope. These more extensive smears, which are sometimes called four-quadrant Pap smears, are also used in the follow-up of DES daughters.

Scrapings from the vaginal wall may also be used to evaluate the estrogen content of cells and to tell whether or not a woman has ovulated. This may be useful in fertility workups.

Pap smears may also reveal the presence of vaginal or cervical infections. Evidence of sexually transmissible infections may also be an incidental finding in a Pap test report; however, the Pap is not used for diagnosing these, as other simpler, more accurate tests are available.

PELVIC EXAM

AKA: gynecological exam, or checkup, bimanual pelvic

Associated Terms: bimanual vaginal exam, rectovaginal exam, digital rectal exam, speculum exam

A pelvic exam is not most women's idea of a good time, but if you know what is happening and what to expect, the procedure becomes a lot more bearable—and perhaps even interesting. Pelvic exams should be done at least once a year, starting at age 16 or 18 or the onset of sexual activity, whichever comes first. They consist of three parts: the speculum exam, the bimanual pelvic and the rectal exam. (Incidentally, the doctor cannot tell whether or not you are a virgin, although s/he may be able to tell if you've had a child or an abortion.) You will be asked to lie on the examining table, with your feet up in stirrups (Illustration 72).

Speculum Exam

Speculum self-exam has been explained in detail in Chapter Two. The procedure is essentially the same when the doctor does it. If you are tense, the exam may feel uncomfortable, but if you are relaxed and the doctor is skilled at it, you shouldn't feel any discomfort unless you have an infection or disease, in which case the vagina may be irritated and tender. The doctor will be looking for any obvious abnormalities or signs of infection. Once the speculum is in place, s/he may use a cotton-tipped applicator or a wooden spatula to take cell samples for a wet smear, a gonorrhea culture or a Pap smear.

Bimanual Pelvic

The doctor inserts two gloved fingers into the vagina and places the fingers of the other hand on the lower abdomen, as shown in Illustration 72, in order to feel for enlargements or abnormalities in the shape and contour of the pelvic organs. If you are tense, your muscles will be rigid, which makes it hard for the doctor to feel for abnormalities, so try to relax. You might ask the doctor to place your hand on your abdomen and help you feel the outline of your uterus.

Rectovaginal Exam

The doctor inserts the index finger into the vagina and the middle finger into the rectum. The fingers of the opposite hand are placed on the lower abdomen to help outline the organs and any enlargements or masses that may be present. This exam allows the doctor to feel areas not accessible by bimanual vaginal exam. Again, you will be more comfortable and the doctor's job will be that much easier if you can relax.

PREGNANCY TESTS

Types: urine tests
blood tests
progesterone-challenge, or progesterone-withdrawal, tests
home pregnancy tests

Most women first become aware of pregnancy because their menstrual period does not begin on time; however, pregnant women may have menstrual-type bleeding, and missed periods are not necessarily an indication of pregnancy. Certain other signs may suggest pregnancy, including breast swelling and tenderness, nausea and vomiting, frequent urination, slightly increased body temperature, weight gain, unusual food cravings, mood swings and possibly an increase in sex drive. Women who practice self-exam may notice a blue

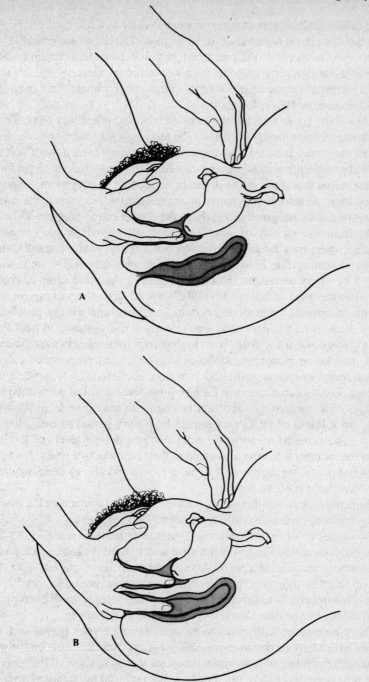

Illustration 72   *Bimanual Pelvic Exam (A) and Rectovaginal Exam (B)*

tinge or hue to the cervix that may appear as early as a few days after conception, but this sign is not obvious in all women. The doctor may be able to feel an enlarged uterus once the pregnancy has progressed to a certain point. But none of these signs or symptoms is entirely reliable. The only reliable tests to detect pregnancy measure levels of the pregnancy hormone, human chorionic gonadotropin, or HCG, for short.

Urine tests: Urine tests are the most widely used pregnancy tests. They are not, however, completely accurate. The tests may give false negative results, that is, they may indicate that you are not pregnant even though you really are. False negative results may be caused by faulty technique in performing the test, urine that is too dilute or has been allowed to sit at room temperature for too long, an ectopic pregnancy or a threatened or incomplete miscarriage. If the urine tests are given too early in the course of the pregnancy (before 6 weeks from the 1st day of your last menstural period) or too late (after 5 months), there may be false negative results. False positive results, that is, results indicating that a woman is pregnant when she really isn't, may be caused by faulty technique, blood or protein in the urine sample, chemical residue in the urine container, thyroid disorders, large doses of aspirin and the use of marijuana, methadone, certain anticonvulsant drugs, psychoactive drugs (such as tranquilizers and antidepressants), drugs used to treat Parkinson's disease and some drugs used to treat hypertension. Physiologic ovarian cysts, premature menopause, tubo-ovarian abscesses, trophoblastic disease, certain forms of cancer and HCG injections for infertility treatments within the past 30 days can also cause false positive results. A test performed within 10 days of a miscarriage, abortion or childbirth may give false positive results, since levels of HCG may remain high for a period of time after pregnancy. The urine of menopausal women contains high levels of luteinizing hormone, as does the urine of women in their reproductive years, for a period of 24 hours around the time of ovulation each month, so these women too may have false positive results.

Urine tests are more likely to be accurate if the test is made on the first urine of the morning, when the concentration of HCG is highest.

Two types of urine tests are the 2-minute urine slide test and the 2-hour tube test. The urine slide test is the most widely used pregnancy test and is 95 percent accurate if used after 42 days, or 6 weeks, have elapsed after the 1st day of your last menstrual period (that is, once your period is about 2 weeks late). One drawback to this test is that you may already have been pregnant for 6 weeks by the time this test confirms the pregnancy.

The 2-hour urine tube test can be accurate once your period is 1 to 1½ weeks late. Many of the do-it-yourself pregnancy test kits now on the market are tube tests. New, ultrasensitive tube tests that rival some of the blood tests have now been developed, but they have not replaced the standard urine tests. No one should rely totally on these home tests, and if you do use one, make

790

sure it measures HCG and not estrogen or progesterone levels, which are not accurate indicators of pregnancy.

Blood tests: New, highly sensitive blood tests can give accurate results within about a week after conception, that is, about a week before your period is due. The original blood tests, called radioimmune assays, were expensive lab tests, but a new blood test called a radioreceptor assay, or a Bio-Cept G Test, is less expensive, about $15 to $20, and is 97 percent to 98 percent accurate eight to ten days after conception. It is 100 percent accurate if you wait until 4 weeks from the 1st day of your last menstrual period or within about 1 day of your missed period. The test is not available everywhere but usually can be obtained at large hospital labs. It often is used in women who have diabetes, hypertension, heart disease, kidney disease or other health problems that can adversely affect pregnancy.

Progesterone-challenge, or progesterone-withdrawal, test: Progestins are given either orally or by injection if a woman's period is late. As the progestin is gradually excreted by the body, the uterine lining will break down and be shed. If you are pregnant, your period will not begin. This test does not stop pregnancy; it merely indicates whether or not pregnancy has occurred. In fact, it is not even a reliable indicator of that, for failure to bleed after this test may be caused by conditions other than pregnancy. Given the availability of other, more reliable tests, we can hardly recommend this procedure for pregnancy testing. Women who do not plan to have an abortion if they discover that they are pregnant should definitely not take this test, for the use of hormones in early pregnancy has been linked to birth defects.[12]

Home Pregnancy Tests

Home pregnancy tests have become extremely popular. If used *precisely as directed,* they can be as accurate as the slide and the tube urine tests used by most doctors and clinics. In one study of women using home tests, the tests were 95 percent accurate in detecting positive test results, that is, if the test result indicated that the woman was pregnant, she was in fact pregnant in 95 percent of cases.[13] However, with negative test results the accuracy was only 77 percent. The inaccuracy of the negative results generally was caused by the woman's using the test too soon. Most manufacturers recommend that the tests not be used until 9 to 15 days after a missed period. Some women apparently were too excited or too anxious to wait the required number of days. Others weren't sure when their menstrual periods should have started.

The manufacturers caution women that negative tests should be redone a week later. Women using the home tests generally have a false negative rate of 20 percent on their first testing, but the rate drops to 9 percent if the women

791

wait a week and do a second test. Only about 10 percent of women with negative results do the second test. Waiting until the 15th day or later, rather than the 9th day, to do the test will increase the accuracy.

Four of the most popular tests on the market are:

☐ *E.P.T.*, which costs about $8 to $12, has a shelf life of 12 months, takes 2 hours to complete and can be used as early as 9 days past the first missed period

☐ *Predictor*, which costs $8 to $10, has a shelf life of 12 months, takes 2 hours to complete and can be used as early as 9 days past the last missed period. The manufacturer has a toll-free user hot line (1-800-821-2111) in case you have questions.

☐ *Acu-Test*, which costs $8 to $10, has a shelf life of 12 months, takes 2 hours to complete and can be used as early as 9 days past the first missed period

☐ *Daisy-2*, which costs $13 to $16, has a shelf life of 18 months, takes 1 hour to complete and can be used as early as 6 to 9 days past the first missed period. The manufacturer maintains a toll-free user hot line (1-800-428-2348).

Some doctors argue that the home tests are a waste of money. If the test is positive, the woman needs to see her doctor anyway to arrange for prenatal care or for an abortion. If the test is negative, she needs to repeat it, and even then she may need to see her doctor, especially if she still "feels" pregnant or misses another period. But many women like the feeling of control over their own bodies that the tests provide.

BASIC BLOOD AND URINE TESTS

AKA: complete blood counts (CBC), serum factors test (SMA 12), urinalysis

Blood Tests

These blood tests, which are also called complete blood counts (CBCs) and serum factor tests (SMA 12s), usually can be done in the doctor's office or lab. Blood is taken from a vein with a needle, and a pinprick is also made on the finger and the blood from there smeared on a slide as well. The blood samples are then subjected to various laboratory analyses. These tests can yield much basic information about your health, including whether or not you are anemic and if there is an infection present. They also can tell the doctor what your clotting time is, which is especially important if you are going to have surgery. The blood tests currently in use cannot indicate whether or not you have cancer, but experimental work is now being done in an effort to devise blood tests that could do so.

Urine Tests

Urinalysis (UA) can also provide a great deal of information. The urine sample usually is collected by having you void into a cup. At other times, in order to collect the urine, the doctor will need to insert a tube called a catheter through the urethra and into the bladder. Urinalysis can detect urinary tract infection, diabetes, kidney damage and urinary obstruction. It can be especially valuable in staging certain forms of gynecological cancer, because it can help the doctor to determine whether or not the cancer has spread to the kidneys, ureters, bladder and so forth.

ANESTHETICS

Types: general anesthetics
   local anesthetics

Associated Terms: regional anesthetics; spinal, saddle, epidural or caudal block; paracervical block

Anesthetics are drugs used to prevent pain during surgery. Basically, there are two types of anesthetics: general and local. General anesthetics put you to sleep or completely block the nerve passageways in large areas of the body (regional anesthetic). Local anesthetics numb a small area of the body temporarily so that you feel little or no pain.

General Anesthetics

General anesthetics are used for operations, such as hysterectomy or laparoscopy. A light anesthetic or a deeper one may be used, depending on the nature of the surgery. The drug may be administered intravenously, by means of a needle that usually is attached to a tube and a hanging bottle called an I.V. bottle. A drug called sodium pentothal is given frequently in this way. A mask may be placed over your face and a mixture of anesthetic gas and oxygen may be administered through a tube attached to the mask. Sometimes sodium pentothal is given first, and once you are out, the gas mask is applied.

793

In any case, once you are asleep, a tube may be inserted into your windpipe to allow the doctor to control your respiration.

Regional anesthetics are used in childbirth, for D&Cs and for other relatively minor procedures. Such terms as "spinal," "saddle," "epidural" and "caudal block" may be used to specify the various types of regionals. Basically, all regionals involve injection of a drug into the space surrounding the vertebral column or the area around a major nerve. The drug blocks nerve messages from the area and causes numbness and temporary paralysis. Since only the area to be operated on is affected, you will not be asleep if a regional is used; however, you may not be fully alert, because a sedative is often given before surgery so that you will not be anxious or feel discomfort.

Most people recover from general anesthesia fairly rapidly, within a period of several hours. It takes about 24 hours before the drugs are excreted fully from the body. Overweight people may take longer to recover, since the drugs are absorbed by fat tissue. The mortality for women who are given anesthetics is about 2.7 per 10,000 operations.[14] Serious problems like stroke and stopping of the heart or lung activity are rare in young, healthy women but are higher for women with such medical problems as heart disease or lung disease. The longer the anesthesia time, the greater the chances of serious complications. Other complications, including headaches, which may persist for days or even weeks, can occur, especially with a spinal. In rare cases injury to or infection of the spinal cord can cause permanent paralysis. Both during and after anesthesia, blood pressure and heart rate must be monitored carefully so that drugs or other measures can be used if problems occur.

Local Anesthetics

Local anesthetics are used for minor operations that are short and technically simple. A drug similar to the Novocain (procaine hydrochloride) used by dentists is injected into the area and usually is effective for a half hour to an hour. When the drug is injected into the area around the cervix the term "paracervical block" is used.

Although locals are less risky than generals, there may be allergic reactions, including rashes, hives, swelling and asthma symptoms. On rare occasions the allergic reactions are so severe that they cause seizures, strokes, heart attacks and death.

ANTIBIOTICS

Types: penicillin
tetracycline
erythromycin
sulfa drugs

Antibiotics are drugs that act against bacteria. They are used in the treatment of infections of the gynecological tract, including vaginitis, pelvic inflammatory disease and sexually transmissible infections. Antibiotics can kill disease-causing organisms but may also destroy the friendly bacteria that help maintain the body's health. Women taking antibiotics may be more susceptible to vaginal infections, particularly yeast infections, and may want to take certain precautions (*see* p. 299).

Types

The four major families of antibiotics are penicillin, tetracycline, erythromycin and sulfa drugs.

Penicillin: This widely used antibiotic can cause serious allergic reactions, but fortunately these are rare (1.5 to 2 per 100,000 users).[15] If you have an allergic reaction, discontinue use and contact the doctor immediately. If you have a reaction to one penicillin drug, you may be allergic to all drugs in this family and should not use any of them.

Ampicillin is a member of the penicillin family, so if you have had a reaction to penicillin, do not use ampicillin. You should also avoid ampicillin if you are using birth control pills, because the drug may diminish the effectiveness of the pills. Diarrhea, which with other antibiotics may be a sign of a serious allergic reaction, is a fairly common side effect with ampicillin. Yeast infections are a common complication.

Tetracycline: Tetracycline may be prescribed for gynecological infections, particularly for women who are allergic to penicillin. Tetracycline should be avoided by pregnant women, infants and preteens, because it can cause permanent tooth discoloration and, sometimes, bone abnormalities in the fetus. Yeast infections and gastrointestinal upsets may also occur, as can skin rashes if you're not careful to avoid prolonged exposure to sunlight (sunbathing). Food, particularly dairy products, may interfere with the absorption of the drug, so it should be taken 1 to 2 hours before eating and should not be taken with milk. Women who are taking the drug should also avoid iron and other mineral-containing preparations.

Erythromycin: This drug is used for people who are allergic to penicillin but cannot take tetracycline. The side effects are relatively few, but safe usage in pregnancy has not been determined.

Sulfa drugs: Sulfa drugs are often used in cream form to treat vaginal infections. Safe use of these drugs during pregnancy has not been established, and since abnormalities in the offspring of laboratory animals treated with those drugs have been noted, they are not recommended for pregnant women. Those with a certain hereditary form of anemia that occurs mostly in black people should not use sulfa drugs.

Preparations containing certain sulfa drugs are still widely used to treat vaginitis, but their effectiveness has been seriously questioned. The Food and Drug Administration rates them, at best, as only "probably effective in the treatment of trich, hemophilus and yeast infections."[16] There are other, more effective medications for treating these conditions, and women should question their doctors about the choice of drugs if a sulfonamide is prescribed. (For more information, *see* p. 304.)

DEPO-PROVERA

AKA: the birth control shot, injectable Provera

Depo-Provera is a progestin, a synthetic (man-made) form of progesterone, the hormone produced during the second half of the menstrual cycle. The drug comes in an oral form (Provera) and in an injectable form, which is Depo-Provera. Although the use of Provera carries certain risks—the same risks associated with the use of any progestin compound—it is the drug in its injectable form that has been the center of a great deal of controversy.

The drug originally was developed as a treatment for endometriosis, threatened miscarriage and repeated miscarriage. It was approved by the Food and Drug Administration (FDA) for these uses in 1960 on the basis of its supposed safety but without an assessment of effectiveness.[17] In 1974 the FDA withdrew its approval, both because the drug had not been shown to be effective and because it may have caused birth defects in children of women who took it while pregnant.[18] In 1972 the FDA approved the drug for use in the treatment of advanced cancer of the endometrial lining. Currently, this is the only approved use of the drug.

Depo-Provera has several effects on the body, including:

☐ Inhibiting ovulation in many women
☐ Increasing the thickness of cervical mucus, so that sperm cannot pass into the uterus

796

☐ Speeding up the time that the egg spends in the fallopian tubes, making fertilization less likely

☐ Changing the endometrial lining of the uterus, so that a fertilized egg cannot implant

These effects suggested that Depo-Provera might be used as a contraceptive. Studies of Depo-Provera as a "birth control shot" given once every 3 months were begun in 1963.[19] In 1967, Upjohn, the company that manufactures the drug, applied for permission to market the drug as a contraceptive.

Permission was denied because of problems with the drug. Some of the women injected with the drug have menstrual irregularities and may even stop menstruating altogether.[20] Even after use is discontinued some women do not regain their periods for some time. Fertility may be impaired, perhaps permanently. Those women who do manage to conceive while on the drug, or who take it without realizing they are pregnant, may unknowingly damage their babies, because the drug is transmitted through breast milk and its effects on infants are unknown. In addition, some statistics suggest, but do not prove, that cervical carcinoma in situ, an early stage of cervical cancer, may occur more often among Depo-Provera users than among nonusers.[21] Beagle dogs treated with both low doses and high doses developed diseases of the endometrial lining of the uterus and malignant breast lumps.[22] The significance of these findings for humans has not been established.

Although the drug is not approved as a contraceptive, some family-planning clinics and private physicians are prescribing the drug for this purpose. In addition, the drug is being given to women in Third World countries despite the fact that Upjohn is restricted from marketing the drug in the United States. Many health-care activists are working to prevent its use on Third World women. In addition, the National Women's Health Network has established a registry to investigate the use of the drug in the United States. Women who received contraceptives by injection can register by writing to Depo-Provera Registry, National Women's Health Network, 2025 I Street NW, Washington, D.C. 20006.

ESTROGEN REPLACEMENT THERAPY

AKA: ERT, hormone replacement therapy (HRT), estrogen and progesterone replacement therapy, replacement therapy.

Estrogen replacement therapy (ERT), as the name implies, involves the administration of estrogen to replace estrogen that for some reason is no longer being made by the body. Nowadays progesterone is given along with the estrogen (for reasons described below), so ERT is now called hormone replacement therapy, or HRT, by many doctors.

Uses

ERT is used most widely in menopausal and postmenopausal women who may no longer be producing large amounts of estrogen in their bodies. It is also given to women who have premature menopause, insufficient amounts of pituitary hormones or congenital abnormalities of the ovary, all of which prevent them from producing the normal ovarian hormones.

Some doctors and many women's health-care activists believe that ERT is a dangerously misused form of therapy.* It first became popular in the late fifties and early sixties as a cure for a wide variety of menopausal symptoms and changes that women of this age are apt to experience. Actually, the only menopausal symptoms on which ERT has any effect are hot flashes, the drying and thinning of vaginal, vulvar and urinary tissues that occur in postmenopausal women as estrogen levels decline; and osteoporosis, a condition that involves loss of bone density and increases a woman's chances of bone fractures. As the result of a clever and well-financed advertising campaign, many women and doctors came to believe that ERT was a sort of magic cure-all that would prevent wrinkles, weight gain and psychological problems and that would keep women "forever young." The stereotyped image of the menopausal woman as an emotionally unstable harpy and the insecurities caused by our youth-worshiping culture made it possible to convince millions of women to use this drug even if they didn't have any of the problems for which it is in fact useful.

Although some studies have indicated that menopausal women have a slightly higher percentage of serious emotional problems—a 7 percent incidence as compared with 6 percent for other age-groups[23]—and a somewhat higher rate of complaints about nervousness, irritability, "feeling blue" and other symptoms of psychological tension,[24] there is no evidence that lack of estrogen per se causes these symptoms or that taking ERT will relieve them. (In fact, some studies don't even show any increase in psychological problems in menopausal women.)

Still, many women believe that estrogen relieves their depression. This erroneous impression is the result of several factors.[25] First, many ERT products also contain antidepressants, tranquilizers or sedatives. It is these added drugs and not the estrogen that have the psychological effects. Second, de-

---

*The dangers associated with ERT may not be the same as those associated with HRT (see "Risks" below).

pression is often self-limiting, which means that it goes away by itself in time. Women suffering from depression who started ERT and found that their depression lifted may mistakenly attribute the relief of their symptoms to the estrogen.

A third reason that women may attribute relief of psychological problems to ERT has to do with hot flashes. Some women have frequent and severe flashes during the night, which causes insomnia. Not surprisingly, these are the women who are most likely to complain of irritability, nervousness and so forth. ERT may eliminate or reduce the flashes, which in turn solves the insomnia and psychological tensions, but it is the reduction of hot flashes, not the estrogen per se, that is responsible for relief of tensions. ERT should not be taken for psychological problems.

ERT was also supposed to prevent skin wrinkling, weight gain and other effects of aging. There is no evidence that any of these conditions are caused by lack of estrogen or that they can be relieved by use of estrogen. In fact, there is some evidence that estrogen can cause drying and wrinkling of the skin.[26]

ERT *is* effective in preventing hot flashes, but once the estrogen is discontinued the hot flashes may come back and may be more severe. Using estrogen may merely delay the occurrence of hot flashes rather than prevent or cure them. Hot flashes normally don't continue for longer than a year or two. There are also alternative treatments that may not involve the serious risks that ERT does (see the section on Menopausal Changes). Some doctors have been experimenting with progesterone and clonidine.[27] Vitamin therapy has proved successful for some women.[28] Vitamins E and C and the B-complex vitamins seem to be particularly helpful. Ginseng, an oriental herb, is also effective for some women.[29] These herbal and vitamin therapies seem to take 4 to 6 weeks to become effective. We suggest that women investigate these alternative therapies. Replacement therapy should not be used merely to treat hot flashes unless the flashes are so severe that the sufferer is willing to take on the risks and side effects that replacement therapy may entail. Many women prefer to try the other medical therapies described above or natural approaches, such as vitamins or herbs, or simply to learn to live with their hot flashes rather than use the replacement therapy. For some women, however, replacement therapy is the only effective treatment for their severe and disabling hot flashes.

ERT is also used to treat postmenopausal vaginitis; postmenopausal vulvitis; prolapses of the uterus, cervix and vagina; rectoceles and cystoceles. Here again there may be other, less risky ways of treating these conditions that are explained under the appropriate headings elsewhere in this book.

ERT is also used to treat the decreased vaginal lubrication that some postmenopausal women experience. Once again, alternative ways of dealing with this problem are discussed under the heading Menopausal Changes. Vaginal lubrication, the postmenopausal shortening and narrowing of the vagina and the postmenopausal thinning and drying of vaginal tissues (which can cause itching, soreness, pain on intercourse, urinary frequency and burning and increased susceptibility to vaginal, vulvar and urinary infections) all respond well to ERT. Within 2 weeks of starting ERT most women notice changes in their vaginal tissues. By 6 weeks, doctors examining women taking ERT will usually notice that the vaginal tissues are more moist and have the pinkish color usually found only in premenopausal women.

Younger women with certain rare congenital abnormalities of the ovary may also be given ERT to stimulate the development of secondary sex characteristics. Sometimes when these young girls see the effect of estrogen on their breasts, they will decide to take extra pills, in hopes of developing larger breasts. Extra estrogen will not further increase their breast size, however, for that is determined by heredity. (Only in those rare instances of young girls whose bodies are not capable of producing estrogen does ERT have any effect on breast development. It will not have any permanent effect on the size of older women's breasts and cannot—and should not—be used, either orally or in the form of creams, for that purpose.)

REPLACEMENT THERAPY AND OSTEOPOROSIS

Replacement therapy is also used to prevent, and at times to treat, osteoporosis, a condition in which so much bone density is lost that the woman's bones become brittle and break easily. Dowager's hump (a rounded upper back resulting in hunched-over posture), often seen in elderly women, may also be a result of osteoporosis owing to compression of the vertebrae in the spine caused by loss of bone density. Backache is a common complaint of women with osteoporosis.

Beginning at about age 30, women begin to lose bone density. After menopause the rate of loss of bone density in most women increases dramatically. Generally, the term ''osteoporosis'' is reserved for those women who actually have such symptoms as bone fractures, dowager's hump and backache. Women who have significant bone loss without any symptoms (which may happen) are not considered to have osteoporosis.

Certain women are more prone to osteoporosis than are others. For example, the condition is more common in Caucasians (whites) and Orientals than in blacks, and more common in small, thin women than in large, heavy women. The following factors also seem to increase a woman's chance of developing osteoporosis: family history of osteoporosis; menopause at an early age; surgically induced menopause or other premature menopause; a diet low in calcium; cigarette smoking; never having had any children; high intake of alcohol; high intake of caffeine and, possibly, low levels of exercise.

The effects of osteoporosis may not be noticeable until many years after menopause. Often a woman is asymptomatic until the first bone fracture occurs. Approximately 25 percent of white women over age 60 have a compression fracture of the vertebrae owing to osteoporosis.[32] This number increases to 50 percent by age 75. But osteoporosis may take its toll in simple fractures at an even earlier age. After age 45 there is a marked increase in the number of forearm fractures in women; the rate of such fractures in women is 10 times greater than in men.[33] Fractures of the forearm or wrist usually are associated with a fall or accident of some sort, whereas spinal compression fractures and hip fractures may occur as a result of normal daily activities.

(Men too suffer from osteoporosis, but they have larger and stronger bones than do women to start with. Male loss of bone density starts 15 to 20 years later than it does in females and progresses at a slower rate. Osteoporosis is uncommon in men under age 70.)

An estimated 35 percent to 40 percent of women will develop some degree of osteoporosis. If osteoporosis were simply a matter of broken bones, it might not be such a problem, but it can have fatal complications, especially in relation to hip fractures. Approximately 120,000 hip fractures occur in elderly women each year, 80 percent of which are thought to be associated with osteoporosis.[34] About 34 percent of women with hip fractures die within 6 months.[35] Deaths after hip fractures generally are related to heart failure, blood clots in the lung or brain and pneumonia as a result of being bedridden or immobile for long periods while the fracture heals.

Osteoporosis normally is not diagnosed until a fracture has occurred, and once it is diagnosed there is no surefire cure for treating it. There is some evidence that ERT may be effective in preventing further fractures in women who have already had at least one osteoporosis fracture.[36] Three studies have pointed directly or indirectly toward an improvement with ERT treatment in women who have already been diagnosed as having osteoporosis.[37] But, to date, there have not been any of the vigorous, thorough scientific studies that research scientists require in order to consider a treatment as having been "proved" effective. Moreover, relatively large doses of estrogen are apparently required if the treatment can even hope to have an effect, and the potential risks and side effects of larger doses in women of this age (generally over age 60) may occur more frequently and be more serious. Other treatments, such as fluoride, anabolic steroids, calcitonin, vitamin D and calcium supplements, are being used alone or with ERT, but the effectiveness of these treatments has not been proved scientifically either.[38]

Because we do not have a surefire cure and often cannot diagnose osteoporosis before a fracture happens, prevention is a key issue. ERT has been shown to retard or halt bone loss and reduce the number of fractures.[39] Some doctors, therefore, believe that *all* women should take ERT to prevent osteoporosis. They prescribe an estrogen, like Premarin, in daily oral doses of at least 0.625 mg, to be taken 25 days a month,* for all their postmenopausal patients. But unlike ERT for hot flashes (in which the smallest dose to control the flashes is given to tide a woman over the worst of her flashes and gradually tapered off over time) or ERT for vaginal thinning and drying (which is given orally or in cream form from time to time to keep the vaginal tissues moist and thick), ERT for prevention of osteoporosis must be given on a long-term basis in order to be effective. In fact, women using ERT to prevent osteoporosis basically need to take it for the rest of their lives. For if they stop, they start losing bone density rapidly.

Taking a pill every day for 3 weeks or more each month for the rest of your life to prevent a disease that does not affect more than 4 out of 10 women and whose major effects would not show up for 10 years after you have passed menopause does not appeal to many women. Also, the possible risks and side effects make many doctors leery of such long-term replacement therapy. Many doctors prefer to use calcium supplements, a diet high in vitamin D and calcium-rich foods and a regular exercise program to prevent osteoporosis. These doctors generally would reserve ERT for women at high risk of developing osteoporosis.

The more natural approach has not definitely been proven to be as effective as ERT in preventing osteoporosis. Some doctors think the natural approach is not effective; others believe it is, although probably not as effective as ERT. No one yet knows who is right on this issue, but there are good reasons for thinking the natural approach may be effective. Our bones are breaking down and being reabsorbed by the body constantly. At the same time new bone formation is taking place continually. As long as the rate of reabsorption and the rate of formation are pretty much equal, our bones retain their density. But as we grow older, and especially after menopause, reabsorption takes place faster than formation. Calcium, which is stored in the bones, is lost from the body during reabsorption. Studies have shown that the average U.S. woman's calcium intake falls significantly below the amount of calcium being lost from her body.[40] It is estimated that the average premenopausal woman has a negative calcium balance of 20 mg a day. Calcium is not only important for bone formation, but also for basic cell needs. If there is not enough calcium for these basic cell needs in the diet, the body will "steal" it from the bones, thus adding to the bone density problem. In some ways, then, osteoporosis is a nutritional disease that is related to a small, but prolonged, calcium deficiency. This small deficiency, over a period of decades, can set the stage for osteoporosis. By taking supplements or eating a calcium-rich diet (1,000 mg a day premenopausal; 1,500 mg a day postmenopausal) you

*Progesterone should be given too; see below.

may be able to prevent such problems. Also, there is reason to think that exercise will help prevent osteoporosis. Muscle stress and strain on the bones can prevent bone density loss, and evidence indicates that it may also stimulate bone mass.[41]

Research to assess the effectiveness of these natural approaches in preventing osteoporosis is now being done, so watch for developments in this area. Other medical approaches are also being studied. Preliminary studies indicate that certain types of progesterone and certain drugs called anabolic steroids may be effective in preventing osteoporosis.[42] Researchers are also attempting to define more clearly who is at high risk and to develop simple, inexpensive, harmless laboratory tests to determine which menopausal women are apt to end up with osteoporosis so preventive medical treatment can be given to the 35 percent to 40 percent who really need it and not to everyone across the board. Until such time as the results of all this research become available, women will have to weigh the contradictory evidence about the risks involved in replacement therapy, assess their chances of being among the 35 percent to 40 percent who will develop osteoporosis, consider whether they have other symptoms that might respond to replacement therapy and, on that basis, make a personal decision as to whether or not to take replacement therapy as a means of preventing osteoporosis. Our personal philosophy is to avoid replacement therapy unless you have such symptoms as hot flashes and vaginal dryness, which cannot be managed by careful attention to diet and exercise, or have risk factors like a family history of osteoporosis and a frail, delicate frame. But each woman must decide for herself.

The Risks of Replacement Therapy

In the past, replacement therapy only involved estrogen (ERT), but now most doctors prescribe *both* estrogen and progesterone (for reasons explained below). When both estrogen and progesterone are given, the term "hormone replacement therapy" (HRT) generally is used. But many doctors still call this therapy ERT, even though they are prescribing both hormones. If you are taking replacement therapy or are considering doing so, be sure to find out if you are taking or will be taking estrogen alone or estrogen *and* progesterone, because this will affect the potential risks.

Unfortunately, we don't have clear-cut information about the potential risks involved in ERT or HRT, partly because most of our information about risks comes from the research done on the risks involved in using birth control pills that contain estrogen and progesterone. But it isn't clear that the risks involved in premenopausal women who are taking these hormones to prevent pregnancy are the same as the risks for menopausal women who are taking these hormones. For one thing, different dosages are used. Moreover, the types of estrogen and progesterone that are used in replacement therapy are not the same types used in birth control pills. We do have some risk information from studies that were done on women taking ERT, but the results of such studies often have been contradictory. What is more, the studies that were done to investigate the risks in menopausal women generally have been done on women taking *estrogen* replacement therapy. Minimal research has been done on women taking both estrogen *and* progesterone (HRT), and the combination of hormones may affect the risks, decreasing them in some instances but perhaps increasing them in others.

The most widely studied risk of ERT use in menopausal women is the risk of endometrial cancer, cancer of the uterine lining, which generally is referred to as uterine cancer.* Studies done in the mid-1970s showed that women who took ERT had about a 4- to 13-fold increased risk of developing uterine cancer.[43] It was this increased risk of developing uterine cancer that led doctors to start giving women progesterone along with the estrogen, that is, to prescribe HRT instead of ERT. Doctors theorized that it wasn't the estrogen per se that was causing the uterine cancer in some of the women who were taking ERT, but the fact that these women were taking what doctors call "unopposed estrogen." Unopposed estrogen is estrogen that is not counterbalanced or "opposed" by progesterone. As you recall from Chapter Four, in premenopausal women, estrogen is produced by the ovary in large quantities during the first half of the menstrual cycle, and it stimulates the uterine lining to grow rich and thick in preparation for a possible pregnancy. After the ripe egg is released from the ovary at ovulation, the ovaries begin to produce the hormone progesterone. If the woman doesn't get pregnant, the ovaries stop making progesterone after about 10 days. Without the support of the progesterone the uterus cannot maintain the rich lining it has built up, so it begins to break down and is shed during the woman's period. If for some reason, such as an illness like polycystic ovarian disease, the woman doesn't ovulate, she doesn't produce any progesterone. Without progesterone to further build up and then break down the lining as the levels of progesterone in the body drop, the uterine lining keeps on growing. A condition known as atypical endometrial hyperplasia (overgrowth of the uterine lining; *see* p. 441) may then develop and, if not treated, can lead to uterine cancer. That's why doctors are careful to induce regular menstrual periods in premenopausal women who aren't ovulating regularly.

Apparently, the same sort of thing happens in menopausal women who are taking ERT. Taking estrogen alone caused the uterine lining to build up in many of these women, which led to atypical endometrial hyperplasia and hence to uterine cancer. By adding progesterone to the ERT, doctors hoped to counterbalance the unopposed estrogen. Women who were on ERT alone

*Women also get cancer of the muscles of the uterus, but such cancers are uncommon.

took a tablet of estrogen each day, usually beginning on the 1st day of the month and continuing for 25 days. Women who are taking HRT also take a tablet of a progesterone preparation on the 16th through 25th day. No tablets are taken on the remaining days of the month, and during that time the woman usually has some menstrual-like bleeding. Studies have shown that this combination of hormones reduces the risk of developing endometrial hyplasia and hence, uterine cancer.[44] As a result of these studies most doctors now believe that the use of both hormones will solve the uterine cancer problem seen in ERT users. Personally, we aren't quite ready to jump on the bandwagon. True, HRT has been shown to reduce the hyperplasia. From what we know of uterine cancer, it seems to develop out of a hyperplasia condition in the uterus, so logically, reducing the hyperplasia will reduce the incidence of cancer. Some short-term studies show a reduced incidence of uterine cancer in women on HRT.[45] But until long-term studies are available we won't feel comfortable in assuring women that the addition of progesterone to ERT will take care of the uterine cancer problem.

One of the things that makes us uneasy is that HRT reminds us of the sequential birth control pill. The sequential pills had to be withdrawn from the market in 1976 because they caused uterine cancer in some of the women who took them.[46] The sequential pills followed the same sort of regimen, that is, taking estrogen pills for so many days and then taking pills that also contained progesterone preparation for so many days.* Of course, the dosages of hormone and the type of hormones used in the sequential pill (see below) were different from those used in HRT. Nonetheless, the similarities between HRT and sequential pills make us uneasy. Based on what we know at this point in time we think that women who are taking replacement therapy should get HRT rather than ERT, but we don't feel comfortable telling women that HRT is guaranteed to protect them from the uterine cancer that is seen in ERT users.

If a woman decides to start on replacement therapy, we often use ERT rather than HRT for the 1st year, because 1 year on ERT isn't enough to cause a woman to develop hyperplasia or cancer. Some women—for example, many of those who are taking hormones for hot flashes—will need replacement therapy only for a year, and most of our women clients are not keen about having menstrual periods again. HRT will cause menstrual-like bleeding on the "pill-free" days at the end of each month in 88 percent of women. Although some women on ERT experience bleeding, the majority do not. At the end of the year, if the woman is going to continue on replacement therapy, we switch to HRT.

*Sequential pills were not like the combination birth control pills now on the market. The combination pills contain both estrogen and progesterone and are taken each day for 21 days.

In general, we encourage women not to use replacement therapy if it is possible to avoid it and, if they do use it, to take the lowest doses possible for the shortest amount of time. Not all doctors would agree with us, but we think it is a potent medication. As explained above, some doctors prescribe HRT for all their menopausal patients, to prevent osteoporosis. Although we think that osteoporosis is indeed a serious problem, at this point in time giving HRT to *all* women in order to prevent osteoporosis in the 35 percent to 40 percent who will eventually develop it, does not seem like a wise idea. For one thing, even if we discount the possibility of uterine cancer, there is the possibility of breast cancer.

The information we have on breast cancer and replacement therapy is contradictory. Two studies showed an increased risk of breast cancer in ERT users; another study also showed an increased risk, but the data from that study was not conclusive.[47] However, the results of at least three other studies have shown that there was no increased risk, and two of these studies showed that ERT actually decreased the risk of breast cancer.[48] Studies of HRT users have indicated no increased risk of breast cancer or even a decreased risk,[49] but HRT is a newer form of treatment and has not been studied for as long a time. It is hoped that the HRT studies will not be as contradictory as the ERT studies have been. The studies done so far certainly are encouraging, but more time and more studies are needed before we can draw any firm conclusions about the relationship between HRT and breast cancer.

Another possible risk of ERT is coronary heart disease. Again, the evidence is contradictory. There is some evidence that ERT increases the risk of coronary heart disease and heart attacks, but there is also evidence to indicate that it decreases the risk.[50] At this time it is unclear whether the addition of progesterone, that is, taking HRT, will increase the risk of coronary heart disease and heart attacks or decrease the risk.[51]

At least one study has shown a two- to threefold increased risk of gallbladder disease requiring surgery in postmenopausal women who are taking ERT.[52] The relationship between HRT and gallbladder disease has not yet been subject to enough study for us to draw any conclusions. Strokes may also be more common in ERT users,[53] but here again, the evidence is contradictory and the relationship between HRT and strokes is unclear.

Contraindications

A contraindication is a condition that makes a form of therapy inadvisable. Because replacement therapy risks have not been clearly defined, contraindications are a subject of some debate, but there are certain, absolute contraindications that everyone accepts, including:

☐ Current or past blood-clotting disorders
☐ Stroke
☐ Cardiovascular disease
☐ Undiagnosed abnormal vaginal bleeding
☐ Cancer of the breast, reproductive organs or skin
☐ Pregnancy

Most doctors would agree that the following are also contraindications:

☐ Impaired liver function
☐ High blood pressure
☐ Diabetes
☐ Fibrocystic disease or fibroadenoma of the breast
☐ Sickle cell disease
☐ High levels of factors called serum lipid levels
☐ Surgery planned in the next 4 weeks

Some doctors would also include the following contraindications, whereas others would prescribe replacement therapy for such women. All would agree that if women with the following conditions take replacement therapy, they must be monitored closely.

☐ Fibroid tumors of the uterus
☐ Family history of diabetes
☐ Epilepsy
☐ Asthma
☐ Varicose veins

Because estrogens can interact with certain other medications, such as anti-coagulants, insulin, promazine hydrochloride, meperidine hydrochloride and tuberculin skin tests, estrogen use may be modified or contraindicated if these are being used. Women on ERT should discuss this issue with their doctors.

Monitoring

Women on ERT therapy should be followed closely. Any vaginal bleeding, chest pain, difficulty in breathing, coughing, headaches, dizziness, faintness, leg pain, breast lumps, vision changes or yellowing of the skin should be reported to the doctor immediately. Should vaginal bleeding occur, a D&C is mandatory to rule out the possibility of cancer. Some doctors recommend that women on ERT have an endometrial biopsy before beginning treatment and that this procedure be repeated annually.

DES

AKA: diethylstilbestrol, stilbestrol

Diethylstilbestrol, or DES, for short, was the first man-made estrogen. Beginning in 1940, DES and similar drugs were given to pregnant women who had histories of premature birth, miscarriage, diabetes or hypertension or who showed signs of bleeding in the early stages of pregnancy. Upward of a million women were given the drug, for it was thought that DES could help prevent miscarriage. DES apparently was also given to healthy women who had none of these problems.[54]

DES Effects

The tragic consequences of DES usage in pregnant women did not become apparent until 1970, when an alert physician, Dr. Arthur Herbst, and his colleagues reported seven cases of a rare form of vaginal cancer, clear cell adenocarcinoma, in women aged 15 to 22.[55] Until this time there had been only three cases of this disease in women under age 35 reported in the worldwide medical literature. As the result of a careful investigation the link between DES exposure and the cancers was established. This led to the creation of a worldwide tumor registry to which such cases could be reported. Thus far more than 500 cases have been reported.[56] The peak incidence seems to occur at about age 19, although DES-related cancer has been reported in girls as young as 7 and women as old as 33. Only a small percentage of DES daughters have actually developed vaginal cancer. The risk is estimated at 1 in 1,000 to 1 in 10,000 DES daughters will develop clear cell adenocarcinoma. Some doctors think this estimate is too high; others think that it is too low and fear that DES daughters are at higher risk for vaginal cancer and other types of cancer as well. For example, some researchers have reported a higher incidence, as much as a fivefold increase, of cervical dysplasia, a possible precursor to cervical cancer, in DES daughters.[57] They fear that as more women reach the age when cervical cancer is most common, ages 35 to 50, more cancer will be seen in DES daughters. Other experts do not believe that there is an increased risk for dysplasia in DES daughters. These issues are discussed more fully under the heading Vaginal Adenosis.

Although only a small percentage of DES daughters have developed vaginal cancer, a much higher number, as many as 90 percent in some studies, have a condition known as vaginal adenosis, in which the glandular-type tissue that normally lines the cervical canal is found growing on the vaginal surface of the cervix and on the walls of the vagina.[58] This abnormal tissue growth can be likened to growth of the tissue that is found inside the mouth and cheeks on the lips and face.

Until DES, vaginal adenosis was uncommon. In most instances it is not thought to have any serious consequences. However, the majority of DES daughters who have vaginal cancer also have had vaginal adenosis, and so it is feared that in a small number of women, adenosis may be a precursor to cancer.

In addition to cancer and adenosis, DES daughters may be more likely to have congenital abnormalities of the cervix, including a peculiarly shaped or strange-looking cervix; ridged cervical or vaginal tissues; a condition called incompetent cervix, in which the cervix dilates prematurely during pregnancy, causing miscarriage; and cervical eversion, a less extensive form of vaginal adenosis.[59] An unusual, T-shaped uterus has been found in the course of fertility workups in some DES daughters.[60] The fallopian tubes may be narrower as well.[61] Studies comparing DES daughters with unexposed women of the same age-group indicate that DES daughters may be more likely to have irregular or infrequent menstrual periods and a lower level of fertility.[62] There have not been any studies indicating that the children of DES daughters or DES sons will have any abnormalities. However, DES sons and daughters may have infertility problems, and DES daughters may have more difficulty in carrying a pregnancy to term.[63] Any DES daughter who becomes pregnant should let her doctor know that she is a DES daughter and should look for a doctor experienced in DES cases (see below).

DES sons have not been studied as extensively as DES daughters, so it is only recently that male problems have been identified. Because of the publicity surrounding DES daughters and vaginal cancer, DES sons seeking medical treatment are often worried about the possibility of developing cancer. Thus far there have been no studies linking DES exposure in males to cancer. However, there are studies that indicate that DES sons may have a higher incidence of hypoplastic (small) testes and undescended testes, a condition in which one or, less frequently, both of the sperm-producing testes fail to descend into the scrotum.[64] These two conditions also occur in males who have not been exposed to DES and may predispose such men to cancer of the testis. Whether these conditions, when they occur in DES sons, may similarly predispose these men to testicular cancer is not known; however, it is suggested that DES sons practice monthly testicular self-examination to detect any lumps or abnormalities.

In addition to the abnormalities stated above, studies have indicated that as many as 40 percent of all DES sons have low sperm counts or abnormally shaped sperm cells.[65] It is not yet known how this will affect the fertility of such men. Moreover, DES sons have a higher incidence of testicular cysts and abnormal placements of the urinary opening. In addition to being examined for abnormalities, DES sons should keep in touch with their doctors and DES Action (see below) to keep abreast of new developments.

Sources and Uses of DES

DES and two similar synthetic estrogens, dienestrol and hexestrol, were the main drugs used. All these drugs are referred to as DES, or DES-type drugs, and all are thought to have similar harmful effects. Table 30 lists some of the names under which DES and similar drugs have been sold.

DES was also given to U.S. cattle to fatten them up before slaughter. This use of DES was the subject of a lengthy battle between drug companies, consumer groups and the Food and Drug Administration (FDA).[66] The drug was first approved for use in animal feed and as pellet implants in 1947. But in 1958 further tests showed that DES caused cancer in laboratory animals. In 1959 newly developed techniques to detect relatively low levels of residues of DES in the tissue of animals that had been given the hormones revealed that the amount of hormone left in poultry was too high, and the FDA withdrew approval of its use with poultry. More sensitive tests to detect DES residue in beef and lamb were developed later, and the use of DES on cows and sheep was banned in November of 1979. However, those who included meat in their diets before that time may have been exposed to DES.

DES is also used as a method of birth control, as described under the heading Morning-After Pill. Some doctors still prescribe DES to dry up a woman's milk after childbirth if she does not plan to breast-feed.

Determining DES Exposure

Any woman who became pregnant between 1941 and 1971* should consider the possibility of DES exposure. Women who had histories of miscarriage, premature birth, hypertension, toxemia during pregnancy or diabetes or who had bleeding problems during their pregnancies are more likely to have received this drug. However, even apparently healthy women were given this drug, sometimes without their consent. Some women apparently were told that it was "just a vitamin pill."[67]

Those who were born during these years should ask their mothers if they remember taking any drug during pregnancy. DES was usually given as a pill but may have been given as a shot. Even small doses of the drug, given for only a few days, have been associated with subsequent cancer. Understand-

---

*Some say 1975, since despite the FDA's 1971 recommendation that DES not be given to pregnant women, some doctors continued to do so.

Table 30
DES-Type Drugs That May Have Been Prescribed to Pregnant Women

Nonsteroidal Estrogens

AVC cream with dienestrol	Estrosyn	Restrol
Benzestrol	Fonatol	Stilbal
Chlorotrianisene	Gynben	Stilbestrol
Comestrol	Gynegen	Stilbestronate
Cyren A	H-Bestrol	Stilbetin
Cyren B	Hexestrol	Stilbinol
Delvinal	Hexoestrol	Stilboestroform
DES	Menocrin	Stilboestrol
DesPlex	Meprane	Stilboestrol DP
Dibestil	Methallenestril	Stilestrate
Dienestrol	Microest	Stilpalmitate
Dienestrol cream	Mikarol	Stilphostrol
Dienoestrol	Mikarol forti	Stil-Rol
Diestryl	Milestrol	Stilronate
Diethylstilbenediol	Monomestrol	Stilrone
Diethylstilbestrol dipalmitate	Neo-Oestranol I	Stils
Diethylstilbestrol diphosphate	Neo-Oestranol II	Synestrin
Diethylstilbestrol dipropionate	Nulabort	Synestrol
Digestil	Oestrogenine	Synthoestrin
Domestrol	Oestromenin	Tace
Estilben	Oestromon	Vallestril
Estrobene	Orestol	Willestrol
Estrobene DP	Pabestrol D	
	Palestrol	

Nonsteroidal Estrogen–Androgen Combinations

Amperone	Teserene
Di-Erone	Tylandril
Estan	Tylosterone
Metystil	

Nonsteroidal Estrogen–Progesterone Combination
Progravidium

SOURCE: This listing is adapted from the U.S. Department of Health, Education and Welfare's *Information for Physicians: DES Exposure in Utero,* Publication No. (NIH) 76-1119, pp. 10–11.

ably, a mother may not recall if she took anything, especially if a number of years have passed, the medication was given for only a few days or she was told that it was just a vitamin pill. Anyone born during the period from 1941 to 1971 should talk with his or her mother about a previous medical history or any complications with pregnancy that may have made her a likely candidate for DES therapy.

Another way to find out about DES exposure is by checking with the doctor or hospital involved. Unfortunately, it may be impossible to get such records, because they may not have been kept correctly or may have been destroyed. Additional difficulty arises from the fact that the medical profession, perhaps from fear of legal problems, has been, by and large, uncooperative about informing DES-exposed women. Details about how to obtain medical records are discussed in Chapter Six.

Medical Care and Follow-Up of DES Daughters

If there is any reason for a woman to think she may have been exposed, she should go to a doctor or clinic experienced in DES screening. It is important to find experienced doctors, for inexperienced ones may not know how to do the correct tests, may miss important signs or may mistreat or dismiss the condition. Table 31 lists DES centers sponsored by the National Cancer Institute that can provide information on proper DES follow-up. Table 32 lists DES Action groups, consumers' groups that can direct women to doctors or clinics experienced in DES exposure.

Females with known or suspected DES exposure should have the diagnostic exam if they have started their first period, if they are age 14 or older or if, at any age, they show any unusual vaginal discharge or irregular bleeding. A

Table 31
DESAD Project Centers and Project Directors

Dr. Duane E. Townsend DESAD Project California Hospital Medical Center 1414 South Hope Street Los Angeles, California 90015 (213) 747-5666	Massachusetts General Hospital 32 Fruit Street Boston, Massachusetts 02114 (617) 726-2780
Dr. Robert Bowser Director, DESAD Project Division of Cancer Control and Rehabilitation National Cancer Institute Blair Building 8300 Colesville Road Silver Spring, Maryland 20910 (301) 496-6641	Dr. David G. Decker DESAD Project Mayo Clinic Rochester, Minnesota 55901 (507) 284-3288 Dr. Raymond H. Kaufman DESAD Project Baylor College of Medicine 1200 Moursand Avenue Houston, Texas (713) 790-4405
Dr. Ann Barnes and Dr. Stanley J. Robboy DESAD Project	

Table 32
DES Action Groups

DES Action National
Long Island Jewish–Hillside Medical
  Center
New Hyde Park, New York 11040
  (516) 775-3450

Regional Offices
DES Action/Massachusetts
P.O. Box 117
Brookline, Massachusetts 02147

DES Action/Northern California
16388 Haight Street
San Francisco, California 94117
(415) 621-8032

DES Action/Oregon
P.O. Box 12092
Portland, Oregon 97212
(503) 282-8868

DES Action/Pennsylvania
Pennsylvania Women's Center
Houston Hall
University of Pennsylvania
Philadelphia, Pennsylvania 19104

DES Action/Sacramento
707 45th Street
Sacramento, California 95819

DES Action/Washington
P.O. Box 5311
Rockville, Maryland 20851
(301) 468-2170

DES Action/Michigan
9146 Greensboro
Detroit, Michigan 48224

DES Action/Connecticut
P.O. Box 49
Mansfield Depot, Connecticut 06251

DES Action/Florida
9586 Portside Drive
Seminole, Florida 33542

few experts believe that even younger females known to have been exposed should be examined, since girls as young as age 7 have developed associated cancer. Some of these doctors have developed special techniques for examining young girls whose vaginal canals may be too small to allow for insertion of the speculum used for diagnosis. A general anesthetic has been used by some doctors, but of course, general anesthesia involves risks of its own. Most doctors, pointing to the fact that 90 percent of exposed daughters who developed cancer were age 14 or older, think that age 14 is young enough. It is true that it is highly unlikely that a girl under age 14 would develop this cancer. Anyone who decides to have a young daughter examined (and if symptoms like excessive vaginal discharge or abnormal vaginal bleeding appear, she *must* be examined, regardless of age) should read the section on psychological aspects below. Even girls age 14 may have vaginal canals too small for comfortable examination. Many doctors suggest that they use tampons for a few months before examination.

DES changes may not show up in the routine pelvic exam and Pap smear.

Special techniques that are quick and usually involve little discomfort are required. First, the doctor will do a careful examination of the vagina by palpating (feeling) the cervix and vagina for rough, sandy or nodular areas. A careful speculum exam of the vaginal walls and cervix to detect red areas or physical abnormalities is also done. The exam should include the special Pap smear known as a four-sided (quadrant) Pap test, in which the vaginal walls as well as the cervix are lightly scraped for cell samples, which should be sent to a lab for analysis by a pathologist, who is familiar with DES-type changes. The walls of the vagina and the cervix are then painted with a special iodine stain (called Schiller's, or Lugol's, stain) that turns normal tissue dark brown. Abnormal tissue will not absorb the stain. Biopsy specimens must be taken of areas that do not stain. The biopsy, which involves cutting away a bit of the suspicious tissue, does not cause too much pain, since there are few nerve endings in the upper vagina, but it may cause some bleeding. The tissue samples are then studied in the lab, to eliminate the possibility of cancer.

A special magnifying instrument called a colposcope, which allows the doctor to see changes not visible to the naked eye, can also be used in diagnosing DES daughters. Colposcopic exam is a simple, safe office procedure; however, there is some controversy about the use of colposcopy to detect DES changes.

There is no doubt that the colposcope is a valuable tool when used by a trained and skilled doctor. The problem lies in interpretation of what is seen. Many private doctors, although they own or have access to colposcopes, may not see enough DES patients to be able to interpret correctly what they see. Another problem is that colposcopes are relatively expensive. A doctor, especially one who sees relatively few DES cases or other conditions requiring a colposcope, may have to charge quite a bit to recover his or her investment in equipment and training. The cost of a colposcopic exam may run as high as $100. Not all insurance plans cover these costs completely. Then, too, colposcopes are not always available, especially to women who live in rural areas, without easy access to medical facilities.

Medical opinion as to the role colposcopy should play in DES follow-up is divided. Some doctors think that the special Pap smear, palpation and visual inspection, staining and, if necessary, biopsy are sufficient. Others think that if the staining indicates abnormality, colposcopy, which will make the biopsy more accurate, should be done, but that unless abnormalities are revealed by staining, colposcopic examination is unnecessary. Still others believe the initial exam of a DES daughter should be done with a colposcope, but if there are no abnormalities, it should not be required in follow-up. Some of the doctors who express these viewpoints are of the opinion that more extensive use of the colposcope is just to make money for the doctor. Still other doctors believe that a colposcope exam should be done on an annual (or even biannual) basis, with careful charts or photos being kept to follow the progress of the disease, since little is known about it. Recently, one doctor reported a case of cancer in a woman who had shown no abnormality during 2 years of routine examination.[68] This doctor thought that without colposcopic examination this woman's cancer would not have been detected as early as it was.

It will probably be some time before the proper role of colposcopic examination of DES women can be determined. Until more research is done the decision about colposcopy lies with the consumer—the daughter or her parents. Availability (either financial or geographic) and age (the incidence of clear cell adenocarcinoma seems to drop dramatically after age 22, although other types of cancer, as noted earlier, may occur later) may influence the decision.

Furthermore, as more information is compiled about uterine abnormalities in DES daughters, hysterograms, special X-ray studies of the uterus, and sonograms, pictures of internal organs taken by means of high-frequency sound waves, may also become part of the medical evaluation. Here again, women can keep abreast of the latest development through DES Action (see below).

After the initial examination, follow-up exams in which all or some of the procedures done in the initial exam are repeated, are scheduled every 3 or 6 months, depending on whether any abnormalities, such as vaginal adenosis, are found and on their extent. If no abnormalities are found, many doctors recommend follow-up exams once a year.

DES Daughters and Sons and Pregnancy

Fertility and pregnancy problems may occur in DES daughters and sons, but most DES-exposed women and children will be able to have children. It has not yet been established how common these problems are, but medical research indicates that, with proper care, about 80 percent of all DES daughters will be able to have children.[69]

More research is needed on DES sons and infertility. What research there is indicates that such problems as poor sperm quality (lack of movement, abnormal structure, low sperm count) and insufficient quantity of sperm may occur more often in DES sons.[70] This may be owing to anatomical abnormalities caused by DES exposure (see above). As yet, there are no studies on how best to treat DES sons who have low sperm counts. Some doctors use Clomid, but there is disagreement among doctors about the effectiveness of this treatment, and the drug carries certain risks (*see* pp. 820–22).

Some studies (but not all) show that DES daughters are more likely to be infertile.[71] The reason for infertility is unclear. It may be related to problems with abnormalities in the shape of the uterus and/or fallopian tubes, problems in ovulation, hormonal imbalances or problems with cervical mucus. As yet, there are no research findings to indicate whether the ovulation problems seen in DES daughters result from the same factors that cause such problems in other women (see the section on infertility). Nor do we know if the treatments commonly used for ovulation-related infertility are as effective or carry more side effects and complications when used by DES daughters. At the present time DES daughters with ovulation problems generally are treated in the same manner as other women with ovulating infertility problems.

In some DES daughters the fallopian tubes are smaller in diameter and abnormally shaped, which may make it difficult for the egg to pass through the tube.[72] So far, corrective surgery of the type used to correct tubal infertility problems in other women has not made a significant difference in pregnancy rates.[73]

The T-shaped uterus problem that is found in some DES daughters may also play a role in the infertility problems. Cervical mucus, which helps to transport the sperm through the cervix and into the uterus (*see* pp. 62), may be the seat of the infertility problem in some DES daughters. Many DES daughters have had conization, which can affect the mucus-producing glands in the cervix. Some DES daughters, even if they have not had such surgery, simply have fewer mucus-producing cervical cells. Some doctors prescribe estrogen to improve cervical mucus. But estrogens *have not* proved to be effective in improving cervical mucus in DES daughters,[74] and such authorities as the World Health Organization and the Federal DES Task Force caution against the use of estrogen by DES daughters.[75]

In addition to problems in *getting* pregnant, DES-exposed women may have problems carrying a pregnancy to term. DES daughters may be more likely to have ectopic pregnancies.[76] DES daughters should familiarize themselves with the signs of ectopic pregnancy (*see* pp. 685–88). They should also have a pregnancy test as soon as they suspect they are pregnant. The routine pregnancy tests used by most doctors are not always effective in detecting ectopics, so DES daughters may want to discuss this with their doctors and ask for the new, highly sensitive tests that can detect pregnancies (including ectopics) before the woman has even missed a menstrual period.

DES daughters may be more apt to miscarry[77] and to have premature births.[78] Although most DES daughters will have normal pregnancies, DES daughters should be under the care of doctors who are knowledgeable about DES problems. For more information on pregnancy problems in DES daughters, you can get a copy of *Fertility and Pregnancy Guide for DES Daughters and Sons* ($5 a copy) from DES Action.

DES Women and the Pill

Many DES daughters and mothers have questions about the advisability of using birth control pills. Medical opinion on this issue is divided. Some doctors point out there is no evidence to date that these women should avoid the Pill or that Pill risks for DES women are higher than they are for other women. Some doctors even use the Pill to treat the menstrual irregularities that may occur in DES daughters. Other doctors believe strongly that DES women should not be given birth control pills or estrogen replacement therapy. They point out that little is known about the long-term effects of the Pill or of DES. Adding another hormone to an already complex hormonal situation may have serious effects. We think that other forms of birth control are preferable for DES mothers and daughters. Indeed, some doctors believe that the diaphragm or spermicidal foams may actually improve DES-related conditions.

Psychological Aspects

One important but often ignored aspect of DES exposure is the psychological impact it may have on both mothers and children. DES mothers are likely to be fearful about the effects on their own health and on their children's health. They may be angry with the medical profession and may also feel terribly guilty. Children may be fearful and angry both at the mother and the medical profession.

The need for a DES exam may come at a time in a young girl's life when she is self-conscious about her genitals. Having a gynecological examination can be a physically and emotionally uncomfortable procedure for a woman of any age and may be especially difficult for a young girl, particularly if she is having her first exam because of possible DES exposure. The fear that some abnormality, perhaps even cancer, might be found makes the situation even more frightening.

Some DES centers have psychological counseling available, and women should take advantage of this if it is offered. DES Action (see below) has local groups across the United States where women can receive support and advice from other DES mothers and daughters who have faced these problems. Some DES clinics and doctors use videotapes and mirrors so that parents and daughters can see what the inside of the vagina looks like. DES-type changes don't, as a rule, produce the striking abnormalities that some people imagine, so "taking a look" can be reassuring. We suggest that DES mothers practice self-exam and, once they are comfortable with the procedure, include their daughters in the process. Young girls who watch their mothers practice speculum exam are more likely to be comfortable with the procedure.

Legal Aspects

Individual DES mothers and daughters have filed lawsuits against drug manufacturers and against their doctors.[79] There have been some legal difficulties with these suits revolving around problems in identifying which company manufactured the DES pills any given woman may have taken (since there were so many manufacturers) and around the fact that, at the time most DES was given, the use of DES was acceptable medical practice and thus not an instance of medical malpractice. However, one lawsuit in New York filed by a DES daughter who developed cancer resulted in a $500,000 award against Eli Lilly Co., as representative of all manufacturers of the drug.

Class-action suits aimed at trying to get the drug companies or the government to pay for the medical care and follow-up of DES daughters have also been filed. For more legal information, contact DES Action (see below) or the National Women's Health Network, 2025 I Street NW, Washington, D.C. 20006.

DES Action

DES Action is a national organization of DES-exposed women and of health-care activists and medical personnel. It has chapters throughout the United States. It is available to help people with questions and concerns about DES. DES Action teaches doctors and nurses about DES, encourages needed medical research, sponsors legislation mandating public information campaigns and the establishment of DES screening clinics and provides referrals and emotional support for those who have been exposed to DES. They have training materials available and information on how to set up a local group. In addition, they publish a quarterly newsletter, *DES Action Voice,* which keeps people up to date on medical and legal developments and other news of interest to anyone concerned about DES exposure. To find out more about DES Action groups or to subscribe to their excellent newsletter (yearly subscription, four issues, costs $15), contact them at the locations listed in Table 32.

FERTILITY DRUGS

Types: estrogen
        human chorionic gonadotropin, or HCG
        clomiphene citrate, or Clomid
        human menopausal gonadotropin, HMG, or Pergonal

Throughout history, humankind has been looking for magic brews—love potions, youth elixirs and fertility concoctions. Thus far we haven't had much luck with the first two, but we now have drugs that can help an infertile woman become pregnant. Although they can't help every woman, they often are effective for women who are unable to conceive because they are not ovulating. Women who are not ovulating regularly are said to have anovulatory cycles. These women may also have a variety of menstrual irregularities, including abnormal uterine bleeding, no menstrual periods (a condition known as amenorrhea) or irregular periods. Certain fertility drugs may be used to treat women who have a luteal phase defect, a condition in which the corpus luteum regresses too soon, depriving the fertilized egg of the necessary support of the rich uterine lining.

Because use of these drugs involves some risk, a woman should first have a complete fertility workup (*see* p. 668) to make sure that her infertility is actually caused by failure to ovulate and not by some other problem. If a woman with an infertility problem also has amenorrhea, she should similarly have a complete diagnostic workup (*see* p. 626) to determine that her amenorrhea is caused by failure to ovulate and that it and her particular infertility problem are of the type that will be responsive to fertility drugs. Moreover, women using these drugs must be monitored carefully for side effects and for the return of ovulation. Pelvic exams must be done frequently. The woman will be asked to keep a basal body temperature chart (BBT) (*see* p. 173), because once she ovulates, her temperature will rise, owing to the progesterone that is produced after ovulation. However, a BBT is not always accurate; a vaginal smear can also be used to detect ovulation, as can an endometrial biopsy, but the latter should not be used on a woman who might be pregnant. Urine and blood tests to measure hormone levels may be necessary in some cases. Pregnancy tests (*see* p. 788) of the most sensitive type must be done before a course of therapy is repeated, because some fertility drugs may be dangerous to a developing fetus and should be discontinued as soon as a woman becomes pregnant.

Estrogen

If the woman's vaginal smear or endometrial biopsy indicates a lack of estrogen, some doctors will prescribe small amounts of this hormone.[80] Too much estrogen may prevent ovulation, so only small amounts are given orally. Premarin, an estrogen taken from the urine of pregnant horses, may be prescribed on days 6 through 15 of the menstrual cycle. If this doesn't cause ovulation, the treatment may be repeated the next month and perhaps again the 3d month. If ovulation does occur, the woman continues treatment each month, timing intercourse so that it occurs just before or during the expected time of ovulation.

Many doctors are hesitant to use estrogen as a fertility drug. First, they find that it is rarely effective, especially in women with amenorrhea. Moreover, they are concerned about the possibility that a woman might ovulate and conceive while taking the estrogen. If, for instance, the woman ovulated on Day 10 or 12, she could still be taking estrogen when conception took place. Or, should a woman get pregnant and still have what appears to be a menstrual period, as occasionally happens, the doctor might inadvertently prescribe another round of estrogen. We know that certain synthetic estrogens, like DES, taken during pregnancy have resulted in a rare form of vaginal cancer in some of the daughters, as well as other abnormalities in both the sons and daughters of the women who took them.[81] Whether Premarin would have similar tragic consequences is not known. However, no one wants to find out the hard way, as we did with DES; so the woman must be given pregnancy tests of the most sensitive type before each course of estrogen.

HCG

Some doctors use HCG, human chorionic gonadotropin, a hormone that is normally produced by the placenta within a few days of conception. HCG behaves much like luteinizing hormone, which is the pituitary hormone whose midcycle surge triggers ovulation. A high-dose injection of HCG, which is obtained from the urine of pregnant women, is given at midcycle. If this does not produce ovulation, a higher-dose injection may be tried the next month. If this is not effective, a third course of treatment may be prescribed.

Many doctors are reluctant to use this form of treatment, for they believe that HCG by itself is rarely effective. Instead, they may use HCG in combination with Clomid or with the more powerful Pergonal (see below).

Clomid

Clomiphene citrate, sold under the brand name Clomid, is also used to treat infertility. The drug is similar in structure to a synthetic estrogen but has only a few, weak estrogen effects. It works on the hypothalamus, which in turn stimulates the pituitary to produce luteinizing hormone (LH) and follicle stimulating hormone (FSH). These hormones cause an egg in the ovary to ripen and to be released at the time of ovulation. Clomid is used, then, in cases where the pituitary gland is normal and capable of producing its hormones but the hypothalamus is not functioning properly. It is used frequently to treat women with Stein-Leventhal disease of the ovaries.

The drug is given on days 5 through 10 of the menstrual cycle. (The period may have to be induced by using progesterone if the woman also has amenorrhea.) It is then continued for 5 days. Most women will ovulate within the next several days. If the woman's BBT does not indicate that she has ovulated, treatment may be attempted again the next month, using higher doses of Clomid. Most women are started with doses of 50 mg to 100 mg a day in successive months. Some doctors will use higher doses, but this is controversial.[82] Some doctors think that if laparoscopic examination has not been done as part of the diagnostic workup, the woman should have one before 200-mg doses are used. Also, it is recommended that women who have Stein-Leventhal disease not receive more than 600 mg of Clomid a month, for they may already have elevated levels of one of these hormones.

HCG may be used in combination with Clomid. It is generally given after Clomid therapy, to trigger ovulation. Estrogen may also be given if the cervical mucus of the woman taking Clomid does not seem to be the proper consistency to allow the sperm to penetrate the cervix, but it should be given only in the early days of the cycle, before ovulation, to eliminate the possibility of its being taken after the woman becomes pregnant.

The most serious complication with Clomid therapy is the formation of multiple ovarian cysts that may rupture and then lead to destruction of the ovary or even death. About 10 percent of women using Clomid will have twins, but other multiple births (triplets and so on) are rare.[83] There may be hot flashes, abdominal pain, soreness, bloating, breast tenderness, nausea, vomiting, headaches and vision problems, including blurring, spots and flashes. These symptoms should be reported to the doctor. If vision problems occur, the medication should be discontinued and the doctor called immediately. Most of these side effects can be prevented if the woman is started on low doses and followed carefully.

Women should be monitored carefully before each course of Clomid, to rule out the possibility of pregnancy and the formation of multiple cysts. Careful pelvic exams and the most sensitive pregnancy tests should be done. Pregnancies conceived after Clomid treatment have not shown an increased incidence of birth defects. However, pregnancies conceived during treatment may have problems. There is no direct evidence that Clomid taken during pregnancy can cause abnormalities in humans, but studies have shown that doses given in early pregnancy can cause birth defects in laboratory animals.[84] Because Clomid is similar in its chemical structure to DES, a synthetic hormone that caused birth defects in the children of the women who took it, most medical personnel are careful to rule out the possibility of pregnancy before giving a second course of the drug. Furthermore, Clomid has been in wide use for only 15 years, and, as with DES, it could be that possible carcinogenic effects will begin to show only after 15 years or more.

Because of these considerations and the fact that Clomid has caused precancerous conditions in the reproductive tract of the mother rats[85] as well as in the offspring exposed during pregnancy, in our opinion a doctor should administer Clomid only to a woman who wants to become pregnant. The doctor who gives it should be experienced in its use and know how to monitor the woman carefully.

About 70 percent of women treated will actually ovulate, and of these about 40 percent will become pregnant.[86] If a woman is going to ovulate with Clomid, she usually will do so within the first three courses of treatment. Most women who ovulate with Clomid will continue to do so with each repeated course. In some cases the response will be erratic. If Clomid is unsuccessful, Pergonal may be used.

Pergonal

Pergonal is used to treat infertility in women who have some sort of problem in the pituitary gland that is preventing the pituitary from producing LH and FSH, but pituitary tumors must first be ruled out. It is also used to treat women who have failed to respond to Clomid. An expensive drug, Pergonal is extracted from the urine of postmenopausal women, and is known as HMB, human menopausal gonadotropin. The urine of these women contains high levels of LH and FSH. Since Pergonal involves greater risks than Clomid, Clomid may be used along with Pergonal so that lower doses of Pergonal can be used. HCG may also be used in combination with Pergonal, to trigger ovulation. The major complications with Pergonal therapy, owing to possible overstimulation of the ovary by the drug, are multiple ovulations, the formation of multiple cysts on the ovary and subsequent multiple pregnancies.[87] These complications have led to death through rupture of the cysts or rupture of the uterus during pregnancy. In less severe cases the rupture of the cysts may still necessitate surgery to remove the ovary. Even where the overstimulation of the ovary by Pergonal doesn't cause these drastic complications, a woman must still be hospitalized and monitored carefully.

About 50 percent of women given Pergonal treatment will actually ovulate.[88] About half these women will get pregnant and about one-fourth of these will have multiple births, usually twins. About 10 percent of women will develop enlarged cystic ovaries. The severe complications occur in about 1 percent of women using this drug; if the doctor administering the drug is inexperienced, however, the complication rate may be higher.

A woman being treated with Pergonal must be monitored carefully with daily tests to measure the amount of estrogen in the blood, and frequent pelvic exams must be done to make sure that not more than one egg follicle is forming. If more than one follicle forms and the estrogen levels rise too high, treatment must be discontinued for that month and the HCG must not be given. Withholding the HCG usually will prevent ovulation.

The trick is in knowing when to stop the Pergonal and when to give the HCG. If too little Pergonal is given and the HCG is given too early, the woman won't ovulate. If too much Pergonal is given, the woman may face serious complications. For this reason it is important that women use Pergonal only under the guidance of an expert who is experienced in the use of this drug. The best place to find such a specialist is through your gynecologist or a fertility clinic connected with a large university hospital or medical center.

Notes

Chapter One: HOW THIS BOOK CAME TO BE WRITTEN

1. Nancy Friday, *My Mother, My Self* (New York: Dell, 1977), p. 141.
2. Friday, p. 141.
3. Friday, p. 141.
4. National Center for Health Statistics, "Surgical Operations, Short-Stay Hospitals, U.S.," *Vital Health Statistics*, Series 13, no. 21, Washington, DC, 1976.
5. Based on a death rate of 0.2 percent.
6. Frank J. Dyck et al., "Effects of Surveillance on the Numbers of Hysterectomies in the Province of Saskatchewan," *New England Journal of Medicine* 296 (1977), pp. 1326–28. Note: The actual rates quoted in this study range from 17 percent to 59 percent. We have used an average figure of 30 percent to 40 percent, which is the figure generally quoted in the literature and by consumer groups.

Chapter Three: BREAST SELF-EXAM

1. P. Greenwald, M.D., et al., "Estimated Effect of Breast Self-Examination on Breast Cancer Mortality," *New England Journal of Medicine* 299 (1978), pp. 271–73.
2. American Cancer Society, *Facts and Figures* (New York: ACS, 1975).

Chapter Four: THE MONTHLY MIRACLE: MENSTRUATION

1. Nancy Friday, *My Mother, My Self* (New York: Dell, 1977). Note: Friday is quoting here from a book review by Anatole Broyard that appeared in the *New York Times* on Sept. 21, 1976.

2. Barbara Seaman and Gideon Seaman, M.D., *Women and the Crisis in Sex Hormones* (New York: Rawson Assoc., Inc., 1977), p. 298.

3. A number of case-control studies report increased risk for endometrial cancer in women using menopausal estrogens. The three most widely cited studies are:

H. K. Ziel and W. C. Finkle, "Increased Risk of Endometrial Carcinoma Among Users of Conjugated Estrogens," *New England Journal of Medicine* 293 (1975), pp. 1167–70;

D. C. Smith et al., "Association of Exogenous Estrogen and Endometrial Carcinoma," *New England Journal of Medicine* 293 (1975), pp. 1164–67; and

T. M. Mack et al., "Estrogens and Endometrial Cancer in a Retirement Community," *New England Journal of Medicine* 294 (1976), pp. 1262–67.

These findings are further supported by the fact that incidence rates of endometrial cancer have increased sharply since 1969, which may be related to the rapidly expanding use of estrogens in the last decade.

4. M. K. McClintock, "Menstrual Syncrony and Suppression," *Nature* 299 (1971), pp. 244–45.

5. James Hassett, "Sex and Smell," *Psychology Today* (March 1978), pp. 40–45.

6. T.A. Holding and K. Minkoff, "Parasuicide and the Menstrual Cycle," *Journal of Psychosomatic Research* 17 (5–6), (Dec. 1973), pp. 365–68.

Chapter Five: BIRTH CONTROL: THE STATISTICAL LIE

1. See the package insert that comes with estrogen products.

2. See the package insert that comes with progesterone products.

3. See the package insert that comes with estrogen products.

4. A.L. Herbst, H. Ulfedler and D.C. Poskanzer, "Adenocarcinoma of the Vagina," *New England Journal of Medicine* 284 (1971), pp. 878–81;

P. Greenwood et al., "Vaginal Cancer After Maternal Treatment with Synthetic Estrogens," *New England Journal of Medicine* 285 (1971), pp. 390–92.

5. A number of abnormalities have been found in DES daughters, including alterations in the shape of the cervix, vaginal adenosis, lowered fertility and irregular menstrual periods. DES sons have been reported as having testis cysts, underdeveloped or undescended testes, abnormally placed urinary openings, low sperm counts, abnormally shaped sperm cells and impaired fertility. For further information see:

R. Mattingly and A. Stafl, "Cancer Risk in DES-Exposed Offspring," *Journal of Obstetrics and Gynecology* 128 (1977), pp. 43–50; R. Kaufman et al., "Upper Genital Tract Changes Associated with Exposure in Utero to Diethylstilbestrol," *Journal of Obstetrics and Gynecology* 128 (1977), pp. 51–59.

M. Bibbo et al., "Follow-up Study of Male and Female Offspring of DES-Exposed Mothers," *Obstetrics and Gynecology* 49:1 (1977), pp. 1–8.

U.S. Dept. of Health, Education and Welfare, Food and Drug Administration, "DES and Breast Cancer," *FDA Drug Bulletin* 8 (March-April 1978), p. 2.

6. H.K. Ziel and W.D. Finkle, "Increased risk of Endometrial Carcinoma Among Users of Conjugated Estrogens," *New England Journal of Medicine* 293 (1975), pp. 1167–70;

D.C. Smith et al., "Association of Exogenous Estrogen and Endometrial Carcinoma," *New England Journal of Medicine* 293 (1975), pp. 1164–67.

7. T.M. Mack et al., "Estrogens and Endometrial Cancer in a Retirement Community," *New England Journal of Medicine* 294 (1976), pp. 1262–67.

These findings are further supported by the fact that incidence rates of endometrial cancer have increased sharply since 1969, which may be related to the rapidly expanding use of estrogens in the last decade. See the FDA-approved package insert for all products containing estrogens for more details.

8. "Sequential Pills Being Withdrawn," *New York Times,* Feb. 26, 1976.

9. Boston Collaborative Drug Surveillance Program, "Oral Contraceptive Use and Venous Thromboembolic Disease, Surgically Confirmed Gallbladder Disease and Breast Tumors," *Lancet* 1 (1973), pp. 1399–404;

M.P. Vessey, R. Dall and P.M. Sutton, "Oral Contraceptives and Breast Neoplasia: A Retrospective Study," *British Medical Journal* 3 (1972), pp. 719–24;

F.G. Arthes, P.E. Sartwell and E.F. Lewison, "The Pill, Estrogens and the Breast: Epidemiologic Aspects," *Cancer* 28 (1971), pp. 1391–94; and

E. Fasal and R.S. Paffenbarger, "Oral Contraceptives as Related to Cancer and Benign Lesions of the Breast," *Journal of the National Cancer Institute* 55 (1975), pp. 767–73.

10. Fasal and Paffenbarger, pp. 767–73.

11. R. Hoover et al., "Menopausal Estrogens and Cancer," *New England Journal of Medicine* 295 (1976), pp. 401–5.

12. Ward Rinehart and Judy C. Felt, "Debate on Oral Contraceptives and Neoplasia Continues; Answers Remain Elusive," *Population Reports,* Series A, no. 4 (May 1977), p. A-80.

13. Elizabeth Stern et al., "Steroid Contraceptive Use and Cervical Dysplasia: Increase in Risk of Progression," *Science* 196 (1977), p. 1460.

14. See the patient package insert and "Is Malignant Melanoma Linked to Oral Contraceptive Use?" *Contraceptive Technology Update,* May 1983, p. 543.

15. Centers for Disease Control, "Long-Term Oral Contraceptive Use and the Risk of Breast Cancer; Oral Contraceptive Use and the Risk of Ovarian Cancer; Oral Contraceptive Use and the Risk of Endometrial Cancer," *Journal of the American Medical Association* 249 (1983), pp. 1591–1604, and S. Ramcharan et al., *"The Walnut Creek Contraceptive Drug Study: A Prospective Study of the Side Effects of Oral Contraceptives* (Washington, DC: NIH, 1981).

16. "OCs Do Not Raise Breast, Endometrium and Ovary Cancer Risks," *Contraceptive Technology Update,* June 1982, pp. 69–73.

17. Stern, p. 1460.

18. Personal communication with Ms. Seaman.

19. M.P. Vessey et al., "Neoplasia of the Cervix Uteri and Contraception: A Possible Adverse Effect of the Pill," *Lancet,* Oct. 22, 1983, pp. 930–34.

20. M.C. Pike et al., "Breast Cancer in Young Women and Use of Oral Contraceptives, Possible Modifying Effect of Formulation and Age at Use," *Lancet,* Oct. 22, 1983, pp. 926–29.

21. Pike, pp. 72–76.

22. Pike, pp. 72–76.

23. R. Gambrell Jr., "Breast Disease in the Postmenopausal Years," *Seminars in Reproductive Endocrinology* 1 (Feb. 1983), pp. 27–40.

24. FDA-approved package insert included with all estrogen products.

25. C.J. Levinson and D.C. Richardson, "The Dalkon Shield Story," *Advances in Planned Parenthood* 11:2 (1976), pp. 53–63.

26. P.T. Piotrow et al., "IUD's Update on Safety, Effectiveness and Research," *Population Reports,* Series B, no. 3 (May 1979), p. B-57 (table).

27. U.S. Dept. of Health, Education and Welfare, "IUD Safety: Report of a Nationwide Physician Survey," *Morbidity and Mortality* 23 (1974), pp. 226–31.

28. J. Balog et al., "Recent Trend in Preference of Contraceptive Methods—Pills Down, Diaphragm on Rise," *Obstetrics and Gynecology Survey* 33:4 (April 1978), pp. 282–83.

29. T.J. Trussell, R. Faden and R.A. Hatcher, "Efficacy and Information in Contraceptive Counseling: Those Little White Lies," *American Journal of Public Health* 66 (1976), pp. 761–67.

30. Robert Hatcher et al., *Contraceptive Technology, 1978–1979,* 9th rev. ed. (New York: Irvington Pub., Inc., 1978), p. 20 (table).

31. G. Carpenter and J. Martin, "Clinical Evaluation of a Contraceptive Foam," *Advances in Planned Parenthood* (New York: Excerpta Medical Foundation, 1970), pp. 170–78.

32. U.S. Dept. of Health, Education and Welfare, *Contraception: Comparing the Options,* HEW Publication no. (FDA) 78,3069.

33. G.W. Beebe, *Contraception and Fertility in the Southern Appalachians* (Baltimore: Williams and Wilkins, 1974), p. 274.

34. Hatcher et al., p. 26 (table).

35. L.J. Latz and E. Reiner, "Failures in Natural Contraception Control and Their Causes," *Illinois Medical Journal* 71 (March 1937), pp. 210–16.

36. Elizabeth B. Connell, M.D., "Contraception," *Current Therapy, 1973* (Philadelphia: W.B. Saunders, 1973), p. 813.

37. U.S. House Select Committee on Population, "Domestic Consequences of United States Population Change," Report to the 95th Congress, Second Session Serial E (Washington, DC: U.S. Govt. Printing Office, Dec. 1978), p. 16 (table).

38. Barbara Seaman and Gideon Seaman, M.D., *Women and the Crisis in Sex Hormones* (New York: Rawson Assoc., Inc., 1977), p. 202. Note: The authors are quoting from a personal communication with Drs. Howard and Joy Osofsky, authorities on abortion and birth control.

39. Ward Rinehart and Phyllis Piotrow, "OC's—Update on Usage, Safety and Side Effects," *Population Reports,* Series A, no. 5 (Jan. 1979), p. A-137 (table).

40. Seaman and Seaman, p. 14.

41. Seaman and Seaman, p. 14.

42. Hatcher et al., p. 126.

43. Judith Wortman, "Vasectomy: What are the Problems?" *Population Reports,* Series D, no. 2 (Jan. 1975), p. D-31.

44. J.R. Neil et al., "Late Complications of Sterilization by Laparoscopy and Tubal Ligation," *Lancet* 1 (Oct. 11, 1975), p. 699.

827

Reference Section: BIRTH CONTROL METHODS

Note to readers: Most of the facts about birth control pills in the text are taken from the FDA-approved package insert that comes with each package of pills and that includes complete reference citations. These facts are given in the text without any specific references. In cases where we have included information that is not from the package insert, we provide specific citations.

1. Ward Rinehart, "Minipill—A Limited Alternative for Certain Women," *Population Reports*, Series A, no. 3 (Sept. 1975), p. A-56.

2. Robert A. Hatcher et al., *Contraceptive Technology, 1978-1979*, 9th rev. ed. (New York: Irvington Pub., Inc., 1978), p. 20 (table)

3. Elizabeth B. Connell, M.D., "Contraception," *Current Therapy, 1973* (Philadelphia: W.B. Saunders, 1973), p. 813.

4. "OC's Provide Non-Contraceptive Benefits, Informs Orly," *Contraceptive Technology Update*, Nov. 1981, pp. 147-48.

5. "OC's Provide Non-Contraceptive Benefits," pp. 147-48.

6. "OC's Provide Non-Contraceptive Benefits," pp. 147-48.

7. "OC's Provide Non-Contraceptive Benefits," pp. 147-48.

8. "OC's Provide Non-Contraceptive Benefits," pp. 147-48.

9. "OC's Provide Non-Contraceptive Benefits," pp. 147-48.

10. R. Rojas et al., "Diagnosis and Management of Post Pill Amenorrhea," *Journal of Family Practice* 3 (1981), pp. 165-69.

11. M.P. Vessey et al., "A Long-Term Follow-Up Study of Women Using Different Methods of Contraception: An Interim Report," *Journal of Biosocial Science* 8 (Oct. 1976), pp. 375-427.

12. Royal College of General Practitioners, *Oral Contraceptives and Health: An Interim Report* (London: Pitman, 1974).

13. "OC Use and Bowel Disease Incidence in Young Women," *Contraceptive Technology Update*, Sept. 1983, pp. 108-9.

14. R.V. Patwardham et al., "Impaired Elimination of Caffeine by Oral Contraceptive Steroids," *Journal of Laboratory and Clinical Medicine* 95 (1980), pp. 603-8.

15. "OC's Linked to Increase of Gingivitis, Dry Socket," *Contraceptive Technology Update*, Dec. 1981, p. 157.

16. S. Ramcharan et al., *The Walnut Creek Contraceptive Drug Study: A Prospective Study of the Side Effects of Oral Contraceptives* (Washington, DC; NIH, 1981).

17. "OC's Have Minimal Effect on Gallbladder Disease," *Contraceptive Technology Update*, Aug. 1981, pp. 105-6.

18. "Study Shows No Link Among OCs, Birth Defects," *Contraceptive Technology Update*, June 1983, and "What Is the Risk of Congenital Defect After OC Failure?" *Contraceptive Technology Update*, Nov. 1981, pp. 141-44.

19. "What Is the Risk,?" pp. 141-44.

20. K.J. Rothman and C. Louick, "Oral Contraceptives and Birth Defects," *New England Journal of Medicine* 299 (Sept. 7, 1978), pp. 522-24.

21. Royal College of General Practitioners, "The Outcome of Pregnancy in Former Oral Contraceptive Users," *British Journal of Obstetrics and Gynecology* 83 (Aug. 1976), pp. 608-16.

22. Vessey et al., pp. 375-427.

23. M.P. Vessey et al., "Fertility After Stopping Different Methods of Contraception," *British Medical Journal* 1 (Feb. 4, 1978), pp. 265–67.

24. B.M. Sherman et al., "Pathogenesis of Prolactin-Secreting Pituitary Adenomas," *Lancet* 2 (1978), pp. 1019–21.

25. R. Maheux et al., "Oral Contraceptives and Prolactinomas: A Case Controlled Study," *American Journal of Obstetrics and Gynecology* 243 (1982), p. 13.

26. A.M. Shojania, "Effect of Oral Contraceptives on Vitamin B_{12} Metabolism," *Lancet* 2 (1971), p. 932.

27. A.S. Prasad et al., "Effect of Oral Contraceptive Agents on Nutrients: II, Vitamins," *American Journal of Clinical Nutrition* 28 (1975), pp. 385–91.

28. M.K. Horwitt, C.C. Harvey and C.H. Dahm, "Relationship Between Levels of Blood Lipids, Vitamins C, A and E, Serum Copper Compound and Urinary Excretions of Tryptophan Metabolites in Women Taking Oral Contraceptive Therapy," *American Journal of Clinical Nutrition* 28 (1975), pp. 403–12.

29. C.J. Levinson and D.C. Richardson, "The Dalkon Shield Story," *Advances in Planned Parenthood* 11:2 (1976), pp. 53–63.

30. L. Liskin and G. Fox, "IUDS: An Appropriate Contraceptive for Many Women," *Population Reports,* Series B, no. 4 (July 1982), p. B-123.

31. U.S. Dept. of Health, Education and Welfare, Food and Drug Administration, "Progestasert IUD and Ectopic Pregnancy," *FDA Drug Bulletin* 8 (Dec. 1978–Jan. 1979), p. 37.

32. J. Jennings, "Report of the Safety and Efficacy of the Dalkon Shield and Other IUDs," FDA Ad Hoc Obstetric–Gynecology Advisory Committee, Oct. 1974.

33. Robert A. Hatcher, "Clinical Challenges," *Contraceptive Technology Update,* Feb. 1981, pp. 20–22.

34. U.S. Dept. of Health, Education and Welfare, Food and Drug Administration, Medical Device and Drug Advisory Committee on Obstetrics and Gynecology, *Second Report on Intrauterine Contraceptive Devices* (Washington, DC: Govt. Printing Office, Dec. 1978), p. 102.

35. P.T. Piotrow et al., "IUDs—Update on Safety, Effectiveness and Research," *Population Reports,* Series B, no. 3 (May 1979), p. B-57 (table).

36. Liskin and Fox, p. B-114.

37. Liskin and Fox, p. B-107.

38. U.S. Dept. of Health Education and Welfare, *Second Report,* p. 102.

39. U.S. Dept. of Health, Education and Welfare, Centers for Disease Control, "IUD Safety: Report of a Nationwide Physician Survey," *Morbidity and Mortality Weekly Report* 23 (July 5, 1974), pp. 226–31.

40. Piotrow et al., pp. B-57 (table) and B-64.

41. Piotrow et al., pp. B-64–67.

42. Piotrow et al., p. B-65.

43. Robert A. Hatcher, *Contraceptive Technology, 1982–1983,* 11th rev. ed. (New York: Irvington Pub., Inc., 1982), p. 85.

44. Robert A. Hatcher, "Commentary," *Contraceptive Technology Update* (April 1980), p. 15.

45. Liskin and Fox, pp. 123–24.

46. Liskin and Fox, pp. 123–24.

47. Liskin and Fox, pp. 123-24.

48. Piotrow et al., pp. B-57 (table) and B-64.

49. C. Tietze and S. Lewit, "Evaluation of Intrauterine Devices: Ninth Progress Report of the Cooperative Statistical Program," *Studies in Family Planning* 55 (July 1970), pp. 1-40.

50. Tietze and Lewit, pp. 1-40.

51. Piotrow et al, p. B-70 (table).

52. Piotrow et al., pp. B-70-72.

53. U.S. Dept. of Health, Education and Welfare, "Progestasert," p. 37.

54. H.J. Tatum et al., "Management and Outcome of Pregnancies Associated with the Copper-T Intrauterine Contraceptive Device," *American Journal of Obstetrics and Gynecology* 126 (Dec. 1, 1976), pp. 869-79.

55. Jennings, p. 19.

56. W. Cates et al., "The Intrauterine Device and Deaths from Spontaneous Abortion," *New England Journal of Medicine* 295 (Nov. 18, 1976), pp. 1155-59.

57. Piotrow et al., p. B-69.

58. J.F. Permutter, "Pregnancy and the IUD," *Journal of Reproductive Medicine* 20 (1978) p. 133.

59. G.T. Alvior, Jr., "Pregnancy Outcome with Removal of the Intrauterine Device," *Obstetrics and Gynecology* 41:6 (June 1973), pp. 894-96.

60. R.M. Shine and J.F. Thompson, "The In Situ IUD and Pregnancy Outcome," *American Journal of Obstetrics and Gynecology* 119:1 (May 1, 1974), pp. 124-30.

61. Permutter, pp. 133-37.

62. H. Barrie, "Congenital Malformation Associated with Intrauterine Contraceptive Device," *British Medical Journal* 1 (1976), pp. 488-90.

63. Tatum et al., pp. 869-79.

64. Tietze and Lewitt, pp. 1-40, and S.J. Segal and C. Tietze, "Contraceptive Technology: Current and Prospective Methods," *Reports on Population/Family Planning*, no. 1 (July 1971), pp. 1-24.

65. Vessey et al., "Fertility," pp. 265-67.

66. A.K. Jain and B. Moots, "Fecundability Following the Discontinuation of IUD Use Among Taiwanese Women," *Journal of Biosocial Science* 9(2) (1977), pp. 135-51.

67. V.E. Johnson and W.H. Masters, "Intravaginal Contraceptive Study, Phase II: Physiology," *Western Journal of Surgery, Obstetrics and Gynecology* 71 (May-June 1963), pp. 144-53.

68. U.S. Dept. of Health, Education and Welfare, Food and Drug Administration, "Comparing the Options," HEW Publication no. (FDA) 78-3069.

69. M. Vessey and P. Wiggins, "Use-Effectiveness of the Diaphragm in a Selected Family-Planning Clinic Population in the United Kingdom," *Contraception* 9:1 (Jan. 1974), pp. 15-21.

70. M. Lane, R. Arleo and A.J. Soberero, "Successful Use of the Diaphragm and Jelly by a Young Population: Report of a Clinical Study," *Family Planning Perspectives* 8:2 (1976), pp. 81-86.

71. Lane, Arleo and Soberero, pp. 81-86.

72. D.W. Beacham and W.D. Beacham, *Synopsis of Gynecology* (St. Louis: C.V. Mosby, 1972), pp. 351–66.

73. M.R. Melamed et al., "Prevalence Rates of Uterine Cervical Carcinoma in Situ for Women Using the Diaphragm or Contraceptive Steroids," *British Medical Journal* 3 (1969), pp. 195–200; and

N.H. Wright et al., "Neoplasia and Dysplasia of the Cervix Uteri and Contraception: A Possible Protective Effect of the Diaphragm," *British Journal of Cancer* 38:2 (Aug. 1978), pp. 273–79.

74. "Seven Year Prospective Study of 17,000 Women Using the Pill, IUD and Diaphragm," *Family Planning Perspectives* 8:5 (1976), pp. 241–48.

75. B. Singh et al., "Studies on the Development of a Vaginal Preparation Providing Both Prophylaxis Against Venereal Disease and Other Genital Infections and Contraception II: Effect in Vitro of Vaginal Contraceptive and Noncontraceptive Preparations on *Treponema pallidum* and *Neisseria gonorrhoeae*," *British Journal of Venereal Diseases* 48 (1972), pp. 51–64.

76. Masters and Johnson, pp. 144–53.

77. Masters and Johnson, pp. 144–53.

78. Hatcher et al.; see addendum in front of the 9th rev. ed.

79. M.E. Panragua, "Field Trial of a Contraceptive Foam in Puerto Rico," *Journal of the American Medical Association* 177 (1961), p. 125.

80. G. Carpenter and J. Martin, "Clinical Evaluation of a Contraceptive Foam," *Advances in Planned Parenthood* (New York: Excerpta Medical Foundation, 1970), pp. 170–78.

81. Seaman and Seaman, p. 202. Note: The authors are quoting from a personal communication with Drs. Howard and Joy Osofsky.

82. G.S. Bernstein, "Clinical Effectiveness of an Aerosol Contraceptive Foam," *Contraception* 3 (1971), pp. 37–43.

83. B. Vaughan et al., "Contraceptive Failure Among Married Women in the United States, 1970–73," *Family Planning Perspectives* 9:6 (Nov.–Dec. 1977), pp. 251–58.

84. N.B. Ryder, "Contraceptive Failure in the United States," *Family Planning Perspectives* 5 (1973), pp. 133–42.

85. S. Coleman and P. Piotrow, "Spermicides—Simplicity and Safety Are Major Assets," *Population Reports*, Series H, no. 5 (Sept. 1979), p. H-95 (table).

86. Singh et al., pp. 57–64.

87. B. Postic et al., "Inactivation of Clinical Isolites of Herpes Virus Hominis, Types 1 and 2, by Chemical Contraceptives," *Sexually Transmitted Diseases* 5 (Jan.–Mar. 1978), pp. 22–24.

88. Hatcher et al., 11th rev. ed., p. 117.

89. H. Jick et al, "Vaginal Spermicides and Congenital Disorders," *Journal of the American Medical Association* 245 (1981), p. 1329.

90. Hatcher et al., 11th rev. ed., p. 117.

91. J.L. Mills et al., "Are Spermicides Peratenatogenic?" *Journal of the American Medical Association* 248 (Nov. 1982), pp. 2148–51.

92. G.W. Beebe, *Contraception and Fertility in the Southern Appalachians* (Baltimore: Williams and Wilkins, 1974), p. 274.

93. J. Peel, "A Male-Oriented Fertility-Control Experiment," *Practitioner* 202 (1969), pp. 677–81.

94. M. Potts and J. McDevitt, "A Use-Effectiveness Trial of Spermicidally Lubricated Condoms," *Contraception* 11:6 (1975), pp. 701–10.

95. U.S. Supreme Court, Decision of June 6, 1977.

96. Press release, Young Drug Products Corporation, Oct. 5, 1978.

97. D. Barlow, "The Condom and Gonorrhea," *Lancet* 2:8042 (Oct. 15, 1977), pp. 811–13.

98. "Condom Sales Rise in Sweden, VD Falls," *Obstetrics and Gynecology News* 8:15 (Aug. 1, 1973), p. 9.

99. Jacqueline D. Shennis, Ph.D., et al., "Update on Condoms," *Population Reports*, Series H, no. 6, (Sept./Oct., 1982) pp. 130–31.

100. A.C. Richardson and J.B. Lyon, "The Effect of Condom Use on Squamous Cell Cervical Intraepithelial Neoplasia," *The American Journal of Obstetrics and Gynecology* 140 (1981), p. 909.

101. Shennis, p. H-130.

102. "FDA Approves Vaginal Sponge as a Contraceptive Device," *Contraceptive Technology Update*, May 1983, pp. 51–53.

103. M. Lane, et al., "Successful use of the Diaphragm and Jelly by a Young Population," *Family Planning Perspectives* 8:2 (1976), pp. 81–86.

104. "FDA Approves Vaginal Sponge . . .", pp. 51–53.

105. "FDA Approves Vaginal Sponge . . .", pp. 51–53.

106. "FDA Prepares Response to Questions on Sponge Safety," *Contraceptive Technology Update*, Sept. 1983, p. 103.

107. "FDA Prepares Response," p. 103.

108. "FDA Prepares Response," p. 103.

109. Planned Parenthood Federation of America, Medical Committee, *Methods of Birth Control in the United States* (New York: Planned Parenthood Federation of America, 1972), p. 41.

110. C. Tietze et al., "The Effectiveness of the Cervical Cap as a Contraceptive Method," *American Journal of Obstetrics and Gynecology* 66 (1953), pp. 904–8.

111. Renee Potick, "Informed Consent," patient handout on the cervical cap.

112. "Consult an Expert: What Is U.S. Status of Cervical Cap?" *Contraceptive Technology Update*, Aug. 1980, pp. 67–68.

113. "Vimule Cap Causes Lesions in Users," *Contraceptive Technology Update*, June 1980, pp. 69–70.

114. "Barrier Methods: Questions Still Need Answers," *Contraceptive Technology Update*, March 1982, pp. 32–33.

115. "Barrier Methods," pp. 32–33.

116. Personal communication with Dr. Robert Goeppe.

117. "Cervical Cap to Undergo New Clinical Trials," *Contraceptive Technology Update*, Nov. 1982, pp. 141–42.

118. Clara Ross and P.T. Piotrow, "Birth Control Without Contraceptives," *Population Reports*, Series I, no. 1 (June 1974), p. I-11 (table).

119. Ross and Piotrow, p. I-12.

120. Ross and Piotrow, p. I-33.

121. Piet H. Jongbloet and Johanna H.J. Van Erkelens-Zwets, "Rhythm Methods: Are

There Risks to Progeny," in *Controversies in Fertility Control,* ed. J. Sciarra, G. Zatuchni and J. Speidel (New York: Harper and Row, 1978), pp. 520–33.

122. Lois Bradshaw, "Vasectomy Reversibility: A Status Report," *Population Reports,* Series D, no. 3 (May 1976), p. D-49 (table).

123. Bradshaw, p. D-159.

124. Judith Wortman, "Vasectomy: What Are the Problems?" *Population Reports,* Series D, no. 2 (Jan. 1975), p. D-32.

125. Wortman, p. D-27.

126. Wortman, p. D-27.

127. Wortman, p. D-25.

128. Wortman, p. D-31, and Hatcher et al., p. 132.

129. Wortman, pp. D-33 and DD-97.

130. "Study Suggests Possible Vasectomy-Impotence Link," *Contraceptive Technology Update,* Sept. 1983, pp. 101–3.

131. "Study Suggests," pp. 101–3.

132. "Study Refutes Atherosclerosis, Vasectomy Link," *Contraceptive Technology Update,* Jan. 1983, pp. 1–3, and "Special Report: The Vasectomy and Atherosclerosis Controversy," *Contraceptive Technology Update,* May 1981, pp. 63–68.

133. Seaman and Seaman, p. 229. Note: The authors are quoting from an article written by Judith Herman, M.D., entitled "Controlling Third World Populations: Forced Sterilization," which appeared in *Sister Courage,* Feb. 1976. Similar statistics are found in literature from the Committee to End Sterilization Abuse, P.O. Box A 244—Cooper Station, NY, NY 10003.

134. Seaman and Seaman, p. 229. Note: The authors are quoting from an article sponsored by the Fund for Investigative Journalism that was written by Claudia Dreifus entitled "Sterilizing the Poor," which appeared in *The Progressive* 39:13–18, 1975.

135. Seaman and Seaman, p. 234.

136. Hatcher et al., p. 20 (table).

137. J.M. Phillips, et al., "Laparoscopic Procedures: A National Survey for 1975," *Journal of Reproductive Medicine* 18 (1975), pp. 219–26.

138. Alice M. Rothchild, M.D., testimony given at public hearings on proposed HEW Sterilization Regulations, Jan. 17, 1978.

139. Hatcher et al., 11th rev. ed., p. 196.

140. "Reasons Given for Sterilization Failures," *Contraceptive Technology Update,* Sept. 1980, pp. 79–81.

141. "Reasons Given," pp. 79–81.

142. "Ectopic Pregnancies Complicate Ligation Failures," *Contraceptive Technology Update,* Sept. 1980, pp. 81–82.

143. "Reasons Given," pp. 79–81.

144. "Half of Sterilization Failures Due to Concurrent Pregnancies," *Contraceptive Technology Update,* Oct. 1982, pp. 124–250.

145. J.R. Neil et al., "Late Complications of Sterilization by Laparoscopy and Tubal Ligation," *Lancet* 1 (Oct. 11, 1975), p. 699.

146. Supreme Court of the United States, *June Roe et al., Appellants, v. Henry Wade,* Jan. 22, 1973.

147. National Women's Health Network, *Abortion* (Washington, DC: NWHN, 1980), p. 8.

148. Supreme Court of the United States, *Planned Parenthood of Missouri v. Danforth*, July 1, 1976.

149. D.T. Liu et al., "Dilation of the Parous Non-Pregnant Cervix," *British Journal of Obstetrics and Gynecology* 82 (1975), p. 246.

150. Emiline Royco Ott, "Cervical Dilation—A Review," *Population Reports*, Series F, no. 6 (Sept. 1977), p. F-92.

151. B.N. Nathanson, "Ambulatory Abortion: Experience with 26,000 Cases," *New England Journal of Medicine* 286 (1972), pp. 403–7.

152. Hatcher et al., p. 119.

153. Centers for Disease Control, *Abortion Surveillance 1976*, HEW Publication no. (CDC) 78-8205, 1978.

154. Ott, p. F-94.

155. Susan L. Chaudry, "Pregnancy Termination in Midtrimester—A Review of the Major Methods," *Population Reports*, Series F, no. 5 (Sept. 1976), p. F-69.

156. Chaudry, pp. F-69–70.

157. Chaudry, pp. F-72–74.

158. Chaudry, pp. F-77–79.

159. Chaudry, p. F-76.

160. Y. Moriyama and O. Hirokawa, "The Relationship Between Artificial Termination of Pregnancy and Abortion of Premature Birth," *Harmful Effects of Induced Abortion*, The Family Planning Federation of Japan, 1966, and L.H. Roht and H. Aoyama, "Induced Abortions and Its Sequels: Prematurity and Spontaneous Abortion," *American Journal of Obstetrics and Gynecology* 120, 1974, pp. 868–74.

161. "Repeat Abortions Increase Risk of Miscarriage, Premature Births and Low-Birth-Weight Babies," *Family Planning Perspectives* 11 (Jan.–Feb. 1979), pp. 39–40.

162. A.A. Levin et al. "Ectopic Pregnancy and Prior Induced Abortion," *American Journal of Public Health* 72 (1982), p. 253, and Emiline Ott, "Pregnancy Termination," *Population Reports*, Series F, no. 6 (Sept. 1977).

163. "Technique, Not Number of Abortions, Affects Future Pregnancy Outcome," *Contraceptive Technology Update*, May 1981, p. 62.

164. "Technique, Not Number, p. 62.

165. "Technique, Not Number," p. 62.

166. "Technique, Not Number," p. 62.

167. "Technique, Not Number," P. 62.

168. "Technique, Not Number," p. 62.

169. Hatcher et al., p. 103.

170. Hatcher et al., p. 103.

171. Ward Rinehart, "Postcoital Contraception—An Appraisal," *Population Reports*, Series J, no. 9 (Jan. 1976), p. J-147.

172. Rinehart, p. J-147.

173. Rinehart, p. J-144.

174. "Ovral Touted as Morning-After Pill," *Contraceptive Technology Update*, May 1980, pp. 11–13, and "Combined Ovral Contraceptive Suggested for Morning After," *Contraceptive Technology Update*, Nov. 1982, pp. 137–38.

175. Seaman and Seaman, p. 42.

176. Rinehart, p. J-150.

Chapter Six: DEALING WITH DOCTORS

1. This bill was signed into law in November 1979. Copies are available from the State House Bookstore, Commonwealth of Massachusetts, Boston, Massachusetts 02133.
2. See Chapter One, notes 4 and 6.

Reference Section: DISEASES

THE VULVA

1. J.R. Willson, C.T. Beacham and E.R. Carrington, *Obstetrics and Gynecology,* 4th ed. (St. Louis: C.V. Mosby, 1971), p. 544.
2. There are a number of case-control studies that report increased risk for endometrial cancer in women using estrogen replacement therapy. The three most widely cited studies are:

H.K. Ziel and W.D. Finkle, "Increased Risk of Endometrial Carcinoma Among Users of Conjugated Estrogens," *New England Journal of Medicine* 293 (1975), pp. 1167–70;

D.C. Smith et al., "Association of Exogenous Estrogen and Endometrial Carcinoma," *New England Journal of Medicine* 293 (1975), pp. 1164–67; and

T.M. Mack et al., "Estrogens and Endometrial Cancer in a Retirement Community," *New England Journal of Medicine* 294 (1976), pp. 1262–67.

These findings are further supported by the fact that incidence rates of endometrial cancer have increased sharply since 1969, which may be related to the rapidly expanding use of estrogens in the past decade. See the FDA-approved package insert for all products containing estrogens for more details.

In addition, one study has indicated that women who used estrogen replacement therapy may be at increased risk for the development of breast cancer; see:

R. Hoover et al., "Menopausal Estrogens and Cancer," *New England Journal of Medicine* 295 (1976), pp. 401–5.
3. Raymond H. Kaufman, "The Management of Benign and Malignant Vulvar Lesions," *Audio-Digest, Obstetrics and Gynecology,* 23:18 (Sept. 14, 1976).
4. Kaufman, *Audio-Digest.*
5. Kaufman, *Audio-Digest.*
6. Personal communication, Dr. Raymond H. Kaufman.
7. Kaufman, *Audio-Digest.*
8. Duane E. Townsend, "Cryosurgery," *Surgical Clinics of North America* 58:1 (Feb. 1978), pp. 97–108.
9. Ernest W. Franklin, III, M.D., "Malignancy of the Vulva," In *Gynecologic Oncology* (Larry McGowan, ed.), (New York: Appleton-Century-Crofts, 1978), pp. 148–68.
10. Phillip J. Krupp, M.D., "Cancer of the Vulva," *Surgical Clinics of North America* 58:1 (Feb. 1978), pp. 19–38.
11. Franklin, pp. 148–68.
12. Franklin, pp. 148–68.

13. E.W. Franklin and F.D. Rutledge, "Epidemiology of Epidermal Carcinoma of the Vulva," *Obstetrics and Gynecology* 39 (1972), p. 165.
14. Franklin and Rutledge, p. 165.
15. Franklin, pp. 148–68.
16. The following discussion is based primarily on two sources: Franklin, pp. 148–68, and Krupp, pp. 19–38.
17. Franklin, pp. 148–68.
18. Franklin, pp. 148–68.
19. Julian P. Smith, "Chemotherapy in Gynecologic Cancer," *Surgical Clinics of North America* 58:1 (Feb. 1978), pp. 202–15.

THE VAGINA

1. K.D. Gunston and P.F. Fairbrother, "Treatment of Vaginal Discharge with Yoghurt," *South African Journal of Medicine* 49:16 (Apr. 12, 1975), pp. 675–76.
2. "Sulfa Cream Efficacy Not Proven Says FDA," *Contraceptive Technology Update* (May, 1980) pp. 28–9.
3. "Sulfa Cream Efficacy," pp. 28–9.
4. *Physician's Desk Reference,* 32nd ed., Charles Baker, ed. (New Jersey: Litton Industries, 1978), pp. 1547–48.
5. Mario Rustia and Philippe Shubik, "Induction of Lung Tumors and Malignant Lymphomas in Mice by Metronidazole," *Journal of the National Cancer Institute* 48 (1972), pp. 721–29.
6. *Physician's Desk Reference,* pp. 1547–48.
7. *Physician's Desk Reference,* pp. 1547–48.
8. Lamon E. V. Ekbladh, "The Expanding Use of Metronidazole (Flagyl)," *Audio-Digest, Obstetrics and Gynecology* 26:11 (June 5, 1979).
9. Herman L. Gardner, M.D., and W. Graham Guerriero, M.D., "Should the Male Sexual Partner Be Treated for Haemophilus or Trichomonas?" *Audio-Digest, Obstetrics and Gynecology* 26:22 (Nov. 20, 1979).
10. Gerald Bernstein, M.D., "Diagnosis and Treatment of Vaginitis," *Audio-Digest, Obstetrics and Gynecology* 26:16 (Aug. 21, 1979).
11. "Sulfa Cream Efficacy," pp. 28–9.
12. "Single Large Dose of Clotrimazole Effective in Treating Vaginal Candidiasis," *Medical World News* 23 (1982), pp. 31–32.
13. "New Success from Old Treatment for Yeast," *Contraceptive Technology Update,* Feb. 1981, pp. 22–3.
14. Bernstein, *Audio-Digest.*
15. J.H. Ferguson, "Effects of Stilbestrol on Pregnancy Compared to the Effect of a Placebo," *American Journal of Obstetrics and Gynecology* 65 (1953), pp. 592–601.
16. A.L. Herbst, H. Ulfedler and D.C. Poskanzer, "Adenocarcinoma of the Vagina," *New England Journal of Medicine* 284 (1971), pp. 878–81; P. Greenwood et al., "Vaginal Cancer After Maternal Treatment with Synthetic Estrogens," *New England Journal of Medicine* 285 (1971), pp. 390–92.
17. A number of different abnormalities have been found in DES daughters, including al-

terations in the shape of the cervix, lowered fertility and irregular menstrual periods. Testis cysts, underdeveloped or undescended testes, abnormally placed urinary openings, low sperm counts, abnormally shaped sperm cells and impaired fertility have been reported in DES sons. For further information, see:

R. Mattingly and A. Stafl, "Cancer Risk in DES-Exposed Offspring," *Journal of Obstetrics and Gynecology* 128 (1977), pp. 43–50;

R. Kaufman et al., "Upper Genital Tract Changes Associated with Exposure in Utero to Diethylstilbestrol," *American Journal of Obstetrics and Gynecology* 128 (1977), pp. 51–59; and

M. Bibbo et al., "Follow-up Study of Male and Female Offspring of DES-Exposed Mothers," *Obstetrics and Gynecology* 49:1 (1977), pp. 1–8.

18. U.S. Dept. of Health, Education and Welfare, Food and Drug Administration, "DES and Breast Cancer," *FDA Drug Bulletin* 8 (Mar.–Apr. 1978), p. 10.

19. Registry for Clear Cell Adenocarcinoma of the Genital Tract in Young Women, Boston, Massachusetts, 1977 Report.

20. Anne P. Lanier et al., "Cancer and Stilbestrol, A Follow-up of 1,719 Persons Exposed to Estrogens in Utero 1943–1959," *Mayo Clinic Proceedings* 48 (1973), p. 793;

A Stafl et al., "Clinical Diagnosis of Vaginal Adenosis," *Journal of Obstetrics and Gynecology* 43 (1974), pp. 118–28;

Sherman et al., "Cervical and Vaginal Adenosis After in Utero Exposure to Synthetic Estrogens," *Journal of Obstetrics and Gynecology* 44 (1974), pp. 531–45; and

A.L. Herbst et al., "Pre-natal Exposure to Stilbestrol," *New England Journal of Medicine* 292 (1975), pp. 334–39.

21. Herbst et al., pp. 334–39.

22. M.S. Singer et al., "Incompetent Cervix in a Hormone-Exposed Offspring," *Obstetrics and Gynecology* 51:5 (May 1978), pp. 625–26.

23. Kaufman et al., pp. 51–59.

24. Bibbo et al., pp. 1–8, and Singer et al., pp. 51–59.

25. Herbst, Ulfedler and Poskanzer, pp. 878–81.

26. Registry for Clear Cell Adenocarcinoma, 1977 Report.

27. H. Ulfedler, "Stilbestrol, Adenosis and Adenocarcinoma," *American Journal of Obstetrics and Gynecology* 117 (1973), p. 795.

28. P.C. O'Brien et al., "Vaginal Epithelial Changes in Young Women Enrolled in the National Cooperative Diethylstilbestrol Adenosis (DESAD) Project," *Obstetrics and Gynecology,* vol. 53:3 (Mar. 1979), pp. 300–8.

29. William C. Fetherston, "Squamous Neoplasia Related to DES Syndrome," *American Journal of Obstetrics and Gynecology* 122 (May 15, 1975), pp. 176–80;
Mattingly and Stafl, p. 543; and
Sherman et al., pp. 531–45.

30. Mattingly and Stafl, p. 543.

31. A.B.P. Ng et al., "Natural History of Vaginal Adenosis in Women Exposed to Diethylstilbestrol in Utero," *Journal of Reproductive Medicine* 18:1 (1977), pp. 1–13.

32. Registry for Clear Cell Adenocarcinoma, 1977 Report.

33. Herbst, Ulfedler and Poskanzer, pp. 878–81.

34. S.N. Hajj and A.L. Herbst, "Evaluation and Management of Diethylstilbestrol Exposed Offspring," *Surgical Clinics of North America* 58:1 (Feb. 1978), pp. 87–96.

35. A case can be made for radiation over surgery in some instances. When the tumor is small, some doctors will remove only the tumor itself. A section of the cervix usually is removed as well, by way of an operation known as conization, a process somewhat akin to removing the core of an apple. The tissue is then examined microscopically. If the lab report indicates that there is no cervical invasion, these doctors will then treat the remaining, hidden disease with a special needle-type of internal radiation, which is less destructive. The ovaries may, in some cases, be preserved. In one case a pregnant woman so treated delivered a baby by cesarean section and also completed two more pregnancies in which apparently normal babies were delivered. However, the radiation damage to the ovaries can produce birth defects, including retardation, so many experts are wary of pregnancy after radiation to the ovaries.

Since less radiation is involved, the risk of radiation-induced cancer should be less, and in some cases the vagina may be able to function normally. The main risk that a woman takes in selecting this form of treatment is that the cancer may have already spread to areas beyond the scope of this more restricted type of treatment. Thus some experts are hesitant about using it.

36. Robert C. Park and Tim H. Parmley, "Vaginal Cancer," in *Gynecologic Oncology,* Larry McGowan, ed. (New York: Appleton-Century-Crofts, 1978), pp. 174–84.

37. Robert D. Hilgers, M.D., "Squamous Cell Carcinoma of the Vagina," *Surgical Clinics of North America* 58:1 (Feb. 1978), pp. 25–38.

38. Hilgers, pp. 25–38.

39. Hilgers, pp. 25–38.

40. Hilgers, pp. 25–38.

41. Park and Parmley, pp. 174–84.

42. Luther W. Brady, M.D., "Radiation Therapy for Carcinoma of the Vagina," in *Gynecologic Oncology,* Larry McGowan, ed. (New York: Appleton-Century-Crofts, 1978), pp. 185–90.

43. Duane E. Townsend, M.D., "Cryosurgery," *Surgical Clinics of North America* 58:1 (Feb. 1978), pp. 97–108.

44. Helmut F. Schellhas, "Laser Surgery in Gynecology," *Surgical Clinics of North America* 58:1 (Feb. 1978), pp. 151–66.

45. Park and Parmley, pp. 174–84, and Julian P. Smith, "Chemotherapy in Gynecologic Cancer," *Surgical Clinics of North America* 58:1 (Feb. 1978), pp. 201–15.

THE CERVIX

1. William L. Benson and Henry J. Norris, "Current Problems in Gynecologic Pathology," in *Gynecologic Oncology,* Larry McGowan, ed. (New York: Appleton-Century-Crofts, 1978), pp. 7–36, and Richard A. Malmgren, "Cytopathology," in *Gynecologic Oncology,* pp. 37–69.

2. In addition to the standard texts used as sources throughout this book (see Chapter Six), the following sources were used in the preparation of this discussion:

William T. Creasman, "Outpatient Management of CIN," *Audio-Digest, Obstetrics and Gynecology* 26:11 (June 5, 1979), Side B;

Henry Clay Frick, II, M.D., "Management of Non-Invasive Carcinoma of the Cervix," *Surgical Clinics of North America* 58:1 (Feb. 1978), pp. 55–60;

Raymond H. Kaufman and John F. Irwin, "The Cryosurgical Therapy of Cervical Intraepithelial Neoplasia," *American Journal of Obstetrics and Gynecology* 131 (1978), p. 381 (Note: This same study is reported in Irwin, *Audio-Digest* 25:1 (Jan. 10, 1978);

John Irwin, "Cryosurgical Therapy of CIN," *Audio-Digest, Obstetrics and Gynecology* 25:1 (Jan. 10, 1978);

George W. Morely et al., "Diagnosis and Treatment of Vulvar and Cervical Lesions," *Audio-Digest, Obstetrics and Gynecology* 23:18 (Sept. 14, 1976), Side B; and

Duane E. Townsend, "Cryosurgery," *Surgical Clinics of North America* 58:1 (Feb. 1978), pp. 97–108.

3. "Physician Recommends Condom for Cervical Dysplasia Therapy," *Contraceptive Technology Update,* Jan. 1983, pp. 10–11.

4. "Physician Recommends," pp. 10–11.

5. See Note 2 above.

6. David M. Mumford, Raymond H. Kaufman and Nancy McCormick, "Immunity, Herpes Simplex Virus and Cervical Carcinoma," *Surgical Clinics of North America* 58:1 (Feb. 1978), pp. 39–54.

7. Mumford, Kaufman and McCormick, pp. 39–54.

8. Robert A. Hatcher et al., *Contraceptive Technology 1982–1983,* 11th rev. ed. (New York: Irvington Publications, 1982), p. 103.

9. Hatcher et al., p. 114.

10. Mumford, Kaufman, McCormick, pp. 39–54. Note: The authors provide an excellent summary of the evidence regarding herpes virus and cervical cancer. Specific citations are included in the article.

11. J. Schachter et al., "Chlamydial Trachomatis and Cervical Dysplasia," *Journal of the American Medical Association* 248 (1982), p. 2134.

12. J.D. Buckley et al., "Case Controlled Study of Husbands of Women with Dysplasia or Carcinoma in Situ of the Cervix Uteri," *Lancet* 2 (1981), pp. 1010–14.

13. Elizabeth Stern et al., "Steroid Contraceptive Use and Cervical Dysplasia," *Science* 196 (1977), p. 1460, and M.D. Vessey et al., "Neoplasia of the Cervix Uteri and Contraception," *Lancet,* Oct. 1983, pp. 930–34.

14. Howard W. Jones, "Recurrent Cervical Cancer," *Audio-Digest, Obstetrics and Gynecology* 26:18 (Sept. 18, 1979).

15. John B. Schlaerth, "Early Invasive Cervical Cancer," *Audio-Digest, Obstetrics and Gynecology* 26:18 (Sept. 18, 1979).

16. Luther W. Brady, "Radiotherapy Treatment of Cervical Cancer," in *Gynecologic Oncology,* Larry McGowan, ed. (New York: Appleton-Century-Crofts, 1978), pp. 217–33.

17. Schlaerth, *Audio-Digest.*

18. Schlaerth, *Audio-Digest.*

19. J.R. van Nagell, Jr., E.S. Donaldson and E.C. Gay, "Evaluation and Treatment of Patients with Invasive Cervical Cancer," *Surgical Clinics of North America* 58:1 (Feb. 1978), pp. 67–86, and Schlaerth, *Audio-Digest.*

20. Hugh R.K. Barber, "Cervical Cancer," in *Gynecologic Oncology,* Larry McGowan, ed. (New York: Appleton-Century-Crofts, 1978), pp. 202–16; and van Nagell, Donaldson and Gay, pp. 67–89.

21. E. Burghardt and E. Holzer, "Diagnosis and Treatment of Microinvasive Carcinoma of the Cervix Uteri," *Journal of the American College of Obstetricians and Gynecologists*

49:6 (June 1977), pp. 641–52; Barber, pp. 202–16; and van Nagell, Donaldson and Gay, pp. 67–89.

22. van Nagell, Donaldson and Gay, pp. 67–89.

23. Burghardt and Holzer, pp. 641–52.

24. The discussion of treatment is based on the discussions in Barber, pp. 202–26, and van Nagell, Donaldson and Gay, pp. 67–89.

25. Barber, pp. 67–89.

THE UTERUS AND THE FALLOPIAN TUBES

1. "Rates of Ectopic Pregnancy, Sterility Follow PID Rise," *Contraceptive Technology Update,* May 1980, pp. 17–19.

2. "Rates of Ectopic Pregnancy," pp. 17–19.

3. "Rates of Ectopic Pregnancy," pp. 17–19.

4. "Rates of Ectopic Pregnancy," pp. 17–19.

5. "Rates of Ectopic Pregnancy," pp. 17–19.

6. "Rates of Ectopic Pregnancy," pp. 17–19.

7. "Rates of Ectopic Pregnancy," pp. 17–19.

8. "Rates of Ectopic Pregnancy," pp. 17–19.

9. Robert A. Hatcher, "Commentary," *Contraceptive Technology Update* June 1980, p. 38.

10. IUD patient package insert.

11. "Contraceptive Choice Can Affect PID Risk," *Contraceptive Technology Update,* June 1980, pp. 35–37.

12. "Contraceptive Choice," pp. 35–37.

13. In addition to the standard medical texts used as references throughout this book (see Chapter Six), the information about the treatment of endometriosis given here is derived primarily from three sources:

    1. A roundtable discussion that involved a number of experts, including John A. Berger (assistant clinical professor, University of California School of Medicine), L. Russell Malinak (associate professor, Baylor College of Medicine), Jaroslav J. Marik (director of the Tyler Medical Clinic and assistant professor, University of California, Los Angeles), George T. Schneider (associate chairman, Ochsner Medical Center, and professor, Louisiana State University School of Medicine) and Samuel B. Ganz (editorial board of *Patient Care*). A version of this discussion, edited by Marion E. Prilook and entitled "Endometriosis: New Views, New Therapies," appeared in *Patient Care,* Nov. 15, 1978, pp. 24–96. (Specific citations are included at the end of this article.)

    2. A talk on infertility problems and endometriosis given by Dr. L. Russell Malinak and recorded on *Audio-Digest, Obstetrics and Gynecology* 26:8 (Apr. 1979).

    3. Product information supplied by the manufacturers of Danocrin that appears in *Physician's Desk Reference,* 32nd ed. (New Jersey: Litton Industries, 1978), p. 1782.

14. J. Phillips et al., "Laparoscopic Procedures: A National Survey for 1975," *Journal of Reproductive Medicine* 18 (1977), pp. 219–26.

15. W.P. Donowski and M.R. Cohen, "Antigonadotropin (danazol) in the Treatment of

Endometriosis—Evaluation of Post-Treatment Fertility and Three Year Follow-up Data,'' *American Journal of Obstetrics and Gynecology* 130 (1978), pp. 41–48.

16. R.S. Schenken and L.R. Malinak, ''Reoperation After Initial Treatment of Endometriosis with Conservative Surgery,'' *American Journal of Gynecology* 131 (1978), pp. 416–21.

17. William Benson and Henry Norris, ''Current Problems in Gynecologic Pathology,'' in *Gynecologic Oncology,* Larry McGowan, ed. (New York: Appleton-Century-Crofts. 1978), p. 20.

18. P. Greenwald, T.A. Caputo and P.E. Wolfgang, ''Endometrial Cancer After the Menopausal Use of Estrogens,'' *Obstetrics and Gynecology* 50 (1977), pp. 239–43.

19. D.W. Cramer and S.J. Cutler, ''Incidence and Histopathology of Malignancies of the Female Genital Organs in the United States,'' *American Journal of Obstetrics and Gynecology* 118 (1974), p. 443.

20. P.K. Silteri, B.E. Schwarz and P.C. MacDonald, ''Estrogen Receptors and Estrone Hypothesis in Relation to Endometrial and Breast Cancer,'' *Gynecologic Oncology* 2 (1974), p. 228.

21. U.S. Department of Health, Education and Welfare, Food and Drug Administration, ''Sequential Oral Contraceptives Removed from the Market,'' *FDA Drug Bulletin* 6 (1976), p. 26, and H.W. Kelley et al., ''Adenocarcinoma of the Endometrium in Women Taking Sequential Oral Contraceptives,'' *Obstetrics and Gynecology* 47 (1976), p. 200.

22. There are a number of case-control studies that report increased risk for endometrial cancer in women using menopausal estrogens. The three most widely cited studies are:

H.K. Ziel and W.D. Finkle, ''Increased Risk of Endometrial Carcinoma Among Users of Conjugated Estrogens,'' *New England Journal of Medicine* 293 (1975), pp. 1167–70;

D.C. Smith et al., ''Association of Exogenous Estrogen and Endometrial Carcinoma,'' *New England Journal of Medicine* 293 (1975), pp. 1164–67; and

T.M. Mack et al., ''Estrogens and Endometrial Cancer in a Retirement Community,'' *New England Journal of Medicine* 294 (1976), pp. 1262–67.

These findings are further supported by the fact that incidence rates of endometrial cancer have increased sharply since 1969, which may be related to the rapidly expanding use of estrogens in the past decade. See the FDA-approved package insert for all products containing estrogens for more details.

23. B. MacMahon, ''Risk Factors for Endometrial Cancer,'' *Gynecologic Oncology* 2 (1974), p. 239, and S.F. Gosberg, ''The Individual at High Risk for Endometrial Carcinoma,'' *American Journal of Obstetrics and Gynecology* 126 (1976), p. 535.

24. The staging scheme here is an adaptation of the classification and staging of malignant tumors from the International Federation of Gynaecology and Obstetrics, 1971, which is accepted by the American College of Obstetricians and Gynecologists.

25. J. Taylor Warton and Gilbert H. Fletcher, ''The Principle of Radiation Therapy for Malignant Pelvic Lesions,'' *Surgical Clinics of North America* 58:1 (Feb. 1978), pp. 181–200.

26. G. Malkasian, T.W. McDonald and J.H. Pratt, ''Carcinoma of the Endometrium,'' *Mayo Clinic Proceedings* 52 (1977), p. 175.

27. Larry McGowan, M.D., ''Endometrial Cancer,'' in *Gynecologic Oncology,* Larry McGowan, ed. (New York: Appleton-Century-Crofts, 1978), pp. 238–57.

28. McGowan, pp. 238–57.

29. John G. Maier, "Radiotherapy Treatment of Endometrial Cancer," in *Gynecologic Oncology,* Larry McGowan, ed. (New York: Appleton-Century-Crofts, 1978), pp. 258–65.

30. Maier, pp. 258–65.

31. John G. Boutselis, "Endometrial Carcinoma: Prognostic Factors and Treatment," *Surgical Clinics of North America* 58:1 (Feb. 1958), pp. 109–19.

32. In addition to the standard medical texts used as references throughout this book (see Chapter Six), the information about the treatment of Stage IA, Grade 2 and 3, Stage IB and Stage II is derived from Boutselis, pp. 109–19; Maier, pp. 258–65; and McGowan, pp. 238–57.

33. In addition to the standard medical texts used as references throughout this book (see Chapter Six), the information about the treatment of Stage III and IV is derived from Boutselis, pp. 109–19; Maier, pp. 258–65; McGowan, pp. 238–57; and Staffan R.B. Nodquist, "Advanced Endometrial Carcinoma," *Audio-Digest, Obstetrics and Gynecology* 26:18 (Sept. 18, 1979).

34. Richard H. Nalick, "Recurrent Endometrial Cancer," *Audio-Digest, Obstetrics and Gynecology* 26:18 (Sept. 18, 1979).

35. Nalick, *Audio-Digest.*

36. Alexander Sedlis, M.D., "Carcinoma of the Fallopian Tube," *Surgical Clinics of North America* 58:1 (Feb. 1978), pp. 121–29.

37. Robert C. Park, M.D., and Tim H. Parmley, M.D., "Fallopian Tube Cancer," in *Gynecologic Oncology,* Larry McGowan, ed. (New York: Appleton-Century-Crofts, 1978), pp. 274–80.

38. Sedlis, pp. 121–29.

39. Sedlis, pp. 121–29.

40. Sedlis, pp. 121–29.

THE OVARIES

1. Richard H. Nalick, "The Pelvic Mass: Diagnosis," *Audio-Digest, Obstetrics and Gynecology,* 26:1 (Jan. 23, 1979).

2. "Should OC's Be Prescribed to Prevent Adnexal Masses?" *Contraceptive Technology Update,* Sept. 1982, pp. 116–18.

3. W.J. Spanos, "Preoperative Hormonal Therapy of Cystic Adnexal Masses," *American Journal of Obstetrics and Gynecology* 116 (1973), pp. 551–58.

4. H. Shapiro and S. Erron, "A Novel Use of Spironolactone," *Journal of Clinical Endocrinology and Metabolism* 51 (1980), pp. 429–32.

5. John J. Mikuta, "Primary Ovarian Cancer," *Audio-Digest, Obstetrics and Gynecology* 24:22 (Nov. 15, 1977).

6. Richard K. Kleppinger, "Ovarian Cyst Fenestration by Laparoscopy," *Audio-Digest, Obstetrics and Gynecology* 26:11 (June 5, 1979).

7. Larry McGowan, "Ovarian Cancer," in *Gynecological Oncology,* Larry McGowan, ed. (New York: Appleton-Century-Crofts, 1978), pp. 283–331.

8. D.W. Cramer and S.J. Cutler, "Incidence and Histopathology of Malignancies of the

Female Genital Organs in the United States," *American Journal of Obstetrics and Gynecology* 118 (1974), p. 443.

9. Brian MacMahon, M.D., Philip Cole, M.D., and Jones Brown, Ph.D., "Etiology of Human Breast Cancer: A Review," *Journal of the National Cancer Institute* 50 (1973), pp. 21–42.

10. C. Paul Morrow, "Advanced Ovarian Cancer: Treatment," *Audio-Digest, Obstetrics and Gynecology* 26:2 (Jan. 23, 1979).

11. C. Paul Morrow, *Audio-Digest.*

12. McGowan, pp. 283–331.

13. McGowan, pp. 283–331.

14. John B. Schlaerth, "Early Ovarian Cancer: Treatment," *Audio-Digest, Obstetrics and Gynecology* 26:2 (Jan. 23. 1979).

15. Ronald R. Reimer et al., "Acute Leukemia After Alkylating Agent Therapy of Ovarian Carcinoma," *New England Journal of Medicine* 297 (July 28, 1977), pp. 177–81.

16. This study found that, overall, a woman with ovarian cancer has 21 times the normal risk of developing acute leukemia, a cancer of the blood-forming tissues. If a woman has ovarian cancer and is treated with an alkylating agent, the risk rises to 36 times normal. If she has ovarian cancer, is treated with an alkylating agent and survives for longer than 2 years, her risk of developing acute leukemia jumps to 171 times normal. Women with those Stage I cancers who have adjuvant therapy are the ones who would have the best chance of surviving for longer than 2 years. They would, then, fall into this highest-risk group.

There are, however, a couple of points to be made about this study. First, if the women studied had not received any radiotherapy, they had received the alkylating agent for long periods of time—46, 84, 90 months. If they had not received the alkylating agent for long periods of time, they had received radiation therapy. Thus it is impossible to say from this data whether the alkylating agents used alone, without radiation therapy, for the shorter periods of 12 to 18 months would be as dangerous. Many doctors believe that the radiation more than the drug may be responsible for the increased rates of leukemia. The question of whether the risks are worth the benefits in Stage I cases cannot be answered at this time. In certain Stage I cases the risk may be worth the benefits. But we know that about 35 percent of women with low-grade Stage IA(1) cancers arising inside a benign ovarian cyst will eventually die of ovarian cancer. In other words, unrecognized microscopic cancer had spread before surgery. These women may have benefited from adjuvant therapy. But according to this study, we could expect that somewhere between 5 percent and 10 percent of these women would develop leukemia as the result of therapy. Further studies may indicate that this form of chemotherapy is worth the risk, but for now, some institutions, in light of this information and preliminary studies showing no increased survival in these cases regardless of whether radiation, chemotherapy, or surgery alone was used, have discontinued the use of chemotherapy in Stage I cases.

17. Schlaerth, *Audio-Digest.*

18. McGowan, pp. 283–331.

19. C. Thomas Griffiths, M.D., and Arlan F. Fuller, M.D., "Intensive Surgical and Chemotherapeutic Management of Advanced Ovarian Cancer," *Surgical Clinics of North America* 58:1 (Feb. 1978), pp. 131–42.

Robert C. Young et al., "Advanced Ovarian Adenocarcinoma: A Prospective Clinical

Trial of Melphalan (C-Pam) Versus Combination Chemotherapy," *New England Journal of Medicine* 299 (1978), p. 1261, and J. Taylor Warton, "Advanced Ovarian Cancer," *Audio-Digest, Obstetrics and Gynecology* 24:22 (Nov. 15, 1977).

Scripps Memorial Cancer Center, 17th Annual Cancer Symposium Proceedings (La Jolla, CA: Scripps Cancer Center, 1983), pp. 159–64.

20. *Scripps Memorial Cancer Center, 17th Annual Cancer Symposium,* pp. 159–64.

21. *Scripps Memorial Cancer Center, 17th Annual Cancer Symposium,*pp. 159–64.

22. Schlaerth, *Audio-Digest.*

23. Schlaerth, *Audio-Digest.*

24. Julian P. Smith, Gregorio Delgado and Felix Rutledge, "Second-Look Operations in Ovarian Carcinoma: Postchemotherapy," *Cancer* 38 (1976), p. 1438.

25. McGowan, pp. 283–331.

26. McGowan, pp. 283–331.

THE BREAST

1. Cancer Information Service, "Diagnosis and Treatment of Breast Cancer," Fact Sheet from CIS.

2. American Cancer Society, *1977 Facts and Figures* (New York: ACS, 1977).

3. P. Greenwald, M.D., et al., "Estimated Effect of Breast Self-Examination on Breast Cancer Mortality," *New England Journal of Medicine* 299 (1978), pp. 271–73.

4. V.K. Frantz et al., "Incidence of Chronic Cystic Disease in So-called Normal Breasts: A Study Based on 225 Postmortem Examinations," *Cancer* 4 (1951), pp. 762–82.

5. Oliver Cope, M.D., *The Breast: Its Problems—Benign and Malignant—and How to Deal with Them* (Boston: Houghton-Mifflin Co., 1977), p. 24.

6. Brian MacMahon, M.D., Philip Cole, M.D., and James Brown, Ph.D., "Etiology of Human Breast Cancer: A Review," *Journal of the National Cancer Institute* 50 (1973), pp. 21–42.

7. Personal Communication, Dr. Peter Schick.

8. Sarah Hainline et al., "Mammographic Patterns and Risk of Breast Cancer," *American Journal of Roentgenology* 130 (June 1978), pp. 1157–58;

John N. Wolfe, M.D., "Breast Parenchymal Patterns: Prevalent and Incident Carcinomas," *Radiology* 131 (April 1979), pp. 267–68; and

John N. Wolfe, M.D., "Risk for Breast Cancer Development," *Cancer* 37:5 (May 1976), pp. 2486–92.

9. J.P. Minton et al., "Response of Fibrocystic Disease to Caffeine Withdrawal and the Correlation of Cystic Nucleotides with Breast Disease," *American Journal of Obstetrics and Gynecology* 135:1 (Sept. 1, 1979), pp. 157–58.

10. M. Blichert-Toft, M.D., et al., "Treatment of Mastagia with Bromocriptive: A Double-Blind Cross-Over Study," *British Medical Journal* 1 (1979), p. 237.

11. Val Davajan, M.D., "Management of Amenorrheas and Galactorrhea," *Audio-Digest, Obstetrics and Gynecology* 26:20 (Oct. 23, 1979).

12. Davajan, *Audio-Digest.*

13. Davajan, *Audio-Digest.*

14. Davajan, *Audio-Digest.*

15. American Cancer Society, *1977 Facts and Figures.*

16. U.S. Department of Health, Education and Welfare, *The Breast Cancer Digest* (Washington, DC: U.S. Govt. Printing Office, 1979), p. 4.

17. Henry P. Lease, "Breast Cancer," *Audio-Digest, Obstetrics and Gynecology* 22:7 (April 8, 1975).

18. Rose Kushner, *Why Me? What Every Woman Should Know About Breast Cancer to Save Her Life* (New York: Signet, 1977), pp. 77–98.

19. MacMahon, Cole and Brown, pp. 21–42. (Unless noted otherwise, the information on risk and cause is derived from this source.)

20. Personal communication, Dr. Peter Schick.

21. Hainline et al., pp. 1157–58; Wolfe, pp. 267–68; and Wolfe, pp. 2486–92.

22. R. Hoover et al., "Menopausal Estrogens and Cancer," *New England Journal of Medicine* 295 (1976), pp. 401–5.

23. U.S. Dept. of Health, Education and Welfare, Public Health Service, National Institutes of Health, *Survival for Cancer of the Breast*, DHEW Publication no. (NIH) 78-1542, p. 5 (table).

24. Greenwald, pp. 271–73.

25. Kushner, p. 153.

26. S. Schwartz, *Textbook of Surgery,* Vol. I (New York: McGraw-Hill, 1974), p. 532.

27. Personal communication, Dr. Peter Schick.

28. Oliver H. Beahrs, M.D., "Report of the Working Group to Review the National Cancer Institute—American Cancer Society Breast Cancer Demonstration Projects," *Journal of the National Cancer Institute* 62:3 (March 1979), pp. 640–709.

29. Sidney M. Wolfe, M.D., and Rebecca Warner, *Mammography: A Case for Informed Consent* (Washington, DC: Health Research Group, Nov. 1976).

30. John C. Bailer, M.D., "Mammography: A Contrary View," *Annals of Internal Medicine* 84 (1976), pp. 72–84.

31. Beahrs, pp. 640–709.

32. George M. Walker II, M.D., et al., "Breast Biopsy: A Comparison of Outpatient and Inpatient Experience," *Archives of Surgery* 113 (1978), pp. 942–46.

33. Schwartz, p. 443.

34. Several studies have supported this conclusion, including C.D. Haagensen, "Role of the Detection of Breast Disease," in *Diseases of the Breast* (Philadelphia: W.B. Saunders Co., 1971), p. 99;

P.P. Jackson and H.H. Pitts, "Biopsy with Delayed Radical Mastectomy for Carcinoma of the Breast," *American Journal of Surgery* 98 (1959), pp. 184–89;

E.H. Pierce et al., "Biopsy of the Breast Followed by Delayed Radical Mastectomy," *Surgery, Gynecology and Obstetrics* 103 (1956), pp. 559–64; and

A. Scheel, "Some Prognostic Factors, Particularly Biopsy, in Carcinoma of the Breast," *Acta Radial* 39 (1953), pp. 249–54.

35. "Special Report: Treatment of Primary Breast Cancer," *New England Journal of Medicine* 301:6 (Aug. 9, 1979), p. 340.

36. Bernard Fisher, M.D., Carol Redmond, Sc.D., and Edwin R. Fisher, M.D., "Clinical Trials and the Surgical Treatment of Breast Cancer," *Surgical Clinics of North America* 58:4 (Aug. 1978), pp. 723–36.

37. Beahrs, pp. 640–709.

38. This figure is perhaps conservative, for it assumes that the other 86 cases (of the 592 minimal cancers) that were not reviewed by the board were diagnosed correctly. On the other hand, it may be a bit high. When it was discovered that 66 cases had been misdiagnosed, yet another pathology review was done. Additional pathology slides were obtained, and it was then decided that 11 of the 66 had been diagnosed correctly in the first place and were indeed cancerous. In 5 of the 66 cases the experts said that they were now unable to decide whether or not the woman had cancer and that 2 of the 66 cases had been included by mistake, leaving only 48 mistaken diagnoses (*Washington Post,* Oct. 24, 1978). Thus the percentage of misdiagnosed cases might have been as low as about 2.5 percent.

Unfortunately, the fact remains that at least 48 women diagnosed at BCDDP projects before June 30, 1976, were misdiagnosed. There are then some women who had unnecessary mastectomies, women who thought, and still think, that they have had breast cancer when in fact they haven't and believe that they and their female relatives—their sisters and daughters—are at higher risk of developing cancer, when in fact they aren't. Moreover, the pathology review reviewed only minimal cases that had been detected at a BCDDP over a certain period. Since that time there may have been others misdiagnosed, both at the BCDDPs and at other places.

Lawyers at the Department of Health, Education and Welfare determined that, legally, the federal government could not notify these women that they did not have cancer. The BCDDPs were set up only as screening centers. If a woman's mammogram was suspicious, notification was sent to her doctor. From that time on, although the BCDDPs collected data on the cases, the NCI, sponsor of the BCDDPs, was out of the picture. The entire matter was seen as a doctor–patient relationship, and, of course, the government couldn't violate this sacred contract. So, the procedure decided on was to inform the individual BCDDP that it had been discovered that Ms. So & So didn't really have cancer after all. Then the director of the center was to inform Ms. So & So's doctor that she had actually had benign disease and not cancer and therefore was not at high risk for recurrent cancer and did not need to have the lifetime follow-up visits. She was also to be told that her daughter and sisters were not at high risk and did not (depending on their age) need annual mammograms.

The NCI cannot, however, force the doctor to pass the word along to those women and thus invite a malpractice suit. (Whether or not such a woman would win a malpractice suit is a moot point, for some pathologists insist that all microscopic diagnoses are a matter of judgment and subject to personal interpretations.) Admittedly, it would take a special kind of courage to call up a woman, especially one who had been treated with a mastectomy, and tell her that she hadn't had cancer after all. As a result, most of those women who have had cancer surgery because of diagnoses from the BCDDPs still don't know whether they did indeed have cancer.

The National Women's Health Network attempted to learn the names of the women involved by way of the Freedom of Information Act, but the information cannot be released to an organization. To do so would be a violation of privacy laws. The individual woman herself may, however, obtain information on her own case. The person to contact is Richard Costlow, Chief, Division of Preventive Medicine, Division of Cancer Control and Rehabilitation, Blair Building/NCI, 8300 Colesville Road, Silver Spring, Maryland 20910.

39. Beahrs, pp. 640–709.

40. Craig Henderson, M.D., and George D. Canellos, M.D., "Cancer of the Breast, the Past Decade, Part One," *New England Journal of Medicine* 302:1 (Jan. 3, 1980), pp. 17–30.

41. Cancer Information Service, *Diagnosis and Treatment of Breast Cancer* (training manual for volunteers), p. 14.

42. Henderson and Canellos, pp. 17–30.

43. Readers interested in a more detailed and academic discussion of the history of breast cancer treatments are referred to Henderson and Canellos, pp. 17–30.

44. Robert E. Hermann, M.D., and Ezra Steiger, M.D., "Modified Radical Mastectomy," *Surgical Clinics of North America* 58:4 (Aug. 1978), pp. 743–54.

45. T. Nemato and T. Dao, "Is Modified Radical Mastectomy Adequate for Axillary Lymph Node Dissection?" *Annals of Surgery* 182 (1975), p. 722.

46. Henderson and Canellos, pp. 17–30, and Nemato and Dao, p. 722.

47. W. Madden et al., "A Randomized Prospective Trial of (Halsted) Mastectomy vs. Radical Mastectomy in 311 Breast Cancer Patients," *Annals of Surgery,* Aug. 1983, pp. 198–207, and Fisher, Redmond and Fisher, pp. 723–36.

48. Fisher, Redmond and Fisher, pp. 723–36.

49. F.W. Foote, Jr., and F.W. Stewart, "Comparative Studies of Cancerous versus Noncancerous Breasts," *Annals of Surgery* 121 (1945), p. 197, and R. Muir, "Evolution of Carcinoma of the Mammary Gland," *Journal of Pathol Bacteriology* 55 (1941), pp. 155–72.

50. Fisher, Redmond and Fisher, pp. 723–36.

51. Avram M. Cooperman, M.D., Janet M. Blanchard, M.D., and Caldwell Esselstyn, Jr., M.D., "Partial Mastectomy," *Surgical Clinics of North America* 58 (Aug. 1978), pp. 737–42.

52. Fisher, Redmond and Fisher, pp. 723–36.

53. U. Veronesi et al., "Comparing Radical Mastectomy with Quadrantectomy, Axillary Dissection and Radiotherapy in Patients with Small Cancers of the Breast," *New England Journal of Medicine* 305 (1981), pp. 6–11.

54. Jay R. Harris, Martin B. Levere and Samuel Hellman, "Results of Treating Stage I and II Carcinoma of the Breast with Primary Radiation Therapy," *Cancer Treatment Reports* 62:7 (July 1978), pp. 985–91, and Martin B. Levere, M.D., Jay R. Harris, M.D., and Samuel Hellman, M.D., "Primary Radiation Therapy for Operable Carcinoma of the Breast," *Surgical Clinics of North America* 58:4 (Aug. 1978), pp. 767–76.

55. Vincent R. Pennises, M.D., Angelo Capozzi, M.D., and F.M. Perez, M.D., "Subcutaneous Mastectomy Data: An Interim Report," *Breast, Diseases of the Breast* 5:2 (1977).

56. Cope, p. 172.

57. Henderson and Canellos, pp. 17–30.

58. Beahrs, table, p. 659.

59. Henderson and Canellos, pp. 17–30.

60. B. Fisher et al., "L-phenylalanine Mustard (L-Pam) in the Management of Primary Breast Cancer: An Update of Earlier Findings and a Comparison with Those Utilizing L-Pam Plus 5-Fluorouracil (5-FU)," *Cancer* 39 (1977), pp. 2883–903, and B. Fisher et al., "Adjuvant Chemotherapy in Breast Cancer," *International Journal of Radiat Oncol Biol Phys* 4 (1978), pp. 295–98.

61. Bernard Fisher and Norman Wolmark, "Systemic Adjuvant Therapy in Primary Breast Cancer," in *Breast Cancer, Advances in Research and Treatment* vol. I, William McGuire, M.D., ed. (New York: Plenum, 1977), pp. 125–63.

62. G. Bonadonna et al., "Are Surgical Adjuvant Trials Altering the Course of Breast Cancer," *Semin Oncology* 5 (1978), pp. 450–64, and G. Bonadonna et al., "Combination Chemotherapy as an Adjuvant Treatment in Operable Breast Cancer," *New England Journal of Medicine* 294 (1976), pp. 405–10.

63. Fisher and Wolmark, pp. 125–163.

64. G.F. Robbins et al., "An Evaluation of Postoperative Prophylactic Radiation Therapy in Breast Cancer," *Surgery, Gynecology and Obstetrics* 122 (1966), pp. 979–82.

65. W.T. Bessler, "Radiotherapy of Metastatic Breast Cancer," in *Breast Cancer,* A. Montague, G. Stonesifer and E. Lewison, eds. (New York: Alan R. Liss, Inc., 1977), pp. 493–504, and Kushner, pp. 277–78.

66. Kushner, pp. 277–78.

67. Henderson and Canellos, pp. 17–30.

68. Data presented at the 25th semi-annual NSABP meeting, Jan. 25, 1984.

69. The information on breast reconstruction is drawn primarily from two sources:

a) a fact sheet, "Breast Reconstruction After Breast Cancer," available from the Cancer Information Service, and

b) a pamphlet, "Breast Reconstruction After Breast Cancer: Some Questions and Answers," prepared by the American Society of Plastic and Reconstructive Surgeons, Inc.

SEXUALLY TRANSMISSIBLE INFECTIONS

1. *V.D. Fact Sheet 1977* and *V.D. Fact Sheet 1978,* Joseph H. Blount, ed., U.S. Dept. of Health, Education and Welfare, Public Health Service, Centers for Disease Control, Venereal Disease Control Division, 1978 and 1979 (respectively).

2. D. Barlow, "The Condom and Gonorrhea," *Lancet* 2:842 (Oct. 15, 1977), pp. 811–13.

3. "Condom Sales Rise in Sweden, VD Falls," *Obstetrics and Gynecology News* 8:15 (Aug. 1, 1973), p. 9.

4. B. Singh et al., "Studies on the Development of a Vaginal Preparation Providing Both Prophylaxis Against Venereal Disease and Other Genital Infections and Contraception II: Effect in Vitro of Vaginal Contraceptive and Noncontraceptive Preparations on *Treponema pallidum* and *Neisseria gonorrhoeae,*" *British Journal of Venereal Disease* 48 (1972), pp. 51–64.

B. Postic et al., "Inactivation of Clinical Isolites of Herpes Viris Hominis, Types 1 and 2, by Chemical Contraceptives," *Sexually Transmitted Diseases* 5 (Jan.–Mar. 1978), pp. 22–24.

5. Boston Women's Health Collective, *Our Bodies, Ourselves,* 2nd ed. (New York: Simon and Schuster, 1976), p. 168.

6. Herman L. Gardner, M.D., "Herpes Genitalis," *Audio-Digest, Obstetrics and Gynecology* 26:3 (Feb. 6, 1979); Raymond H. Kaufman, "Herpes Genitalis, Clinical Features and Laboratory Diagnosis," *Audio-Digest, Obstetrics and Gynecology* 26:3 (Feb. 6, 1979); and Erwin Adam, M.D., et al., "Asymptomatic Virus Shedding After Herpes Genitalis," *American Journal of Obstetrics and Gynecology* 137:7 (Aug. 1, 1980), pp. 827–30.

7. Dr. William E. Josey, "Herpes Genitalis, Effects on Infants," *Audio-Digest, Obstetrics and Gynecology* 26:3 (Feb. 6, 1979), and Anne S. Yeager, M.D., "Genital Herpes Simplex Virus (HSV), Infections and Pregnancy," *The Helper* 1:2 (Oct. 1979), pp. 1–2.

8. *V.D. Fact Sheet, 1978.*

9. The information on gonorrhea treatment is based on the Centers for Disease Control's guidelines. For a summary of these guidelines, see "CDC Writes First Guidelines for Sexually Transmitted Diseases," *Contraceptive Technology Update,* Oct. 1982, pp. 129–34.

10. Centers for Disease Control, "Herpes Genital Infection," Information Sheet.

11. Kaufman, *Audio-Digest.*

12. Kaufman, *Audio-Digest.*

13. Adam et al., pp. 827–30.

14. "Patient Information Sheet, Herpes Simplex Infection," UCLA School of Medicine, Center for Health Sciences.

15. David K. Mumford, Raymond H. Kaufman and Nancy McCormick, "Immunity, Herpes Simplex Virus and Cervical Carcinoma," *Surgical Clinics of North America* 58:1 (Feb. 1958), pp. 39–54.

16. A.J. Nahmias, "Significance of Herpes Simplex Virus During Pregnancy," *Clinical Obstetrics and Gynecology* 15:4 (1972), p. 929.

17. Josey, *Audio-Digest.*

18. Josey, *Audio-Digest.*

19. Yeager, pp. 1–2.

20. Kaufman, *Audio-Digest.*

21. Robert A. Hatcher, "Commentary," *Contraceptive Technology Update,* (Feb. 1983), pp. 20–22.

22. This list was adapted from "How, Where, When or What to Tell a Sex Partner About Genital Herpes," available from HELP.

23. Julius Schachter, Ph.D., "Chlamydia Trachomatis Infections," *Medical Times,* (Dec. 1982), pp. 67–69.

24. Schachter, pp. 67–69.

25. Michael F. Rein, M.D., "Recent Developments in Sexually Transmitted Chlamydial Infections," *Medical-Times* 109 (March 1981), pp. 29–35.

26. David A. Eschenbach, M.D., "Recognizing Chlamydial Infections," *Contemporary OB/GYN* 1G (Aug. 1980), pp. 15–30.

27. King K. Helmes, "The Chlamydia Epidemic," *Journal of the American Medical Association* 245 (May 1, 1981), pp. 1718–23.

28. Helmes, pp. 1718–23.

29. Helmes, pp. 1718–23.

30. Eschenbach, pp. 15–30.

31. Rein, pp. 29–35.

32. Helmes, pp. 1718–23.

33. Eschenbach, pp. 15–30.

34. *V.D. Fact Sheet, 1977.*

35. J.H. Newson et al., "Treatment of Infestation with Pthirus Pubis: Comparative Efficiencies of Synergized Pyrethrins and Gamma-Benzene Hexachlorophene," *American Veneral Disease Journal* 6, (July–Sept. 1979), pp. 203–5.

36. "Treatment of Genital Warts Is Involved, Often Neglected," *Contraceptive Technology Update*, July 1983, pp. 77–79.

37. "Treatment of Genital Warts," pp. 77–79.

38. "Treatment of Genital Warts," pp. 77–79.

39. "Treatment of Genital Warts," pp. 77–79.

40. *V.D. Fact Sheet, 1977.*

41. *V.D. Fact Sheet, 1977.*

42. *V.D. Fact Sheet, 1977.*

PROBLEMS RELATED TO THE MENSTRUAL CYCLE

1. Edmund R. Novak, M.D., Georgeanna Seegar Jones, M.D. and Howard W. Jones, Jr., M.D., *Novak's Textbook of Gynecology,* 9th ed. (Baltimore, Williams & Wilkins Co., 1975), p. 652.

2. Ellen Switzer, "PMS, the Return of Raging Hormones," *Working Woman,* Oct. 1983, pp. 123–27.

3. Switzer, p. 126.

4. Switzer, pp. 126–27.

5. This classification scheme was first developed by Dr. Guy Abraham.

6. Dr. G.E. Abraham has published a number of articles on PMS, including "Premenstrual Tension," which appears in *Current Problems in OB/GYN* (Chicago: Yearbook Medical Publishers, 1980); G.E. Abraham and J.T. Hargrove, "Effect of Vitamin B-6 on Premenstrual Symptomology in Women with Premenstrual Tension Syndrome: A Double-Blind Crossover Study," *Infertility* 3 (1980), p. 155; and G.E. Abraham et al., "Hormonal and Behavioral Changes During the Menstrual Cycle," *Senolgia* 3 (1978), pp. 33–38.

7. K. Dalton, *The Premenstrual Syndrome* (Springfield, IL: Charles C. Thomas, 1964).

8. Switzer, p. 125.

9. See the patient package insert that comes with all progesterone preparations, for details.

10. See the patient package insert that comes with all progesterone preparations, for details.

11. Personal communication, Diane Burr, R.N., N.P.

12. A. Schwartz et al., "Primary Dysmenorrhea, Alleviation by an Inhibitor of Prostaglandin Synthesis," *Obstetrics and Gynecology* 44 (1974), pp. 709–12.

13. F.H. Boehm and H. Sarralt, "Indomethacin for the Treatment of Dysmenorrhea, A Preliminary Report," *Journal of Reproductive Medicine* 15 (1975), pp. 84–86.

14. M.R. Henzl et al., "The Treatment of Dysmenorrhea with Naproxen Sodium: A Report on Two Independent Double-Blind Trials," *American Journal of Obstetrics and Gynecology* 127 (1977), pp. 818–23.

15. P.W. Budoff, "Use of Mefenamic Acid in the Treatment of Primary Dysmenorrhea," *Journal of the American Medical Association* 241:25 (June 22, 1979), pp. 2713–16.

16. K.T. Witty et al., "Dysmenorrhea, Quelling Severe Menstrual Cramps," *Patient Care,* April 15, 1978, pp. 198–216.

17. Witty, pp. 198–216.

18. Val Davajan, M.D., "Management of Amenorrheas and Galactorrhea," *Audio-Digest, Obstetrics and Gynecology* 26:20 (Oct. 23, 1979).

19. Davajan, *Audio-Digest.*

20. Davajan, *Audio-Digest.*

21. Davajan, *Audio-Digest.*

22. Lorraine C. King, M.D., "Dysfunctional Uterine Bleeding: Medical vs. Surgical Treatment," *Audio-Digest, Obstetrics and Gynecology* 26:21 (Nov. 6, 1979).

23. Subcommittee of Council of Medical Women's Federation of England, "Investigation of Menopause in 1000 Women," *Lancet* 1 (1933), p. 106, quoted in W.H. Utian, "The Symptom Complex Associated with Menopause," *Seminars in Reproductive Endocrinology* 1 (Feb. 1983), pp. 1–9.

24. Penny Wise Budoff, M.D., *No More Hot Flashes and Other Good News* (New York: Putnam, 1983), p. 16.

25. M. McGuire and D. Labby, "Sexuality and the Menopausal and Postmenopausal Woman," *Seminars in Reproductive Endocrinology,* Feb. 1983, pp. 69–73.

26. G. Winokur, "Depression in the Menopause," *American Journal of Psychiatry* 130 (1973), pp. 92–93.

27. B. Neugarten and R.K. Kraines, "Menopausal Symptoms in Women of Various Ages," *Psychosomatic Medicine* 27 (1965) pp. 266–73.

28. Budoff, p. 54.

29. R. Lindsay and B.S. Herrington, "Estrogens and Osteoporosis," *Seminars in Reproductive Endocrinology* 1 (Feb. 1983), pp. 55–67.

30. Barbara Seaman and Gideon Seaman, M.D., *Women and the Crisis in Sex Hormones* (New York: Rawson, 1977), pp. 283–84.

31. See the section on ERT for details and references.

32. David R. Meldrum, M.D., "The Pathophysiology of Postmenopausal Symptoms," *Seminars on Reproductive Endocrinology* 1 (Feb. 1983), pp. 11–17.

33. Meldrum, pp. 11–17.

34. Meldrum, pp. 11–17.

35. W. Masters and V. Johnson, *Human Sexual Response* (Boston: Little, Brown, 1966), quoted in M. McGuire and D. Labby, p. 70.

36. Information on TSS in this section is derived from *Toxic Shock Syndrome: Assessment of Current Information and Research Needs* (Washington, DC: National Academic Press, 1982), and the package insert that comes with Tampax tampons.

37. *Toxic Shock Syndrome,* p. 7.

38. Nancy Friedman, "The Truth About Tampons," *New West,* Oct. 20, 1980, pp. 33–42.

39. "Virus Villain in TSS," *Contraceptive Technology Updates,* Aug. 1983, pp. 89–90.

40. *Toxic Shock Syndrome,* p. 7.

41. Friedman, pp. 33–42.

42. *Toxic Shock Syndrome,* p. 5.

PROBLEMS RELATED TO PREGNANCY AND FERTILITY

1. Tracy Hotchner, *Pregnancy and Childbirth* (New York: Avon Books, 1979), p. 41.
2. Langdon Parsons, M.D. and Sheldon Sommers, M.D., *Gynecology,* 2nd ed. (Philadelphia: W.B. Saunders Co., 1978), p. 494.
3. A.L. Herbst, H. Ulfedler and D.C. Poskanzer, "Adenocarcinoma of the Vagina," *New England Journal of Medicine* 284 (1971), pp. 878–81.
4. Howard A. Zacur and John Rock, "Diagnosis and Treatment of Infertility," *The Female Patient* 8 (June 1983), pp. 52/15–52/23.
5. Zacur and Rock, pp. 52/15–52/23.
6. Zacur and Rock, pp. 52/15–52/23.
7. Michael Leviton, Commentary, broadcast on KPFK, Nov. 7, 1979. NOVA, the public television show, also did an expose of the Agent Orange problem. Additional information on Agent Orange is available from the Citizen Soldier, Suite 1010, 175 Fifth Avenue, New York, NY 10160.
8. Robert A. Hatcher et al., *Contraceptive Technology, 1982–1983,* 11th rev. ed. (New York: Irvington Publishers, 1982), p. 225.
9. "Study Shows Vitamin C Quickly Restores Fertility," *Contraceptive Technology Update,* Aug. 1980, p. 94.
10. Hatcher et al., p. 219.
11. Hatcher et al., p. 219.
12. J.B. Van Dijk, M.D., et al., "The Treatment of Unexplained Fertility with Danazol," *Fertility and Sterility* 31 (May, 1979), pp. 481–85.
13. Hotchner, pp. 440–41.
14. Jennie Kline et al., "Smoking: A Risk Factor for Spontaneous Abortion," *New England Journal of Medicine* 297 (Oct. 13, 1977), pp. 793–96.
15. See Note 7 above.
16. "Repeat Abortions Increase Risk of Miscarriage, Premature Births and Low-Birth-Weight-Babies," *Family Planning Perspectives* 2 (Jan.–Feb. 1979), pp. 39–40.
17. I. Gal, B. Kirman and J. Stern, "Hormonal Pregnancy Tests and Congenital Malformation," *Nature* 216 (1967), p. 83;

  E.P. Levy, A. Cohen and F.C. Fraser, "Hormone Treatment During Pregnancy and Congenital Heart Defects," *Lancet* 1 (1973), p. 611;

  D.T. Janevich, J.M. Piper and D.M. Glebatis, "Oral Contraceptives and Congenital Limb-reduction Effects," *New England Journal of Medicine* 291 (1974), pp. 697–700; and

  L. Wilkins, "Masculization of Female Fetus Due to Use of Orally Given Progestins," *Journal of the American Medical Association* 172 (1960), p. 1028.
18. See Note 17 above.
19. Kline et al., pp. 793–96.
20. Martin M. Quigley, "Trophoblastic Disease: Diagnosis and Treatment," *Audio-Digest, Obstetrics and Gynecology* 24:5 (March 3, 1977).
21. Charles B. Hammond, M.D., Herbert J. Schmidt, M.D. and Roy T. Parker, M.D.,

"Gestational Trophoblastic Disease," in *Gynecologic Oncology*, Larry McGowan, ed. (New York: Appleton-Century-Crofts, 1978), pp. 359–81.

22. Quigley, *Audio-Digest.*

23. Quigley, *Audio-Digest.*

24. Quigley, *Audio-Digest.*

25. Quigley, *Audio-Digest.*

26. Hammond, Schmidt and Parker, pp. 359–81, and Walter B. Jones, M.D., "Gestational Trophoblastic Neoplasms," *Surgical Clinics of North America* 58:1 (Feb. 1978), pp. 167–79.

27. Quigley, *Audio-Digest.*

CANCER

1. A.L. Herbst, H. Ulfedler and D.C. Poskanzer, "Adenocarcinoma of the Vagina," *New England Journal of Medicine* 284 (1971), pp. 878–81.

2. B. MacMahon, "Risk Factors for Endometrial Cancer," *Gynecologic Oncology* 2 (1974), p. 239.

3. There are a number of case-control studies that report increased risk for endometrial cancer in women using menopausal estrogens. The three most widely cited studies are:

H.K. Ziel and W.D. Finkle, "Increased Risk of Endometrial Carcinoma Among Users of Conjugated Estrogens," *New England Journal of Medicine* 293 (1975), pp. 1167–70.

D.C. Smith et al., "Association of Exogenous Estrogen and Endometrial Carcinoma," *New England Journal of Medicine* 294 (1976), pp. 1164–67.

T.M. Mack et al., "Estrogens and Endometrial Cancer in a Retirement Community," *New England Journal of Medicine* 294 (1976), pp. 1262–67.

These findings are further supported by the fact that incidence rates of endometrial cancer have increased sharply since 1969, which may be related to the rapidly expanding use of estrogens in the past decade. See the FDA-approved package insert for all products containing estrogens for more details.

4. David M. Mumford, Raymond H. Kaufman and Nancy McCormick, "Immunity, Herpes Simplex Virus and Cervical Carcinoma," *Surgical Clinics of North America* 58:1 (Feb. 1978), pp. 39–54.

5. Bernard Fisher, M.D., Carol Redmond, Sc.D., and Edwin R. Fisher, M.D., "Clinical Trials and the Surgical Treatment of Breast Cancer," *Surgical Clinics of North America* 58:4 (Aug. 1978), pp. 723–36.

6. J.P. Minton et al., "Response of Fibrocystic Disease to Caffeine Withdrawal and the Correlation of Cystic Nucleotides with Breast Disease," *American Journal of Obstetrics and Gynecology* 135:1 (Sept. 1, 1979), pp. 157–58.

7. William L. Broad, "New Laetrile Study Leaves Cancer Institute in the Pits," *Science* 202:4363 (Oct. 6, 1978), pp. 33–36, and William L. Broad, "Upton OK's Laetrile Test on Humans," *Science* 202:4364 (Oct. 13, 1978), p. 196.

8. John Elliott, "Clinical Trials of Laetrile May Soon Be Under Way," *Journal of the American Medical Association* 243:6 (Feb. 8, 1980), pp. 505–6.

Chapter Seven: GYNECOLOGICAL OPERATIONS, TESTS, PROCEDURES AND DRUGS

1. William Nolen, M.D., "The Big Knives," *Esquire* 93:4 (April 1980), pp. 58–60.

2. See p. 824, Note 6.

3. Barbara Caress, "Womb Bomb," *Health/PAC Bulletin,* July–Aug. 1977.

4. Caress, "Womb Bomb."

5. S. Schwartz, *Textbook of Surgery,* vol. I (New York: McGraw-Hill, 1974), p. 443.

6. A.L. Herbst, H. Ulfedler and D.C. Poskanzer, "Adenocarcinoma of the Vagina," *New England Journal of Medicine* 284 (1971), pp. 878–81.

7. A number of abnormalities have been found in DES daughters, including alterations in the shape of the cervix, vaginal adenosis, lowered fertility and irregular menstrual periods. Testis cysts, underdeveloped or undescended testes, abnormally placed urinary openings, low sperm counts, abnormally shaped sperm cells and impaired fertility have been reported in DES sons.

For further information, see:

R. Mattingly and A. Stafl, "Cancer Risk in DES-exposed Offspring," *Journal of Obstetrics and Gynecology* 128 (1977), pp. 43–50;

R. Kaufman et al., "Upper Genital Tract Changes Associated with Exposure in Utero to Diethylstilbestrol," *American Journal of Obstetrics and Gynecology* 128 (1977), pp. 51–59; and

M. Bibbo et al., "Follow-up Study of Male and Female Offspring of DES-Exposed Mothers," *Obstetrics and Gynecology* 49:1 (1977), pp. 1–8.

8. Food and Drug Administration, Department of Health, Education and Welfare, "DES and Breast Cancer," *FDA Drug Bulletin* 8 (March–April 1978), p. 2.

9. There are a number of case-control studies that report increased risk for endometrial cancer in women using menopausal estrogens. The three most widely cited studies are:

H.K. Ziel and W.D. Finkle, "Increased Risk of Endometrial Carcinoma Among Users of Conjugated Estrogens," *New England Journal of Medicine* 293 (1975), pp. 1167–70;

D.C. Smith et al., "Association of Exogenous Estrogen and Endometrial Carcinoma," *New England Journal of Medicine* 293 (1975), pp. 1164–67; and

T.M. Mack et al., "Estrogens and Endometrial Cancer in a Retirement Community," *New England Journal of Medicine* 294 (1976), pp. 1262–67.

These findings are further supported by the fact that incidence rates of endometrial cancer have increased sharply since 1969, which may be related to the rapidly expanding use of estrogens in the past decade. See the FDA-approved package insert for all products containing estrogens for more details.

10. R. Hoover et al., "Menopausal Estrogens and Cancer," *New England Journal of Medicine* 295 (1976), pp. 401–5.

11. *Physician's Desk Reference,* 32nd ed., Charles Baker, ed. (New Jersey: Litton Industries, 1978), p. 624.

12. Hoover et al., pp. 401–5.

13. Ward Rinehart and Jane Winter, "Injectable Progestogens—Officials Debate, but Use Increases," *Population Reports,* Series K. no. 1 (March 1975), pp. K1–K9.

14. Rinehart and Winter, pp. K1–K9.

15. Rinehart and Winter, pp. K1–K9.

16. Rinehart and Winter, pp. K1–K9.

17. Center for Medical Consumers and Health Care Information "Informed Consent," vol. IV, no. 22 (July–Aug. 1980), pp. 1–8.

18. *Physician's Desk Reference,* p. 1661.

Reference Section: OPERATIONS, TESTS, PROCEDURES AND DRUGS

1. J.P. Bunker, K. McPherson and P.C. Henneman, "Elective Hysterectomy," in *Costs, Risks and Benefits of Surgery* (New York: Oxford University Press, 1977), pp. 262–76.

2. W. Ledger and M. Child, "The Hospital Care of Patients Undergoing Hysterectomy: An Analysis of 12,026 Patients from the Professional Activity Study," *American Journal of Obstetrics and Gynecology* 117 (1973), pp. 423–33.

3. Ledger and Child, pp. 423–33.

4. There are a number of case-control studies that report increased risk for endometrial cancer in women using menopausal estrogens. The three most widely cited studies are:

H.K. Ziel and W.D. Finkle, "Increased Risk of Endometrial Carcinoma Among Users of Conjugated Estrogens," *New England Journal of Medicine* 293 (1975), pp. 1167–70;

D.C. Smith et al., "Association of Exogenous Estrogen and Endometrial Carcinoma," *New England Journal of Medicine* 293 (1975), pp. 1164–67; and

T.M. Mack et al., "Estrogens and Endometrial Cancer in a Retirement Community," *New England Journal of Medicine* 294 (1976), pp. 1262–67.

These findings are further supported by the fact that incidence rates of endometrial cancer have increased sharply since 1969, which may be related to the rapidly expanding use of estrogens in the past decade. See the FDA-approved package insert for all products containing estrogens for more details.

5. Robert Hoover et al., "Menopausal Estrogens and Cancer," *New England Journal of Medicine* 295 (1976); pp. 401–5.

6. W. Gifford Jones, *What Every Woman Should Know About Hysterectomy* (New York: Funk & Wagnalls, 1977), p. 175.

7. H. Judd et al., "Endocrine Function of the Post-Menopausal Ovary," *Journal of Clinical Endocrinology and Metabolism* 39 (1974), p. 1020.

8. L. Moses, "Comparison of Crude and Standardized Anesthetic Death Rates," in *The National Halothane Study: Report of the Subcommittee on the National Halothane Study,* J.P. Bunker et al., eds. (Washington, DC: U.S. Government Printing Office, 1969), Chapter IV-2.

9. Barbara J. Culliton and Walter K. Waterfall, "Low-Dose Radiation," *British Medical Journal* 1:6177 (June 9, 1979), pp. 1545–46.

10. Culliton and Waterfall, pp. 1545–46.

11. "The X-Raying of America," *FDA Consumer,* Dec. 1979–Jan. 1980, pp. 13–17.

12. I. Gal, B. Kirman and J. Stern, "Hormonal Pregnancy Tests and Congenital Malformation," *Nature* 216 (1967), p. 83;

E.P. Levy, A. Cohen and F.C. Fraser, "Hormone Treatment During Pregnancy and Congenital Heart Defects," *Lancet* 1 (1973), p. 611.

D.T. Janevich, J.M. Piper and D.M. Glebatis, "Oral Contraceptives and Congenital Limb-reduction Effects," *New England Journal of Medicine* 291 (1974), pp. 697–700, and

L. Wilkins, "Masculinization of Female Fetus Due to Use of Orally Given Progestins," *Journal of the American Medical Association* 172 (1960), p. 1028.

13. "Users Fail to Repeat Negative Home Pregnancy Tests," *Contraceptive Technology Update,* April 1982, pp. 45–47.

14. J.C. Phillips, "Public Health Aspects of Critical Care Medicine: Anesthesia Mortality," *Clinical Anesthesia* 10 (1974), pp. 220–44.

15. O. Idose, "Nature and Extent of Penicillin Side Reactions with Particular Reference to the Fatalistic Form: Anaphylactic Shock," *World Health Organization Bulletin* 38 (1968), p. 159.

16. *Physician's Desk Reference,* 32nd ed., Charles Baker, ed. (New Jersey: Litton Industries, 1978), p. 1166.

17. Ward Rinehart and Jane Winter, "Injectable Progestogens—Officials Debate, but Use Increases," *Population Reports,* Series K, no. 1 (March 1975), pp. K1–K16.

18. Rinehart and Winter, pp. K1–K16.

19. Rinehart and Winter, pp. K1–K16.

20. Rinehart and Winter, pp. K1–K16.

21. Rinehart and Winter, pp. K1–K16.

22. Rinehart and Winter, pp. K1–K16.

23. G. Winokur, "Depression in the Menopause," *American Journal of Psychiatry* 130 (1973), pp. 92–93.

24. B. Neugarten and R.J. Kraines, "Menopausal Symptoms in Women of Various Ages," *Psychosomatic Medicine* 27 (1965), pp. 266–73.

25. Barbara Seaman and Gideon Seaman, M.D., *Women and the Crisis in Sex Hormones* (New York: Rawson Associates, 1977), pp. 283–84.

26. Seaman and Seaman, pp. 300–2.

27. "Progesterone Therapy for Hot Flashes?" *Medical World News,* July 23, 1979, pp. 18–19.

28. Seaman and Seaman, pp. 363–70.

29. Seaman and Seaman, pp. 351–62.

30. R. Lindsay, M.D. and B.S. Herrington, "Estrogens and Osteoporosis," *Seminars in Reproductive Endocrinology* 1 (Feb. 1983), pp. 55–67.

31. Lindsay and Herrington, pp. 55–67.

32. Penny Wise Budoff, M.D., *No More Hot Flashes and Other Good News* (New York: Putnam, 1983), pp. 53–54.

33. Budoff, p. 54.

34. Budoff, p. 54.

35. Budoff, p. 54.

36. Lindsay and Herrington, pp. 62–63.

37. Lindsay and Herrington, p. 63.

38. Lindsay and Herrington, pp. 64–65.

39. Lindsay and Herrington, p. 60.

40. Lindsay and Herrington, p. 59.

41. Lindsay and Herrington, p. 59.

42. Lindsay and Herrington, pp. 60–61.

43. There are a number of case control studies that report an increased risk for endometrial cancer in women using menopausal estrogens, including H.K. Ziel and W.D. Finkle, "Increased Risk of Endometrial Carcinoma Among Users of Conjugated Estrogens, "*New England Journal of Medicine* 293 (1975), pp. 1167–70; D.C. Smith et al., "Association of Exogenous Estrogen and Endometrial Carcinoma," *New England Journal of Medicine* 293 (1975), pp. 1164–67; and T.M. Mack et al., "Estrogens and Endometrial Cancer in a Retirement Community," *New England Journal of Medicine* 294 (1975), pp. 1262–67.

44. Malcolm Whitehead, et al., "Avoidance of Endometrial Hyper Stimulation in Estrogen-treated Postmenopausal Women," *Seminars in Reproductive Endocrinology* 1 (Feb. 1983), pp. 41–53.

45. Whitehead et al., p. 440.

46. "Sequential Pills," *New York Times*, Feb. 26, 1976.

47. R. Don Gambrell, Jr., M.D., "Breast Disease in Postmenopausal Years," *Seminars in Reproductive Endocrinology*, 1 (Feb. 1983), pp. 27–40.

48. Gambrell, pp. 27–40.

49. Gambrell, pp. 27–40.

50. R.K. Ross and A. Paganini-Hill, "Estrogen Replacement Therapy and Coronary Heart Disease," *Seminars in Reproductive Endocrinology*, 1 (Feb. 1983), pp. 19–25.

51. Ross and Paganini-Hill, pp. 19–25 and Budoff, pp. 43–47.

52. The Boston Collaborative Drug Surveillance Program, "Surgically Confirmed Gall Bladder Disease, Venous Thromboembolism and Breast Tumors in Relation to Post Menopausal Estrogen Therapy," *New England Journal of Medicine*, 290 (1974), pp. 15–19.

53. R.I. Pfeiffer and S. Van den Noort, "Estrogen Use and Stroke Risk in Postmenopausal Women," *American Journal of Epidemiology*, 103 (1976), pp. 445–46.

54. Seaman and Seaman, p. 34.

55. A.L. Herbst, H. Ulfedler and D.C. Poskanzer, "Adenocarcinoma of the Vagina," *New England Journal of Medicine* 284 (1971), pp. 878–81.

56. Nancy Adess et al., *Fertility and Pregnancy Guide for DES Daughters and Sons* (New York: DES Action National, 1983), p. 2.

57. R. Mattingly and A. Stafl, "Cancer Risk in DES-Exposed Offspring," *Journal of Obstetrics and Gynecology* 128 (1977), pp. 43–50.

58. Anne P. Lanier et al., "Cancer and Stilbestrol, a Follow-Up of 1,719 Persons Exposed to Estrogens in Utero, 1943–1959," *Mayo Clinic Proceedings* 48 (1973), p. 793;

   A. Stafl et al., "Clinical Diagnosis of Vaginal Adenosis," *Journal of Obstetrics and Gynecology* 43 (1974), pp. 118–28; and

   Sherman et al., "Cervical Vaginal Adenosis After in Utero Exposure to Synthetic Estrogens," *Journal of Obstetrics and Gynecology* 44 (1974), pp. 531–45.

59. R. Kaufman et al., "Upper Genital Tract Changes Associated with Exposure in Utero to Diethylstilbestrol," *American Journal of Obstetrics and Gynecology* 128 (1977), pp. 51–59, and M.S. Singer et al., "Incompetent Cervix in Hormone-Exposed Offspring," *Obstetrics and Gynecology* 51:5 (May 1978), pp. 625–26.

60. See note 59.

61. Adess et al., p. 6.

62. Kaufman et al., pp. 51–59.

63. M. Bibbo et al., "Follow-Up Study of Male and Female Offspring of DES-Exposed Mothers," *Obstetrics and Gynecology* 49:1 (1977), pp. 1–8, and Singer et al, pp. 625–26.

64. Bibbo et al., pp. 1–8, and W. Gill, G. Schumacher and M. Bibbo, "Genital and Semen Abnormalities in Adult Males Two and One Half Decades After in Utero Exposure to Diethylstilbestrol," in *Intrauterine Exposure to Diethylstilbestrol in the Human*, A. Herbst, ed., Proceedings of Symposium on DES, Chicago, Feb. 1977, American College of Obstetricians and Gynecologists (Monograph).

65. Bibbo et al., pp. 1–8, and Gil, Schumacher and Bibbo, monograph.

66. Seaman and Seaman, pp. 49–59.

67. Seaman and Seaman, p. 6.

68. Personal communication, Nancy Adess, DES Action.

69. Adess et al., p. 2.

70. Adess et al., p. 8.

71. Adess et al., p. 9.

72. Adess et al., p. 11.

73. Adess et al., p. 12.

74. Adess et al., pp. 12–13.

75. Adess et al., p. 11.

76. Adess et al., p. 18.

77. Adess et al., p. 23.

78. Adess et al., pp. 24–25.

79. Fay A. Saber, "The DES Problem Revisited: On Whose Shoulders Should the Legal Responsibility Fall?," *DES Action Voice* 1:2 (Spring 1979).

80. Abraham E. Rakoff, "Ovarian Failure," *Audio-Digest, Obstetrics and Gynecology* 24:10 (May 17, 1977).

81. See Notes 55 and 57–63 above.

82. Rakoff, *Audio-Digest*.

83. Rakoff, *Audio-Digest*.

84. Shirley McCormack and James H. Clark, "Clomid Administration to Pregnant Rats Causes Abnormalities of the Reproductive Tract in Offspring and Mothers," *Science* 204 (May 11, 1979), pp. 629–31.

85. McCormack and Clark, pp. 629–31.

86. Rakoff, *Audio-Digest*.

87. Rakoff, *Audio-Digest*.

88. Rakoff, *Audio-Digest*.

Table of Measurements

Measurements in medicine are given in terms of centimeters. A doctor might, for instance, refer to a tumor as being 2 cm, which means that it is 2 cm in diameter at its greatest width. One inch equals 2.54 centimeters (cm). The following table will help you understand the measurements used in this book.

Centimeters	Inches	Approximate Diameter
1 cm	.3937 inch, or about ⅓″	Slightly larger than a pea
2 cm	.7874 inch, or about ¾″	About the same as a cherry or a nickel
3 cm	1.811 inch, or about 1-⅕″	About the same as a Ping-Pong ball or a half dollar
4 cm	1.5748 inch, or about 1-½″	About the same as a golf ball
5 cm	1.9685 inch, or about 2″	About the same as a chicken's egg
6 cm	2.3622 inch, or about 2-⅓″	About the same as a plum
7 cm	2.7559 inch, or about 2-¾″	About the same as a peach
8 cm	3.1496 inch, or about 3-⅙″	About the same as a tomato
9 cm	3.5432 inch, or about 3-½″	About the same as a baseball
10 cm	3.937 inch, or about 4″	About the same as a navel orange
11 cm	4.3307 inch, or about 4-⅓″	About the same as a softball
12 cm	4.7244 inch, or about 4-¾″	About the same as a grapefruit

Women's Clinics Where You Can Obtain a Speculum*

CALIFORNIA

Berkeley Women's Health Collective
2908 Ellsworth
Berkeley, CA 94705
(415) 843-6194 or 843-6195

Chico Feminist Women's Health Center
330 Flume Street
Chico, CA 95926
(916) 891-1911

Oakland Feminist Women's Health Center
2930 McClure Street
Oakland, CA 94609
(415) 444-5676

Our Health Center
270 Grant Avenue
Palo Alto, CA 94306
(415) 327-8717

Everywoman's Clinic
1936 Linda Drive
Pleasant Hill, CA 94532
(415) 825-7900

Womancare, A Feminist Women's Health Center
424 Pennsylvania Avenue
San Diego, CA 92103
(714) 298-9352

Buena Vista Women's Medical Services
Buena Vista Counseling Center
2000 Van Ness Avenue
San Francisco, CA 94109
(415) 771-5000 or 441-1204

San Francisco Women's Health Center
3789 24th Street
San Francisco, CA 94114
(415) 282-6999

Women's Needs Center
1698 Haight Street
San Francisco, CA 94117
(415) 621-1003

Women's Community Clinic
696 East Santa Clara Street
San Jose, CA 95112
(408) 287-4322

*Some of these organizations have self-help groups; some provide instruction on an individual basis; still others will refer you to local sources.

861

Santa Cruz Women's Health Collective
250 Locust Street
Santa Cruz, CA 95060
(408) 427-3500

COLORADO

Women's Health Service Clinic
111 East Dale
Colorado Springs, CO 80903
(303) 471-9492

FLORIDA

Gainesville Women's Health Center
805 South West 4th Avenue
Gainesville, FL 32601
(904) 377-5055

Feminist Women's Health Center
540 West Brevard Street, Suite C
Tallahassee, FL 32301
(904) 224-9600

GEORGIA

Feminist Women's Health Center
580 14th Street, North West
Atlanta, GA 30318
(404) 874-7551

HAWAII

Women's Health Center of Hawaii, Inc.
2500 Pali Highway
Honolulu HI 96815
(808) 595-2506

Mailing address:
P.O. Box 17652
Honolulu, HI 96817

ILLINOIS

Chicago Women's Health Center
3435 North Sheffield
Chicago, IL 60657
(312) 935-6126

Emma Goldman Women's Health Center
1628 West Belmont
Chicago, IL 60657
(313) 528-4310

IOWA

Cedar Rapids Clinic for Women
86½ 16th Avenue, South West
Cedar Rapids, IA 52404
(319) 365-9527

Emma Goldman Clinic for Women
715 North Dodge
Iowa City, IA 52240
(319) 337-2111

MASSACHUSETTS

Everywoman's Center
Wilder Hall
University of Massachusetts
Amherst, MA 01003
(413) 545-0883

Women's Health Project
73 Union Avenue
Framingham, MA 01701
(617) 872-0711

Women's Community Health Center, Inc.
639 Massachusetts Avenue
Cambridge, MA 02139
(617) 547-2302

Family Planning of Hyannis
Cape Cod Medical Center
Hyannis, MA 02601
(617) 771-8010

Health Information Referral Service, Inc.
  (H.I.R.S.)
P.O. Box 160
Marlboro, MA 01752
(617) 481-8290

New Bedford Women's Center
  —Health Project
252 County Street
New Bedford, MA 02740
(617) 996-3341

862

MICHIGAN

Woman's Health and Information Project
Box 110 Warriner Hall
Central Michigan University
Mt. Pleasant, MI 48858
(517) 774-3151

MONTANA

Blue Mountain Women's Clinic
218 East Front
Missoula, MT 59801
(406) 542-0029

NEW HAMPSHIRE

New Hampshire Feminist Health Center
38 South Main Street
Concord, NH 03301
(603) 225-2739
and
232 Court Street
Portsmouth, NH 03801
(603) 436-7588

NEW JERSEY

Livingston Self-Help Group
Livingston College
Rutgers University
New Brunswick, NJ 08903
(201) 932-4333

NEW MEXICO

Women's Health Services
316 East Marcy Street
Santa Fe, NM 87501
(505) 988-8869

NEW YORK

Binghamton Women's Health Care Project
c/o Women's Center
P.O. Box 354
Binghamton, NY 13902
(607) 723-3200

Ithaca Women's Resource Center
112 The Commons
Ithaca, NY 14850
(607) 272-6922

Feminist Health Works
487-A Hudson Street
New York, NY 10014
(212) 929-7886

The Lesbian Health Collective
St Marks Clinic
44 St. Marks Place
New York, NY 10003
(212) 533-9500/9501

Women's Health Alliance
of Long Island, Inc.
Health House
555 North Country Road
St. James, NY 11780
(516) 862-6743

OREGON

Ashland Community Health Center
295 East Main Street, No. 15
Ashland, OR 97520
(503) 482-9741

Portland Women's Health Center
6510 South East Foster
Portland, OR 97206
(503) 777-7044

PENNSYLVANIA

Elizabeth Blackwell Health Center for
    Women
112 South 16th Street
Philadelphia, PA 19102
(215) 563-7577

Cindy Goldstein
258 Toftrees, No. 213
State College, PA 16801
(814) 234-8430

863

RHODE ISLAND

The Rhode Island Health Collective
2 Stimson Avenue
Providence, RI 02906
(401) 274-9264

TEXAS

Brookside Women's Medical Center
1902 South 1 H 35
Austin, TX 78704
(512)443-9595

Houston Women's Health Collective
c/o Nancy Kern
2804 Morrison Street
Houston, TX 77009
(713)523-6494

VERMONT

Planned Parenthood of Vermont
—Barre Center
24 Spauling Street
Barre, VT 05641
(802) 476-6696

Vermont Women's Health Center
P.O. Box 29
336 North Avenue
Burlington, VT 05401
(802) 863-1388

WASHINGTON

Blackwell Women's Health Resource Center
1520 North State Street
Bellingham, WA 98225
(206) 734-8592

Aradia Women's Health Center
1827 12th Avenue
Seattle, WA 98122
(206) 323-9388

Abortion and Birth Control Referral Service
4224 University Way, North East
Seattle, WA 98105
(206) 634-3460

Freemont Women's Clinic
6817 Greenwood Avenue North
Seattle, WA 98103
(206) 789-0773

WASHINGTON, D.C.

Washington Free Clinic
16th and Newton Streets, North West
Washington, DC 20010
(202) 667-1106

WISCONSIN

Bread & Roses Women's Health Center
238 West Wisconsin Avenue, No. 700
Milwaukee, WI 53203
(414) 278-0260

Planned Parenthood Regional Offices

Western Region

(Alaska, Arizona, California, Colorado, Hawaii, Idaho, Montana, Nevada, New Mexico, North Dakota, Oregon, South Dakota, Utah, Washington, Wyoming)

150 Green Street, Suite 3A
San Francisco, CA 94111
(415) 956-8856

Southern Region

(Alabama, Arkansas, Florida, Georgia, Kentucky, Louisiana, Mississippi, North Carolina, Oklahoma, South Carolina, Tennessee, Texas, Virginia)

3030 Peachtree Road, N.W., Room 303
Atlanta, GA 30305
(404) 262-1128

Northern Region

(Connecticut, Delaware, District of Columbia, Illinois, Indiana, Iowa, Kansas, Maine, Maryland, Massachusetts,

Michigan, Minnesota, Missouri, Nebraska, New Hampshire, New Jersey, New York, Ohio, Pennsylvania, Rhode Island, Vermont, West Virginia, Wisconsin)

2625 Butterfield Road
Oak Brook, IL 60521
(312) 986-9270

Planned Parenthood— Washington, DC Office

Planned Parenthood Federation of America
2010 Massachusetts Avenue, N.W., Suite 500
Washington, DC 20036
(202) 785-3351

Planned Parenthood Affiliates and Chapters

ALABAMA
Birmingham
Planned Parenthood of Alabama (M)
1108 S. 20th Street (35256)
(205) 933-8444

(M) = Medical   (E) = Educational   (P) = Provisional

Mobile
Planned Parenthood of the Mobile Bay
  Area (E,P)
2004 Airport Boulevard (36606)
(205) 479-5363

ALASKA

Anchorage
Planned Parenthood of Alaska (M)
100 W. 13th Street (99501)
(907) 279-2576 (Clinic)/ 279-9581
  (Admin.)

ARIZONA

Phoenix
Planned Parenthood of Central & Northern
  Arizona (M)
1301 S. Seventh Avenue (85007)
(602) 257-1515 (Clinic)/ 258-4299
  (Admin.)

Tucson
Planned Parenthood of Southern Arizona,
  Inc. (M)
127 S. Fifth Avenue (85007)
(602) 624-1761

ARKANSAS

For information call:
Planned Parenthood of Eastern Oklahoma
  & Western Arkansas
Tulsa, OK
(918) 587-1101

CALIFORNIA

Eureka
Planned Parenthood of Humboldt County
  (M)
2316 Harrison Avenue (95501)
(707) 442-5709 (Admin.)

Fresno
Planned Parenthood of Central California
  (M)
633 N. Van Ness (93728)
(209) 486-2411

Los Angeles
Planned Parenthood—World Population
  Los Angeles (M)
3100 W. Eighth Street (90005)
(213) 380-9300

Monterey
Planned Parenthood of Monterey County,
  Inc. (M)
5 Via Joaquin (93940)
(408) 373-1691 (Clinic)/373-1709
  (Admin.)

Pasadena
Pasadena Planned Parenthood Committee,
  Inc. (M)
1045 N. Lake Avenue (91104)
(213) 798-0706 (Clinic)/681-7202
  (Admin.)

Sacramento
Planned Parenthood of Sacramento Valley
  (M)
1507 21st Street, Suite 100 (95814)
(916) 446-5034 (Clinic)/446-5037
  (Admin.)

San Diego
Planned Parenthood of San Diego County
  (M)
2100 Fifth Avenue (92101)
(619) 231-2941

San Francisco
Planned Parenthood Alameda–San
  Francisco (M)
1660 Bush Street (94109)
(415) 441-5454

San Jose
Planned Parenthood Assn. of Santa Clara
  County Inc. (M)
17 N. Pedro (95110)
(408) 287-7526 (Clinic)/287-7532
  (Admin.)

(M)=Medical   (E)=Educational   (P)=Provisional

San Mateo
Planned Parenthood Assn. of San Mateo
County (M)
2211 Palm Avenue (94403)
(415) 574-2622 (Clinic)/574-5823
(Admin.)

San Rafael
Planned Parenthood of Marin and Sonoma
(M)
20 H Street (94901)
(415) 454-0471 (Clinic)/454-0476
(Admin.)

Santa Ana
Planned Parenthood Assn. of Orange
County Inc. (M)
1801 N. Broadway (92706)
(714) 973-1727 (Clinic)/973-1733
(Admin.)

Santa Barbara
Planned Parenthood of Santa Barbara
County (M)
518 Garden Street (93101)
(805) 963-5801

Santa Cruz
Planned Parenthood of Santa Cruz County
(M)
212 Laurel Street (95060)
(408) 426-5550 (Clinic)/425-1553
(Admin.)

Stockton
Planned Parenthood of San Joaquin County
(M)
19 N. Pilgrim Street (95205)
(209) 466-2081 (Clinic)/466-9220
(Admin.)

Walnut Creek
Planned Parenthood: Butte, Contra Costa,
Napa, Solano (M)
1291 Oakland Boulevard (94596)
(415) 935-3010 (Clinic)/935-4066
(Admin.)

COLORADO

Aurora
Rocky Mountain Planned Parenthood (M)
1537 Alton Street (80010)
(303) 360-0006

Springfield, MO (Associate)
The Greater Springfield Planned
Parenthood Assn., Inc. (M)
1918 E. Meadowmere, (65804)
(417) 883-3800

Parkersburg, WV (Associate)
Planned Parenthood of Parkersburg (M)
1100 Market Street, P.O. Box 1095
(26101)
(304) 485-1144

CONNECTICUT

New Haven
Planned Parenthood League of
Connecticut, Inc. (M)
129 Whitney Avenue (06510)
(203) 865-0595 (Clinic)/865-5158
(Admin.)

Bridgeport Chapter
1067 Park Avenue (06604)
(203) 366-0664

Danbury Chapter
44 Main Street (06810)
(203) 743-2446

Greater Hartford Chapter
Hilda Standish Center
1030 New Britain Avenue
West Hartford (06110)
(203) 522-6201

Manchester Chapter
1 Haynes Street (06040)
(203) 643-1607

Middletown Chapter
45 Broad Street (06457)
(203) 347-5255

New Haven Chapter
Griswold–Buxton Clinic
129 Whitney Avenue (06510)
(203) 865-0595

(M)=Medical   (E)=Educational   (P)=Provisional

867

New London Chapter
420 Williams Street (06320)
(203) 443-5820

Norwich Chapter
12 Case Street (06360)
(203) 889-5211

Norwalk Chapter
20 N. Main Street
South Norwalk (06854)
(203) 853-2605

Stamford Chapter
80 Lincoln Avenue (06902)
(203) 327-2722

Waterbury Chapter
125 Grove Street (06710)
(203) 423-0336

Willimantic Chapter
872 Main Street (06226)
(203) 423-0336

DELAWARE

Wilmington
Delaware League for Planned Parenthood,
   Inc. (M)
625 Shipley Street (19801)
(302) 655-7293

DISTRICT OF COLUMBIA

Washington
Planned Parenthood of Metropolitan
   Washington, DC, Inc. (M)
1108 16th Street, N.W. (20036)
(202) 347-8500

Washington, DC Chapter
1108 16th Street, N.W. (20036)
(202) 347-8512

Montgomery County Chapter
Randolph Medical Center, Suite 209
4701 Randolph Road
Rockville, MD 20852
(301) 468-7676

Prince George County Chapter
Landover Mall, E. Tower Suite 203
Landover, MD 20785
(301) 773-5601

Northern Virginia Chapter
5622 Columbia Pike
Falls Church, VA 22041
(703) 820-3335

FLORIDA

Boca Raton
Planned Parenthood of South Palm Beach
   & Broward Counties Inc. (M)
160 N.W. 4th Street (33432)
(305) 368-1023

Coral Gables
Planned Parenthood Assn. of Greater
   Miami, Inc. (M)
351 Altara Avenue (33146)
(305) 443-0774

Gainesville
Planned Parenthood of North Central
   Florida, Inc. (M)
P.O. Box 12385 (32604)
(904) 377-0881/0856

Jacksonville
Planned Parenthood of Northeast Florida,
   Inc. (M)
603 N. Market Street (32202)
(904) 358-2244

Lakeland
Planned Parenthood of Central Florida,
   Inc. (M)
1104 N. Dakota Avenue (33805)
(813) 688-2646

Sarasota
Planned Parenthood of Southwest Florida,
   Inc. (M)
1958 Prospect Street (33579)
(813) 953-4060/1 (Clinic)/365-3913/4
   (Admin.)

Naples Chapter
482 Tamiami Trail N. (33940)
(813) 262-0301

(M) = Medical   (E) = Educational   (P) = Provisional

868

Tallahassee
Planned Parenthood of Tallahassee, Inc. (M)
201 S. Bronough (32301)
(904) 222-0471/0472

West Palm Beach
Planned Parenthood Palm Beach Area, Inc.
(M)
5312 Broadway (33407)
(305) 848-6300

GEORGIA

Atlanta
Planned Parenthood Assn. of the Atlanta
Area, Inc. (M)
100 Edgewood Avenue, N.E. Suite 1604
(30303)
(404) 688-9300

Augusta
Planned Parenthood of East Central
Georgia, Inc. (M)
1289 Broad Street (30902)
(404) 724-5557

HAWAII

Honolulu
Hawaii Planned Parenthood (M)
1164 Bishop Street (96813)
(808) 521-6991

IDAHO

Boise
Planned Parenthood Assn. of Idaho (M)
4301 Franklin Road (83705)
(208) 345-0760

ILLINOIS

Bloomington
Planned Parenthood of Mid Central
Illinois, Inc. (M)
McBarnes Memorial Building
201 E. Grove Street, 2nd Fl. (61701)
(309) 827-8025

Champaign
Planned Parenthood of Champaign County
(M)
314 S. Neil Street (61820)
(217) 359-8022

Chicago
Planned Parenthood Assn.—Chicago Area
(M)
17 N. State Street, 15th Fl. (60602)
(312) 781-9550

Decatur
Planned Parenthood of Decatur, Inc. (M)
988–990 S. Main Street (62521)
(217) 429-9211

Peoria
Planned Parenthood Assn. of Peoria Area
(M)
705 N.E. Jefferson (61603)
(309) 673-0907/6911

Springfield
Planned Parenthood—Springfield Area (M)
500 E. Capitol, 3rd Fl. (62701)
(217) 544-2744

INDIANA

Bloomington
Planned Parenthood of South Central
Indiana, Inc. (M)
421 S. College Avenue (47401)
(812) 336-0219 (Clinic)/336-7050
(Admin.)

Evansville
Planned Parenthood of Southwestern
Indiana (M)
1610 S. Weinbach Avenue (47714)
(812) 473-8800

Fort Wayne
Planned Parenthood of Northeastern
Indiana (M)
347 W. Berry, Suite 300 (46802)
(219) 423-1322

(M) = Medical   (E) = Educational   (P) = Provisional

Indianapolis
Planned Parenthood Assn. of Central
  Indiana, Inc. (M)
3209 N. Meridian Street (46208)
(317) 926-4662

Lafayette
Tecumseh Area Planned Parenthood
  Assn., Inc. (M)
P.O. Box 1159
1016 E. Main (47902)
(317) 742-9073

Merrillville
Planned Parenthood of Northwest Indiana,
  Inc. (M)
8645 Connecticut (46410)
(219) 769-3500

Muncie
Planned Parenthood of East Central
  Indiana, Inc. (M)
110 N. Cherry at W. Main (47305)
(317) 282-3546

South Bend
Planned Parenthood of North Central
  Indiana (M)
201 S. Chapin (46625)
(219) 289-7062

Terre Haute
Planned Parenthood Assn. of Wabash
  Valley, Inc. (M)
330 S. 6th Street (47808)
(812) 238-2636 (Clinic)/232-0183
  (Admin.)

IOWA

Burlington
Planned Parenthood of Southeast Iowa (M)
413 Tama Building (52601)
(319) 753-6209

Des Moines County Chapter
413 Tama Building
Burlington (52601)
(319) 753-2281

Henry County Chapter
125 ½ W. Monroe
Mount Pleasant (52641)
(319) 385-4310

North Lee County Chapter
631 Avenue H
Fort Madison (52627)
(319) 372-1130

South Lee County Chapter
206 ½ N. 7th Street
Keokuk (52632)
(319) 524-1820

Washington County Chapter
P.O. Box 44
McCreedy & 4th
Washington (52353)
(319) 653-3525

Cedar Rapids
Planned Parenthood of Linn County, Inc.
  (M)
1500 Second Avenue, S.E., Suite 100
  (52403)
(319) 363-8572

Des Moines
Planned Parenthood of Mid–Iowa (M)
P.O. Box 4557 (50306)
(515) 280-7000

Sioux City
Planned Parenthood Committee of Sioux
  City (M)
2831 Douglas Street (51104)
(712) 277-3332

KANSAS

Wichita
Planned Parenthood of Kansas (M)
2226 E. Central (67214)
(316) 263-7575

Hays Chapter
115 E. 6th Street (67601)
(913) 628-2434

(M)=Medical   (E)=Educational   (P)=Provisional

KENTUCKY

Berea
Mountain Maternal Health League, Inc. (M)
P.O. Box 429 (40403)
(606) 986-2326

Lexington
Lexington Planned Parenthood Center,
Inc. (M)
508 W. Second Street (40507)
(606) 252-8494

Louisville
Planned Parenthood of Louisville, Inc. (M)
834 E. Broadway, Suite 506 (40204)
(502) 584-2471

LOUISIANA

New Orleans
Planned Parenthood of Louisiana (E,P)
620 Governor Nichols (70116)
(504) 524-8265

MARYLAND

Baltimore
Planned Parenthood Assn. of Maryland,
Inc. (M)
610 N. Howard Street (21201)
(301) 752-0131

Maryland County Chapter—Rockville,
MD
(See District of Columbia)

Prince George County Chapter
—Landover, MD
(See District of Columbia)

MASSACHUSETTS

Cambridge
Planned Parenthood League of
Massachusetts (M)
99 Bishop Richard Allen Drive (02139)
(617) 492-0518

MICHIGAN

Ann Arbor
Planned Parenthood of Mid–Michigan (M)
912 N. Main Street (48104)
(313) 996-4000

Benton Harbor
Planned Parenthood Assn. of Southwestern
Michigan, Inc. (M)
785 Pipestone (49022)
(616) 925-1306

Detroit
Planned Parenthood League, Inc. (M)
13100 Puritan (48227)
(313) 861-6704

Flint
Flint Community Planned Parenthood
Assn. (M)
310 E. Third Street, YWCA (48503)
(313) 238-3631

Shiawassee County Chapter
P.O. Box 542
826 W. King, 3rd Fl.
Owosso (48867)
(517) 723-6420

Grand Rapids
Planned Parenthood Centers of West
Michigan (M)
425 Cherry, S.E. (49503)
(616) 774-7005

Ionia County Chapter
111 Kidd Street, N. (48846)
(616) 527-3250

Kalamazoo
Reproductive Health Care Center of South
Central Michigan, An Affiliate of
PPFA, Inc. (M)
P.O. Box 1069
4201 W. Michigan Avenue (49005)
(616) 372-1200

Marquette
Marquette–Alger Planned Parenthood (M)
228 W. Washington, Suite 1 (49855)
(906) 225-5070

(M)=Medical   (E)=Educational   (P)=Provisional

871

Muskegon
Muskegon Area Planned Parenthood
  Assn., Inc. (M)
1642 Peck (49441)
(616) 722-2928

Petoskey
Northern Michigan Planned Parenthood
  Assn. Lockwood Division, N.M.H. (M)
820 Arlington (49770)
(616) 347-9692

MINNESOTA

St. Paul
Planned Parenthood of Minnesota, Inc. (M)
1965 Ford Parkway (55116)
(612) 698-2401

Bemidji Chapter
411 ½ Beltrami (56601)
(218) 751-8683

Brainerd Chapter
507 Washington (56401)
(218) 829-1469

Duluth Chapter
Arrowhead Place
211 W. 2nd, 4th Fl. (55802)
(218) 722-0833

Mankato Chapter
104 E. Liberty, Room 203 (56001)
(507) 378-5581

Minneapolis Chapter
127 S. 10th Street (55403)
(612) 332-8931

Rochester Chapter
1202 ½ 7th Street, Suite C
Box 7117 (55901)
(507) 288-5186

St. Paul Chapter
110 Hamm Building
408 St. Peter Street (55102)
(612) 224-1361

Willmar Chapter
Bonde Building, 2nd Fl.
Fourth Street & Litchfield Avenue (56201)
(612) 235-9150

MISSISSIPPI

Jackson
Mississippi Planned Parenthood (E,P)
P.O. Box 16092 (39206)
(601) 354-0095

MISSOURI

Columbia
Planned Parenthood of Central Missouri (M)
800 N. Providence Road, Suite 5 (65201)
(314) 443-0427 (Clinic)/449-2475
  (Admin.)

Kansas City
Planned Parenthood of Greater Kansas City
  (M)
1001 E. 47th Street (64110)
(816) 756-2277

Kirksville
Planned Parenthood of Northeast Missouri,
  Inc. (M)
P.O. Box 763 (63501)
(816) 665-5672

Rolla
Planned Parenthood of the Central Ozarks
  (M)
Box 359, 1032B Kings Highway (65401)
(314) 364-1509

Springfield
See Rocky Mountain Planned Parenthood,
  Aurora, CO.

St. Louis
Planned Parenthood Assn. of St. Louis,
  Inc. (M)
2202 S. Hanley Road (63144)
(314) 781-3800

MONTANA

Billings
Planned Parenthood of Billings (M)
721 N. 29th (59101)
(406) 248-3636

(M) = Medical (E) = Educational (P) = Provisional

Missoula
Planned Parenthood of Missoula, Inc. (M)
235 E. Pine (59802)
(406) 728-5490

NEBRASKA

Lincoln
Planned Parenthood of Lincoln (M)
3830 Adams Street (68504)
(402) 467-4691

Omaha
Planned Parenthood of Omaha—Council
Bluffs (M)
4610 Dodge (68132)
(402) 554-1040 (Clinic)/554-1045
(Admin.)

NEVADA

Las Vegas
Planned Parenthood of Southern Nevada,
Inc. (M)
601 S. 13th Street (89101)
(702) 385-3451

Reno
Planned Parenthood of Northern Nevada (M)
455 W. Fifth Street (89503)
(702) 329-1781

NEW HAMPSHIRE

Lebanon
Planned Parenthood Assn. of the Upper
Valley (M)
127 Mascoma Street (03766)
(603) 448-1214

NEW JERSEY

Camden
Planned Parenthood—Greater Camden
Area (M)
590 Benson Street (08103)
(609) 365-3519

Hackensack
Planned Parenthood Center of Bergen
County (M)
575 Main Street (07601)
(201) 489-1140 (Clinic)/489-1420
(Admin.)

Morristown
Planned Parenthood of Northwest New
Jersey, Inc. (M)
197 Speedwell Avenue (07960)
(201) 539-9580

Newark
Planned Parenthood—Essex County (M)
151 Washington Street (07102)
(201) 622-3900

New Brunswick
Planned Parenthood League of Middlesex
County (M)
211 Livingston Avenue (08901)
(201) 246-2411

Paterson
Passaic County Planned Parenthood Center
(M)
175 Market Street (07505)
(201) 345-3883

Plainfield
Planned Parenthood of Union County
Area, Inc. (M)
203 Park Avenue (07060)
(201) 756-3765

Shrewsbury
Planned Parenthood of Monmouth County,
Inc. (M)
69 Newman Springs Road (07701)
(201) 842-9300

Trenton
Planned Parenthood Assn. of the Mercer
Area (M)
437 E. State Street (08608)
(609) 599-4881 (Clinic)/599-3736
(Admin.)

(M)=Medical   (E)=Educational   (P)=Provisional

873

NEW MEXICO

Albuquerque
Rio Grande Planned Parenthood (M)
113 Montclaire, S.E. (87108)
(505) 265-5976

Las Cruces
Planned Parenthood of South Central New
 Mexico (M)
302 W. Griggs Avenue (88001)
(505) 524-8516 (Clinic)/524-4471
 (Admin.)

Silver City
Planned Parenthood of Southwest New
 Mexico (M)
110 E. 11th (88061)
(505) 388-1553

NEW YORK

Albany
Upper Hudson Planned Parenthood, Inc. (M)
259 Lark Street (12210)
(518) 434-2182/4979

Binghampton
Planned Parenthood of Broome &
 Chenango Counties, Inc. (M)
710 O'Neill Building (13901)
(607) 723-8306

Buffalo
Planned Parenthood Center of Buffalo (M)
210 Franklin Street (14202)
(716) 853-1771

Elmira
Planned Parenthood of the Southern Tier,
 Inc. (M)
200 E. Market Street (14901)
(607) 734-3313

Geneva
Planned Parenthood of the Finger Lakes,
 Inc. (M)
435 Exchange Street (14456)
(315) 781-1092

Glens Falls
Southern Adirondack Planned Parenthood
 (M)
144 Ridge Street (12801)
(518) 798-8999

Huntington
Planned Parenthood of Suffolk County (M)
17 E. Carver Street (11743)
(516) 427-7154

Ithaca
Planned Parenthood of Tompkins County
 (M)
314 W. State Street (14850)
(607) 273-1513 (Clinic)/273-1526
 (Admin.)

Mineola
Planned Parenthood of Nassau County,
 Inc. (M)
107 Mineola Boulevard (11501)
(516) 742-0144

Newburgh
Planned Parenthood of Orange–Sullivan,
 Inc. (M)
91 DuBois Street (12550)
(914) 562-5748

New York
Planned Parenthood of New York City,
 Inc. (M)
380 Second Avenue, 3rd Fl. (10010)
(212) 777-2002

Niagara Falls
Planned Parenthood of Niagara County (M)
The Haeberle Plaza
Pine Avenue & Portage Road (14301)
282-1221 (Clinic)/282-2501 (Admin.)

Oneonta
Planned Parenthood Assn. of Delaware &
 Otsego Counties (M)
48 Market Street (13820)
(607) 432-2250

Plattsburgh
Northern Adirondack Planned Parenthood,
 Inc. (M)
66 Brinkerhoff Street (12901)
(518) 561-4430

(M)=Medical   (E)=Educational   (P)=Provisional

Poughkeepsie
Planned Parenthood of Dutchess–Ulster,
   Inc. (M)
85 Market Street (12601)
(914) 471-1540

Rochester
Planned Parenthood of Rochester &
   Monroe County, Inc. (M)
24 Windsor Street (14605)
(716) 546-2595

Schenectady
Planned Parenthood of Schenectady &
   Affiliated Counties, Inc. (M)
414 Union Street (12305)
(518) 374-5353

Syracuse
Planned Parenthood Center of Syracuse,
   Inc. (M)
1120 E. Genesee Street (13210)
(315) 374-5532

Utica
Planned Parenthood Assn. of the Mohawk
   Valley, Inc. (M)
1424 Genesee Street (13502)
(315) 724-6146

Watertown
Planned Parenthood of Northern New
   York, Inc. (M)
220 Sherman Street (13601)
(315) 782-1818

West Nyack
Planned Parenthood of Rockland County (M)
37 Village Square (10994)
(914) 358-1145/2155

White Plains
Planned Parenthood of Westchester, Inc. (M)
Administrative Office—Upper Level
88 E. Post Road (10601)
(914) 428-7876

NORTH CAROLINA

Asheville
Planned Parenthood of
   Asheville/Buncombe County, Inc. (M)
131 McDowell Street (28801)
(704) 252-7928

Chapel Hill
Planned Parenthood of Orange County,
   Inc. (E,P)
P.O. Box 3258 (27514)
(919) 942-7762 (Clinic)/929-5402
   (Admin.)

Charlotte
Planned Parenthood of Greater Charlotte (M)
East Independence Plaza Building
951 S. Independence Boulevard, Suite 430
   (28202)
(704) 377-0841

Raleigh
Planned Parenthood of Greater Raleigh,
   Inc. (M,P)
Bryan Building, Suite 230
Cameron Village (27605)
(919) 833-7526 (Clinic)/833-7534
   (Admin.)

Winston-Salem
Planned Parenthood of the Triad, Inc. (M)
823 Reynolds Road, Suite 102 (27104)
(919) 761-1052 (Clinic)/761-1058
   (Admin.)

OHIO

Akron
Planned Parenthood of Summit, Portage &
   Medina Counties (M)
39 E. Market Street (44308)
(216) 535-2674

Athens
Planned Parenthood of Southeast Ohio (M)
306 Security Building
8 N. Court Street (45701)
(614) 593-3375

(M) = Medical   (E) = Educational   (P) = Provisional

Canton
Planned Parenthood of Stark County (M)
626 Walnut Avenue, N.E. (44702)
(216) 456-7191

Cincinnati
Planned Parenthood Assn. of Cincinnati (M)
2406 Auburn Avenue (45219)
(513) 721-7993

Cleveland
Planned Parenthood of Cleveland, Inc. (M)
Bulkley Building
1501 Euclid Avenue, Suite 300 (44115)
(216) 781-0410

Lorain County Chapter
502 Middle Avenue
Elyria (44035)
(216) 322-9874

Columbus
Planned Parenthood of Central Ohio, Inc.
  (M)
206 E. State Street (43215)
(614) 224-2235

Dayton
Planned Parenthood Assn. of Miami
  Valley (M)
224 N. Wilkinson Street (45402)
(513) 226-0780

Hamilton
Planned Parenthood Assn. of Butler
  County, Inc. (M)
P.O. Box 631
11 Ludlow Street (45012)
(513) 894-3875 (Clinic)/894-8335
  (Admin.)

Mansfield
Planned Parenthood of North Central Ohio
  (M)
35 N. Park Street (44902)
(419) 525-3075
Crawford County Chapter
777 Portland Way N.
Galion (44833)
(419) 468-9926

Wayne County Chapter
2680 ½ Cleveland Road
Wooster (44691)
(216) 345-7798

Newark
Planned Parenthood Assn. of East Central
  Ohio (M)
Newark Medical Center
843 N. 21st Street (43055)
(614) 366-3377

Springfield
Planned Parenthood of West Central Ohio
  (M)
Arcue Building, 5th Fl.
6 W. High Street (45502)
(513) 325-6416/7

Toledo
Planned Parenthood of Northwest Ohio,
  Inc. (M)
1301 Jefferson (43624)
(419) 255-1115

Youngstown
Planned Parenthood of Mahoning Valley (M)
105 E. Boardman Street (44503)
(216) 746-5662

OKLAHOMA

Oklahoma City
Planned Parenthood Assn. of Oklahoma
  City (M)
619 N.W. 23rd Street (73103)
(415) 528-2157

Tulsa
Planned Parenthood of Eastern Oklahoma
  & Western Arkansas, Inc. (M)
1007 S. Peoria (74120)
(918) 587-1101

OREGON

Eugene
Planned Parenthood Assn. of Lane County
  (M)
134 E. 13th Avenue (97401)
(503) 344-9411

(M)=Medical   (E)=Educational   (P)=Provisional

Medford
Planned Parenthood of Southern Oregon (M)
650 Royal Avenue, Suite 18 (97501)
(503) 773-8285

Portland
Planned Parenthood Assn., Inc. (M)
3231 S.E. 50th (97206)
(503) 775-0861 (Clinic)/775-4931
(Admin.)

PENNSYLVANIA

Allentown
Planned Parenthood of Lehigh Valley (M)
112 N. 13th Street (18102)
(215) 439-1033

Bristol
Planned Parenthood Assn. of Bucks
County (M)
721 New Rodgers Road (19007)
(215) 785-4591

Harrisburg
Tri–County Planned Parenthood (M,P)
1910 N. Second Street (17102)
(717) 234-2479

Johnstown
Planned Parenthood Cambria/Somerset (M)
502 Main Street (15901)
(814) 535-5545

Lancaster
Planned Parenthood of Lancaster (M)
37 S. Lime Street (17602)
(717) 299-2891

Philadelphia
Planned Parenthood Assn. of Southeastern
Pennsylvania (M)
1220 Sansom Street (19107)
(215) 592-4100

Pittsburgh
Planned Parenthood Center of Pittsburgh,
Inc. (M)
102 9th Street (15222)
(412) 434-8950

Reading
Planned Parenthood Center of Berks
County, Inc. (M)
48 S. 4th Street (19602)
(215) 376-8061

Scranton
Planned Parenthood of Lackawanna &
Wyoming Counties (M)
207 Wyoming Avenue, Suite 322 (18503)
(717) 344-2626

Stroudsburg
Monroe County Planned Parenthood Assn.
(M)
28 N. 7th Street (18360)
(717) 424-8306

West Chester
Planned Parenthood of Chester County (M)
202 N. Church Street (19380)
(215) 436-8645

Wilkes–Barre
Planned Parenthood Assn. of Luzerne
County Inc. (M)
63 N. Franklin Street (18701)
(717) 824-8921

York
Planned Parenthood of Central
Pennsylvania (M)
728 S. Beaver Street (17403)
(717) 845-9681

RHODE ISLAND

Providence
Planned Parenthood of Rhode Island (M)
187 Westminster Mall (02903)
(401) 421-9620

SOUTH CAROLINA

Columbia
Planned Parenthood of Central South
Carolina, Inc. (M)
3101 Carlisle at Butler Street (29205)
(803) 256-4908

(M)=Medical   (E)=Educational   (P)=Provisional

TENNESSEE

Memphis
Memphis Assn. for Planned Parenthood,
, Inc. (M)
1407 Union Avenue (38104)
(901) 725-1717

Nashville
Planned Parenthood Assn. of Nashville,
Inc. (M)
University Plaza
112 21st Avenue S. (37203)
(615) 327-1066 (Clinic)/327-1095
(Admin.)

Oak Ridge
Planned Parenthood Assn. of East
Tennessee, Inc. (M)
162 Ridgeway Center (37830)
(615) 482-3406

TEXAS

Amarillo
Panhandle Planned Parenthood Assn. (M)
604 W. Eighth Street (79101)
(806) 372-8731

Austin
Planned Parenthood Center of Austin (M)
1309 E. 12th Street (78702)
(512) 477-5846 (Clinic)/472-0868
(Admin.)

Brownsville
Planned Parenthood of Cameron & Willacy
Counties (M)
15 E. Levee Street (78520)
(512) 546-4571

Corpus Christi
South Texas Planned Parenthood Center (M)
801 Elizabeth Street (78404)
(512) 884-4352

Dallas
Planned Parenthood of Greater Dallas, Inc.
(M,P)
One Glen Lakes Park
8140 Walnut Hill, Suite 501 (75231)
(214) 363-2004

El Paso
Planned Parenthood Center of El Paso (M)
2817 E. Yandell (79903)
(915) 566-6707 (Clinic)/566-1613
(Admin.)

Fort Worth
Planned Parenthood of North Texas, Inc.
(M)
1101 University (76107)
(817) 332-7966

Houston
Planned Parenthood of Houston and
Southeast Texas (M)
3601 Fannin (77004)
(713) 522-3976 (Clinic)/522-6240
(Admin.)

Kingsville
Planned Parenthood Assn. of Chaparral
County (M)
P.O. Box 1070 (78363)
(512) 592-2201

Lubbock
Planned Parenthood Center of Lubbock (M)
3821 22nd Street
P.O. Box 6193 (79413)
(806) 795-7123

McAllen
Planned Parenthood Assn. of Hidalgo
County (M)
1017 Pecan (78501)
(512) 686-0585

Odessa
Planned Parenthood of the Permian Basin,
Inc. (M)
910-B S. Grant Street (79763)
(915) 333-4133/35

San Angelo
Planned Parenthood Center of San Angelo
(M)
122 W. Second Street (76901)
(915) 655-9141

(M)=Medical   (E)=Educational   (P)=Provisional

878

San Antonio
Planned Parenthood Center of San Antonio (M)
104 Babcock at Fredricksburg Road (78201)
(512) 736-2244

Waco
The Central Texas Planned Parenthood Assn. (M)
P.O. Box 6308
1121 Ross Avenue (76706)
(817) 754-2392

UTAH

Salt Lake City
Planned Parenthood Assn. of Utah (M)
70 S. 900 E. #13 (84102)
(801) 322-5571 (Clinic)/532-1586 (Admin.)

VERMONT

Burlington
Planned Parenthood of Vermont (M)
State Office
23 Mansfield Avenue (05401)
(802) 862-9637

VIRGINIA

Falls Church
(See District of Columbia)

Hampton
Planned Parenthood of Southeastern Virginia, Inc. (M)
1520 Aberdeen Road, Room 101 (23666)
(804) 826-2079

Richmond
Virginia League for Planned Parenthood, Inc. (M)
1218 W. Franklin Street (23220)
(804) 353-5516 (Clinic)/353-5518 (Admin.)

Tri County Area Chapter
P.O. Box 1400
Suffolk (23434)
(804) 539-3456

Roanoke
Planned Parenthood of Southwest Virginia, Inc. (M)
309 Luck Avenue S.W. (24016)
(703) 342-6741 (Clinic)/982-7621 (Admin.)

WASHINGTON

Bellingham
Mount Baker Planned Parenthood (M)
500 Grand Avenue (98225)
(206) 734-9095 (Clinic)/734-9007 (Admin.)

Everett
Planned Parenthood of Snohomish County (M)
2730 Hoyt Avenue (98201)
(206) 339-3389

Kennewick
Planned Parenthood of Benton–Franklin Counties
P.O. Box 6842 (99336)
(509) 586-2164

Seattle
Planned Parenthood of Seattle—King County (M)
2211 E. Madison (98112)
(206) 447-2364

Spokane
Planned Parenthood of Spokane (M)
W. 521 Garland Avenue (99205)
(509) 326-2142 (Clinic)/326-6292 (Admin.)

Tacoma
Planned Parenthood of Pierce County (M)
813 S. K Street, Suite 200 (98405)
(206) 572-6955

(M) = Medical   (E) = Educational   (P) = Provisional

Walla Walla
Planned Parenthood of Walla Walla (M)
136 E. Birch Street (99362)
(509) 529-3570

Yakima
Planned Parenthood Assn. of Yakima
County (M)
208 N. 3rd Avenue (98902)
(509) 248-3625

WEST VIRGINIA

Parkersburg
(See Rocky Mountain Planned Parenthood,
Aurora, CO.)

WISCONSIN

Wilwaukee
Planned Parenthood of Wisconsin, Inc. (M)
744 N. Fourth Street (53203)
(414) 271-8045

Bay-Lakes Chapter
302 N. Adams Street
Green Bay (54301)
(414) 432-0031/4421

Central Wisconsin Chapter
214 W. Grand Avenue, P.O. Box 941
Wisconsin Rapids (54494)
(715) 423-9610

Dane-Sauk-Columbia Chapter
1050 Regent Street
Madison (53715)
(608) 256-7257/7705

Fox Valley Chapter
508 W. Wisconsin Avenue
Appleton (54911)
(414) 731-6304/6064

Kenosha-Walworth Chapter
2002 63rd Street
Kenosha (53140)
(414) 654-0491

Kettle Moraine Lakeshore Chapter
814 Plaza 8
Sheboygan (53081)
(414) 458-9401

Lakeland Area Chapter
138 Front Street
Beaver Dam (53916)
(414) 885-3528/3791

Greater Milwaukee Chapter
1135 W. State Street
Milwaukee (53233)
(414) 271-8116/8181

WYOMING

For information call:
Rocky Mountain Planned Parenthood
Aurora, CO
(303) 360-0006

State Public Affairs Offices

CALIFORNIA

Planned Parenthood Affiliates of California
(PPAC)
1317-A 15th Street
Sacramento (95814)
(916) 446-5247

FLORIDA

Florida Assn. of Planned Parenthood
Affiliates
5312 Broadway
West Palm Beach (33407)
(305) 848-6300

ILLINOIS

Planned Parenthood Illinois Council
104 N. Fourth Street
Springfield (62701)
(217) 522-6776

(M) = Medical   (E) = Educational   (P) = Provisional

INDIANA

Indiana Planned Parenthood Affiliates
Planned Parenthood Assoc. of
  Indianapolis, Inc.
3209 N. Meridan
Indianapolis (46208)
(317) 926-4662

MICHIGAN

Planned Parenthood Affiliates of Michigan
c/o YWCA
217 Townsend Street, Room 102
Lansing (48901)
(517) 482-1080

MISSOURI

Missouri Assn. of Planned Parenthood
  Affiliates
129 E. High Street, Suite B
Jefferson City (65101)
(314) 634-2761

NEW JERSEY

Family Planning Advocates of New Jersey
Planned Parenthood Affiliates of N.J.
154 W. State Street
Trenton (08608)
(609) 393-8423

NEW MEXICO

Planned Parenthood Assn. of New Mexico
  Affiliates
Suite 318A
4001 Indian School Road, N.E.
Albuquerque (87110)
(505) 265-8181

NEW YORK

Family Planning Advocates of New York
  State
284 State Street
Albany (12210)
(518) 436-8408

OHIO

Planned Parenthood Affiliates of Ohio,
  Inc. (PPAO)
16 E. Broad Street, Room 915
Columbus (43215)
(614) 224-0761

OREGON

Family Planning Advocates of Oregon
  (FPAO)
3231 S.E. 50th Avenue
Portland (97206)
(503) 233-1131

PENNSYLVANIA

Planned Parenthood Pennsylvania
  Affiliates/Pennsylvania Advocates for
  Reproductive Health
227 State Street, 3rd Fl.
Harrisburg (17102)
(717) 234-3024

TENNESSEE

Tennessee Assn. of Planned Parenthood
  Affiliates
P.O. Box 2567, Suite 123
162 Fourth Avenue, N.
Nashville (37219)
(615) 255-9032

881

TEXAS

Texas Family Planning Assn.
P.O. Box 5571
Austin (78763)
(512) 474-7427

VIRGINIA

Assn. of Virginia Planned Parenthood
   Affiliates
1001 E. Main
Suite 522
Richmond (23219)
(804) 643-3353

This list reprinted Courtesy of Planned Parenthood Federation of America, Inc.

National Surgical Adjuvant Project for Breast and Bowel Cancers Institutional Headquarters Staff and Major Participants

NSABP Headquarters Office
3550 Terrace Street
Room 914, Scaife Hall
Pittsburgh, PA 15261
Phone: (412/624-2671)

Bernard Fisher, M.D., Project Chairman

1. Albany Regional Cancer Center, NY
    (108)

    St. Peter's Professional Building
    317 S. Manning Boulevard
    Suite 330
    Albany, NY 12208
    (518/489-2607)
    *Dr. Thomas J. Cunningham (Med.
      Oncol.)
    Dr. Robert W. Sponzo (Med.
      Oncol.)
    Ms. Michele Trombly, R.N.
    Ms. Angela Viana, R.N.
    Ms. Barbara Demyan
    Ms. Maureen Baxter, R.N.

    St. Peter's Hospital

*Principal Investigator

632 New Scotland Avenue
Albany, NY 12208
(518/471-1550)
Dr. Thomas J. Cunningham
  (NSABP Program Dir.)
Dr. Maureen Archambault (Rad.
  Oncol.)
Dr. Russell Newkirk (Pathol.)
Dr. Nathan Reed (Surg. Oncol.)
Dr. David O'Keeffe (Surg. Oncol.)
Dr. Robert Jordan (Surg. Oncol.)
Dr. James Otto (Surg. Oncol.)

Putnam Memorial Hospital
Bennington, VT 05201
(802/442-6361)
Dr. Mark Donavan (Med. Oncol.)

Samaritan Hospital
2215 Burdett Avenue
Troy, NY 12180
(518/271-3300)
Dr. Thomas J. Cunningham
    (NSABP Program Dir.)
Dr. Ancieto Lomotan (Pathol.)
Dr. E. Carl Quinlan (Surg. Oncol.)
Mrs. Sherry Simpson–Root, R.N.
Mrs. Lynn Wheland, R.N.
Mrs. Linda Dobransky, R.N.

Columbia Memorial Hospital
71 Prospect Avenue
Hudson, NY 12534
(518/828-7601)
Dr. Thomas J. Cunningham
    (NSABP Program Dir.)
Ms. Jane Meicht, R.N.

2. Albert Einstein College of
    Medicine, NY (1)

Van Ettan Hospital, Room 5021
1300 Morris Park Avenue
Bronx, NY 10461
(212/430-3063)
*Dr. Herbert Volk (Surg. Oncol.)
Dr. George Escher (Med. Oncol.)
Dr. Barry Kaplan (Med. Oncol.)
Ms. Giovanna Cavasotto
Ms. Margot Wulf

Jacobi Hospital
Pelham Parkway & Eastchester
    Road
Bronx, NY 10461
(212/430-5000)
Dr. Nino Carnevaie (Surg. Oncol.)

Hospital of the Albert Einstein
    College of Medicine
1825 Eastchester Road, I–92
Bronx, NY 10461
(212/430-2000)
Dr. Michael S. Gold
    (Surgeon–in–Chief)
Dr. Sam Lan (Surg. Oncol.)
Dr. Andre Abitol (Rad. Oncol.)

*Principal Investigator

3. Albert Einstein Medical Center,
    PHILA. (109)

Medical Oncology Hematology
    Associates, PC
1335 W. Tabor Road
Philadelphia, PA 19141
(215/927-3900)
*Dr. Stanley N. Levick (Med.
    Oncol.)
*Dr. Ajit M. Desai (Med. Oncol.)
Dr. Leonard J. Levick (Med.
    Oncol.)
Ms. Elizabeth Meyer, R.N.
Ms. Joy Andreas, R.N.

1335 W. Tabor Road
Philadelphia, PA 19141
(215/924-2723)
Dr. John Robertson (Surg. Oncol.)

Northern Division
York & Tabor Roads
Philadelphia, PA 19141
(215/456-7890)
Dr. Sucha Asbell (Rad. Oncol.)
Dr. Stanton Carroll (Surg. Oncol.)
Dr. E. A. Cohen (Surg. Oncol.)
Dr. Alexander Labe (Surg. Oncol.)
Dr. Robert Solit (Surg. Oncol.)
Dr. Robert Somers (Surg. Oncol.)
Dr. David White (Surg. Oncol.)
Dr. Robert B. Sklaroff (Med.
    Oncol.)
Dr. Phillip Kim (Pathol.)

1301 W. Tabor Road
Philadelphia, PA 19141
(215/333-0432)
Dr. Leonard Cohen (Surg. Oncol.)

John F. Kennedy Memorial Hospital
Langdon Street & Cheltenham
    Avenue
Philadelphia, Pa. 19124
(215/831-7000)
*Dr. Stanley N. Levick (Med.
    Oncol.)
*Dr. Ajit M. Desai (Med. Oncol.)
Dr. John Robertson (Surg. Oncol.)
Dr. Alexander Labe (Surg. Oncol.)
Dr. James Williams (Pathol.)

4. Allentown Hospital/Allentown
   Sacred Heart Hospital Center, PA
   (64)

   1730 Chew Street
   Allentown, PA 18104
   (215/433-6691)
   *Dr. David Prager (Med. Oncol.)
   Dr. Robert Post (Med. Oncol.)
   Dr. Lloyd E. Barron II (Med.
     Oncol.)
   Mrs. Rhoda Prager
   Ms. Mary Boyle, R.N.

   Lehigh Valley Hospital Center
   1200 S. Cedar Crest Boulevard
   Allentown, PA 18104
   (215/821-3770)
   Mr. Richard Attilio, R.Ph.

   121 N. Cedar Crest Boulevard
   Allentown, PA 18104
   (215/439-4055)
   Dr. Joseph Prorok (Surg. Oncol.)
   Dr. George Hartzell (Surg. Oncol.)
   Dr. Mark Gittleman (Surg. Oncol.)

   1627 Chew Street
   Allentown, PA 18102
   (215/433-6691)
   Dr. Nathaniel Silon (Rad. Oncol.)
   Dr. Alexander Nedwich (Pathol.)
   Dr. John Young (Rad. Oncol.)

   2200 Hamilton Street
   Allentown, PA 18104
   Dr. Milton Friedberg (Surg. Oncol.)

   Allentown Sacred Heart Hospital
     Center
   1200 S. Cedar Crest Boulevard
   Allentown, PA 18105
   (215/821-2050)
   Dr. John Shane (Pathol.)
   Dr. Michael Scarlotto (Pathol.)
   Dr. Raymond Rachman (Pathol.)

   1736 Hamilton Street
   Allentown, PA 18104
   Dr. Robinson Fry (Surg. Oncol.)
   Dr. Willard Noyes (Surg. Oncol.)

   175 E. Brown Street
   East Stroudsburg, PA 18301
   Dr. Jean Golden (Surg. Oncol.)
   Dr. John DeBoer (Surg. Oncol.)
   Dr. William Jordan (Surg. Oncol.)
   Dr. William Rogers (Surg. Oncol.)

   1532 Park Avenue
   Quakertown, PA 18951
   (215/536-1133)
   Dr. Wendell Eicher (Surg. Oncol.)
   Dr. T. Wistar Brown (Surg. Oncol.)

   1275 S. Cedar Crest Boulevard
   Allentown, PA 18103
   (215/433-7571)
   Dr. Indru Khubchandani (Surg.
     Oncol.)
   Dr. James Sheets (Surg. Oncol.)
   Dr. John Stasik (Surg. Oncol.)
   Dr. Lester Rosen (Surg. Oncol.)
   Dr. Robert Reither (Surg. Oncol.)

   239 E. Brown Street
   East Stroudsburg, PA 18301
   (717/421-4000)
   Dr. Theodore Kowalyshyn
     (Hematol./Oncol.)
   Dr. Elmo Lilli (Fam. Practice)

   Wallenpaupack Medical Foundation
   Tafton, PA 18464
   (717/266-2151)
   Dr. William Dewar (Internist)

   40 W. Catawissa Street
   Nesquehoning, PA 18240
   (717/669-6133)
   Dr. John Evans (Surg. Oncol.)

   Grandview Hospital
   Nurses Home
   724 Lawn Avenue
   Sellersville, PA 18960
   (215/257-8858)
   Dr. Alan Kaufman
     (Hematol./Oncol.)

5. Baptist Medical Center, OK (165)

   Baptist Medical Center of Oklahoma
   3300 Northwest Expressway
   Oklahoma City, OK 73112

*Principal Investigator

885

(405/949-6711)
*Dr. Karl K. Boatman (Surg.
   Oncol.)
Dr. Stan Shrago (Pathol.)
Dr. Michael Sartin (Rad. Oncol.)
Ms. Jan Prestwood, R.N.
Ms. Carl Elder, Data

6. Baptist Memorial Hospital,
   Pensacola, FL (159)

   1000 Moreno Street
   Pensacola, FL 32501
   (904/434-4785)
   *Dr. Allan Patton (Med. Oncol.)
   Dr. Paul Meadows (Rad. Oncol.)
   Dr. Albert Drlicka (Pathol.)
   Ms. Harriet Barrington

   5140 N. 9th Avenue
   Pensacola, FL 32504
   (904/434-4785)
   Dr. Russell Lowery (Surg. Oncol.)
   Dr. Manuel Lopez (Clin. Immunol.)

7. Baylor University Medical Center

   3500 Gaston Avenue
   Dallas, TX 75246
   (214/820-3445)
   *Dr. Leon Dragon (Med. Oncol.)
   Dr. Robert Pickett Scruggs, III
      (Rad. Oncol.)
   Dr. J. Harold Cheek (Surg. Oncol.)
   Dr. William B. Kingsley (Patho.)
   Dr. George Peters (Surg. Oncol.)

   (214/820-2657)
   Ms. Mari Lewis (Data Manager)

8. Berkshire Medical Center,
   Pittsfield, MA (86)

   725 North Street
   Pittsfield, MA 01201
   (413/49904161)
   *Dr. Jesse Spector
      (Hematol./Oncol.)
   *Dr. Harvey Zimbler
      (Hematol./Oncol.)
   Dr. Jeffrey Ross (Pathol.)
   Ms. Judith Tremblay, R.N.

*Principal Investigator

886

276 South Street
Pittsfield, MA 01201
Dr. Michael Giborski (Surg. Oncol.)

9. Billings Interhospital Oncology
   Project, MT (125)

   Yellowstone Medical Building
   1145 N. 29th Street
   Suite 400
   Billings, MT 59101
   (406/245-6378)
   *Dr. David B. Myers (Surg. Oncol.)
   Ms. Lois Miller, R.N.

   Poly Drive & N. 28th Street
   Billings, MT 59101
   (406/248-2212)
   Dr. Fred Deigert (Rad. Oncol.)
   Dr. Ted Reinke (Rad. Oncol.)

   1230 N. 30th Street
   Billings, MT 59101
   (406/252-2147)
   Dr. Neel Hammond (Med. Oncol.)
   Dr. Benjamin T. Marchello (Med.
      Oncol.)
   Ms. Judy Lohrenz, R.N.
   Ms. Marion Tebay, R.N.

   P.O. Box 2505
   Billings, MT 59103
   (406/657-7733)
   Dr. Kenneth Mueller (Pathol.)
   Mrs. Sandy Kassion, R.N.

10. Boston University (91)

   75 E. Newton Street
   Boston, MA 02118
   (617/247-5219)
   *Dr. Peter J. Deckers (Surg. Oncol.)
   *Dr. Merrill I. Feldman (Rad.
      Oncol.)
   Dr. Peter Mozden (Surg. Oncol.)
   Dr. Richard J. Elkort (Surg. Oncol.)
   Dr. Maureen Kavanah (Surg.
      Oncol.)
   Dr. Bernard E. Kreger (Internal
      Med.)
   Dr. Michael O'Brien (Pathol.)
   Ms. Judy Cook, R.N.

Mrs. Lin Mason, Cancer Control
Coord.

32 South Street
Waltham, MA 02154
(617/894-0097)
Dr. Edward Kondi (Surg. Oncol.)
Dr. Alphonse Gallitano (Surg.
Oncol.)

Boston City Hospital
Ambulatory Care Center
818 Harrison Avenue
Boston, MA 02118
(617/424-4961)
Dr. Dennis Devereux (Surg. Oncol.)

St. Anne's Hospital
495 Middle Street
Fall River, MA 02722
(617/674-5741)
Dr. Richard Hellwig
(Hematol./Oncol.)
Dr. Simon Kim. (Rad. Med.)
Ms. Mary Jane Rimmer-Doherty,
R.N., B.S.

Jordan Hospital
Sandwich Street
Plymouth, MA 02360
(617/746-2000)
Dr. Dominic Zazzarino (Surg.
Oncol.)
Dr. Stephan Hochstin (Med.
Oncol.)
Mrs. Judy Aldrovandi, R.N., B.S.

Brockton Hospital/Cardinal Cushing
Hospital
Medical Oncology & Hematology,
P.C.
225 Quincy Avenue
Brockton, MA 02401
(617/586-1410)
Dr. Richard Samaha
(Hematol./Oncol.)
Dr. Harvey Neitlich
(Hematol./Oncol.)

Malden Hospital
Hospital Road
Malden, MA 02148

*Principal Investigator

(617/322-7560, ext. 5504)
Dr. Roberto Mattii
(Hematol./Oncol.)
Mrs. Susan Bleiden, R.N., B.S.

South Shore Hospital
55 Fogg Road
South Weymouth, MA 02190
(617/337-7011)
Dr. James Everett (Med. Oncol.)

Brockton Hospital
61 Libby Street
Brockton, MA 02402
(617/587-5000)
Dr. David Marcello (Surg. Oncol.)

CDMS
720 Harrison Avenue
Boston, MA 02118
(617/247-5016)
Ms. Theresa C. Trapilo

11. Bowman Gray School of Medicine,
NC (124)

300 S. Hawthorne Road
Winston-Salem, NC 27103
(919/748-4241)
*Dr. John Michael Sterchi (Surg.
Oncol.)
Dr. Richard B. Marshall (Pathol.)
Dr. Carolyn Ruth Ferree (Rad.
Oncol.)
Dr. Hyman B. Muss (Med.
Oncol./Hematol.)
Dr. Frederick Richards, II (Med.
Oncol./Hematol.)
Ms. Donna Morris, R.N.
(Surg./Hematol.)
Ms. Marie Polkinhorn (Data
Coordinator)

12. Brentwood Hospital, Warrensville
Heights, OH (122)

2166 Middlefield Road
Cleveland Heights, OH 44106
(216/321-8630)
*Dr. B. L. Horvat (Pathol./Med.
Oncol.)

4110 Warrensville Center Road
Warrensville Heights, OH 44122
(216/283-2900)
Dr. Roger F. Classen (Surg. Oncol.)
Dr. T. F. Classen (Surg. Oncol.)
Dr. Charles V. Gemma (Surg.
  Oncol.)
Dr. C. Russell Zachem (Surg.
  Oncol.)
Dr. W. B. Grigg (Ob/Gyn. Surgeon)
Dr. William Settlemire (Rad.
  Oncol.)
Dr. V. Rapp (Rad. Oncol.)
Dr. W. Swenfurth (Rad. Oncol.)
Dr. S. Lie (Rad. Oncol.)
Dr. Chi–Hoon Lee (Pathol.)
Dr. Nevanka Horvat (Pathol.)
Dr. John J. Mizenko
  (Gastroenterol.)
Dr. James E. Coan (Gen. Practice)
Dr. Robert G. DeRue (Internal
  Med.)
Dr. Ernest Lewandowski (Gen.
  Practice)
Dr. John P. Sevastos (Gen. Practice)
Dr. Jerome R. Vidd (Internal Med.)
Ms. Nancy Palumbo, R.N.

St. Vincent Charity Hospital
2351 E. 22 Street
Cleveland, OH 44115
(216/861-6200)
Dr. Robert Porter (Rad. Oncol.)
Dr. Dong Kim (Rad. Oncol.)

14055 Cedar Road
South Euclid, OH 44118
(216/371-3181)
Dr. Franklin B. Price (Med. Oncol.)
Dr. David Fishman (Med. Oncol.)

619 Northfield Road
Bedford, OH 44146
(216/232-2395)
Dr. Robert G. Tupa (Fam. Practice)

7689 Sagamore Hills Blvd.
Northfield, OH 44067
(216/467-8101)
Dr. James C. Lenox (Gen. Practice)

Cleveland Clinic Foundation
950 Euclid Avenue
Cleveland, OH 44106
(216/444-5576)
Dr. Gwynn Jelden (Rad. Oncol.)

St. Luke's Hospital
11311 Shaker Boulevard
Cleveland, OH 44104
(216/368-7783)
Dr. Carl W. Groppe, Jr., (Med.
  Oncol.)

13. Brookdale Hospital Medical Center
    (164)

Linden Boulevard at Brookdale
  Plaza
Brooklyn, NY 11212
(212/240-5653)
*Dr. Stanley L. Lee (Med. Oncol.)
Dr. Fakhiuddin Ahmed (Med.
  Oncol.)
Dr. Neal M. Friedberg (Med.
  Oncol.)
Dr. Kyung Ja Hong (Med. Oncol.)
Dr. Stephen Lichter (Med. Oncol.)
Dr. Allan D. Novetsky (Med.
  Oncol.)
Dr. William Steier (Med. Oncol.)
Dr. Jen C. Wang (Med. Oncol.)
Dr. Yale Rosen (Pathol.)
Ms. Rose Ann Block (Data
  Manager)

14. Brookwood Medical Center

2010 Brookwood Medical Center
  Drive
Birmingham, AL 35209
(205/877-1000)
*Dr. John Hankins (Med. Oncol.)
Dr. Lee Chapman (Surg. Oncol.)
Dr. Robert Jones (Pathol.)
Dr. John Glover (Rad. Oncol.)
Ms. Sheila Pegram, R.N. (Data)

15. Bryn Mawr Hospital, PA (129)

600 Haverford Road
Haverford, PA 19041

*Principal Investigator

(215/649-4017)
*Dr. Thomas G. Frazier (Surg.
  Oncol.)
Dr. David Rose (Surg. Oncol.)
Ms. Sally Ryan, R.N. (Coordinator)

933 Haverford Road
Bryn Mawr, PA 19010
(215/525-4511)
Dr. Patrick M. Growney (Med.
  Oncol.)
Dr. James P. Bond (Med. Oncol.)
Dr. Abigail A. Silvers (Med.
  Oncol.)

The Bryn Mawr Hospital
Bryn Mawr, PA 19010
(215/896-3000)
Dr. Robert L. Ravel (Rad. Oncol.)
Dr. David Moylan (Rad. Oncol.)
Dr. Charlott W. Rowland (Pathol.)
Dr. Ann M. Ainsworth (Pathol.)
Dr. Paul V. Strumia (Pathol.)
Dr. Vincent J. DePillis (Pathol.)
Dr. Harvey F. Watts (Pathol.)
Dr. Richard J. Carella (Rad. Oncol.)

844 County Line Road
Rosemont, PA 19010
(215/527-1290)
Dr. John Garofalo (Med. Oncol.)

16. Camden–Clark Memorial Hospital,
    WV (119)

    800 Garfield Avenue
    Parkersburg, WV 26101
    (304/424-2276)
    *Dr. Nikunj Shah (Med.
      Oncol./Hematol.)
    Dr. Chandra Sekar (Rad. Oncol.)
    Dr. S. W. Thacker (Pathol.)
    Dr. Gilberto Ramierz (Pathol.)
    Mrs. Janet Packard, R.N.
    Ms. Martha Butler, R.N.

    1122 Market Street
    Parkersburg, WV 26101
    (304/485-5531)
    Dr. Joseph L. Boggs (Surg. Oncol.)
    Dr. Ghassan A. Khalil (Surg.
      Oncol.)

*Principal Investigator

Dr. Gary W. Miller (Surg. Oncol.)
Dr. Paul G. Modie (Surg. Oncol.)
Dr. Harry L. Shannon (Urol.)

935 Market Street
Parkersburg, WV 26101
(304/485-3836)
Dr. William E. Barnes (Surg.
  Oncol.)

3803 Emerson Avenue
Parkersburg, WV 26101
(304/485-5041)
Dr. Humberto Escandon
  (Neurosurgeon)
Dr. Charles R. Loar (Neurosurgeon)

1812 Garfield Avenue
Parkersburg, WV 26101
(304/485-3891)
Dr. Eric L. David (Surg. Oncol.)

1815 Murdoch Avenue
Parkersburg, WV 26101
(304/485-4489)
Dr. Manuel G. Magno (Surg.
  Oncol.)

2910 Emerson Avenue
Parkersburg, WV 26101
(304/485-3836)
Dr. Q. Santiago (Surg. Oncol.)

17. Catholic Medical Center (162)

    Catholic Medical Center of
      Brooklyn & Queens, Inc.
    88-25 153rd Street
    Jamaica, NY 11432
    (212/291-3300)
    *Dr. I. Joseph Aprile (Surg. Oncol.)
    Dr. John Klavins (Pathol.)
    Dr. John Butler (Med. Oncol.)
    Dr. Steven Alderman (Rad. Oncol.)

18. CCOP, Allegheny–Singer Research
    Corp.

    Allegheny General Hospital
    320 E. North Avenue
    Pittsburgh, PA 15212
    (412/359-3630)

*Dr. Reginald P. Pugh (Med. Oncol.)
Dr. Bernard L. Zidar (Med. Oncol.)
Dr. Robert N. Raju (Med. Oncol.)
Dr. Kalpana A. Vaidya (Med. Oncol.)

Dr. T. K. Dutta (Rad. Oncol.)
Dr. Prabha Bansal (Rad. Oncol.)
Dr. Julian W. Proctor (Rad. Oncol.)
Dr. Robert J. Hartsock (Pathol.)
Dr. Reuben Zemel (Surg. Oncol.)
Dr. Sergio Betancourt (Surg. Oncol.)
Dr. Arthur I. Murphy (Surg. Oncol.)
Dr. Alan J. Kunschner (Gynecol. Oncol.)
Dr. Ronald Sapiente (Rad. Oncol.)
Dr. Stanley E. Shackney (Med. Oncol.)

Allegheny Hematology/Oncology Assoc.
Suite 208—APB
490 E. North Avenue
Pittsburgh, PA 15212
(412/359-5400)
Dr. Stanley Marks (Med. Oncol.)
Dr. Wayne J. Pfrimmer (Med. Oncol.)
Dr. Theodore L. Crandall (Med. Oncol.)

Beaver County Medical Center
1000 Dutch Ridge Road
Beaver, PA 15009
(412/728-7000)
Dr. Joseph Concannon (Rad. Oncol.)
Dr. James M. Hughes, (Rad. Oncol.)

Sandy Lane & Fourth Street
Lewistown, PA 17044
(717/248-5411)
Dr. Duilio Valdivia (Med. Oncol.)

423 Jenkins Building
Pittsburgh, PA 15222
(412/281-4387)
Dr. Raimund Rueger (Med. Oncol.)

19. CCOP, Billings Interhospital Oncology Project (902)

1145 N. 29th Street
Yellowstone Medical Building, Suite 1B
Billings, MT 59101
(406/252-2147)
Dr. David Myers (Surg. Oncol.)

1230 N. 30th Street
Billings, MT 59101
(406/252-2147)
*Dr. Neel Hammond (Med. Oncol.)
Dr. Benjamin Marchello (Med. Oncol.)

28th Street & Poly Drive
Billings, MT 59101
(406/248-2212
Dr. Fred Deigert (Rad. Oncol.)
Dr. Ted Reinke (Rad. Oncol.)

20. CCOP. Grand Rapids Community Clinical Oncology Program (906)

Butterworth Hospital
100 Michigan N.E.
Grand Rapids, MI 48503
(616/774-1230)
Dr. Richard E. Dean (Surg. Oncol.)
Dr. Hohn H. Edlund (Rad. Oncol.)
Dr. Robert W. Gillies (Rad. Oncol.)
Dr. Joseph D. Mann (Pathol.)
Mr. Galen Beverly (Data Coordinator)

Grand Rapids Oncology Group
1001 Medical Park Drive S.E.
Grand Rapids, MI 49506
(616/949-5260)
*Dr. Edward L. Moorhead, II (Med. Oncol.)
Dr. James R. Borst (Med. Oncol.)
Dr. Raymond L. Gonzalez (Med. Oncol.)
Dr. Thomas V. Murray (Med. Oncol.)
Dr. Lawrence E. Pawl (Med. Oncol.)
Dr. Emiliana L. SanDiego (Med. Oncol.)

*Principal Investigator

245 State Street
Grand Rapids, MI 49503
(616/774-2414)
Dr. Jerry W. Anderson (Med.
  Oncol.)
Dr. John O'Donnel (Med. Oncol.)
Dr. David Oviatt (Med. Oncol.)

3934 Cascade Road S.E.
Grand Rapids, MI 49506
(616/942-1310)
Dr. Mark G. Campbell (Med.
  Oncol.)
Dr. Richard K. Rotman (Med.
  Oncol.)

4550 Cascade Road S.E.
Suite 101
Grand Rapids, MI 49506
(616/942-9712)
Dr. Calvin J. Dykstra (Med. Oncol.)

Blodgett Memorial Medical Center
1840 Wealthy S.E.
Grand Rapids, MI 49503
(616/774-7845)
Dr. Wilma Ewald (Rad. Oncol.)

Saint Mary's Hospital
200 Jefferson S.E.
Grand Rapids, MI 49503
(616/774-6385)
Dr. Andre V. Jubert (Med. Oncol.)
Dr. Michael Kie Seng Tay (Rad.
  Oncol.)

Blodgett Professional Bldg. 1900
  Wealthy S.E.,
Suite 220
Grand Rapids, MI 49506
(616/459-3254)
Dr. F. Raymer Lovell (Surg.
  Oncol.)

Blodgett Professional Bldg. 1900
  Wealthy S.E.,
Suite 330
Grand Rapids, MI 49506
(616/774-0700)
Dr. Richard T. Upton (Gynecol.
  Oncol.)

*Principal Investigator

Ferguson Hospital
72 Sheldon S.E.
Grand Rapids, MI 49503
(616/456-0202)
Dr. John M. MacKeigan (Surg.
  Oncol.)

155 W. 27th Street
Holland, MI 49423
(616/396-5286)
Dr. Bruce A. Masselink

Leila Hospital and Health Center
300 N. Avenue
Battle Creek, MI 49016
(616/962-8551)
Dr. Stephen L. Smiley (Med.
  Oncol.)

515 Lakeside Drive S.E., Suite 112
Grand Rapids, MI 49506
(616/451-2933)
Dr. Enrico Sobong (Med. Oncol.)
Kenneth A. Stoutenborough (Med.
  Oncol.)

2355 E. Paris S.E.
Grand Rapids, MI 49506
(616/949-6421)
Dr. James R. White (Surg. Oncol.)

21. CCOP, Marshfield Medical
    Foundation (905)

Quadrant 3-C
1000 N. Oak Avenue
Marshfield, WI 54449
(715/387-5511)
Dr. James L. Hoehn (Surg. Oncol.)
Dr. Constante Avecilla (Surg.
  Oncol.)
Dr. Jerry Hardacre (Surg. Oncol.)
Dr. Marvin Kuehner (Surg. Oncol.)
Dr. Mark Swanson (Surg. Oncol.)
Dr. Gail Williams (Surg. Oncol.)
Dr. Efstathios Beltaos (Pathol.)
Dr. Robert H. Greenlaw (Rad.
  Oncol.)
Dr. Homer H. Russ (Rad. Oncol.)
Mr. David Eisberner, R.N.
Ms. Darlene Koontz, R.N.
Ms. Mary Krueger, R.N.

Ms. Della Rudolf, R.N.

Quadrant 3-A
1000 N. Oak Avenue
Marshfield, WI 54449
(715/387-5416)
*Dr. Tarit K. Banerjee (Med.
  Oncol.)
Dr. J. L. Ousley (Med. Oncol.)
Dr. Y. G. Lin (Med. Oncol.)
Dr. Daniel Rushing (Med. Oncol.)
Dr. Jane Gehlsen (Med. Oncol.)
Dr. William Friedenberg (Hematol.)
Ms. Nancy Goldbach, R.N.

Radiation Therapy Department
St. Joseph Hospital
Marshfield, WI 54449
(715/387-7637)
Ms. Ann Heiman (Data
  Doordinator)
Marshfield Foundation

510 N. St. Joseph Avenue
Marshfield, WI 54449
(715/387-5241)
Ms. Cherri Jacoby (Data
  Coordinator)

Quadrant 5A
1000 N. Oak Avenue
Marshfield, WI 54449
(715/387-5416)
Dr. Stuart J. Tipping (Med. Oncol.)

22. CCOP, Newark Beth Israel Medical
    Center (904)

201 Lyons Avenue
Newark, NJ 07112
(201/926-7000)
*Dr. Frederick B. Cohen (Med.
  Oncol.)
Dr. Alan J. Lippman (Med. Oncol.)
Dr. Marcelito C. Custodio (Med.
  Oncol.)
Dr. Fred L. Steinbaum (Med.
  Oncol.)
Dr. Andrea M. Ruiz (Med. Oncol.)
Dr. Julian A. Decter (Med.
  Oncol./Hematol.)
Dr. Alkinviadis Campbell (Pathol.)

Dr. Viera Schweitzer (Rad. Oncol.)
Ms. Janice Beinsky, R.N.
Ms. Ina Yalof

159 Millburn Avenue
Millburn, NJ 07041
(201/379-5888)
Dr. Donald Brief (Surg. Oncol.)
Dr. Bruce Brener (Surg. Oncol.)

23. City of Faith Medical and Research
    Center, Tulsa, OK (146)

8181 S. Lewis
P.O. Box 3600
Tulsa, OK 74171
(918/493-1000)
*Dr. Arther Hoge (Med. Oncol.)
Dr. John Lewis (Pathol.)
Dr. D. Lewis Moore (Surg. Oncol.)
Dr. Anthony Murgo (Med. Oncol.)
Dr. Phillip Jones (Rad. Oncol.)
Dr. Nadim Nimeh (Med. Oncol.)
Ms. Rita Scanlon (Data Manager)

St. John Medical Center
1823 S. Utica Street
Tulsa, OK 74104
(918/744-2345)
Dr. Abraham Rosenthal (Rad.
  Oncol.

24. City of Hope Medical Center,
    Duarte, CA (123)

1500 Duarte Road
Duarte, CA 91010
(213/359-8111)
*Dr. Jose J. Terz (Surg. Oncol.)
Dr. Daniel U. Riihimaki (Surg.
  Oncol.)
Dr. Michael Meguid (Surg. Oncol.)
Dr. Margaret Kemeny (Surg.
  Oncol.)
Dr. John R. Benfield (Surg. Oncol.)
Dr. J. David Beatty (Surg. Oncol.)
Dr. Richard Pezner (Rad. Oncol.)
Dr. Hector Battifora (Pathol.)
Dr. Marcelle Bertrand (Med.
  Oncol.)

*Principal Investigator

Dr. Scott M. Browning (Med. Oncol.)
Dr. Kim Allyson Margolin (Med. Oncol.)
Dr. Douglas W. Blayney (Med. Oncol.)
Dr. David A. Goldberg (Med. Oncol.)
Dr. Lucille A. Leong (Med. Oncol.)
Ms. Anita Mackie

25. Cross Cancer Institute, Edmonton (112)

11560 University Avenue
Edmonton, Alberta T6G 1Z2
(403/432-8771)
*Dr. A. H. G. Paterson (Med. Oncol.)
Dr. Alan Lees (Rad. Oncol.)
Miss Jane Boskill, R.N.

51 - 6th Street, S.E.
Medicine Hat, Alberta TIA 1G5
CANADA
(403/527-2281)
Dr. A. R. McClelland (Surg. Oncol.)
Dr. B. Bose (Surg. Oncol.)

26. Dana–Farber Cancer Institute (160)

44 Binney Street
Boston, MA 02115
(617/732-3472)
*Dr. I. Craig Henderson (Med. Oncol.)
Ms. Diane Ascoli (Data Manager)

Beth Israel Hospital
300 Brookline Avenue
Boston, MA 02115
(617/735-4344)
Dr. Jim Connelly (Pathol.)

St. Elizabeth Hospital
736 Cambridge Street
Brighton, MA 02135
(617/782-7000, ext. 2405)
Dr. Nelson Burnstein (Pathol.)

27. Daniel Freeman Hospital, Inglewood, CA (56)

333 N. Prairie Avenue, Suite 222
Inglewood, CA 90301
(213/674-7050)
Dr. Richard Small (Rad. Oncol.)
Dr. Raouf Yuja (Pathol.)

301 N. Prairie Avenue, Suite 311
Inglewood, CA 90301
(213/674-0050)
*Dr. Elliott Hinkes (Med. Oncol.)
Dr. Allan A. Orenstein (Med. Oncol.)
Dr. John L. Barstis (Hematol./Oncol.)
Ms. Eileen M. McAndrew, R.N.

28. Dekalb General Hospital, GA (88)

2701 N. Decatur Road
Decatur, GA 30022
(404/292-4444)
Dr. Frank Matthews (Pathol.)
Dr. Frank Critz (Rad. Oncol.)
Dr. Jack Manfredi (Med. Oncol./Hematol.)
Ms. Linda Sheivlhud, R.N.
Miss Sara Fensterer
Ms. Faye Sophy

755 Columbia Drive
Decatur, GA 30030
(404/373-3196)
*Dr. S. Angier Wills (Surg. Oncol.)

29. Denver General Hospital (76)

750 Cherokee Street
Denver, CO 80204
(303/893-7024)
*Dr. George E. Moore (Surg. Oncol.)
Dr. Don Clarke (Pathol.)
Dr. Adam Myers (Med. Oncol./Hematol.)
Ms. Mona Bernaiche, R.N.

4200 E. Ninth Avenue
Denver, CO 80220
(303/394-8613)

*Principal Investigator

Dr. Robert Gerner (Surg. Oncol.)
Dr. Franklin B. Johnson (Rad. Oncol.)

University of Colorado Medical Center
E. 9th Street
Denver, CO 80206
(303/394-8614, Ext. 272)
Ms. Jenny Vance, R.N.

30. Downstate Medical Center, SUNY (2)

450 Clarkson Avenue
Brooklyn, NY 11203
(212/270-1552)
*Dr. C. Julian Rosenthal (Med. Oncol.)
Dr. Jose Marti (Surg. Oncol.)
Dr. Albert Broverman (Med. Oncol.)
Dr. Julian Rosenthal (Med. Oncol.)
Dr. Marvin Rotman (Rad. Oncol.)
Dr. Anthony Nicastri (Pathol.)
Dr. Javier Domingo (Pathol.)
Ms. Karen Britt, R.N.
Ms. Regina DeVita, R.N.
Ms. Elizabeth Manzione

Methodist Hospital
506 Sixth Street
Brooklyn, NY 11215
Dr. Sameer Rafla (Rad. Oncol.)

9920 Fourth Avenue
Brooklyn, NY 11209
(212/238-9090)
Dr. Joseph Newman (Med. Oncol.)

31. Ellis Fischel State Cancer Hospital, MO (24)

Business Loop 70 & Garth Avenue
Columbia, MO 65201
(314/875-2214)
*Dr. William G. Kraybill (Surg. Oncol.)
Dr. Ronald Vincent (Surg. Oncol.)
Dr. Marvin Lopez (Surg. Oncol.)
Dr. Carlos Perez–Mesa (Pathol.)
Dr. Ralph Reynolds (Med. Oncol.)

Dr. Ali Khojasteh (Med. Oncol.)
Ms. Donna Meyer
Ms. Mona Laird, R.N.

32. Geisinger Medical Center, Danville, PA (4)

Danville, PA 17822
(717/271-6362)
*Dr. James Evans (Surg. Oncol.)
Dr. John E. Deitrick (Surg. Oncol.)
Dr. John C. West (Surg. Oncol.)
Dr. Philip C. Breen (Surg. Oncol.)
Dr. James C. Pierce (Surg. Oncol.)
Dr. Robert C. Eyerly (Surg. Oncol.)
Dr. Bert Bernath (Med. Oncol.)
Dr. James G. Gallagher (Med. Oncol.)
Dr. Neil M. Ellison (Med. Oncol.00
Dr. David Beiler (Rad. Oncol.)
Dr. John A. Clement (Rad. Oncol.)
Dr. Nita Natividad (Rad. Oncol.)
Dr. C. James Favino (Pathol.)
Dr. M. Fleetwood (Clin. Immunol.)
Ms. Patricia Porter, R.N.
Ms. Kathy Rine, R.N.
Mrs. May Fallon (Data Manager/Coordinator)

33. Good Samaritan Hospital, Cincinnati, OH (121)

317 Howell Avenue
Cincinnati, OH 45220
(513/961-4335)
*Dr. Richard E. Welling (Surg. Oncol.)
Ms. Mindy Davis (Data)

Clifton & Dyxmyth Avenue
Cincinnati, OH 45220
(513/872-2636)
Dr. Wagih Shehata (Rad. Oncol.)
Dr. Harry Boss (Pathol.)

71 E. Hollister Street
Cincinnati, OH 45219
(513/381-8440)
Dr. Richard Meyer (Med. Oncol.)
Mr. Charles Cook, P.A.

*Principal Investigator

34. Good Samaritan Hospital,
    Lexington, KY (94)

    310 S. Limestone
    Lexington, KY 40504
    (606/252-6612)

    2366 Nicholasville Road
    Lexington, KY 40503
    (606/278-0589)
    *Dr. William R. Meeker (Surg.
      Oncol.)

    Good Samaritan Hospital
    310 S. Limestone Street
    Lexington, KY 40508
    (606/252-6612)
    Dr. Leonard E. Wallace (Pathol.)
    Ms. Jettie Woodward, R.N.
    Ms. Cynthia Leedham

    2370 Nicholasville Road
    Lexington, KY 40503
    (606/277-5716)
    Dr. Claude H. Farley (Med. Oncol.)

    (606/278-2354)
    Dr. James E. Ross (Surg. Oncol.)

    1517 S. Lime
    Lexington, KY 40508
    (606/278-5479)
    Dr. Juan Reusche (Rad. Oncol.)
    Dr. Jose A. Avila (Rad. Oncol.)

    1800 S. Lime
    Lexington, KY 40503
    (606/278-6031)
    Dr. John M. Fox (Surg. Oncol.)

    135 E. Maxwell
    Lexington, KY 40508
    (606/254-6572)
    Dr. William T. Swartz (Surg.
      Oncol.)

    (606/255-0831)
    Dr. Allen E. Grimes, Jr. (Surg.
      Oncol.)

    1221 S. Broadway
    Lexington, KY 40504
    (606/255-6841)

*Principal Investigator

Dr. Lawrence C. Maguire
  (Hematol.)
Dr. John D. Cronin (Hematol.)

1725 Harrodsburg Road
Lexington, KY 40503
(606/278-2334)
Dr. Michael Daugherty (Surg.
  Oncol.)

35. Grant Hospital, Columbus, OH
    (144)

    323 E. Town Street
    Columbus, OH 43215
    (614/461-3232)
    *Dr. Leslie Laufman (Med. Oncol.)
    Dr. William Hicks (Med. Oncol.)
    Dr. Bernard J. Silver (Med. Oncol.)

    309 E. State Street
    Columbus, OH 43215
    (614/461-3232)
    Dr. Jerry Guy (Med. Oncol.)
    Dr. Thomas Nims (Surg. Oncol.)
    Dr. Gerald Penn (Pathol.)
    Dr. Syed Rahman (Rad. Oncol.)
    Dr. Jack Tetirick (Surg. Oncol.)

    300 E. Town Street
    Columbus, OH 43215
    (614/221-2643)
    Dr. James McCaughan (Surg.
      Oncol.)

    283 E. State Street
    Columbus, OH 43215
    (614/221-4541)
    Dr. Kathleen Musser (Surg. Oncol.)
    Dr. John Schwarzell (Surg. Oncol.)

    Grant Hospital
    Department of Oncology Services
    311 S. Grant Avenue
    Columbus, OH 43215
    (614/461-3045)
    Ms. Jennifer File Guy, R.N.
    Ms. Patricia M. Dunn, R.N.
    Ms. Suzanne Courter, R.N.
    Ms. Linda Rae Frush

36. Group Health Medical Center,
    Seattle (45)

895

200 15th Avenue, E.
Seattle, WA 98112
(206/326-6262)
*Dr. Robert Bourdeau (Surg.
Oncol.)
Dr. S.W. Douglas (Med. Oncol.)
Dr. I. L. Schuldberg (Pathol.)
Dr. Robert Tobe (Hematol./Oncol.)
Dr. Thomas W. Johnson (Rad.
Oncol.)

Group Health Medical Center
200 15th Avenue, E.
CX3 Research
Seattle, WA 98112
(206/326-6632)
Ms. Janice Mahloch
Ms. Sheri Ann Strite

37. Harbor UCLA Medical Center,
Torrance, CA (5)

100 W. Carson Street
Torrance, CA 90509
(213/533-2768)
*Dr. David State (Surg. Oncol.)
Dr. Frank Hirose (Pathol.)
Dr. Jerome Block (Med. Oncol.)
Dr. Joseph Scallon (Rad. Oncol.)
Ms. Karen Schlotzhauer, R.N.
Ms. Susan Rizzo
Ms. Lynn Scheffler

38. Hennepin County Medical Center,
MN (21)

701 Park
Minneapolis, MN 54415
(612/347-2810)
*Dr. Calude R. Hitchcock (Surg.
Oncol.)
Dr. Michael B. Belzer (Med.
Oncol.)
Dr. John I. Coe (Pathol.)
Ms. Phyllis Muzzy

900 S. 8th Street
Minneapolis, MN 55404
(612/347-4187)
Dr. Manucher Azad (Rad. Oncol.)

39. Hopital Avicenne (20)

93000 Bobigny
France
(830-04-19)
*Professor Lucien Israel (Med.
Oncol.)
Dr. Jean Luc Breau (Med. Oncol.)
Dr. Jenri Amouroux (Pathol.)
Dr. Jacques Aguilera (Med. Oncol.)
Pr. G. de Saint Florent (Surg.
Oncol.)

Hopital Boucicaut
75015 Paris
France
Dr. Jacques Reynier (Surg. Oncol.)

40. Hotel–Dieu de Levis (166)

143, Rue Wolfe
Levis, Quebec
Canada
(418/837-7121)
*Dr. Yvan Drolet
(Hematol./Oncol.)
Dr. Rene Blouin (Hematol./Oncol.)
Dr. Arthur Langford (Surg. Oncol.)
Dr. Jacques Smith (Surg. Oncol.)
Dr. Hubert Falanga (Pathol.)
Ms. Lise Bilodeau, R.N.
Ms. Marie Fortin, R.N.

41. Hotel–Dieu, Montreal (55)

3840 St. Urban Street
Montreal, Quebec
Canada
(514/844-0161)
*Dr. Andre Robidoux (Surg.
Oncol.)
Dr. Jacques Cantin (Surg. Oncol.)
Dr. Claude Potvin (Surg. Oncol.)
Dr. Paul Simard (Rad. Oncol.)
Dr. Yvan Boivin (Pathol.)
Ms. Sylvie Christine Michaud,
(Data)

11, Cote due Palais
Quebec, G1R 2J6 Canada
(418/694-5352)
*Dr. Louis Dionne (Surg. Oncol.)

*Principal Investigator

Dr. Antoine Kibrite (Surg. Oncol.)
Dr. Jacques Laverdiere (Rad. Oncol.)
Dr. Andre Girard (Rad. Oncol.)
Dr. Rene Blouin (Hematol.)
Dr. Leonard Bernier (Pathol.)
Dr. Michael Plante (Pathol.)
Ms. Marjolaine Berube

43. Jewish General Hospital, Montreal (22)

3755 Cote St. Catherine Road
Montreal, Quebec H3T 1E2
Canada
(514/342-3111)
*Dr. Richard Margolese (Surg. Oncol.)
Dr. Philip H. Gordon (Surg. Oncol.)
Dr. Claude LaChance (Pathol.)
Dr. Louis Begin (Pathol.)
Dr. Mark Wainberg (Immuno.)
Dr. Carolyn Freeman (Rad. Oncol.)
Dr. Laurence Panasci (Med. Oncol.)
Ms. Linda Nemerofsky
Ms. Janet Burghart

1650 Cedar Avenue
Montreal, Quebec H3G 1A4
Canada
(514/937-6011)
Dr. Julio Guerra (Rad. Oncol.)

44. Kaiser Permanente, Harbor City (93)

25825 Vermont Avenue
Harbor City, CA 90710
(213/325-5111)
*Dr. Eugene Pollack (Surg. Oncol.)
Dr. Irving Applebaum (Surg. Oncol.)
Dr. John Rowe (Pathol.)
Dr. James Grossman (Med. Oncol.)
Dr. Allen Rosen (Med. Oncol.)
Mrs. Toni Cabalse, R.N.
Ms. Barbara Wolfe, R.N.
Mrs. Catherine Lang, R.N.
Mrs. Ethel Richardson
Mrs. Barbara Wolfe, R.N.

*Principal Investigator

45. Kaiser Permanente, Portland (73)

5055 N. Greeley Avenue
Portland, OR 97232
(503/282-8421)
Dr. Robert McFarlane (Surg. Oncol.)
Dr. Edward Ariniello (Surg. Oncol.)
Dr. Richard Davis (Surg. Oncol.)
Dr. Peter Feldman (Surg. Oncol.)
Dr. John Brown (Surg. Oncol.)

Montana Medical Offices
3414 N. Montana
Portland, OR 97227
(503/249-8555)
*Dr. Andrew Glass (Med. Oncol.)
Dr. J. T. Leimert (Med. Oncol.)
Ms. Marge Erwin, R.N.
Ms. Nancy Hayes
Ms. Alice Gemmet
Ms. Drudy Seifuddin

700 N.E. 47th Avenue
Portland, OR 97213
(503/234-8211)
Dr. John Molendyk (Rad. Oncol.)
Dr. Frederick Wagner (Rad. Oncol.)

9205 S.W. Barnes Road
Portland, OR 97229
(503/297-4411)
Dr. Richard Lowy (Rad. Oncol.)
Dr. Jerald Algrich (Rad. Oncol.)

2801 N. Gantenbein
Portland, OR 97227
(503/280-4161)
Dr. Norman Willis (Rad. Oncol.)
Dr. Michael Goldman (Rad. Oncol.)

1501 N.E. Medical Center Way
Bend, OR 97701
(503/382-2811)
Dr. Richard Woods (Med. Oncol.)
Ms. Janet Knapp, R.N.

Vancouver Memorial Hospital
3400 Main Street
Vancouver, WA 98661
(206/693-6391)
Dr. Norman Helgason (Rad. Oncol.)

897

Dr. Lynn Dawson (Rad. Oncol.)

175 W. B Street
Springfield, OR 97447
(503/726-6829)
Dr. Stuart Markwell (Med. Oncol.)

46. Kaiser Permanente, San Diego (84)

4647 Zion Avenue
San Diego, CA 92120
(619/563-3186)
*Dr. Thomas Campbell (Med.
Oncol.)
Dr. Marvin Nicola (Pathol.)
Dr. Kirby Browns (Surg. Oncol.)
Ms. Barbara House, P.A.

1510 N. Edgemont
Los Angeles, CA 90027
(213/667-5495)
Dr. A. Robert Kagan (Rad. Oncol.)

47. Kaiser Permanente, West Los
Angeles (148)

6041 Cadillac Avenue
Los Angeles, CA 90034
(213/857-2000)
*Dr. Ivan S. Shulman (Surg.
Oncol.)
Dr. Joan Chlebowski (Med. Oncol.)
Dr. Ren Ridolfi (Pathol.)

1510 N. Edgemont
Los Angeles, CA 90027
(213/667-5495)
Dr. A. Robert Kagan (Rad. Oncol.)

48. Lancaster County Medical Center
(161)

2966 O Street
Lincoln, NE 68510
(402/474-2405)

Gateway Professional Building
600 N. Cotner Boulevard, Suite 600
Lincoln, NE 68505
(402/467-2395)
*Dr. William T. Griffin (Gen.
Surgeon)

*Principal Investigator

St. Elizabeth Community Health
Center
555 S. 70th Street
Lincoln, NE 68510
(402/489-7181)
Dr. John Casey (Pathol.)

Lincoln General Hospital
2300 S. 16th Street
Lincoln, NE 68502
(402/475-1114)
Dr. Prentiss Dettman (Rad. Oncol.)

Lincoln Medical Education
Foundation
4600 Valley Road
Lincoln, NE 68510
(402/483-4591)
Ms. Barbara Morton (Data
Coordinator)

49. Letterman Army Medical Center,
CA (46)

Presidio of San Francisco, CA
94129
(415/561-2232)
*Dr. David Gandara (Med. Oncol.)
Dr. Geoffrey Chapman (Med.
Oncol.)
Dr. Christopher George (Med.
Oncol.)
Dr. Joseph Homann (Surg. Oncol.)
Dr. Myron Whitehead (Pathol.)
Dr. Nerqesh Surti (Rad. Oncol.)
Dr. Ranu Bohl (Rad. Oncol.)
Capt. Patricia O'Rourke, R.N.
Ms. L. Gourley, P.A.-C (Data
Coordinator)

(415/561-4386)
Dr. Pat Cornett (Med. Oncol.)

P.O. Box 118
Presidio of San Francisco, CA
94129
(415/561-2232)
Dr. William Phillips (Med. Oncol.)

50. Louisiana State University, New
Orleans (6)

1542 Tulane Avenue
New Orleans, LA 70112
(504/568-4750)
*Dr. Isidore Cohn, Jr. (Surg.
   Oncol.)
*Dr. Charles Dictzen (Surg. Oncol.)
Dr. John Brown (Rad. Oncol.)
Dr. Ronald Welsh (Pathol.)
Ms. Carolyn Crucia, R.N.
Ms. Connie Carter

Earl K. Long Memorial Hospital
5825 Airline Highway
Baton Rouge, LA 70805
(504/356-3361)
Dr. Shaista Faruqui (Med. Oncol.)

51. Louisiana State University,
    Shreveport (110)

Department of Surgery
School of Medicine
P.O. Box 33932
Shreveport, LA 71130
(318/674-5000)
*Dr. Don M. Morris (Surg. Oncol.)
Dr. Leonard I. Goldman (Surg.
   Oncol.)
Dr. Darryl Williams
   (Hematol./Oncol.)
Dr. Warren D. Grafton (Pathol.)
Dr. Louis H. Barr (Surg. Oncol.)
Ms. Jacqueline Anderson Edwards,
   R.N.

1035 Creswell Avenue
Highland Clinic
Shreveport, LA 71130
(318/227-7544/7246)
Dr. Charles D. Knight (Surg.
   Oncol.)
Dr. F. D. Griffen (Surg. Oncol.)

1509 Doctors Drive
Bossier City, LA 71111
(318/746-8538)
Dr. E. B. Robinson, Jr. (Surg.
   Oncol.)

2748 Virginia
Shreveport, LA 71103
(318/277-4801)

*Principal Investigator

Dr. A. A. Bullock (Surg. Oncol.)
Dr. Alan Grosbach (Hematol.)

Louisiana State University Medical
Ctr.
P.O. Box 33932
Shreveport, LA 71130
(318/674-5970)
Dr. F. S. Bahrassa (Rad. Oncol.)

52. Madigan Army Medical Center
    (149)

P.O. Box 241
Tacoma, WA 98431
(206/967-6398)
*Dr. Preston L. Carter (Surg.
   Oncol.)

53. Manitoba Cancer Foundation (54)

100 Olivia Street
Winnipeg, Manitoba R3E OV9
Canada
(204/787-2128)
*Dr. David Bowman (Med. Oncol.)
Dr. Martin Levitt (Med. Oncol.)
Dr. H. Yazdi (Pathol.)
Dr. Wayne Beecroft (Surg. Oncol.)
Dr. James Gillies (Rad. Oncol.)
Ms. Janice Lutz, R.N.
Mrs. Kerry McDonald, R.N.
Mrs. Elaine Janke, A.R.T. (Data
   Manager)
Ms. Heidi Funk (Data Manager)

St. Boniface Hospital
409 Tache Avenue
Winnipeg, Manitoba R2H 2A6
Canada
(204/237-2128)
Dr. Harvey Schipper (Med. Oncol.)
Ms. Anne McMurray (Data
   Manager)
Mrs. Erna Stiles, A.R.T. (Data
   Manager)

54. Marin General Hospital, GA (113)

250 Bon Air Road, Greenbrae
Box 2129
San Rafael, CA 94902

(415/461-0100)
Dr. Robert Cohen (Pathol.)
Dr. Richard Evans (Rad. Oncol.)

599 Sir Francis Drake Boulevard,
 Suite 303
Greenbrae, CA 94904
(415/461-2933)
*Dr. Peter D. Eisenberg
 (Hematol./Oncol.)
Ms. Diane Wrona

599 Sir Francis Drake Boulevard,
 Suite 206
Greenbrae, CA 94904
(415/461-7955)
Dr. Michael D. Osborne (Surg.
 Oncol.)
Dr. Scott Strathairn (Surg. Oncol.)

1615 Hill Road
Novato, CA 94947
(415/897-2626)
Dr. Palmer H. White (Surg. Oncol.)
Dr. Jacques Couacaud (Surg.
 Oncol.)

1300 S. Elisieo Drive
Greenbrae, CA 94904
(415/461-2262)
Dr. James Dahl (Med. Oncol.)
Dr. Mervyn F. Burke (Surg. Oncol.)

1350 S. Eliseo Drive
Greenbrae, CA 94904
(415/461-1350)
Dr. Bruce Manheim (Surg. Oncol.)
Dr. Chester Noyes (Surg. Oncol.)
Dr. William H. Stamps (Surg.
 Oncol.)

1000 S. Eliseo Drive
Greenbrae, CA 94904
(415/461-0535)
Dr. Albert Hall (Surg. Oncol.)

1540 Fifth Avenue
San Rafael, CA 94901
(415/454-9100)
Dr. Robert Celli (Surg. Oncol.)

*Principal Investigator

55. Marshfield Clinic, WI (140)

Quadrant 3-C
1000 N. Oak Avenue
Marshfield, WI 54449
(715/387-5511)
*Dr. James L. Hoehn (Surg. Oncol.)
Dr. Constante Avecilla (Surg.
 Oncol.)
Dr. Jerry Hardacre (Surg. Oncol.)
Dr. Marvin Kuehner (Surg. Oncol.)
Dr. Mark Swanson (Surg. Oncol.)
Dr. Gail Williams (Surg. Oncol.)
Dr. Efstathios Beltaos (Pathol.)
Dr. Robert H. Greenlaw (Rad.
 Oncol.)
Dr. Homer H. Russ (Rad. Oncol.)
Dr. Stuart J. Tipping (Med. Oncol.)
Mr. David Eisberner, R.N.
Ms. Darlene Koontz, R.N.
Ms. Mary Krueger, R.N.
Ms. Della Rudolf, R.N.

Quadrant 3-A
1000 N. Oak AVenue
Marshfield, WI 54449
(715/387-5416)
Dr. Tarit K. Banerjee (Med. Oncol.)
Dr. J. L. Ousley (Med. Oncol.)
Dr. Y. G. Lin (Med. Oncol.)
Dr. Daniel Rushing (Med. Oncol.)
Dr. Jane Gehlsen (Med. Oncol.)
Dr. William Friedenberg (Hematol.)
Ms. Nancy Goldbach, R.N.

Radiation Therapy Department
St. Joseph Hospital
Marshfield, WI 54449
(715/387-7637)
Ms. Ann Heiman (Data
 Coordinator)
Marshfield Foundation

510 N. St. Joseph Avenue
Marshfield, WI 54449
(715/387-5241)
Ms. Cherri Jacoby (Data
 Coordinator)

56. McLeod Regional Medical Center
 (168)

Pee Dee Medical Associates, P.A.
506 E. Cheves Street, Suite 202
P.O. Box 1905
Florence, SC 29503
(803/667-0816)
*Dr. Robert McNutt (Med. Oncol.)
*Dr. Michael Pavy (Med. Oncol.)
Ms. Gladys Ann Black, R.N.

Pee Dee Medical Associates, P.A.
555 E. Cheves Street
P.O. Box F-8700
Florence, SC 29501
(803/667-2000)
Dr. Louis D. Wright, Jr. (Pathol.)

McLeod Regional Medical Center
555 E. Cheves Street
Florence, SC 29501
(803/667-2015)
Dr. Arthur Woodward (Rad.
  Oncol.)

4708 Oleander Drive
Myrtle Beach, SC 29577
(803/449-9415)
Dr. Kent Woodward (Rad. Oncol.)

57. McMaster University, Hamilton
     (115)

St. Joseph Hospital
50 Charlton Avenue E.
Hamilton, Ontario L8N 1Y4
Canada
(416/528-5403)
*Dr. S.E. O'Brien (Surg. Oncol.)
Dr. P. R. Knight (Surg. Oncol.)
Dr. W. R. Matthews (Surg. Oncol.)
Dr. A. R. C. Butson (Surg. Oncol.)

Ontario Cancer Foundation
Hamilton Clinic
711 Concession Street
Hamilton, Ontario L8V 1C3
Canada
(416/387-94q5)
Dr. William Hryniuk (Med. Oncol.)
Dr. William Muirhead (Rad.
  Oncol.)
Dr. T. D'Souza (Pathol.)
Ms. Sue Rendell, R.N.

Mrs. Carole Thompson
Ms. Maurene Mamone, R.N.

58. Medical College of Pennsylvania
     (35)

3300 Henry Avenue
Philadelphia, PA 19129
(215/842-6000)
*Dr. James Bassett (Surg. Oncol.)
Dr. John Clarke (Surg. Oncol.)
Dr. Donald R. Cooper (Surg.
  Oncol.)
Dr. Harry L. Thomas (Surg. Oncol.)
Dr. Leon E. Clarke (Surg. Oncol.)
Dr. Ajit K. Sachdeva (Surg. Oncol.)
Dr. Pamela Scott (Surg. Oncol.)
Dr. Anne U. Barnes (Surg. Oncol.)
Dr. Janet Parker (Rad. Oncol.)
Dr. William D. Johnson (Pathol.)
Dr. Sally Lane (Med. Oncol.)
Ms. Maureen Brunetti, R.N.,
  B.S.N.
Ms. Phyllis Brehm, R.N.
Ms. Eleanor Cairns

59. Medical College of Virginia (7)

1200 E. Broad Street
Richmond, VA 23298
(804/786-9323)
*Dr. Walter Lawrence (Surg.
  Oncol.)
Dr. J. Shelton Horsley (Surg.
  Oncol.)
Dr. James Neifeld (Surg. Oncol.)
Dr. George A. Parker (Surg.
  Oncol.)
Dr. Robert Diasio (Med. Oncol.)
Dr. Richard Belgrad (Rad. Oncol.)
Dr. Saul Kay (Pathol.)
Ms. Linda Keener, R.N.

60. Medical College of Wisconsin (38)

8700 W. Wisconsin Avenue
Milwaukee, WI 53226
(414/257-5226)
Dr. James Cox (Rad. Oncol.)
Dr. Lawrence Clowry (Pathol.)
Dr. Tom Anderson (Med. Oncol.)

*Principal Investigator

Dr. Richard Hansen (Med. Oncol.)
Ms. Julie Jensen, R.N. (Nurse
 Oncol.)
Ms. Maureen Koehler (Data
 Manager)

Mt. Sinai Medical Center
950 N. 12th Street
Milwaukee, WI 53233
(414/289-8022)
*Dr. William Donegan (Surg.
 Oncol.)

61. Memorial Cancer Research
 Foundation, CA (72)

Brotman Medical Center
3828 Hughes Avenue
Culver City, CA 90230
(213/836-7600)
Dr. Irwin Grossman (Rad. Oncol.)
Dr. Victor Rosen (Pathol.)
Dr. Jacob Terner (Pathol.)
Dr. Gerald Glantz (Surg. Oncol.)

9808 Venice Boulevard
Culver City, CA 90230
(213/559-3550)
*Dr. David Plotkin (Med. Oncol.)
Dr. Peter Schick (Surg. Oncol.)
Ms. Leanne Fernando (Data
 Manager)
Ms. Donna Deering (Administrator)
Ms. Zena Woo, R.N.

Oncology Medical Group of Orange
 County
18102 Irvine Boulevard
Tustin, CA 92680
(714/838-8151)
Dr. David Margileth (Med. Oncol.)
Ms. Nancy Scaglione

2840 Long Beach Boulevard
Long Beach, CA 90806
(213/427-3108)
Dr. Leroy Fass (Med. Oncol.)
Dr. Herman Kattlove (Med. Oncol.)
Ms. Karen Byczynski, R.N.

540 N. Central Avenue
Glendale, CA 91203

(213/247-5440)
Dr. Donald Bogdon (Med. Oncol.)
Dr. John Gunnell (Med. Oncol.)
Dr. Gary Gota (Med. Oncol.)
Ms. Tanya Rieth, R.N.

2625 W. Alameda, Suite 326
Burbank, CA 91505
(213/247-5440)
Dr. Gilbert Hum (Med. Oncol.)
Ms. Mary P. McEntee, R.N.

3440 Lomita
Torrance, CA 90505
(213/530-3813)
Dr. Stephen Lemkin (Med. Oncol.)
Dr. Malin R. Dollinger (Med.
 Oncol.)
Dr. Lowell Greenberg (Med.
 Oncol.)
Dr. Stuart Wong (Med. Oncol.)
Ms. Hilary Price, R.N.

Rees–Stealy Medical Group
2001 4th Avenue
San Diego, CA 92101
(619/234-6261)
Dr. Thomas Lehar (Med. Oncol.)
Dr. Donald Newman (Med. Oncol.)
Dr. Donald Balfour (Med. Oncol.)
Ms. Georgia Nally, R.N.
Ms. Toni Georgian, L.V.N.

St. Joseph's Hospital
c/o Tumor Registry
1100 W. Stuart Drive
Orange, CA 92627
(714/633-9111, ext. 7859)
Ms. Elaine Blake

c/o Drs. Paroly & Smith
3925 Waring Road, Suite C
Oceanside, CA 92054
(714/758-5770)
Ms. Corene Toner

c/o J. W. Allgood, M.D.
625 E. Grand Avenue
Escondido, CA 92025
(714/745-1551)
Ms. Bobbi Siebert

*Principal Investigator

62. Methodist Hospital of Indiana, Inc.
(167)

1604 N. Capitol Avenue
Indianapolis, IN 46206
(317/929-8288)
*Dr. William M. Dugan, Jr. (Med.
Oncol.)
Dr. William Sobat (Surg. Oncol.)
Dr. Randal Strate (Pathol.)
Ms. Terri Ades, R.N.

63. Michael Reese Hospital, Chicago
(26)

29th & Ellis Avenue
Chicago, IL 60616
(312/791-2000)
*Dr. Richard Desser (Med. Oncol.)
Dr. Richard Evans (Surg. Oncol.)
Dr. Arthur Michel (Surg. Oncol.)
Dr. Richard Shapiro (Surg. Oncol.)
Dr. Raman Kaul (Rad. Oncol.)
Dr. Wendy Recant (Pathol.)
Ms. Rhonda Shackelford
Mrs. Anne Solarski, R.N.
Ms. Carol Berkhart, R.N.
Ms. Sandy Purl, R.N.

64. Michigan State University, East
Lansing (90)

Department of Medicine
B-220 Life Sciences
East Lansing, MI 48824
(517/353-6625)
*Dr. Nikolay Dimitrov (Med.
Oncol.)
*Dr. Leif Suhrland (Med. Oncol.)
Dr. Harrold Bowman (Pathol.)
Dr. Ralph Edminster (Pathol.)
Dr. Raphael de los Santos (Surg.
Oncol.)
Ms. Maureen Chojnacki, R.N.
Ms. Judith Munson, R.N.
Ms. Debra Trogu–Barbour, R.N.

Foote Hospital
502 Lansing Avenue
Jackson, MI 49201
(517/789-7123)

*Principal Investigator

Dr. Ray Clark (Med. Oncol.)
Dr. John Axelson (Med. Oncol.)
Dr. N. D. Munro (Surg. Oncol.)
Dr. Stewart Miller (Pathol.)
Ms. Marlene Sebastian, R.N. (Data
Manager)

Ingham Medical Professional Center
405 W. Greenlawn
Lansing, MI 48909
(517/372-5177)
Dr. Richard Meinke (Surg. Oncol.)
Dr. L. Rao Kareti (Surg. Oncol.)
Dr. Kurt Carter (Surg. Oncol.)

Saginaw Cooperative Hospitals,
Inc.
1000 Houghton Avenue
Saginaw, MI 48602
(517/771-6800)
Dr. Paul Calligan (Pathol.)
Dr. Charles Koucky (Surg. Oncol.)
Dr. Thomas O'Callaghan (Surg.
Oncol.)
Dr. Robert S. Powers (Surg. Oncol.)
Dr. William Knapp (Rad. Oncol.)

Michigan Avenue Professional
Center
1320 N. Michigan Avenue
Saginaw, MI 48605
(517/753-1002)
Dr. Ernie Balcueva (Med. Oncol.)
Ms. Nancy Sollner, R.N. (Data
Manager)

St. Joseph Hospital
302 Kensington Avenue
Flint, MI 48502
(313/762-8000)
Dr. George Kovak (Med. Oncol.)
Dr. Wayne Eaton (Pathol.)
Dr. William Dwyer (Surg. Oncol.)
Dr. Heedong Park (Surg. Oncol.)
Dr. Haesook Kim (Rad. Oncol.)
Ms. Valinda Rowe, R.N.
Ms. Mary Kay Spleet, L.P.N.

Butterworth Hospital
100 Michigan, N.E.
Grand Rapids, MI 49503
(616/774-1774)

Dr. Joseph Mann (Pathol.)
Dr. Robert Gillis (Rad. Oncol.)
Dr. Lowell Bursch (Surg. Oncol.)
Dr. John Rienstra (Surg. Oncol.)

Grand Rapids Clinical Oncology
  Program
100 Michigan, N.E.
Grand Rapids, MI 49503
(616/774-1230)
Ms. Diane Van Ostenberg, R.N.
  (Director)

Marquette Medical Arts
414 W. Fair Avenue
Marquette, MI 49855
(906/228-3608)
Dr. Aaron P. Scholnik (Med.
  Oncol.)
Dr. Daniel Arnold (Med. Oncol.)
Ms. Anna Curry Sanford, R.N.

Grand Rapids Oncology Group
1001 Medical Park Drive, Suite 100
Grand Rapids, MI 49506
(616/949-5260)
Dr. James Borst (Med. Oncol.)
Dr. Edward L. Moorhead, II (Med.
  Oncol.)
Dr. Steven Smiley (Med. Oncol.)
Ms. Linda Pool, L.P.N. (Data
  Manager)

Marquette General Hospital
323 Wallace Building
420 W. Magnetic
Marquette, MI 49855
(906/228-9440, ext. 464)
Dr. John Weiss (Pathol.)
Dr. Phillip Dennis (Surg. Oncol.)
Dr. James Keplinger (Surg. Oncol.)
Dr. Eric Lincke (Surg. Oncol.)
Dr. Thomas Mudge (Surg. Oncol.)
Ms. Diane Gordon, R.N. (Data
  Manager)

McLarren Hospital
401 S. Ballenger Highway
Flint, MI 48502
(313/762-2000)
Dr. T. T. Singh (Med. Oncol.)
Dr. Traver Sighng (Med. Oncol.)

Dr. R. Hutson (Surg. Oncol.)
Mrs. Dee Buchholy, R.N.

Owosso Memorial Hospital
826 W. King Street
Owosso, MI 48867
(517/723-5211)
Dr. Christopher Wiseman (Pathol.)
Dr. James MacGregor (Surg.
  Oncol.)
Dr. Garson Tishkoss (Med. Oncol.)

2243 W. Grand River
Okemos, MI 48864
(517/349-3250)
Dr. Richard Collier (Surg. Oncol.)

65. Montefiore Hospital & Medical
    Center, NY (8)

111 E. 210th Street
Bronx, NY 10467
(212/920-5411)
*Dr. Richard G. Rosen (Surg.
  Oncol.)
Dr. Edward Greenwald (Med.
  Oncol.)
Dr. Mark Markham (Med. Oncol.)
Dr. Flora Mincer (Rad. Oncol.)
Dr. Norwin Becker (Pathol.)
Ms. Beatrice Markham (Secretary)
Ms. Diane de la Flor, R.N.
Ms. Karen DiFalco, R.N.

Montefiore Hospital & Medical
  Center
c/o Oncology Department
111 E. 210th Street
DCT, Room 360
Bronx, NY 10467
(212/920-5589)
Ms. Anna Hayes, R.N.

89-06-135 Street
Apartment 5-A
Jamaica, Long Island, NY 11478
(212/658-8188)
Dr. Delifino Crescenzo (Med.
  Oncol.)

*Principal Investigator

66. Montreal General Hospital (87)

    1650 Cedar Avenue
    Montreal, Quebec H3G 1A4
    Canada
    (514/937-7813)
    *Dr. John MacFarlane (Surg.
      Oncol.)
    Dr. J.D. Palmer (Surg. Oncol.)
    Dr. Michael Thirlwell (Med.
      Oncol.)
    Dr. G. A. Boileau (Med. Oncol.)
    Dr. Francisco Dexeus (Med.
      Oncol.)
    Dr. Julio Guerra (Rad. Oncol.)
    Dr. Carolyn Freeman (Rad. Oncol.)
    Dr. Joseph Hazel (Rad. Oncol.)
    Dr. Lawrence Hampson (Surg.
      Oncol.)
    Dr. W.P. Duguid (Pathol.)
    Dr. D.M.P. Thomson (Clin.
      Immunol.)
    Ms. Mary Chadsey
    Ms. Azra Sareen (Network
      Coordinator)

67. Mount Sinai Medical Center,
    Milwaukee (114)

    950 N. Twelfth Street
    P.O. Box 342
    Milwaukee, WI 53201
    (414/289-8200)
    *Dr. William Donegan (Surg.
      Oncol.)
    Dr. Thomas C. Anderson
      (Hematol./Oncol.)
    Dr. Hugh Davis (Hematol./Oncol.)
    Dr. Alberto Lopes Da Conceicao
      (Rad. Oncol.)
    Dr. Reuben Eisenstein (Pathol.)
    Ms. Nancy Stoerzbach, R.N.
    Ms. Jean Zimmermann, R.N.
    Ms. Jude Groniger, R.N.
    Ms. Julie Cukic

    c/o Stein Medical Home Care
    3724 W. Wisconsin Avenue
    Milwaukee, WI 53208
    (414/342-7755)
    Ms. Diane Ross, R.N.

68. Mount Sinai Medical Center,
    Cleveland (58)

    University Circle
    Cleveland, OH 44106
    (216/421-4829)
    *Dr. Richard Bornstein (Med.
      Oncol.)
    Dr. Jeffrey L. Ponsky (Surg.
      Oncol.)
    Dr. Edward Siegler (Pathol.)
    Dr. Norman Berman (Rad. Oncol.)
    Dr. Uri Mintz (Med. Oncol.)
    Dr. Ram Goyal (Rad. Oncol.)
    Ms. Sherrie Reynolds, R.N.,
      B.S.N.
    Ms. Nancy Urbancic, R.N., B.S.N.
    Ms. Joanne Markiewicz (Data
      Coordinator)
    Ms. Brenda Maddox

    2690 Cedar Road
    Cleveland, OH 44122
    (216/831-5656)
    *Dr. Lawrence Levy (Surg. Oncol.)

    (216/831-2890)
    Dr. Isadore Lidsky, M.D. (Surg.
      Oncol.)

    3609 Park East
    Beachwood, OH 44122
    (216/831-4206)
    Dr. James Sampliner (Surg. Oncol.)

69. Naval Regional Medical Center,
    Oakland (36)

    8750 Mountain Boulevard
    Oakland, CA 94627
    (415/639-2418)
    *Dr. Michael A. Crucitt
      (Hematol./Oncol.)
    Dr. Stephen E. Campbell (Med.
      Oncol.)
    Dr. Douglas Cameron (Surg.
      Oncol.)
    Dr. David Karp (Rad. Oncol.)
    Dr. Phillip Voght (Pathol.)
    Ms. Mickey Burns, B.S.
    Ms. Patricia Acord, B.A.

*Principal Investigator

70. NCOG, Central California Cancer Council (404)

2940 N. Fresno Street
Fresno, CA 93703
(209/226-1881)
Ms. Debra Butler (Protocol
  Administrator)

3636 N. First, #120
Fresno, CA 93726
(209/226-1881)
*Dr. Marshall Flam (Med. Oncol.)
Dr. Peter Wittlinger (Med. Oncol.)
Dr. A. Padmanabhan (Med. Oncol.)
Dr. Edward Felix (Surg. Oncol.)

Fresno Community Hospital
PO Box 1232
Fresno, CA 93715
(209/442-3959)
Dr. Phyllis Mowry, (Rad. Oncol.)
Dr. Madhu John (Rad. Oncol.)
Dr. William Podolsky (Rad. Oncol.)
Ms. DeAnn Lazovich (Protocol
  Administrator)

1187 E. Herndon, #106
Fresno, CA 93710
(209/432-0350)
Dr. Victor Medrano (Med. Oncol.)

4420 N. First, #116
Fresno, CA 93726
(209/222-4866)
Dr. Klaus Hoffmann (Med. Oncol.)

Veterans Administration
2615 E. Clinton
Fresno, CA 93703
(209/225-6100)
Dr. Michael Jensen–Akula (Med.
  Oncol.)
Dr. Lawrence Stolberg

3730 N. First
Fresno, CA 93726
(209/226-7717)
Dr. Richard Wolk (Med. Oncol.)

1149 E. Warner
Fresno, CA 93710
(209/224-2821)

Dr. Dix Morgan (Rad. Oncol.)
Dr. Charles Prather (Rad. Oncol.)

1201 E. Herndon, #101
Fresno, CA 93710
(209/435-5570)
Dr. B. Peck Lau

1383 E. Herndon
Fresno, CA 93710
(209/435-5690)
Dr. Paul Frye (Surg. Oncol.)
Dr. Jack Snauffer (Surg. Oncol.)

1735 N. Fresno Street
Fresno, CA 93703
(209/237-9171)
Dr. Thomas Glenchur (Surg.
  Oncol.)

4134 E. Clinton
Fresno, CA 93703
(209/233-9785)
Dr. Anthony Cheng (Surg. Oncol.)

3821 N. Clark
Fresno, CA 93726
(209/224-7453)
Dr. Phillip Hinton (Surg. Oncol.)

2828 Fresno Street
Fresno, CA 93721
(209/485-6440)
Dr. James Kemp (Surg. Oncol.)
Dr. James Sung (Surg. Oncol.)

5359 N. Fresno
Fresno, CA 93710
(209/225-0311)
Dr. Michael Maruyama (Surg.
  Oncol.)

2155 Divisadero
Fresno, CA 93701
(209/442-1343)
Dr. Walter Ruminson (Surg.
  Oncol.)

71. NCOG, David Grant USAF
Medical Center

Travis Air Force Base, CA 84535
(707/438-5052)

*Principal Investigator

*Dr. Edith P. Mitchell, Major
(Med. Oncol.)
Ms. Susan Armstrong (Data
Manager)

(707/438-5705)
Dr. Armando San Diego (Pathol.)

(707/438-2140)
Dr. Douglas Johnson (Rad. Oncol.)

72. NCOG, East Bay Oncology Group
(401)

2023 Vale Road, Suite 102
San Pablo, CA 94806
(415/234-1084)
*Dr. Eli Richman (Med. Oncol.)
Dr. Douglas Kaufman (Med.
Oncol.)

Suite 210
(415/237-2203)
Dr. Mark Silvert (Urol.)

East Bay Oncology Group
Bay Area Tumor Institute
2844 Summit Street, Suite 204
Oakland, CA 94609
(415/465-8570)
Ms. Jeanne Hoek (Protocol
Administrator)

Eden Hospital
20103 Lake Chabot Road
Castro Valley, CA 94546
(415/889-5084)
Dr. Joseph Beck (Rad. Oncol.)
Dr. Michael Forrest (Rad. Oncol.)
Dr. Carl Van Wey (Rad. Oncol.)

Peralta Hospital
450-30th Street
Oakland, CA 94609
(415/451-4900)
Dr. Melvin Borowsky (Pathol.)
Dr. Anthony Engelbrecht (Rad.
Oncol.)
Dr. John Salzman (Rad. Oncol.)

Kaiser Permanente Medical Center
280 W. MacArthur Boulevard
Oakland, CA 94611

(415/428-5000)
Dr. Richard Burnett (Internist)
Dr. Frederick Byl (Surg. Oncol.)
Dr. Thomas Ewing (Gynecol.)
Dr. Raymond Hilsinger (Surg.
Oncol.)
Dr. Leonard Morgenstern (Pathol.)
Dr. David Baer (Med. Oncol.)

Alta Bates Hospital
3001 Colby Street at Ashby
Berkeley, CA 94705
(415/845-7110)
Dr. Michael Cassidy (Med. Oncol.)
Dr. William Palmer (Pathol.)
Dr. Theodore Purcell (Rad. Oncol.)
Dr. Jeffrey Wolf (Med. Oncol.)

2191 Mowry Avenue, #600A
Fremont, CA 94536
(415/791-1115)
Dr. David Cheng (Med. Oncol.)

Brookside Hospital
2000 Vale Road
San Pablo, CA 94806
(415/236-7000)
Dr. Stanley Chism (Rad. Oncol.)
Dr. Allan Rosenberg (Rad. Oncol.)
Dr. Joseph Sabella (Pathol.)

2999 Regent Street
Berkeley, CA 94705
(415/848-9023)
Dr. Norman Cohen (Med. Oncol.)

(415/845-7417)
Dr. Robert Fowler (Surg. Oncol.)

Highland General Hospital
1411 E. 31st Street
Oakland, CA 94602
(415/534-8055)
Dr. Hunter Cutting (Med. Oncol.)

Providence Hospital
3012 Summit Street
Oakland, CA 94609
(415/835-4500)
Dr. Justin Dorgeloh (Pathol.)

3324 Webster Street
Oakland, CA 94609

*Principal Investigator

(415/465-6508)
Dr. Owen Ellington (Med. Oncol.)

3000 Colby Street, #203
Berkeley, CA 94705
(415/849-2636)
Dr. Jon Hollander (Med. Oncol.)

3300 Webster Street, #1100
Oakland, CA 94609
(415/452-3424)
Dr. Charles Jenkins (Surg. Oncol.)

3300 Webster Street, #608
Oakland, CA 94609
(415/763-9611)
Dr. Phyllis Klein (Med. Oncol.)

3300 Webster Street, #1010
Oakland, CA 94609
(415/839-2650)
Dr. James Mooney, Jr. (Urol.)

Merritt Hospital
Hawthorne & Webster Streets
Oakland, CA 94609
(415/655-4000)
Dr. Albert Keller (Pathol.)
Dr. M. Donald Merrill (Rad.
  Oncol.)
Dr. Rollin Odell (Rad. Oncol.)
Dr. Jeffrey Demanes (Rad. Oncol.)

433 Estudillo Avenue
San Leandro, CA 94577
(415/483-3565)
Dr. Harvey Freedman (Surg.
  Oncol.)

Kaiser Permanente Medical Center
27400 Hesperian Boulevard
Hayward, CA 94545
(415/784-5000)
Dr. Howard Kleckner (Med.
  Oncol.)

13847 E. 14th Street
San Leandro, CA 94578
(415/483-2555)
Dr. Thomas Leavitt (Med. Oncol.)
Dr. Ravi Arora (Med. Oncol.)

3232 Elm Street
Oakland, CA 94609
(415/653-5375)
Dr. Tom Lee (Med. Oncol.)

Dr. Lionel Schour (Surg. Oncol.)
Dr. Robert Schweitzer (Surg.
  Oncol.)

3010 Colby Street
Berkeley, CA 94705
(415/845-7751)
Dr. David Miller (Med. Oncol.)

2006 Dwight Way, #204
Berkeley, CA 94704
(415/548-3200)
Dr. John Norton (Urol.)

2101 Vale Road
San Pablo, CA 94806
(415/237-4773)
Dr. Joel Ross (Surg. Oncol.)
Dr. Mark Saberman (Surg. Oncol.)

3017 Summit Street
Oakland, CA 94609
(415/452-3375)
Dr. Mervyn Sahud (Med. Oncol.)

828 Harrison Street, #102
Oakland, CA 94612
(415/451-3900)
Dr. Betty Shen (Med. Oncol.)

2929 Summit Street, #210
Oakland, CA 94609
(415/465-1961)
Dr. John Simmons (Med. Oncol.)

426-17th Street
Oakland, CA 94609
(415/451-0793)
Dr. James Smyth (Med. Oncol.)

2500 Milvia Street
Berkeley, CA 94704
(415/548-8888)
Dr. Anthony Somkin (Med. Oncol.)

3043 Summit Street
Oakland, CA 94609
(415/834-6923)
Dr. Larry Strieff (Med. Oncol.)

1330 Terra Hills Drive, Suite J
Pinole, CA 94564
(415/758-0365)
Dr. Steven Turman (Med. Oncol.)

20055 Lake Chabot Road, #130
Castro Valley, CA 94546

(415/886-0535)
Dr. Peter Wong (Med. Oncol.)

2324 Santa Rita Road
Pleasanton, CA 94566
(415/462-8181)
Dr. Kenneth Roth (Urol.)

515-30th Street
Oakland, CA 94609
(415/465-9206)
Dr. Thierno Diallo (Med. Oncol.)

2500 Milvia, #108
Berkeley, CA 94704
(415/548-9812)
Dr. Martha Tracy (Med. Oncol.)

2089 Vale Road, #21
San Pablo, CA 94806
(415/232-3603)
Dr. Walter Rohlfing (Surg. Oncol.)

400-30th Street
Oakland, CA 94609
(415/834-8121)
Dr. William Sullivan (Surg. Oncol.)

27225 Calaroga
Hayward, CA 94545
(415/782-3133)
Dr. Charles Feldstein (Surg. Oncol.)

20257 Redwood Road
Castro Valley, CA 94546
(415/881-8445)
Dr. Ernest Kundert (Surg. Oncol.)

73. NCOG, Greater Sacramento Cancer
Council, Inc. (402)

3130 L Street
Sacramento, CA 95816
(916/446-4606)
*Dr. Robert F. Bohnen (Med.
Oncol.)
Ms. Liz Linn (Protocol
Administrator)

3625 Mission Avenue
Carmichael, CA 95608
(916/446-6406)
Dr. Bernard Levinson (Med.
Oncol.)

*Principal Investigator

Dr. Paul Jacquin (Med. Oncol.)

5301 F Street, Suite 307
Sacramento, CA 95819
(916/736-3391)
Dr. Mary Retzer (Med. Oncol.)
Dr. Paul Rosenberg (Med. Oncol.)
Dr. Neil Culp (Med. Oncol.)

3939 J Street, Suite 300
Sacramento, CA 95816
(916/739-8216)
Dr. Bruce Chosney (Med. Oncol.)
Dr. David Harrison (Med. Oncol.)
Dr. Jack Fisher (Med. Oncol.)

Division of Hematology/Oncology
Kaiser Permanente Medical Center
2025 Morse Avenue
Sacramento, CA 95825
(916/486-6417)
Dr. Pam Oster (Med. Oncol.)
Dr. Sidney Crain (Med. Oncol.)
Dr. Edward Hearn (Med. Oncol.)

Woodland Clinic Medical Group
1207 Fairchild Court
Woodland, CA 95695
(916/666-1631)
Dr. Robert Edmondson (Med.
Oncol.)
Dr. Edward Hoppin (Med. Oncol.)
Dr. William Keane (Med. Oncol.)

1133 Coloma Way
Roseville, CA 95678
(916/969-0292)
Dr. Chia Yian Chou (Med. Oncol.)

333 Sunrise
Roseville, CA 95678
(916/969-4422)
Dr. Saul Silverman (Rad. Oncol.)
Dr. James Andras (Rad. Oncol.)

5271 F Street
Sacramento, CA 95819
(916/453-8653)
Dr. Edward Ordorica (Rad. Oncol.)
Dr. Gerald Hanks (Rad. Oncol.)
Dr. Scotte Doggett (Rad. Oncol.)
Dr. Steve Sorgen (Rad. Oncol.)
Dr. John Mesic (Rad. Oncol.)

Department of Radiology
4001 J Street
Sacramento, CA 95816
(916/453-4414)
Dr. Franklin Banker (Rad. Oncol.)

74. NCOG, Northern Nevada Cancer
Council (407)

236 W. Sixth Street
Reno, NV 89503
(702/329-0873)
*Dr. Stephen A. Schiff (Med.
Oncol.)

Washoe Medical Center
77 Pringle Way
Reno, NV 89520
(702/785-5638)
Dr. Roger Miercort (Rad. Oncol.)
Dr. Samuel Parks (Pathol.)

75 Kirman Avenue
Reno, NV 89502
(702/784-4954)
Ms. Mel Holderman, R.N.
Ms. Connie Gleason (Data
Manager)
Ms. Margo Kennedy (Data
Manager)

75. NCOG, South Bay Oncology
Program (405)

El Camino Hospital
2500 Grant Road
Mountain View, CA 94042
(415/965-8465)
*Dr. Richard Borrison (Rad.
Oncol.)
Ms. Patricia Cheney (Data)

Valley Medical Center
750 S. Bascom
San Jose, CA 95128
(408/279-5635)
Dr. Thomas J. Barclay (Rad.
Oncol.)

Valley Medical Center
751 S. Bascom
San Jose, CA 95128
(408/279-5638)

Dr. John Frenster (Med. Oncol.)

851 Fremont Avenue, Suite 107
Los Altos, CA 94022
(408/948-3513)
Dr. William Buchholz (Hematol.)

15899 Los Gatos–Almaden Road,
#10
Los Gatos, CA 95030
(408/358-1827)
Dr. Rakesh Bhutani (Med. Oncol.)

281 E. Hamilton Avenue
Campbell, CA 95008
(408/379-8436)
Dr. Edward Cahn
(Hematol./Oncol.)

25 N. 14th Street, Suite 150
San Jose, CA 95112
(408/998-3212, ext. 241)
Dr. Dan Clark (Rad. Oncol.)

2410 Samaritan Drive, #202
San Jose, CA 95124
(408/371-6262)
Dr. James Cohen (Med. Oncol.)

45 S. 17th Street
San Jose, CA 95112
(408/998-5551)
Dr. Donald Brennan (Hematol./
Oncol.)

14981 National Avenue, #3
Los Gatos, CA 95030
(408/356-4128)
Dr. Eric Chevlen (Hematol./
Oncol.)

125 South Drive
Mountain View, CA 94040
(408/961-6600)
Dr. James Heckmann (Hematol.)

OCH
2105 Forest Avenue
San Jose, CA 95128
(408/298-3900)
Dr. Joseph Kraut (Rad. Oncol.)

2101 Forest Avenue, #226
San Jose, CA 95128
Dr. Klaus Porzig (Med. Oncol.)

*Principal Investigator

515 South Drive, #10
Mountain View, CA 94040
(408/961-5548)
Dr. Wallace Sampson (Hematol./
  Oncol.)
Dr. Lawrence William (Med.
  Oncol.)

2101 Forest Avenue
San Jose, CA 95128
(408/292-4175)
Dr. Jonathan Schechter (Med.
  Oncol.)
Dr. Martin Rubenstein (Hematol.)

2066 Clarmar Way, Suite A
San Jose, CA 95128
(408/279-1212)
Dr. Anne Smith (Hematol./Oncol.)

700 W. Parr
Los Gatos, CA 95030
(408/374-3306)
Dr. Richard Steffen
  (Hematol./Oncol.)

2520 Samaritan Drive
San Jose, CA 95124
(408/358-1827)
Dr. Gail Yip (Rad. Oncol.)

Sequoia Hospital
Whipple & Alameda de las Pulgas
Redwood City, CA 94062
Dr. Roy Deffebach (Rad. Oncol.)

1100 Laurel Avenue, "A"
San Jose, CA 94070
Dr. Michael Turbow (Med. Oncol.)

2900 Whipple Avenue
Redwood City, CA 94062
San Jose, CA 94062
(408/369-5861)
Dr. Frederic Marcus (Med. Oncol.)

29 Baywood Drive, #2
San Mateo, CA 94402
Dr. Brian Henderson (Hematol./
  Oncol.)

76. NCOG, University of California,
     Davis (406)

*Principal Investigator

Division of Hematology/Oncology
4301 X Street
Sacramento, CA 95817
(916/453-3772)
*Dr. Jerry P. Lewis (Med. Oncol.)
Dr. Henry Tesluk (Pathol.)
Dr. Edward Odorico (Rad. Oncol.)
Dr. Lois O'Grady (Med. Oncol.)
Dr. Fred Meyers (Med. Oncol.)
Dr. E. J. Watson–Williams (Med.
  Oncol.)
Ms. Deborah Armstrong (Protocol
  Administrator)

77. New England Deaconess Hospital,
     Boston (138)

185 Pilgrim Road
Boston, MA 02215
(617/732-8541)
*Dr. Jacob J. Lokich (Med. Oncol.)
Dr. Blake Cady (Surg. Oncol.)
Dr. William McDermott (Surg.
  Oncol.)
Dr. Merle Legg (Pathol.)
Ms. Natalie E. Fossati (Data
  Coordinator)
Ms. Cheryl L. Moore, R.N.
  (Coordinator)

St. Luke's Hospital
101 Page Street
New Bedford, MA 02741
(617/997-1515)
Dr.Thomas Zipoli (Med. Oncol.)
Dr. J. Greer McBratney (Surg.
  Oncol.)
Dr. William Jenney (Surg. Oncol.)
Dr. James Tierney (Surg. Oncol.)
Dr. Robert Greene (Surg. Oncol.)

Wentworth–Douglass Hospital
789 Central Avenue
Dover, NH 03820
(603/749-3019)
Dr. Paul Butler (Surg. Oncol.)
Dr. Paul Young (Pathol.)

Doctors' Park
Dover, NH 03820
(603/742-9226)

Dr. Jack Myers (Surg. Oncol.)
Dr. Roger Temple (Surg. Oncol.)

230 Lafayette Road
Portsmouth, NH 03801
(603/436-9241)
Dr. Stephen Paul (Med. Oncol.)
Dr. Henry Sonneborn (Med.
  Oncol.)

Frisbie Memorial Hospital
78 Wakefield Street
Rochester, NH 03867
(603/332-4371)
Dr. Donald Phillips (Hematol./
  Oncol.)

78. New York Medical College

240 First Avenue
New York, NY 10009
(212/473-6100)
*Dr. Norman Bloom (Surg. Oncol.)

Lincoln Hospital
Mental Health Center
237 E. 149th Street
Bronx, NY 10041
(212/579-5000)
Dr. Umhra Mishra (Rad. Oncol.)

North General Hospital
1919 Madison Avenue
New York, NY 10035
(212/650-4000)
Dr. Peter Yeung (Rad. Oncol.)

Metropolitan Hospital Center
1901 18th Avenue
New York, NY 10035
(212/360-6262)
Dr. John McCreavey (Med. Oncol.)

79. Newark Beth Israel Medical Center
  (43)

201 Lyons Avenue
Newark, NJ 07112
(201/926-7000)
*Dr. Frederick B. Cohen (Med.
  Oncol.)
Dr. Alan J. Lippman (Med. Oncol.)

*Principal Investigator

Dr. Marcelito C. Custodio (Med.
  Oncol.)
Dr. Fred L. Steinhaum (Med.
  Oncol.)
Dr. Andrea M. Ruiz (Med. Oncol.)
Dr. Julian A. Decter (Med.
  Oncol./Hematol.)
Dr. Alkinviadis Campbell (Pathol.)
Dr. Viera Schweitzer (Rad. Oncol.)
Ms. Janice Belsky, R.N.
Ms. Ina Yalof

159 Millburn Avenue
Millburn, NJ 07041
(201/379-5888)
Dr. Donald Brief (Surg. Oncol.)
Dr. Bruce Brener (Surg. Oncol.)

80. Novato Community Hospital (169)

1625 Hill Road
Novato, CA 94948
(415/897-3111)
*Dr. Charles B. Engelberg (Med.
  Oncol.)
Dr. Palmer White (Surg. Oncol.)
Dr. Jacques Couacaud (Surg.
  Oncol.)
Ms. Terry Guy, R.N.

Marin General Hospital
250 Bon Air Road
Greenbrae, CA 94904
(415/461-0100)
Dr. Wayne Torigoe (Rad. Oncol.)
Dr. Robert Schneider (Pathol.)

81. Ohio State University (53)

Univesity Hospital N-723
410 W. 10th Avenue
Columbus, OH 43210
(614/421-8890)
*Dr. William B. Farrar (Surg.
  Oncol.)

University Hospital N-1022
410 W. 10th Avenue
Columbus, OH 43210
(614/421-8727)
*Dr. James A. Neidhart
  (Hematol./Oncol.)

University Hospital N-1025
Columbus, OH 43210
(614/421-8728)
Dr. John J. Rinehart
  (Hematol./Oncol.)
Dr. Michael R. Grever
  (Hematol./Oncol.)
Dr. Eric H. Kraut
  (Hematol./Oncol.)

University Hospital N-1014
Columbus, OH 43210
(614/421-8723)
Dr. Robert L. Wall
  (Hematol./Oncol.)

(614/421-8722)
Dr. Henry E. Wilson
  (Hematol./Oncol.)

University Hospital N-1003
Columbus, OH 43210
(614/421-8719)
Dr. Bertha A. Bouroncle
  (Hematol./Oncol.)

University Hospital
Means Hall 259
Columbus, OH 43210
(614/421-8725)
Dr. Earl N. Metz (Hematol./Oncol.)

University Hospital N-1035
Columbus, OH 43210
(614/421-8729)
Dr. Stanley P. Balcerzak
  (Hematol./Oncol.)

University Hospital N0729
Columbus, OH 43210
(614/421-8700)
Dr. John P. Minton (Surg. Oncol.)

University Hospital N-724
Columbus, OH 43210
(614/421-8540)
Dr. Arthur G. James (Surg. Oncol.)

University Hospital N-716
Columbus, OH 43210
(614/421-8538)
Dr. Peter J. Fabri (Surg. Oncol.)

University Hospital N-717
Columbus, OH 43210
(614/421-8701)
Dr. Larry C. Carey (Surg. Oncol.)

University Hospital N-717
Columbus, OH 43210
(614/421-8542)
Dr. Marc Cooperman (Surg.
  Oncol.)

(614/421-8843)
Dr. Edward W. Martin, Jr. (Surg.
  Oncol.)

University Hospital N-1012
Columbus, OH 43210
(614/421-8704)
Dr. John J. Ferrara (Surg. Oncol.)

450 W. 10th Avenue S-1095 RH
Columbus, OH 43210
(614/421-4976)
Ms. Patti Kessler (Data Manager)

University Hospital N-082B
Columbus, OH 43210
(614/421-8413)
Dr. Shelin Hodgson (Rad. Oncol.)

University Hospital N-312
Columbus, OH 43210
(614/421-8473)
Dr. Joel Lucas (Surg. Oncol.)

University Hospital N-723
410 W. 10th Avenue
Columbus, OH 43210
(614/421-8890)
Ms. Joyce Bennett, R.N.
Ms. Penny Ekegren, R.N.

82. Ottawa Civic Hospital (57)

Division of Ontario Cancer
  Foundation
190 Melrose Avenue
Ottawa, Ontario K1Y 4K7
Canada
(613/725-6300)
*Dr. Rebecca McDermot (Rad.
  Oncol.)
*Dr. Leo Stolbach (Med. Oncol.)

*Principal Investigator

913

Dr. C.E. Catton (Rad. Oncol.)
Dr. James Devitt (Surg. Oncol.)
Dr. E. Leipa (Pathol.)
Dr. Wolfgang E. Hirte (Med. Oncol.)
Dr. D. J. Perrault (Med. Oncol.)
Dr. D. J. Stewart (Med. Oncol.)
Dr. J. A. Maroun (Med. Oncol.)
Dr. C. M. Cripps (Med. Oncol.)
Dr. V. P. Young (Med. Oncol.)
Mrs. Lori O'Connor (Data Manager)
Ms. Terry Clayton
Ms. Christine McNulty
Ms. Brenda Waterfield
Ms. Mary Stewart, R.N.
Ms. Joan Robertson, R.N.
Ms. Suzie Joanisse–Lesage, R.N.

Ottawa General Clinic
501 Smyth Road
Ottawa, Ontario K1G 8L6
Canada
(613/737-8723)
Ms. Joanne Walker (Data Manager)

83. Pennsylvania Hospital (60)

330 S. 9th Street
Philadelphia, PA 19107
(215/829-3583)
*Dr. Harvey Lerner (Surg. Oncol.)
Ms. Kate Godwin, R.N.

8th & Spruce Streets
Philadelphia, PA 19107
(215/829-3000)
Dr. Dominic DeLaurentis (Surg. Oncol.)
Dr. Howard Zaren (Surg. Oncol.)
Dr. John Glassburn (Rad. Oncol.)
Dr. Else Olen (Pathol.)
Dr. Edward Burka (Hematol./Oncol.)

2 Bala Plaza, Suite IL-20
Bala Cynwyd, PA 19004
(215/839-4162)
Dr. Steven Katz (Surg. Oncol.)

84. Presbyterian Hospital, Oklahoma City, OK (141)

N.E. 13th at Lincoln Boulevard
Oklahoma City, OK 73104
(405/271-5100)
*Dr. Daniel Carmichael (Surg. Oncol.)
Dr. Stephen Remine (Surg. Oncol.)
Dr. William L. Hughes (Med. Oncol.)
Dr. Richard Ishmael (Med. Oncol.)
Dr. Ted Clemens, Jr. (Med. Oncol.)
Dr. Ralph Ganick (Med. Oncol.)
Dr. Thomas A. Hosty (Pathol.)
Dr. Michael R. Harkey (Pathol.)
Dr. Stephen Acker (Rad. Oncol.)
Mrs. Barbara Baxter (Data Manager)
Ms. Ann Denyer, R.N.
Ms. Velma Harrison, R.N.
Ms. Diane Kirk, R.N.
Ms. Pat Tobin, R.N.
Sammie Wier, R.N.

701 N.E. Tenth Street
Oklahoma City, OK 73104
(405/271-2731)
Dr. Mark E. King (Med. Oncol.)

85. Richmond Heights General Hospital (154)

27100 Chardon Road
Richmond Heights, OH 44143
(216/585-6500)
*Dr. Prabha Murthy (Pathol.)
Dr. Doug Zinni (Surg. Oncol.)
Dr. Jerry Zinni (Surg. Oncol.)
Dr. Frank Hocka (Surg. Oncol.)
Dr. Thomas Warren (Gastrointerol.)
Dr. Gregg Arko (Rad. Oncol.)
Ms. Jan Wallace, R.N. (Oncol. Coordinator)

Medical Oncology Association, Inc.
Mt. Sinai Medical Building
26900 Cedar Road, Suite 122
Beachwood, OH 44122
(216/831-6434)
Dr. Richard Bornstein (Med. Oncol.)
Dr. Uri Mintz (Med. Oncol.)

*Principal Investigator

Mt. Sinai Radiologist Group
26900 Cedar Road, Suite 129
Beachwood, OH 44122
(216/464-5222)
Dr. Norman Berman (Rad. Oncol.)
Dr. Ram Goyal (Rad. Oncol.)

86. Royal Melbourne Hospital,
Australia (139)

Royal Melbourne Hospital
Private Consulting Room, Suite 2
Parkville, 3050
Melbourne, Australia
(011/613/347-0122)
*Dr. Ian Russell (Surg. Oncol.)
Dr. John Collins (Surg. Oncol.)
Dr. R. Brown (Pathol.)

Peter MacCallum Hospital
481 Little Lonsdale Street
Vic 3000
Melbourne, Australia
(011/613/602-1333)
Dr. Peter Jeal (Rad. Oncol.)

Chief, Medical Record
    Administrator
VCCG Trial Secretariat
Anti-Cancer Council of Victoria
90 Jolimont Street
East Melbourne, Australia 3002
(011/613/654-2411)
Ms. Andrienne Mursell (Data
    Coordinator)

87. Royal Victoria Hospital, Montreal
(85)

687 Pine Avenue W.
Montreal, Quebec H3A 1A1
Canada
(514/842-1231)
*Dr. Henry Schibata (Surg. Oncol.)
Dr. Catherine Milne (Surg. Oncol.)
Dr. N. Belliveau (Surg. Oncol.)
Dr. A. Loutfi (Surg. Oncol.)
Dr. M. Wexler (Surg. Oncol.)
Dr. A. Peter H. McLean (Surg.
    Oncol.)
Dr. G. Tremblay (Pathol.)

*Principal Investigator

Dr. Jocelyne Arseneau (Pathol.)
Dr. Guerin Dorval (Clin. Immunol.)
Dr. Samuel Solomon (Endocrino.)
Dr. Roger Hand (Med. Oncol.)
Dr. C. Freeman (Rad. Oncol.)
Ms. Nicki Sellitto, R.N.
Ms. Josie Pepe

88. Rush Presbyterian-St. Luke's
Medical Center, IL (65)

1753 W. Congress Parkway
830 Professional Building
Protocol Office
Chicago, IL 60612
(312/942-5000)
*Dr. Janet Wolter (Med. Oncol.)
*Dr. Steven Economou (Surg.
    Oncol.)
Dr. Frank Hendrickson (Rad.
    Oncol.)
Dr. Elizabeth Wiley (Pathol.)
Dr. Jules Harris (Med. Oncol.)
Dr. Arthur Rossof (Clin. Immunol.)
Ms. Sharon Nisius, R.N., M.S.
Ms. Jean Busby, R.N., M.S.
Mr. Tom Philpot

Department of Medical Oncology
1725 W. Harrison
Chicago, IL 60612
(312/942-5906)
Dr. John Showel (Med. Oncol.)

89. Rutgers Medical School (156)

Academic Health Science Center
CN 19
New Brunswick, NJ 08903
(201/937-7761)
*Dr. Ralph S. Greco (Surg. Oncol.)
Ms. Ellen Fynan

(201/937-7680)
Dr. Hugh C. Kim (Med. Oncol.)
Dr. Parvin Saidi (Med. Oncol.)

(201/937-7682)
Dr. Edward F. Schnipper (Med.
    Oncol.)

Middlesex General Hospital
180 Somerset Street
New Brunswick, NJ 08903
(201/937-8651)
Dr. Paul C. Smilow (Pathol.)

St. Peter's Medical Center
254 Easton Avenue
New Brunswick, NJ 08903
(201/745-8590)
Dr. Alexander Haas (Rad. Oncol.)

7 Wirt Street
New Brunswick, NJ 08903
(201/828-9570)
Dr. Michael Nissenblatt (Med.
  Oncol.)

c/o RCHP
57 U.S. Highway #1
New Brunswick, NJ 08901
(201/249-5700)
Dr. Julia Ladd Smith (Med. Oncol.)

90. St. Joseph Hospital, Lancaster, PA
(132)

Professional Building
250 College Avenue, Suite 109
Lancaster, PA 17604
(717/291-8904)
*Dr. H. P. DeGreen
  (Hematol./Oncol.)
Dr. Ross B. Moquin
  (Hematol./Oncol.)
Ms. Cindy Ulmer, R.N.

(717/291-8025)
Dr. E. Eisenhower (Pathol.)

(717/291-8211)
Dr. Paul Gachwend (Surg. Oncol.)

Lancaster General Hospital
555 N. Duke Street
Lancaster, PA 17603
(717/295-8302)
Dr. Terry Moore (Rad. Oncol.)

Lancaster Osteopathic Hospital
1175 Clark Street
Lancaster, PA 17604
(717/397-3711)

*Principal Investigator

916

Dr. Norman Axelrod (Surg. Oncol.)
Dr. Robert Scott (Surg. Oncol.)

91. St. Luc Hospital, Montreal (97)

1058 St. Denis Street
Montreal, Quebec
Canada
(514/285-1525)
*Dr. Roger Poisson (Surg. Oncol.)
*Dr. Sandra
  LegaultLegault–Poisson (Surg.
  Oncol.)
Dr. Denis Bernard (Surg. Oncol.)
Dr. Steve Morgan (Surg. Oncol.)
Dr. Romeo Lafrance (Surg. Oncol.)
Dr. Pierre Franche Bois (Surg.
  Oncol.)
Dr. Jean Cote (Pathol.)
Dr. Andre Dumont (Pathol.)
Dr. Claude Thuot (Hematol.)
Dr. Louis Perron (Hematol.)
Dr. Raymond Guevin (Hematol.)
Dr. Anne Marie Nutini
  (Hematol./Oncol.)
Ms. Linda Bisaillon (Secretary)
Ms. Odette Rivard Sergerie, R.N.
Ms. Suzanne Bisaillon, R.N.
Ms. Mimi Fortin (Data Coordinator)

Maisonneuve Hospital
Montreal, Canada
(514/254-8341)
Dr. Jean Philip Mercier (Rad.
  Oncol.)

92. St. Luke's Hospital, Kansas City
(83)

44th & Wornall Road
Kansas City, MO 64111
(816/932-2000)
Dr. John Rippey (Pathol.)
Dr. Joe L. Rector (Rad. Oncol.)
Ms. Peggy Brinkman, R.N.
Ms. Mary Follis, R.N.

4320 Wornall Road
308 Medical Plaza
Kansas City, MO 64111
(816/753-7460)
*Dr. Paul Koontz (Surg. Oncol.)

4320 Wornall Road
308 Medical Plaza, Suite 212
Kansas City, MO 64111
(816/753-7460)
Dr. Karl H. Hanson (Med. Oncol.)

4320 Wornall Road, Suite 624
Kansas City, MO 64111
(816/531-2992)
Dr. Richard Mundis (Med. Oncol.)

4240 Blue Ridge Boulevard, Suite
500
Kansas City, MO 64133
(816/356-8877)
Dr. Larry Rosen (Med. Oncol.)

Independence Sanitarium and
Hospital
1515 W. Truman Road
Independence, MO 64050
(816/836-8100)
Dr. Raymond J. Caffrey (Pathol.)

1515 W. Truman Road, Suite 402
Independence, MO 64050
(816/254-9292)
Dr. John H. Nesselrode (Surg.
Oncol.)

93. St. Mary's Hospital Center, Quebec
(157)

3830 Avenue Lacombe
Montreal, Quebec H3T 1M5
Canada
(514/344-3395)
*Dr. John Keyserlingk (Surg.
Oncol.)
Dr. Jose Rodriguez (Surg. Oncol.)
Dr. R. Moralejo (Surg. Oncol.)
Dr. I. Kulcyzcki (Surg. Oncol.)
Dr. Charles Pick (Med. Oncol.)
Dr. Peter Gruner (Med. Oncol.)
Dr. B. Lipowski (Med. Oncol.)
Dr. J. Hazel (Rad. Oncol.)
Dr. R. Murphy (Pathol.)
Dr. G. Berry (Pathol.)
Mrs. Judy Montesano, R.N.
Miss Monique Michaud, R.N.
Mrs. Claire Desrosiers (Data
Collector)

*Principal Investigator

Mrs. Diana D'Angelo

200 Jefferson, S.E.
Grand Rapids, MI 49503
(616/774-6385)
*Dr. Andre V. Jubert (Surg. Oncol.)
Dr. Keh–Ming Sun (Pathol.)
Dr. Michael Kie Seng Tay (Rad.
Oncol.)
Ms. Glenda Didion, R.N.

260 Jefferson, S.E.
Grand Rapids, MI 49503
(616/459-5091)
Dr. William J. Passinault (Gen.
Surgeon)
Dr. Robert A. Vanderploeg (Gen.
Surgeon)

26 Sheldon Avenue, S.E.
Grand Rapids, MI 49503
(616/459-7169)
Dr. Anthony M. Kam (Gen.
Surgeon)

50 College, S.E.
Grand Rapids, MI 49503
(616/774-8365)
Dr. Denis Alix (Gen. Surgeon)

515 Lakeside Drive, S.E.
Grand Rapids, MI 49506
(616/461-2933)
Dr. Enrico C. Sobong (Med.
Oncol.)

95. St. Michael's Hospital, Toronto
(11)

30 Bond Street
Toronto, M5B 1W8
Canada
(416/864-5851)
Dr. Ken R. Butler (Med. Oncol.)
Dr. M.B. Garvey (Med. Oncol.)
Dr. Ara Chalvardjian (Pathol.)
Dr. Arthur Leznoff (Clin.
Immunol.)
Ms. Karen Connelly, R.N.
Ms. Gloria Scherer, R.N.
Ms. Tarcila Soropia, R.N.
Ms. Linda DeCoste

St. Michael's Hospital
30 Bond Street
Day Care Unit - 2 DS
Toronto, Ontario M5B 1WB
Canada
(416/864-5127)
Dr. Robert Myers (Med. Oncol.)

55 Queen Street E.
Toronto, M5C 1R5
Canada
(416/367-9670)
*Dr. Leo Mahoney (Surg. Oncol.)
Dr. Dennis Jirsch (Surg. Oncol.)
Dr. Nicholas Colapinto (Surg.
   Oncol.)
Dr. Donald Currie (Surg. Oncol.)

Princess Margaret Hospital
500 Sherbourne Street
Toronto, M4X 1K9
Canada
(416/924-0671)
Dr. Roy Clark (Rad. Oncol.)

96. St. Sacrement Hospital, Quebec
     City (145)

1050 Chemin Ste-Foy
Quebec P.Q. G1S 4LB
(418/688-7676)
*Dr. Jean Couture (Surg. Oncol.)
Dr. Luc Deschenes (Surg. Oncol.)
Dr. Jean Robert (Surg. Oncol.)
Dr. Simon Jacob (Pathol.)
Dr. Pierre Leblond (Med. Oncol.)
Ms. Edith Picard Marcoux, R.N.

Hotel–Dieu, Quebec City
11, Cote due Palais
Quebec, G1R 2J6 Canada
(418/694-5352)
Dr. Andre Girard (Rad. Oncol.)
Dr. Jacques Laverdiere (Rad.
   Oncol.)

97. St. Vincent's Hospital, IN (82)

2001 W. 86th Street
Indianapolis, IN 46260
(317/871-2345)
Dr. James Sullivan (Pathol.)

Dr. Marvin Melton (Pathol.)
Dr. J. Horvath (Rad.)

8220 Naab Road
Indianapolis, IN 46260
(317/872-4359)
*Dr. John A. Cavins (Med. Oncol.)
Ms. Nancy Keefe, R.N.

8330 Naab Road, Suite 213
Indianapolis, IN 46260
(317/872-9586)
Dr. E. D. Habegger (Surg. Oncol.)
Dr. D. Price (Surg. Oncol.)

Suite 301
(317/872-3355)
Dr. J. George (Surg. Oncol.)

8402 Harcourt Road
Indianapolis, IN 46260
(317/872-0041)
Dr. Bud McDougal (Surg. Oncol.)

Suite 602
(317/872-1161)
Dr. Charles Johnson (Gastrointrol.)

Suite 810
(317/871-2194)
Ms. Marsha Eagan (Data)

98. St. Vincent's Hospital, NY (10)

Cronin 802
153 W. 11th Street
New York, NY 10011
(212/790-8344)
*Dr. Thomas Nealon (Surg. Oncol.)
Dr. Carlo E. Grossi (Surg. Oncol.)
Dr. William R. Grace (Med.
   Oncol.)
Dr. Barbara Johnston (Med. Oncol.)
Dr. George Schwarz (Rad. Oncol.)
Dr. John F. Gillooley (Pathol.)
Dr. Ilona Toth (Pathol.)
Mrs. Rosalie McCauley, R.N. (Data
   Coordinator)

99. Scranton Hematology/Oncology
     Associates (155)

*Principal Investigator

918

Mercy General Service Building
743 Jefferson Avenue, Suite 205
Scranton, PA 18510
(717/342-3675)
*Dr. William Heim (Med.
  Oncol./Hematol.)
Dr. Robert Wright (Med.
  Oncol./Hematol.)
Dr. Francis LaLuna (Med.
  Oncol./Hematol.)
Dr. Salvatore Scialla (Med.
  Oncol./Hematol.)
Ms. Diane Shebaugh, R.N. (Data
  Manager)

Mercy Hospital
746 Jefferson Avenue
Scranton, PA 18510
(717/348-7898)
Dr. James J. O'Connor (Pathol.)
Dr. Harmar Brereton (Rad. Oncol.)

100. SECSG, CCOP, Alton Ochsner
      Medical Foundation (561)

      1516 Jefferson Highway
      New Orleans, LA 70121
      (504/838-3910)
      *Dr. Carl G. Kardinal (Med.
        Oncol.)
      Ms. Marilyn Bateman (Data
        Manager)

      Ochsner Clinic
      1514 Jefferson Highway
      New Orleans, LA 70121
      (504/838-3910)
      Dr. Don M. Samples (Med. Oncol.)
      Dr. Archie W. Brown, Jr. (Med.
        Oncol.)
      Dr. Morris A. Flaum (Med. Oncol.)

      Baton Rouge Clinic
      8415 Goodwood Boulevard
      Baton Rouge, LA 70806
      (504/923-1515)
      Dr. Henry O. Williams (Rad.
        Oncol.)
      Dr. Frederi T. Billings, III (Med.
        Oncol.)

Dr. Joseph Benton Dupont (Surg.
  Oncol.)
Dr. David D. Kahn (Med. Oncol.)
Dr. Richard F. Burroughs (Med.
  Oncol.)
Dr. James E. Hancock (Rad.
  Oncol.)
Dr. Sheldon A. Johnson (Rad.
  Oncol.)

Southern Louisiana Medical Center
1978 Industrial Boulevard
Houma, LA 70360
(504/868-8140)
Dr. Harry J. McGaw (Med. Oncol.)
Dr. John O. Dampeer (Surg.
  Oncol.)

Hattiesburg Clinic
415 S. 28th Avenue
Hattiesburg, MS 39401
(601/264-6000)
Dr. David M. Owen (Med. Oncol.)
Dr. Walton E. Stevens (Rad.
  Oncol.)
Dr. Carl R. Hale (Rad. Oncol.)

101. SECSG, Emory University, CA
      (596)

      Hematology–Oncology
      Emory University
      Box AR
      Atlanta, GA 30322
      (404/329-7016)
      *Dr. James W. Keller (Med.
        Oncol.)
      Ms. Lorraine Johnson
        (Hematol./Oncol.)

      Emory University Clinic
      Surgical Oncology
      Atlanta, GA 30322
      (404/321-0111, ext. 3300)
      Ms. Jean Bried, P.A.

      Winship Clinic
      Emory University Clinic
      Atlanta, GA 30322
      (404/321-0111)
      Dr. John Coleman (Surg. Oncol.)
      Dr. Douglas Murray (Surg. Oncol.)

*Principal Investigator

Dr. R. Waldo Powell (Surg. Oncol.)

Department of Anatomical
Pathology
Emory University Hospital
1364 Clifton Road, N.E.
Atlanta, GA 30322
(404/329-7001)
Dr. Whitaker Sewell (Pathol.)

Division of Radiation Oncology
Emory University Clinic
Atlanta, GA 30322
(404/321-0111)
Dr. John McLaren (Rad. Oncol.)

102. SECSG, Georgetown University
(531)

Georgetown University Hospital
Division of Medical Oncology
3800 Reservoir Road, N.W.
Washington, DC 20007
(202/625-7081, 7082)
*Dr. Patrick J. Bryne (Med. Oncol.)
Dr. James Ahlgren (Med. Oncol.)
Dr. John Neefe (Med. Oncol.)
Dr. Frederick Smith (Med. Oncol.)
Dr. Paul Woolley (Med. Oncol.)

(202/625-7706)
Ms. Mary McCabe, R.N.
Ms. Marilyn Ayoob, R.N.
Ms. Connie Hinds, R.N.

Vincent T. Lombardi Cancer Center
Georgetown University Medical
Center
Data Management Office
Washington, DC 20007
(202/625-7900)
Ms. Mary Wyatt Bowers, M.A.
(Data Manager)

103. SECSG, St. Louis University
Medical Center (746)

School of Medicine
1325 S. Grand Boulevard
St. Louis, MO 63104
(314/771-7600, ext. 3895)

*Principal Investigator

920

*Dr. G. O. Brown, Jr. (Med.
Oncol.)
Dr. N. I. Gallagher
(Hematol./Oncol.)
Dr. N. I. Gallagher
(Hematol./Oncol.)
Dr. N. I. Gallagher (Hematol.)
Dr. D. W. Luedke (Med. Oncol.)
Dr. S. L. Luedke (Med. Oncol.)
Dr. P. J. Petruska (Med. Oncol.)
Ms. Linda Hackney, R.N.
Ms. Kathleen Merlo, R.N.
Ms. Jean Schlueter (Data Manager)

104. SECSG , University of Alabama
(501)

638 Zeigler Building
University Station
Birmingham, AL 35294
(205/934-3204)
*Dr. George A. Omura
(Hematol./Oncol.)
Ms. Linda G. Miles (Data Manager)

University of Alabama School of
Medicine
University Station, CSB-320
Birmingham, AL 35294
(205/934-3028)
Dr. Charles M. Balch (Surg.
Oncol.)

University of Alabama School of
Medicine
University Station, CSB-320
Birmingham, AL 35294
(205/934-2306)
Dr. William Maddox (Surg. Oncol.)
Ms. Marie McGregor, R.N., M.S.
Ms. Karen Ford, R.N.
Ms. Lynn Watkins, R.N.
Ms. Judy Smith (Data Manager)

University of Alabama School of
Medicine
University Station, LBWIT-114
Birmingham, AL 35294
(205/934-5670)
Dr. Merle M. Salter (Rad. Oncol.)

University of Alabama School of
Medicine
University Station, Zeigler-643
Birmingham, AL 35294
(205/934-2084)
Dr. John T. Carpenter, Jr.
(Hematol./Oncol.)

105. SECSG, University of Cincinnati,
OH (556)

231 Bethesda Avenue
Cincinnati, OH 45267
(513/872-4233)
*Dr. Orlando J. Martelo
(Hematol./Oncol.)
Dr. M. Drue Denton
(Hematol./Oncol.)
Dr. Herbert C. Flessa
(Hematol./Oncol.)
Dr. Thomas L. Wright
(Hematol./Oncol.)
Dr. David C. Zellner
(Hematol./Oncol.)
Dr. Robert Hummel (Surg. Oncol.)

231 Bethesda Avenue
Cincinnati, OH 45267
(513/872-4233)
Dr. Donna L. Stahl (Surg. Oncol.)
Dr. Martin Popp (Surg. Oncol.)
Dr. Mark Weiss (Surg. Path.)
Dr. Bernard S. Aron (Rad. Oncol.)
Dr. Paul Hurtubisc (Diag. Immunol.
Lab)
Ms. JoAnn Hake, R.N.
Ms. Denise Barlag (Data
Doordinator)
Ms. Peggy Cordons, R.N.

106. SECSG, University of Florida,
Gainesville (629)

Box J 277
Gainesville, FL 32610
(904/392-3431)
*Dr. Roy S. Weiner (Med. Oncol.)
Ms. Mary Monahan, R.N.

107. SECSG, University of Kentucky,
Lexington (661)

VA Medical Center
Lexington, KY 40511
(606/233-4511)
*Dr. Philip DeSimone (Hematol.)
Dr. Michael Ram (Surg. Oncol.)

University of Kentucky Medical
Center
Lexington, KY 40536
(606/233-6602)
Dr. Daniel Kenady (Surg. Oncol.)
Dr. Oscar Mendiondo (Rad. Oncol.)

VA Medical Center
Lexington, KY 40511
(606/233-4511)
Dr. Ralph Powell (Pathol.)

VA Hospital
Hematology–Oncology (111E)
Lexington, KY 40511
(606/233-4511)
Ms. Phyllis Arnold
Ms. Marsha Oakley, R.N.

University of Kentucky Medical
Center
Division of Hematology/Oncology
MS681
Lexington, KY 40536
(606/233-5292)
Juanita Garrison, R.N.
Mary Morrison, R.N.

108. SECSG, University of Tennessee,
Knoxville (766)

University of Tennessee
Memorial Research Center
1924 Alcoa Highway
Knoxville, TN 37920
(615/971-3160)
*Dr. Stephen Krauss (Med. Oncol.)
Dr. Anthony Kattine, (Pathol.)
Dr. Frank Comos, (Rad. Oncol.)
Ms. Cindy Hansard, R.N. (Data
Manager)

106. SECSG, University of Florida,
Gainesville (629)

*Principal Investigator

921

Box J 277
Gainesville, FL 32610
(904/392-3431)
*Dr. Roy S. Weiner (Med. Oncol.)
Ms. Mary Monahan, R.N.

107. SECSG, University of Kentucky, Lexington (661)

VA Medical Center
Lexington, KY 40511
(606/233-4511)
*Dr. Philip DeSimone (Hematol.)
Dr. Michael Ram (Surg. Oncol.)

University of Kentucky Medical Center
Lexington, KY 40536
(606/233-6602)
Dr. Daniel Kenady (Surg. Oncol.)
Dr. Oscar Mendiondo (Rad. Oncol.)

VA Medical Center
Lexington, KY 40511
(606/233-4511)
Dr. Ralph Powell (Pathol.)

VA Hospital
Hematology–Oncology (111E)
Lexington, KY 40511
(606/233-4511)
Ms. Phyllis Arnold
Ms. Marsha Oakley, R.N.

University of Kentucky Medical Center
Division of Heamtology/Oncology
MS681
Lexington, KY 40536
(606/233-5292)
Juanita Garrison, R.N.
Mary Morrison, R.N.

108. SECSG, University of Tennessee, Knoxville (766)

University of Tennessee
Memorial Research Center
1924 Alcoa Highway
Knoxville, TN 37920
(615/971-3160)
*Dr. Stephen Krauss (Med. Oncol.)

Dr. Anthony Kattine, (Pathol.)
Dr. Frank Comos, (Rad. Oncol.)
Ms. Cindy Hansard, R.N. (Data Manager)

109. SECSG, University of Tennessee Center for the Health Sciences (773)

800 Madison Avenue
Memphis, TN 38163
(901/528-5817)
*Dr. Charles L. Neely (Hematol./Oncol.)

(901/528-7730)
Dr. Subir Nag (Rad. Oncol.)

(901/528-5798)
Dr. Luther Burkett (Hematol.)

Division of Hematology/Oncology
800 Madison Avenue
N201 Van Vleet
Memphis, TN 38163
(901/528-5817)
Ms. Mara F. Jones (Med. Tech.)

1331 Union Avenue, Suite 1220
Memphis, TN 38104
(901/725-1921)
Dr. Raza A. Dilawari (Surg. Oncol.)

Baptist Memorial Hospital
899 Madison Avenue
Memphis, TN 38146
(901/522-7574)
Dr. Rodger C. Haggitt (Pathol.)

110. SECSG, Washington University, St. Louis (804)

Jewish Hospital
216 S. Kingshighway
St. Louis, MO 63110
(314/454-7170)
*Dr. Gordon W. Philpott (Surg. Oncol.)
Ms. Patty Flynn, R.N.
Ms. Patricia M. Scannell

(314/454-8462)
Dr. John S. Meyer (Pathol.)

*Principal Investigator

(314/454-7182)
Dr. Ralph Graff (Surg. Oncol.)

(314/454-7463)
Dr. Alan Lyss (Med. Oncol.)

4910 Forest Park Boulevard, Suite 202
St. Louis, MO 63108
(314/361-7786)
Dr. Gary A. Ratkin (Med. Oncol.)
Dr. Albert VanAmburg (Med. Oncol.)

Mallinckrodt Institution of Radiology
4511 Forest Park
St. Louis, MO 63108
(314/454-3381)
Dr. John Bedwinek (Rad. Oncol.)
Dr. Todd H. Wasserman (Rad. Oncol.)
Dr. Miljenko V. Pilepich (Rad. Oncol.)
Dr. Joseph Simpson (Rad. Oncol.)
Dr. Patrick Thomas (Rad. Oncol.)
Dr. Bruce Walz (Rad. Oncol.)

(314/454-2134)
Dr. Carlos A. Perez (Rad. Oncol.)

Wohl Hospital Building
Cancer Center
4960 Audubon, 3rd Fl.
St. Louis, MO 63110
(314/454-5000)
Dr. Alex E. Denes (Med. Oncol.)
Dr. Geoffrey P. Herzig (Med. Oncol.)
Dr. Gordon Phillips (Med. Oncol.)
Dr. Jay Marion (Med. Oncol.)

Wohl Clinic Building
4950 Audubon Avenue, 9th Fl.
St. Louis, MO 63110
(314/454-2870)
Dr. Samuel Wells (Surg. Oncol.)

Barnes Hospital
East Pavilion, Suite 16422
St. Louis, MO 63110
(314/367-9595)

Dr. Robert E. Kraetsch (Med. Oncol.)

522 N. New Ballas Road
St. Louis, MO 63141
(314/569-0160) or (314/946-2388)
Dr. Morton A. Levy (Med. Oncol.)

4989 Barnes Hospital Plaza
Queeny Tower, Suite 3103
St. Louis, MO 63110
(314/454-5360)
Dr. Virgil Loeb (Med. Oncol.)

510 S. Kingshighway
Division of Radiation Oncology
St. Louis, MO 63110
(314/454-3638)
Dr. Gilbert H. Nussbaum (Rad. Oncol.)
Dr. Glenn P. Glasgow (Rad. Oncol.)

111. South Nassau Communities Hospital, NY (96)

2445 Oceanside Road
Oceanside, NY 11572
(516/536-1600)
*Dr. Nicholas LiCalzi (Surg. Oncol.)
Dr. Salvatore Noto (Surg. Oncol.)
Dr. Bong Kim (Rad. Oncol.)
Dr. Ahmed Khapra (Pathol.)
Dr. Ivan Rothman (Med. Oncol.)
Dr. Ronald Primis (Med. Oncol.)
Dr. Leonard Kessler (Med. Oncol.)
Dr. Sanford Pariser (Med. Oncol.)
Mrs. Dorothy S. Rece
Ms. Carole Potter, R.N.

112. Tacoma General Hospital, WA (147)

314 S. K Street
Tacoma, WA 98405
(206/272-5378)
*Dr. A. Robert Thiessen (Med. Oncol.)
Dr. H. Irving Pierce (Med. Oncol.)
Dr. J. Gale Katterhagen (Med. Oncol.)

*Principal Investigator

Dr. Ronald S. Goldberg (Med. Oncol.)

314 S. K Street, Suite 501
Tacoma, WA 98405
(206/383-5949)
Dr. William Martin (Surg. Oncol.)

314 S. K Street, Suite 11
Tacoma, WA 98405
(206/627-6171)
Dr. Michael Soronen (Rad. Oncol.)

314 S. K Street, Suite 104
Tacoma, WA 98405
(206/272-5378)
Ms. Carolyn Mitchell (Data Coordinator)

315 S. K Street
Tacoma, WA 98405
(206/597-6640)
Dr. L. Cargol (Pathol.)

113. Texas Tech Medical School, Amarillo (130)

1400 Wallace Boulevard
Amarillo, TX 79106
(806/358-3101)
*Dr. Edwin Savlov (Surg. Oncol.)
Dr. Robert Justice (Med. Oncol.)
Dr. Brian Pruitt (Med. Oncol.)

1600 Wallace Boulevard
Amarillo, TX 79106
(806/355-9151)
Dr. Ralph R. Mennemeyer (Pathol.)

Northwest Texas Hospital
P.O. Box 1110
Amarillo, TX 79105
(806/374-9912)
Dr. John Denko (Pathol.)

5211 W. 9th Avenue, Suite 203
Amarillo, TX 79106
(806/355-9248)
Dr. Karim Nawaz (Med. Oncol.)

1501 Arizona Building 16
El Paso, TX 79902
(915/532-4626)
Dr. Thomas Twele (Med. Oncol.)

Health Science Center
4800 Alberta Avenue
El Paso, TX 79905
(915/533-3020)

Texas Tech University
School of Medicine
Department of Surgery
3A-133 Health Science Center
Building
Lubbock, TX 70430
(806/743-2370)
Dr. Gerald Woolam (Surg. Oncol.)
Dr. Lowell Larson (Pathol.)
Dr. Ali ElDomeire (Surg. Oncol.)

Don and Sybil Harrington Cancer Center
1500 Wallace Boulevard
Amarillo, TX 79106
(806/353-3571)
Dr. Phillip Periman (Med. Oncol.)
Dr. Daniel Epley (Rad. Oncol.)
Ms. Sandee Rodene, R.N.
Ms. Kathy Rolfe, R.N.
Ms. Melva Fowler, R.N.
Ms. Mary C. Smith, R.N.
Ms. Joh Cheatham, R.N.
Ms. Diane Ash, R.N.
Ms. Lyn York (Data Manager)

114. Tom Baker Cancer Centre, Calgary (104)

1331 29th Street, N.W.
Calgary, Alberta T2N 4N2
Canada
(403/270-1701)
*Dr. L. Martin Jerry (Clin. Immunol.)
Dr. John Berry (Med. Oncol.)
Dr. Peter Geggie (Med. Oncol.)
Dr. J.R. Francis (Surg. Oncol.)
Dr. R.E. Pow (Surg. Oncol.)
Dr. Keith Arthur (Rad. Oncol.)
Dr. Fred Alexander (Pathol.)
Mr. Simone Coombes, R.N.
Ms. Earlyne Weaver, R.N.

Calgary General Hospital
841 Center Avenue E.

*Principal Investigator

Calgary, Alberta T2E OA1
Canada
(403/268-7511)
Dr. M. A. Andersen (Pathol.)

115. Trumbull Memorial Hospital,
      Warren, OH (126)

      1350 E. Market Street
      Warren, OH 44482
      (216/841-9011)
      *Dr. Jerome J. Stanislaw (Surg.
        Oncol.)
      Dr. Engleburt Hecker (Rad. Oncol.)
      Dr. Robert E. Pence (Pathol.)
      Ms. Anna Marie Holt, R.N.
      Ms. Cheryl Garrett, R.N.

      Youngstown Hospital Association
      500 Gypsy Lane
      Youngstown, OH 44501
      (216/747-1431)
      Dr. Masud R. Bhatti (Med. Oncol.)
      Dr. Lawrence M. Pass (Med.
        Oncol.)
      Dr. Renwick N. Goldberg (Med.
        Oncol.)

116. Tufts University-New England
      Medical Center(66)

      New England Medical Center
        Hospital
      171 Harrison Avenue
      P.O. Box 245
      Boston, MA 02111
      (617/956-5144)
      *Dr. David R. Parkinson (Med.
        Oncol.)
      Dr. Richard A. Rudders (Med.
        Oncol.)
      Dr. Henry Wagner (Rad. Oncol.)
      Dr. Steven Papish (Med. Oncol.)
      Dr. James Mier (Hematol./Oncol.)
      Dr. Thomas Smith (Surg. Oncol.)
      Dr. Hywel Madoc-Jones (Rad.
        Oncol.)

      Tufts Cancer Clinical Studies
      New England Medical Center
      171 Harrison Avenue

*Principal Investigator

Box 452
Boxton, MA 02111
(617/956-5558)
Ms. Stephanie Hunter
Ms. Donna Casey (Data Manager)
Ms. Christine Sigrist, B.A. (Data
  Manager)
Ms. Nancy Guccione, R.N.
Ms. Valerie Hoynacki, R.N.
Ms. Jane Stockman, R.N. (Data
  Manager)

Southwood Community Hospital
111 Dedham Street
Norfolk MA 02056
(617/668/0385)
Dr. Vinubhai Patel (Rad. Oncol.)
Dr. Gerald M. Reid (Surg. Oncol.)
Dr. Mona Kaddis (Med. Oncol.)
Dr. Paula McBrine (Med. Oncol.)
Dr. Ock S. Choi (Med. Oncol.)
Dr. Lee Parker (Med. Oncol.)
Ms. Mary Jane Scannell (Data)

Lemuel Shattuck Hospital
170 Morton Street
Jamaica Plain, MA 02130
(617/522-8400)
Dr. Joseph Cohen (Med. Oncol.)
Dr. Carol Amick (Pathol.)

Norwood Hospital
Ambulatory Care Center
800 Washington Street
Norwood, MA 02062
(617/769-4000 ext. 350)
Dr. Ausma Wright (Med. Oncol.)
Ms. Paulette Meyer, R.N.

Newton–Wellesley Hospital
Ambulatory Oncology Center
2000 Washington Street
Newton Lower Falls, MA 02162
(617/964-7260)
Dr. Timothy P. O'Connor (Med.
  Oncol.)
Ms. Viola Pollock, R.N.

Goddard Memorial Hospital
Sumner Street
Stoughton, MA 02072
(617/344-5100)

Dr. Ruth McLain (Med. Oncol.)
Ms. Marcie Belanger, R.N.

St. Elizabeth's Hospital
736 Cambridge Street
Brighton, MA 02135
(617/782-7000)
Dr. Leslie A. Martin
  (Hematol./Oncol.)

Lawrence Memorial Hospital
170 Governors Avenue
Medford, MA 02155
(617/396-9250, ext. 223)
Dr. C. Douglas Taylor (Med.
  Oncol.)
Ms. Ellen Kapito, R.N.

Faulkner Hospital
1153 Centre Street
Jamaica, MA 02130
(617/522-5800)
Dr. Arthur L. DeLoca (Med.
  Oncol.)
Ms. Mean LeClair, R.N.

117. Tulane University, New Orleans
     (49)

     1430 Tulane Avenue
     New Orleans, LA 70112
     (504/588-5110)
     *Dr. Carl Sutherland (Surg. Oncol.)
     Dr. Edward Krementz (Surg.
       Oncol.)
     Dr. D. Carter (Surg. Oncol.)
     Dr. H. Nina Dhurandhar (Pathol.)
     Dr. Joseph Schlosser (Rad. Oncol.)
     Ms. Sara Lother (Data Coordinator)

     7th Ward Hospital
     P.O. Box 2668
     Hammond, LA 70404
     (504/345-2700)
     Dr. Paul Vega (Surg. Oncol.)
     Dr. Alan Manning (Surg. Oncol.)

     Methodist Hospital
     5620 Read Boulevard
     New Orleans, LA 70127
     (504/241-2400)
     Dr. James E. Brown (Surg. Oncol.)

Dr. Donald J. Palmisano (Surg.
  Oncol.)
Dr. Jan T. McClanahan (Surg.
  Oncol.)

Touro Infirmary
1401 Foucher Street
New Orleans, LA 70115
(504/897-7011)
Dr. Elmo Cerise (Surg. Oncol.)

Southern Baptist Hospital
2700 Napolean Avenue
New Orleans, LA 70115
(504/899-9311)
Dr. Edward S. Lindsey (Surg.
  Oncol.)

West Jefferson General Hospital
4500 Eleventh Street
Marrero, LA 70072
(504/347-5511)
Dr. Douglas A. Haddow (Surg.
  Oncol.)
Dr. Charles Silver (Surg. Oncol.)

Jo Ellen Smith Memorial Hospital
4444 General Meyer Avenue
New Orleans, LA 70114
(504/363-7011)
Dr. John L. Overby (Surg. Oncol.)
Dr. Mark Kappelman (Surg. Oncol.)
Dr. Akio Kitahama (Surg. Oncol.)

Singing River Hospital
Denny Avenue
Pascagoula, MS 39567
(601/762-4483)
Dr. Dewey Lane (Surg. Oncol.)
Dr. David Spencer (Surg. Oncol.)

118. U.S . Naval Hospital, San Diego
     (37)

     San Diego, CA 92134
     (714/233-2746)
     *Dr. Jim Guzik (Surg. Oncol.)
     Dr. John Koval (Rad. Oncol.)
     Dr. J.W. Lea (Hematol./Oncol.)
     Dr. Dan Masys (Hematol./Oncol.)
     Dr. S. H. Myster (Pathol.)
     Ms. Monica Stopak, R.N.

*Principal Investigator

119. University of California, Los
Angeles (137)

John Wayne Cancer Clinic
Factor Building, 9th Fl.
10833 Le Conte Avenue
Los Angeles, CA 90024
(213/825-7081)
*Dr. Armando Giuliano (Surg.
Oncol.)
Dr. Robert G. Parker (Rad. Oncol.)
Dr. Allstair Cochran (Pathol.)
Dr. Charles Haskell (Med. Oncol.)
Ms. Karen Patterson, R.N.

120. University of California, San Diego
(12)

University Hospital
225 Dickinson Street H891B
San Diego, CA 92103
(619/294-6840)
*Dr. Yosef Pilch (Surg. Oncol.)
Dr. John Mendelsohn (Med.
Oncol.)
Dr. Joella F. Utley (Rad. Oncol.)
Dr. Sidney Saltzstein (Pathol.)
Ms. M. Jeanne Bingman, R.N.
Ms. Ellen Hammersley

3930 Fourth Avenue, Suite 301
San Diego, CA 92103
(714/299-3121)
Dr. Robert M. Barone (Surg.
Oncol.)
Dr. Paul M. Goldfarb (Surg.
Oncol.)

121. University of California, San
Francisco (128)

San Francisco, CA 94143
(415/666-9000)
*Dr. William H. Goodson (Surg.
Oncol.)
Dr. Ruth Grobstein (Rad. Oncol.)
Dr. Mike Freedman (Med. Oncol.)
Dr. Jim McKerrow (Pathol.)

400 Parnassus Avenue, Room
A-680
San Francisco, CA 94143

*Principal Investigator

(415/666-3282)
Ms. Rachel Mailman, R.N.

122. University of Chicago (136)

950 E. 59th Street
Chicago, IL 60637(312/947-5012,
1000)
*Dr. Harvey M. Golomb
(Hematol./Oncol.)
Dr. Philip Hoffman
(Hematol./Oncol.)
Dr. Peter Dawson (Pathol.)
Dr. Donald J. Ferguson (Surg.
Oncol.)
Dr. Harold Sutton (Rad. Oncol.)
Ms. Maureen Ruane, R.N.

123. University of Florida, JHEP (44)

820 Prudential Drive, Suite 511
Jacksonville, FL 32207
(904/399-0818)
*Dr. Neil Abramson (Med. Oncol.)
Dr. Thomas A. Marsland (Med.
Oncol.)
Mrs. Betty Benfield (Data Manager)
Ms. Donna Bird, L.P.N.

(904/398-8484)
Dr. Warren M. Barrett (Surg.
Oncol.)

(904/398-0033)
Dr. Ernest R. Kimball, III (Surg.
Oncol.)

(904/398-5629)
Dr. Curtis M. Phillips (Surg.
Oncol.)

820 Prudential Drive, Suite 510
Jacksonville, FL 32207
(904/399-7390)
Dr. Barbara Bradley (Surg. Oncol.)

800 Prudential Drive
Jacksonville, FL 32207
(904/393-2000
Dr. Bhojraj Paryani (Rad. Oncol.)
Dr. Brian Vitsky (Pathol.)

Baptist Medical Center
800 Prudential Drive
Jacksonville, FL 32207
(904/393-2077)
Dr. Shyam Paryani (Rad. Oncol.)

University Hospital
655 W. 8th Street
Jacksonville, FL 32209
(904/350-6899)
Dr. Alan Marks (Med. Oncol.)
Ms. Debbie Kennedy, R.N.

1820 Barrs Street, Suite 310
Jacksonville, FL 32204
(904/388-2619)
Dr. Joel A. Stone (Med. Oncol.)

1842 King Street
Jacksonville, FL 32204
(904/388-5452)
Dr. Harry W. Reinstine (Surg.
  Oncol.)

124. University of Hawaii (118)

Cancer Center of Hawaii
1236 Lauhala Street, Room 301
Honolulu, HI 96813
(808/548-8400)
*Dr. Robert Oishi (Surg. Oncol.)
*Dr. Noboru Oishi
  (Hematol./Oncol.)
Dr. Ben Lin Hom (Pathol.)
Dr. Melvin S. Inamasu
  (Hematol./Oncol.)
Dr. Glenn M. Kokame (Surg.
  Oncol.)
Dr. Clarence S. Sakai (Surg.
  Oncol.)
Dr. Victor Mori (Surg. Oncol.)
Dr. Edward Quinlan (Rad. Oncol.)
Ms. Dorothy Coleman, R.N.
Ms. Sharon Shigemasa, R.N.
Ms. Lois Nakamoto
Ms. Paula Waterman

125. University of Iowa (13)

University of Iowa Hospitals &
  Clinics
Iowa City, IA 52242

(319/356-2778)
*Dr. Peter Jochimsen (Surg. Oncol.)
Dr. Luis Urdaneta (Surg. Oncol.)
Dr. Adel Al-Jurf (Surg. Oncol.)
Dr. Michael Corder (Med. Oncol.)
Dr. Barry Sherman (Med. Oncol.)
Dr. Hamed Tewfik (Rad. Oncol.)

University of Iowa Hospitals &
  Clinics
Iowa City, IA 52242
(319/356-2778)
Dr. Frederick Stamler (Pathol.)
Ms. Mary Spaight, R.N.
Ms. Judith Gust, R.N.
Ms. Kathleen Full, R.N.
Ms. Lara Miller
Ms. Paula Landgraf, R.N.

McFarland Clinic
12th & Douglas
Ames, IA 50010
(515/239-4400)
Dr. S. Donald Zaentz (Internist)

717 A Avenue, NE
Cedar Rapids, IA 52402
(319/364-0255)
Dr. Reuben Keegan (Surg. Oncol.)
Dr. Campbell F. Watts (Surg.
  Oncol.)

St. Francis Professional Building
Waterloo, IA 50702
(319/235-9331)
Dr. Cornelius P. Addison (Surg.
  Oncol.)

927 S. 4th Street
Waterloo, IA 50702
(319/291-5950)
Dr. Robert J. Cak (Surg. Oncol.)
Dr. Andrew Devine (Surg. Oncol.)
Dr. P. Thomas McGarvey (Surg.
  Oncol.)

1005 E. Pennsylvania
Ottumwa, IA 52501
(515/682-4594)
Dr. Peter Reiter (Internist)
Dr. Winn Gregory (Surg. Oncol.)

*Principal Investigator

Allen Memorial Hospital
Waterloo, IA 50703
(319/234-7561)
Dr. James C. Collins (Pathol.)

3319 Spring Street
Davenport, IA 52807
(319/359-1637)
Dr. Charles Fesenmeyer (Surg.
Oncol.)

412 W. 4th Street
Waterloo, IA 50702
(319/234-7769)
Dr. Russell S. Gerard II (Surg.
Oncol.)
Dr. Heins D. Jacobi (Surg. Oncol.)

600 Black
Waterloo, IA 50702
(319/233-3044)
Dr. Robert T. Guthrie (Rad. Oncol.)

Buena Vista Clinic
620 NW Drive
Storm Lake, IA 50588
(712/732-5030)
Dr. K. M. Johannsen (Surg. Oncol.)

Sartori Hospital
W. 6th & College
Cedar Falls, IA 50613
(319/277-5763, 268-0461)
Dr. Robert L. Savereide (Surg.
Oncol.)
Dr. M. Neil Williams (Surg.
Oncol.)

Leon Clinic
1012 N. Church
Leon, IA 50144
(515/446-4863)
Dr. Vince Sullivan (Internist)

330 South Street
Waterloo, IA 50702
(319/232-3714)
Dr. Richard D. Wells (Surg. Oncol.)

Ackley Medical Center
Ackley, IA 50601
(515/847-2625)
Dr. G. E. Lawrence (Gen. Practice)

2942 Brady Street
Davenport, IA 52803

(319/326-5161)
Dr. Cecil Zuckerman (Internist)

204 E. 8th Avenue, S.E.
Oelwein, IA 50662
(319/283-2651)
Dr. H. C. Hallberg (Gen. Practice)

206 N. 7th Street
Keokuk, IA 52632
(319/524-5734)
Dr. Robert R. Kemp (Gen. Practice)

Medical Arts Building
408 S. Maple
Fairfield, IA 52556
(515/472-4156)
Dr. Gene E. Egli (Gen. Practice)

1605 Cedar Street
Muscatine, IA 52761
(319/263-4334)
Dr. Victor W. Swayze (Surg.
Oncol.)

Hall Radiation Center
603 10th Street, S.E.
Cedar Rapids, IA 52403
(319/366-5401)
Dr. A. Curtiss Hass (Rad. Oncol.)

Masonic Building
7th & Blondeau
Keokuk, IA 52632
(319/524-5401)
Dr. Billy J. Williamson (Fam.
Practice)

811 First Street
Keosauqua, IA 52601
(319/293-3181)
Dr. Kiyoshi Furumoto (Fam.
Practice)

610 N. 4th Street
Burlington, IA 52601
(319/753-5444)
Dr. Robert L. Kent (Gen. Practice)

820 N. Franklin Street
Manchester, IA 52057
(319/927-2629)
Dr. Richardson E. Clark (Gen.
Practice)

929

1615 Young Avenue
Muscatine, IA 52671
(319/263-8502)
Dr. G. Patrick Kealey (Surg.
  Oncol.)

1225 C Avenue, E.
Oskaloosa, IA 52577
(515/672-2571)
Dr. Sidney A. Smith (Gen. Practice)

115 1st Street, S.E.
Clarion, IA 50525
(515/532-2836)
Dr. Richard Young (Gen. Pract.)

1005 E. Pennsylvania
Ottumwa, IA 52501
(515/682-8709)
Dr. Gerald Paluska (Surg. Oncol.)
Dr. Alan Anderson (Surg. Oncol.)

Medical Arts
2nd & Burns
Ida Grove, IA 51445
(712/364-3195)
Dr. Alan Vasher (Gen. Practice)

1307 S. Broadway Street
Toledo, IA 52342
(515/484-4953)
Dr. Ted J. Akers (Gen. Practice)

910 N. Eisenhower Avenue
Mason City, IA 50401
(515/421-5294)
Dr. John K. MacGregor (Surg.
  Oncol.)

Gilfilan Clinic
505 W. Jefferson
Bloomfield, IA 52537
(515/664-2357)
Dr. James R. Mincks (Surg. Oncol.)

7 Professional Arts Building
Davenport, IA 52803
(319/326-6273)
Dr. George River (Internist)

126. University of Louisville (78)

James Graham Brown Cancer
  Center

529 S. Jackson Street, Room 229
Louisville, KY 40292
(502/588-5245)
*Dr. Joseph C. Allegra (Med.
  Oncol.)
Marilyn Allegra, R.N. (Data Base
  Devel. Specialist)
Dr. Thomas M. Woodcock (Med.
  Oncol.)
Dr. Stephen P. Richman (Med.
  Oncol.)
Dr. Martin S. Blumenreich (Med.
  Oncol.)
Dr. Thomas T. Kubota (Med.
  Oncol.)
Dr. Patrick S. Gentile (Med.
  Oncol.)
Dr. Condict Moore (Surg. Oncol.)
Dr. Hiram C. Polk, Jr. (Surg.
  Oncol.)
Dr. Kirby I. Bland (Surg. Oncol.)
Dr. Baby Jose (Therapeutic Rad.)
Beverly Shields, R.N. (Oncol. Res.
  Nurse)
Mariesa Jones, R.N. (Oncol. Res.
  Nurse)
Susan Kitchen, R.N.
Joyce DiBlasi, R.N. (Data
  Manager)

University of Louisville School of
  Medicine
Department of Pathology
323 E. Chestnut
Louisville, KY 40292
(502/588-5341)
Dr. George H. Barrows (Pathol.)

Helmwood Medical Center
914 N. Dixie
Elizabeth Town, KY 42701
(502/769-6665)
Dr. Yusuf Khan Deshmukh (Med.
  Oncol.)

127. University of Maryland (39)

22 S. Greene Street
Baltimore, MD 21201
(301/528-5224)
*Dr. E. George Elias (Surg. Oncol.)

*Principal Investigator

Dr. Mukund S. Didolkar (Surg.
Oncol.)
Dr. William P. Reed (Surg. Oncol.)
Dr. Pradip Amin (Rad. Oncol.)
Dr. Vinita Patanaphan (Rad.
Oncol.)
Dr. Mohammad A. Hafiz (Pathol.)
Dr. Elizabeth A. Poplin (Med.
Oncol.)
Ms. Mary Ellen Jonas R.N.
Ms. Barbara Buda, R.N.
Ms. Sally Brown, R.N.
Ms. Linda A. McDonnell
Ms. Geraldine Messina

128. University of Massachusetts,
Worcester (127)

University of Massachusetts
Medical Center
55 Lake Avenue N.
Worcester, MA 01605
(617/856-3902)
*Dr. Mary E. Costanza (Med.
Oncol.)
*Dr. Michael Wertheimer (Surg.
Oncol.)
Dr. Nilima Patwardhan (Surg.
Oncol.)
Dr. Wayne Silva (Surg. Oncol.)
Dr. Thomas Dodson (Surg. Oncol.)
Dr. Thomas W. Griffin (Med.
Oncol.)
Dr. Harry L. Greene (Med. Oncol.)
Dr. Marcia Liepman (Med. Oncol.)
Dr. Frank Reale (Pathol.)
Ms. Donna M. Antonelli (Data
Manager)
Ms. Sherrie Coval (Data Manager)

Memorial Hospital
119 Belmont Street
Worcester, MA 01605
(617/793-6216)
*Dr. Robert Quinlan (Surg. Oncol.)
*Dr. Andrew Cederbaum (Med.
Oncol.)
Dr. Robert Harper (Pathol.)
Dr. Won Kyun Tak (Rad. Oncol.)

St. Vincent Hospital

25 Winthrop Street
Worcester, MA 01604
(617/798-6093)
Dr. Joel Schwartz (Med. Oncol.)
Dr. Gary Strauss (Med. Oncol.)
Dr. Sidney Kadish (Rad. Oncol.)
Dr. David Sherman (Rad. Oncol.)

Worcester City Hospital
26 Queen Street
Worcester, MA 01610
(617/756-1551)
Dr. MichaelEntmacher (Med.
Oncol.)

119 Belmont Street
Worcester, MA 01605
(617/752-7470)
Dr. David L. Dykhuizen (Surg.
Oncol.)

Hahnemann Hospital
281 Lincoln Street
Worcester, MA 01606
(617/757-7751)
Dr. Allen Ward (Med. Oncol.)

129. University of Miami, FL (688)

University of Miami School of
Medicine
P.O. Box 016310
Miami, FL 33101
(305/547-6364)
*Dr. Alfred Ketcham (Surg. Oncol.)
Dr. David Robinson (Surg. Oncol.)
Dr. Rene Lafreniere (Surg. Oncol.)
Dr. David Robinson (Surg. Oncol.)
Ms. Janice W. Vogel, P.A.

Jackson Memorial Hospital
North Wing 1
1611 N.W. 12th Avenue
Miami, FL 33136
(305/325-6674)
Dr. Juan Fayos (Rad. Oncol.)

South Wing 2
(305/325-7244)
Dr. Sharon Thomsen (Pathol.)

1475 N.W. 12th Avenue
Miami, FL 33136

*Principal Investigator

(305/545-7707)
Dr. Grace Wang (Med. Oncol.)

130. University of North Carolina (117)

3018 Old Clinic Building-226H
Chapel Hill, NC 27514
(919/966-4431)
*Dr. Stephen Bernard (Med. Oncl..)
Dr. Don Gabriel (Med. Oncol.)
Dr. Stephen Tremont (Med. Oncol.)

210 Clinical Sciences
  Building-229H
Chapel Hill, NC 27514
(919/962-2211)
Dr. Stanley R. Mandel (Surg.
  Oncol.)

215 Clinical Sciences
  Building-229H
Chapel Hill, NC 27514
(919/962-2211)
Dr. H.J. Proctor (Surg. Oncol.)

North Carolina Memorial Hospital
Department of Radiation Therapy
Chapel Hill, NC 27514
(919/966-1101)
Dr. Julian Roseman (Rad. Oncol.)
Dr. Jan Halle (Rad. Oncol.)
Dr. Mehesh A. Varia (Rad. Oncol.)

University of North Carolina at
  Chapel Hill
Department of Surgery
Burnett–Womack Building 229-H
Chapel Hill, NC 27514
(919/966-5221)
Dr. Charles Herbst (Surg. Oncol.)
Dr. James K. Newsome (Surg.
  Oncol.)
Dr. Robert D. Croom, III (Surg.
  Oncol.)
Ms. Jean Ayer, R.N.

University of North Carolina School
  of Medicine
1009 Old Clinic Building
226H
Chapel Hill, NC 27514
(919/966-1392)

Dr. Fred Askin (Pathol.)
Ms. Candice Singletary

131. University of Pittsburgh (14)

3550 Terrace Street
Pittsburgh, PA 15261
(412/624-2671)
*Dr. Bernard Fisher (Surg. Oncol.)
Dr. Norman Wolmark (Surg.
  Oncol.)
Ms. Mary Ketner, R.N. (Exec.
  Clin. Coordinator)
Ms. Colleen Murphy (Network
  Coordinator)
Dr. D. Lawrence Wickerham
  (NSABP Fellow)
Dr. Samuel Jacobs (Med. Oncol.)
Dr. Ronald Stoller (Med. Oncol.)
Dr. Melvin Deutsch (Rad. Oncol.)

Adjuvant Therapy Center
3515 Fifth Avenue, Suite 500
Pittsburgh, PA 15213
(412/624-6221)
Ms. Debra Pollak, R.N., B.S.
Ms. Ann Schirnhofer, R.N.
Ms. Marilyn Holmes, R.N.
Ms. Mary Ann Gerdis
Ms. Wendy Kramer

Shadyside Hospital
5230 Centre Avenue
Pittsburgh, PA 15232
(412/622-2121)
Dr. Edwin R. Fisher (Pathol.)
Dr. Alka Sharad Palekar (Pathol.)
Dr. Remigio Gregorio (Pathol.)
Dr. Morgan McCoy II (Pathol.)
Ms. Marion Siebert

Allegheny General Hospital
320 E. North Avenue
Pittsburgh, PA 15212
(412/359-3630)
Dr. Reginald Pugh (Med. Oncol.)
Dr. Bernard Zidar (Med. Oncol.)
Dr. Robert Hartsock (Pathol.)
Ms. Carol Noonan, R.N.

Jameson Hospital
W. Leasure Avenue

*Principal Investigator

New Castle, PA 15105
(412/658-9001)
Ms. Pauline Gargasz, R.N.
Ms. Norene Koscevic, R.N.

Sewickley Valley Hospital
700 Broad Street
Sewickley, PA 15143
(412/7412700)
Dr. Alfred P. Doyle (Med. Oncol.)
Dr. Clarence Miller (Pathol.)

Allegheny Valley Hospital
1301 Carlisle Street
Natrona Heights, PA 15065
(412/337-3531)
Dr. James G. Lichter (Med. Oncol.)
Dr. S. J. C. Miller (Pathol.)

Forbes Regional Health Center
2570 Haymaker Road
Monroeville, PA 15146
(412/273-2424)
Dr. George H. Benz (Surg. Oncol.)
Dr. Richard L. Myerowitz (Pathol.

South Hills Health System
Jefferson Center
Coal Valley Road
Pittsburgh, PA 15236
(412/665-5000)
Dr. Edward W. Jew, Jr. (Surg.
 Oncol.)
Dr. Manuel DeLeon (Pathol.)

Montefiore Hospital
3458 Fifth Avenue
Pittsburgh, PA 15213
(412/683-1100, ext. 448)
Dr. Thomas Julian (Surg. Oncol.)
Dr. Harvey Mendelow (Pathol.)

Medical Center of Beaver County
Cancer Treatment Center
1000 Dutch Ridge Road
Beaver, PA 15009
(412/728-7000, ext. 1617)
Dr. Thomas McCreary (Med.
 Oncol.)
Dr. John Baska (Med. Oncol.)
Dr. Edward W. Heinle (Med.
 Oncol.)

*Principal Investigator

Dr. George W. Brett (Med. Oncol.)
Dr. Joseph P. Concannon (Rad.
 Oncol.)
Dr. James R. Hughes (Rad. Oncol.)
Dr. Vincent Cuddy (Surg. Oncol.)
Dr. Bradford Thompson (Surg.
 Oncol.)
Ms. Dorothy Kowal, R.N.

132. University of Rochester Cancer
      Center (67)

The Genesee Hospital
224 Alexander Street
Rochester, NY 14607
(716/263-6028)
*Dr. Sidney Sobel (Rad. Oncol.)
Ms. Marlene Manning (Data
 Manager)

Highland Hospital
South Avenue at Bellevue Drive
Rochester, NY 14620
(716/473-2200)
Dr. Raman Qazi (Med. Oncol.)
Dr. Jonathan Rubins (Med. Oncol.)
Dr. Davie Platt (Pathol.)
Dr. Donald Duckles (Surg. Oncol.)
Ms. Jean Bost, R.N.
Ms. Jean Rotoli, R.N.
Ms. Karen Gerella

St. Mary's Hospital
89 Genesee Street
Rochester, NY 14611
(716/464-3000)
Dr. N. Nadaraja (Surg. Oncol.)
Dr. K. Pandya (Med. Oncol.)

Rochester General Hospital
1421 Portland Avenue
Rochester, NY 14621
(716/338-4032)
Dr. Eileen Paterson (Rad. Oncol.)
Dr. Raymond Hinshaw (Surg.
 Oncol.)

133. University of Texas, Galveston (16)

Department of Surgery
Galveston, TX 77550
(713/765-1283)

933

*Dr. Edward B. Rowe (Surg.
Oncol.)
Ms. Diane Smith (Data)

134. University of Texas, San Antonio
(17)

7703 Floyd Curl Drive
San Antonio, TX 78284
(512/691-7473)
*Dr. A.B. Cruz (Surg. Oncol.)
*Dr. J. Bradley Aust (Surg. Oncol.)
Dr. Cary P. Page (Surg. Oncol.)
Dr. Ken Osborne (Med. Oncol.)
Dr. James Robinson (Pathol.)
Dr. Thomas C. Pomeroy (Rad.
Oncol.)
Ms. Mary Lou Guerrero
Ms. Tomas Gaitan, R.N.

Rugeley & Blasingame Clinic
Association
2100 N. Fulton Street
Wharton, TX 77488
(713/532-1700)
Dr. William C. Yankowsky (Surg.
Oncol.)
Dr. Robert Bruce Carraway, Jr.
(Surg. Oncol.)

135. University of Vermont (18)

Given Building
Burlington, VT 05405
(802/656-2563)
*Dr. Roger Foster (Surg. Oncol.)
Dr. Carleton Haines (Surg. Oncol.)
Dr. Richard Albertini (Clin.
Immunol.)
Ms. Marilyn Driscoll
Ms. Ruth LeBlanc, R.N.
Ms. Louise D. Flower

Vermont Regional Cancer Center
Burlington, VT 05401
(802/656-4414)
Dr. James Stewart (Med. Oncol.)
Ms. Marilyn Rinker, R.N.

Medical Alumni Building
Burlington, VT 05401
(802/656-2210)

Dr. Roy Korson (Pathol.)

Mary Fletcher Unit
Burlington, VT 05401
(802/656-3506)
Dr. Jack A. Abarbanel (Rad.
Oncol.)

136. VA Medical Center, Boston (135)

150 S. Huntington Avenue
Boston, MA 02130
(617/232-9500)
*Dr. Waun Ki Hong (Med. Oncol.)
Dr. Richard Bromer (Med. Oncol.)
Dr. Harold Bush (Surg. Oncol.)
Dr. Bernard L. Willett (Rad.
Oncol.)
Dr. Leonard Berman (Lab Service)
Ms. Susan Hoffer, R.N.
Ms. Darisse Paquette (Data
Manager)

137. Valley Hospital, Ridgewood, NJ
(42)

Linwood & N. Van Dien Avenues
Ridgewood, NJ 07451
(201/447-8285)
*Dr. Hugh Auchincloss (Surg.
Oncol.)
Dr. Paul Hartman (Rad. Oncol.)
Dr. William Green (Pathol.)
Ms. Wanda Borgen (Med. Librarian
& Tumor Registrar

127 Union Street
Ridgewood, NJ 07540
(201/445-2725)
Dr. Allen Chinitz (Med. Oncol.)

385 S. Maple
Ridgewood, NJ 07540
(201/652-2800)
*Dr. Harold Bruck (Surg. Oncol.)

174 Union Street
Ridgewood, NJ 07450
(201/444-2528)
Dr. Barry R. Fernbach (Med.
Oncol.)

130 Prospect Street

*Principal Investigator

Ridgewood, NJ 07450
(201/444-4526)
Dr. Thomas J. Rakowski (Med.
Oncol.)

138. Washington Regional Medical
Center, AR (120)

No. 6 Halsted Circle
Rogers, AR 72756
(501/636-5411)
*Dr. James H. Bledsoe (Surg.
Oncol.)
Dr. R. Pearson (Surg. Oncol.)
Dr. Mario Costaldi (Surg. Oncol.)
Dr. Frank J. Panettiere (Med.
Oncol.)
Ms. Donna Ruffer, L.P.N.
Ms. Regina Beckford, L.P.N.

1749 N. College
Fayetteville, AR 72701
(501/521-3300)
Dr. Warren Murry (Surg. Oncol.)
Dr. Charles H. Miller (Surg.
Oncol.)
Dr. Jack Wood (Surg. Oncol.)

3000 Market
Fayetteville, AR 72701
(501/521-6780)
Dr. Michaek Rudko (Surg. Oncol.)

651 N. Spring
Harrison, AR 72601
(501/741-8275)
Dr. Jean Gladden (Surg. Oncol.)
Dr. Rhys Williams (Surg. Oncol.)

651 N. Spring
Harrison, AR 72601
(501/741-6418)
Dr. Tom Bell (Surg. Oncol.)
Dr. Tom Hoberock (Surg. Oncol.)

160-A Poplar
Fayetteville, AR 72701
(501/521-1484)
Dr. William McNair (Surg. Oncol.)
Dr. C. R. Magness (Surg. Oncol.)

675 Lollar Lane
Fayetteville, AR 72701

(501/521-8200)
Dr. William C. Martin (Internist)
Dr. Malcolm Hayward (Med.
Oncol.)
Ms. Hazel Freely, L.P.N.

1617 N. College
Fayetteville, AR 72701
(501/521-6480)
Dr. Earl B. Riddick, Jr. (Rad.
Oncol.)

Springdale Memorial Hospital
Springdale, AR 72764
(501/751-5711)
Dr. John Boyce (Pathol.)

Robers Memorial Hospital
Rogers, AR 72756
(501/636-0200)
Dr. William McKnight
(Gastroenterol. Internist)

Dr. David Denman (Pathol.)
Dr. Eva Litton (Pathol.)

1019 W. Cypress
Rogers, AR 72756
(501/636-6551)
Dr. Bruce Waldon (Internal Med.)
Dr. Richard Miles (Internal Med.)
Dr. William Swindell (Internal
Med.)
Dr. Wallace Rolniak (Internal Med.)

1040 W. Walnut
Rogers, AR 72756
(501/636-2711)
Dr. Larry Wright (Internal Med.)
Dr. Robert W. Donnell (Internal
Med.)

139. Washington University, St. Louis
(19)

Barnard Cancer Center
3rd Fl. Wohl
4960 Audubon Avenue
St. Louis, MO 63110
(314/454-2919)
*Dr. Jay Marion (Med. Oncol.)
Ms. Diane Bohner, R.N.
Ms. Mary Griffin, R.N.

*Principal Investigator

516 S. Kingshighway
St. Louis, MO 63110
(314/454-7170)
Dr. Gordon Philpott (Surg. Oncol.)

4948 Barnes Hospital
St. Louis, MO 63110
(314/454-3420)
Dr. Harvey Butcher (Surg. Oncol.)
Dr. Walter Bauer (Pathol.)

4948 Barnes Hospital
St. Louis, MO 63110
(314/454-5000)
Dr. Alex Denes (Med. Oncol.)

4511 Forest Park Boulevard
St. Louis, MO 63110
(314/454-2134)
Dr. John Bedwinek (Rad. Oncol.)

140. Wayne State University, Detroit,
MI (28)

540 E. Canfield Avenue
Detroit, MI 48201
(313/494-8775)
*Dr. Alexander J. Walt (Surg.
Oncol.)

Harper Grace Hospital
Department of Surgery
3990 John R. Street
Detroit, MI 48201
313/494-8776)
Mr. Keith W. Goodchild (Data
Manager)

141. West Suburban Hospital Medical
Center, Oak Park, IL (48)

Erie at Austin
Oak Park, IL 60302
(312/383-6200)
Dr. Sheldon Krasnow (Med.
Oncol./Hematol.)
Dr. John Showel (Med. Oncol.)
Dr. Stanley V. Hoover (Rad.
Oncol.)
Dr. Frederick I. Volini (Pathol.)
Ms. Laima Berzins, R.N.

One Erie Court, Suite 7050

W. Suburban Plaza
Oak Park, Il 60302
(312/386-2400)
*Dr. Everett Nicholas (Surg.
Oncol.)

142. West Virginia University,
Morgantown (133)

School of Medicine
Medical Center
Morgantown, WV 26506
(304/293-3311)
*Dr. Alvin Watne (Surg. Oncol.)
Dr. LeLand Foshag (Surg. Oncol.)
Dr. Winfield Morgan (Surg.
Pathol.)
Dr. Frederick Avis (Surg. Oncol.)
Dr. Thomas Vargish (Surg. Oncol.)
Dr. John Frich (Rad. Oncol.)
Dr. Peter Raich (Med. Oncol.)
Ms. Sharon Bartholomew

United Hospital Center
#3 Hospital Plaza
Clarksburg, WV 26301
(304/624-2281)
Dr. James Knost (Med. Oncol.)

143. White Memorial Medical Center,
Los Angeles (70)

1710 Brooklyn Avenue
Los Angeles, CA 90033
(213/264-2633)
*Dr. Matthew Tan (Surg. Oncol.)
Dr. Ernest Braun (Rad. Oncol.)
Dr. Oluwole Odujinrin (Med.
Oncol.)
Dr. George Kypridakis (Pathol.)
Ms. Janice Campos, L.V.N.
Ms. Marlene Hensel

1700 Brooklyn Avenue
Los Angeles, CA 90030
(213/262-5157)
Dr. Robert Sullivan (Med. Oncol.)

144. Wilmington Medical Center, DE
(52)

Carpenter Memorial Clinic

*Principal Investigator

936

Chestnut & Broom Streets
Wilmington, DE 19899
(302/428-4743)
*Dr. Timothy F. Wozniak (Med.
  Oncol.)
Dr. Leslie Whitney (Surg. Oncol.)
Dr. Siamak Samil (Med. Oncol.)
Dr. Irving Berkowitz (Med. Oncol.)
Dr. Timothy Wozniak (Med.
  Oncol.)
Dr. Donald Tilton (Rad. Oncol.)
Dr. Patrick Ashley (Pathol.)
Dr. Yogi Patel (Med. Oncol.)
Dr. Carlo Cuccia (Rad. Oncol.)
Dr. Anita Hodson (Clin. Immunol.)
Dr. Emerson Gledhill (Surg.
  Oncol.)
Ms. Alice Kyle, R.N.
Ms. Mary Balascio, R.N.

Beebe Hospital
Patient Registry
424 Savannah Road
Lewes, DE 19958
(302/645-3510)
Ms. Doris Hatfield, R.N.

Nanticoke Memorial Hospital
801 Middleford Road
Seaford, DE 19973
(302/629-6611)
Ms. Dawn Simmons, R.N.
Ms. Beverly Morthole, R.N.

Kent General Hospital
Medical Records
640 S. State Street
Dover, DE 19901
(302/734-4701)
Ms. Hazel Thompson

145. Women's College Hospital, Toronto
    (134)

Henrietta Banting Breast Centre
Women's College Hospital
60 Grosvenor Street, Room 506

Toronto, Ontario M5S 1B6
Canada
(416/961-8968)
*Dr. Edward B. Fish (Surg. Oncol.)
Dr. G. Y. Hirski (Surg. Oncol.)
Dr. H. Lavina Lickley (Surg.
  Oncol.)
Dr. Ted M. Ross (Surg. Oncol.)
Mrs. Gladys Oldfield, R.N.
  (Surgical Research Coordinator
Dr. Kathleen I. Pritchard (Med.
  Oncol.)
Dr. George Kutas (Med. Oncol.)
Dr. Donald Ryder (Pathol.)
Dr. W. M. Hanna (Pathol.)

Princess Margaret Hospital
500 Sherbourne Street
Toronto, Ontario M4X 1K9
Canada
(416/9140671 ext. 259)
Dr. Roy Clark (Rad. Oncol.)

146. Wuesthoff Memorial Hospital,
    Rockledge, FL (131)

107 Longwood Avenue
Rockledge, FL 32955
(305/636-2111)
*Dr. Edward W. Knight (Med.
  Oncol.)
Ms. Neena Tennant, P.A.

110 Longwood Avenue
Rockledge, FL 32955
(305/636-2211)
Dr. Robert I. Sakolsky (Pathol.)

1033 S. Florida Avenue
Rockledge, FL 32995
(305/632-0352)
Dr. James C. Glebink (Rad. Oncol.)

1007 Beverly Drive
Rockledge, FL 32955
(305/636-8241)
Dr. Kenneth W. Korey (Surg.
  Oncol.)

*Principal Investigator

APPENDIX V

Cancer Information Services Hot Lines

The Cancer Information Service (CIS) operates a hot line staffed by trained volunteers. In most states the number to call is 1–800–4–6237. In Oahu, Hawaii, the number is 524–1234 (neighbor islands can call collect). In Washington, DC and suburbs in Maryland and Virginia the number is 636–5700. In Alaska call 1–800–638–6070.

The calls are toll free and there is no charge for the information. If you call between 9:00 A.M. and 4:30 P.M., your call is automatically routed to the CIS office nearest you. After regular hours (until midnight Eastern Time) and on weekends, calls are routed to the central office at the National Cancer Institute.

CIS provides information in clear, simple language about cancer causes, prevention, detection, diagnosis, treatment, and rehabilitation. Information about medical facilities and community resources can be provided, as well as information about patient referrals to physicians. In some cases CIS staff may help by translating into lay language information provided by a physician but not understood by the caller. Staff members may also provide emotional support.

Personally, we have found that the hot line staff does well with general kinds of questions, but in-depth or complicated questions are generally beyond the volunteers. Still, it's a valuable resource and well worth a call.

Comprehensive Cancer Centers

ALABAMA

Dr. Albert F. LoBuglio, Director
Comprehensive Cancer Center
University of Alabama in Birmingham
University Station
Birmingham (35294)
205/934-5077

CALIFORNIA

Dr. Brian E. Henderson, Director
Kenneth Norris, Jr. Cancer Research
  Institute
University of Southern California
  Comprehensive Cancer Center
P.O. Box 33804
1441 Eastlake Avenue
Los Angeles (90033-0804)
213/224-6416

Dr. Richard J. Steckel, Director
Jonsson Comprehensive Cancer Center
University of California, Los Angeles
Louis Factor Health Sciences Building
10833 Le Conte Avenue
Los Angeles (90024)
Tel: 213/825-1532/5268

CONNECTICUT

Dr. Jack W. Cole, Director
Yale University Comprehensive Cancer
  Center
333 Cedar Street
New Haven (06510)
203/785-4095

DISTRICT OF COLUMBIA

Georgetown Univ./Howard Univ.
  Comprehensive Cancer Center
Dr. John F. Potter, Director
Vincent T. Lombardi Cancer Research
  Center
Georgetown Univ. Medical Center
3800 Reservoir Road, N.W.
Washington, DC 20007
202/625-7066

Dr. Jack E. White, Director
Cancer Research Center
Howard University Hospital
2400 Sixth Street, N.W.
Washington, DC 20059
202/636-7697

FLORIDA

Dr. C. Gordon Zubrod, Director
Comprehensive Cancer Center for the State
 of Florida
Univ. of Miami Hospital & Clinics
1475 N.W. 12th Avenue
P.O. Box 016960 (D8-4)
Miami (33101)
305/545-7707, ext. 103

ILLINOIS

Illinois Cancer Council (includes the
 institutions listed and several other
 health organizations)
Dr. Shirley B. Lansky, Acting Director
Illinois Cancer Council
36 S. Wabash Avenue, Suite 700
Chicago (60603)
312/346-9813

Dr. Nathaniel I. Berlin, Director
Northwestern University Cancer Center
Health Sciences Building
303 E. Chicago Avenue
Chicago (60611)
312/266-5250

Dr. John E. Ultmann, Director
University of Chicago Cancer Research
 Center
905 E. 59th Street
Chicago (60637)
312/962-6180

MARYLAND

Dr. Albert H. Owens, Jr., Center Director
Professor of Oncology & Medicine
Johns Hopkins Oncology Center
600 North Wolfe Street, Room 157
Baltimore (21205)
301/955-8822

MASSACHUSETTS

Dr. Emil Frei, III, Director
Dana-Farber Cancer Institute
44 Binney Street
Boston (02115)
617/732-3555

MICHIGAN

Dr. Michael J. Brennan, Director
Comprehensive Cancer Center of
 Metropolitan Detroit
110 E. Warren Street
Detroit (48201)
313/833-1083

MINNESOTA

Dr. Charles G. Moertel, Director
Mayo Comprehensive Cancer Center
200 First Street Southwest
Rochester (55901)
507/284-2511

NEW YORK

Dr. Gerald P. Murphy
Institute Director
Roswell Park Memorial Institute
666 Elm Street
Buffalo (14263)
716/845-5770

Dr. Paul Marks, President
Memorial Sloan–Kettering Cancer Center
1275 York Avenue
New York (10021)
212/794-6561
Dr. Harold S. Ginsberg, Acting Director
Columbia University Cancer Center
College of Physicians & Surgeons
701 W. 168th Street
New York (10032)
212/694-3647

NORTH CAROLINA

Dr. William W. Shingleton, Director
Comprehensive Cancer Center
Duke University Medical Center
Durham (27710)
919/684-2282

942

OHIO

Dr. David S. Yohn, Director
Ohio State Univ. Comprehensive Cancer
  Center
410 W. 12th Avenue, Suite 302
Columbus (43210)
614/422-5022

PENNSYLVANIA

Fox Chase/Univ. of Pennsylvania
  Comprehensive Cancer Center
Dr. John R. Durant, President
Fox Chase Cancer Center
7701 Burholme Avenue
Philadelphia (19111)
215/728-2781

Dr. Richard A. Cooper, Director
University of Pennsylvania Cancer
  Center
7 Silverstein Pavilion
3400 Spruce Street
Philadelphia (19104)
215/662-3910

TEXAS

Dr. Charles A. LeMaistre, President
University of Texas System Cancer Center
M. D. Anderson Hospital & Tumor
  Institute
6723 Bertner Avenue
Houston (77030)
713/792-6000

WASHINGTON

Dr. Robert W. Day, Director
Fred Hutchinson Cancer Research Center
1124 Columbia Street
Seattle (98104)
206/292-7545

WISCONSIN

Dr. Paul P. Carbone, Director
University of Wisconsin Clinical Cancer
  Center
600 Highland Avenue
Madison (53792)
608/263-8610

Listing prepared by:
Cancer Centers Branch
Division of Resources, Centers, and
  Community Activities, NCI
Blair Building/Room 714
Silver Spring, MD 20205
301/427-8663

Clinical and Nonclinical Cancer Centers

ARIZONA

Dr. Sydney E. Salmon, Director
University of Arizona Cancer Center
University of Arizona
College of Medicine
Tucson (85724)
602/626-6044

CALIFORNIA

Dr. Saul A. Rosenberg, Director*
Northern California Cancer Program
1801 Page Mill Road
Building B, Suite 200
P.O. Box 10144
Palo Alto (94303)
415/497-7431

Dr. William H. Fishman, Director†
Cancer Research Center
La Jolla Cancer Research Foundation
10901 North Torrey Pines Road
La Jolla (92037)
619/455-6480

*Clinical Cancer Center
†Nonclinical Cancer Center

Dr. John Mendelsohn, Director*
UCSD Cancer Center
University of California at San Diego
School of Medicine
La Jolla (92093)
619/294-6930

Dr. Henry S. Kaplan, Director†
Cancer Biology Research Laboratory
Stanford University Medical Center
Stanford (94305)
415/497-7311/5055

Dr. Charles Mittman, Director*
Cancer Research Center
City of Hope Research Institute
1450 East Duarte Road
Duarte (91010)
213/357-9711, x 2705

Dr. Walter Eckhart†
Professor and Director
Armand Hammer Center for Cancer
  Biology
The Salk Institute
P.O. Box 85800

San Diego (92138)
619/453-4100, ext. 386

Dr. Leroy E. Hood, Director†
Cancer Center
California Institute of Technology
Biology Division 156-29
Pasadena (91125)
213/356-4951

HAWAII

Dr. Lawrence H. Piette, Director*
Cancer Center of Hawaii
University of Hawaii at Manca
1236 Lauhala Street
Honolulu (96813)
808/548-8415/8416

INDIANA

Dr. D. James Morre, Director†
Cancer Research Center
Purdue University
Pharmacy Building
West Lafayette (47907)
317/494-1388

IOWA

Dr. Richard L. DeGowin, Director*
University of Iowa Cancer Center
College of Medicine
20 Medical Laboratories
Iowa City (52242)
319/353-6595

MAINE

Dr. Barbara H. Sanford, Director†
The Jackson Laboratory
Bar Harbor (04609)
207/288-3371 X206

*Clinical Cancer Center
†Nonclinical Cancer Center

946

MASSACHUSETTS

Dr. Thoru Pederson, Director†
Cancer Center
Worcester Foundation for Experimental
   Biology
222 Maple Avenue
Shrewsbury (01545)
617/842-8921

Dr. Salvador E. Luria, Director†
Massachusetts Institute of Technology,
   Room E17-113
77 Massachusetts Avenue
Cambridge (02139)
617/253-6401

NEW HAMPSHIRE

Dr. O. Ross McIntyre, Director*
Norris Cotton Cancer Center
Dartmouth-Hitchcock Medical Center
Hanover (03755)
603/646-5505

NEW YORK

Dr. James F. Holland, Chairman*
Department of Neoplastic Diseases
Mount Sinai School of Medicine
Fifth Avenue at 100th Street
New York (10029)
212/650-6361

Dr. Enrico Mihich, Director†
Grace Cancer Drug Center
Roswell Park Memorial Institute
666 Elm Street
Buffalo (14263)
716/845-5759

Dr. Harry Eagle, Director*
Cancer Research Center
Albert Einstein College of Medicine
1300 Morris Park Avenue
Bronx (10461)
212/430-2302
212/792-2233

Dr. Vittorio Defendi, Director*
Cancer Center
New York University Medical Center
550 First Avenue
New York (10016)
212/340-5349

Dr. Robert A. Cooper, Jr., Director*
University of Rochester Cancer Center
601 Elmwood Avenue, Box 704
Rochester (14642)
716/275-4865

Dr. Arthur C. Upton†
Professor and Chairman, Department of
  Environmental Medicine
Director, Institute of Environmental
  Medicine
New York University Medical Center
550 First Avenue
New York (10016)
212/340-5280

Dr. Ernst L. Wynder†
President and Medical Director
American Health Foundation
320 E. 43d Street
New York (10017)
212/953-1900

NORTH CAROLINA

Dr. Joseph S. Pagano, Director*
Cancer Research Center
University of North Carolina
Box 30, MacNider Building 202H
Chapel Hill (27514)
919/966-1183/3036

Dr. Robert L. Capizzi, Director*
Oncology Research Center
Bowman Gray School of Medicine
300 S. Hawthorne Road
Winston-Salem (27103)
919/748-4606

OHIO

Dr. Ralph J. Alfidi†

*Clinical Cancer Center
†Nonclinical Cancer Center

Director of Specialized Cancer Research
  Center
Case Western Reserve University
University Hospitals
2074 Abington Road
Cleveland (44106)
216/444-3858

PENNSYLVANIA

Dr. Fred Rapp, Director†
Specialized Cancer Research Center
Pennsylvania State University
College of Medicine
Hershey (17033)
717/534-8253

Dr. Hilary Koprowski, Director†
Wistar Institute of Anatomy and Biology
36th Street at Spruce
Philadelphia (19104)
215/898-3703

Dr. Peter N. Magee, Director†
Fels Research Institute
Temple University School of Medicine
3420 N. Broad Street
Philadelphia (19140)
215/221-4312

PUERTO RICO

Dr. Angel A. Roman-Franco, Director*
Puerto Rico Cancer Center
University of Puerto Rico
Medical Sciences Campus
G.P.O. Box 5067
San Juan (00936)
809/763-2443

RHODE ISLAND

Dr. Paul Calabresi*
Professor and Chairman
Department of Medicine

947

Brown University
Roger Williams General Hospital
825 Chalkstone Avenue
Providence (02908)
401/456-2070

TENNESSEE

Dr. Joseph V. Simone, Director*
St. Jude Children's Research Hospital
332 N. Lauderdale
Memphis (38101)
301/522-0301

TEXAS

Dr. John J. Costanzi, Director*
UTMB Cancer Center
University of Texas Medical Branch
Galveston (77550)
713/761-2981/1862

VERMONT

Dr. John McCormack, Acting Director*
Vermont Regional Cancer Center
University of Vermont
1 S. Prospect Street

Burlington (05401)
802/656-4414

VIRGINIA

Dr. Walter Lawrence, Jr., Director*
Massey Cancer Center
Medical College of Virginia
Virginia Commonwealth University
MCV Station, Box 37
Richmond (23298)
804/786-9322/9323/0448

WISCONSIN

Dr. Henry C. Pitot, Director†
McArdle Laboratory for Cancer Research
University of Wisconsin
450 N. Randall Avenue
Madison (53706)
608/262-2177

*Listing prepared by:*Cancer Centers Branch
Division of Resources, Centers, and
    Community Activities, NCI
Blair Building/Room 714
Silver Spring, MD 20205
301/427-8663

*Clinical Cancer Center
†Nonclinical Cancer Center

Community Clinical Oncology Programs (CCOPs) and Their Research Bases

ARIZONA

Phoenix
Greater Phoenix CCOP; David K. King, M.D.

Internists, Oncologists, Ltd.
1010 E. McDowell, Suite 201 (85006)
602-258-4875

H ospitals
Good Samaritan Medical Center
John C. Lincoln Hospital and Health Center
Maricopa Medical Center
Maryvale Samaritan Hospital
St. Joseph's Hospital and Medical Center

Offices
Internists, Oncologists, Ltd.
Dr. Palo Verde
Affiliated Medical Specialists, P.C.
Hematology Associates Ltd.
Baranko, Wood & McCallister

ARKANSAS

Little Rock
Arkansas Oncology Clinic CCOP; Billy L. Tranum, M.D.

Arkansas Oncology Clinic, P.A.
500 S. University, Suite 401 (72205)
501-664-2262

Hospital
Arkansas Oncology Clinic

CALIFORNIA

Fresno
San Joaquin Valley CCOP; Phyllis Ager Mowry, M.D.

Medical Director, Radiation Oncology
Fresno Community Hospital and Medical Center
P.O. Box 1232 (93715)
209-442-6000, ext. 5156

Hospital
Fresno Community Hospital and Medical Center

Offices
Nagen Bellare, M.D.
Hematology–Medical Oncology Group of Fresno
Michael Jensen–Akula, M.D.
B. Peck Lau, M.D.

949

Victor Medrano, M.D.
Morgan & Prather, M.D.s
Radiation Oncology Dept.
Richard W. Wolk, M.D.
Klaus Hoffman, M.D.

Los Angeles
Greater Los Angeles CCOP; Jim S.
   Bonorris, M.D.

Hospital of the Good Samaritan
1245 Wilshire Boulevard, Suite 207
   (90017)
213-481-3948

Hospitals
Hospital of the Good Samaritan
Los Angeles Orthopedic Hospital

Central Los Angeles CCOP; Armand
   Bouzaglou, M.D.

St. Vincent Medical Center
2131 W. Third Street
P.O. Box 57992 (90057)
213-483-2700/484-7052

Hospital
St. Vincent Medical Center

Pasadena
San Gabriel Valley CCOP; Michael R.
   Kadin, M.D.

Vice President Administration
Huntington Memorial Hospital
100 Congress Street (91105)
213-440-5140

Hospitals
Community Hospital of San Gabriel
Huntington Memorial Hospital
Methodist Hospital of Southern California
St. Luke's Hospital

Sacramento
Kaiser Foundation Research Institute; Scott
   S. Johnson, M.D.

Kaiser Foundation Research Institute
Department of Pediatrics, Station D
2025 Morse Avenue (95825)
916-486-5919

Hospitals
David Grant Medical Center
Sacramento Medical Center

Office
Kaiser–Permanente Medical Group

COLORADO

Denver
Presbyterian/St. Luke's Cancer Study
   Group; Robert F. Berris, M.D.

Presbyterian/St. Luke's Medical Center
2005 Franklin Street, Suite 150 (80205)
303-388-4876

Hospital
Presbyterian/St. Luke's Medical Center

CONNECTICUT

Newington
Greater Hartford CCOP; Dominick N.
   Pasquale, M.D.

St. Francis Hospital & Medical Center
114 Woodland Street
Hartford, 06105
203-548-4680

Hospitals
Hartford Hospital
Mount Sinai Hospital
St. Francis Hospital and Medical Center

New Haven
Hospital of St. Raphael CCOP; Leonard R.
   Farber, M.D.

Main 238
1450 Chapel Street (06511)
203-789-2050

Hospital
Hospital of St. Raphael

Offices
Hematology–Oncology, P.C.
Medical Oncology and Hematology, P.C.

FLORIDA

Daytona Beach
Halifax Hospital Medical Center; Herbert
   D. Kerman, M.D.

950

303 N. Clyde Morris Boulevard
P.O. Box 1990 (32015)
904-258-1598

Hospital
Regional Oncology Center, Halifax
  Hospital Medical Center

Gainesville
Florida Pediatric CCOP; James L. Talbert,
  M.D.

President, Florida Assn. of Pediatric
  Tumor Programs, Inc.
P.O. Box 13372, University Station
  (32604)
904-375-6848

Hospitals
All Children's Hospital
Jacksonville Wolfson Children's Hospital
Orlando Regional Medical Center
Sacred Heart Children's Hospital

GEORGIA

Augusta
University Hospital CCOP; Stephen M.
  Shlaer, M.D.

University Hospital Medical Center
820 St. Sebastian Way (10), Suite 5B
  (30910)
404-722-4245

Hospitals
University Hospital
Medical College of Georgia

HAWAII

Honolulu
Hawaii CCOP; Reginald C. S. Ho,
  M.D.QL Hawaii Medical Association
320 Ward Avenue, Suite 200 (96814)
808-536-7702

Hospitals
Fronk Clinic
Kaiser Foundation
Straub Clinic
Hilo Hospital

Kapiolani/Children's Medical Center
Kauai Veterans Memorial Hospital
Kona Hospital
Kuakini Medical Center
St. Francis Hospital
The Queen's Medical Center
Tripler Hospital
Wahiawa General Hospital

Offices
Honolulu Medical Group
Kauai Medical Group
Maui Medical Group

ILLINOIS

Chicago
Saint Mary of Nazareth Hospital Center;
  Korathu Thomas, M.D.

2233 W. Division Street (60622)
312-770-3205

Hospital
St. Mary of Nazareth Hospital Center

Evanston
Evanston Hospital; Janardan D.
  Khandekar, M.D.

Associate Professor of Medicine
Evanston Hospital
2650 Ridge Avenue (60201)
312-492-3989

Hospital
Evanston Hospital Corporation

Peoria
Methodist Medical Center of Illinois;
  Stephen A. Cullinan, M.D.

Oncology/Hematology Associates
Physicians Medical Plaza, Suite 605
214 N.E. Glen Oak (61603)
309-672-5783

Hospital
The Methodist Medical Center of Illinois

Offices
Oncology/Hematology Associates
Midwest Radiation Therapy Consultants

Urbana
Carle Cancer Center CCOP; Alan Kramer
  Hatfield, M.D.

951

Carle Clinic Association
Head, Department of
  Hematology/Oncology
602 W. University Avenue (61801)
217-337-3010

Hospital
Carle Clinic Association

IOWA

Des Moines
Iowa Oncology Research Association; S.
  Fred Brunk, M.D.

c/o Sharon Kuebler
Iowa Oncology Research Association
1048 4th Avenue (50314)
515-244-7586

Hospitals
Iowa Methodist Medical Center
Iowa Luthern Hospital
Mercy Hosital Medical Center
Des Moines General Hospital
Northwest Community Hospital

KANSAS

Wichita
Wichita CCOP; Henry E. Hynes, M.D.

929 N. St. Francis
Box 1358 (67201)
316-268-5784

Hospitals
St. Francis Regional Medical Center
St. Joseph Medical Center
Wesley Medical Center

LOUISIANA

New Orleans
Alton Ochsner Medical Foundation; Carl
  G. Kardinal, M.D.

Ochsner Clinic
1514 Jefferson Highway (70121)
504-838-3910

Hospitals
Ochsner Clinic and Ochsner Foundation
  Hospital
Baton Rouge Clinic
Hattiesburg Clinic
South Louisiana Medical Center

MAINE

Bangor
Eastern Maine Medical Center; Alan W.
  Boone, M.D.

489 State Street (04401)
207-947-3711

Hospital
Eastern Maine Medical Center

Portland
Southern Maine CCOP; Ronald J. Carroll,
  M.D.

Maine Medical Center
22 Bramhall Street (04102)
207-871-2213

Hospitals
Maine Medial Center
Mid–Maine Medical Center

Offices
O ncology/Hematology Associates
Marjorie Boyd, M.D.
Louis Bove, M.D.
Stephen Blattner, M.D.
Eugene Beaupre
Joseph Hiebel

MASSACHUSETTS

Boston
New England Collaborative CCOP; Jacob
  J. Lokich, M.D.

New England Deaconess Hospital
185 Pilgrim Road (02215)
617-732-8540

Hospitals
New England Deaconess Hospital
St. Luke's Hospital
Wentworth–Douglass Hospital
Frisbie Hospital

Elliot Hospital
Portsmouth Hospital
Symmes Hospital
Choate Hospital

MICHIGAN

Kalamazoo
Kalamazoo CCOP; Phillip Stott, M.D.
Borgess Medical Center

1521 Gull Road (49001)
517-383-4829

Hospitals
Borgess Medical Center
Bronson Methodist Hospital

Grand Rapids
Grand Rapids CCOP; Edward L.
  Moorhead II, M.D.
Butterworth Hospital

100 Michigan N.E. (49503)
616-774-1230

Hospitals
Blodgett Memorial Medical Center
Butterworth Hospital
Ferguson Hospital
Grand Rapids Osteopathic Hospital
Saint Mary's Hospital

MINNESOTA

Duluth
Duluth Clinic, Ltd.; James E. Krook,
  M.D.

Chairman, Duluth Clinic
400 E. Third Street (55805)
218-722-8364

Hospitals
The Duluth Clinic, Ltd.
Miller-Dwan Hospital & Medical Center
  Radiation Unit

St. Louis Park
W. Metro-Minneapolis CCOP; Joseph M.
  Ryan, M.D.
St. Louis Park Medical Center Research
  Foundation

St. Louis Park Medical Center
5000 W. 39th Street (55416
612-927-3248

Hospitals
Abbott-Northwestern Hospital
Fairview-Southdale Hospital
Mercy Medical Center
Methodist Hospital
Metropolitan Medical Center
North Memorial Medical Center
Unity Medical Center

MISSISSIPPI

Tupelo
North Mississippi CCOP; Julian B. Hill,
  M.D.

North Mississippi Medical Center
806 Garfield (38801)
601-844-9166

Hospital
North Mississippi Medical Center

Office
North Mississippi Hematology and
  Oncology Association, Ltd.

MISSOURI

Kansas City
Midwest CCOP; Karl H. Hanson, Jr.,
  M.D.
St. Luke's Hospital

St. Luke's Hospital of Kansas City
4320 Wornall Road, Suite 212 (64111)
816-513-0930

Hospitals
St. Luke's Hospital of Kansas City
Bethany Medical Center
The Children's Mercy Hospital

Offices
University of Health Sciences
Larry Rosen, M.D.
Richard Morrison, M.D.

Kansas City CCOP; Robert J. Belt, M.D.

953

Baptist Memorial Hospital
6601 Rockhill Road (64131)
816-361-3500, ext. 7224

Hospitals
Baptist Memorial Hospital
Menorah Medical Center
Research Medical Center
Shawnee Mission Medical Center
St. Mary Hospital
Trinity Lutheran Hospital

St. Louis
St. Louis CCOP
St. John's Mercy Medical Center; Patrick
  H. Henry, M.D.

Mercy Doctors Building
621 S. New Ballas Road (63141)
314-569-6959

Hospitals
Christian Hospitals
DePaul Health Center
Missouri Baptist Hospital
St. Anthony's Medical Center
St. John's Mercy Medical Center

MONTANA

Billings
Billings Interhospital Oncology Project;
  Neel Hammond, M.D.

1230 N. 30th Street (59101)
1-406-252-2147

Hospitals
St. Vincent's Hospital
Billings Deaconess Hospital
Northern Rockies Cancer Center

Offices
Neel Hammond, M.D.
Benjamin T. Marchello, M.D.
David B. Myers, M.D.

NEVADA

Las Vegas
Southern Nevada Cancer Research
  Foundation; John A. Ellerton, M.D.

650 Shadow Lane, Suite 5 (89106)
702-384-0808

Hospitals
Nevada Radiation Oncology Center
Southern Nevada Memorial Hospital
Valley Hospital Medical Center

Offices
Robert Belliveau, M.D.
B. Norman Brown, MD.
Kirk Cammack, M.D.
Cancer Care Consultants
Ann Marie Hoye, R.N.
Stephen Kollins, M.D.
Dermot O'Rourke, M.D.
William Rydell, M.D.

NEW JERSEY

Hackensack
Bergen–Passaic CCOP; Allan N. Krutchik,
  M.D.

Hackensack Medical Center
Hospital Place (07601)
201-441-2355

Hospitals
Beth Israel Hospital
Hackensack Medical Center
Holy Name Hospital

Livingston
Essex County Cancer Consortium; Rodger
  J. Winn, M.D.

St. Barnabas Medical Center
Old Short Hill Road (07039)
201-533-5905

Hospitals
St. Barnabas Medical Center
The Hospital Center at Orange
The Mountainside Hospital

Newark
Medical Center CCOP Consortium;
  Frederick B. Cohen, M.D.

Newark Beth Israel Medical Center
201 Lyons Avenue (07112)
201-926-7230

Hospitals
Newark Beth Israel Medical Center
Christ Hospital
West Hudson Hospital
Memorial General Hospital

Summit

Northern New Jersey CCOP; James A. Wolff, M.D.

Director, Valerie Fund Children's Center
Overlook Hospital
193 Morris Avenue (07901)
201-543-2353

Hospitals
Overlook Hospital
Morristown Memorial Hospital
Elizabeth General Medical Center

NEW YORK

Binghamton

Twin Tiers CCOP; Robert E. Enck, M.D.

Our Lady of Lourdes Hospital;
169 Riverside Drive (13905)
607-798-5431

Hospitals
Our Lady of Lourdes Hospital
Robert Packer Hospital

Brooklyn

Lutheran Medical Center; Hosny Selim, M.D.

Radiotherapy Department
150 55th Street (11220)
212-630-7065

Hospitals
Lutheran Medical Center
Maimonides Medical Center
Methodist Hospital

Cooperstown

Mary Imogene Bassett Hospital CCOP; Richard J. Horner, M.D.

Mary Imogene Bassett Hospital (13326)
607-547-3336

Hospital
Mary Imogene Bassett Hospital

Manhasset

North Shore University Hospital; Vincent P. Vinciguerra, M.D.

Associate Professor of Clinical Medicine
Cornell University Medical College
North Shore University Hospital

300 Community Drive (11030)
516-562-4160

Hospital
North Shore University Hospital

Offices
Philip Schulman, M.D.
Klaus Dittmar, M.D.
Frank Tomao, M.D.
Francis X. Moore, M.D.
Robert Levy, M.D.
Jakow Diener, M.D.
Jerome Appelbaum, M.D.
Inyoung Chung, M.D.
John Lovecchio, M.D.
Samuel Packer, M.D.
Jay Bosworth, M.D.

Mineola

Nassau Regional Cancer Program; Larry Nathanson, M.D.

Nassau Hospital Professional Building
222 Station Plaza North (11501)
516-663-2310

Hospitals
Lydia Hall Hospital
Nassau Hospital

Rochester

St. Mary's Hospital CCOP; Kishan J. Pandya, M.D.

St. Mary's Hospital
89 Genesee Street (14611)
716-464-3591

Hospital
St. Mary's Hospital

Syracuse

CCOP of Central New York; Kenneth E. Gale, M.D.

East Genesee Medical Building
1200 E. Genesee Street (13210)
315-476-5388

Hospitals
St. Joseph's Hospital
Upstate Medical Center
Crouse–Irving Memorial Community General

Offices
Henry R. Bartos, M.D.
Manuel G. Dalope, M.D.
Nabila A. Elbadawai, M.D.
Abdul G. Musa, M.D.
J. Robert Smith, M.D.
Richard W. Weiskopf, M.D.

NORTH DAKOTA

Fargo
St. Luke's Hospitals CCOP; Lloyd
  Everson, M.D.

Fargo Clinic, Ltd.
737 Broadway (58123)
701-237-2439

Hospitals
St. Luke's General Hospital
Fargo Clinic
The Neuropsychiatric Institute
St. John's Hospital
St. Ansgar Hospital

OHIO

Cincinnati
Tri-State CCOP; Albert W. Schreiner,
  M.D.

The Christ Hospital
Department of Internal Medicine
2139 Auburn Avenue (45219)
513-369-2532

Hospitals
Bethesda Hospital
The Christ Hospital
Good Samaritan Hospital
The Jewish Hospital
St. Luke Hospital

Columbus
Columbus CCOP; Jerry T. Guy, M.D.

c/o Grant Hospital
300 E. Towns Street, 5th Fl. (43215)
614-461-3295

Hospitals
Grant Hospital
St. Anthony Hospital
Doctors Hospital

Kettering
Dayton CCOP; James S. Ungerleider,
  M.D.

c/o Charlene Luciane
3525 Southern Boulevard (45429)
513-293-1117

Hospitals
Good Samaritan Hospital
Grandview Hospital
Kettering Medical Center
Miami Valley Hospital
St. Elizabeth Medical Center

Toledo
Toledo CCOP; Charles D. Cobau, M.D.

Toledo Clinic, Inc.
4235 Secor Road (43623)
419-473-3561

Hospitals
Flower Hospital
St. Charles Hospital
St. Joseph Mercy Hospital
The Toledo Hospital
The Toledo Clinic, Inc.

PENNSYLVANIA

Danville
Geisinger Clinic CCOP; Albert M.
  Bernath, M.D.

Geisinger Medical Center (17822)
717-271-6413

Hospital
Geisinger Clinic and Medical Center

Pittsburgh
Allegheny CCOP; Reginald P. Pugh,
  M.D.

Allegheny General Hospital
Division of Medical Oncology
320 E. North Avenue (15212)
412-359-3630

Hospitals
Allegheny General Hospital
Jameson Memorial Hospital

956

SOUTH CAROLINA

Spartanburg
Spartanburg CCOP; John H. McCulloch, M.D.

1776 Skylyn Drive
P.O. Box 2768 (29304)
803-585-8343

Hospitals
Spartanburg General Hospital
Mary Black Memorial Hospital
Doctor's Memorial Hospital

SOUTH DAKOTA

Sioux Falls
Sioux Falls Community Cancer Consortium; Robert F. Marschke, Jr., M.D.

Hematology–Oncology
1301 S. 9th Avenue, Suite 501 (57105)
605-331-3160

Hospitals
McKennan Hospital
Central Plains Clinic
Sioux Valley Hospital
Veterans Administration Hospital

Office
Medical Oncology Associates

TENNESSEE

Memphis
Memphis CCOP; Ronald D. Lawson, M.D.

Methodist Central Hospital
1265 Union Avenue (38104)
901-726-7780

Hospitals
Methodist Central Hospital
Methodist North Hospital
Methodist South Hospital
St. Francis Hospital

TEXAS

Fort Worth
Fort Worth/Arlington CCOP; John L. E. Nugent, M.D.

Radiation Therapy & Chemotherapy Association
800 5th Avenue, #319 (76104)
817-339-4333

Hospital
St. Joseph's Hospital

Offices
Radiation Therapy & Chemotherapy Associates, Fort Worth
Radiation Therapy & Chemotherapy Associates, Arlington

VERMONT

Rutland
Green Mountain Oncology Group; H. James Wallace, M.D.

The Rutland Hospital, Inc. (05701)
802-775-7111, x207

Hospitals
Rutland Hospital, Inc.
Putnam Memorial Hospital

Offices
Mildred Reardon, M.D.
John Valentine, M.D.

VIRGINIA

Roanoke
CCOP of Roanoke; Stephen H. Rosenoff, M.D.

2013 S. Jefferson Street (24014)
703-981-7424

Hospitals
Roanoke Memorial Hospitals
Community Hospital of Roanoke
Lewis–Gale Hospital
Veterans Administration Medical Center

957

WASHINGTON

Seattle
Virginia Mason Medical Center CCOP;
  Albert B. Einstein, Jr., M.D.

The Mason Clinic
1100 Ninth Avenue (98111)
206-223-6945

Hospitals
Virginia Mason Medical Center
Valley General Hospital

Tacoma
Southwest Washington CCOP; Joseph G.
  Katterhagen, M.D.

409 S. J Street
P.O. Box 5277 (98405)
206-597-6964

Hospitals
Auburn General Hosital
Good Samaritan Hospital
St. Joseph Hospital
Allenmore Community Hospital
VA Medical Center
Mary Bridge Children's Health Center
St. Peter Hospital
Community Hospital
St. Joseph Hospital in Aberdeen
Tacoma General Hospital

WEST VIRGINIA

Charleston
West Virginia Cooperative CCOP; Steven
  J. Jubelirer, M.D.

Department of Medicine
Charleston Division, WVU Medical
  School
3110 MacCorkle Avenue, S.E. (25304)
304-347-1318

Hospitals
West Virginia University Hospital
Camden–Clark Hospital
United Hospital Center
Charleston Area Medical Center
Veterans Administration Medical Center
Ohio Valley Medical Center
Raleigh General Hospital
City Hospital of Martinsburg
St. Mary's Hospital
Cabell–Huntington Hospital

WISCONSIN

Marshfield
Marshfield CCOP; Tarit K. Banerjee,
  M.D.

Marshfield Medical Foundation
1000 N. Oak Avenue (54449)
715-387-5416

Hospitals
Marshfield Clinic
St. Joseph's Hospital

Research Bases
and Principal Investigators

Clinical Trials Groups

ECOG	*Eastern Cooperative Oncology Group*—Chairman: Paul Carbone, M.D. University of Wisconsin Clinical Cancer Center, Madison, WI
SWOG	*Southwest Oncology Group*—Chairman: Charles Coltman, Jr., M.D. Cancer Therapy and Research Center, San Antonio, TX
NCCTG	*North Central Cancer Treatment Group*—Charles Moertel, M.D.
GITSG	*Gastrointestinal Tumor Study Group*—Elliot Livstone, M.D. Yale University, New Haven, CT
RTOG	*Radiation Therapy Oncology Group*— Associate Chairman: Lawrence W. Davis, M.D. American College of Radiology, Philadelphia
CALGB	*Cancer and Leukemia Group B*—Chief of Staff: W. Bradford Patterson, M.D. Dana-Farber Cancer Institute, Boston
SCSG	*Southeastern Cancer Study Group*—Chairman: George Omura, M.D. University of Alabama, Birmingham
NSABP	*National Surgical Adjuvant Project for Breast and Bowel Cancers*— Chairman: Bernard Fisher, M.D. University of Pittsburgh
GOG	*Gynecologic Oncology Group*—Chairman: George C. Lewis, M.D. American College of Obstetricians and Gynecologists, Philadelphia
CCSG	*Children's Cancer Study Group*— Chairman: Denman Hammond, M.D. University of Southern California, Los Angeles

MAOP	*Mid-Atlantic Oncology Program* Georgetown University Medical Center, Washington, DC
POG	*Pediatric Oncology Group*—Chairman: Teresa J. Vietti, M.D. Washington University, St. Louis
POA	*Piedmont Oncology Association*—Charles Shurr, M.D. Bowman Gray School of Medicine, Winston-Salem, NC
NCOG	*Northern California Oncology Group*— Acting Chairman, Byron W. Brown, Jr., Ph.D. Palo Alto, CA

NCI-Supported Cancer Centers

Comprehensive Cancer Center of Metropolitan Detroit—Melvin L. Reed, M.D.
Wayne State University School of Medicine, Detroit

Dana–Farber Cancer Institute—W. Bradford Patterson, M.D.
Boston

Yale University Comprehensive Cancer Center—Joseph Bertino, M.D.
New Haven, CT

Memorial Sloan-Kettering Cancer Center—David Kelsen, M.D.
New York

Comprehensive Cancer Center, University of Alabama in Birmingham—Richard H. Wheeler, M.

University of Wisconsin Clinical Cancer Cancer—Donald Trump, M.D.
Madison, WI

University of Southern California Comprehensive Cancer Center—Brian Henderson, M.D.
Los Angeles

Columbia University Cancer Center—Rose Ruth Ellison, M.D.
New York

University of Rochester Cancer Center—John M. Bennett, M.D.

Illinois Cancer Council—Shirley B. Lansky, M.D.
Chicago

Fred Hutchinson Cancer Research Center—Frederick Appelbaum, M.D.
Seattle

Ohio State University Comprehensive Cancer Center—David S. Yohn, Ph.D.
Columbus

University of Arizona Cancer Center—Thomas E. Moon, Ph.D.
Tucson

Cancer Center of Hawaii, University of Hawaii at Manoa—Noboru Oishi, M.D.

Vermont Regional Cancer Center, University of Vermont— James A. Stewart, M.D.
Burlington

Vincent T. Lombardi Cancer Research Center, Georgetown University Medical Center—
Paul V. Woolley, M.D.
Washington, DC

University of California, San Diego, Cancer Center— Mark R. Green, M.D.

960

Cancer Programs Approved by the Commission on Cancer of the American College of Surgeons

ALABAMA

Birmingham
Baptist Medical Center—Princeton
Brookwood Medical Center
Carraway Methodist Medical Center
Cooper Green Hospital
University of Alabama Hospitals
Veterans Admin. Medical Center

Gadsden
Baptist Memorial Hospital

Mobile
University of South Alabama Medical
   Center

Tuskegee
Veterans Admin. Medical Center

ALASKA

Anchorage
Humana Hospital
PHS Alaska Native Medical Center

ARIZONA

Flagstaff
Flagstaff Hospital and Medical Center

Mesa
Desert Samaritan Hospital
Mesa Lutheran Hospital

Phoenix
Good Samaritan Hospital
Maricopa Medical Center
Memorial Hospital
Veterans Admin. Medical Center

Scottsdale
Scottsdale Memorial Hospital

Tucson
Tucson Medical Center
University Hospital

ARKANSAS

Fayetteville
Washington Regional Medical Center

Fort Smith
Sparks Regional Medical Center
St. Edward Mercy Medical Center

Little Rock
Veterans Admin. Medical Center

Rogers
St. Mary–Rogers Memorial Hospital

CALIFORNIA

Alhambra
Alhambra Community Hospital

Anaheim
Anaheim Memorial Hospital
Martin Luther Hospital Medical Center
West Anaheim Community Hospital

Apple Valley
St. Mary Desert Valley Hospital

Arcadia
Methodist Hospital of South California

Bakersfield
Kern Medical Center
San Joaquin Community Hospital

Bellflower
Bellwood General Hospital
Kaiser Foundation Hospital (ROS)

Berkeley
Alta Bates Hospital
Herrick Hospital and Health Center

Burbank
St. Joseph Medical Center

Burlingame
Peninsula Hospital and Medical Center

Canoga Park
West Hills Medical Center

Castro Valley
Eden Hospital

Chico
N. T. Enloe Memorial Hospital

Concord
Mt. Diablo Hospital Medical Center

Covina
Inter-Community Medical Center

Culver City
Brotman Medical Center

Duarte
City of Hope National Medical Center
Santa Teresita Hospital

Escondido
Palomar Memorial Hospital

Fontana
Kaiser Foundation Hospital (SIE)

Fountain Valley
Fountain Valley Community Hospital

Fresno
Fresno Community Hospital Medical
  Center
Valley Children's Hospital
Veterans Admin. Medical Center

Fullerton
St. Jude Hospital and Rehabilitation Center

Glendale
Glendale Adventist Medical Center
Memorial Hospital of Glendale

Glendora
Foothill Presbyterian Hospital
Glendora Community Hospital

Granada Hills
Granada Hills Community Hospital

Harbor City
Kaiser Foundation Hospital (VER)

Hawthorne
Hawthorne Community Hospital

Imola
Napa State Hospital

Indio
Indio Community Hospital

Inglewood
Centinela Hospital Medical Center
Daniel Freeman Memorial Hospital

Laguna Hills
Saddleback Community Hospital

La Jolla
Green Hospital of Scripps Clinic
Scripps Memorial Hospital

La Mesa
Grossmont District Hospital

Livermore
Veterans Admin. Medical Center

Loma Linda
Loma Linda University Medical Center

Long Beach
Long Beach Community Hospital
Los Altos Hospital
Memorial Hospital Medical Center
St. Mary Medical Center—Bauer Hospital
Veterans Admin. Medical Center

Los Angeles
California Hospital Medical Center
Cedars–Sinai Medical Center
Childrens Hospital of Los Angeles
Hollywood Presbyterian Medical Center
Hospital of the Good Samaritan
Kaiser Foundation Hospital (CAD)
Kaiser Foundation Hospital (SUN)
Los Angeles County—USC Medical
    Center
Martin Luther King Jr. General Hospital
Orthopaedic Hospital Medical Center
Queen of Angels Medical Center
UCLA Hospital and Clinics
White Memorial Medical Center

Lynwood
St. Francis Medical Center

Martinez
Veterans Admin. Medical Center

Mission Viejo
Mission Community Hospital

Modesto
Memorial Hospitals Association

Montebello
Beverly Hospital

Monterey Park
Garfield Medical Center

Napa
Queen of the Valley Hospital

Newport Beach
Hoag Memorial Hospital Presbyterian

Northridge
Northridge Hospital Foundation

Oakland
Naval Hospital
Samuel Merritt Hospital

Oceanside
Tri-City Hospital

Orange
Childrens Hospital of Orange County
St. Joseph Hospital
University of California Irvine Medical
    Center

Oxnard
St. John's Hospital

Palm Springs
Desert Hospital

Palo Alto
Palo Alta Medical Foundation
Veterans Admin. Medical Center

Panorama City
Kaiser Foundation Hospital (CAN)
Panorama Community Hospital

Pasadena
Huntingdon Memorial Hospital
St. Luke Hospital of Pasadena

Pomono
Pomono Valley Community Hospital

Poway
Pomerado Hospital

Rancho Mirage
Eisenhower Medical Center

Redlands
Redlands Community Hospital

Redondo Beach
South Bay Hospital

Redwood City
Sequoia Hospital District

Riverside
Parkview Community Hospital
Riverside Community Hospital
Riverside General Hospital—UN Medical
    Center

963

Sacramento
Mercy Hospital
Sutter Community Hospitals of Sacramento
University of California Davis Medical
  Center

San Bernardino
San Bernardino Community Hospital
San Bernardino County Medical Center
St. Bernardine Hospital

San Clemente
San Clemente General Hospital

San Diego
Childrens Hospital and Health Center
Donald N. Sharp Memorial Community
  Hospital
Kaiser Foundation Hospital (ZIO)
Mercy Hospital and Medical Center
Naval Regional Medical Center
University Hospital

San Dimas
San Dimas Community Hospital

San Francisco
Childrens Hospital of San Francisco
French Hospital/Medical Center
Letterman Army Medical Center
Mount Zion Hospital and Medical Center
Ralph K. Davis Medical Center
San Francisco General Hospital Medical
  Center
St. Francis Memorial Hospital
St. Luke's Hospital
St. Mary's Hospital and Medical Center
University of California Hospitals and
  Cinics

San Gabriel
Community Hospital of San Gabriel

San Jose
Good Samaritan Hospital
O'Connor Hospital
San Jose Hospital
Santa Clara Valley Medical Center

San Pablo
Brookside Hospital

San Pedro
San Pedro Peninsula Hospital

Santa Ana
Western Medical Center

Santa Barbara
Goleta Valley Community Hospital
Santa Barbara Cottage Hospital
St. Francis Hospital

Santa Monica
Santa Monica Hospital Medical Center
St. John's Hospital and Health Center

South Laguna
South Coast Medical Center

Stockton
Dameron Hospital Association
St. Joseph's Hospital

Tarzana
Medical Center of Tarzana Hospital

Thousand Oaks
Los Robles Regional Medical Center

Torrance
Los Angeles County Habor—UCLA
  Medical Center
Little Company of Mary Hospital
Torrance Memorial Hospital Medical
  Center

Travis AFB
David Grant USAF Medical Center

Upland
San Antonio Community Hospital

Van Nuys
Valley Presbyterian Hospital

Victorville
Victor Valley Community Hospital

Visalia
Kaweah Delta District Hospital

Walnut Creek
John Muir Memorial Hospital

West Covina
West Covina Hospital

Whittier
Presbyterian Intercommunity Hospital

964

COLORADO

Aurora
Fitzsimons Army Center

Colorado Springs
Penrose Hospital

Denver
Porter Memorial Hospital
Presbyterian Denver Hospital
Rose Medical Center
Saint Joseph Hospital
Saint Luke's Hospital
St. Anthony Hospital Systems
University Hospital—University of
    Colorado
Veterans Admin. Medical Center

Englewood
Swedish Medical Center

Fort Carson
U.S. Army Community Hospital

Fort Collins
Poudre Valley Hospital

Greeley
North Colorado Medical Center

Lakewood
AMC Cancer Research Center

Longmont
Longmont United Hospital

Montrose
Montrose Memorial Hospital

Pueblo
St. Mary—Corwin Hospital

Wheat Ridge
Lutheran Medical Center

CONNECTICUT

Bridgeport
Bridgeport Hospital
Park City Hospital
St. Vincent's Medical Center

Danbury
Danbury Hospital

Derby
Griffin Hospital

Farmington
University of Connecticut Health
    Center/Jack Dempsey Hospital

Greenwich
Greenwich Hospital Association

Hartford
Hartford Hospital
Mount Sinai Hospital
Saint Francis Hospital and Medical Center

Meriden
Meriden–Wallingford Hospital

Middletown
Middlesex Memorial Hospital

New Haven
Hospital of St. Raphael
Yale–New Haven Hospital

Norwalk
Norwalk Hospital

Stamford
St. Joseph Hospital
Stamford Hospital

Torrington
Charlotte Hungerford Hospital

Waterbury
St. Mary's Hospital
Waterbury Hospital

DELAWARE

Lewes
Beebe Hospital of Sussex County

Wilmington
St. Francis Hospital
Veterans Admin. Medical Center
Wilmington Medical Center

DISTRICT OF COLUMBIA

Washington
Georgetown University Hospital
Greater Southeast Community Hospital
Howard University Hospital

Veterans Admin. Medical Center
Walter Reed Army Medical Center

FLORIDA

Daytona Beach
Halifax Hospital Medical Center

Dunedin
Mease Hospital and Clinic

Gainesville
Shands Teaching Hospital and Clinics

Jacksonville
Naval Regional Medical Center
St. Vincent's Medical Center
University Hospital of Jacksonville

Largo
Medical Center Hospital

Miami
Cedars of Lebanon Health Center
Jackson Memorial Hospital

Miami Beach
Mount Sinai Medical Center

Naples
Naples Community Hospital

Ocala
Marion Community Hospital
Munroe Regional Medical Center

Pensacola
Baptist Hospital
Naval Aerospace and Regional Medical
   Center
West Florida Hospital

Tallahassee
Tallahassee Memorial Regional Medical
   Center

Tampa
St. Joseph's Hospital
Tampa General Hospital

GEORGIA

Albany
Phoebe Putney Memorial Hospital

Americus
Americus and Sumter County Hospital

Atlanta
Crawford W. Long Memorial Hospital
Emory University Hospital
Georgia Baptist Medical Center
Grady Memorial Hospital
Northside Hospital
Piedmont Hospital
St. Joseph's Hospital
West Paces Ferry Hospital

Augusta
Eugene Talmadge Memorial Hospital

Austell
Cobb General Hospital

Columbus
The Medical Center

Dalton
Hamilton Memorial Hospital

Decatur
DeKalb General Hospital
Veterans Admin. Medical Center—Atlanta

East Point
South Fulton Hospital

Fort Benning
Martin Army Community Hospital

Fort Gordon
Dwight D. Eisenhower Army Medical
   Center

Gainesville
Northeast Georgia Medical Center

La Grange
West Georgia Medical Center/E. Callaway
   C.C.

Macon
Medical Center of Central Georgia

Marietta
Kennestone Hospital

Savannah
Memorial Medical Center

Tifton
Tift General Hospital

Toccoa
Stephens County Hospital

Valdosta
South Georgia Medical Center

HAWAII

Honolulu
Kaiser Foundation Hospital
Kuakini Medical Center
Queen's Medical Center
St. Francis Hospital
Straub Clinic and Hospital
Tripler Army Medical Center

Lihue
G. N. Wilcox Memorial Hospital and
  Health Center

Wailuku
Maui Memorial Hospital

Waimea
Kauai Veterans Memorial Hospital

IDAHO

Blackfoot
Bingham Memorial Hospital

Boise
St. Luke's Hospital/Mountain States Tech.
  Inst.

Burley
Cassia Memorial Hospital and Medical
  Center

Lewiston
St. Joseph's Hospital

Nampa
Mercy Medical Center

Pocatello
Bannock Memorial Hospital

Twin Falls
Magic Valley Regional Medical Center

ILLINOIS

Arlington Heights
Northwest Community Hospital

Aurora
Copley Memorial Hospital
Mercy Center for Health Care Services

Berwyn
MacNeal Memorial Hospital

Blue Island
St. Francis Hospital

Carbondale
Memorial Hospital of Carbondale

Champaign
Burnham Hospital

Chicago
Bethesda Hospital
Central Community Hospital
Children's Memorial Hospital
Columbus Hospital
Cook County Hospital
Edgewater Hospital
Franklin Boulevard Community Hospital
Holy Cross Hospital
Illinois Masonic Medical Center
Jackson Park Hospital
Louis A. Weiss Memorial Hospital
Mary Thompson Hospital
Mercy Hospital and Medical Center
Michael Reese Hospital and Medical
  Center
Mount Sinai Hospital Medical Center
Northwestern Memorial Hospital
Ravenswood Hospital Medical Center
Resurrection Hospital
Rush–Presbyterian–St. Luke's Medical
  Center
St. Elizabeth's Hospital
St. Joseph Hospital
St. Mary of Nazareth Hospital Center
Swedish Covenant Hospital
University of Chicago Hospitals and
  Clinics
University of Illinois Hospital
Veterans Admin. West Side Medical
  Center

Chicago Heights
St. James Hospital

967

Danville
Lakeview Medical Center
St. Elizabeth Hospital

Decatur
Decatur Memorial Hospital

De Kalb
Kishwaukee Community Hospital

Effingham
St. Anthony's Memorial Hospital

Elgin
Saint Joseph Hospital
Sherman Hospital

Elk Grove Village
Alexian Brothers Medical Center

Elmhurst
Memorial Hospital of Dupage County

Evanston
Evanston Hospital
St. Francis Hospital

Evergreen Park
Little Company of Mary Hospital

Galesburg
St. Mary's Hospital

Great Lakes
Naval Regional Medical Center

Harvey
Ingalls Memorial Hospital

Highland Park
Highland Park Hospital

Hinsdale
Hinsdale Sanitarium and Hospital

Joliet
Saint Joseph Hospital

Kankakee
St. Mary's Hospital of Kankakee

Lake Forest
Lake Forest Hospital

Libertyville
Condell Memorial Hospital

McHenry
McHenry Hospital

Macomb
McDonough District Hospital

Maywood
F. G. McGaw Hospital, Loyola University
    Med. Center

Moline
Lutheran Hospital

Oak Lawn
Christ Hospital

Oak Park
West Suburban Hospital Medical Center

Olney
Richland Memorial Hospital

Park Ridge
Lutheran General Hospital

Peoria
Methodist Medical Center of Illinois
St. Francis Hospital Medical Center

Quincy
Blessing Hospital
St. Mary Hospital

Rockford
Rockford Memorial Hospital
St. Anthony Hospital Medical Center
Swedish–American Hospital

Skokie
Skokie Valley Community Hospital

Springfield
Memorial Medical Center
St. John's Hospital

Sterling
Community General Hospital

Streator
St. Mary's Hospital

Urbana
Carle Foundation Hospital
Mercy Hospital

Winfield
Central Dupage Hospital

968

INDIANA

Bluffton
Caylor—Nickel Hospital

Columbus
Bartholomew County Hospital

East Chicago
St. Catherine Hospital of East Chicago

Evansville
Deaconess Hospital
St. Mary's Medical Center
Welborn Memorial Baptist Hospital

Gary
Methodist Hospital of Gary

Hammond
St. Margaret Hospital

Indianapolis
Community Hospital of Indianapolis
Methodist Hospital of Indiana
St. Vincent Hospital and Health Center

Terre Haute
Terre Haute Regional Hospital
Union Hospital

Vincennes
Good Samaritan Hospital

IOWA

Des Moines
Iowa Methodist Medical Center
Mercy Hospital Medical Center
Veterans Admin. Medical Center

Iowa City
University of Iowa Hospitals and Clinics

Mason City
North Iowa Medical Center
St. Joseph Mercy Hospital

Sioux City
Marian Health Center

KANSAS

Fort Riley
Irwin Army Hospital

Hays
Hadley Regional Medical Center
St. Anthony Hospital

Kansas City
Bethany Medical Center
University of Kansas Medical Center

Topeka
St. Francis Hospital and Medical Center

Wichita
St. Francis Regional Medical Center
St. Joseph Medical Center
Wesley Medical Center

KENTUCKY

Fort Campbell
F. A. Blanchfield Army Community
  Hospital

Lexington
Central Baptist Hospital
Good Samaritan Hospital
University Hospital

Louisville
Highlands Baptist Hospital
Humana Hospital University
Kosair–Childrens Hospital Medical Center
Norton Hospital
Veterans Admin. Medical Center

Madisonville
Regional Medical Center of Hopkins
  County

LOUISIANA

Alexandria
Rapides Regional Medical Center
St. Frances Cabrini Hospital

Lake Charles
St. Patrick Hospital of Lake Charles

New Orleans
Charity Hospital of Louisiana at New
  Orleans
Touro Infirmary
Veterans Admin. Medical Center

969

Shreveport
Louisiana State University Hospital
Veterans Admin. Medical Center

MARYLAND

Annapolis
Anne Arundel General Hospital

Baltimore
Franklin Square Hospital
Greater Baltimore Medical Center
Johns Hopkins Hospital
Sinai Hospital of Baltimore
South Baltimore General Hospital
University of Maryland Hospital
Wyman Park Health System, Inc.

Bethesda
Naval Hospital

Camp Springs
Malcolm Grow USAF Medical Center

Cumberland
Sacred Heart Hospital

Leonardtown
St. Mary's Hospital

Olney
Montgomery General Hospital

Salisbury
Peninsula General Hospital Medical Center

Towson
St. Joseph Hospital

MAINE

Augusta
Kennebec Valley Medical Center

Bangor
Eastern Maine Medical Center

Lewiston
Central Maine Medical Center
St. Mary's General Hospital

Portland
Maine Medical Center

Presque Isle
The Aroostook Medical Center

Rockland
Penobscot Bay Medical Center

Rumford
Rumford Community Hospital

Togus
Veterans Admin. Medical Center

Waterville
Mid-Maine Medical Center

MASSACHUSETTS

Arlington
Symmes Hospital

Beverly
Beverly Hospital

Boston
Boston City Hospital
Brigham and Women's Hospital
Carney Hospital
Children's Hospital Medical Center
Faulkner Hospital
Massachusetts General Hospital
New England Deaconess Hospital
New England Medical Center
St. Elizabeth's Hospital of Boston
University Hospital

Brockton
Brockton Hospital
Cardinal Cushing General Hospital

Burlington
Lahey Clinic Hospital

Cambridge
Mount Auburn Hospital

Chelsea
Quigley Memorial Hospital/Soldiers Home

Concord
Emerson Hospital

Danvers
Hunt Memorial Hospital

Fall River
St. Anne's Hospital

Framingham
Framingham Union Hospital

Holyoke
Holyoke Hospital
Providence Hospital

Hyannis
Providence Hospital

Jamaica Plain
Veterans Admin. Medical Center

Lynn
Lynn Hospital

Medford
Lawrence Memorial Hospital of Medford

Melrose
Melrose–Wakefield Hospital

Needham
Glover Memorial Hospital

Newton Lower Falls
Newton–Wellesley Hospital

North Adams
North Adams Regional Hospital

Northampton
Cooley Dickinson Hospital

Norwood
Norwood Hospital

Pittsfield
Berkshire Medical Center

Plymouth
Jordan Hospital

Salem
Salem Hospital

South Weymouth
South Shore Hospital

Springfield
Baystate Medical Center
Mercy Hospital

Stoughton
Goddard Memorial Hospital

Waltham
Waltham Hospital

Winchester
Winchester Hospital

Worcester
St. Vincent Memorial Hospital

MICHIGAN

Ann Arbor
St. Joseph Mercy Hospital
University Hospital

Battle Creek
Leila Hospital and Health Center

Dearborn
Oakwood Hospital

Detroit
Harper–Grace Hospital
Henry Ford Hospital

Flint
Hurley Medical Center
St. Joseph Hospital

Grand Rapids
Blodgett Memorial Hospital
Butterworh Hospital
Ferguson–Droste–Ferguson Hospital
St. Mary's Hospital

Kalamazoo
Borgess Medical Center
Bronson Methodist Hospital

Lansing
Edward W. Sparrow Hospital

Marquette
Marquette General Hospital

Menominee
Menominee County Lloyd Hospital

Muskegon
Hackley Hospital and Medical Center

Rochester
Crittenton Hospital

Royal Oak
William Beaumont Hospital

Saginaw
St. Mary's Hospital

Southfield
Providence Hospital

MINNESOTA

Grand Rapids
Itasca Memorial Hospital

971

Hibbing
Central Mesabi Medical Center

Mankato
Immanuel–St. Joseph's Hospital

Minneapolis
Abbott–Northwestern Hospital
Children's Health Center
Hennepin County Medical Center
Methodist Hospital
Metropolitan Medical Center
St. Mary's Hospital
University of Minnesota Hospitals and
  Clinics
Veterans Admin. Medical Center

Moorhead
St. Ansgar Hospital

Rochester
Mayo Clinic

St. Paul
St. Paul–Ramsey Medical Center

Virginia
Virginia Regional Medical Center

MISSISSIPPI

Biloxi
Howard Memorial Hospital
Veterans Admin. Medical Center

Gulfport
Memorial Hospital at Gulfport

Hattiesburg
Forrest County General Hospital
Methodist Hospital

Jackson
University of Mississippi Medical Center
Veterans Admin. Medical Center

Keesler AFB
USAF Medical Center Keesler

Pascagoula
Singing River Hospital

Tupelo
North Mississippi Medical Center

Vicksburg
Mercy Regional Medical Center

MISSOURI

Cape Girardeau
Southeast Missouri Hospital
St. Francis Medical Center

Columbia
Boone County Hospital
Columbia Regional Hospital
Ellis Fischel St. Cancer Hospital
University of Missouri Hospital and
  Clinics

Fort Leonard Wood
General Leonard Wood Army Hospital

Kansas City
Baptist Medical Center
Children's Mercy Hospital
Menorah Medical Center
St. Luke's Hospital
Trinity Lutheran Hospital

Poplar Bluff   .
Doctors Regional Medical Center

Sikeston
Missouri Delta Community Hospital

St. Joseph
Methodist Medical Center

St. Louis
Christian Hospital Northeast/Northwest
Deaconess Hospital
Incarnate Word Hospital
Jewish Hospital of St. Louis
St. Anthony's Medical Center
St. John's Mercy Medical Center
St. Louis Children's Hospital
St. Mary's Health Center
Veterans Admin. Medical Center—JC Div.

MONTANA

Butte
St. James Community Hospital

Great Falls
Columbus Hospital

NEBRASKA

Hastings
Mary Lanning Memorial Hospital

Kearney
Good Samaritan Hospital

Lincoln
Bryan Memorial Hospital
Lincoln General Hospital
St. Elizabeth Community Health Center
Veterans Admin. Medical Center

Omaha
Archbishop Bergan Mercy Hospital
Bishop Clarkson Memorial Hospital
Immanuel Medical Center
Lutheran Medical Center
Nebraska Methodist Hospital
Saint Joseph Hospital
University of Nebraska Hospital and
  Clinics

NEVADA

Las Vegas
Southern Nevada Memorial Hospital
Sunrise Hospital Medical Center

NEW HAMPSHIRE

Dover
Wentworth–Douglass Hospital

Exeter
Exeter Hospital

Hanover
Mary Hitchcock Memorial Hospital

Keene
Cheshire Hospital

Laconia
Lakes Region General Hospital

Littleton
Littleton Hospital

Manchester
Catholic Medical Center
Elliot Hospital

Portsmouth
Portsmouth Hospital

Rochester
Frisbie Memorial Hospital

NEW JERSEY

Atlantic City
Atlantic City Medical Center

Belleville
Clara Maass Medical Center

Camden
West Jersey Hospital

Denville
St. Clare's Hospital

East Orange
Veterans Admin. Medical Center

Elizabeth
Elizabeth General Medical Center

Englewood
Englewood Hospital

Hackensack
Hackensack Medical Center

Hackettstown
Hackettstown Community Hospital

Livingston
St. Barnabas Medical Center

Long Branch
Monmouth Medical Center

Montclair
The Mountainside Hospital

Morristown
Morristown Memorial Hospital

Mount Holly
Burlington County Memorial Hospital

Neptune
Jersey Shore Medical Center—Fitkin
  Hospital

Newark
Newark Beth Israel Medical Center

New Brunswick
Middlesex General—University Hospital

973

Newton
Newton Memorial Hospital

Orange
The Hospital Center at Orange

Passaic
Beth Israel Hospital

Paterson
St. Joseph's Hospital and Medical Center

Phillipsburg
Warren Hospital

Plainfield
Muhlenberg Hospital

Princeton
Medical Center at Princeton

Red Bank
Riverview Hospital

Somerville
Somerset Medical Center

Sussex
Wallkill Valley Hospital

Teaneck
Holy Name Hospital

Trenton
St. Francis Medical Center

NEW MEXICO

Albuquerque
Lovelace Medical Center
St. Joseph Hospital
University of New Mexico Hospital
Veterans Admin. Medical Center

NEW YORK

Albany
Veterans Admin. Medical Center

Amityville
Brunswick Hospital Center

Binghamton
Our Lady of Lourdes Memorial Hospital

Bronx
Bronx–Lebanon Hospital Center
Misericordia Hospital Medical Center
Veterans Admin. Medical Center

Brooklyn
Brookdale Hospital
Caledonian Hospital
Coney Island Hospital
Jewish Hospital and Medical Center
Kings County Hospital Center/SUNY
 Downstate
Long Island College Hospital
Lutheran Medical Center
Maimonides Medical Center
Methodist Hospital
SUNY Downstate/Kings County Hospital
 Center
The Brooklyn Hospital
Wyckoff Heights Hospital

Buffalo
Erie County Medical Center
Roswell Park Memorial Institute
Veterans Admin. Medical Center

Cobleskill
Community Hospital Schoharie County

Cooperstown
Mary Imogene Bassett Hospital

East Meadow
Nassau County Medical Center

Elmhurst
St. Johns Queens Hospital Div. of CMC

Elmira
Arnot–Ogden Memorial Hospital

Flushing
Booth Memorial Center
Flushing Hospital and Medical Center

Forest Hills
La Guardia Hospital

Glen Cove
Community Hospital at Glen Cove

Jamaica
Jamaica Hospital
Mary Immaculate Hospital Div. of CMC
Queens Hospital Center

Jamestown
Woman's Christian Association Hospital

Johnson City
Charles S. Wilson Memorial Hospital

Kenmore
Kenmore Mercy Hospital

Manhasset
North Shore University Hospital

Mineola
Nassau Hospital

Mount Kisco
Northern Westchester Hospital Center

New Hyde Park
LI Jewish–Hillside Medical Center

New Rochelle
New Rochelle Hospital Medical Center

New York
Bellevue Hospital Center
Beth Israel Medical Center
Cabrini Medical Center
Harlem Hospital Center
Manhattan EET Hospital
Memorial Sloan–Kettering Cancer Center
Montefiore Medical Center
New York University Medical Center
New York Infirmary—Beekman
  Downtown Hospital
Presbyterian Hospital in New York City
St. Clare's Hospital and Health Center
St. Luke's—Roosevelt Hospital Center
St. Vincent's Hospital and Medical Center
Veterans Admin. Medical Center

Nyack
Nyack Hospital

Oceanside
South Nassau Communities Hospital

Patchogue
Brookhaven Memorial Hospital Medical
  Center

Plainview
Central General Hospital

Port Jefferson
John T. Mather Memorial Hospital
St. Charles Hospital

Port Jervis
Mercy Community Hospital

Poughkeepsie
Vassar Brothers Hospital

Rochester
Genesee Hospital
Highland Hospital of Rochester
Park Ridge Hospital
Rochester General Hospital
St. Mary's Hospital
Strong Memorial Hospital

Rockville Centre
Mercy Hospital

Schenectady
Ellis Hospital

Staten Island
Bayley Seton Hospital
Doctors' Hospital of Staten Island
St. Vincent's Medical Center of Richmond
Staten Island Hospital

Syracuse
St. Joseph's Hospital Health Center
University Hospital of Upstate Medical
  Center

Valley Stream
Franklin General Hospital

Walton
Delaware Valley Hospital

NORTH CAROLINA

Camp LeJeune
Naval Regional Medical Center

Chapel Hill
North Carolina Memorial Hospital

Durham
Duke University Medical Center

Shelby
Cleveland Memorial Hospital

Valdese
Valdese General Hospital

Winston–Salem
North Carolina Baptist Hospital

975

NORTH DAKOTA

Fargo
Dakota Hospital
St. John's Hospital
St. Luke's Hospitals

Grand Forks
United Hospitals

Minot
St. Joseph's Hospital

Rugby
Good Samaritan Hospital Association

Williston
Mercy Hospital

OHIO

Akron
Akron City Hospital
Akron General Medical Center

Chardon
Geauga Community Hospital

Cincinnati
Bethesda Hospital/Oak
Children's Hospital Medical Center
Good Samaritan Hospital
Jewish Hospital of Cincinnati
The Christ Hospital
University of Cincinnati Hospital

Cleveland
Cleveland Clinic Hospital
Deaconess Hospital of Cleveland
Huron Road Hospital
Lutheran Medical Center
St. Alexis Hospital

Columbus
Children's Hospital
Hawkes Hospital of Mount Carmel
Ohio State University Hospitals
Riverside Methodist Hospital

Dayton
Good Samaritan Hospital and Health
  Center
Miami Valley Hospital
St. Elizabeth Medical Center

Dover
Union Hospital Association

Kettering
Kettering Medical Center

Marion
Marion General Hospital

Mayfield Heights
Hillcrest Hospital

Parma
Parma Community General Hospital

Ravenna
Robinson Memorial Hospital

Sandusky
Good Samaritan Hospital

Springfield
Community Hospital of Springfield
Mercy Medical Center

Sylvania
Flower Hospital

Toledo
Medical College of Ohio Hospital
Toledo Hospital

Urbana
Mercy Memorial Hospital

Wright–Patterson AFB
USAF Medical Center Wright–Patterson

Youngstown
St. Elizabeth Hospital Medical Center
Youngstown Hospital Association

OKLAHOMA

Ada
Valley View Hospital

Bartlesville
Jane Phillips Episcopal–Memorial Medical
  Center

Chickasha
Grady Memorial Hospital

Muskogee
Muskogee General Hospital

Oklahoma City
Baptist Medical Center
Mercy Health Center
Oklahoma Children's Memorial Hospital
Oklahoma Memorial Hospital
Presbyterian Hospital
South Community Hospital
St. Anthony Hospital

Okmulgee
Okmulgee Memorial Hospital Authority

Shattuck
Newm an Memorial Hospital

Shawnee
Shawnee Medical Center Hospital

Tulsa
Hillcrest Medical Center
St. Francis Hospital
St. John Medical Center

OREGON

Albany
Albany General Hospital

Bend
St. Charles Medical Center

Clackamas
Sunnyside Medical Center—Kaiser
  Foundation

Corvallis
Good Samaritan Hospital

Eugene
Sacred Heart General Hospital

Grants Pass
Josephine Memorial Hospital

Klamath Falls
Merle West Medical Center

La Grande
Grande Ronde Hospital

Medford
Providence Hospital
Rogue Valley Memorial Hospital

Oregon City
Willamette Falls Community Hospital

Pendleton
Pendleton Community Hospital
St. Anthony Hospital

Portland
Bess Kaiser Medical Center
Emanuel Hospital
Good Samaritan Hospital and Medical
  Center
Oregon Health Sciences University
Physicians and Surgeons Hospital
Portland Adventist Medical Center
Providence Medical Center
St. Vincent Hospital and Medical Center
Veterans Admin. Medical Center

Salem
Salem Hospital

Springfield
McKenzie–Willamette Memorial Hospital

Tualatin
Meridian Park Hospital

PENNSYLVANIA

Allentown
Lehigh Valley Hospital Center
Sacred Heart Hospital
The Allentown Hospital

Altoona
Mercy Hospital
The Altoona Hospital

Bethlehem
St. Luke's Hospital of Bethlehem

Bryn Mawr
Bryn Mawr Hospital

Danville
Geisinger Medical Center

Drexel Hill
Delaware County Memorial Hospital

Easton
Easton Hospital

Erie
Hamot Medical Center

Franklin
Franklin Regional Medical Center

977

Greensburg
Westmoreland Hospital

Greenville
Greenville Hospital

Johnstown
Conemaugh Valley Memorial Hospital

Lancaster
Lancaster General Hospital
St. Joseph Hospital

Latrobe
Latrobe Area Hospital

Lewistown
Lewistown Hospital

Natrona Heights
Allegheny Valley Hospital

New Castle
Jameson Memorial Hospital

Norristown
Montgomery Hospital
Sacred Heart Hospital

Paoli
Paoli Memorial Hospital

Philadelphia
Albert Einstein Medical Center—Northern Div.
American Oncologic Hospital
Childrens Hospital of Philadelphia
Episcopal Hospital
Graduate Hospital
Hahnemann University Hospital
Hospital of the University of Pennsylvania
Jeanes Hospital
Mercy Catholic Medical Center
Pennsylvania Hospital
Temple University Hospital
Thomas Jefferson University Hospital

Pittsburgh
Allegheny General Hospital
Childrens Hospital of Pittsburgh
Magee–Women's Hospital
Mercy Hospital of Pittsburgh
Presbyterian–University Hospital
St. Francis General Hospital

Pottsville
Pottsville Hospital and Warne Clinic

Quakertown
Quakertown Community Hospital

Reading
Reading Hospital and Medical Center
Saint Joseph Hospital

Sayre
Robert Packer Hospital

Scranton
Mercy Hospital

Sellersville
Grand View Hospital

State College
Centre Community Hospital

West Chester
Chester County Hospital

Wilkes-Barre
Veterans Admin. Medical Center

Williamsport
Divine Providence Hospital

York
York Hospital

PUERTO RICO

Ponce
Clinica Oncologica Grillasca
Hospital Damas

San German
Hospital de la Concepcion

San Juan
I. Gonzalez Martinez Onco Hospital
University Hospital

RHODE ISLAND

Newport
Naval Regional Medical Center

SOUTH CAROLINA

Aiken
Aiken Community Hospital

Charleston
Medical University of South Carolina

Columbia
Baptist Medical Center at Columbia
Richland Memorial Hospital
William Jennings Bryan Dorn Vets
  Hospital

Florence
McLeon Regional Medical Center

Fort Jackson
Moncrief Army Hospital

Greenville
Greenville General Hospital
Greenville Memorial Hospital

Greenwood
Self Memorial Hospital

Orangeburg
Orangeburg Regional Hospital

Spartanburg
Spartanburg General Hospital

SOUTH DAKOTA

Aberdeen
St. Luke's Hospital

Rapid City
Rapid City Regional Hospital

Watertown
Memorial Medical Center
St. Ann's Hospital

Yankton
Sacred Heart Hospital

TENNESSEE

Bristol
Bristol Memorial Hospital

Chattanooga
Erlanger Medical Center

Johnson City
Johnson City Medical Center Hospital

Knoxville
East Tennessee Baptist Hospital

Fort Sanders Regional Medical Center
University of Tennessee Memorial
  Hospital

Memphis
Baptist Memorial Hospital
Methodist Hospital—Central Unit
Regional Medical Center at Memphis
St. Francis Hospital
St. Jude Children's Res. Hospital
University of Tennessee Medical Center

Millington
Naval Regional Medical Center—Memphis

Mountain Home
Veterans Admin. Medical Center

Nashville
Hubbard Hospital Meharry Medical
  College
Metropolitan Nashville General Hospital
Vanderbilt University Hospital

TEXAS

Amarillo
High Plains Baptist Hospital
Northwest Texas Hospital
St. Anthony's Hospital
Veterans Admin. Medical Center

Big Spring
Veterans Admin. Medical Center

Carswell AFB
U.S. Air Force Regional Hospital

Corpus Christi
Memorial Medical Center
Naval Regional Medical Center
Spohn Hospital

Dallas
Baylor University Medical Center
Methodist Hospitals of Dallas
Parkland Memorial Hospital/Dallas City
  Hospital
Presbyterian Hospital of Dallas
St. Paul Hospital

El Paso
R. E. Thomason General Hospital
Williams Beaumont Army Medical Center

Fort Sam Houston
Brooke Army Medical Center

Fort Worth
John Peter Smith Hospital
St. Joseph Hospital

Galveston
University of Texas Medical Branch
  Hospitals

Hereford
Deaf Smith General Hospital

Houston
Ben Taub General Hospital
M D. Anderson Hospital and Tumor
  Institute
Park Plaza Hospital
St. Joseph Hospital

Lackland AFB
Wilford Hall USAF Medical Center

Lubbock
Highland Hospital
Methodist Hospital

McAllen
McAllen Methodist Hospital

Midland
Midland Memorial Hospital

Odessa
Medical Center Hospital

Plainview
Central Plains Regional Hospital

San Angelo
Angelo Community Hospital

San Antonio
Medical Center Hospital
Santa Rosa Medical Center
Southwest Texas Methodist Hospital

Stephenville
Stephenville Hospital

Temple
King's Daughers Hospital
Olin E. Teague Veterans' Center
Scott and White Memorial Hospital

Tyler
University of Texas Health Center

Waco
Hillcrest Baptist Hospital
Providence Hospital

Wharton
Gulf Coast Medical Center

UTAH

Ogden
St. Benedict's Hospital

Salt Lake City
Holy Cross Hospital
LDS Hospital
University of Utah Hospital
Veterans Admin. Medical Center

VERMONT

Bennington
Putnam Memorial Hospital

Burlington
Medical Center Hospital of Vermont

Randolph
Gifford Memorial Hospital

VIRGINIA

Alexandria
The Alexandria Hospital

Arlington
Arlington Hospital
Northern Virginia Doctors Hospital

Big Stone Gap
Lonesome Pine Hospital

Charlottesville
University of Virginia Hospital

Chesapeake
Chesapeake General Hospital

Danville
The Memorial Hospital

Fairfax
Commonwealth Hospital

Falls Church
Fairfax Hospital

Fredericksburg
Mary Washington Hospital

Hampton
Veterans Admin. Medical Center

Harrisonburg
Rockingham Memorial Hospital

Leesburg
Loudoun Memorial Hospital

Low Moor
Alleghany Regional Hospital

Lynchburg
Lynchburg General—Marshall Lodge
   Hospital
Virginia Baptist Hospital

Newport News
Riverside Hospital

Norfolk
DePaul Hospital
Norfolk General Hospital Div./Medical
   Center Hospital

Portsmouth
Naval Regional Medical Center

Richmond
Medical College of Virginia Hospitals
St. Luke's Hospital
St. Mary's Hospital

Roanoke
Community Hospital of Roanoke Valley
Roanoke Memorial Hospitals

Salem
Lewis–Gale Hospital
Veterans Admin. Medical Center

Winchester
Winchester Memorial Hospital

WASHINGTON

Aberdeen
Grays Harbor Community Hospital
St. Joseph Hospital

Anacortes
Island Hospital

Bellevue
Overlake Hospital

Bellingham
St. Joseph Hospital
St. Luke's General Hospital

Bremerton
Harrison Memorial Hospital
Naval Hospital

Coupeville
Whidbey General Hospital

Everett
General Hospital of Everett
Providence Hospital

Kennewick
Kennewick General Hospital

Kirkland
Evergreen General Hospital

Longview
Monticello Medical Center
St. John's Hospital

Mount Vernon
Skagit Valley Hospital

Olympia
St. Peter Hospital

Pasco
Our Lady of Lourdes Hospital

Seattle
Childrens Ortho. Hospital and Medical
   Center
Group Health Coop Central Hospital
Northwest Hospital
Providence Medical Center
Swedish Hospital Medical Center
Virginia Mason Hospital

Sedro Woolley
United General Hospital

Spokane
Deaconess Hospital
Sacred Heart Medical Center

Tacoma
Madigan Army Medical Center
Tacoma General Hospital

Vancouver
Southwest Washington Hospitals

Walla Walla
St. Mary Community Hospital
Walla Walla General Hospital

Wenatchee
Wenatchee Valley Clinic

Yakima
St. Elizabeth Hospital
Yakima Valley Memorial Hospital

WEST VIRGINIA

Charleston
Charleston Area Medical Center

Clarksburg
Veterans Admin Medical Center

Elkins
Davis Memorial Hospital
Memorial Center Hospital Association

Huntington
Saint Mary's Hospital
Veterans Admin. Medical Center

Montgomery
Montgomery General Hospital

Morgantown
West Virginia University Hospital

Wheeling
Ohio Valley Meeical Center

WISCONSIN

Appleton
St. Elizabeth Hospital

Cudahy
Trinity Memorial Hospital

Eau Claire
Luther Hospital
Sacred Heart Hospital

Fond du Lac
St. Agnes Hospital

Green Bay
St. Vincent Hospital

Janesville
Mercy Hospital

La Crosse
La Crosse Lutheran Hospital
St. Francis Medical Center

Madison
Madison General Hospital
St. Mary's Hospital Medical Center
University of Wisconsin Hospital and
    Clinics

Manitowoc
Holy Family Hospital

Marinette
Marinette General Hospital

Marshfield
Marshfield Clinic/St. Joseph's Hospital

Milwaukee
Columbia Hospital
Good Samaritan Medical
    Center/Deaconess Hospital Campus
Mount Sinai Medical Center
St. Francis Hospital
St. Joseph's Hospital
St. Luke's Hospital
St. Mary's Hospital
St. Michael Hospital

Milwaukee (Wood)
Veterans Admin. Medical Center

Monroe
St. Clare Hospital of Monroe

Oshkosh
Mercy Medical Center

Wausau
Wausau Hospital Center

West Allis
West Allis Memorial Hospital

WYOMING

Cheyenne
De Paul Hospital
Memorial Hospital of Laramie County

WOMANCARE

INDEX

A

Abdominal pain, 201, 228
  conditions that may cause, 259–60, 397,
    405, 434, 489, 515, 565, 608
  IUD and, 125, 127, 131
Abdominal pregnancy, 691
Abdominal surgery, 277, 333–34
Abdominal swelling:
  ectopic pregnancy and, 489
  ovarian cancer and, 489
Abdominal X-rays, 498
Abortion(s), 87, 93–94, 103, 111, 112,
    133, 205–25, 321, 322, 400
  birth control method selection after, 225
  cervical lacerations and, 353, 356, 361,
    362, 363
  costs of, 216, 217
  future developments, 224
  incomplete, 216, 223, 676, 680, 688
  legalization of, 93, 206–207, 321
  making the decision, 207–208
  multiple, 205–206, 216, 224, 225
  opponents of, 206–207
  septic, 132, 133
  spontaneous, *see* Miscarriage

subsequent pregnancies, 224–25, 675
test and examinations before, 208–10
types of, 205
  amniocentesis abortion (16–24
    weeks), 219–23
  dilation and curettage, 216
  dilation and evacuation (13–20
    weeks), 218–19
  early vacuum abortion (4–12 weeks),
    210–16, 224
  hysterectomy and hysterotomy, 223
  menstrual extraction, 217–18
  prostaglandin vaginal suppositories,
    223
Abortion Action Coalition, 207
Abortion clinics, 209, 215, 222
Abrahams, Guy, 604
Abstinence, *see* Natural Family Planning
Accessory ovaries, 467
Acid/alkaline balance, *see* pH balance of
  the vagina
Acidophilic adenoma, 622
Acne, 70, 104, 106
Acromegaly, 515, 622
Actinomyces, 126, 127, 128, 396, 400
Acupressure, 613

Strokes, 79, 87, 109, 115, 228, 794, 806, 807
Stukane, Eileen, 609
Submucous fibroids, 433, 434–35, 436–37
Subserous or subperitoneal fibroids, 433, 435
Suction curettage, see Vacuum abortion
Suction machine, 214
Sufamal, 742
Sugar, 299, 302, 313, 506, 609
  metabolism of, 114
Sulfabenzamide, 304
Sulfacetamide, 304
Sulfa drugs, 103, 304, 312, 316, 319, 353, 595, 796
Sulfanilamide, 304, 742–43
Sulfa Tablets, 304
Sulfathiazole, 304
Sulfisoxazole, 304
Sulfonamide, 796
Sultrin, 304
Sunlight, sensitivity to, 106, 795
Supernumerary ovaries, 467
Supreme Court, 206, 207
Surgeon, choosing a, 733–35
Surgery, 13–14, 353, 730–37
  after the operation, 736–37
  before, what may occur, 735–36
  for cancer, 715, 717–19
    see also specific forms of cancer
  choosing a surgeon, 733–35
  in the operating room, 736
  overly extensive, 731–33
  on Pill users, 109
  previous, noted in medical history, 194
  questions to ask before, 732
  unnecessary, 730–33
  see also specific surgical procedures,
    e.g. Dilation and curettage;
    Hysterectomy(ies)
Surgical oncologist, 496, 718–19, 733
Surgilube, 648
Symptoms Index, 13, 14–15, 37, 243
  abdominal or pelvic pain, 259–60
  how to use, 14, 245–46
  infertility and sterility, 259
  symptoms related to breast, 256–57

symptoms related to cervix, 254–55
symptoms related to menstrual cycle, 257–59
symptoms related to vagina, 248–54
symptoms related to vulva, 246–48
Syphilis, 73, 156, 352, 582–87
  cause and transmission, 583
  diagnosis of, 585–86
  getting treatment, 559–61
  incidence, 557, 582
  pregnancy and, 585
  reporting, 561–62
  symptoms of, 583–85
  treatment of, 586–87
  see also Sexually transmissible diseases

T

"Tailless" IUD, 127
Tamoxifen, 550
Tampons, 19, 29, 30, 59–60, 301, 356
  toxic shock syndrome and, 651–52, 653
Tea, 506, 575
Teenagers, 226, 795
  abortion decision, 208
  dilation and curettage and, 637–68
  with sexually transmissible diseases, 561
Temperature, body, 76, 215
  after ovulation, 68
  rhythm method and basal, 173–79, 184
    effectiveness, 183
    interpreting the chart, 174–79
    taking and recording temperature, 174
  see also Basal body temperature,
    charting
Tenaculum, 762
Terramycin, 312
Testes, 53, 54, 188, 189, 466
  cancer of the, 809
  of DES sons, 809–10
  male infertility and, 664–65
  undescended, 664, 809
Testicular biopsy, 670
Testicular cysts, 809